AF903472

LUNG DISEASES – SELECTED STATE OF THE ART REVIEWS

Edited by **Elvis Malcolm Irusen**

Lung Diseases – Selected State of the Art Reviews
Edited by Elvis Malcolm Irusen

Published by InTech
Janeza Trdine 9, 51000 Rijeka, Croatia

Copyright © 2012 InTech
All chapters are distributed under the Creative Commons Attribution 3.0 license, which allows users to download, copy and build upon published articles even for commercial purposes, as long as the author and publisher are properly credited, which ensures maximum dissemination and a wider impact of our publications. After this work has been published by InTech, authors have the right to republish it, in whole or part, in any publication of which they are the author, and to make other personal use of the work. Any republication, referencing or personal use of the work must explicitly identify the original source.

As for readers, this license allows users to download, copy and build upon published chapters even for commercial purposes, as long as the author and publisher are properly credited, which ensures maximum dissemination and a wider impact of our publications.

Notice
Statements and opinions expressed in the chapters are these of the individual contributors and not necessarily those of the editors or publisher. No responsibility is accepted for the accuracy of information contained in the published chapters. The publisher assumes no responsibility for any damage or injury to persons or property arising out of the use of any materials, instructions, methods or ideas contained in the book.

Publishing Process Manager Romana Vukelic

Technical Editor Teodora Smiljanic

Cover Designer InTech Design Team

Additional hard copies can be obtained from orders@intechopen.com

Lung Diseases – Selected State of the Art Reviews, Edited by Elvis Malcolm Irusen
p. cm.
ISBN 978-953-51-0180-2

We are IntechOpen, the first native scientific publisher of Open Access books

3,250+
Open access books available

106,000+
International authors and editors

112M+
Downloads

151
Countries delivered to

Our authors are among the
Top 1%
most cited scientists

12.2%
Contributors from top 500 universities

BOOK CITATION INDEX
CLARIVATE ANALYTICS
INDEXED

WEB OF SCIENCE™

Selection of our books indexed in the Book Citation Index in Web of Science™ Core Collection (BKCI)

Interested in publishing with us? Contact book.department@intechopen.com

Numbers displayed above are based on latest data collected.
For more information visit www.intechopen.com

For EU product safety concerns:
IN TECH d.o.o., Prolaz Marije Krucifikse Kozulić 3, 51000 Rijeka, Croatia,
info@intechopen.com or visit our website at intechopen.com.

Meet the editor

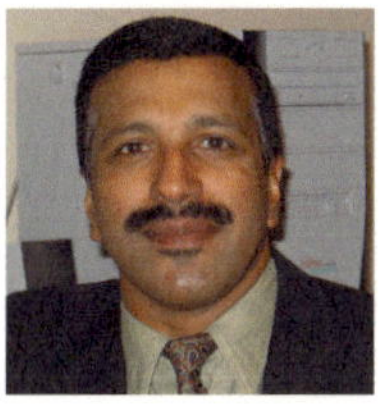

Professor E. M. Irusen, FCP(SA), Pulmonology, PhD, is a principal specialist and Clinical Head of the Pulmonology and Critical Care Division of the Department of Internal Medicine, Faculty of Health Sciences, University of Stellenbosch and Tygerberg Academic Hospital in Cape Town, South Africa. He is widely published and has tremendous experience in these speciality fields. His PhD training in molecular immunology and biology related to asthmatic inflammation was undertaken under the supervision of Professors Fan Chung and Peter Barnes at the Royal Brompton Hospital and the Unit of Thoracic Medicine of the National Heart and Lung Institute at Imperial College. He has won numerous awards for his research, both local and international. He has served on the Council of SA Thoracic Society and is the immediate former president. He is currently the South African national representative in the European Respiratory Society, GOLD and on the international executive of the International COPD Coalition.

Contents

Preface

The developments in molecular medicine are leading to important insights with regard to lung diseases. Leading clinicians and scientists in the world have brought their considerable knowledge and experience, and focused research in their contributions to this book. Clinicians and researchers will learn about the most recent advances in a variety of lung diseases that will enable them to better understand respiratory disorders. The book presents state-of-the-art essays on airways disease, neoplastic diseases, and pediatric respiratory conditions. Additionally, aspects of immune regulation, respiratory infections, acute lung injury/ ARDS, pulmonary oedema, functional evaluation in respiratory disorders, and a variety of other conditions are also expounded upon. The compilation and availability of the book online has also ensured that information is as current as possible, which is an advantage over the printed editions.

The book will be invaluable for clinicians who appreciate the pathogenetic basis and current concepts in lung diseases and improve their diagnostic and therapeutic skills. Scientists will also gain something from the detailed applied molecular techniques and descriptions that could potentially open a plethora of new research avenues for exploration.

Professor E.M. Irusen
Department of Medicine,
Faculty of Health Sciences,
University of Stellenbosch,
Western Cape Province,
South Africa

Part 1

Airways Disease

1

Airway Smooth Muscle in Asthma Symptoms: Culprit but Maybe Innocent

Ynuk Bossé[1], Peter D. Paré[1] and Yohan Bossé[2]
[1]*James Hogg Research Center, University of British Columbia, Vancouver*
[2]*Institut Universitaire de Cardiologie et de Pneumologie de Québec and Department of Molecular Medicine, Laval University, Quebec City*
Canada

1. Introduction

The main function of smooth muscle found in either the airways or in other hollow organs is to contract. Once stimulated to contract, the smooth muscle strives to shorten. In turn, smooth muscle shortening narrows the lumen of the organ it surrounds. Contraction usually serves a physiological purpose, such as increasing arterial tension for vascular smooth muscle, micturition for the detrusor muscle or parturition for the uterus muscle. However, for the airway smooth muscle (ASM), the shortening narrows the airway lumen, which concomitantly increases the resistance to airflow. So it seems that every time ASM manifests its function it causes respiratory distress. This had raised the question of whether its existence is the problem (65, 162)?

One common respiratory disorder in which the symptoms are greatly engendered by ASM contraction is asthma. In fact, a proper asthma diagnosis involved testing the reversibility of airway obstruction with a bronchodilator, a drug relaxing ASM (usually a β_2-adrenoceptor agonist). A positive test is indicated by complete or partial reversibility, which simultaneously confirms the implication of ASM shortening in asthma symptoms. However, we know that a judge will never blame the gun for a murder. She/he would rather blame the assassin that pulled the trigger. Thus, the ASM could simply be an obeisant effector tissue that responds to external cues that are asking it to contract. So despite being culprit in the elaboration of asthma symptoms it may still be 'innocent'.

Hence, for asthma symptoms (at least the one mediated by airway narrowing) to be provoked, contractile stimuli need to be present. There is no doubt about the increased expression of spasmogens (i.e., contractile agonists) into asthmatic airways. Histamine (251), leukotrienes (125), endothelin-1 (148), prostaglandin D_2 (170), thromboxane A_2 (249), adenosine (61), bradykinin (136), anaphylatoxin C3a and C5a (121), substance P (231) and others, are all inflammatory mediators capable of stimulating ASM contraction and were all shown to be overexpressed in asthmatic lungs. These spasmogens are secreted/synthesized following exposure to environmental asthma triggers, such as allergens, viruses, bacteria, fungi, air pollutants, exercise, aspirin and/or cold dry air. The nature of the environmental trigger involved obviously varies among asthmatics but all of them ultimately lead to a type of airway inflammation with inflammation-derived spasmogens. However, not everyone who gets inflammation into her/his airways because of a cold, because they are exposed to an allergen to which they are sensitized (atopic), because they do exercise, etc… gets asthma symptoms. So it might not be enough to have airway inflammation to get asthma symptoms. If you try to kill a moose with a pellet gun, you may have the gun and you may pull the trigger, but you are more likely to have no responsiveness. Saying that it may also be necessary to be responsive, or maybe hyperresponsive, to these inflammation-derived spasmogens to get asthma symptoms.

In fact, one of the pathognomonic feature of asthma is airway hyperresponsiveness (AHR). AHR is defined as an increased sensitivity and maximal narrowing in response to an inhalational challenge with a spasmogen (methacholine is the most commonly used). Whether AHR is a prerequisite to suffer from asthma or whether asthma is the cause of AHR is a contemporaneous debate and will be slightly addressed in this chapter. Some can argue that asthma can affect the degree of airway responsiveness and others would be just as right by arguing that AHR is a predisposing factor to be diagnosed with asthma. What is clear is that the degree of responsiveness is a good surrogate for the airway narrowing that will take place *in vivo* in response to endogenously produced spasmogens that are released either in normal state or during asthma exacerbation.

In a syndrome like asthma, understanding the factors involved in AHR may give important clues concerning the pathogenesis of asthma and the generation of asthmatic symptoms. As aforementioned, this is because the symptoms of asthma are caused, to a great extent, by airway narrowing induced by ASM shortening. Due to its unequivocal role in airway responsiveness, it is clear that the ASM plays an important role in AHR; without responsiveness there would be no hyperresponsiveness. However, whether the ASM is intrinsically different in asthma and responsible for AHR is still unclear. Several ASM dysfunctions, but also many other defects in non-muscle factors have been suggested to play a role in the manifestation of AHR. Whether these defects are genetically inherited or acquired as a result of disease processes is also a question of great interest. This chapter is an attempt to outline the current state of comprehension regarding the alterations in muscle and non-muscle factors that may contribute to the hyperresponsive phenotype seen in asthmatics.

2. Muscle factors

Studying ASM mechanics involves more than measuring its force-generating capacity. Many other ASM contractile properties may play a role in determining the degree of airway responsiveness *in vivo*, such as shortening amount and velocity, stiffness, ability to relax and to tolerate and/or recover from the decline in contractility induced by length perturbations. The term 'contractility' in this chapter is vague and refers to any contractile properties. So a hypercontractile ASM phenotype can mean one or all of the following: the muscle is stronger (increased force-generating capacity), it shortens more and/or shortens faster, it is stiffer, it has an attenuated ability to relax either spontaneously or in response to bronchodilators, or has an increased ability to tolerate and/or to recover from a drop in contractility caused by length perturbations. In the following section, these contractile properties are discussed individually and the rationale for their respective involvement in determining the degree of airway responsiveness *in vivo* is described. The published evidences suggesting that alterations to some of these contractile properties contribute to AHR in asthma are also briefly reviewed. The premise, here, is that AHR would be due to an inherited ASM hypercontractility; not one that would be acquired due to defects in non-muscle factors. Some of the factors discussed were addressed in a previous review (24).

It is worth-mentionning that the ASM has also been shown to proliferate, to migrate, to express adhesion molecules and receptors interacting with immune cells, as well as to synthesize extracellular matrix components, cytokines and chemokines. Most of these ASM functions were studied in monolayers of ASM cells in culture. More evidences are eagerly needed to confirm the existence of these ASM functions *in vivo*. However, if they happen *in vivo*, their relevance to asthma pathogenesis is unquestionable. These subjects have been reviewed lately and will not be addressed in the present chapter (18, 50, 72).

2.1 Force

The load impeding ASM shortening is auxotonic; i.e., it increases progressively as the muscle shortens. It is thus logical that greater force would lead to more shortening and concomitantly more airway narrowing. That is the reason why the force-generating capacity of ASM is such an important determinant of airway responsiveness.

The force-generating capacity also matters because it influences other ASM contractile properties. The relationship between the load and the velocity can be fitted with an exponential decay equation; so that increasing the load decreases the shortening velocity exponentially. This implies that a stronger muscle would counteract a given load faster and would thus shorten faster. In a context where the muscle is subjected to contract under a progressively increasing load, as it occurs *in vivo*, a stronger muscle would also shorten further. This is because a muscle able to produce more force at any given length would allow the shortening to progress further before reaching a load equal to its force. A stronger muscle would also increase ASM stiffness, which, as discussed below (subsection 2.2), can have an important impact on *in vivo* airway responsiveness.

The force or stress, which is the force per cross-sectional area, produced by the ASM depends on the potency and the concentration of the contractile stimulus involved. The relationship between spasmogen concentration and ASM-force can be described by a sigmoidal equation. So, *in vivo*, the amount of spasmogen reaching the ASM is one of the main determinants of the force produced by the muscle. The force produced by the ASM is also dictated by its length. Longer muscle generally generates more force in response to a given contractile stimulus (86, 154, 259, 261). In fact, the decrease in ASM-force caused by length reduction is proportional to he magnitude of the length change (103). Hence, *in situ* factors affecting the operating length of the ASM can be of considerable importance in the understanding of AHR, but that will be discussed later in this chapter (subsection 4.1.5).

Regardless of the aforementioned factors, the force can also be determined by the muscle's intrinsic capacity to generate force. So for a given concentration of a chosen spasmogen and a given length, the stress produced by the muscle can be different. This has led some to suggest that ASM derived from asthmatics may produce more stress than ASM derived from non-asthmatics, and that might be the cause of AHR. This hypothesis has been tested by several groups now and, although still debatable, the bulk of evidence suggests that the stress-generating capacity of asthmatic and non-asthmatic ASM is the same (reviewed in (153)). Taken together, the force-generating capacity of the ASM is certainly an important determinant of airway responsiveness, but no data published thus far convincingly demonstrate that this contractile property is altered in asthma.

2.2 Stiffness

In the field of ASM the term 'stiffness' certainly has different connotations. By definition stiffness is the amount of force required to cause a given change in length. The stiffness of

ASM can be either passive or active depending on whether the resistance to stretch stems from relaxed or activated components of ASM, respectively. Passive stiffness relies predominantly on the cell cytoskeleton. In fact, ablation of the cytoskeleton protein vimentin was shown to reduce passive stiffness by 3-fold (243). However, it came to experts' attention that the ASM is relatively compliant. The resting tension observed along the range of *in situ* operating lengths, even when the ASM is stretched to a level comparable to the one observed in a lung inflated to total lung capacity (TLC), is almost neglectable. On the other hand, the amount of tension generated by the same stretch in the presence of an active tone (i.e., in the presence of spasmogens) is disproportionally greater. For this reason, we focus here on ASM active stiffness, since it would be the principal component affecting airway responsiveness. Passive stiffness can also have a broader connotation if one considers the other components of the airway wall and the extracellular matrix (ECM) surrounding the ASM cells. These other passive elements obviously impact the overall stiffness of the airway wall and will be addressed later in this chapter (subsections 4.1.4 and 4.1.6).

Active stiffness is related to the level of ASM activation by spasmogenic stimuli. Its magnitude has always been thought to be dictated by the number of myosin heads bound to the actin filaments (i.e., number of cross-bridges). However, an emerging field in ASM suggests that other factors might play a part in active siffness. That is the level of interconnectivity between the ECM, the plasma membrane and the cell's cytoskeleton. These points of junction are excessively important for mechanotransduction efficiency; i.e., the transfer of individual resistive forces to the overall stiffness of the tissue during a stretch. Once considered as passive, recent studies rather suggested that the structures responsible for this interconnectivity can rearrange extensively upon ASM cell activation (reviewed in (264)). For example, Zhang and coworkers (263) have shown that α-actinin translocates to the plasmalemma and binds to β_1-integrin early after acetylcholine (ACh) activation, and blocking this interaction reduces active tension in response to ACh (263). This and other recent findings (105, 188, 265) confirmed that this interconnectivity between intracellular proteins, the plasma membrane proteins (integrins) and the ECM relies on dynamic processes that are activated by spasmogens. We shall henceforth consider this level of interconnectivity as an integral part of the active stiffness component of ASM.

ASM stiffness has captured the eyes of many scientists in the field recently because of its influence on airway responsiveness. To understand the link between stiffness and airway responsiveness, it is important to emphasize that ASM operates in a dynamic environment. The swings in transpulmonary pressure required for ventilation cause oscillating stresses on the airway wall, which, in turn, cause continuous variations of airway caliber. The effects of these oscillating strains (a strain is a change in length caused by a change in stress) on ASM mechanics are not small (Fredberg). In fact, in was predicted that the bronchodilating effect of oscillating strains at an amplitude that is thought to prevail *in vivo* due to tidal breathing is just as potent as high concentrations of a β_2-adrenoceptor agonist (isoproterenol) to reverse airway constriction induced by different contractile stimuli (84). In fact, a single stretch of the airway wall at greater amplitude seems to be sufficient. Stretching the airway wall by taking a deep inspiration (DI) has been recognized as a powerful way to induce bronchodilatation and bronchoprotection (171, 222). Inversely, refraining from taking regular DIs has been shown to increase AHR in normal (i.e., non-asthmatic) subjects (117, 118, 221). In the same vein, cessation of tidal breathing during breath-holding caused a decrease in tracheal and central bronchial diameter (165). This later observation suggests that the bronchodilating effect of breathing is omnipresent *in vivo,* and that removing the oscillating airway wall strains caused by breathing allows the baseline level of ASM activation (tone) to constrict the airways. Finally, breathing at low lung volume has been shown to increase airway responsiveness (56), suggesting that not only the presence but also the amplitude of the airway wall strains induced by breathing impacts on the subsequent degree of airway narrowing provoked by a given spasmogenic challenge. Therefore, identifying the factors decreasing airway lumen expansion during a DI, or the factors limiting fluctuating strains of the airway wall during tidal breathing, such as passive and active ASM stiffness, are relevant to the understanding of airway narrowing and AHR.

The decrease in airway responsiveness induced by a DI has also been mimicked *ex vivo* on isolated porcine (178) and human (177) airways. In these studies, the liquid-filled airways were subjected to luminal volume changes reproducing the changes in transmural pressure occurring during tidal breathing (from 5 to 10 cmH_2O) and DIs (from 5 to 30 cmH_2O). The authors showed that the presence of DI simulations reduces the active pressure or the decrease in luminal volume produced by ASM in response to different concentrations of ACh.

Oscillations of airway caliber by breathing maneuvers seem to have a bronchodilating effect because they stretch the ASM. It was estimated that tidal breathing, sigh and DI, stretch the relaxed ASM by 4, 12 and 25% of its initial length, respectively (66). This is probably an overestimation since it was calculated based on changes in lung volume occurring during these breathing maneuvers while considering the lungs as isotropic material. Nevertheless, these length oscillations are known to decrease ASM stiffness, even during supra-maximal activation with ACh (66, 84, 128, 198). Importantly, the maximal force-generating capacity of ASM during or immediately following these oscillations is also reduced (66, 84, 85, 128, 186, 198, 242). The decline in isometric force that ensues length oscillations has been shown to be proportional to the amplitude and the duration of the stretch, but not to the frequency (242). These results demonstrated that the force produced by ASM in response to a given stimulus is greater in a static environment than a dynamic environment.

Oscillating strains at amplitude that is thought to prevail *in vivo* during breathing maneuvers also caused elongation of the contracted muscle (128, 130, 160). This later phenomenon is now referred to as force fluctuation-induced relengthening (FFIR). It also occurred in experimental settings more closely mimicking the *in situ* environment, where the ASM was subjected to an auxotonic load (186). Therefore, oscillating strains not only reduce the stiffness and the force-generating capacity of ASM in response to a given stimulus but also cause ASM relengthening. *In vivo*, this ASM relengthening will be translated into airway dilatation. The mechanisms underlying FFIR are not well understood but the length of the actin filaments seems to play a role (160).

Collectively, these studies have shown that the force (66, 84, 85, 128, 186, 198, 242) and the stiffness (66, 84, 128, 198) of ASM, as well as the length of the contracted ASM (128, 130, 160, 186), are affected by length oscillations (66, 84, 85, 128, 130, 160, 186, 198, 242) or simply by an acute stretch (242). Considering these phenomena together, one can envision the following *in vivo* vicious cycle. With exposure to spasmogens and the development of stiffer ASM, the same fluctuating stresses of breathing will cause less airway wall strains. This will allow the muscle to operate in a more static environment, where it will be able to produce more force and will be subjected to less FFIR. By producing more force, the muscle becomes stiffer, which further decreases the airway wall strains induced by breathing, and so on. Because the load impeding muscle shortening increases with the amount of airway narrowing, ASM shortening will eventually stop (when the force generated by the muscle is equal to the load opposing its contraction). However, the repetitive sequence of events described above allows greater ASM shortening and consequently greater airway narrowing for any level of ASM activation. The link between stiffer ASM and AHR is thus indirect and explained by the fact that stiffening of ASM reduces the magnitude of airway wall strains (i.e., ASM stretches) caused by breathing maneuvers. In conjunction, these studies also suggest that the bronchodilating and bronchoprotective effect of breathing maneuvers seen *in vivo* may be due to he fact that ASM contractile properties are malleable and affected by straining forces.

Having said that, the bronchodilating effect of tidal breathing does not make unanimity (reviewed in (176)). In systems that more closely imitate the *in vivo* situation, such as in a liquid-filled airway segment subjected to transmural pressure oscillations mimicking the swings in transpulmonary pressure occurring *in vivo* due to breathing maneuvers, only the DI (but not tidal breathing) was shown to attenuate the increase in pressure (178) or the reduction in luminal volume (177) caused by ACh stimulation. Nevertheless, it will be important to determine whether the stiffness of the ASM is different between asthmatics and non-asthmatics. So far, the only evidence to support the conjecture that an increased ASM stiffness causes AHR comes from a study using animal cells. The ASM cells derived from the inherently hyperresponsive Fisher rats were shown to exhibit a higher stiffening response to a panel of spasmogens compared to the cells derived from the hyporesponsive Lewis rats (6).

2.3 Tolerance to oscillating stretches and rate of recovery following length perturbations

In the previous subsection, we have seen that length perturbations can greatly affect ASM contractility. From now on, by length perturbations we meant any of the following: a length change, either elongation or length reduction; a single stretch or release with an immediate return to the initial length; oscillating strains (length oscillations); or oscillating stresses (force oscillations) that is sufficient to modulate ASM length. The ability to tolerate and recover from these length perturbations are thus important ASM contractile properties that may influence the degree of airway responsiveness. The ASM's ability to maintain its force-generating capacity during shortening could also be important in determining the degree of airway narrowing. It is well-known that the ASM becomes 'weaker' as it shortens. So that the instantaneous capacity to produce force during (or immediately after a) length reduction is inversely proportional to the magnitude of the length change (103). This suggests that the force-generating capacity of ASM at shorter lengths is an important factor determining the extent of airway narrowing; simply because it dictates the remaining force available to counteract the loads which limit further airway narrowing at these new shorter lengths. There is currently no data comparing the decline in force caused by given reductions of ASM length between asthmatics and non-asthmatics.

Since we just came to realize the potentially important role of these contractile properties in airway responsiveness, it is not surprising that not enough comparisons were made between asthmatic and non-asthmatic tissues. The only evidence that we are aware of comes from our group (Leslie *et al.*, accepted in the European Respiratory Journal). In that study, tracheal ASM strips derived from asthmatics and non-asthmatics were isolated and their ability to tolerate length perturbations and to recover from them was studied *ex vivo*. We found that the decline in force caused by length perturbations was attenuated in asthmatic tissues. The length perturbations used were a 60% length oscillations for 10 min, which are way beyond the length changes that would occur *in vivo*. The physiologic meaning of this finding may thus be questioned. However, since all tissues were exposed to the same oscillating strains, it still means that there is an intrinsic difference between asthmatic and non-asthmatic ASM tissues in their ability to tolerate length oscillations. Interestingly, other ASM contractile properties were also compared in that study, such as the stress-generating capacity in response to electrical field stimulation (EFS), the velocity of shortening, the amount of shortening and the ability to relax. Among all the contractile properties tested, only the ability to tolerate length oscillations was clearly different between asthmatic and non-asthmatic ASM. These results suggested that the influence of disparate ASM in determining the different degree of airway responsiveness observed between asthmatics and non-asthmatics would only be manifested in certain circumstances… such as in a human that is breathing?? These results would need to be confirmed by other investigators.

The speed and the extent of force recovery following an initial decline in force induced by length perturbations could also contribute to the manifestation of AHR. In the aforementioned study using human tracheal ASM strips (Leslie *et al.*, accepted in the European Respiratory Journal), no difference in the rate and extent of recovery was observed between asthmatic and non-asthmatic tissues. Since the decline in force induced by length oscillations was greater in non-asthmatic ASM, this implies that the force produced by the non-asthmatic ASM was lower during the entire recovery period (which was measured for 30 min). Also worth-mentioning is that this time period was sufficient for the asthmatic ASM to come back to its force before oscillations, which was not the case for non-asthmatic tissues. Other studies have used animal models to study the recovery of ASM-force following length oscillations. Wang and coworkers (241) measured the effect of length oscillations on isometric force-generating capacity of tracheal ASM strips from guinea pigs of different age groups. The force was assessed before and immediately after length oscillations, as well as at 6-min intervals thereafter to follow both the change and the recovery of force following oscillations. All age groups showed a similar decline in force immediately following length oscillations. However, whereas the force produced by tissues from older animals (3 week-old and adult) recovered to pre-oscillations levels over a time course of ~30 min, the force produced by the tissues from the youngest animals (1 week-old) rapidly rose above baseline (i.e., force before oscillations) and remained at this higher value for the entire time-window over which force recovery was measured. The increase in force over baseline induced by length oscillations was called 'force potentiation'. The molecular mechanisms underlying force potentiation are not well understood, but differential synthesis of prostaglandins seems to explain this age-dependent phenomenon in the guinea pig (44)).

A phenomenon closely related to force potentiation, which was dubbed the 'myogenic response', has also been suggested as a possible contributor to AHR in humans. Marthan and Woolcock (144) studied asthmatic patients in whom a DI induced a decrease in specific airway conductance. As discussed earlier, this paradoxical response is not uncommon in severe asthmatics and is an indicator of marked AHR (134). They found that nifedipine, a L-type calcium channel blocker, prevented the decrease in specific airway conductance induced by the DI (144). They suggested that the stretch of the ASM caused by the DI provoked a calcium-dependent bronchoconstriction (myogenic response).

Taken together, it seems clear that the tolerance to the decrease in contractility induced by length perturbations and the ability to recover from them may play a role in determining the degree of airway responsiveness. However, more data are warranted to confirm that these contractile properties can discriminate normo-responsiveness from AHR. Studying these contractile properties also unveiled other phenomena, such as force potentiation and the myogenic response, which can also be significant in the understanding of AHR.

2.4 Amount of shortening and velocity of shortening

The amount of ASM shortening is of major importance because it ultimately determines the amount of airway narrowing. As discussed earlier, the amount (as well as the velocity) of shortening depends on the ASM-force relative to the load. Therefore, all the factors influencing ASM-force, such as the potency and the concentration of the contractile stimulus involved, the quantity of spasmogens reaching the ASM, the muscle's intrinsic capacity to generate force, and its length, as well as all the factors influencing the load impeding muscle shortening affect the amount and velocity of shortening. However, the intrinsic ability to shorten may also be different between asthmatics and non-asthmatics. So that under the same load and despite producing the same stress, the amount of shortening achieved may be different. Interestingly, this has been shown in isolated ASM cells (140). In that study, the authors showed that unloaded ASM cells derived from asthmatics shorten more at room temperature in response to EFS. However, this observation, which now has a decade old, still awaits confirmation. The underlying mechanisms involved are also unclear but decreased resistance to shortening due to reduction in either internal resistive load (214, 226) or stiffness (44) has been proposed.

The shortening velocity of ASM could also be a critical determinant of the amount of airway narrowing. Again, to comprehend the potential implication of ASM shortening velocity in determining the degree of airway responsiveness, it is important to understand that ASM operates in a dynamic environment. The load impeding its shortening is continuously fluctuating due to swings in transpulmonary pressure caused by ventilatory maneuvers (e.g., tidal breathing and DI). The amount of ASM shortening *in vivo* is determined by a balance between the rate of cross-bridge cycling on the actin filaments causing muscle shortening versus the rate and the magnitude of stretch-induced disruption of cross-bridges causing muscle elongation (67). A faster cycling rate of the cross-bridges with a commensurate increased velocity of shortening would lead to more shortening during exhalation, when the load opposing muscle shortening is lowering. A faster rate of cycling would also lead to more cross-bridges being attached at the end of expiration, rendering the ASM and the entire airway wall stiffer. In turn, the stiffer airway wall would be less vulnerable to the stress imposed by the subsequent inspiration; i.e., the airway wall would be exposed to the same stress of breathing but the strain of the airway wall and, consequently, the stretch of the ASM would be attenuated in an airway with stiffer ASM. The combination of more shortening and more cross-bridge attachments during exhalation with less stretch and less cross-bridge detachments during inhalation means that the ASM with an increased shortening velocity would eventually reach a new equilibrium where the size of the airway lumen would be smaller than with a slower ASM. In addition, the airway wall that has reached this equilibrium becomes more static. Since ASM operating in a static environment produces more force in response to the same stimulus (as discussed above), it is possible that a faster muscle would not only cause more shortening and more cross-bridges during exhalation, but would also becomes stronger (i.e. able to produce more force for the same level of activation). By acquiring more force the ASM would then be able to narrow the airway further during the next exhalation and… the cycle can perpetuate itself. This vicious cycle is likely to happen in airways possessing ASM with faster shortening velocity and this is the rationale behind the idea that the speed of ASM contraction could be the cause of AHR.

Experimental evidences exist to support the hypothesis that a faster ASM velocity of shortening can contribute to AHR. The velocity of ASM shortening was shown to be greater in animal models in which there is innate AHR (reviewed in (132)). Similarly, there is greater maximal shortening velocity in human ASM cells derived from asthmatics (140). Whether this increased velocity of shortening is innate or acquired due to asthma in humans remains to be determined. Two mechanisms have been suggested to be responsible for the observed increased velocity of shortening in asthmatic ASM: 1-The increased expression of myosin light chain kinase (MLCK) (3, 16, 133); and 2-a preponderant expression of the faster cycling smooth muscle myosin heavy chain (smMHC) isoform B over the slower cycling smMHC isoform A (reviewed in (132)).

MLCK is a enzyme capable of phosphorylating the regulatory myosin light chain (rMLC), which is a necessary step required for actin-activation of myosin ATPase activity and the subsequent binding and pivotal of the cross-bridges on the actin filaments. The rationale is that faster rMLC phosphorylation caused by the increased amount of MLCK would lead to the activation of more cross-bridges and a faster onset and velocity of shortening at early time-points following ASM stimulation. However, increased expression of MLCK in asthma is not a unanimous finding (147, 256). An alternate explanation for the increased velocity of shortening of asthmatic ASM is a differential expression of smMHC isoforms. The so called B isoform (also called the (+) insert isoform because of the presence of a 7-amino acid insert in the loop 1 of the protein) shows a greater rate of cross-bridge cycling *in vitro* (129). Its preponderant expression over the A isoform would likely increase the velocity of ASM shortening and, therefore, contributes to AHR. In accordance to this assertion, the ratio of the isoforms correlates with the level of airway responsiveness in rats; i.e., hyperresponsive animals expressed more of the B than the normo-responsive animals (73). The mRNA expression of the B isoform is also overexpressed in human asthmatics (133). Taken together, the amount and the velocity of shortening are potentially important factors determining the level of airway responsiveness. However, more data are needed to confirm that derangements in these contractile properties are involved in the manifestation of asthmatic AHR.

2.5 Ability to relax

ASM relaxation can also affect airway luminal diameter and the degree of airway responsiveness (reviewed in (69) and (44)). Just as stiffness, relaxation can have different connotations. It could refer to the relaxation either during or following the removal of the spasmogenic stimulation, as well as the relaxation induced by a relaxing agonist (bronchodilator). The time of onset, the rate and the extent of relaxation following stimulation with a relaxing agonist, or during or after the removal of the spasmogen, can also impact airway patency. The potential implication of impaired relaxation in asthma is clear. Incomplete or slower relaxation could keep the airways narrowed and, thus, prolong the respiratory distress experienced by asthmatics during an asthma attack. However, the mechanism by which impaired relaxation could contribute to AHR is not as obvious. It relies on the assumption that spontaneous relaxation occurs rapidly following airway narrowing induced by inhalational challenge with a spasmogen. Increased time for the muscle to relax following a spasmogenic stimulation certainly means that the airway luminal size will remain smaller for an extended period of time following a bronchoprovocative challenge and, consequently, will limit airflow during a forced expiratory maneuver (which is often used to assess airway responsiveness).

The following studies provide some evidences that impaired relaxation may play a role in determining the degree of airway responsiveness. Altered relaxation of ASM has been proposed to play a role in determining inherent differences in the degree of airway responsiveness observed between guinea pigs of different ages (reviewed in (44)). The absence or presence of spontaneous relaxation in response to continuous EFS has also been proposed to be a factor explaining innate differences of airway responsiveness seen in different strains of mice (44). The role of impaired relaxation of ASM in AHR seen in human asthmatics needs further investigations.

To reiterate, contractility is defined here as a vague term that may imply different contractile properties. So a hypercontractile ASM phenotype may imply one or all of the following: the muscle may be stronger (increased force-generating capacity), it may shorten more and/or shorten faster, it may be stiffer, it may have an attenuated ability to relax either spontaneously or in response to bronchodilators, or it may have an increased ability to tolerate or recover from a drop in force caused by length perturbations. As seen in this last chapter's section, there are currently evidences suggesting that some intrinsic defects of ASM can contribute to asthmatic AHR. This also suggests that being hyperresponsive could be a prerequisite, or at least a predisposing factor, to be diagnosed with athma. However, whether these intrinsic defects are genetically inherited or acquired as a result of other defects seen in asthmatics is still unknown. One might expect that if asthmatic AHR is due to inherited ASM hypercontractility, it should be encrypted into the genome? The next section shall explore this question.

3. Interrogating the genome for asthma susceptibility genes

Genetics has evolved tremendously in the last decades and is now endowed with powerful tools to ask questions on the etiology of complex human traits (77). Asthma and the degree of airway responsiveness are irrefutably complex traits. Based on genetic epidemiology studies, the heritability of asthma was estimated to be 40 to 60% (22). However, finding genes and genetic variants responsible for this important genetic component is still very challenging. Not only asthma is a complex trait because of its heterogeneous nature, but also because its manifestation relies on the exposure of an (or many) environmental trigger(s). Thus, a lot of noise in genetic analyses of asthma may stand from the fact that some non-asthmatics (control cohort) are carriers of susceptibility alleles, but are not asthmatics because they never encountered the environmental trigger(s). In addition, maybe more than a single complex trait is required to develop clinical manifestations of asthma. For example, both AHR and airway inflammation may be required to suffer from asthma. If true, the noise in genetic analyses may arise from people with airway inflammation (e.g., atopy) that are protected from asthma symptoms because they are normo- or hypo-responsive. In fact, ~50% of the population is atopic but most of the affected individuals are non-asthmatics. On the other hand, some people may be carrier of alleles that confer susceptibility to AHR, which also confer susceptibility to asthma, but will always be free of asthma symptoms because they will never develop airway inflammation. In fact, it is estimated that roughly 15% of the population is hyperresponsive. Some of these people are asymptomatic, will never be diagnosed with asthma, and are counted in the control (non-asthmatic) group in most genetic studies despite being carriers of alleles conferring susceptibility to asthma.

Despite these challenges, recent progress in genetics of asthma was made by genome-wide association studies (GWAS). These studies consist of testing hundreds of thousands of single-nucleotide polymorphisms (SNPs) distributed across the human genome for association with a disease in hundreds or thousands of individuals. This genomic approach was particularly successful to identify robustly replicated genetic variants involved in complex diseases and biological traits (142). Asthma and asthma-related phenotypes are no exception and a number of GWAS were performed in the field (83, 104, 163, 164, 223).

Before the era of GWAS, more than 100 genes have been associated with asthma and related phenotypes (22, 183). Figure 1 shows these genes classified by their most likely pathobiological implication in asthma. Most of these genes were found using a candidate gene strategy (in blue), while fewer were found using genome-wide linkage studies (in green). Eleven genes were specifically studied for their possible involvement in bronchoconstriction and it is suspected that the risk conferred by genetic variants in these genes may act directly through ASM. However, for all these genes the functional demonstration remains to be made. In addition, candidate gene studies were plagued with

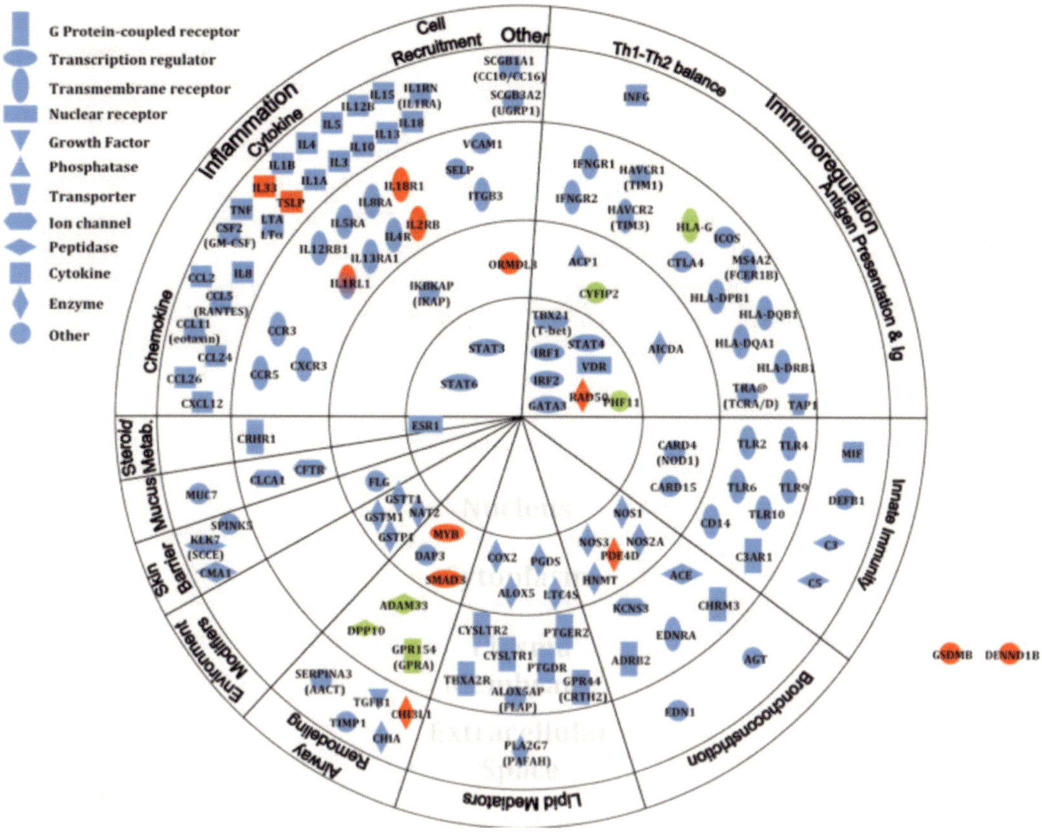

Fig. 1. Overview of asthma susceptibility genes. Genes illustrated are reported to be associated with asthma or asthma-related phenotypes in at least one published study. Each gene is categorized according to what we believe is its major role in the pathogenesis of asthma. In blue and green are genes identified using candidate gene and genome-wide linkage studies, respectively. The latest and more robust asthma susceptibility genes are illustrated in red and identified using a genome-wide association approach. Complete references for genes in blue and green can be found in Ober & Hoffjan (183). References for genes in red are in the text (see section 3). The shapes and subcellular localizations are taken from the Ingenuity System (http://www.ingenuity.com). Genes are labeled with official Entrez Gene symbols, and common alias names are shown in parentheses for some genes. The figure is updated from Bossé & Hudson (Annu Rev Med 2007; 58: 171-84).

inconsistency and genetic associations illustrated in Figure 1 require validation in large population samples.

In contrast to candidate gene studies, susceptibility genes derived from GWAS on asthma were confirmed in multiple and larger set of samples. These genes include ORMDL3, GSDMB, IL33, TSLP, IL18R1, IL1RL1, IL2RB, RAD50, MYB, SMAD3, CHI3L1, PDE4D, and DENND1B (illustrated in red in Figure 1). The specific cells and tissues that are molecularly altered by the risk variant in these genes are still unknown. Most of these genes are not known as regulators of airway responsiveness, suggesting that the genetic predisposition to suffer from asthma do not originate from genes altering ASM function. In fact, most of the GWAS-nominated asthma genes are expressed in the airway epithelium or in inflammatory cells, which is consistent with the growing body of evidences that asthma originates in subjects whose epithelium has altered response to environmental triggers and whose immune system is susceptible to the development of inflammation. The exception is the PDE4D gene found to be associated with asthma in multiple white and Hispanic populations (104). PDE4D is expressed in ASM and can potentially alter ASM contractile function, suggesting that this tissue, in addition to the epithelium and inflammatory cells, may influence susceptibility to asthma.

It should be noted that we cannot rule out the contribution of other GWAS-nominated genes acting on ASM. We know from our previous whole-genome gene expression experiment in bronchial smooth muscle cells (23) that approximately half of the genes in the human genome are expressed in non-stimulated ASM cells (nearly 10,000 genes). Obviously other genes might be inducible and expressed only in a 'sick' environment. However, at baseline, in a monolayer of ASM cells, many GWAS-nominated asthma genes are expressed including ORMDL3, GSDMB, IL33, TSLP, RAD50, SMAD3, CHI3L1, and DENND1B. Although what is known about the biological functions of these genes is not pointing toward ASM as the primary pathobiological target, their expression in this tissue suggests that they may play a role. The characterization of asthma susceptibility genes derived from GWAS is currently a priority in the field of genetics of asthma (182). The functions of these genes in ASM, if any, will need to be investigated, as are the consequences of the risk variants on these functions.

4. Non-muscle factors

In contrast to the above, AHR may also be secondary to the asthmatic syndrome. In fact, many causes of AHR in asthma are attributed to alterations in the lung environment; implying that the ASM can be absolutely normal but would lead to AHR upon activation because it operates in a 'bad' environment. Two scenarios here are envisaged: First, AHR may develop in asthmatic individuals because inflammatory or remodeling changes alter ASM contractile properties. In those instances, AHR still relies on a defect in ASM contractile properties, as discussed in section 2, but they are acquired as a result of an altered environment. Parenthetically, the phenomena that lead to an acquired increase in contractility will be called here an 'ASM behavior' (see Figure 2). Thus, a behavior is a normal ASM's ability to adapt to its surrounding environment. Some ASM behaviors are addressed in the non-muscle factors section of this chapter because their appearance is attributable to lung defects. This didactic distinction between ASM contractile properties and behaviors would become clearer along the remaining of this chapter. In the second scenario, certain causes of AHR are unrelated to genetically or acquired abnormalities of ASM but are rather due, exclusively, to lung alterations. In those instances, the abnormal milieu is sufficient to cause AHR in a setting where none of the ASM contractile properties are altered. In the following section, we will describe the non-muscle factors that are potentially involved in asthmatic AHR by affecting, or not, the contractile properties of ASM. Four broad themes will be discussed; that is remodeling, airway inflammation, ASM-tone and ventilation heterogeneity. Some of the factors discussed below were addressed in previous reviews (24, 26).

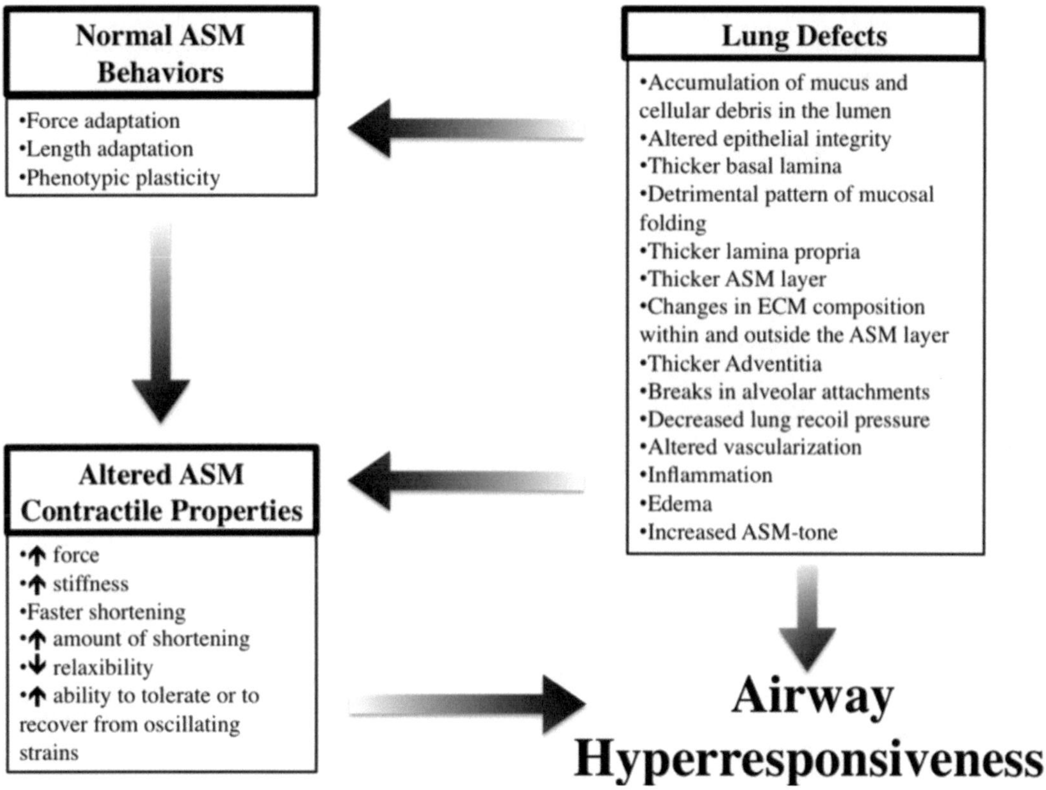

Fig. 2. Muscle and non-muscle mechanisms potentially involved in airway hyperresponsiveness (AHR) seen in asthmatic patients. Any alterations in airway smooth muscle (ASM) contractile properties, which can be innate or acquired as a result of lung defects, may participate in the development and manifestation of AHR. Lung defects can also contribute to AHR either directly or by fostering normal ASM behaviors, such as force adaptation. See text for further details.

4.1 Remodeling

The term 'remodeling' refers to any structural changes occurring in the lungs. It could be any alteration in the quantity, the distribution and the composition of the molecular, cellular and tissular constituents of the lungs. It can affect, or not, the physical and mechanical properties of the lung constituents. The term 'remodeling' is also usually reserved for structural changes that are permanent or fixed (relatively), such as the deposition of extra ECM components. So even if edema and inflammatory cell infiltrates fit into the definition of remodeling given above, these changes are not usually perceived as remodeling changes. They are rather the results of inflammatory processes that are transient and reversible in nature. Generally speaking, remodeling can designate any or all of the following: epithelial metaplasia, such as zone of denudation, deciliated areas and goblet cell hyperplasia; fibrosis of all the airway wall layers but especially the *lamina reticularis* (the third layer of the basal lamina); vascular alterations, such as vessel enlargement and angiogenesis; thickening of all the layers of the airway wall including the epithelium, the basal lamina, the lamina propria, the ASM and the adventitia; and parenchymal changes, such as emphysema and breaks of alveolar attachments on the outer edge of the airway wall (Figure 3). Lung remodeling, especially airway remodeling, has been reviewed by many in the past (25). In the present chapter, we focus on the structural changes that have been shown or suggested to alter the level of airway responsiveness.

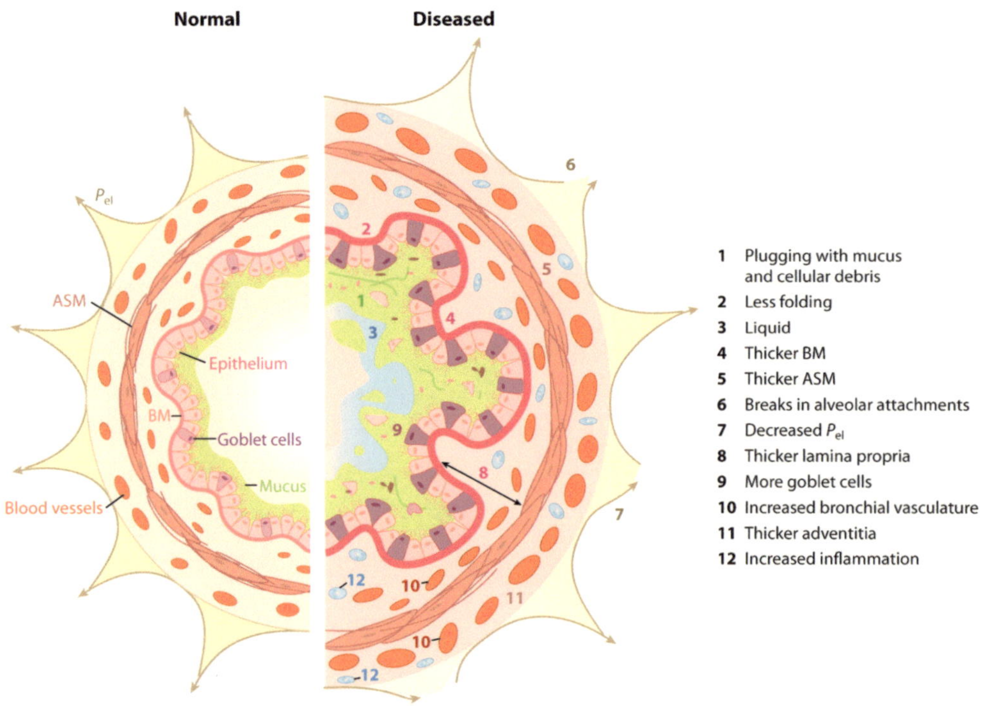

AR Bossé Y, et al. 2010.
Annu. Rev. Physiol. 72:437–62

Fig. 3. A cartoon of an airway half normal (on the left) and half asthmatic (on the right) to illustrate the various features of airway remodeling in asthma. Airway responsiveness can be influenced by (1) an increase in volume of mucus and/or cellular debris in the airway lumen, (2) fewer but deeper folds in the mucosal membrane, (3) increased volume or altered surface tension of the liquid layer, (4) thickening and stiffening of the basement membrane (BM), (5) increased ASM mass embedded in an increased fibrous network, (6) decreased integrity and/or (7) decreased number of alveolar tethers to the adventitia contributing to decreased elastic recoil, (8) increased thickness of the lamina propria, (9) increased goblet cell number, (10) increased vascularity and/or vascular dilatation in the lamina propria and adventitia, (11) increased thickness of the adventitia, and (12) increased inflammatory cell infiltration throughout the airway wall. From Bossé *et al*. Annu Rev Physiol 2010; 72: 437-62.

4.1.1 Epithelium integrity

Researchers working with isolated airway segments *ex vivo* have long recognized that the concentration of spasmogens required for a given response is orders of magnitude greater (30 to 300-fold) when a chosen spasmogen is delivered on the mucosal side (within the lumen) compared to when it is delivered on the adventitial side (179). Mechanical removal of the epithelium in bronchial segments of dogs has also been shown to increase ACh sensitivity by 100 to 716-fold (159, 187). These observations suggested that the epithelium acts as a cellular barrier and establishes a large concentration gradient across the airway wall. A breach in the integrity of the epithelium would disrupt its barrier function and, consequently, increases airway responsiveness by facilitating the delivery of spasmogens to the ASM. In fact, association between epithelial permeability and airway responsiveness in humans has been previously reported (108); albeit this finding is not unanimous (197). Increased leakiness of the epithelium can be due to cellular damage and desquamation, which can be induced, for example, by eosinophil mobilization and activation into the airways. Disruption of cell-cell connectivity, by interrupting E-cadherin adhesion for example, can equally facilitate the delivery of spasmogens to the ASM by increasing the paracellular conductance (254). Many asthma stressors, such as allergens, ozone, particulate matters, smoke and occupational triggers have been shown to affect airway epithelial integrity, which may underlie their link with AHR. Alterations in epithelium integrity by these asthma stressors can be mediated directly, or indirectly by fostering inflammatory cell infiltration into the epithelium or by increasing the release of endogenous proteases (187).

In addition to act as a physical barrier, the airway epithelium can also play a direct role in controlling ASM contractility. The airway epithelium has been shown to produce several bronchoactive substances, such as lipooxygenase and cyclooxygenase products as well as nitric oxide. This subject was reviewed in the past (225) and will not be discussed in detail here. Briefly, the combined effect of these mediators seems to be bronchodilatory and may thus play a protective role against airway narrowing. Collectively, these observations suggest that any alteration in the lungs affecting the integrity of the epithelium or the release of epithelium-derived bronchoactive substances may influence airway responsiveness.

4.1.2 Vascular remodeling

The number and size of blood vessels, as well as the vascular area, are increased in asthmatic airways (reviewed in (55)). Signs of dilation, congestion, endothelium leakiness and abnormal wall thickness of the airway vessels have also been noted, which all alter by different manner and different extent the normal function of these vessels. The space occupied by the vessels conspicuously increases airway wall thickness, but may also do so by changing its turgidity. It may also modify the mechanical properties of the airway wall and affect the pattern of airway wall folding during airway narrowing. The detrimental effects of these structural changes are discussed in the following subsections (4.1.3 and 4.1.4).

Chronic vascular alterations also have the potential to exacerbate edematous changes occurring in the face of inflammation (discussed in section 4.2.2). It may also alter the clearance of spasmogens into the airways, which can greatly affect the degree of airway responsiveness (151). Taken together, these results suggest that changes in number, size, structure and integrity of the vascular bed interwinding the airway wall can have direct or indirect repercussions on airway responsiveness.

4.1.3 Increased amount of material inner the ASM layer

As aforementioned, all the layers of the airway wall were shown to be thicker in asthma. An increased amount of material inner the ASM layer amplifies the luminal airway narrowing for any given degree of ASM shortening. This is because of a geometrical effect. Airway resistance is inversely related to the luminal radius at the fourth power. So small decreases in radius can cause huge increases in airflow resistance. This effect is more pronounced when the thickening encroaches the lumen (inwardly-directed remodeling) prior constriction. This is because the airway lumen will be smaller to begin with. Thus, the same amount of ASM shortening (or the same decrease in luminal radius) would increase further the resistance to airflow. However, this geometric effect would also occur if the thickening does not encroach the lumen (outwardly-directed remodeling) prior constriction. This is because the luminal area decreases as the ASM shortens, but the area of the material inner the ASM does not; assuming that this material is uncompressible. With a greater fraction of the total area occupied by uncompressible material to begin with, a thicker airway wall would exaggerate the changes in the luminal area during ASM shortening. In other words, for a given change in total area (i.e., area inner the ASM layer), if more area is occupied by uncompressible material, more changes in the compressible area (i.e., lumen) would have to occur. Importantly, filling the airway lumen by inflammatory cells, mucus accumulation or by plasma extravasation would have the same detrimental consequence.

In vivo, even if the material inner the ASM would be somewhat compressible, an increased amount of material inner the ASM layer would still contribute to AHR, unless the compressibility of this material is severely affected in asthma. Computation models of the human bronchial tree confirmed that thicker airway wall inner the ASM increases airflow resistance caused by any given degree of ASM activation (126). This effect may not be small. Wagers and coworkers have developed a computational model based on morphometric and functional data derived from a mouse model of allergic airway inflammation to address this question. They predicted that thickening of the airway wall combined with an increased propensity for airway closure (discussed later in subsection 4.4.2) in the 'asthmatic' mice were sufficient to explain entirely AHR, without the need of increasing ASM shortening (237). Taken together, any lung defect that increase the volume of material inner the ASM layer leads to more luminal narrowing for any given degree of ASM shortening. This is a good example showing that AHR may be present despite normal ASM contractility.

4.1.4 Reduced ASM-load due to remodeling

The load impeding muscle shortening is just as important as the force-generating capacity of the ASM. A weaker load will allow the ASM to shorten more but also to shorter faster for the same reasons as a stronger ASM would shorten more and faster against a given load (discussed in subsection 2.1).

The loads impeding ASM shortening originate from different airway wall and lung elements. One of the most important load is the parenchymal recoil; i.e., the radial tethering force offered by the parenchymal attachments on the outer edge (adventitia) of the airway wall. In fact, this load seems to be crucial for the maintenance of intraparenchymal airway patency. In condition where the ASM would be fully relaxed, this load is totally counterbalanced by the circumferential tension of the airway wall; an inwardly-directed force equal to the force of recoil but acting in opposite direction. To overcome a greater recoil, more strain within the airway wall would be required to reach a circumferential tension equal but opposite to the recoil, which would mean more airway dilatation. Therefore, greater parenchymal recoil leads to greater airway caliber. The extent of the recoil depends on lung volume, the elasticity of the parenchymal tissue and the strength of the connection between the airway wall and the parenchyma (the later is sometimes called the force of interdependence). Any lung defect affecting these parameters may influence the strength of the recoil at a given lung volume and, concomitantly, change airway caliber. The parenchymal recoil also offers an additional load during airway narrowing because the lung parenchyma is progressively distorted as the ASM shortens. This load can be calculated from the shear modulus (μ) of the lung parenchyma, which was estimated to be 0.7 time the transpulmonary pressure (124), and the changes in adventitial diameter during airway narrowing, which is geometrically related to the changes in ASM length during shortening (126). So in addition to keep the intraparenchymal airways patent prior constriction, the lung recoil imposes an after-load that further limits airway narrowing once the ASM begins to shorten. Lung defects previously observed in asthma, such as alveolar breaks (149) and adventitial thickening (190), were shown to decouple the airways from the parenchyma and affect the extent of both the pre- and the after-load offered by the recoil. These lung defects may contribute to AHR.

The ECM within and surrounding the ASM bundle also affects the after-load impeding muscle shortening. In conditions where the muscle is fully relaxed, the circumferential tension (which is carrying the load of the recoil) would be born from the passive elements of the airway wall, including the resting tension of the ASM. However, during narrowing induced by ASM shortening, the load carried by the parallel elastic elements is progressively transferred to the ASM. This transfer proceeds until these parallel elastic elements are no longer in tension but in compression. At that time, they become a direct load impeding muscle shortening. So whether these parallel elastic elements are in tension and progressively transfer the load to the ASM during airway narrowing or whether they pass the transition from being in tension to become in compression, they still limit ASM shortening by increasing the after-load. If this material is stiffer for example, it would be carrying more load for less strain (i.e., for a given lung recoil pressure there will be less airway dilatation). In those conditions, while the ASM begins to shorten upon activation, a greater load would be transferred to the ASM for a given amount of airway narrowing. It will also be harder to compress this material if airway narrowing proceeds until the parallel elastic elements are no longer in tension but in compression. In addition, when a cell or a bundle of ASM shortens, its center tempts to bulge. Anything that would prevent the modification of cell shape required for shortening may limit airway narrowing. This load has been called radial constraint (190). Together, this suggests that the quantity and the mechanical properties of the ECM, but also any other wall constituents, within and surrounding the ASM cells or bundles may affect the degree of airway narrowing. In support of this contention, pre-treatment of airway wall strips with collagenase was shown to increase ASM shortening in response to a given contractile stimulus (29). This result suggested that degradation of the collagenous matrix in the airway wall reduces the load, allowing the ASM to shorten further in response to a given level of activation.

Epithelial buckling pressure and airway wall corrugation that occur during airway narrowing are also believed to provide an after-load hampering ASM shortening. The number of mucosal folds developing during narrowing seems to be of major importance. The number of folds, in turn, may be determined by the flexibility, stiffness and thickness of the airway wall, by the stiffness and thickness ratios of the different layers composing the airway wall, or by structural features such as longitudinal elastic bundles (37) or blood and lymphatic vessels (239), which could dictate the location of the folds. More studies are warranted to establish a consensus concerning the factors influencing the pattern of mucosal folding and how it affects ASM-load. Current evidences suggested that the number of folds is not different between asthmatic and non-asthmatic airways (37).

The load impeding ASM shortening may either decrease or increase due to airway remodeling. Thickening and/or fibrosis of the airway wall, for instance, may protect against airway narrowing. Accordingly, airway reactivity was shown to correlate negatively with airway wall thickness in humans with asthma (155, 175). Similar observations were made in a mouse model of asthma (2). Therefore, even if thickening due to fibrosis can theoretically increase airway narrowing in response to spasmogens because of geometrical effects, airway wall stiffening due to thicker or more fibrotic wall may well protect against AHR. Clearly, it is not just the geometric effects of wall thickening that influence airway narrowing (189). The mechanical properties of the material that causes the thickening are also important since ASM has to deform this material to narrow the lumen. The composition of the ECM may also affect the ASM phenotype (discussed in subsection 4.1.6).

Taken together, we have seen that the caliber of the airways embedded in the parenchyma is determined by the dilating force of the lung elastic recoil and the stiffness of the airway wall. Anything affecting the parenchymal recoil, the airway-parenchymal interdependence, the parallel elastic elements, the radial constraint and the pattern of mucosal folding may reduce (or augment) the load and, consequently, causes more (or less) ASM shortening for any given degree of ASM activation.

4.1.5 Length adaptation

A decrease in airway caliber caused by any lung defect attenuating the pre-load would cause a reduction in ASM length. Because the force-generating capacity of the ASM is proportional to its length, decreasing ASM length simultaneously decreases its force-generating capacity. However, the ASM is endowed with an intrinsic ability to adapt to length changes (reviewed in (27)). This phenomenon was called length adaptation and is defined as the recovery of ASM force-generating capacity that was loss following length perturbations. Adaptation of ASM to a shorter length is particularly relevant to the understanding of AHR. This is because a muscle adapted to shorten length is able to generate more force at any given length during shortening comparatively to a muscle adapted to a longer length. In contradistinction, adaptation to longer length would have a protective effect in terms of airway responsiveness. This is a good example to show how a normal ASM behavior (i.e., length adaptation), may contribute to AHR by increasing a contractile property of the ASM (herein force).

Length adaptation is likely to occur in different situations. Emphysema, for example, decreases airway caliber by reducing lung recoil, which will allow the ASM to adapt to shorter length. Other factors reducing lung volume such as recumbent posture (247), high spinal cord injury (201) and obesity could have a similar effect. However, a recent review on obesity and AHR (206) rather concludes that obesity has little direct effect on airway caliber despite reducing functional residual capacity (FRC) and expiratory reserve volume. Based on the authors, the expiratory flow limitation observed in individuals with low lung volume (like the obese) is due to an increased propensity for airway closure (discussed in subsection 4.4.2). That may also apply to other conditions affecting lung volume.

Another contractile property that is affected by length adaptation is the ASM-passive stiffness. It was shown that the passive stiffness initially declines following a length reduction but slowly re-develops over time (28). However, since the contribution of ASM-passive stiffness to the overall stiffness of the airway wall is neglectable, it is insignificant to the understanding of AHR in asthma.

4.1.6 Alterations in the composition to the ECM

It was suggested that the phenotype of ASM cells can be switched around from a contractile phenotype to a synthetic/proliferative phenotype (95). ECM components are thought to play an important role in determining ASM phenotypes. Laminin, for example, was shown to be required for the transformation of ASM cells into a more contractile phenotype (233). The existing interplay between ECM and ASM phenotypes and functions has been the subject of other reviews (232). It is known that the composition of the ECM is altered in asthma due to either a change in the rate of ECM component synthesis or a change in the rate of their degradation, the later being controlled by a balance between proteases and their inhibitors. Taken together, this suggests that a fine balance of ECM components is required to keep the ASM phenotype in check. Any alteration in this balance may affect ASM contractility and airway responsiveness.

4.1.7 Enlargement of ASM mass

We came to realize that the mass of ASM is increased in asthmatic airways almost a century ago (106). This structural change was one of the first hypothesis advanced to explain AHR in asthma and has not been refuted yet. Although a recent study suggested that the increased ASM mass is related predominantly to cellular hyperplasia rather than hypertrophy (199), the exact origin of ASM enlargement is still a matter of debate. In addition to the possibilities of cellular hyperplasia and hypertrophy, alternative hypotheses have been proposed, such as myositis (i.e., inflammation of the ASM) and increased ECM deposition. The origin of hyperplasia is also unclear but could stem from increased proliferation, decreased rate of apoptosis and/or migration of ASM progenitors into the ASM bundle with their subsequent differentiation into ASM cells (reviewed in (25)). The role of proliferation in ASM hyperplasia has gained credibility recently when Hassan and coworkers (100) provided data suggestive of an increased rate of ASM cell proliferation in humans with severe asthma. Irrespective of the mechanism of ASM thickening, the increased mass could lead to a greater total force generation for any given level of ASM activation; assuming that the ASM from asthmatics produce the same stress (force per cross-sectional area) as non-asthmatic ASM. *In vivo,* that would be translated into increased airway narrowing for any given dose of inhaled spasmogen and, therefore, AHR.

To reiterate, asthmatic remodeling is characterized by relatively permanent changes in the architecture of the airways, the lung parenchyma and their interconnection. Many of these changes can affect, positively or negatively, the degree of airway responsiveness. The integrity of the epithelium and vascular remodeling may influence the delivery and the clearance of spasmogens toward and away from the ASM, respectively. Increased amount of material inner the ASM layer can increase airway narrowing by a geometrical effect. Decremented load impeding ASM shortening can cause more ASM shortening for any given degree of ASM activation. Remodeling can also promote ASM hypercontractility by fostering normal ASM behaviors such as length adaptation or phenotype switching. Finally, factors fostering the growing of the ASM mass encircling the airways may increase ASM-force per unit of airway length. Those are all different ways by which a normal ASM may account for AHR in a remodeled environment.

4.2 Airway inflammation

Airway inflammation is a hallmark of asthma. The use of the term 'airway inflammation' is vague though. Asthma can be characterized by different types of inflammation, which may be useful to distinguish for diagnosis purposes and to offer patients the optimal therapeutic strategy (248). There is clearly a link between airway inflammation and AHR. Interventions altering airway inflammation are effective in changing the degree of airway responsiveness. For example, AHR can be increased in asthmatics following the induction of acute inflammation by inhalation of allergens (47, 143) or IL-5 (218). On the other hand, reducing inflammation by the use of glucocorticoids attenuates AHR (reviewed in (30)).

Airway inflammation can affect airway responsiveness by many means. It is sometime hard to dissociate the effect of inflammatory changes from remodeling changes, since both can affect features of the airway wall, such as its thickness, that participate to AHR. It is also hard to dissociate because of the interplay that exists between inflammation and remodeling. Many believe that inflammation is the cause of remodeling, as the damage caused by inflammation may lead to impaired repair, scaring and loss of function. For the sake of this chapter, we considered inflammation as the transient and potentially reversible changes occurring in the lungs of asthmatics following exposure to the triggering agent. We also consider the direct influence of asthma triggers and inflammation-derived molecules on ASM contractile properties.

4.2.1 Mucus accumulation

Any encroachment of the airway lumen, whether it is provoked by narrowing or by filling the lumen, causes airway obstruction, increases airway resistance and contributes to AHR. The mucus layer is required for normal lung homeostasis. It is recognized as a physical and immunological barrier protecting the host against inhaled pathogens, particulates and pollutants. However, its hyper-secretion can encroach the lumen and causes airway obstruction. Goblet cell hyperplasia (1), as well as enlargement and hyperplasia of the submucosal glands (16), can contribute to mucus hyper-secretion. These are remodeling changes but their contribution to lung dysfunction is only manifested upon exposure to airway stresses. In the extreme cases, mucus can also cause complete occlusion by forming mucus plugs, which contain, in addition to mucus, proteinaceous exudate, inflammatory cells and isolated epithelial cells and creola bodies (123). Complete occlusion of some airways severely compromises airflow into the lungs, and may thus be an important player in the manifestation of AHR. It also has severe repercussions on ventilation.

The accumulation of mucus can also originate from improper clearance. Mucociliary clearance was shown to be slower in asthmatics (108). The cephalad transport of mucus into the lungs is motored by a synchronized rotational beating of the epithelial cils and by cough when necessary. It also relies on the integrity of a low-viscosity solution lying atop the epithelial cells called the periciliary liquid layer (PCL), which prevents the shear friction between the epithelial surface glycocalyx and the mucus layer (120). Any alteration in mucus clearance, such as cil diskinesia, changes in mucus consistency, overly thin PCL and problems associated with cough reflex can all lead to mucus accumulation and airway obstruction. In addition, stagnant mucus can increase the risk of infection (120).

Mucus accumulation also increases the surface tension. It was estimated that replacing the normal fluid lining the epithelium of peripheral airways by mucus would increase surface tension by 5 folds (141). Surface tension is sometime overlook but can play an important role in determining the degree of airway responsiveness. This was well demonstrated when we came to realize that the pressure required to achieve a given lung volume is significantly higher when the lung is inflated with a gas compare to when it is filled with a liquid. In addition to its great impact on airway resistance, surface tension also increases the propensity for airway closure. In fact, a 5-fold increase in surface tension was predicted to be sufficient to cause airway instability and collapse (141). The influence of airway closure in airway responsiveness is discussed further in subsection 4.4.2. The role of surfactant in controlling surface tension is thus of major importance. Any alteration in surfactant caused by allergen exposure (51) or plasma exudation (238) is likely to affect surface tension and, concomitantly, lung functions (257). Finally, combined with ASM constriction, the baseline airway obstruction induced by mucus accumulation can synergistically increase airway responsiveness for geometric reasons mentioned in section 4.1.3.

4.2.2 Edema

Edema is a characteristic feature of inflammation. It is due to an increased permeability of the vessels. This increased leakiness of the vascular endothelium swells the tissue by fostering extravasation of inflammatory cells, as well as plasmatic fluid and proteins, into the interstitial tissue. It may also encroach the airway lumen. Plasma exudation onto the epithelial lining is increased in asthma and the extent of it is associated with the level of airway responsiveness (235). Many inflammatory molecules that are overexpressed in asthma were shown to increase vascular permeability, such as substance P, histamine and many others. Newly formed blood vessels are also more permeable than the existing vessels (10). Angiogenic remodeling seen in asthma may thus render the airways more prone to tumefaction.

Edema can alter the degree of airway responsiveness by many means. Plasma exudation induced experimentally by infusion of saline in dogs was shown to increase airway wall thickness and to decrease the caliber of the airway lumen over the level achieved simply by increasing the vascular pressure (35). This model of airway edema suggested that both the airway wall thickness and the size of the lumen are affected at baseline by airway turgidity. These changes in lumen and airway wall geometry can severely increase the degree of airway responsiveness as discussed in section 4.1.3. In fact, using this dog model of airway engorgement by saline infusion, it was shown that airway responsiveness to histamine increases for the same level of ASM shortening (34). Leakage of plasma protein in the epithelial lining fluid can also be detrimental for airway narrowing and closure. Fibrin, for example, inactivates the surfactant and can increase airway responsiveness by increasing the surface tension (238).

4.2.3 Inflammatory cells and molecules

In addition to mucus accumulation and edema, which increase airway responsiveness mainly by changing the luminal and airway wall geometry, other inflammatory changes may increase directly ASM contractility.

At the cellular level, mast cells have been linked to increased ASM contractility. The number of mast cells has been shown to be elevated in ASM tissues of asthmatics compared to non-asthmatic subjects with or without other inflammatory disorders (31). The participation of mast cells in AHR has been suggested based on correlations observed between the percentage of mast cells recovered in the bronchoalveolar lavage fluid (BALF) (64) or interspersed in the ASM tissue (113) and the degree of airway responsiveness. Interestingly, the later correlation was even stronger when the mast cells with a fibroblastoid phenotype, which spontaneously produce more histamine, were counted (113). It was also demonstrated using immunohistological sections of human airways that ASM cells that localized in vicinity of mast cells express higher levels of α-smooth muscle actin (α-SMA), suggesting a paracrine influence of mast cells that increases ASM contractility (255). Taken together, these results suggest that the release of mast cell-derived mediators or direct mast cell-ASM contact could contribute to AHR by making the ASM stronger.

An earlier study also suggested that a short period of mast cell activation alone is sufficient to induce AHR in mice. In that study, it was shown that acute activation of mast cells by an anti-IgE antibody 20 min prior to methacholine (MCh) challenge increases airway responsiveness in wild-type naïve (i.e., non-sensitized and challenged) animals but not in mast cell-deficient naïve animals (146). Apart from histamine, mast cells can release a plethora of inflammatory mediators upon activation. As it is the case for histamine, some of these mediators increase ASM-tone directly by triggering ASM contraction, such as prostaglandin D_2 and leukotrienes. It would be a hard task to distinguish the effect of inflammation from the effect of increased ASM-tone on airway responsiveness. This is because a lot of molecules that are part of the asthmatic inflammatory processes are spasmogens. The increase ASM-tone caused by inflammation-derived spasmogens will be discussed separately in a following subsection (4.3). In the present subsection, the focus is on the inflammatory mediators that are not spasmogenic but have been shown to increase ASM contractility.

At the molecular level, several asthma triggers have been shown to increase ASM contractility *ex vivo*. For example, ASM contractility has been shown to be enhanced following prolong (at least 16 h) incubation with atopic serum (15, 19, 78, 89, 91, 161, 211, 245, 246), IgE immune complex (80, 89, 250) and exogenous asthma triggers such as the house dust mite allergen *Der p 1* (82), the bacterial endotoxin lipopolysaccharide (LPS) (8, 166, 216, 220) and the rhinovirus (serotype 16) (78, 81) or the virus mimetic toll-like receptor (TLR)3 ligand polyinosinic polycytidylic acid (poly-IC) (8). Most of these studies assessed ASM contractility by measuring its force-generating capacity. However, some studies also reported that some of these inflammatory insults change the velocity and amount of shortening of the ASM in response to a spasmogen (161), as well as its ability to relax in response to bronchodilators (8, 15, 78, 81, 89, 216). The half-time of relaxation after short EFS-induced tetani has also been shown to increase (double) in ASM strips derived from dogs sensitized to ragweed (109).

The effect of asthma triggers on *ex vivo* ASM contractility can be indirect; i.e., due to an autocrine loop of mediators that are produced by the ASM in response to asthma triggers (79, 80, 91, 166). *In vivo*, the paracrine influence of other cells that are responsive to asthma triggers can also impact ASM contractility. Ultimately, all the inflammatory mediators overexpressed in asthma, whether they originate from other cells or from the ASM itself, can contribute individually or in combination to ASM hypercontractility and AHR. Supports for this contention are accumulating. Cytokines such as interleukin (IL)-1β (11, 92, 200, 250), tumor necrosis factor (TNF)α (4, 7, 167, 168, 172, 191, 193, 200, 227), the combination of TNFα and IL-1β (90, 92), IL-13 (41, 62, 80, 228), IL-5 (93, 250), IL-10 (79), granulocyte-macrophage colony-stimulating factor (GM-CSF) (94), interferon (IFN)γ (5), leukemia inhibitory factor (LIF) (63, 119) and transforming growth factor (TGF)β (75, 255), as well as the protease β-tryptase (212, 255) were shown to increase ASM contractility. In turn, the effect of these mediators is not always direct. For example, the potentiating effect of IL-1β on bradykinin-induced contraction is due to a greater release of thromboxane (Tx)A_2 in response to bradykinin (166). As for the asthma triggers, most of these studies assessed ASM contractility by measuring its force-generating capacity. However, inflammatory mediators found in asthmatic airways can also impair ASM relaxation. For example TNFα (90, 92), IL-1β (90, 92), IL-13 (127), IL-10 (79), IL-5 (79) and lysophosphatidic acid (LPA) (230) have all been shown to attenuate ASM relaxation elicited by β_2-adrenoceptor agonists. In addition, TNFα (9, 92) and IL-1β (92) were shown to attenuate the relaxant effect of prostaglandin (PG)E_2.

The molecular mechanisms governing the transformation of ASM into a hypercontractile phenotype may differ from one inflammatory mediator to another. In the case of TGFβ, increased expression of the contractile protein α-SMA and actin filamentogenesis have been proposed (75, 76). On the other hand, many inflammatory mediators increase ASM contractility through shared mechanisms related to alterations in calcium handling; either by Ca^{2+} sensitization via the Rho-ROCK pathway or by increasing the intracellular mobilization of Ca^{2+} via the CD38/cADPR/RyR pathway (both briefly described below and illustrated in Figure 4).

Ca^{2+} sensitization is a phenomenon that allows the ASM to produce more force in response to a given mobilization of intracellular calcium concentration ($[Ca^{2+}]_i$). Ca^{2+} sensitization seems to rely mainly on a signaling pathway running in parallel to canonical Ca^{2+} signaling pathways (inositol 3-phosphate receptor (IP_3R)-dependent and entry from the extracellular compartment). The pathway is referred to as the Rho-Rho-associated, coiled coil-containing kinase (ROCK) pathway and is activated by certain G protein-coupled receptors (GPCRs) following ligation with their cognate spasmogen (see Figure 4). Rho is a small G (GTPase) protein activated by the exchange of GDP for GTP. The identity of the guanine exchange factor (GEF) that is activated by the GPCR and involved in Rho activation is unclear, and is probably receptor specific. However, one of the downstream signals mediated by Rho that leads to Ca^{2+} sensitization is well characterized. GTP-bound (active) Rho initially activates ROCK, which then inhibits myosin light chain (MLC) phosphatase (MLCP) both directly, via phosphorylation of the myosin phosphatase-targeting subunit 1 (MYPT1) of MLCP, and indirectly, via CPI-17 (17-kDa PKC-potentiated inhibitory protein of PP1; PP1 stands for protein phosphatase 1, which is the catalytic subunit of the heterotrimeric MLCP). Since the level of MLC phosphorylation depends on a balance between its phosphorylation by MLCK and its dephosphorylation by MLCP, direct or indirect inhibition of MLCP by ROCK causes more MLC phosphorylation for the same degree of MLCK activation. Therefore, when the Rho-ROCK pathway is activated, the same degree of MLCK activation induced by a given sarcoplasmic Ca^{2+} mobilization leads to more MLC phosphorylation and sequentially more activated cross-bridges and more force.

AHR in animal models of airway inflammation has been attributed to an increased ASM-sensitivity to Ca^{2+} (40, 43). Ca^{2+} sensitization is more typically triggered by inflammation-derived spasmogens (discussed in section 4.3.1), which bind to GPCRs capable of activating the Rho-ROCK pathway. However, non-spasmogenic inflammatory mediators such as TNFα have also been shown to potentiate ASM-force by fostering Ca^{2+} sensitization (107, 172, 191). In addition, the extent of Ca^{2+} sensitization can be regulated by mediators affecting the levels of expression or activation of key regulatory proteins involved in the Rho-ROCK pathway. For example, IL-13 (41) increases the level of RhoA expression in ASM, which consequently increases the proficiency of Rho-ROCK signaling pathway to induce Ca^{2+}

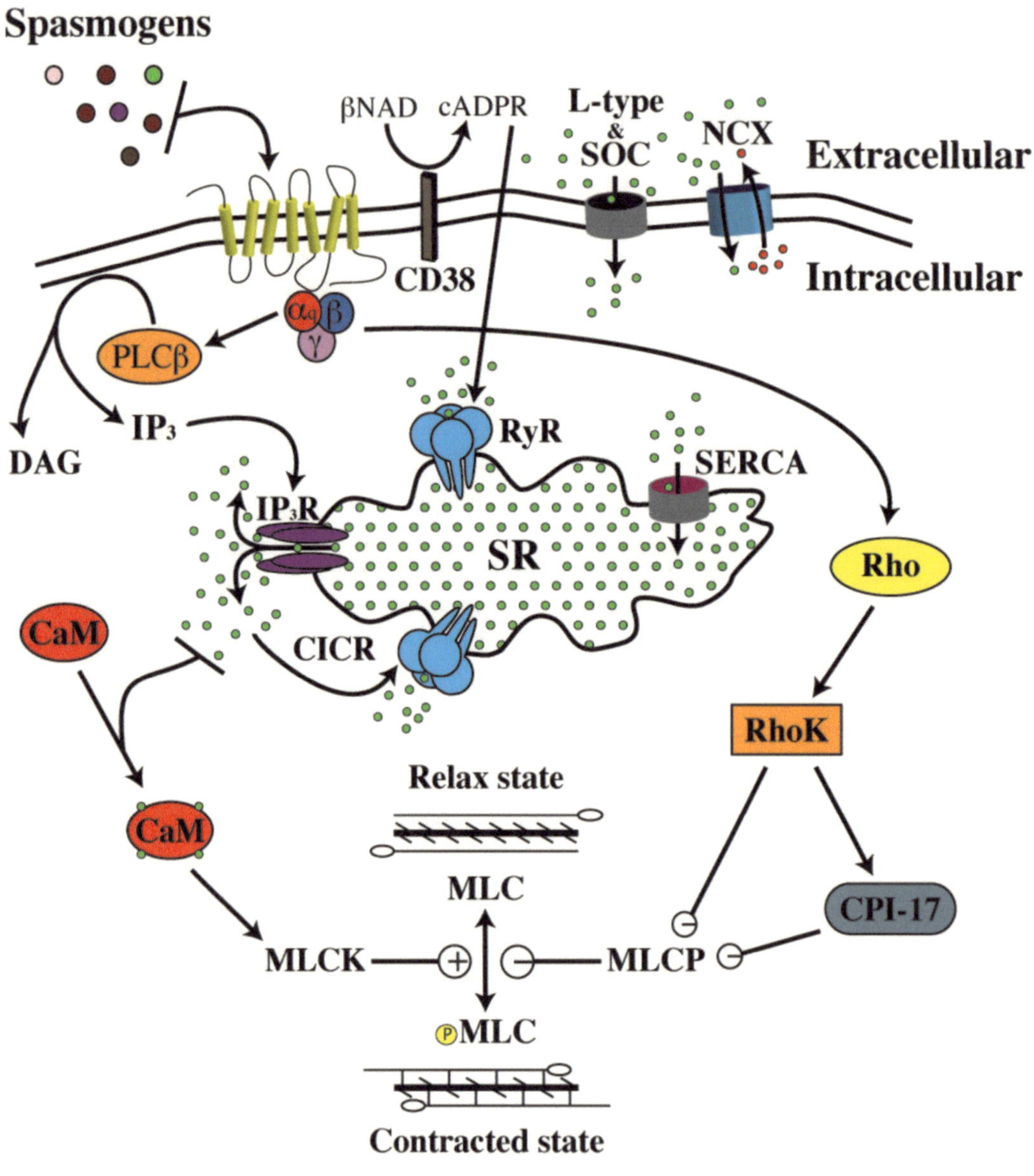

Fig. 4. Pathways transducing the extracellular signal of the spasmogens from their cognate cell-surface receptor to the contractile apparatus. See text for descriptions and abbreviations. The green and red dots represent Ca^{2+} and Na^{+}, respectively. The reverse mode of the Na^{+}/Ca^{2+} exchanger (NCX) is shown. Reproduced with permission from: Bossé and Paré. Airway smooth muscle responsiveness: The origin of airway hyperresponsiveness in asthma? Current Respiratory Medicine Reviews. 7(4): 289-301, 2011.

sensitization. On the other hand, mediators capable of reducing the expression/activity of intermediate proteins involved in this pathway may have therapeutic potential for diminishing Ca^{2+} sensitization and AHR. One example is the effect of glucocorticoids in reducing the expression of RhoA, which concomitantly attenuates antigen-induced ASM hyperresponsiveness in a rat model of allergic airway inflammation (40).

In addition to canonical Ca^{2+} signaling pathways, at least one other Ca^{2+} signaling pathway contributes to the release of Ca^{2+} into the sarcoplasm (see Figure 4). This pathway is referred to as the CD38/cyclic adenosine-5'-diphosphate (ADP) ribose (cADPR) signaling pathway and has received significant attention recently in regard to its potential role in AHR. CD38 is a type II transmembrane protein of 45-kDa with dual ecto-enzymatic activity. It possesses an ADP-ribosyl cyclase activity, converting β-NAD into cADPR and a cADPR hydrolase activity, converting the cADPR into ADPR. The product of the ADP-ribosyl cyclase activity, cADPR, sensitizes the ryanodine receptor (RyR) for Ca^{2+} release and, more specifically, potentiates Ca^{2+}-induced Ca^{2+} release (CICR) (70). Whether cADPR binds directly to RyR or requires other intermediates to open the RyR channel is still a matter of debate (54). What is sure is that cADPR increases the open probability of the RyR, liberating more Ca^{2+} from the sarcoplasmic reticulum (SR) (196). As is the case for IP_3R-dependent Ca^{2+} release, the CD38 pathway is also activated by binding of specific spasmogens to their cognate receptors (252). Thus, this pathway acts in parallel with the canonical Ca^{2+} signaling pathways to amplify the mobilization of Ca^{2+} into the sarcoplasm following spasmogenic stimulation.

The amplitude of Ca^{2+} release by the CD38/cADPR/RyR pathway, as well as its contribution in ASM-force generation, is influenced by CD38 expression. CD38 expression and/or activity were shown to be upregulated by many of the pro-inflammatory cytokines present in asthmatic airways, such as IFNβ (229), IFNγ (53), TNFα (53, 229), IL-1β (53) and IL-13 (52). Therefore, in the presence of inflammation, the proficiency of this signaling pathway to liberate the Ca^{2+} from the internal stores may be enhanced. Consequently, higher force generation would be attained for a given contractile stimulus since more Ca^{2+} would be released. The influence of inflammatory mediators on the CD38/cADPR/RyR pathway may thus play a role in AHR seen in asthma.

Taken together, these results suggested that the contractile properties of ASM are not fixed but rather plastic; i.e., they can change rapidly in the face of external (inflammatory) cues. So in an inflammatory lung disorder such as asthma, the ASM may be stronger or faster, for example, because of the 'bad' environment in which it is embedded. This increased contractility may only be present *in vivo* when the muscle is exposed to inflammation-derived mediators, but might be lost once the muscle is removed from the airways and washed repetitively before being studied *ex vivo*. These results may offer an explanation for the failure of *ex vivo* studies to show an increased strength of ASM from asthmatics (reviewed in (153)). The ability of ASM to rapidly change its contractile capacity in response to inflammatory molecules can also contribute to changes in airway responsiveness observed in response to interventions altering airway inflammation (30, 47, 143, 218). Those are all different ways by which a normal ASM may account for AHR in an inflamed environment. Another way by which inflammation can increase airway responsiveness is by producing spasmogens, which increases ASM-tone.

4.3 Increased ASM-tone

The responsiveness of asthmatics to bronchodilators, together with more direct evidence (165), indicate that ASM-tone is increased in asthmatic airways. The origin of this augmented ASM-tone is not clear and likely varies between asthmatic individuals. Nonetheless, asthmatic lungs are characterized by the overexpression of inflammation-derived spasmogens. These spasmogens trigger sustained ASM contraction and, acting individually or collectively, are a likely cause of increased ASM-tone in asthma. In the present subsection, we discuss the mechanisms by which inflammation-derived spasmogens, together with the attendant increase in ASM-tone, can contribute to AHR.

The rationale is that the amount of airway narrowing in response to a given concentration of a chosen spasmogen (e.g., MCh) is due to the combined effect of this extrinsically delivered spasmogen plus the baseline tone, which is caused by the endogenous spasmogens already present. In other words, it is the cooperative effect of all the spasmogens present at the time of the challenge that determines the total level of ASM activation and, ultimately, the amount of airway narrowing achieved. In addition, one of the causes of AHR can be the contractile synergistic interactions that are often observed when different spasmogens are used in combination. In this regard, a sizable literature exists documenting contractile synergisms between different spasmogens (Table 1). The mechanisms involved in these synergistic interactions have been debated in the last few decades and it is now clear that all the mechanisms that may be involved are not mutually exclusive. The nature of these interplays can give us important clues regarding the role of baseline airway tone in determining the degree of airway responsiveness.

4.3.1 Interactive synergisms between spasmogens

Initial studies in that area begin in the late 1970s and have started by looking at the combined effect of spasmogens on different measures of lung function in animals (45, 46, 57, 99, 102, 112, 131, 152, 180, 181, 192, 208, 209, 224, 244), as well as in humans (49, 68, 97, 101, 110, 156, 158, 194, 202, 240). Apart from an interactive synergism at the level of ASM contraction, many other factors can account for these *in vivo* interactive synergisms. In fact, although these synergistic interactions can be extremely relevant to the understanding of AHR, the mechanisms involved are sometime impossible to delineate.

First, the interactions between spasmogens were assessed *in vivo* by measuring airway resistance (or conductance) and/or flow parameters (flow rate at different lung volumes, forced expiratory volume in 1 sec (FEV1), etc...). All of these measurements are geometry-dependent. As mentioned earlier, airway resistance is inversely proportional to the luminal radius at the 4th power. The potentiation of the effect of one spasmogen by another spasmogen (or an increased baseline tone) might be related to a geometrical effect more than a true synergistic interaction of spasmogens on ASM-force. In other words, an additive effect at the level of muscle activation that may result in an additive effect in terms of ASM-force generation and shortening can be perceived as a synergistic effect when looking at airway resistance.

To circumvent these limitations, others have used *in situ* preparations allowing the assessment of tracheal smooth muscle-isometric force (12, 33, 131) or have measured airway caliber using tantalum bronchography (17). Some of these studies confirmed the synergistic effect of spasmogens on airway narrowing and ASM-force generation. However, these results are also confounded by the acute effect of some spasmogens on vessels and nerves, or by the effect of some spasmogens on airway inflammation and the epithelium. In regard to the vessels, many airway spasmogens also have vasoactive properties. Both vasoconstrictors and vasodilators have significant impact on the degree of airway

Mediators	*in vivo*	*ex vivo*	*in vitro*
ET-1	CCh (180) in sheep; HIST (112) in pigs		
Muscarinic agonists (ACh, MCh or CCh)	HIST (158) in humans; HIST (131) and NE (33) in dogs	HIST (71), 5-HT (71) and NE (87, 185) in canine tracheal SM strips	
HIST	MCh (158) and HIST (97) in humans MCh (131), ACh (33) and NE (12, 33, 131) in dogs	MCh (71), ACh (87), 5HT (87) and NE (12, 87) in canine tracheal SM strips; CCh (135) in bovine tracheal strips	
AII	MCh (156) in humans; MCh (244) in guinea pigs	MCh (156) in human bronchi; ET-1 (32, 173, 174, 195) in bovine bronchi; CCh (203, 204), K^* (204) and NaF (204) in rat bronchial rings	
5-HT	NE (12, 33), HIST (57), ACh (57) in dogs	MCh (71), ACh (87) and NE (12, 87) in canine tracheal SM strips; CCh (135) in bovine tracheal strips	
NE (in the presence of β-adrenoceptor brockade)	HIST (131) in dogs; HIST (208) and bombesin (208) in guinea pigs		
ATP		MCh (184) in guinea pig tracheal strips	
Adenosine	HIST (224) in guinea pigs		
Dopamine	HIST (208) and bombesin (208) in guinea pigs		
TXA_2 (or its pharmacological analog U46619)	MCh (110) in humans		
PGD_2	HIST (68, 97) and MCh (68) in humans		
PGE_2		CCh (38) in bovine tracheal strips	
$PGF_{2\alpha}$	HIST (101, 210) in humans	CCh (38) in bovine tracheal	
8-isoprostanes	MCh (102) in mice	K^+ (38), CCh (38, 135) and histamine (38) in bovine tracheal SM	
PAF	MCh (49, 202) in humans; LTD_4 (192) in rhesus monkeys; ACh (46) in dogs; HIST (45) in sheep; HIST (152) and bombesin (209) in guinea pigs		

Mediators	*in vivo*	*ex vivo*	*in vitro*
LTB_4	ACh (181) in dogs		
Cys-LTs	HIST (194) and PGD_2 (194) in humans; PAF (192) in rhesus monkeys	K^+ (215) and CCh (215) in porcine tracheal strips; ET-1 (195) in bovine bronchial rings; ACh (48) and HIST (48) in guinea pig tracheal rings	
S1P		MCh (122) in guinea pig tracheal strips; K^+ in bronchial rings from normal but not antigen-challenged mice (42)	
LPA		MCh (230), 5-HT (230), SP (230) in rabbit tracheal rings; MCh (230) in cat tracheal rings; ACh (98) in guinea pig tracheal rings	ATP (205) and K^+ (205) in bovine tracheal SM cells (205)
PA		MCh (230) in rabbit tracheal rings	

Abbreviations in the table: AII, angiotensin II; ACh, acetylcholine; ATP, adenosine triphosphate; BK, bradykinin; CCh, carbachol; Cys-LTs, cysteinyl-leukotrienes; ET-1, endothelin-1; HIST, histamine; 5-HT, 5-hydroxytryptamine (also called serotonine); K^+, potassium; LPA, lysophosphatidic acid; LTB_4, leukotriene B_4; MCh, methacholine; NaF, sodium fluoride; NE, norepinephrine; PA, phosphatidic acid; PAF, platelet activating factor; PGD_2, prostaglandin D_2; PGE_2, prostaglandin E_2; $PGF_{2\alpha}$, prostaglandin $F_{2\alpha}$; SM, smooth muscle; SP, substance P; S1P, sphingosine-1-phosphate; TXA_2, thromboxane A_2.

Table 1. Interactions between spasmogens increasing ASM contractility

responsiveness (151). The potentiating effect of histamine on the responsiveness to muscarinic agonists (33, 131), for example, can likely be due to its vasodilating effect, especially when the drugs are administered intravenously or via the tracheal vasculature. This is because vasodilatation facilitates the delivery of the bronchoactive substance (ACh) to the ASM. Histamine also increases airway epithelium permeability by altering E-cadherin-based adhesions (262). The effect of a second inhaled spasmogen may thus be potentiated by histamine pre-treatment because the second spasmogen will have easier access to the ASM.

In regard to the nerves, many studies have shown synergistic interactions between spasmogens and electrical stimulation of the vagal nerves (17, 33, 57, 88, 114, 137, 217, 258). Similarly, a decrease in responsiveness to spasmogens (other than ACh (88)) was observed following vagotomy (59, 137, 157, 258), cooling of the vagal nerves (58, 88), or treatments with either atropine (59, 219), tetrodotoxin (219) or hexamethonium (59). These results suggest that the basal cholinergic tone synergistically interacts with the exogenously delivered spasmogen. These studies are not included in Table 1 because it is not clear whether the potentiating effect is due to a true synergistic effect at the level of ASM-force generation or due to the ability of the spasmogens to either trigger a vagal reflex (36, 58, 74, 157) or to increase cholinergic neurotransmission and/or synaptic transmission at the ganglia (217). These latter phenomena would lead to more ACh release and concomitantly higher ASM activation for the same neural input. On the other hand, the bronchoconstricting effect of spasmogens is known to decrease the vagal tone (13, 210). This is because of their indirect effect on the slowly adapting stretch receptors (SARs), which, upon an enhanced discharge, relax the ASM by reducing parasympathetic tone to the airways. However, other spasmogens, such as bradykinin, would synergize with the effect of these mechanoreceptors via C-fibers activation to initiate the bronconconstricting reflex (150). Together, the influence of the nervous system is intricate and certainly a major confounding factor *in vivo* when one tries to elucidate the synergistic interaction between spasmogens.

Finally, thickening of the airway wall by edema and inflammatory infiltrates, encroachment of the airway lumen by mucus hypersecretion and cellular debris, and reduction in the forces of interdependence between the airway wall and the lung parenchyma by the accumulation of inflammatory exudates in the adventitial layer are all means by which airway inflammation can increase airway responsiveness without affecting ASM-force (reviewed in (26)). Therefore, the hyperresponsiveness observed in response to the second spasmogen, when the first spasmogen is administered hours before the second spasmogen (180), may be due to the inflammation provoked by the initial spasmogen.

To avoid these confounding factors and to investigate whether the synergistic action of two spasmogens on airway responsiveness relies on mechanisms operating at the level of ASM, the only solution is to study the ASM tissue in isolation. Many investigators have focused on this strategy. Most studies were performed using freshly dissected ASM strips or bronchial rings from which isometric force was measured *ex vivo* (12, 32, 38, 48, 71, 87, 98, 122, 135, 156, 173, 174, 184, 185, 195, 203, 204, 215, 230). *In vitro* preparations (i.e., cell culture) have also been used on occasions (205). These reported synergisms are also enumerated inTable 1.

The molecular mechanisms involved in contractile synergisms observed between different pairs of spasmogens have been extensively studied. The synergisms involve the co-activation of ASM by two spasmogens acting on two distinct GPCRs. The activation of two distinct GPCRs can lead to intracellular signaling synergisms that ultimately potentiate ASM-force. The more commonly discussed mechanism is Ca^{2+} sensitization, defined as an increased ASM-force generation in response to a given amount of intracellular Ca^{2+} mobilization (as discussed in subsection 4.2.3). Many spasmogenic mediators, such as leukotriene C_4 (215), isoprostanes (135), ATP (184), endothelin-1 (260), LPA (205), TxA_2 (167) and S1P (122), have been shown to increase the responsiveness of the contractile apparatus to Ca^{2+}.

However, these synergisms in terms of force generation can also be related to an additive effect in terms of ASM activation, especially when the concentrations of spasmogens used are low. This is because the dose-response curve to any spasmogen is sigmoidal, regardless of whether the response is measured in terms of ASM-force or shortening. That means that initially, a threshold concentration is needed before any response can be measured, but then there is a progressive increase toward a steeper, relatively linear slope followed by a progressive decrease in slope to reach a plateau. When two different spasmogens are used in combination, their additive effect on ASM-activation could be erroneously interpreted as being synergistic because sub-threshold concentrations of two spasmogens could have a measurable effect on ASM-force or shortening. Similarly, if one uses a concentration just above the response threshold, the subsequent addition of a different or the same spasmogen will have more effect simply because it is now acting on the steeper part of the dose-response curve. In fact, many of the previously documented examples of 'synergism' performed either *in vivo* (110, 112, 131, 158, 244) or *ex vivo* (38, 71, 87, 135) were involving low concentrations of spasmogens, and were unable to demonstrate a synergism at higher concentrations for at least some of the reported spasmogenic interactions (71, 87, 131). So the level of basal tone, even if low, can seemingly synergize with the extrinsically delivered spamogen to cause AHR simply by an additive effect at the level of ASM activation

Collectively, the force potentiation of one spasmogen (or baseline tone) on another spasmogen can be due to many factors such as: 1-use of sub-threshold or barely active concentrations of spasmogens, which simply act additively in terms of ASM activation but will be perceived as being synergistic in terms of ASM-force, ASM shortening, airway narrowing or airway resistance; 2-use of geometry-dependent measurements such as airway resistance; so that the effect of the second spasmogen is augmented by the reduced airway caliber caused by the first spasmogen; 3-a synergistic effect due to the contribution of vascular, neural or inflammatory effects when tested *in vivo* or *in situ*, which can be observed when the spasmogens used have vasoactive and inflammatory activities or when they can trigger either a vagal reflex and/or an increase in the efferent cholinergic traffic; and 4-a true synergistic effect on myosin cross-bridge cycling due to the convergence of intracellular signaling pathways that are activated by the ligation of two distinct GPCRs (such as Ca^{2+} sensitization).

4.3.2 Force adaptation

There is an additional, more subtle way by which the tone can contribute to AHR. Recent studies from our laboratory have demonstrated that a short period (~30 min) of increased ASM-tone augments ASM strength over time (20, 21). Specifically, ASM was exposed to ACh and ASM-force generation in response to EFS was monitored both before and after the induction of the ACh-induced tone. The first EFS in the presence of tone was given 1 min post ACh administration and then at 5-min intervals thereafter. Addition of ACh immediately increased the total force (ACh-induced tone + EFS-induced force), suggesting that ASM generates more force in response to two sub-maximal stimuli (ACh + EFS) compared with EFS alone. More surprisingly, while the EFS-induced force decreased immediately following the administration of ACh, it recovered significantly over time. Since the tone produced by the exogenous ACh remained relatively constant, the total force increased over time. We termed this phenomenon 'force adaptation' (20). The potential significance of force adaptation on airway narrowing based on a computational model has been demonstrated recently (Bossé *et al.*, in press in the journal of Respiratory Physiology & Neurobiology).

Force adaptation is distinct from the synergisms in force that were attributed to the convergence of intracellular signaling pathways described above, which occur as a result of activation of two distinct GPCRs. This form of synergism cannot occur when ACh is combined with activation of the ASM by EFS, which was the experimental setting that was used to describe force adaptation. This is because EFS triggers ASM contraction by releasing ACh from the nerve endings (145), which, in turn, binds on the same M_3 receptor as the exogenously administered ACh. In fact, all studies investigating the acute effect of a muscarinic agonist on EFS-induced force have failed to show a synergistic effect (57, 114). Therefore, despite abundant literature reporting synergistic effects between spasmogens on ASM strength, force adaptation is a phenomenon with no precedent.

The molecular mechanisms involved in force adaptation are also likely to be different from those described above because it occurs over minutes. This time-course would be too fast for *de novo* gene expression; so it is not likely due to transcriptional activation of genes involved in ASM contraction induced by the initial tone. On the other hand, if it was due to biochemical events such as increased phosphorylation of MLC due MLCP deactivation leading to Ca^{2+} sensitization (as described in subsection 4.2.3), the potentiating effect would be very fast and seen at the first EFS following ACh administration (1 min). Taken together, the kinetic of force adaptation is too slow to be explained by fast biochemical reactions, such as protein phosphorylation, but too fast for *de novo* gene expression. We thus suggest that this time-dependent increase in ASM-force is due to post-translational mechanisms. All the necessary machinery responsible for this increased ASM-force might be present within the cell prior to activation, but it is only upon stimulation (i.e., induction of tone) that this protein machinery re-organizes to optimize generation of force. Processes such as actin (264) or myosin (213) filamentogenesis and/or re-arrangement of the cytoskeleton and its connectivity with the contractile apparatus, the plasmalemma and the ECM (264) are likely possibilities. However, these remain pure speculations as the mechanisms underlying force adaptation have never been investigated.

4.3.3 Increased tone on airway wall stiffness

Apart from ASM-force, increased ASM-tone can also impact other ASM contractile properties. For instance, stiffness is greatly enhanced upon ASM activation. By increasing ASM stiffness, an increased tone would reduce the strains experienced by the airway wall due to the cyclical stresses of breathing. Interestingly, Noble and coworkers (178) have demonstrated that the amount of airway wall strain induced by a DI is proportional to its bronchodilating effect (178). They also showed that the main factor limiting the strain was the magnitude of ASM-tone, which was controlled by delivering different concentrations of ACh. These observations suggested that the ASM needs not only to be stressed but to be stretched for a DI to be effective in reducing ASM contractility. They concluded by saying that a stiffer airway caused by an increased ASM-tone reduces the strain induced by the dynamic load associated with DI and, for this reason, reduces the bronchodilating effect of a DI.

Taken all together, these observations suggest that baseline tone is of crucial importance in determining the degree of airway responsiveness to an inhalational challenge with a spasmogen. The increased tone observed in asthma can be from inflammatory and/or vagal origin. In both cases, this increased tone acts additively with the extrinsically delivered spamogen in terms of ASM activation, force generation, ASM shortening and airway diameter narrowing. This can also be translated into a synergistic effect when geometry-dependent measurements are taken, such as airway cross-sectional area of the lumen or airflow resistance (or other measurements relying on it, such as peak expiratory flow (PEF), FEV_1, ...). In cases where the increased tone is mediated by inflammation-derived spasmogens, the potentiating effect of increased tone on airway responsiveness can also be due to a vascular effect, a neural effect, an inflammatory effect and/or an increase in ASM-force caused by either Ca^{2+} sensitization or force adaptation. Finally, augmented tone also increases ASM stiffness and, concomitantly, airway wall stiffness, which can further enhance airway responsiveness by many ways as discussed in subsections 2.2 and 2.3.

4.4 Heterogeneity

To assess airway responsiveness airway resistance is measured at the mouth using the forced oscillation technique or, alternatively, flow parameters are measured using standard spirometry. These measurements take into account airway resistance but also lung tissue and chest wall resistance. Since chest wall resistance does not change during bronchoprovocation, and lung tissue resistance does not change by much, the progressive increase of resistance occurring in response to increasing doses of a spasmogen is thought to reflect changes of airway caliber. In other words, the change of resistance along the course of a challenge is viewed as being due to airway narrowing caused by ASM shortening. However, even this change of resistance is intricate. This is because this resistance represents represents the combined resistance of all generations of airways arranged in series and in parallel. Therefore, simply looking at the factors affecting resistance in a single airway, as we have done since the beginning of this chapter, may not be sufficient to understand the full nature of airway responsiveness.

4.4.1 Mathematical link between airway narrowing heterogeneity and airway responsiveness

The link between heterogeneity and AHR was initially though as being simply due to geometric considerations. As aforementioned, the relationship between airway luminal radius and resistance to airflow is not linear. A decrease in radius causes an exponential increase in airway resistance. For this reason, even if the total cross sectional area within a given airway generation is the same, inhomogeneous airway caliber increases airway resistance. In other words, the increase in resistance caused by narrowing of some airways is not compensated for by the decrease in resistance caused by dilation of other airways. Airway narrowing heterogeneity upon a bronchoprovocative challenge with a spasmogen will have the same consequence. So that the increases in resistance caused by augmented narrowing in some airways are not compensated for by the attenuated increases in resistance caused by reduced narrowing happening in other airways.

The consequences of baseline heterogeneity on baseline resistance and of non-homogeneous airway narrowing on airway responsiveness were predicted based on computational models. Bates (14) was one of the first to address the issue of heterogeneity. He developed a stochastic model of the airway tree in which the values of airway radii within every airway generation were chosen randomly according to a probability distribution function. The mean values were based on realistic values (morphometric data of human lungs). He found that, while the mean values were kept the same, increasing the standard deviations progressively leads to greater airway resistance. This suggested that the simple presence of heterogeneity increases airway resistance. The model further predicted that, upon ASM activation, both baseline airway caliber heterogeneity and ASM shortening heterogeneity increase airway responsiveness. Obviously, this is only true if one assumes that the flow is not redistributed into more patent airways.

More sophisticated computational models have then been developed and brought additional insights about the origin of this increased resistance evoked by baseline or airway narrowing heterogeneity. The main contributor to this increased resistance comes from nearly closed peripheral airways, especially when resistance is measured at frequency near the breathing frequency (138). These airway closures (or near closed) ultimately lead to ventilation defects and attendant flow limitation. They might be the link between ventilation heterogeneity and AHR.

4.4.2 Non-uniform ventilation with air trapping and AHR

Using the forced oscillation technique, several groups noticed that the frequency-dependence of resistance and elastance was increased at baseline in asthmatics (139) and upon MCh challenge in both asthmatics and non-asthmatics (111, 139). In accordance to the computational models discussed above, this is indicative of a heterogenous pattern of constriction that includes randomly distributed airway closures or near closures (138). These observations are supported by ventilation imaging studies such as hyperpolarized ^{3}He MRI (39, 207, 234), single-photon emission computed tomography (116) and positron emission tomography (169). These studies showed that asthmatics have increased ventilation heterogeneity at baseline and, even if heterogeneous airway response to a spamogen is also observed in non-asthmatics, the level of ventilation heterogeneity achieved is greater in asthmatics (39, 207, 234). This heterogeneous pattern of ventilation is characterized by relatively large zone of non-ventilated area, which supports the presence of airway closure. These ventilations defects represent zones of air trapping, which are characteristic of obstructive diseases and known to contribute to airflow limitation. Ventilation heterogeneity can thus be one of the sources of AHR seen in asthmatics. This is consistent with recent reports showing that baseline ventilation heterogeneity measured by nitrogen washouts correlates with the severity of AHR in both younger (60) and older (96) asthmatic subjects.

The increase in ventilation heterogeneity in response to a spasmogenic challenge may simply be due to an amplifying effect over the baseline heterogeneity. However, upon induced bronchoconstriction, airway narrowing heterogeneity can also contribute to ventilation heterogenetity. King and coworkers (115) have used high resolution computed tomography (HRCT) to measure the heterogeneity of airway narrowing in response to MCh challenge in human subjects. The heterogeneity was measured by the standard deviations of the changes in luminal airway caliber caused by MCh. They showed that in airways of ≥ 2 mm of diameter that the variability of airway narrowing was greater than the measure of repeatability (the variability in the changes in luminal airway caliber when two pre-MCh scans were compared), suggesting that airways narrow heterogeneously. They also shown that for the same level of bronchoconstriction achieved, asthmatic airways narrowed more heterogeneously than non-asthmatics. Together, these observations suggest that the larger and more numerous ventilation defects observed in asthmatics during a spasmogenic challenge are due to both greater baseline heterogeneity and greater airway narrowing heterogeneity.

4.4.3 Mechanistic link between airway narrowing heterogeneity and airway responsiveness

As aforementioned, the emergence of ventilation defects during bronchoconstriction is essentially the link between ventilation heterogeneity and AHR. In other words, simple heterogeneity without airway closure (or near closure) does not seem to cause AHR. It is true that for the same mean level of bronchoconstriction, heterogeneity would increase resistance but only if the flow is still evenly distributed among the different airways. However, during heterogeneous constriction, the flow is more likely to be redirected into more conductant (patent) airways and correspondingly less flow would be redirected into more resistant (constricted) airways. Consequently, the overall resistance would rather decrease with heterogeneity. On the other hand, when the airways are closed (or nearly), the volume of air subtended by these airways is trapped and will not be able to be expelled (at least not as fast) upon maximal expiratory flow maneuvers and that would be the cause of AHR.

It is also unlikely that the ventilation defects are due to random closure of single peripheral airways. Based on the size of these ventilation defects, they are more likely due to clustering of constricted peripheral airways. In a computational model developed by Venegas and coworkers (236, 253), it was shown that airway closure occurs in cluster. In their model, the bronchial tree branches dichotomously, where every bifurcation is composed of one parent airway and two daughter airways with slight heterogeneity between them. During bronchoconstriction, the flow is redistributed according to divergence of patency among daughter airways. The model predicted that all the airways shorten uniformly when the level of ASM activation is low. However, passed a certain threshold of ASM activation, daughter airways develop a dichotomic response. Whereas one constricts excessively the other one dilates. This is because the initial heterogeneity between the two daughter airways fosters the redistribution of flow into the more conductant airway. The insufflation pressure thus rises in the hyperventilated areas subtended by this airway, which increases the load impeding ASM shortening. In fact, the model predicted that this airway dilates despite the rise in ASM activation. On contrary, diminution of flow in the other daughter airway causes regional lung deflation and loss of parenchymal tethering recoil. The load impeding muscle shortening thus decreases and, for the same level of ASM activation, more narrowing occurs. Because of axial interdependence of pathways in series, all the smaller airways downstream of the excessively closed airways are also affected. The size of the ventilation defects depends on the first airway generation afflicted by this dichotomic response. Since more ASM activation is required to close larger airways, this dichotomic response begins in more peripheral airways. But as the ASM activation progressively rises, the model predicted that larger and larger airways are affected and larger and larger patches of lung become non-ventilated.

Taken together, Venegas and colleagues suggested that only a slight degree of heterogeneity at baseline can trigger a self-perpetuating feedback loop when a certain level of ASM activation is achieved; such that the redistribution of flow in slightly more patent airways, makes the other airways and their downstream pathways unstable because of the loss of elastic recoil. This ultimately leads to clustering of peripheral airway constriction and the emergence of large ventilation defects, which, in turn, cause flow limitation. The chase for the factors determining this baseline heterogeneity, which was heretofore ignored, is now on.

4.4.4 Factors potentially involved in determining baseline heterogeneity

The amplifying effect described by Venegas and coworkers (236), which can lead to large ventilation defects and attendant AHR, relies on subtle structural and/or functional changes that were already present prior the inhalation of the spasmogen. Therefore, the identification of factors responsible for this baseline airway wall heterogeneity is of major interest.

Remodeling can certainly impact heterogeneity and can potentially discriminate the different levels of heterogeneity observed between asthmatics and non-asthmatics. Remodeling occurs non-uniformly throughout the tracheobronchial tree. The occurrence of epithelium desquamation or inflammatory infiltrates for example is patchy in nature. The extent of subepithelial fibrosis, ASM enlargement, and other structural changes present in asthmatic lungs could also vary at different locations in the lung. Together, these disparities alter the mechanical properties of the airway wall non-uniformly along the bronchial tree. It can also modify airway geometry and sometimes lead to the formation of bottlenecks, a characteristic feature found in terminal bronchioles of chronic obstructive pulmonary disease (COPD) patients (McDonough *et al.*, provisionally accepted in the New England Journal of Medicine). The effect of a bottleneck is treacherous because not only it increases the resistance to airflow in an airway that otherwise may look normal but also because it reduces ventilation in the parenchymal tissue subtended by this airway. This ultimately fosters the development of a ventilation defect due to a decrease in the force of airway-parenchymal interdependence. Greater ventilation defects at baseline seen in asthmatics can thus be attributed to remodeling. However, ventilation heterogeneity is mainly attributable to the fact that airways narrow heterogeneously. So, it is upon bronchoconstriction that the functional consequences of these disparities (localized remodeling changes) along the length of a pathway are exacerbated. For example, remodeling heterogeneity can affect locally the initial geometry, which has a huge influence on airway responsiveness (as discussed in subsection 4.1.3). It can also modify locally the after-load impeding ASM shortening. Another example would be the patchiness of ASM mass enlargement, which can potentially amplify regional differences in airway narrowing upon ASM activation.

Gain in contractile properties (e.g., force-generating capacity) due to ASM behaviors could also be patchy within the lungs. For example, acquisition of supplemental force by length adaptation can occur in an area where the airway caliber is smaller because of a localized decrease in the force of airway-parenchymal interdependence. The baseline ASM-tone also likely differs in different areas of the lung. Its magnitude may be spatially correlated with zones of inflammation, where inflammation-derived spasmogens are produced/released. That would also lead to force adaptation and the attendant gain in force-generating capacity in those areas. All these factors can affect ASM contractile properties in a localized manner and contribute to narrowing heterogeneity and AHR.

Hence, remodeling and inflammatory changes seen in asthmatic lungs can give rise to a greater baseline level of airway wall heterogeneity. It can also cause inhomogeneity of narrowing upon a bronchoprovocative challenge with a spasmogen by changing the load impeding ASM shortening or by fostering the development of increased ASM contractility. Together with the strong interplay between the parenchymal tethering and airway patency, this increased level of heterogeneity can be sufficient to trigger a self-perpetuating loop leading to patches of hypo- or non-ventilated area and the appearance of AHR in asthmatics.

5. Conclusion

Despite abundant evidence implicating the ASM as the culprit of AHR in asthma, the latest genetic studies are relatively weak to support the role of asthma susceptibility gene risk variants in causing ASM dysfunction. The more reliable genetic analyses performed to date have instead suggested that the well-recognized genetic predisposition to suffer from asthma may be related to polymorphisms in genes that are predominately involved in immunology and/or epithelial integrity and functions. Even if we cannot rule out the contribution of genetic alterations affecting the ASM in AHR at the present time, the bulk of evidence rather suggests that if alterations in ASM mechanics contribute to AHR, these alterations are acquired as a result of inflammatory mediators and/or extracellular matrix remodeling that are present in asthmatic lungs. For example, lung defects can foster the appearance of normal ASM behaviors that render the muscle hypercontractile, such as length adaptation, force adaptation and changes in ASM cell's phenotype. These ASM behaviors are the testimony that he contractile properties of the ASM are not fixed but rather plastic (adaptable).

On the other hand, alterations in ASM contractile properties are not necessarily a prerequisite to suffer from AHR. Many lung defects are sufficient alone (i.e., without the need of increased ASM contractility) to cause AHR. These include but are not restricted to: 1-alterations in epithelial integrity, which increase the bioavailability of the inhaled spasmogen onto the ASM; 2-increased ASM-tone (due to the preponderance of inflammation-derived spasmogens, an augmented vagal input and/or decreased expression of relaxant factors), which acts additively with the extrinsically-delivered spasmogen in terms of ASM activation and ASM shortening, and synergistically in terms of narrowing of the cross-sectional area of the lumen and airway resistance; 3-obstruction of the vessels irrigating the ASM, which prevents clearance of the spasmogens into the circulation and concomitantly sequesters the spasmogens in the vicinity of ASM; 4-increased mass of the material inner the ASM layer, which increases airway narrowing for any given degree of ASM shortening; 5-decreased ASM-load (due to adventitial thickening, detachment of the parenchymal tethers from the outer edge of the airway wall, decrease in lung recoil, reduction in lung volume, diminution of the radial constraint limiting ASM bulging during shortening, other changes in ECM constitution which may change the mechanical properties of the airway wall to make it easier to compress by affecting, or not, its pattern of folding), which increases ASM shortening for any given degree of ASM activation; and 6-ventilation heterogeneity with airway closure, which affects flow measurements (such as FEV_1, PEF and others) because of air trapping. For all of these reasons, some asthmatics can be hypperresponsive even when their ASM operates as normal. In conclusion, we think that the ASM is often 'blamed' for the AHR seen in asthma simply because of its unequivocal role in airway responsiveness. We would like to propose that without further or more convincing proofs to incriminate ASM in AHR, this obeisant tissue should still be considered 'innocent'.

6. References

[1] Aikawa T, Shimura S, Sasaki H, Ebina M, and Takishima T. Marked goblet cell hyperplasia with mucus accumulation in the airways of patients who died of severe acute asthma attack. *Chest* 101: 916-921, 1992.

[2] Alcorn JF, Rinaldi LM, Jaffe EF, van Loon M, Bates JH, Janssen-Heininger YM, and Irvin CG. Transforming growth factor-beta1 suppresses airway hyperresponsiveness in allergic airway disease. *Am J Respir Crit Care Med* 176: 974-982, 2007.

[3] Ammit AJ, Armour CL, and Black JL. Smooth-muscle myosin light-chain kinase content is increased in human sensitized airways. *Am J Respir Crit Care Med* 161: 257-263, 2000.

[4] Amrani Y, Chen H, and Panettieri RA, Jr. Activation of tumor necrosis factor receptor 1 in airway smooth muscle: a potential pathway that modulates bronchial hyper-responsiveness in asthma? *Respir Res* 1: 49-53, 2000.

[5] Amrani Y, Moore PE, Hoffman R, Shore SA, and Panettieri RA, Jr. Interferon-gamma modulates cysteinyl leukotriene receptor-1 expression and function in human airway myocytes. *Am J Respir Crit Care Med* 164: 2098-2101, 2001.

[6] An SS, Fabry B, Trepat X, Wang N, and Fredberg JJ. Do biophysical properties of the airway smooth muscle in culture predict airway hyperresponsiveness? *Am J Respir Cell Mol Biol* 35: 55-64, 2006.

[7] Anticevich SZ, Hughes JM, Black JL, and Armour CL. Induction of human airway hyperresponsiveness by tumour necrosis factor-alpha. *Eur J Pharmacol* 284: 221-225, 1995.

[8] Bachar O, Adner M, Uddman R, and Cardell LO. Toll-like receptor stimulation induces airway hyper-responsiveness to bradykinin, an effect mediated by JNK and NF-kappa B signaling pathways. *Eur J Immunol* 34: 1196-1207, 2004.
[9] Bachar O, Rose AC, Adner M, Wang X, Prendergast CE, Kempf A, Shankley NP, and Cardell LO. TNF alpha reduces tachykinin, PGE2-dependent, relaxation of the cultured mouse trachea by increasing the activity of COX-2. *Br J Pharmacol* 144: 220-230, 2005.
[10] Baluk P, Bowden JJ, Lefevre PM, and McDonald DM. Upregulation of substance P receptors in angiogenesis associated with chronic airway inflammation in rats. *Am J Physiol* 273: L565-571, 1997.
[11] Barchasz E, Naline E, Molimard M, Moreau J, Georges O, Emonds-Alt X, and Advenier C. Interleukin-1beta-induced hyperresponsiveness to [Sar9,Met(O2)11]substance P in isolated human bronchi. *Eur J Pharmacol* 379: 87-95, 1999.
[12] Barnes PJ, Skoogh BE, Brown JK, and Nadel JA. Activation of alpha-adrenergic response in tracheal smooth muscle: a postreceptor mechanism. *J Appl Physiol* 54: 1469-1476, 1983.
[13] Baroffio M, Barisione G, Crimi E, and Brusasco V. Noninflammatory mechanisms of airway hyper-responsiveness in bronchial asthma: an overview. *Ther Adv Respir Dis* 3: 163-174, 2009.
[14] Bates JH. Stochastic model of the pulmonary airway tree and its implications for bronchial responsiveness. *J Appl Physiol* 75: 2493-2499, 1993.
[15] Ben-Jebria A, Marthan R, Rossetti M, and Savineau JP. Effect of passive sensitization on the mechanical activity of human isolated bronchial smooth muscle induced by substance P, neurokinin A and VIP. *Br J Pharmacol* 109: 131-136, 1993.
[16] Benayoun L, Druilhe A, Dombret MC, Aubier M, and Pretolani M. Airway structural alterations selectively associated with severe asthma. *Am J Respir Crit Care Med* 167: 1360-1368, 2003.
[17] Benson MK, and Graf PD. Bronchial reactivity: interaction between vagal stimulation and inhaled histamine. *J Appl Physiol* 43: 643-647, 1977.
[18] Bentley JK, and Hershenson MB. Airway smooth muscle growth in asthma: proliferation, hypertrophy, and migration. *Proc Am Thorac Soc* 5: 89-96, 2008.
[19] Black JL, Marthan R, Armour CL, and Johnson PR. Sensitization alters contractile responses and calcium influx in human airway smooth muscle. *J Allergy Clin Immunol* 84: 440-447, 1989.
[20] Bosse Y, Chin LY, Pare PD, and Seow CY. Adaptation of airway smooth muscle to basal tone: relevance to airway hyperresponsiveness. *Am J Respir Cell Mol Biol* 40: 13-18, 2009.
[21] Bosse Y, Chin LY, Pare PD, and Seow CY. Chronic activation in shortened airway smooth muscle: a synergistic combination underlying airway hyperresponsiveness? *Am J Respir Cell Mol Biol* 42: 341-348, 2010.
[22] Bosse Y, and Hudson TJ. Toward a Comprehensive Set of Asthma Susceptibility Genes. *Annu Rev Med* 2006.
[23] Bosse Y, Maghni K, and Hudson TJ. 1alpha,25-dihydroxy-vitamin D3 stimulation of bronchial smooth muscle cells induces autocrine, contractility, and remodeling processes. *Physiol Genomics* 29: 161-168, 2007.
[24] Bosse Y, and Pare PD. Airway Smooth Muscle Responsiveness: The Origin of Airway Hyperresponsiveness in Asthma? *Curr Respir Med Rev* In Press, 2010.

[25] Bosse Y, Pare PD, and Seow CY. Airway wall remodeling in asthma: from the epithelial layer to the adventitia. *Curr Allergy Asthma Rep* 8: 357-366, 2008.
[26] Bosse Y, Riesenfeld EP, Pare PD, and Irvin CG. It's not all smooth muscle: Nonsmooth muscle elements in control of resistance to airflow. *Annu Rev Physiol* 72: 437-462, 2010.
[27] Bosse Y, Sobieszek A, Pare PD, and Seow CY. Length adaptation of airway smooth muscle. *Proc Am Thorac Soc* 5: 62-67, 2008.
[28] Bosse Y, Solomon D, Chin LY, Lian K, Pare PD, and Seow CY. Increase in passive stiffness at reduced airway smooth muscle length: potential impact on airway responsiveness. *Am J Physiol Lung Cell Mol Physiol* 298: L277-287, 2010.
[29] Bramley AM, Roberts CR, and Schellenberg RR. Collagenase increases shortening of human bronchial smooth muscle in vitro. *Am J Respir Crit Care Med* 152: 1513-1517, 1995.
[30] Brannan JD. Bronchial hyperresponsiveness in the assessment of asthma control: Airway hyperresponsiveness in asthma: its measurement and clinical significance. *Chest* 138: 11S-17S, 2010.
[31] Brightling CE, Bradding P, Symon FA, Holgate ST, Wardlaw AJ, and Pavord ID. Mast-cell infiltration of airway smooth muscle in asthma. *N Engl J Med* 346: 1699-1705, 2002.
[32] Brown AJ, and Nally JE. Hydrocortisone abolishes the angiotensin II-mediated potentiation of endothelin-1 in bovine bronchi. *Clin Sci (Lond)* 100: 19-23, 2001.
[33] Brown JK, Shields R, Jones C, and Gold WM. Augmentation of alpha-adrenergic contractions in the trachealis muscle of living dogs. *J Appl Physiol* 54: 1558-1566, 1983.
[34] Brown RH, Zerhouni EA, and Mitzner W. Airway edema potentiates airway reactivity. *J Appl Physiol* 79: 1242-1248, 1995.
[35] Brown RH, Zerhouni EA, and Mitzner W. Visualization of airway obstruction in vivo during pulmonary vascular engorgement and edema. *J Appl Physiol* 78: 1070-1078, 1995.
[36] Canning BJ, Reynolds SM, and Mazzone SB. Multiple mechanisms of reflex bronchospasm in guinea pigs. *J Appl Physiol* 91: 2642-2653, 2001.
[37] Carroll NG, Perry S, Karkhanis A, Harji S, Butt J, James AL, and Green FH. The airway longitudinal elastic fiber network and mucosal folding in patients with asthma. *Am J Respir Crit Care Med* 161: 244-248, 2000.
[38] Catalli A, and Janssen LJ. Augmentation of bovine airway smooth muscle responsiveness to carbachol, KCl, and histamine by the isoprostane 8-iso-PGE2. *Am J Physiol Lung Cell Mol Physiol* 287: L1035-1041, 2004.
[39] Chen BT, and Johnson GA. Dynamic lung morphology of methacholine-induced heterogeneous bronchoconstriction. *Magn Reson Med* 52: 1080-1086, 2004.
[40] Chiba Y, Goto K, Hirahara M, Sakai H, and Misawa M. Glucocorticoids ameliorate antigen-induced bronchial smooth muscle hyperresponsiveness by inhibiting upregulation of RhoA in rats. *J Pharmacol Sci* 106: 615-625, 2008.
[41] Chiba Y, Nakazawa S, Todoroki M, Shinozaki K, Sakai H, and Misawa M. Interleukin-13 augments bronchial smooth muscle contractility with an up-regulation of RhoA protein. *Am J Respir Cell Mol Biol* 40: 159-167, 2009.

[42] Chiba Y, Suzuki K, Uechi M, Kurihara E, Goto K, Sakai H, and Misawa M. Downregulation of sphingosine-1-phosphate receptors in bronchial smooth muscle of mouse experimental asthma. *Pharmacol Res* 62: 357-363, 2010.
[43] Chiba Y, Takada Y, Miyamoto S, MitsuiSaito M, Karaki H, and Misawa M. Augmented acetylcholine-induced, Rho-mediated Ca2+ sensitization of bronchial smooth muscle contraction in antigen-induced airway hyperresponsive rats. *Br J Pharmacol* 127: 597-600, 1999.
[44] Chitano P, Wang L, and Murphy TM. Three paradigms of airway smooth muscle hyperresponsiveness in young guinea pigs. *Can J Physiol Pharmacol* 85: 715-726, 2007.
[45] Christman BW, Lefferts PL, and Snapper JR. Effect of platelet-activating factor on aerosol histamine responsiveness in awake sheep. *Am Rev Respir Dis* 135: 1267-1270, 1987.
[46] Chung KF, Aizawa H, Leikauf GD, Ueki IF, Evans TW, and Nadel JA. Airway hyperresponsiveness induced by platelet-activating factor: role of thromboxane generation. *J Pharmacol Exp Ther* 236: 580-584, 1986.
[47] Cockcroft DW, Ruffin RE, Dolovich J, and Hargreave FE. Allergen-induced increase in non-allergic bronchial reactivity. *Clin Allergy* 7: 503-513, 1977.
[48] Creese BR, and Bach MK. Hyperreactivity of airways smooth muscle produced in vitro by leukotrienes. *Prostaglandins Leukot Med* 11: 161-169, 1983.
[49] Cuss FM, Dixon CM, and Barnes PJ. Effects of inhaled platelet activating factor on pulmonary function and bronchial responsiveness in man. *Lancet* 2: 189-192, 1986.
[50] Damera G, and Panettieri RA, Jr. Does airway smooth muscle express an inflammatory phenotype in asthma? *Br J Pharmacol* 163: 68-80, 2011.
[51] Deb R, Shakib F, Reid K, and Clark H. Major house dust mite allergens Dermatophagoides pteronyssinus 1 and Dermatophagoides farinae 1 degrade and inactivate lung surfactant proteins A and D. *J Biol Chem* 282: 36808-36819, 2007.
[52] Deshpande DA, Dogan S, Walseth TF, Miller SM, Amrani Y, Panettieri RA, and Kannan MS. Modulation of calcium signaling by interleukin-13 in human airway smooth muscle: role of CD38/cyclic adenosine diphosphate ribose pathway. *Am J Respir Cell Mol Biol* 31: 36-42, 2004.
[53] Deshpande DA, Walseth TF, Panettieri RA, and Kannan MS. CD38/cyclic ADP-ribose-mediated Ca2+ signaling contributes to airway smooth muscle hyper-responsiveness. *Faseb J* 17: 452-454, 2003.
[54] Deshpande DA, White TA, Dogan S, Walseth TF, Panettieri RA, and Kannan MS. CD38/cyclic ADP-ribose signaling: role in the regulation of calcium homeostasis in airway smooth muscle. *Am J Physiol Lung Cell Mol Physiol* 288: L773-788, 2005.
[55] Detoraki A, Granata F, Staibano S, Rossi FW, Marone G, and Genovese A. Angiogenesis and lymphangiogenesis in bronchial asthma. *Allergy* 65: 946-958, In press.
[56] Ding DJ, Martin JG, and Macklem PT. Effects of lung volume on maximal methacholine-induced bronchoconstriction in normal humans. *J Appl Physiol* 62: 1324-1330, 1987.
[57] Dixon M, Jackson DM, and Richards IM. The effects of 5-hydroxytryptamine, histamine and acetylcholine on the reactivity of the lung of the anaesthetized dog. *J Physiol* 307: 85-96, 1980.

[58] Dixon M, Jackson DM, and Richards IM. The effects of histamine, acetylcholine and 5-hydroxytryptamine on lung mechanics and irritant receptors in the dog. *J Physiol* 287: 393-403, 1979.
[59] Douglas JS, Dennis MW, Ridgway P, and Bouhuys A. Airway constriction in guinea pigs: interaction of histamine and autonomic drugs. *J Pharmacol Exp Ther* 184: 169-179, 1973.
[60] Downie SR, Salome CM, Verbanck S, Thompson B, Berend N, and King GG. Ventilation heterogeneity is a major determinant of airway hyperresponsiveness in asthma, independent of airway inflammation. *Thorax* 62: 684-689, 2007.
[61] Driver AG, Kukoly CA, Ali S, and Mustafa SJ. Adenosine in bronchoalveolar lavage fluid in asthma. *Am Rev Respir Dis* 148: 91-97, 1993.
[62] Eum SY, Maghni K, Tolloczko B, Eidelman DH, and Martin JG. IL-13 may mediate allergen-induced hyperresponsiveness independently of IL-5 or eotaxin by effects on airway smooth muscle. *Am J Physiol Lung Cell Mol Physiol* 288: L576-584, 2005.
[63] Fayon M, Rebola M, Berger P, Daburon S, Ousova O, Lavrand F, Moukaila B, Pujol W, Taupin JL, Labbe A, Molimard M, and Marthan R. Increased secretion of leukemia inhibitory factor by immature airway smooth muscle cells enhances intracellular signaling and airway contractility. *Am J Physiol Lung Cell Mol Physiol* 291: L244-251, 2006.
[64] Flint KC, Leung KB, Hudspith BN, Brostoff J, Pearce FL, and Johnson NM. Bronchoalveolar mast cells in extrinsic asthma: a mechanism for the initiation of antigen specific bronchoconstriction. *Br Med J (Clin Res Ed)* 291: 923-926, 1985.
[65] Fredberg JJ. Counterpoint: airway smooth muscle is not useful. *J Appl Physiol* 102: 1709-1710; discussion 1710-1701, 2007.
[66] Fredberg JJ, Inouye D, Miller B, Nathan M, Jafari S, Raboudi SH, Butler JP, and Shore SA. Airway smooth muscle, tidal stretches, and dynamically determined contractile states. *Am J Respir Crit Care Med* 156: 1752-1759, 1997.
[67] Fredberg JJ, Inouye DS, Mijailovich SM, and Butler JP. Perturbed equilibrium of myosin binding in airway smooth muscle and its implications in bronchospasm. *Am J Respir Crit Care Med* 159: 959-967, 1999.
[68] Fuller RW, Dixon CM, Dollery CT, and Barnes PJ. Prostaglandin D2 potentiates airway responsiveness to histamine and methacholine. *Am Rev Respir Dis* 133: 252-254, 1986.
[69] Fust A, and Stephens NL. Relaxation of canine airway smooth muscle. *Can J Physiol Pharmacol* 85: 672-678, 2007.
[70] Galione A, Lee HC, and Busa WB. Ca(2+)-induced Ca2+ release in sea urchin egg homogenates: modulation by cyclic ADP-ribose. *Science* 253: 1143-1146, 1991.
[71] Gerthoffer WT. Agonist synergism in airway smooth muscle contraction. *J Pharmacol Exp Ther* 278: 800-807, 1996.
[72] Gerthoffer WT. Migration of airway smooth muscle cells. *Proc Am Thorac Soc* 5: 97-105, 2008.
[73] Gil FR, Zitouni NB, Azoulay E, Maghni K, and Lauzon AM. Smooth muscle myosin isoform expression and LC20 phosphorylation in innate rat airway hyperresponsiveness. *Am J Physiol Lung Cell Mol Physiol* 291: L932-940, 2006.
[74] Gold WM, Kessler GF, and Yu DY. Role of vagus nerves in experimental asthma in allergic dogs. *J Appl Physiol* 33: 719-725, 1972.

[75] Goldsmith AM, Bentley JK, Zhou L, Jia Y, Bitar KN, Fingar DC, and Hershenson MB. Transforming growth factor-beta induces airway smooth muscle hypertrophy. *Am J Respir Cell Mol Biol* 34: 247-254, 2006.
[76] Goldsmith AM, Hershenson MB, Wolbert MP, and Bentley JK. Regulation of airway smooth muscle alpha-actin expression by glucocorticoids. *Am J Physiol Lung Cell Mol Physiol* 292: L99-L106, 2007.
[77] Green ED, and Guyer MS. Charting a course for genomic medicine from base pairs to bedside. *Nature* 470: 204-213, 2011.
[78] Grunstein MM, Hakonarson H, Hodinka RL, Maskeri N, Kim C, and Chuang S. Mechanism of cooperative effects of rhinovirus and atopic sensitization on airway responsiveness. *Am J Physiol Lung Cell Mol Physiol* 280: L229-238, 2001.
[79] Grunstein MM, Hakonarson H, Leiter J, Chen M, Whelan R, Grunstein JS, and Chuang S. Autocrine signaling by IL-10 mediates altered responsiveness of atopic sensitized airway smooth muscle. *Am J Physiol Lung Cell Mol Physiol* 281: L1130-1137, 2001.
[80] Grunstein MM, Hakonarson H, Leiter J, Chen M, Whelan R, Grunstein JS, and Chuang S. IL-13-dependent autocrine signaling mediates altered responsiveness of IgE-sensitized airway smooth muscle. *Am J Physiol Lung Cell Mol Physiol* 282: L520-528, 2002.
[81] Grunstein MM, Hakonarson H, Whelan R, Yu Z, Grunstein JS, and Chuang S. Rhinovirus elicits proasthmatic changes in airway responsiveness independently of viral infection. *J Allergy Clin Immunol* 108: 997-1004, 2001.
[82] Grunstein MM, Veler H, Shan X, Larson J, Grunstein JS, and Chuang S. Proasthmatic effects and mechanisms of action of the dust mite allergen, Der p 1, in airway smooth muscle. *J Allergy Clin Immunol* 116: 94-101, 2005.
[83] Gudbjartsson DF, Bjornsdottir US, Halapi E, Helgadottir A, Sulem P, Jonsdottir GM, Thorleifsson G, Helgadottir H, Steinthorsdottir V, Stefansson H, Williams C, Hui J, Beilby J, Warrington NM, James A, Palmer LJ, Koppelman GH, Heinzmann A, Krueger M, Boezen HM, Wheatley A, Altmuller J, Shin HD, Uh ST, Cheong HS, Jonsdottir B, Gislason D, Park CS, Rasmussen LM, Porsbjerg C, Hansen JW, Backer V, Werge T, Janson C, Jonsson UB, Ng MC, Chan J, So WY, Ma R, Shah SH, Granger CB, Quyyumi AA, Levey AI, Vaccarino V, Reilly MP, Rader DJ, Williams MJ, van Rij AM, Jones GT, Trabetti E, Malerba G, Pignatti PF, Boner A, Pescollderungg L, Girelli D, Olivieri O, Martinelli N, Ludviksson BR, Ludviksdottir D, Eyjolfsson GI, Arnar D, Thorgeirsson G, Deichmann K, Thompson PJ, Wjst M, Hall IP, Postma DS, Gislason T, Gulcher J, Kong A, Jonsdottir I, Thorsteinsdottir U, and Stefansson K. Sequence variants affecting eosinophil numbers associate with asthma and myocardial infarction. *Nat Genet* 41: 342-347, 2009.
[84] Gump A, Haughney L, and Fredberg J. Relaxation of activated airway smooth muscle: relative potency of isoproterenol vs. tidal stretch. *J Appl Physiol* 90: 2306-2310, 2001.
[85] Gunst SJ. Contractile force of canine airway smooth muscle during cyclical length changes. *J Appl Physiol* 55: 759-769, 1983.
[86] Gunst SJ, and Stropp JQ. Pressure-volume and length-stress relationships in canine bronchi in vitro. *J Appl Physiol* 64: 2522-2531, 1988.
[87] Gunst SJ, Stropp JQ, and Flavahan NA. Interaction of contractile responses in canine tracheal smooth muscle. *J Appl Physiol* 63: 514-520, 1987.
[88] Hahn HL, Wilson AG, Graf PD, Fischer SP, and Nadel JA. Interaction between serotonin and efferent vagus nerves in dog lungs. *J Appl Physiol* 44: 144-149, 1978.

[89] Hakonarson H, and Grunstein MM. Autologously up-regulated Fc receptor expression and action in airway smooth muscle mediates its altered responsiveness in the atopic asthmatic sensitized state. *Proc Natl Acad Sci U S A* 95: 5257-5262, 1998.

[90] Hakonarson H, Halapi E, Whelan R, Gulcher J, Stefansson K, and Grunstein MM. Association between IL-1beta/TNF-alpha-induced glucocorticoid-sensitive changes in multiple gene expression and altered responsiveness in airway smooth muscle. *Am J Respir Cell Mol Biol* 25: 761-771, 2001.

[91] Hakonarson H, Herrick DJ, Serrano PG, and Grunstein MM. Autocrine role of interleukin 1beta in altered responsiveness of atopic asthmatic sensitized airway smooth muscle. *J Clin Invest* 99: 117-124, 1997.

[92] Hakonarson H, Herrick DJ, Serrano PG, and Grunstein MM. Mechanism of cytokine-induced modulation of beta-adrenoceptor responsiveness in airway smooth muscle. *J Clin Invest* 97: 2593-2600, 1996.

[93] Hakonarson H, Maskeri N, Carter C, Chuang S, and Grunstein MM. Autocrine interaction between IL-5 and IL-1beta mediates altered responsiveness of atopic asthmatic sensitized airway smooth muscle. *J Clin Invest* 104: 657-667, 1999.

[94] Hakonarson H, Maskeri N, Carter C, and Grunstein MM. Regulation of TH1- and TH2-type cytokine expression and action in atopic asthmatic sensitized airway smooth muscle. *J Clin Invest* 103: 1077-1087, 1999.

[95] Halayko AJ, Tran T, and Gosens R. Phenotype and functional plasticity of airway smooth muscle: role of caveolae and caveolins. *Proc Am Thorac Soc* 5: 80-88, 2008.

[96] Hardaker KM, Downie SR, Kermode JA, Farah CS, Brown NJ, Berend N, King GG, and Salome CM. The predictors of airway hyperresponsiveness differ between old and young asthmatics. *Chest.*

[97] Hardy CC, Bradding P, Robinson C, and Holgate ST. The combined effects of two pairs of mediators, adenosine with methacholine and prostaglandin D2 with histamine, on airway calibre in asthma. *Clin Sci (Lond)* 71: 385-392, 1986.

[98] Hashimoto T, Nakano Y, Ohata H, and Momose K. Lysophosphatidic acid enhances airway response to acetylcholine in guinea pigs. *Life Sci* 70: 199-205, 2001.

[99] Hashimoto T, Nakano Y, Yamashita M, Fang YI, Ohata H, and Momose K. Role of Rho-associated protein kinase and histamine in lysophosphatidic acid-induced airway hyperresponsiveness in guinea pigs. *Jpn J Pharmacol* 88: 256-261, 2002.

[100] Hassan M, Jo T, Risse PA, Tolloczko B, Lemiere C, Olivenstein R, Hamid Q, and Martin JG. Airway smooth muscle remodeling is a dynamic process in severe long-standing asthma. *J Allergy Clin Immunol* 125: 1037-1045 e1033, In press.

[101] Heaton RW, Henderson AF, Dunlop LS, and Costello JF. The influence of pretreatment with prostaglandin F2 alpha on bronchial sensitivity to inhaled histamine and methacholine in normal subjects. *Br J Dis Chest* 78: 168-173, 1984.

[102] Held HD, and Uhlig S. Mechanisms of endotoxin-induced airway and pulmonary vascular hyperreactivity in mice. *Am J Respir Crit Care Med* 162: 1547-1552, 2000.

[103] Herrera AM, McParland BE, Bienkowska A, Tait R, Pare PD, and Seow CY. 'Sarcomeres' of smooth muscle: functional characteristics and ultrastructural evidence. *J Cell Sci* 118: 2381-2392, 2005.

[104] Himes BE, Hunninghake GM, Baurley JW, Rafaels NM, Sleiman P, Strachan DP, Wilk JB, Willis-Owen SA, Klanderman B, Lasky-Su J, Lazarus R, Murphy AJ, Soto-Quiros ME, Avila L, Beaty T, Mathias RA, Ruczinski I, Barnes KC, Celedon JC, Cookson WO, Gauderman WJ, Gilliland FD, Hakonarson H, Lange C, Moffatt MF,

O'Connor GT, Raby BA, Silverman EK, and Weiss ST. Genome-wide association analysis identifies PDE4D as an asthma-susceptibility gene. *Am J Hum Genet* 84: 581-593, 2009.

[105] Huang Y, Zhang W, and Gunst SJ. Activation of vinculin induced by cholinergic stimulation regulates contraction of tracheal smooth muscle tissue. *J Biol Chem* 286: 3630-3644, 2011.

[106] Huber HL, and Koessler KK. The pathology of bronchial asthma. *Archs Intern Med* 30: 689, 1922.

[107] Hunter I, Cobban HJ, Vandenabeele P, MacEwan DJ, and Nixon GF. Tumor necrosis factor-alpha-induced activation of RhoA in airway smooth muscle cells: role in the Ca2+ sensitization of myosin light chain20 phosphorylation. *Mol Pharmacol* 63: 714-721, 2003.

[108] Ilowite JS, Bennett WD, Sheetz MS, Groth ML, and Nierman DM. Permeability of the bronchial mucosa to 99mTc-DTPA in asthma. *Am Rev Respir Dis* 139: 1139-1143, 1989.

[109] Jiang H, and Stephens NL. Isotonic relaxation of sensitized bronchial smooth muscle. *Am J Physiol* 262: L344-350, 1992.

[110] Jones GL, Saroea HG, Watson RM, and O'Byrne PM. Effect of an inhaled thromboxane mimetic (U46619) on airway function in human subjects. *Am Rev Respir Dis* 145: 1270-1274, 1992.

[111] Kaminsky DA, Irvin CG, Lundblad L, Moriya HT, Lang S, Allen J, Viola T, Lynn M, and Bates JH. Oscillation mechanics of the human lung periphery in asthma. *J Appl Physiol* 97: 1849-1858, 2004.

[112] Kanazawa H, Kurihara N, Hirata K, Fujiwara H, Matsushita H, and Takeda T. Low concentration endothelin-1 enhanced histamine-mediated bronchial contractions of guinea pigs in vivo. *Biochem Biophys Res Commun* 187: 717-721, 1992.

[113] Kaur D, Saunders R, Hollins F, Woodman L, Doe C, Siddiqui S, Bradding P, and Brightling C. Mast cell fibroblastoid differentiation mediated by airway smooth muscle in asthma. *J Immunol* 185: 6105-6114.

[114] Kikuchi Y, Okayama H, Okayama M, Sasaki H, and Takishima T. Interaction between histamine and vagal stimulation on tracheal smooth muscle in dogs. *J Appl Physiol* 56: 590-595, 1984.

[115] King GG, Carroll JD, Muller NL, Whittall KP, Gao M, Nakano Y, and Pare PD. Heterogeneity of narrowing in normal and asthmatic airways measured by HRCT. *Eur Respir J* 24: 211-218, 2004.

[116] King GG, Eberl S, Salome CM, Young IH, and Woolcock AJ. Differences in airway closure between normal and asthmatic subjects measured with single-photon emission computed tomography and technegas. *Am J Respir Crit Care Med* 158: 1900-1906, 1998.

[117] King GG, Moore BJ, Seow CY, and Pare PD. Airway narrowing associated with inhibition of deep inspiration during methacholine inhalation in asthmatics. *Am J Respir Crit Care Med* 164: 216-218, 2001.

[118] King GG, Moore BJ, Seow CY, and Pare PD. Time course of increased airway narrowing caused by inhibition of deep inspiration during methacholine challenge. *Am J Respir Crit Care Med* 160: 454-457, 1999.

[119] Knight D, McKay K, Wiggs B, Schellenberg RR, and Bai T. Localization of leukaemia inhibitory factor to airway epithelium and its amplification of contractile responses to tachykinins. *Br J Pharmacol* 120: 883-891, 1997.

[120] Knowles MR, and Boucher RC. Mucus clearance as a primary innate defense mechanism for mammalian airways. *J Clin Invest* 109: 571-577, 2002.

[121] Krug N, Tschernig T, Erpenbeck VJ, Hohlfeld JM, and Kohl J. Complement factors C3a and C5a are increased in bronchoalveolar lavage fluid after segmental allergen provocation in subjects with asthma. *Am J Respir Crit Care Med* 164: 1841-1843, 2001.

[122] Kume H, Takeda N, Oguma T, Ito S, Kondo M, Ito Y, and Shimokata K. Sphingosine 1-phosphate causes airway hyper-reactivity by rho-mediated myosin phosphatase inactivation. *J Pharmacol Exp Ther* 320: 766-773, 2007.

[123] Kuyper LM, Pare PD, Hogg JC, Lambert RK, Ionescu D, Woods R, and Bai TR. Characterization of airway plugging in fatal asthma. *Am J Med* 115: 6-11, 2003.

[124] Lai-Fook SJ, Hyatt RE, and Rodarte JR. Effect of parenchymal shear modulus and lung volume on bronchial pressure-diameter behavior. *J Appl Physiol* 44: 859-868, 1978.

[125] Lam S, Chan H, LeRiche JC, Chan-Yeung M, and Salari H. Release of leukotrienes in patients with bronchial asthma. *J Allergy Clin Immunol* 81: 711-717, 1988.

[126] Lambert RK, Wiggs BR, Kuwano K, Hogg JC, and Pare PD. Functional significance of increased airway smooth muscle in asthma and COPD. *J Appl Physiol* 74: 2771-2781, 1993.

[127] Laporte JC, Moore PE, Baraldo S, Jouvin MH, Church TL, Schwartzman IN, Panettieri RA, Jr., Kinet JP, and Shore SA. Direct effects of interleukin-13 on signaling pathways for physiological responses in cultured human airway smooth muscle cells. *Am J Respir Crit Care Med* 164: 141-148, 2001.

[128] Latourelle J, Fabry B, and Fredberg JJ. Dynamic equilibration of airway smooth muscle contraction during physiological loading. *J Appl Physiol* 92: 771-779, 2002.

[129] Lauzon AM, Tyska MJ, Rovner AS, Freyzon Y, Warshaw DM, and Trybus KM. A 7-amino-acid insert in the heavy chain nucleotide binding loop alters the kinetics of smooth muscle myosin in the laser trap. *J Muscle Res Cell Motil* 19: 825-837, 1998.

[130] Lavoie TL, Dowell ML, Lakser OJ, Gerthoffer WT, Fredberg JJ, Seow CY, Mitchell RW, and Solway J. Disrupting actin-Myosin-actin connectivity in airway smooth muscle as a treatment for asthma? *Proc Am Thorac Soc* 6: 295-300, 2009.

[131] Leff AR, and Munoz NM. Cholinergic and alpha adrenergic augmentation of histamine-induced contraction of canine airway smooth muscle. *J Pharmacol Exp Ther* 218: 582-587, 1981.

[132] Leguillette R, and Lauzon AM. Molecular mechanics of smooth muscle contractile proteins in airway hyperresponsiveness and asthma. *Proc Am Thorac Soc* 5: 40-46, 2008.

[133] Leguillette R, Laviolette M, Bergeron C, Zitouni N, Kogut P, Solway J, Kachmar L, Hamid Q, and Lauzon AM. Myosin, transgelin, and myosin light chain kinase: expression and function in asthma. *Am J Respir Crit Care Med* 179: 194-204, 2009.

[134] Lim TK, Ang SM, Rossing TH, Ingenito EP, and Ingram RH, Jr. The effects of deep inhalation on maximal expiratory flow during intensive treatment of spontaneous asthmatic episodes. *Am Rev Respir Dis* 140: 340-343, 1989.

[135] Liu C, Tazzeo T, and Janssen LJ. Isoprostane-induced airway hyperresponsiveness is dependent on internal Ca2+ handling and Rho/ROCK signaling. *Am J Physiol Lung Cell Mol Physiol* 291: L1177-1184, 2006.

[136] Liu MC, Hubbard WC, Proud D, Stealey BA, Galli SJ, Kagey-Sobotka A, Bleecker ER, and Lichtenstein LM. Immediate and late inflammatory responses to ragweed antigen challenge of the peripheral airways in allergic asthmatics. Cellular, mediator, and permeability changes. *Am Rev Respir Dis* 144: 51-58, 1991.
[137] Loring SH, Drazen JM, Snapper JR, and Ingram RH, Jr. Vagal and aerosol histamine interactions on airway responses in dogs. *J Appl Physiol* 45: 40-44, 1978.
[138] Lutchen KR, and Gillis H. Relationship between heterogeneous changes in airway morphometry and lung resistance and elastance. *J Appl Physiol* 83: 1192-1201, 1997.
[139] Lutchen KR, Jensen A, Atileh H, Kaczka DW, Israel E, Suki B, and Ingenito EP. Airway constriction pattern is a central component of asthma severity: the role of deep inspirations. *Am J Respir Crit Care Med* 164: 207-215, 2001.
[140] Ma X, Cheng Z, Kong H, Wang Y, Unruh H, Stephens NL, and Laviolette M. Changes in biophysical and biochemical properties of single bronchial smooth muscle cells from asthmatic subjects. *Am J Physiol Lung Cell Mol Physiol* 283: L1181-1189, 2002.
[141] Macklem PT. The physiology of small airways. *Am J Respir Crit Care Med* 157: S181-183, 1998.
[142] Manolio TA. Genomewide association studies and assessment of the risk of disease. *N Engl J Med* 363: 166-176, 2010.
[143] Mapp CE, Polato R, Maestrelli P, Hendrick DJ, and Fabbri LM. Time course of the increase in airway responsiveness associated with late asthmatic reactions to toluene diisocyanate in sensitized subjects. *J Allergy Clin Immunol* 75: 568-572, 1985.
[144] Marthan R, and Woolcock AJ. Is a myogenic response involved in deep inspiration-induced bronchoconstriction in asthmatics? *Am Rev Respir Dis* 140: 1354-1358, 1989.
[145] Martin JG, and Collier B. Acetylcholine release from canine isolated airway is not modulated by norepinephrine. *J Appl Physiol* 61: 1025-1030, 1986.
[146] Martin TR, Takeishi T, Katz HR, Austen KF, Drazen JM, and Galli SJ. Mast cell activation enhances airway responsiveness to methacholine in the mouse. *J Clin Invest* 91: 1176-1182, 1993.
[147] Matsumoto H, Moir LM, Oliver BG, Burgess JK, Roth M, Black JL, and McParland BE. Comparison of gel contraction mediated by airway smooth muscle cells from patients with and without asthma. *Thorax* 62: 848-854, 2007.
[148] Mattoli S, Soloperto M, Marini M, and Fasoli A. Levels of endothelin in the bronchoalveolar lavage fluid of patients with symptomatic asthma and reversible airflow obstruction. *J Allergy Clin Immunol* 88: 376-384, 1991.
[149] Mauad T, Silva LF, Santos MA, Grinberg L, Bernardi FD, Martins MA, Saldiva PH, and Dolhnikoff M. Abnormal alveolar attachments with decreased elastic fiber content in distal lung in fatal asthma. *Am J Respir Crit Care Med* 170: 857-862, 2004.
[150] Mazzone SB, and Canning BJ. Synergistic interactions between airway afferent nerve subtypes mediating reflex bronchospasm in guinea pigs. *Am J Physiol Regul Integr Comp Physiol* 283: R86-98, 2002.
[151] Mazzone SB, Lim LH, Wagner EM, Mori N, and Canning BJ. Sympathetic nerve-dependent regulation of mucosal vascular tone modifies airway smooth muscle reactivity. *J Appl Physiol* 109: 1292-1300, 2010.
[152] Mazzoni L, Chapman ID, and Morley J. Changes in airway sensitivity to histamine are not necessarily paralleled by changed sensitivity to acetylcholine. *Agents Actions Suppl* 34: 257-266, 1991.

[153] McParland BE, Macklem PT, and Pare PD. Airway wall remodeling: friend or foe? *J Appl Physiol* 95: 426-434, 2003.
[154] Mehta D, Wu MF, and Gunst SJ. Role of contractile protein activation in the length-dependent modulation of tracheal smooth muscle force. *Am J Physiol* 270: C243-252, 1996.
[155] Milanese M, Crimi E, Scordamaglia A, Riccio A, Pellegrino R, Canonica GW, and Brusasco V. On the functional consequences of bronchial basement membrane thickening. *J Appl Physiol* 91: 1035-1040, 2001.
[156] Millar EA, Nally JE, and Thomson NC. Angiotensin II potentiates methacholine-induced bronchoconstriction in human airway both in vitro and in vivo. *Eur Respir J* 8: 1838-1841, 1995.
[157] Mills JE, and Widdicombe JG. Role of the vagus nerves in anaphylaxis and histamine-induced bronchoconstrictions in guinea-pigs. *Br J Pharmacol* 39: 724-731, 1970.
[158] Mitchell C, and Bouhuys A. Interaction between bronchoconstrictor stimuli on human airway smooth muscle. *Yale J Biol Med* 49: 317-325, 1976.
[159] Mitchell HW, Fisher JT, and Sparrow MP. The integrity of the epithelium is a major determinant of the responsiveness of the dog bronchial segment to mucosal provocation. *Pulm Pharmacol* 6: 263-268, 1993.
[160] Mitchell RW, Dowell ML, Solway J, and Lakser OJ. Force Fluctuation induced Relengthening of Acetylcholine-contracted Airway Smooth Muscle. *Proc Am Thorac Soc* 5: 68-72, 2008.
[161] Mitchell RW, Ruhlmann E, Magnussen H, Leff AR, and Rabe KF. Passive sensitization of human bronchi augments smooth muscle shortening velocity and capacity. *Am J Physiol* 267: L218-222, 1994.
[162] Mitzner W. Airway smooth muscle: the appendix of the lung. *Am J Respir Crit Care Med* 169: 787-790, 2004.
[163] Moffatt MF, Gut IG, Demenais F, Strachan DP, Bouzigon E, Heath S, von Mutius E, Farrall M, Lathrop M, and Cookson WO. A large-scale, consortium-based genomewide association study of asthma. *N Engl J Med* 363: 1211-1221, 2010.
[164] Moffatt MF, Kabesch M, Liang L, Dixon AL, Strachan D, Heath S, Depner M, von Berg A, Bufe A, Rietschel E, Heinzmann A, Simma B, Frischer T, Willis-Owen SA, Wong KC, Illig T, Vogelberg C, Weiland SK, von Mutius E, Abecasis GR, Farrall M, Gut IG, Lathrop GM, and Cookson WO. Genetic variants regulating ORMDL3 expression contribute to the risk of childhood asthma. *Nature* 448: 470-473, 2007.
[165] Molfino NA, Slutsky AS, Julia-Serda G, Hoffstein V, Szalai JP, Chapman KR, Rebuck AS, and Zamel N. Assessment of airway tone in asthma. Comparison between double lung transplant patients and healthy subjects. *Am Rev Respir Dis* 148: 1238-1243, 1993.
[166] Molimard M, Naline E, Boichot E, Devillier P, Lagente V, Begaud B, and Advenier C. In vitro-induced human airway hyperresponsiveness to bradykinin. *Eur Respir J* 12: 1301-1306, 1998.
[167] Morin C, Sirois M, Echave V, Gomes MM, and Rousseau E. EET displays anti-inflammatory effects in TNF-alpha stimulated human bronchi: putative role of CPI-17. *Am J Respir Cell Mol Biol* 38: 192-201, 2008.
[168] Morin C, Sirois M, Echave V, and Rousseau E. CPI-17 silencing-reduced responsiveness in control and TNF-alpha-treated human bronchi. *Am J Respir Cell Mol Biol* 39: 638-643, 2008.

[169] Murata K, Itoh H, Senda M, Todo G, Yonekura Y, and Torizuka K. Ventilation imaging with positron emission tomography and nitrogen 13. *Radiology* 158: 303-307, 1986.
[170] Murray JJ, Tonnel AB, Brash AR, Roberts LJ, 2nd, Gosset P, Workman R, Capron A, and Oates JA. Release of prostaglandin D2 into human airways during acute antigen challenge. *N Engl J Med* 315: 800-804, 1986.
[171] Nadel JA, and Tierney DF. Effect of a previous deep inspiration on airway resistance in man. *J Appl Physiol* 16: 717-719, 1961.
[172] Nakatani Y, Nishimura Y, Nishiuma T, Maeda H, and Yokoyama M. Tumor necrosis factor-alpha augments contraction and cytosolic Ca(2+) sensitivity through phospholipase A(2) in bovine tracheal smooth muscle. *Eur J Pharmacol* 392: 175-182, 2000.
[173] Nally JE, Bunton DC, Martin D, and Thomson NC. The role of cyclooxygenase and 5-lipoxygenase metabolites in potentiated endothelin-1-evoked contractions in bovine bronchi. *Pulm Pharmacol* 9: 211-217, 1996.
[174] Nally JE, Clayton RA, Wakelam MJ, Thomson NC, and McGrath JC. Angiotensin II enhances responses to endothelin-1 in bovine bronchial smooth muscle. *Pulm Pharmacol* 7: 409-413, 1994.
[175] Niimi A, Matsumoto H, Takemura M, Ueda T, Chin K, and Mishima M. Relationship of airway wall thickness to airway sensitivity and airway reactivity in asthma. *Am J Respir Crit Care Med* 168: 983-988, 2003.
[176] Noble PB, Hernandez JM, Mitchell HW, and Janssen LJ. Deep inspiration and airway physiology: human, canine, porcine, or bovine? *J Appl Physiol* 109: 938-939; author reply 940-931, 2010.
[177] Noble PB, Jones RL, Needi ET, Cairncross A, Mitchell HW, James AL, and McFawn PK. Responsiveness of the human airway in vitro during deep inspiration and tidal oscillation. *J Appl Physiol* 110: 1510-1518, 2011.
[178] Noble PB, McFawn PK, and Mitchell HW. Responsiveness of the isolated airway during simulated deep inspirations: effect of airway smooth muscle stiffness and strain. *J Appl Physiol* 103: 787-795, 2007.
[179] Noble PB, McLaughlin RA, West AR, Becker S, Armstrong JJ, McFawn PK, Eastwood PR, Hillman DR, Sampson DD, and Mitchell HW. Distribution of airway narrowing responses across generations and at branching points, assessed in vitro by anatomical optical coherence tomography. *Respir Res* 11: 9, 2010.
[180] Noguchi K, Ishikawa K, Yano M, Ahmed A, Cortes A, and Abraham WM. Endothelin-1 contributes to antigen-induced airway hyperresponsiveness. *J Appl Physiol* 79: 700-705, 1995.
[181] O'Byrne PM, Leikauf GD, Aizawa H, Bethel RA, Ueki IF, Holtzman MJ, and Nadel JA. Leukotriene B4 induces airway hyperresponsiveness in dogs. *J Appl Physiol* 59: 1941-1946, 1985.
[182] Ober C, Butte AJ, Elias JA, Lusis AJ, Gan W, Banks-Schlegel S, and Schwartz D. Getting from genes to function in lung disease: a National Heart, Lung, and Blood Institute workshop report. *Am J Respir Crit Care Med* 182: 732-737, 2010.
[183] Ober C, and Hoffjan S. Asthma genetics 2006: the long and winding road to gene discovery. *Genes Immun* 7: 95-100, 2006.
[184] Oguma T, Ito S, Kondo M, Makino Y, Shimokata K, Honjo H, Kamiya K, and Kume H. Roles of P2X receptors and Ca(2+) sensitization in extracellular adenosine

triphosphate-induced hyperresponsiveness in airway smooth muscle. *Clin Exp Allergy* 37: 893-900, 2007.
[185] Ohno Y, Watanabe M, and Kasuya Y. Manifestation of latent alpha-excitatory response in the canine tracheal smooth muscle preparation--relation to basal tone. *Arch Int Pharmacodyn Ther* 251: 205-216, 1981.
[186] Oliver MN, Fabry B, Marinkovic A, Mijailovich SM, Butler JP, and Fredberg JJ. Airway hyperresponsiveness, remodeling, and smooth muscle mass: right answer, wrong reason? *Am J Respir Cell Mol Biol* 37: 264-272, 2007.
[187] Omari TI, and Sparrow MP. Epithelial disruption by proteases augments the responsiveness of porcine bronchial segments. *Clin Exp Pharmacol Physiol* 19: 785-794, 1992.
[188] Opazo Saez A, Zhang W, Wu Y, Turner CE, Tang DD, and Gunst SJ. Tension development during contractile stimulation of smooth muscle requires recruitment of paxillin and vinculin to the membrane. *Am J Physiol Cell Physiol* 286: C433-447, 2004.
[189] Pare PD. Airway hyperresponsiveness in asthma: geometry is not everything! *Am J Respir Crit Care Med* 168: 913-914, 2003.
[190] Pare PD, McParland BE, and Seow CY. Structural basis for exaggerated airway narrowing. *Can J Physiol Pharmacol* 85: 653-658, 2007.
[191] Parris JR, Cobban HJ, Littlejohn AF, MacEwan DJ, and Nixon GF. Tumour necrosis factor-alpha activates a calcium sensitization pathway in guinea-pig bronchial smooth muscle. *J Physiol* 518 (Pt 2): 561-569, 1999.
[192] Patterson R, Bernstein PR, Harris KE, and Krell RD. Airway responses to sequential challenges with platelet-activating factor and leukotriene D4 in rhesus monkeys. *J Lab Clin Med* 104: 340-345, 1984.
[193] Pennings HJ, Kramer K, Bast A, Buurman WA, and Wouters EF. Tumour necrosis factor-alpha induces hyperreactivity in tracheal smooth muscle of the guinea-pig in vitro. *Eur Respir J* 12: 45-49, 1998.
[194] Phillips GD, and Holgate ST. Interaction of inhaled LTC4 with histamine and PGD2 on airway caliber in asthma. *J Appl Physiol* 66: 304-312, 1989.
[195] Pitt CM, and Nally JE. Angiotensin II-mediated potentiation of endothelin-1-evoked bronchial contractions: a role for leukotrienes? *Pulm Pharmacol Ther* 12: 7-12, 1999.
[196] Prakash YS, Kannan MS, Walseth TF, and Sieck GC. Role of cyclic ADP-ribose in the regulation of [Ca2+]i in porcine tracheal smooth muscle. *Am J Physiol* 274: C1653-1660, 1998.
[197] Que LG, Stiles JV, Sundy JS, and Foster WM. Pulmonary Function, Bronchial Reactivity, and Epithelial Permeability are Response Phenotypes to Ozone and Develop Differentially in Healthy Humans. *J Appl Physiol* In press.
[198] Raboudi SH, Miller B, Butler JP, Shore SA, and Fredberg JJ. Dynamically determined contractile states of airway smooth muscle. *Am J Respir Crit Care Med* 158: S176-178, 1998.
[199] Regamey N, Ochs M, Hilliard TN, Muhlfeld C, Cornish N, Fleming L, Saglani S, Alton EW, Bush A, Jeffery PK, and Davies JC. Increased airway smooth muscle mass in children with asthma, cystic fibrosis, and non-cystic fibrosis bronchiectasis. *Am J Respir Crit Care Med* 177: 837-843, 2008.
[200] Reynolds AM, Holmes MD, and Scicchitano R. Cytokines enhance airway smooth muscle contractility in response to acetylcholine and neurokinin A. *Respirology* 5: 153-160, 2000.

[201] Roth EJ, Nussbaum SB, Berkowitz M, Primack S, Oken J, Powley S, and Lu A. Pulmonary function testing in spinal cord injury: correlation with vital capacity. *Paraplegia* 33: 454-457, 1995.

[202] Rubin AH, Smith LJ, and Patterson R. The bronchoconstrictor properties of platelet-activating factor in humans. *Am Rev Respir Dis* 136: 1145-1151, 1987.

[203] Sakai H, Nishimura A, Watanabe Y, Nishizawa Y, Hashimoto Y, Chiba Y, and Misawa M. Involvement of Src family kinase activation in angiotensin II-induced hyperresponsiveness of rat bronchial smooth muscle. *Peptides* 31: 2216-2221.

[204] Sakai H, Nishizawa Y, Nishimura A, Chiba Y, Goto K, Hanazaki M, and Misawa M. Angiotensin II induces hyperresponsiveness of bronchial smooth muscle via an activation of p42/44 ERK in rats. *Pflugers Arch* 460: 645-655.

[205] Sakai J, Oike M, Hirakawa M, and Ito Y. Theophylline and cAMP inhibit lysophosphatidic acid-induced hyperresponsiveness of bovine tracheal smooth muscle cells. *J Physiol* 549: 171-180, 2003.

[206] Salome CM, King GG, and Berend N. Physiology of obesity and effects on lung function. *J Appl Physiol* 108: 206-211, 2010.

[207] Samee S, Altes T, Powers P, de Lange EE, Knight-Scott J, Rakes G, Mugler JP, 3rd, Ciambotti JM, Alford BA, Brookeman JR, and Platts-Mills TA. Imaging the lungs in asthmatic patients by using hyperpolarized helium-3 magnetic resonance: assessment of response to methacholine and exercise challenge. *J Allergy Clin Immunol* 111: 1205-1211, 2003.

[208] Sanjar S, Kristersson A, Mazzoni L, Morley J, and Schaeublin E. Increased airway reactivity in the guinea-pig follows exposure to intravenous isoprenaline. *J Physiol* 425: 43-54, 1990.

[209] Sanjar S, Smith D, Schaeublin E, Kristersson A, Chapman I, Mazzoni L, and Morley J. The effect of prophylactic anti-asthma drugs on PAF-induced airway hyperreactivity. *Jpn J Pharmacol* 51: 151-160, 1989.

[210] Schelegle ES. Functional morphology and physiology of slowly adapting pulmonary stretch receptors. *Anat Rec A Discov Mol Cell Evol Biol* 270: 11-16, 2003.

[211] Schmidt D, Ruehlmann E, Branscheid D, Magnussen H, and Rabe KF. Passive sensitization of human airways increases responsiveness to leukotriene C4. *Eur Respir J* 14: 315-319, 1999.

[212] Sekizawa K, Caughey GH, Lazarus SC, Gold WM, and Nadel JA. Mast cell tryptase causes airway smooth muscle hyperresponsiveness in dogs. *J Clin Invest* 83: 175-179, 1989.

[213] Seow CY. Myosin filament assembly in an ever-changing myofilament lattice of smooth muscle. *Am J Physiol Cell Physiol* 289: C1363-1368, 2005.

[214] Seow CY, Schellenberg RR, and Pare PD. Structural and functional changes in the airway smooth muscle of asthmatic subjects. *Am J Respir Crit Care Med* 158: S179-186, 1998.

[215] Setoguchi H, Nishimura J, Hirano K, Takahashi S, and Kanaide H. Leukotriene C(4) enhances the contraction of porcine tracheal smooth muscle through the activation of Y-27632, a rho kinase inhibitor, sensitive pathway. *Br J Pharmacol* 132: 111-118, 2001.

[216] Shan X, Hu A, Veler H, Fatma S, Grunstein JS, Chuang S, and Grunstein MM. Regulation of Toll-like receptor 4-induced proasthmatic changes in airway smooth muscle function by opposing actions of ERK1/2 and p38 MAPK signaling. *Am J Physiol Lung Cell Mol Physiol* 291: L324-333, 2006.

[217] Sheller JR, Holtzman MJ, Skoogh BE, and Nadel JA. Interaction of serotonin with vagal- and ACh-induced bronchoconstriction in canine lungs. *J Appl Physiol* 52: 964-966, 1982.

[218] Shi HZ, Xiao CQ, Zhong D, Qin SM, Liu Y, Liang GR, Xu H, Chen YQ, Long XM, and Xie ZF. Effect of inhaled interleukin-5 on airway hyperreactivity and eosinophilia in asthmatics. *Am J Respir Crit Care Med* 157: 204-209, 1998.

[219] Shore S, Irvin CG, Shenkier T, and Martin JG. Mechanisms of histamine-induced contraction of canine airway smooth muscle. *J Appl Physiol* 55: 22-26, 1983.

[220] Simonsson BG, Svedmyr N, Skoogh BE, Anderson R, and Bergh NP. In vivo and in vitro studies on alpha-receptors in human airways; potentiation with bacterial endotoxins. *Chest* 63: Suppl:3S-4S, 1973.

[221] Skloot G, Permutt S, and Togias A. Airway hyperresponsiveness in asthma: a problem of limited smooth muscle relaxation with inspiration. *J Clin Invest* 96: 2393-2403, 1995.

[222] Skloot G, and Togias A. Bronchodilation and bronchoprotection by deep inspiration and their relationship to bronchial hyperresponsiveness. *Clin Rev Allergy Immunol* 24: 55-72, 2003.

[223] Sleiman PM, Flory J, Imielinski M, Bradfield JP, Annaiah K, Willis-Owen SA, Wang K, Rafaels NM, Michel S, Bonnelykke K, Zhang H, Kim CE, Frackelton EC, Glessner JT, Hou C, Otieno FG, Santa E, Thomas K, Smith RM, Glaberson WR, Garris M, Chiavacci RM, Beaty TH, Ruczinski I, Orange JM, Allen J, Spergel JM, Grundmeier R, Mathias RA, Christie JD, von Mutius E, Cookson WO, Kabesch M, Moffatt MF, Grunstein MM, Barnes KC, Devoto M, Magnusson M, Li H, Grant SF, Bisgaard H, and Hakonarson H. Variants of DENND1B associated with asthma in children. *N Engl J Med* 362: 36-44, 2010.

[224] Smith N, and Broadley KJ. Adenosine receptor subtypes in the airways responses to 5'-adenosine monophosphate inhalation of sensitized guinea-pigs. *Clin Exp Allergy* 38: 1536-1547, 2008.

[225] Sparrow MP, Omari TI, and Mitchell HW. The epithelial barrier and airway responsiveness. *Can J Physiol Pharmacol* 73: 180-190, 1995.

[226] Stamenovic D, Mijailovich SM, Tolic-Norrelykke IM, Chen J, and Wang N. Cell prestress. II. Contribution of microtubules. *Am J Physiol Cell Physiol* 282: C617-624, 2002.

[227] Sukkar MB, Hughes JM, Armour CL, and Johnson PR. Tumour necrosis factor-alpha potentiates contraction of human bronchus in vitro. *Respirology* 6: 199-203, 2001.

[228] Tliba O, Deshpande D, Chen H, Van Besien C, Kannan M, Panettieri RA, Jr., and Amrani Y. IL-13 enhances agonist-evoked calcium signals and contractile responses in airway smooth muscle. *Br J Pharmacol* 140: 1159-1162, 2003.

[229] Tliba O, Panettieri RA, Jr., Tliba S, Walseth TF, and Amrani Y. Tumor necrosis factor-alpha differentially regulates the expression of proinflammatory genes in human airway smooth muscle cells by activation of interferon-beta-dependent CD38 pathway. *Mol Pharmacol* 66: 322-329, 2004.

[230] Toews ML, Ustinova EE, and Schultz HD. Lysophosphatidic acid enhances contractility of isolated airway smooth muscle. *J Appl Physiol* 83: 1216-1222, 1997.

[231] Tomaki M, Ichinose M, Miura M, Hirayama Y, Yamauchi H, Nakajima N, and Shirato K. Elevated substance P content in induced sputum from patients with asthma and patients with chronic bronchitis. *Am J Respir Crit Care Med* 151: 613-617, 1995.

[232] Tran T, Gosens R, and Halayko AJ. Effects of extracellular matrix and integrin interactions on airway smooth muscle phenotype and function: It takes two to tango! *Curr Respir Med Rev* 3: 193-205, 2007.

[233] Tran T, McNeill KD, Gerthoffer WT, Unruh H, and Halayko AJ. Endogenous laminin is required for human airway smooth muscle cell maturation. *Respir Res* 7: 117, 2006.

[234] Tzeng YS, Lutchen K, and Albert M. The difference in ventilation heterogeneity between asthmatic and healthy subjects quantified using hyperpolarized 3He MRI. *J Appl Physiol* 106: 813-822, 2009.

[235] Van de Graaf EA, Out TA, Roos CM, and Jansen HM. Respiratory membrane permeability and bronchial hyperreactivity in patients with stable asthma. Effects of therapy with inhaled steroids. *Am Rev Respir Dis* 143: 362-368, 1991.

[236] Venegas JG, Winkler T, Musch G, Vidal Melo MF, Layfield D, Tgavalekos N, Fischman AJ, Callahan RJ, Bellani G, and Harris RS. Self-organized patchiness in asthma as a prelude to catastrophic shifts. *Nature* 434: 777-782, 2005.

[237] Wagers S, Lundblad LK, Ekman M, Irvin CG, and Bates JH. The allergic mouse model of asthma: normal smooth muscle in an abnormal lung? *J Appl Physiol* 96: 2019-2027, 2004.

[238] Wagers SS, Norton RJ, Rinaldi LM, Bates JH, Sobel BE, and Irvin CG. Extravascular fibrin, plasminogen activator, plasminogen activator inhibitors, and airway hyperresponsiveness. *J Clin Invest* 114: 104-111, 2004.

[239] Wagner EM, and Mitzner W. Effects of bronchial vascular engorgement on airway dimensions. *J Appl Physiol* 81: 293-301, 1996.

[240] Walters EH, Parrish RW, Bevan C, and Smith AP. Induction of bronchial hypersensitivity: evidence for a role for prostaglandins. *Thorax* 36: 571-574, 1981.

[241] Wang L, Chitano P, and Murphy TM. Length oscillation induces force potentiation in infant guinea pig airway smooth muscle. *Am J Physiol Lung Cell Mol Physiol* 289: L909-915, 2005.

[242] Wang L, Pare PD, and Seow CY. Effects of length oscillation on the subsequent force development in swine tracheal smooth muscle. *J Appl Physiol* 88: 2246-2250, 2000.

[243] Wang R, Li Q, and Tang DD. Role of vimentin in smooth muscle force development. *Am J Physiol Cell Physiol* 291: C483-489, 2006.

[244] Watanabe K, Myou S, Fujimura M, Tachibana H, Kita T, and Nakao S. Importance of the angiotensin type 1 receptor in angiotensin II-induced bronchoconstriction and bronchial hyperresponsiveness in the guinea pig. *Exp Lung Res* 30: 207-221, 2004.

[245] Watson N, Bodtke K, Coleman RA, Dent G, Morton BE, Ruhlmann E, Magnussen H, and Rabe KF. Role of IgE in hyperresponsiveness induced by passive sensitization of human airways. *Am J Respir Crit Care Med* 155: 839-844, 1997.

[246] Watson N, Ruhlmann E, Magnussen H, and Rabe KF. Histamine hypersensitivity induced by passive sensitization of human bronchus: effect of serum IgE depletion. *Clin Exp Allergy* 28: 679-685, 1998.

[247] Watson RA, and Pride NB. Postural changes in lung volumes and respiratory resistance in subjects with obesity. *J Appl Physiol* 98: 512-517, 2005.

[248] Wenzel SE. Asthma: defining of the persistent adult phenotypes. *Lancet* 368: 804-813, 2006.

[249] Wenzel SE, Westcott JY, and Larsen GL. Bronchoalveolar lavage fluid mediator levels 5 minutes after allergen challenge in atopic subjects with asthma: relationship to the development of late asthmatic responses. *J Allergy Clin Immunol* 87: 540-548, 1991.

[250] Whelan R, Kim C, Chen M, Leiter J, Grunstein MM, and Hakonarson H. Role and regulation of interleukin-1 molecules in pro-asthmatic sensitised airway smooth muscle. *Eur Respir J* 24: 559-567, 2004.

[251] White J, and Eiser NM. The role of histamine and its receptors in the pathogenesis of asthma. *Br J Dis Chest* 77: 215-226, 1983.

[252] White TA, Kannan MS, and Walseth TF. Intracellular calcium signaling through the cADPR pathway is agonist specific in porcine airway smooth muscle. *Faseb J* 17: 482-484, 2003.

[253] Winkler T, and Venegas JG. Complex airway behavior and paradoxical responses to bronchoprovocation. *J Appl Physiol* 2007.

[254] Winter MC, Shasby SS, Ries DR, and Shasby DM. PAR2 activation interrupts E-cadherin adhesion and compromises the airway epithelial barrier: protective effect of beta-agonists. *Am J Physiol Lung Cell Mol Physiol* 291: L628-635, 2006.

[255] Woodman L, Siddiqui S, Cruse G, Sutcliffe A, Saunders R, Kaur D, Bradding P, and Brightling C. Mast cells promote airway smooth muscle cell differentiation via autocrine up-regulation of TGF-beta1. *J Immunol* 181: 5001-5007, 2008.

[256] Woodruff PG, Dolganov GM, Ferrando RE, Donnelly S, Hays SR, Solberg OD, Carter R, Wong HH, Cadbury PS, and Fahy JV. Hyperplasia of smooth muscle in mild to moderate asthma without changes in cell size or gene expression. *Am J Respir Crit Care Med* 169: 1001-1006, 2004.

[257] Wright SM, Hockey PM, Enhorning G, Strong P, Reid KB, Holgate ST, Djukanovic R, and Postle AD. Altered airway surfactant phospholipid composition and reduced lung function in asthma. *J Appl Physiol* 89: 1283-1292, 2000.

[258] Yanta MA, Loring SH, Ingram RH, Jr., and Drazen JM. Direct and reflex bronchoconstriction induced by histamine aerosol inhalation in dogs. *J Appl Physiol* 50: 869-873, 1981.

[259] Yoo J, Ellis R, Morgan KG, and Hai CM. Mechanosensitive modulation of myosin phosphorylation and phosphatidylinositol turnover in smooth muscle. *Am J Physiol* 267: C1657-1665, 1994.

[260] Yoshimura H, Jones KA, Perkins WJ, Kai T, and Warner DO. Calcium sensitization produced by G protein activation in airway smooth muscle. *Am J Physiol Lung Cell Mol Physiol* 281: L631-638, 2001.

[261] Youn T, Kim SA, and Hai CM. Length-dependent modulation of smooth muscle activation: effects of agonist, cytochalasin, and temperature. *Am J Physiol* 274: C1601-1607, 1998.

[262] Zabner J, Winter MC, Shasby S, Ries D, and Shasby DM. Histamine decreases E-cadherin-based adhesion to increase permeability of human airway epithelium. *Chest* 123: 385S, 2003.

[263] Zhang W, and Gunst SJ. Dynamic association between alpha-actinin and beta-integrin regulates contraction of canine tracheal smooth muscle. *J Physiol* 572: 659-676, 2006.

[264] Zhang W, and Gunst SJ. Interactions of airway smooth muscle cells with their tissue matrix: implications for contraction. *Proc Am Thorac Soc* 5: 32-39, 2008.

[265] Zhang W, Wu Y, Wu C, and Gunst SJ. Integrin-linked kinase regulates N-WASp-mediated actin polymerization and tension development in tracheal smooth muscle. *J Biol Chem* 282: 34568-34580, 2007.

2

Polymerization and Oxidation of Alpha-1-Antitrypsin in Pathogenesis of Emphysema

Aleksandra Topic[1] and Dragica Radojkovic[2]
[1]*University of Belgrade, Faculty of Pharmacy, Department of Medical Biochemistry,*
[2]*University of Belgrade, Institute of Molecular Genetics and Genetic Enginieering,*
Belgrade
Serbia

1. Introduction

The last two decades efforts have been made in investigation of genes that encode proteins involved in pathogenesis of emphysema and chronic obstructive pulmonary disease (COPD). So far, SERPINA1 gene which encodes protein alpha-1-antitrypsin (A1AT) is the only defined genetic risk factor associated with early development of emphysema.

The A1AT is dominant protein of α_1 electrophoretic fraction of serum proteins, whose main physiological role is to inhibit neutrophil elastase (NE) in the lower respiratory tract, and protect pulmonary connective tissue from NE released from triggered neutrophiles. Neutrophil elastase is serine protease that degrades elastin of the alveolar walls as well other structural proteins of a variety of tissues.

Hereditary alpha-1-antitrypsin deficiency (A1ATD) is associated with retention of mutant A1AT polymers in hepatocytes which leads to decrease of circulating A1AT with less than 15% of normal level in A1ATD homozygotes. Since the integrity of lung alveoli is maintained by proper circulating level of A1AT, severe deficiency of this protein was identified as genetic risk factor for emphysema and COPD. Clinical manifestation of emphysema in patients with A1ATD occurs in 3th decade in smokers and in the 5th decade in non-smokers (Larsson, 1978; Janus et al., 1985) and requires replacement therapy with purified A1AT pooled from donor plasma.

Genetic epidemiologic studies show that A1ATD may affect 1 in about 1,500 individuals in Europe (De Serres, 2002). Approximately 3.4 million individuals of all racial subgroups are affected by A1ATD worldwide (De Serres, 2002).

Liver disease in early childhood is second clinically significant consequence resulting from retention of mutant A1AT polymers in hepatocytes (Eriksson, 1986; Sveger, 1976). Clinically it is presents as neonatal cholestasis which may progress to juvenile chirosis or slowly progress to the liver disease in adults (Mahadeva and Lomas, 1998).

In the early sixties of the last century, Laurell and Eriksson discovered that the absence of the electrophoretic α_1-globulin pattern of serum is associated with A1AT deficiency (Laurell and Eriksson, 1963). At the same time was discovered an association between A1ATD and emphysema in relatively young patients in fourth decade of life (Eriksson, 1964; Lieberman,

1969). These observations suggested a significant role of A1ATD in pathogenesis of emphysema. The proteinase-antiproteinase hypothesis, established by Janoff (Janoff, 1985) still remains central in our understanding of the pathogenesis of lung disease. According to this hypothesis, emphysema in A1ATD arises from an imbalance of neutrophil elastase and A1AT as antielastase, which leads to inappropriate antielastase defense and the relatively excessive activity of neutrophil elastase and consequent degradation of elastin and other extracellular matrix components of the lower respiratory tract.

However, only 1% of patients with COPD are A1ATD (Lieberman, et al., 1986), indicating that A1ATD alone is not sufficient to induce emphysema (Silverman, et al., 1989). The additional factor which may induce emphysema in A1ATD is inflammation, when elastin repair mechanisms are overwhelmed by a massive attack of elastase from triggered neutrophils and cigarette smoke. Studies of the genetic and environmental factors have shown a difference in the reduction of pulmonary function in A1ATD, indicating that additional genetic factors (modifier genes) may influence the pulmonary function in A1ATD subjects (Silverman et al., 1990). Also, the single-nucleotide polymorphisms (SNPs) were identified in the six haplotypes of the SERPINA1 gene, which controls synthesis of A1AT (Chappell, et al., 2006). Several environmental factors that accelerate the onset of symptoms in A1ATD patients, such as personal and second hand exposure to tobacco smoke in childhood, respiratory infections (Mayer et al., 2006), and higher exposures to ozone (Wood et al., 2009) have been also identified.

In addition to the low circulating levels of A1AT in hereditary A1ATD, the risk of emphysema includes reduced antielastase activity. Functional inactivation of A1AT by oxidants present in cigarette smoke could impair antielastase defence in lower respiratory tract, and represent acquired A1AT inactivation. Furthermore, in hereditary A1ATD smoking could impair the function of A1AT both quantitatively and qualitatively.

2. Alpha-1-antitrypsin

Alpha-1-antitrypsine (A1AT) is the archetype of the serpin family of proteins. SERPINs (SER*ine* P*roteinase* IN*hibitors*) are the superfamily of structurally related proteins that control many physiological processes. A1AT is a highly polymorphic, acute-phase glycoprotein, synthesised in hepatocytes (Koj et al., 1978) and subsequently secreted into the plasma. Hepatic synthesis of this acute phase protein by SERPINA1 gene is under control of different cytokines, such as interleukin-1 (IL-1), tumour necrosis factors α (TNFα) and most effectively the interleukin-6 family of cytokines (interleukin-6, leukaemia inhibitory factor, oncostatin M) (Richards and Gauldie, 1991). Besides liver, the small quantities of A1AT are produced by alveolar macrophages, circulating monocytes and intestinal, renal and lung-derived epithelial cells (Mornex et al., 1986; Carlson et al., 1988; Molmenti et al., 1993; Cichy et al., 1997; Mulgrew et al., 2004). Extra hepatic synthesis of A1AT is important in preventing tissue damage in the site of inflammation or injury. For instance, synthesis of A1AT in monocytes is up-regulated by inflammatory mediators such as IL-1 and TNFα in lung tissue (Knoell et al., 1998). Serum level of A1AT is elevated in inflammation, trauma, and pregnancy.

Healthy individuals produce 34 mg of A1AT per kilogram of body weight per day (Jones, 1978). Normal reference interval for antigenic concentration of serum A1AT measured by nephelometry is 15-40 μM (0.83-2.20 g/L) (ATS/ERS Statement, 2003). The threshold level of 11 μM (0.59 g/L) provides relevant antielastase protection of lower respiratory tract (WHO Meeting, 1996.). As a relatively small protein (52 kD), the mature A1AT is capable to diffuse into many organs. The concentration of A1AT in organs is lower than in plasma. Thus,

Olsen et al. (Olsen et al., 1975) reported that A1AT level in a bronchoalveolar lavage fluid of non-smokers is 7% of serum level, with a higher value (11%) in smokers. Also, total amount of A1AT in the lavage fluid of smokers was significantly greater than in non-smokers. The same authors reported about five times higher A1AT concentration in pulmonary alveolar macrophages in smokers in comparison to non-smokers. All these results suggest an increased A1AT concentration in the air spaces of the cigarette smokers.

2.1 Structure and function of alpha-1-antitrypsin

The mature A1AT protein is a single chain composed of 394 amino acids. The main characteristics of the protein are: Met^{358} residue at the active site, isoelectric point ranging from 4.4 to 4.6, and a total molecular weight of 52 kDa. Crystalographic analysis of the mature protein reveals that A1AT is a globular protein with tree N asparigynil-linked carbohydrate side chains on the external surface of the one end of the molecule (Loebermann et al., 1984). The side chains are composed of N-acetylglukosamine, mannose, galactose and sialic acid and they are N-linked to amino acids Asn^{46}, Asn^{83} and Asn^{247}. These carbohidrate side chains are on the outside surface of one-half of the elongated structure. The difference in carbohydrate side chains at position of Asn^{83} is responsible for the two major bands of A1AT when serum focused at pH 4-4.9 on thin-layer polyacrilamide gel. The internal structure of A1AT is highly ordered with 30 percent α-helices and 40 percent β-pleated sheets. There are nine α-helices (A$\rightarrow$I) and three β-sheets (A$\rightarrow$I).
Similar to other inhibitory serpins, A1AT is „suicide" or „single use" inhibitor that employs a unique and extensive conformational change in the process of inhibition of target proteases (Figure 1.). The hallmark of serpins is the reactive centre loop (RCL) that presents the key P1-P'1 methionine–serine bond as a pseudosubstrate for the cognate proteinase, neutrophil elastase (Johnson and Travis, 1978). The reactive centre loop of A1AT is highly stressed external loop protruding from the molecule with Met^{358}-Ser^{359} in the active center. Inhibitory process begins by docking of the serpin and the protease, and formation of Michaelis complex. Like the other inhibitory serpins, the structure of the RCL is crucial for the ability of the inhibitor to undergo a „stressed to relaxed" (S$\rightarrow$R) conformational change. The active A1AT is in metastable or „stressed form", which is essential for inhibition of proteases. During the process of inhibition, A1AT is like mousetrap with spring-like shift from a metastable to a hyperstable state (Hunington et al., 2000; Carrell and Lomas, 2002). After the formation of Michaelis complex there are two possible different ending of the reaction. One is inactivation of protease, where serpin has undergone the S $\rightarrow$ R transition, and the protease hangs distorted at the base of the molecule. The other possibility is A1AT substrate-like behavior, where RCL forms the fourth β sheet, providing the opportunity for the protease to escape the conformational trap, leaving active protease and inactive cleaved serpin. Thus, *in vivo*, A1AT can exist in: native inhibitory conformation with an exposed RCL, latent conformation with a partially inserted RCL and non-inhibitory conformation.
Non-inhibitory conformation of A1AT occurs in certain circumstances: when A1AT is in complex with neutrophil elastase, when the reactive center loop of A1AT is cleaved by non-target proteinases, when reactive oxygen species oxidized A1AT, and when A1ATD variants form polymers.
Moreover, A1AT non-inhibitory conformations show other biological effects. For instance, oxidized A1AT and the cleaved peptide fragment of A1AT stimulate monocyte activation, and A1AT-elastase complexes and polymeric A1AT are chemotactic for neutrophils (Banda et al., 1988; Dabbagh et al., 2001; Moraga and Janciauskiene, 2000; Moraga et al., 2001).

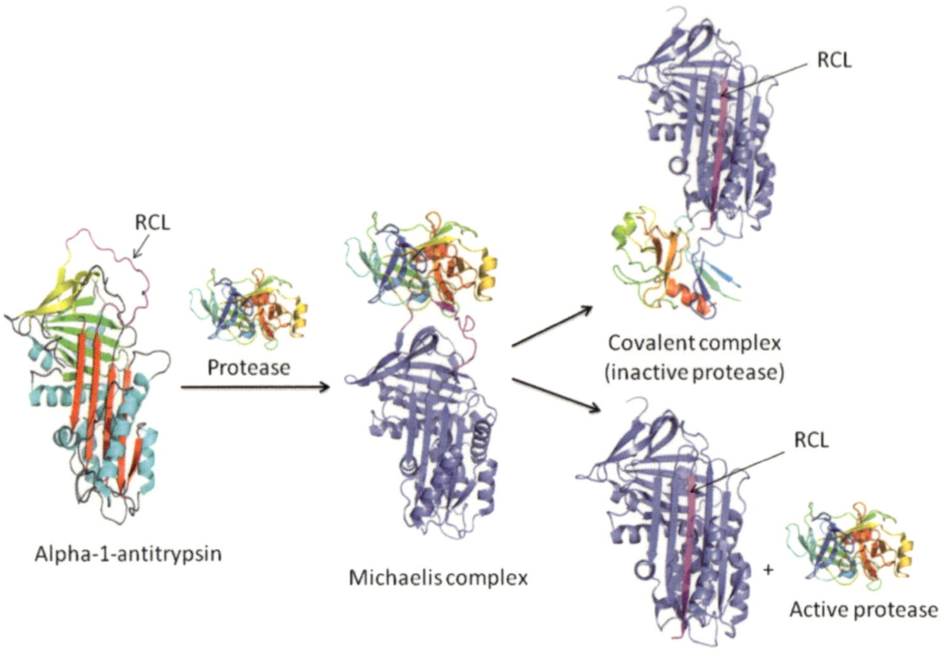

Fig. 1. Structure of alpha-1antitrypsin and reaction with target protease (modified from Law, et al., 2006)

2.2 Physiological roles of alpha-1-antitrypsin

The main physiological role of A1AT is protection of lower respiratory tract by inhibiting proteases released from triggered neutrophiles including neutrophil elastase, cathepsin G, and proteinase-3 (Carrell, 1986). The target proteases of A1AT derive from azurophilic granules of polymorphonuclear neutrophils which participate in lysosomal bacterial digestion and neutrophil migration through the extracellular matrix at the sites of inflammation. This protective role of A1AT occurs primarily extracellular. A1AT enters the lung from the circulation by passive diffusion (Stockley, 1984). Besides direct inhibition of NE, there are evidences that A1AT exhibits anti-inflammatory properties to suppress cigarette smoke induced production of tumor necrosis factor α (TNFα) and matrix metalloproteinase 12 (MMP12) by alveolar macrophages, and subsequent inflammatory cell infiltration (Churg et al., 2007). Furthermore, studies have shown that native A1AT modulates function of immune cells, such as neutrophils (Bergin et al., 2010), monocytes (Janciauskiene et al., 2007), and T cells (Lu et al., 2006). *Ex vivo* and *in vitro* experiments have shown that endogenous A1AT in blood contributes to the suppression of proinflammatory cytokine synthesis (Pott et al., 2009). Thus, A1AT is an endogenous inhibitor of proinflammatory cytokine production in whole blood, and may participate in innate immune response to an inflammation-inducing stimulus. The recently discovered role of A1AT in prevention of emphysema is the inhibition of lung endothelial cell apoptosis due to inactivation of intracellular caspase-3 (Petrache et al., 2006a; Petrache et al., 2006b). Antiapoptotic role of A1AT in the lung *in vivo* and *in vitro* in micro vascular endothelial cells is associated with intracellular presence of A1AT. Lung endothelial cells don't produce

A1AT and they take it. Sohrab et al. (Sohrab et al., 2009) showed that clathrin-mediated endocytosis predominantly regulates A1AT intracellular function in the lung endothelium, and might represent an important determinant of the serpin's protection against development of cigarette smoke-induced emphysema. The uptake is severely affected by exposure to cigarette smoke extract *in vitro* and *in vivo*, probably directly influencing clathrin-mediated endocytosis. Furthermore, polymers of A1AT exhibit a marked decrease in lung endothelial cell uptake. Inhibition of A1AT uptake by cigarette smoke may further weaken the A1AT protective role in the lung.

In the last decade other physiological roles of A1AT have been discovered, such as roles in atherogenesis (Talmud et al., 2003), angiogenesis (Huang et al., 2004), fibroblast proliferation, and procollagen synthesis (Dabbagh et al., 2001).

2.3 Genetics of alpha-1-antitrypsin

The alpha-1-antitrypsin is encoded by SERPINA1 gene (serpin peptidase inhibitor, clade A) located in proteinase inhibitor (Pi) locus on the long arm of chromosome 14q32.1 (Schroeder et al., 1985; Billingsley et al., 1993). The Pi locus is 12.2 kb long and consists of 4 coding exons, 3 non-coding exons and 6 introns (Figure 2.). At the 5′ region of the SERPINA1 gene there are three non-protein coding exons (I_A, I_B, I_C) which control gene transcription. Exons referred as exons II-V are coding and containing the sequence information that defines the protein itself. The start codon (ATG) for translational of the mRNA and the signal peptide are in exon II, and the stop codon (TAA) is in exon V, followed by the polyadenilatyon signal (ATTAA). The carbohydrate attachmnent site (Asn^{46}, Asn^{83}, Asn^{247}) are coded for in exon II and III. The region coding for the reactive loop with the active inhibitory centre Met^{358} is within exon V.

Following transcription, A1AT mRNA is translated on ribosome bound to the the rough endoplasmatic reticulum, producing a preprotein of 418 amino acids. The signal peptide of 24 residues is removed during secretion into the cisterne of the rough endoplasmatic reticulum where the protein is glycosylated with high-mannose type carbohydrates, and folds into appropriate globular tree-dimensional configuration. Complete protein maturation is accomplished within the Golgi apparatus and protein is secreted.

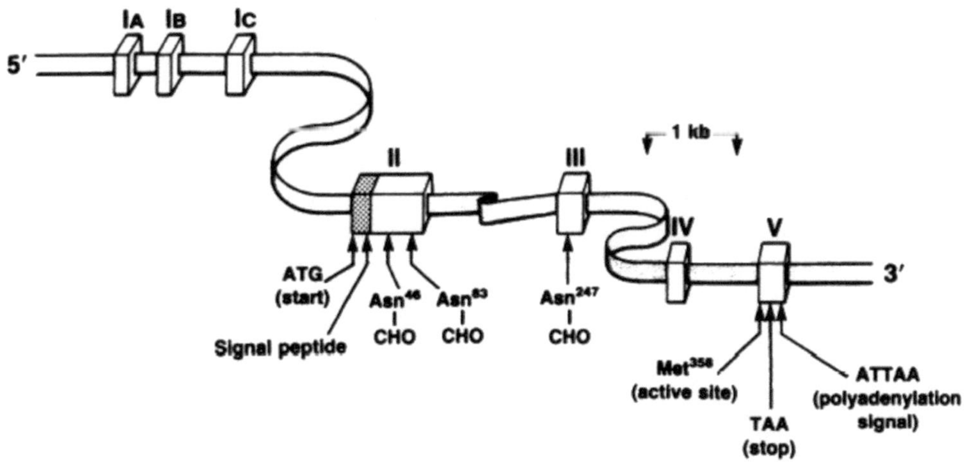

Fig. 2. Structure of the SERPINA1 gene (Crystal et al., 1989)

Hepatocytes and monocytes have two different promotors (Perlino et al., 1987) that operate via different mechanisms. The SERPINA1 gene in macrophages is transcribed from a macrophags-specific promoter located about 2,000 bp upstream of the hepatocyte-specific promoter. Transcription from the two SERPINA1 promoters is mutually exclusive; the macrophage promoter is silent in hepatocytes, and the hepatocyte promoter is silent in macrophages. In macrophages, two distinct mRNAs are generated by alternative splicing. In addition, Hafeez et al. (Hafeez et al., 1992) demonstrated that the SERPINA1 gene has 3 monocyte-specific transcriptional initiation sites upstream from a single hepatocyte-specific transcriptional initiation site. Macrophages use these sites during basal and modulated expression. Hepatoma cells use the hepatocyte-specific transcriptional initiation site during basal and modulated expression, but also switch to transcription from the upstream macrophage transcriptional initiation sites during modulation by the acute phase mediator interleukin-6 (IL-6).

2.4 Polymorphism of alpha-1-antitrypsin

The A1AT coding gene SERPINA1 is a highly polimorphic, with more than 125 SNPs reported in public SNP databases (Entrez SNP). Protein variants of A1AT are classified by the Pi (P*rotese* i*nhibitor*) system and each variant is identified by migration on agarose gel electrophoresis. These differences in migration relate to variations in protein charge resulting from amino acid alterations (Fagerhol and Laurell, 1970; Cox, 1978). Isoelectric focusing in the narrow range of pH (4.2-4.9) has enabled identification of more A1AT variants then in agarose gel electrophoresis. The alleles were given symbols according to the relative electrophoretic mobility of the allele product, so anodal variants are marked with the first letters, and cathodal with last letters. All A1AT variants are categorized according to the serum level and functional activity as normal, deficient, null and dysfunctional.

2.4.1 Normal A1AT variants

Normal A1AT variants have normal serum level and functional activity to inhibit neutrophil elastase. More than 95% of normal variants are the „common" M1 (Ala^{213}), M1 (Val^{213}), M2 and M3. Among Caucasians, M1 (Val^{213}) is the most common, and M1 (Ala^{213}), M2 and M3 are less frequent. The „rare" normal variants with frequencies less than 1% are: M4, $B_{alhambra}$, F, $P_{StAlbans}$ and $X_{Chirstchurch}$. Usually, rare variants are named by the birthplace of the oldest individual tested in pedegree. PiM homozygotes and heterozygotes are characterized by normal serum level of A1AT (20-50 μM) and normal functional activity (ATS/ERS Statement, 2003).

2.4.2 Deficient A1AT variants

Deficient variants are associated with lower serum level of A1AT than normal variants. Several mutations associated with A1ATD have been identified, and the most common are Z and S alleles. Rare A1ATD variants are M_{Malton}, $M_{MineralSprings}$, $M_{Nichinan}$, $M_{Procida}$, P_{Lowell}, S_{Iiyama} and others.

Gene-mapping studies have shown that the PiZ allele probably arose in Northern Europe (Cox et al., 1985). Age estimates of A1AT variants based on microsatellite variation, suggest that the Z deficiency allele appeared 107 to 135 generations ago and could have been spread in neolithic times. Frequency of the Z allele shows a large variation in Caucasians, but is rare or absent in Asians and Africans (De Croo et al., 1991; Hutchison, 1998.).

The PiS deficiency allele has an older 279-generation to 470-generation age and from its high incidence on the Iberia peninsula it has been suggested that it could have originated in this region (Seixas et al., 2001).

2.4.2.1 Z variant

The Z variant represents a „classic" A1ATD variant and derives from M1 (Ala^{213}) following a point mutation which is the same for the all Z individuals who are probably descendants of a single ancestral progenitor. The result of mutation is the substitution of a *GAG* that codes for Glu^{342} with an *AAG* that code for Lys^{342} (Nukiwa et al., 1987). The Z mutation perturbs the folding (Yu et al., 1995.) and structure of the protein (Lomas et al., 1993a). It distorts the relationship between the reactive centre loop and β-sheet A, and the consequent perturbation in structure allows opening of β-sheet A to favor partial loop insertion and formation of an unstable intermediate (M*) (Figure 3.). Then the patent β-sheet A accepts the loop of another A1AT molecule to form a dimer (D) which then extends to form chains of loop-sheet polymer (P) (Lomas, et al., 1992; Elliott et al., 1996a; Lomas, 2000).

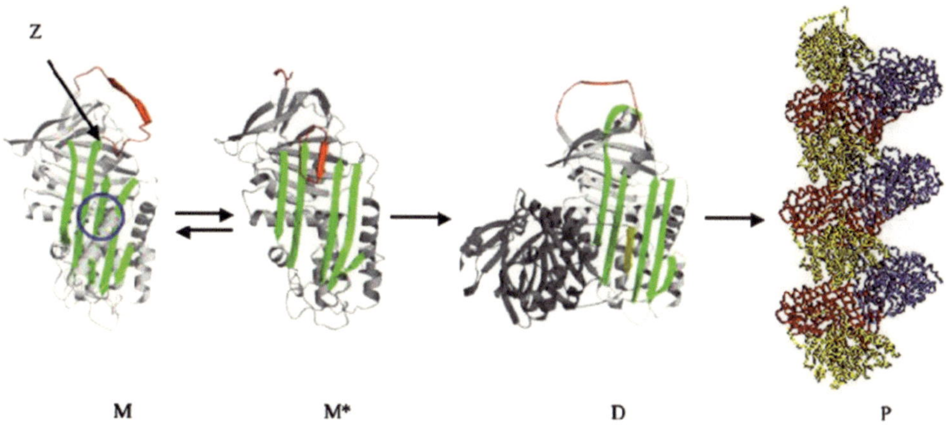

Fig. 3. Formation of Z polymers (Lomas, 2005)

Process of polymerization depends on concentration and temperature. Abnormality in posttranslational modification of protein causes accumulation of the A1AT polymers in the cisterna of the rough endoplsmatic reticulum with a drastic reduction in secretion rates. The abnormal protein accumulates in hepatocytes and forms inclusion bodies (aggregates) that are positive to diastase-resistant periodic acid Schiff (PAS-D) staining and visible on microscopy. The retained A1AT polymers are cytotoxic for hepatocytes and can cause a diverse liver damages, ranging from neonatal hepatitis to juvenile cirrhosis, and hepatocellular carcinoma in adults (Eriksson, et al., 1986). As a consequence of polymer accumulation, hepatocytes of PiZZ homozygote secrete only 10–15 % of normal quantity. PiMZ heterozygotes have about 50 % of normal A1AT circulating level.

Besides low circulation level, the Z protein also less efficiently inhibits elastase (Ogushi, et al., 1987). Consequently, in PiZZ individuals, quantitative and qualitative defects of A1AT lead to early-onset COPD including emphysema and chronic bronchitis.

A similar form of loop-sheet polymers *in vivo* with hepatic inclusions and plasma deficiency was found in two other variants, M_{Malton} (Phe^{52} deleted) (Lomas et al., 1995) and S_{Iiyama} (Ser^{53}→Phe) (Lomas et al., 1993b.), that are common in Sardinia and Japan, respectively.

A1AT polymers were also detected in bronchoalveolar lavage fluid (BALF) from PiZ homozygotes with emphysema. This conformational transition may further reduce the levels of functional proteinase inhibitor in the lungs, and consequently exacerbate lung tissue damage (Elliott et al., 1998).

Studies of Parmar et al. (Parmar et al., 2002) and Mulgrew et al. (Mulgrew et al., 2004) showed that Z A1AT locally produced on the epithelial surface of the lung polymerizes and A1AT polymers demonstrate proapoptotic and proinflammatory effects. These studies also revealed that unlike M A1AT protein, Z A1AT protein polymerized at body temperature, and in addition of being an ineffective antiprotease inhibitor, might become a strong neutrophil chemoattractant, thus representing an ongoing source of inflammation in the lungs of individuals with A1ATD. Thus, polymerization of locally produced ZA1AT is a contributory factor to the lung inflammation experienced by those with A1AT deficiency and that standard antiprotease therapies may not address this problem. Other studies reported that even PiZZ patients with near-normal lung function had high concentrations of neutrophils on respiratory epithelial surfaces (Rouhani et al., 2000). Neutrophil burden in PiZZ and in PiMZ (on a lesser extent) is attributed to leukotriene B4 or IL-8 released from neutrophils or epithelial cells (Woolhouse et al., 2002; Malerba et al., 2006). Neutrophil accumulation in the lung of PiZZ deficient individuals is multifactorial and chemoattraction due to polymerized Z protein represents another potential cause of neutrophil dominated inflammation. These findings suggest a novel mechanism in pathogenesis of emphysema associated with Z antitrypsin deficiency.

Lomas (Lomas, 2006) highlighted a possible role of Z mutant in systemic response to infection. In the case of invasion of pathogens, organism initiates a systemic inflammatory response that results in increased secretion of Z A1AT as acute phase protein, by hepatocytes. Factors such as: elevation of body temperature, increased concentration of mutant Z A1AT, and lower pH at the site of bacterial invasion of lung (Stockley and Burnett, 1979) favor polymerization of mutant Z A1AT. Polymers possess chemotactic properties, which in turn amplify inflammatory response and enhance the recruitment of neutrophils. Excessive burden of neutrophils may cause increase of proinflamatory and proxidative factors.

Therefore, a rational approach in therapy of A1ATD would be to inhibit the polymerization of the Z protein (intracellularly and extracellularly), accompanied by standard augmentation therapy. It is clear that in addition to increased level of A1AT above a putative therapeutic threshold, it is necessary to increase the secretion of active non-polymerized form of Z protein. This approach could potentially ameliorate the liver disease, and defend respiratory epithelial surface, providing antielastase protection and avoiding the proinflammatory effects of polymerized Z A1AT.

Currently, there is some progress in development of synthetic peptide designed to selectively inhibit Z polymerisation (Mahadeva et al., 2002; Parfrey et al., 2004; Chang et al., 2006; Mallya et al., 2007; Chang et al., 2009).

2.4.2.2 S variant

In contrast to the Z allele, S causes only mild plasma deficiency. The genetic sequence of the S variant derives from M1 (Val^{213}) as a result of a mutation which cause substitution of *GAA* that codes for Glu^{264} with an *GTA* that codes for Val^{264} (Owen et al., 1976; Yoshida et al., 1977).

The single mutation of the S variant leads to spontaneous polymer formation, but slower than the Z variant, without affecting the ability to inhibit neutrophil elastase (Elliott, et al.,

1996b; Mahadeva et al., 1999; Dafforn et al., 1999). The slower polymerization causes less retention of S variant in the liver, and hence the plasma levels are 60% of the normal M allele. Thus, carriers of S allele (PiSS, PiSZ and PiMS) have levels of 52%, 32% and 75% of normal level, respectively. Furthermore, Z A1AT forms heteropolymers with S A1AT (Mahadeva et al., 1999), which explains cases of hepatic cirrhosis in PiSZ patients (Cruz et al., 1975; Campra et al., 1973; Craig et al., 1975.). Also, PiSZ smokers are at significant risk of the development of COPD, while in nonsmoking individuals the PiSZ phenotype may confer little or no risk to develop COPD (Turino et al., 1996).

2.4.2.3 Null A1AT variants

Null variants are characterized by the modification of an important part of the gene with no detectable mRNA. Although extremely rare, they have been found in all populations. Frequencies of null variants among Caucasians are estimated to be less than 0.1%. Null-allelic variants are denoted as Q0 rather than Pi. The Null mutations do not result in secreted protein or the formation of polymers. Subjects with Null mutations show significantly lower lung function values than PiSZ and PiZZ individuals, and they are at particularly high risk to develop emphysema (Cox and Levison, 1988; Fregonese et al., 2008). Early detection of Null carriers is important for preventive and therapeutic interventions.

The $PiNull_{Bellingham}$ differs from the normal M1 (Val^{213}) gene by the mutation in exon II, where the codon for Lys^{217} (*A*AG) is altered to Stop codon (*T*AG) (Satoh et al., 1988). Homozygotes for $PiNull_{Bellingham}$ have complete absence of A1AT, and develop premature emphysema much earlier than more common PiZZ individuals (Cook et al., 1994). The $Null_{isola\ di\ procida}$ is caused by complete deletion of exons II-V of SERPINA1 gene (Takahashi and Crystal, 1990). The $Null_{granite\ falls}$ allele derives from the M1 (Ala^{213}) by the deletion of a single base in exon II in the codon for Tyr^{160} (TA*C*) with deletion of the *C*. Consequently, there is 5' frame shift of the downstream nucleotides, moving the G form the next codon, Val^{161} *G*TC in place of the normal Tyr^{160} (Holmes et al., 1989).

The $Null_{mattawa}$ allele is a consequence of the insertion of a single nucleotide within the coding region of exon V, causing a 3' frameshift with generation of a premature stop signal (Curiel et al., 1989).

Prins et al. (Prins et al., 2008) performed genotyping by direct sequencing of the SERPINA1 gene coding region in patients with A1AT concentrations ≤1.0 g/L, and this approach allowed them to discover $Q0_{soest}$ and $Q0_{amersfoort}$ null alleles.

2.4.2.4 Dysfunctional variants

Dysfunctional A1AT variants are synthesized in normal quantities, but have altered protein function. The PiPittsburgh allele is a mutation which occurs at the A1AT active site, and represents an example of a mutation responsible for altered function of the gene product. A1AT becomes a potent inhibitor of thrombin and factor XI rather than of elastase, which results in a bleeding disorder (Lewis et al., 1978; Owen et al., 1983).

3. Hereditary alpha-1-antitrypsin deficiency and emphysema

The risk of developing early-onset emphysema caused by hereditary A1ATD is inversely correlated with the serum A1AT level (ATS/ERS Statement, 2003). Only PiZ homozygotes with severe decreased A1AT serum level, or carriers of M-like or Null alleles are at significant risk to develop panlobular emphysema with typical dilatation or destruction of all lower lobules. However, the risk of COPD in PiMZ individuals is still controversial. Heterozygous, PiMZ individuals have moderately reduced serum levels A1AT, but whether they have increased risk of COPD is uncertain. Tarjan et al. (Tarjan et al., 1994) in longitudinal lung function study in heterozygous PiMZ subjects observed a decrease in elasticity and deterioration lung function parameters in comparison to those without A1ATD, which supports the concept of PiMZ phenotype being a risk factor for pulmonary emphysema development at a younger age. Dahl et al. (Dahl et al., 2002) found that PiMZ heterozygotes had a slightly greater rate of decrease in FEV_1. Meta analysis by Hersh et al. (Hersh et al., 2004) has shown an increased odd of COPD in PiMZ individuals with suggestion that variability in study design and quality limits interpretation. Recent study (Sørheim et al., 2010) suggests that PiMZ individuals may be slightly more susceptible to the development of the airflow obstruction than PiMM individuals.

3.1 Epidemiology of A1ATD

The majority of the data regarding frequency and geographical distribution of severe A1ATD genotypes refer to the most frequent deficient variants PiZZ and PiSZ. Considering that severe A1ATD predisposes the development of emphysema that requires expensive diagnostic methods and treatment, it would be very useful to determine prevalence of severe A1ATD in every population.

The most comprehensive study that has been performed on 200,000 Swedish newborns revealed the prevalence rate of PiZZ phenotype of approximately 1 in 1,600 newborns (Sveger, 1976). Despite the lack of reliable epidemiological studies and marked differences between countries, Blanco et al. (Blanco et al., 2006) estimated numbers of individuals carrying two most common deficiency alleles, Z and S in Europe. Highest prevalence of the PiZZ phenotype is in the Scandinavian Peninsula, Latvia and Denmark and progressively decreases towards the South and the East of Europe. While the highest prevalence of the PiSZ is in the Iberian Peninsula and it gradually decreases towards the North, South and East of the continent. Prevalence of the moderate PiMZ is highest in the South of the Scandinavian Peninsula, Baltic Republics, Denmark and the UK, and progressively decreases towards the East, South and North of the continent. The estimated prevalence of PiZZ, PiSZ and PiMZ in European adults was 1/4727, 1/1051 and 1/36 respectively, with large variation in different countries. In this regard, it was estimated that there are 124,594 PiZZ, 560,515 PiSZ, and even 16 million PiMZ individuals in all Europe. Globally, A1ATD affects all major racial subgroups, and there are at least 116 million carriers (PiMZ and PiMS) and 3.4 million deficiency allele's combinations (PiSS, PiSZ and PiZZ) worldwide (De Serres, 2002). According to these data, frequency of the Z allele is lowest in Far East Asia (0.04%), and highest in Northern Europe (1.53%), while the S allele is lowest in Far East Asia (0.07%), and highest in Southern Europe (5.64%).

Although the epidemiological data indicate a large of number of A1ATD individuals worldwide, this condition is largely undiagnosed and exact prevalence of A1ATD in most population remains unknown. Owing to data from international registry of A1ATD, established in several countries, it was estimated that only 0.35% of severe A1ATD (PiZZ and PiSZ) are actually recognized (Luisetti and Seersholm, 2004). One of the reasons may be significantly delayed onset of symptoms. In 1994 Stoller at al. (Stoller et al., 1994) reported a mean interval of 7.2 years between initial symptom and first diagnosis. A decade later, a decrement in the overall diagnostics of 5.6 years was noted (Stoller et al., 2005a), which was attributed to the better education of physicians about recognising A1ATD. Authors concluded that despite this decrement in the overall diagnostics, underrecognition of individuals with A1ATD persisted. Under-recognition of A1ATD may be a part of a larger phenomenon of under-recognition of individuals with COPD. The second reason could be a low penetrance of the PiZ gene, so that the relationship between genotype and clinical phenotype is not strong.

There are many benefits of early detection of A1ATD, such as avoidance of exposures to cigarette smoke and air pollution in prevention of pulmonary emphysema. Also, measure of prevention is protection from pneumonia, which is frequently reported in medical history of A1ATD patients with emphysema (McElvaney et al., 1997). In A1ATD patients, pulmonary infection further increases the risk of developing emphysema. Pulmonary infection favors increasing of elastase activity with subsequent destruction of lung due to compromised antiprotease defenses, and promotion of A1AT polymers due to elevated body temperature in inflammation. In this regard, it is very important to protect lung function of A1ATD individuals trough aggressive treatment of pulmonary infections and by vaccination with pneumococcal and influenza A vaccines.

Data concerning genetic epidemiology of the rare A1ATD variants are incomplete, and therefore raise a suspicion that the prevalence of these variants might be higher than 2-4%, as previously considered, due to misclassification as Z variant (Luisetti and Seersholm, 2004). Phenotyping by isoelectric focusing is often used to characterize α_1AT deficiency, but this method may lead to misdiagnosis (e.g., by missing null alleles). Zorzetto et al. (Zorzetto et al., 2008) sequenced exons II, III, IV, and V of subjects whose are negative for Z and S alleles, and detected even 7% rare A1ATD alleles. Moreover, Prins et al. (Prins et al., 2008) have analyzed patients with A1ATD by sequencing of exons II, III, and V of the SERPINE1 gene and reported that up to 22% of deficiency variants were missed by conventional diagnostic methods.

3.2 Emphysema caused by A1ATD

The main lung manifestations of severe A1ATD are emphysema and COPD (ATS/ERS Statement, 2003). In A1ATD-smokers, the first symptoms usually occur between 32 and 41 years, with considerable variability in the time of onset of symptoms (Larsson, 1978; Tobin et al., 1983).

Panlobular emphysema is dominant clinical manifestation in A1ATD patients, and affects the lower half of the lungs. Pulmonary vessels of the emphysematous lung appear fewer and smaller than normal (Stein et al., 1971). In severe A1ATD changes at the level of bronchioli such as bronchiolitis obliterans, bronchiolectasia, acute and chronic bronchiolitis and bronchiolitis with organizing pneumonia are more frequent than in emphysema without A1ATD (Theegarten et al., 1998).

First representative study that included 124 patients with A1ATD and symptomatic emphysema (Brantly et al., 1988) showed predominance of male gender, ex-smoke status, levels of A1AT $\leq$ 5.5 μM (0.3 g/L), and abnormalities in a lower zone distribution. About one third of patients had pulmonary hypertension. The lung function tests were typical for emphysema: the FEV_1 and DL_{CO} were dramatically reduced, and their annual rate of decline was greater than in general population. The cumulative probability of survival of the patients indicated a significantly shortened lifespan with a mean survival of 16% at 60 yr of age compared with 85% for normal persons.

The largest study ever conducted has been included 1,129 patients who participated in the National Heart, Lung, and Blood Institute (NHLBI) Registry of Individuals with Severe Deficiency of A1AT (McElvaney et al., 1997). Most frequent were PiZZ (97%), and very few PiSZ (1%), and rare variants (2%). Pulmonary function test results were consistent with emphysema. The pulmonary function impairment was moderate to severe, frequently associated with a bronchodilator response, but generally with preservation of the $PaCO_2$ until the development of severe airway obstruction. Medical history of lung function revealed that initial diagnoses included asthma (in 35% of participants), respiratory tract allergies (28%), pneumonia (43%), and chronic bronchitis (36%). The most frequent symptoms in A1ATD patients were dyspnea on exertion (in 84% of participants), self-reported wheezing during respiratory tract infections (76%), and wheezing independent of infections (65%), usual cough (45%), and „annual" cough in phlegm episodes (52%). Significant number of patients who initially diagnosed as asthma had symptoms that suggest airway hyper-responsiveness such as cough and wheezing, responded to aerosol bronchodilator moderately (Eden et al., 1997). It is interesting that a subgroup of individuals in the Registry with relatively normal lung function was younger, more likely to have never smoked and more likely to have come to medical attention owing to a family history of A1ATD.

Cigarette smoking is associated with more accelerated decline of lung function and early development of emphysema in PiZZ individuals leading to a considerably reduced life expectancy (Larsson, 1978). A mortality study showed that emphysema was a major determinant of mortality in population of severe A1ATD patients (Stoller et al., 2005b). Negative impact of smoking on survival of A1ATD patients was demonstrated in two recently published studies. Tanassh et al. (Tanash et al., 2008) reported that PiZZ individuals who have never smoked and have been identified trough screening do not have an increased mortality risk in comparison to general Swedish population. Larger study which included 1,349 PiZZ individuals selected from the Swedish National AATD Registry showed that smokers with severe A1ATD had a significantly higher mortality risk than the general Swedish population (Tanash et al., 2010). The pulmonary emphysema has been more common in PiZZ smokers (78%) than in PiZZ never smokers (47%), and respiratory diseases have been main cause of death among PiZZ smokers (58%).

3.3 Laboratory diagnosis of hereditary A1ATD

Although being one of the most prevalent and potentially severe hereditary disorders, A1ATD still remains under-recognized. Affected individuals often visit several physicians before obtaining the correct diagnosis. The main reason is generally low knowledge about A1ATD among internists and respiratory therapists (Taliercio et al., 2010). Clinically relevant A1ATD is often caused by homozygous inheritance of the Z allele, but A1ATD can also be due to the combination of other rare deficient or null alleles at the Pi locus. Even moderate A1ATD in PiMZ heterozygote is associated with reduced pulmonary functions in individuals with clinically established COPD (Dahl et al., 2001).

The guidelines of the American Thoracic Society and the European Respiratory Society (ATS/ERS Statement, 2003) recommend quantitative and qualitative laboratory testing for A1ATD for all patients with COPD, asthma, unexplained liver disease, and necrotizing panniculitis, as well as for asymptomatic subjects with persistent airflow limitation and siblings of A1ATD individuals. Laboratory testing of suspected A1ATD individuals involve

analysis of A1AT concentrations in serum and identification of specific alleles by genotyping or phenotyping. Therefore it is important to identify appropriate cutoff that balances costs of testing identification of deficiency alleles in the general population.
Diagnostic algorithms for laboratory testing of the A1AT deficiency that were proposed (Snyder et al., 2006; Bornhorst et al., 2007; Miravitlles et al., 2010) should lead to improve diagnostics of A1ATD (Figure 4.). Initial testing involves quantification of A1AT concentrations and genotyping. Quantification of A1AT alone is not sufficient to diagnose genetic causes of A1ATD due to secondary causes of reduced concentration of A1AT in severe liver diseases, protein-losing enteropathies or nephrotic syndrome which may cause a general decrease of serum proteins. If serum level of A1AT lay in the expected range for the certain genotype, than the results and interpretation should be reported to physician. Qualitative analyses of A1ATD include two complementary methods, genotyping and phenotyping, each with advantages and disadvantages. Using conventional phenotyping of the A1AT by isoelectic focusing (IEF) necessarily leads to misdiagnoses of the null alleles (Klaassen et al., 2001). Therefore, the replacement of IEF with direct sequencing of the relevant parts of the SERPINA1 gene enables an efficient and reliable approach to reveal A1ATD patient. Direct sequencing of exons II, III and V of the SERPINA1 gene is the preferred method in initial phase of diagnostic algorithm for laboratory testing of A1ATD (Prins et al., 2008), as it allows detection of disease-associated A1AT allele combinations, including null alleles.
However if quantitative result are in discrepancy with obtained genotype, laboratory should perform phenotype assay. Determination of phenotypes serve as complementary to the genetic assay, in order to clarify cases that cannot be detected by genotyping. Besides phenotyping, other techniques that can be considered as complementary include whole-gene sequencing and the addition of other alleles to the melting curve genotype assay (Rodriguez et al., 2002).
There are two approaches to assess the complementarity between serum level of A1AT and genotype result. Previously, the estimate was based on established threshold of A1AT serum levels for the most frequent A1AT phenotypes/genotypes in the general population. The various ranges for A1AT serum level of the most common phenotypes, which can be found in the literature, are results of different methods of quantification, different commercially available standards of A1AT, and samples size. (Brantly et al., 1991; Lee et al., 2002; ATS/ERS Statement, 2003). Additional difficulty is the estimation of the ranges for rare phenotypes because it is difficult to collect a representative number of samples in a given population.
In the context of these concerns, particular problem is the presence of inflammation in examined population. The A1AT is an acute phase protein and its production and secretion increases with inflammation. Thus, serum levels might be „falsely elevated" and are not reflecting the genotype, especially in moderate A1ATD. This was confirmed in a recent study which found that PiMZ individuals with a higher level of C-reactive protein (CRP, a sensitive marker of inflammation) had higher level of A1AT than those with lower level of CRP (Zorzetto et al., 2008). Also, we should bear in mind that in healthy blood donors only 26% of the variance of circulating A1AT level is explained by known SERPINA1 gene variants (Oakeshott et al., 1985). Recently, large population-based study on the Swiss SAPALDIA cohort (Senn et al., 2008) revealed that female gender, hormone intake, systolic blood pressure, age in men and in postmenopausal women, as well active and passive smoking were positively, whereas alcohol intake and body mass index (BMI) were

inversely correlated with serum A1AT levels, independent of CRP adjustment. The results of this study reflect a complexity of relationship between tobacco exposures, gender, circulating A1AT, systemic inflammatory status and lung function.

Nowadays, the efforts are directed towards determination of the cut-off values with high specificity and sensitivity, in order to separate normal from deficient phenotypes. The value of A1AT serum level of 22 μM (1, 2 g/L) has been determined as a reliable cut-off able to identify A1ATD with a specificity of 73% and a sensitivity of 97% (Corda et al., 2006). The lower value of 18.5 μM (1.00 g/L) was able to detect heterozygous A1ATD (Simsek et al., 2011), while cut-off value of 14.7 μM (0.8 g/L) was proposed for detection of all patients who are at risk of A1ATD (Prins et al., 2008).

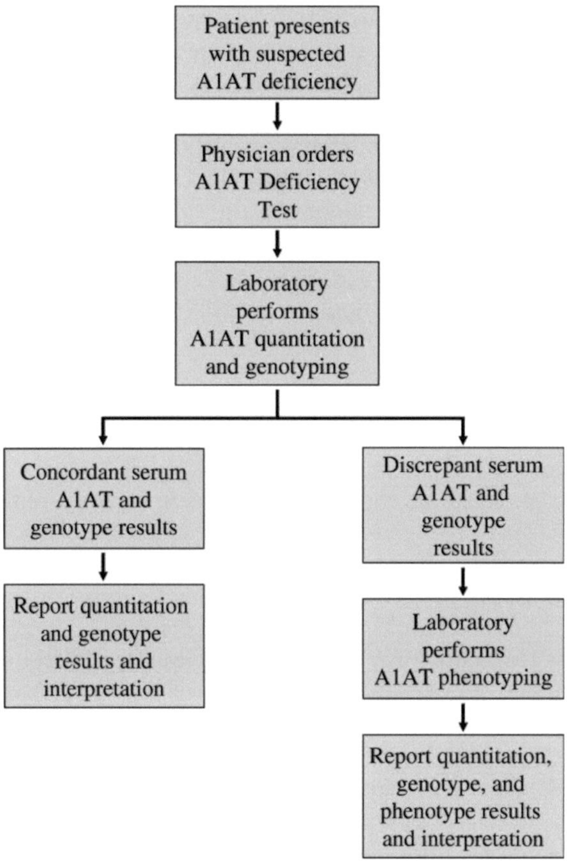

Fig. 4. Alpha-1-antitrypsin deficiency−testing algorithm (Snyder et al., 2006)

4. Oxidation of alpha-1-antitrypsin and emphysema

Cigarette smoke and lung inflammation leads to proteolytic destruction of the lung parenchyma with characteristic loss of alveolar integrity and an enlargement of alveolar space (reviewed in: Sharafkhaneh et al., 2008). Oxidative stress, as a result of an imbalance between oxidants and antioxidants, plays a critical role in the pathogenesis of emphysema (Rahman, 2005; Janoff et al., 1983). There are two main significant sources of oxidants:

exogenous from cigarette smoke or air pollutants and endogenous from activated neutrophils and macrophages.
Oxidative stress caused by cigarette smoke and airway inflammation together form a vicious circle. It has been shown that cigarette smoke-mediated oxidative stress induces the release of proinflammatory cytokine by activation of NF-kappaB and posttranslational modifications of histone deacetylase in macrophages (Yang et al., 2006). Chronic inflammation that persists in emphysema leads to the activation of macrophages and neutrophils (Finkelstein et al., 1995), which are a significant source of reactive oxygen species (ROS). When ROS overwhelm lung antioxidant defenses, the oxidative stress arises. Thus, cigarette smoke and activated macrophages/neutrophils represent considerable source of reactive oxygen species in emphysema.
Cigarette smoke contains free radicals with tremendous oxidative power which serve as direct damaging agents and/or precursor of the other damaging substances. The main free radicals in cigarette smoke are superoxide ($O_2^{-}\bullet$), hydroxyl radical ($\bullet OH$), and hydrogen peroxide (H_2O_2) (Pryor, 1997).
Harmful effects of oxidative stress are numerous: inactivation of antiproteases, disregulation of cell proliferation, induction of apoptosis, modulation the immune system, direct damages of proteins, lipids, and nucleic acids. The products of lipid peroxidation, protein oxidation, and nucleic acid oxidation have been shown in emphysema (Mohsenin, 1991; Sahin et al., 2001; Hackett et al., 2010; Torres-Ramos et al., 2009; Deslee et al., 2009; Deslee et al., 2010).

4.1 Oxidation of A1AT - structural and functional consequences

A1AT is a protein susceptible to oxidation, and its exposure to pro-oxidative enzymes and chemicals results in their oxidation. Exposure of one A1AT molecule to oxidants results in oxidation of Met^{358} and Met^{351} residues to methionine sulfoxide (Johnson and Travis, 1979). Oxidation of both Met^{358} and Met^{351} significantly reduces the ability of A1AT to inhibit neutrophil elastase (Beatty et al., 1980; Taggart et al., 2000). Oxidation of Cys^{232} is far more likely to occur in oxidizing environments comparing with oxidation of exposed and reactive methionine residues (Griffiths et al., 2002). The structural and biological aspects of Cys^{232} oxidation are still unknown.
Methionine residues can be oxidized by cigarette smoke-derived oxidants (Pryor et al., 1984), produced *in vivo* such as peroxide, hydroxyl radicals, chloramines, hypochloride, inducible nitric oxide, and peroxynitrite (Vogt, 1995), or with mineral dust (coal, amosite asbestos, silica, or titanium dioxide) (Li et al., 1997). Thus the oxidation of A1AT by cigarette smoke or free radicals *in vivo* could lead to a functional deficiency of A1AT and has been suggested as a mechanism contributing to the development of emphysema in non-deficient PiM individuals. Cigarette smoke-mediated oxidation of the Z mutant accelerates process of polymerization, which further reduces defense of lung, increases neutrophil influx into the lungs (Alam et al., 2011), and contributes to premature emphysema in PiZZ homozygotes who smoke.
It has been reported that cigarette smoke oxidize A1AT (oxyA1AT), and reduces inhibitory activity of A1AT against elastase (Janoff et al., 1979) and caspase-3 (Petrache et al., 2006a). Substantial constituents of cigarette smoke that oxidise and inactivate A1AT include hydrogen peroxyde, nitrogen dioxide, transition metals, and products of lipid peroxidation initiated by cigarette smoke (reviewed in: Evans and Pryor, 1994). Inactivation of antielastase activity of A1AT is reversible and phenolic antioxidants prevented the suppression of serum elastase-inhibition by cigarette smoke (Carp and Janoff, 1978).

Another mechanism of A1AT oxidation is its oxidative inactivation in the microenvironment of inflammatory cells, at sites of acute or chronic inflammation. The lower airways of smokers are infiltrated with phagocitic cells. Induced neutrophils and alveolar macrophage release a spectrum of oxidants and pro-oxidative enzymes that may inactivate A1AT in their local environment. Increased release of proteases from triggered phagocytes and reduced antiprotease defense leads to damage of lung tissue (Carp and Janoff, 1980). Myeloperoxidase-dependent production of oxidants from neutrophils is increased in inflammation, and can cause significant damage of A1AT. Myeloperoxidase (MPO) is located in the azurophilic granules of the neutrophils, and plays an important role in the human immune system by killing bacteria and invading pathogen. Under certain circumstances, a MPO can be released into the extracellular space. In the presence of hydrogen peroxide and chloride ions, MPO produces hypochlorous acid (HOCl), the major strong oxidant which reacts readily with free amino groups to form N-chloramines. *In vitro* studies show that MPO inactivates purified A1AT trough oxidation of two methionine residues (Matheson et al., 1979; Summers et al., 2008). Hydrogen peroxide released from macrophages in the small airways of smokers synergistically with hydrogen peroxide from tobacco may contribute to the oxidative inhibition of A1AT (Cohen and James, 1982). Moreover, A1AT oxidized by the myeloperoxidase-hydrogen peroxide system (MPO-H_2O_2), in inflammation, promotes the formation of IgA-A1AT complexes, and consequently the elastase inhibitory activity of A1AT is reduced (Scott et al., 1999).
Recent studies have shown that although oxyA1AT loses antielastase activity it gets new biological properties that may be important in the pathogenesis of certain diseases. Several studies have shown that oxyA1AT behaves as a proinflammatory stimulus. Moraga et al. (Moraga and Janciauskiene, 2000) revealed that oxyA1AT activates monocytes, which is reflected in significant elevation in monocyte chemoattractant protein-1, cytokine IL-6, and TNFα expression, as well in increased activity of NADPH oxidase. Furthermore, oxyA1AT by activation of pro-oxidative NADPH oxidase may promote its own formation and thereby contributes to inflammation. OxyA1AT generated in the airway interacts directly with epithelial cells to release chemokines IL-8 and MCP-1, which in turn attracts macrophages and neutrophils into the airways (Li et al., 2009). The release of oxidants by these inflammatory cells could oxidize A1AT, perpetuating the cycle and potentially contributing to the pathogenesis of COPD.

4.2 Oxidation of A1AT - clinical aspects

Centrolobular emphysema in smokers as a clinical manifestation is strongly associated with functional deficiency caused by oxidation of A1AT. Several studies supported the mechanism by which tobacco smoke increased the risk of developing emphysema. According to this mechanism, cigarette smoke reduces protease inhibitory capacity, causing the increase of the lung vulnerability to elastolytic destruction and thereby increasing the risk for the development of emphysema (Carp et al., 1982; Janoff et al., 1983; Ogushi et al., 1991). By losing the antiprotease ability and becoming pro-inflammatory stimulus, the oxyA1AT favors the development of clinical emphysema.
OxyA1AT has a potential clinical significance in atherogenesis. Mashiba et al. (Mashiba et al., 2001) have revealed that A1AT produced and oxidized by macrophages, attaches to low density lipoprotein (LDL) in the intima of the arterial wall and contributes to the lipid accumulation in arterial wall cells in the early stage of atherogenesis.

In addition, reduction of antielastase activity was observed in hemodialysis patients (Hashemi et al., 2009). Furthermore, Honda et al. (Honda, et al., 2009) reported that serum levels of oxyA1AT positively correlated with myeloperoxidase in patients on hemodialysis, and could represent a useful marker for the estimation of the increasing carotid intima-media thickness. They also found that oxyA1AT might be an independent predictor of protein-energy wasting in patients on hemodialysis. Oxidized A1AT was also detected in patients with Alzheimer's disease, heart failure, and in premature rupture of the fetal membrane (Choi et al., 2002; Banfi et al., 2008; Izumi-Yoneda et al., 2009).

4.3 Perspective of the determination of oxidized A1AT

Determination of oxyA1AT as biomarker is not used in routine practice, although it may be useful in assessment of pulmonary emphysema risk, and other pathological conditions associated with oxidative stress and inflammation. Our knowledge of the clinical significance of oxyA1AT is still insufficient, as well the optimal quantification of oxyA1AT.
Previously used method for quantification of oxyA1AT was based on determination of elastase- (EIC) and trypsin inhibitory capacity (TIC) (Beatty et al., 1982). As oxyA1AT loses its ability to inhibit porcine elastase but retains antitrypsin activity, the increased TIC/EIC ratio correlates with degree of A1AT oxidation. Progress in oxyA1AT methodology includes development of immunochemical method (Ueda et al., 2002).
Advanced methodology of quantification of oxyA1AT should be developed as a sensitive, specific method which would be suitable for routine practice.

5. Conclusion

The only proven genetic risk factor in pathogenesis of emphysema is severe alpha-1-antitrypsin deficiency. However, several known and unknown genetic and environmental factors contribute to the differences in the susceptibility of A1ATD individuals to develop lung disease. Among the most important are cigarette smoke and air pollutants that could provoke oxidative stress and inflammatory response.
So far, a lot of attention and efforts in A1ATD research was given to the deficient A1AT variants and A1AT polymerization, while the oxidation of A1AT protein has been generally overlooked. Non-deficient, heavy smokers may have normal serum level of A1AT, but with reduced functional activity due to functional deficiency caused by oxidation. The physiological role of oxyA1AT could be particularly important regarding growing evidence of different biological functions of A1AT that go beyond those usually linked to its antiprotease activities. Future studies will elucidate the role of A1AT oxidation in modulation of inflammation and tissue destruction which represent landmarks of emphysema, as well in modulation of augmentation therapy.
The early recognition and diagnostics of A1ATD is the most important in terms of prevention and delay of the onset of symptoms of emphysema. The optimal approach in therapy of A1ATD would be to inhibit the polymerization of the Z protein (intracellular and extracellular) and prevent oxidative stress, accompanied by standard augmentation therapy.

6. Acknowledgment

This work was supported by grants 173008 from the Ministry of Education and Science, Republic of Serbia.

7. References

Alam, S., Li, Z, Janciauskiene, S. & Mahadeva, R. (2011). Oxidation of Z α_1-antitrypsin by cigarette smoke induces polymerization: a novel mechanism of early-onset emphysema. *Am J Respir Cell Mol Biol* 45, 261-269.

American Thoracic Society/European Respiratory Society Statement. (2003). Standards for the diagnosis and management of individuals with alpha-1 antitrypsin deficiency. *Am J Respir Crit Care Med* 168, 818-900.

Banda, M.J., Rice, A.G., Griffin, G.L. & Senior, R.M. (1988). The inhibitory complex of human α_1-proteinase inhibitor and human leukocyte elastase is a neutrophil chemoattractant. *J Exp Med* 167, 1608-1615.

Banfi, C., Brioschi, M., Barcella, S., Veglia, F., Biglioli, P., Tremoli, E. & Agostoni, P.G. (2008). Oxidized proteins in plasma of patients with heart failure: Role in endothelial damage. *Eur J Heart Fail* 10, 244-251.

Beatty, K., Robertie, P, Senior, R.M. & Travis J. (1982). Determination of oxidized alpha-1-proteinase inhibitor in serum. *J Lab Clin Med* 100, 186-192.

Beatty, K., Bieth, J. & Travis, J. (1980). Kinetics of association of serine proteinases with native and oxidized α-1-proteinase inhibitor and α-1-antichymotrypsin. *J Biol Chem* 255, 3931-3934.

Bergin, D.A., Reeves, E.P., Meleady, P., Henry, M., McElvaney, O.J., Carroll, T.P., Condron, C., Chotirmall, S.H., Clynes, M., O'Neill, S.J. & McElvaney, N.G. (2010). α-1 antitrypsin regulates human neutrophil chemotaxis induced by soluble immune complexes and IL-8. *JClin Invest* 120, 4236-4250.

Billingsley, G.D., Walter, M.A., Hammond, G.L. & Cox, D.W. (1993). Physical mapping of four serpin genes: α1 -antitrypsin, α1 -antishymotrypsin, corticosteroid-binding globulin, and proteinC inhibitor, within a 280-kb region on chromosome 14q32.1. *Am J Hum Genet* 52, 343-353.

Blanco, I., De Serres, F.J., Fernandez-Bustillo, E., Lara, B. & Miravitlles, M. (2006). Estimated numbers and prevalence of PI*S and PI*Z alleles of α_1-antitrypsin deficiency in European countries. *Eur Respir J* 27, 77-84.

Bornhorst, J.A., Procter, M., Meadows, C., Ashwood, E.R. & Mao, R. (2007). Evaluation of an integrative diagnostic algorithm for the identification of people at risk for α_1-antitrypsin deficiency. *Am J Clin Pathol* 128, 482-490.

Brantly M.L., Paul, L.D., Miller, B.H., Falk, R.T., Wu, M. & Crystal, R.G. (1988). Clinical features and history of the destructive lung disease associated with alpha-1-antitrypsin deficiency of adults with pulmonary symptoms. *Am Rev Respir Dis* 138, 327-336.

Brantly, M.L., Wittes, J.T., Vogelmeier, C.F., Hubbard, R.C., Fells, G.A. & Crystal, R.G. (1991). Use of a highly purified alpha 1-antitrypsin standard to establish ranges for the common normal and deficient alpha 1-antitrypsin phenotypes. *Chest* 100, 703-708.

Campra, J.L., Craig, J.R., Peters, R.L. & Reynolds, T.B. (1973). Cirrhosis aassociated with partial deficiency of alpha-1-antitrypsn in an adult. *Ann Intern Med* 78, 233-238.

Carlson, J. A., Rogers B.B., Sifers R.N., Hawkins H.K., Finegold M.J. & Woo, S.L. (1988). Multiple tissues express alpha 1-antitrypsin in transgenic mice and man. *J Clin Invest* 82, 26-36.

Carp, H. & Janoff, A. (1978). Possible mechanisms of emphysema in smokers. In vitro suppression of serum elastase-inhibitory capacity by fresh cigarette smoke and its prevention by antioxidants. *Am Rev Respir Dis* 118, 617-621.

Carp, H. & Janoff, A. (1980). Potential mediator of inflammation. Phagocyte-derived oxidants suppress the elastase-inhibitory capacity of alpha 1-proteinase inhibitor in vitro. *J Clin Invest* 66, 987-995.

Carp, H., Miller, F., Hoidal, J.R. & Janoff, A. (1982). Potential mechanism of emphysema: alpha 1-proteinase inhibitor recovered from lungs of cigarette smokers contains oxidize ethionine and has decreased elastase inhibitory capacity. *PNAS* 79, 2041-2045.

Carrell, R.W. (1986). Alpha 1-antitrypsin: molecular pathology, leukocytes, and tissue damage. *J Clin Invest* 78, 1427-1431.

Carrell, R.W. & Lomas, D.A. (2002). Alpha1-antitrypsin deficiency-a model for conformational diseases. *N Engl J Med* 346, 45-53.

Chang, Y.P., Mahadeva, R., Chang, W.S., Lin, S.C. & Chu, Y.H. (2009). Small-molecule peptides inhibit Z alpha1-antitrypsin polymerization. *J Cell Mol Med* 13, 2304-2316.

Chang, Y.P., Mahadeva, R., Chang, W.S., Shukla, A., Dafforn, T.R. & Chu, Y.H. (2006). Identification of a 4-mer peptide inhibitor that effectively blocks the polymerization of pathogenic Z alpha1-antitrypsin. *Am J Respir Cell Mol Biol* 35, 540-548.

Chappell, S., Daly, L, Morgan, K, Baranes, G.T., Rosa, J., Rabinovich, R., Millar, A., Donnelly, S.C., Keatings, V., MacNee, W., Stolk, J., Hiemstra, P., Miniati, M., O`Connor, C.M. & Kalsheker, N. (2006). Cryptic haplotypes of SERPINA1 confer susceptibility to chronic obstructive pulmonary disease. *Hum Mutat* 27, 103-109.

Choi, J., Malakowsky, C.A., Talent, J.T, Conrad, C.C. & Gracy, R.W. (2002). Identification of oxidized plasma proteins in Alzheimer's disease. *Biochem Biophys Res Commun* 293, 1566-1570.

Churg, A., Wang, X., Wang, R.D., Meixner, S.C., Pryzdial, E.L.G. & Wright, J.L. (2007). α_1-antitrypsin suppresses TNF-α and MMP-12 production by cigarette smoke-stimulated macrophages. *Am J Respir Cell Mol Biol* 37, 144-151.

Cichy, J., Potempa, J. & Travis, J. (1997). Biosynthesis of α_1-proteinase inhibitor by human lung-derived epithelial cells. *J Biol Chem* 272, 8250-8255.

Cohen, A.B. & James, H.L. (1982). Reduction of the elastase inhibitory capacity of alpha 1-antitrypsin by peroxides in cigarette smoke: an analysis of brands and filters. *Am Rev Respir Dis* 126, 25-30.

Cook, L., Janus, E.D., Brenton, S., Tai, E. & Burdon; J. (1994). Absence of alpha-1-antitrypsin (Pi Null Bellingham) and the early onset of emphysema. *Aust N Z J Med* 24, 263-269.

Corda, L., Bertella, E., Pini, L., Pezzini, A., Medicina, D., Boni, E., Guerini, M., Trivella, S., Grassi, V. & Tantucci, C. (2006). Diagnostic flow chart for targeted detection of alpha1-antitrypsin deficiency. *Respir Med* 100, 463-470.

Cox, D.W. & Levison, H. (1988). Emphysema of early onset associated with a complete deficiency of α_1 antitrypsin (null homozygotes). *Am Rev Respir Dis* 137, 371-375.

Cox, D.W. Genetic variation in α_1 antitrypsin. (1978). *Am J Hum Genet* 30, 660-662.

Cox, D.W., Woo, S.L. & Mansfield, T. (1985). DNA restriction fragments associated with α_1-antitrypsin indicate a single origin for deficiency allele PI Z. *Nature* 316, 79-81.

Craig, J.R., Dunn, A.E. & Peters, R.L. (1975). Cirrhosis associated with partial deficiency of alpha-1- antitrypsin: a clinical and autopsy study. *Hum Pathol* 6, 113-120.

Cruz, M., Molina, J.A., Pedrola, D. & Muñoz-López, F. (1975). Cirrhosis and heterozygous α1-antitrypsin deficiency in a 4 year old girl. *Helv Paediatr Acta* 30, 501-507.

Crystal, R.G., Brantly, M.L., Hubbard, R.C., Curiel, D.T, States, D.J. & Holmes. M.D. (1989). The α_1-antitrypsin gene and its mutations. Clinical consequences and strategies for therapy. *Chest* 95, 196-208.

Curiel, D., Brantly, M., Curiel, E., Stier, L. & Crystal, R.G. (1989). α_1-antitrypsin deficiency caused by the α1-antitrypsin $Null_{mattawa}$ gene. An insertion mutation rendering the α_1-antitrypsin gene incapable of producing α_1-antitrypsin. *J Clin Invest* 83, 1144-1152.

Dabbagh, K., Laurent, G.J., Shock, A., Leoni, P., Papakrivopoulou, J. & Chambers, R.C. (2001). α_1 antitrypsin stimulates fibroblast proliferation and procollagen production and activates classical MAP kinase signalling pathways. *J Cell Physiol* 186, 73-81.

Dafforn, T.R., Mahadeva R., Elliott, P.R. Sivasothy, P. & Lomas, D.A. (1999). A kinetic mechanism for the polymerization of α_1-antitrypsin. *J Biol Chem* 274, 9548-9555.

Dahl, M., Nordestgaard, B.G., Lange P., Vestbo, J. &Tyjærg-Hansen, A. (2001). Molecular diagnosis of intermediate and severe α_1-antitrypsin deficiency: *MZ* individuals with chronic obstructive pulmonary disease may have lower lung function than *MM* individuals. *Clin Chem* 47, 56-62.

Dahl, M.,Tybjærg-Hansen, A., Lange, P., Vestbo, J. & Nordestgaar, B.G. (2002). Change in lung function and morbidity from chronic obstructive pulmonary disease in α_1-antitrypsin *MZ* heterozygotes: a longitudinal study of the general population. *Ann Intern Med* 136, 270-279.

De Croo, S., Kamboh, M.I. &Ferrell, R.E. (1991). Population genetics of alpha-1-antitrypsin polymorphism in US whites, US blacks and African blacks. *Hum Hered* 41, 215- 221.

De Serres, FJ. (2002). Worldwide racial and ethnic distribution of α_1-antitrypsin deficiency: summary of an analysis of published genetic epidemiologic surveys. *Chest* 122, 1818-1829.

Deslee, G., Woods, J.C., Moore, C., Conradi, S.H., Gierada, D.S., Atkinson, J.J., Battaile, J.T., Liu, L., Patterson, G.A., Adair-Kirk, T.L., Holtzman, M.J. & Pierce, R.A. (2009). Oxidative damage to nucleic acids in severe emphysema. *Chest* 135, 965-974.

Deslee, G., Adair-Kirk, T.L., Betsuyaku, T., Woods, J.C., Moore, C.H., Gierada, D.S., Conradi, S.H., Atkinson, J.J., Toennies, H.M., Battaile, J.T., Kobayashi, D.K., Patterson, G.A, Holtzman M,J. & Pierce, R.A. (2010). Cigarette smoke induces nucleic-acid oxidation in lung fibroblasts. *Am J Respir Cell Mol Biol* 43, 576-584.

Eden, E., Mitchell, D., Mehlman, B., Khouli, H., Mejat, M., Grieco, M.H. & Turino, G.M. (1997). Atopy, asthma and emphysema in patients with severe $\alpha_1$antitrypsin deficiency. *Am J Respir Crit Care Med* 156, 68-74.

Elliott, P.R., Lomas, D.A., Carrell, R.W. & Abrahams, J.P. (1996a). Inhibitory conformation of the reactive loop of α_1-antitrypsin. *Nat Struct Biol* 3, 676-681.

Elliott, PR., Stein, P.E., Bilton, D., Carrell, R.W. & Lomas, D.A. (1996b). Structural explanation for the deficiency of S α_1-antitrypsin. *Nat Struct Biol* 3, 910-911.

Elliott, P.R., Bilton, D. & Lomas, D.A. (1998). Lung Polymers in Z α_1-antitrypsin deficiency-related emphysema. *Am J Respir Cell Mol Biol* 18, 670-674.

Entrez SNP, http://www.ncbi.nlm.nih.gov/projects/SNP.

Eriksson, S., Carlson, J. & Velez, R. (1986). Risk of cirrhosis and primary liver cancer in α_1 antitrypsin deficiency. *N Engl J Med* 314, 736-739.

Eriksson, S. (1964). Pulmonary emphysema and alpha-1-antitrypsin deficiency. *Acta Med Scand* 175, 197-205.

Evans, M.D. & Pryor, W.A. (1994). Cigarette smoking, emphysema, and damage to α_1 proteinase inhibitor. *Am J Physiol Lung Cell Mol Physiol* 266, L593-L611.

Fagerhol, M.K. & Laurell, C.B. (1970). The Pi system-inherited variants of serum $\alpha_1$antitrypsin. *Prog Med Genet* 7, 96-111.

Finkelstein, R., Fraser, R.S., Ghezzo, H. & Cosio, M.G. (1995). Alveolar inflammation and its relation to emphysema in smokers. *Am J Respir Crit Care Med* 152, 1666-1672.

Fregonese, L., Stolk, J., Frants, R.R. & Veldhuisen, B. (2008). $\alpha_1$antitrypsin Null mutations and severity of emphysema. *Respir Med* 102, 876-884.

Griffiths, S.W., King, J. & Cooney, C.L. (2002). The reactivity and oxidation pathway of cysteine 232 in recombinant human α_1-antitrypsin. *J Biol Chem* 277, 25486-25492.

Hackett, T.L., Scarci, M., Zheng, L., Tan, W., Treasure, T. & Warner, J.A. (2010). Oxidative modification of albumin in the parenchymal lung tissue of current smokers with chronic obstructive pulmonary disease. *Respir Res* 11, 180.

Hafeez, W., Ciliberto, G. & Perlmutter, D. H. (1992). Constitutive and modulated expression of the human α1antitrypsin gene: different transcriptional initiation sites used in three different cell types. *J Clin Invest* 89, 1214-1222.

Hashemi, M., Mehrabifar, H., Homayooni, F., Naderi, M., Montazerifar, F. & Ghavami, S. (2009). Serum trypsin inhibitory capacity in hemodialysis patients. *Saudi J Kidney Dis Transpl* 20, 604-607.

Hersh, C.P., Dahl, M., Ly, N.P., Berkey, C.S., Nordestgaard, B.G. & Silverman, E.K. (2004). Chronic obstructive pulmonary disease in $\alpha_1$antitrypsin PI MZ heterozygotes: meta-analysis. *Thorax* 59, 843-849.

Honda, H., Ueda, M., Kojima, S., Mashiba, S., Hirai, Y., Hosaka, N., Suzuki, H., Mukai, M., Watanabe, M., Takahashi, K., Shishido, K. & Akizawa, T. (2009). Assessment of myeloperoxidase and oxidative α_1-antitrypsin in patients on hemodialysis. *Clin J Am Soc Nephrol* 4: 142-151.

Holmes, M., Curiel, D., Brantly, M. & Crystal, R.G. (1989). Characterization of the intracellular mechanism causing the alpha-1-antitrypsin $\text{Null}_{\text{granite falls}}$ deficiency state. *Am Rev Respir Dis* 140, 1662-1667.

Huang, H., Campbell, S.C., Nelius, T., Bedford, D.F., Veliceasa, D., Bouck, N.P. & Volpert, O.V. (2004). Alpha1-antitrypsin inhibits angiogenesis and tumor growth. *Int J Cancer,* 112, 1042-1048.

Hunington, J.A., Read, R.J. & Carrell, R.W. (2000). Structure of a serpin-protease complex shows inhibition by deformation. *Nature* 407, 923-926.

Hutchison, D.C.S. (1998). α_1-antitrypsin deficiency in Europe: geographical distributionof Pi types S and Z. *Resp Med* 92, 367-377.

Izumi-Yoneda, N., Toda, A., Okabe, M., Koike, C., Takashima, S., Yoshida, T., Konishi, I., Saito, S. & Nikaido, T. (2009). Alpha 1 antitrypsin activity is decreased in human amnion in premature rupture of the fetal membranes. *Mol Hum Reprod* 15, 49-57.

Janciauskiene, S.M., Nita, I.M. & Stevens, T. (2007). α_1-antitrypsin, old dog, new tricks. α_1-antitrypsin exerts in vitro anti-inflammatory activity in human monocytes by elevating cAMP. *J Biol Chem* 282, 8573-8582.

Janoff, A., Carp, H., Laurent, P. & Raju. L. (1983). The role of oxidative processes in emphysema. *Am Rev Respir Dis* 127, S31-S38.

Janoff, A., Carp, H., Lee, D. K. & Drew, R.T. (1979). Cigarette smoke inhalation decreases α1-antitrypsin activity in rat lung. *Science* 206, 1313-1314.

Janoff, A. (1985). Elastases and emphysema. Current assessment of the protease-antiprotease hypothesis. *Am Rev Respir Dis* 132, 417-433.

Janus, E.D., Phillips, N.T. & Carrell, R.W. (1985). Smoking, lung function and α_1-antitrypsin deficiency. *Lancet* 1, 152-154.

Johnson, D. & Travis, J. (1979). The oxidative inactivation of human alpha-1-proteinase inhibitor. Further evidence for methionine at the reactive center. *J Biol Chem* 254, 4022-4026.

Johnson, D. & Travis, J. (1978). Structural evidence for methionine at the reactive site of human α-1-proteinase inhibitor. *J Biol Chem* 253, 7142-7144.

Jones, E.A., Vergalla, J., Steer, C.J., Bradley-Moore, P.R. & Vierling, J.M. (1978). Metabolism of intact and desialylated α_1 antitrypsin. *Clin Sci Mol Med* 55, 139-148.

Klaassen, C.H.W., de Metz, M., van Aarssen, Y. & Janssen, J. (2001). α_1 antitrypsin deficiency as a result of compound heterozygosity for the Z and $M_{Heerlen}$ alleles. *Clin Chem* 47, 978-979.

Knoell, D.L., Ralston, D.R., Coulter, K.R. & Wewers, M.D. (1998). α_1-antitrypsin and protease complexation is induced by lipopolysaccharide, interleukin-1β, and tumor necrosis factor-α in monocytes. *Am J Respir Crit Care Med.*, Jan 157, 246-255.

Koj, A., Regoeczi, E., Toews, C.J., Leveille, R. & Gauldie, J. (1978). Synthesis of antithrombin III and α_1 antitrypsin by the perfused rat liver. *Biochim Biophys Acta* 539, 496-504.

Lai, E.C., Kao, F.T., Law, M.L. & Woo, S.L. (1983). Assignment of the α_1-antitrypsin gene and a sequence-related gene to human chromosome 14 by molecular hybridization. *Am J Hum Genet* 35, 385-392.

Larsson, C. (1978). Natural history and life expectancy in severe α_1-antitrypsin deficiency, Pi Z. *Acta Med Scand* 204, 345-351.

Laurell, C.B. & Eriksson, S. (1963). The electrophoretic α_1-globulin pattern of serum in α_1-antitrypsin deficiency. *Scand J Clin Lab Invest*, 15, 132-140.

Law, R.H., Zhang, Q., McGowan, S., Buckle, A.M., Silverman, G.A., Wong, W., Rosado, C.J., Langendorf, C.G, Pike, R.N., Bird, P.I. & Whisstock, J.C. (2006). An overview of the serpin superfamily. *Genome Biol* 7, 216.

Lee. P., Gildea, T.R. & Stoller, J.K. (2002). Emphysema in nonsmokers: α_1-antitrypsin deficiency and other causes. *Cleve Clin J Med* 69, 928-946.

Lewis, J. H., Iammarino, R. M., Spero, J. A. & Hasiba, U. (1978). Antithrombin Pittsburgh: an alpha1-antitrypsin variant causing hemorrhagic disease. *Blood* 51, 129-137.

Li, K., Zay, K. & A. Churg. (1997). Mineral dusts oxidize methionine residues: probable mechanism of inactivation of alpha-1-antitrypsin. *Ann Hyg* 41, 379-383.

Li, Z., Alam, S., Wang, J., Sandstrom, C.S., Janciauskiene, C. & Mahadeva, R. (2009). Oxidized α_1-antitrypsin stimulates the release of monocyte chemotactic protein-1 from lung epithelial cells: potential role in emphysema. *Am J Physiol Lung Cell Mol Physiol* 297, L388-L400.

Lieberman, J. (1969). Heterozygous and homozygous α_1-antitrypsin deficiency in patients with pulmonary emphysema. *N Engl J Med* 281, 279-284.

Lieberman, J; Winter, B. & Sastre, A. (1986). α_1-antitrypsin Pi types in 956 COPD patients. *Chest* 89, 370-373.

Loebermann, H., Tokuoka, R., Deisenhofer, J. & Huber, R. (1984). Human α_1-proteinase inhibitor: crystal modifications, molecular model and preliminary analysis of the implications for function. *J Mol Biol* 177, 531-556.

Lomas, D.A. (2005). Molecular mousetraps, α_1-antitrypsin deficiency and the serpinopathies. *Clin Med* 5, 249-257.

Lomas, D.A., Elliott, P.R., Sidhar, S.K., Foreman R.C., Finch, J.T., Cox, D.W., Whisstock, J.C. & Carrell, R.W. (1995). α_1-antitrypsin Mmalton (Phe^{52}-deleted) forms loop-sheet polymers in vivo. Evidence for the C sheet mechanism of polymerization. *J Biol Chem* 14, 16864-16870.

Lomas, D. A., Evans, D.L., Stone, S.R., Chang, W.S. & Carrell. R.W. (1993a). Effect of the Z mutation on the physical and inhibitory properties of α_1-antitrypsin. *Biochemistry* 32, 500-508.

Lomas, D.A., Finch, J.T., Seyama, K., Nukiwa, T. & Carrell, R.W. (1993b). α1-antitrypsin Siiyama ($Ser^{53}\rightarrow$Phe). Further evidence for intracellular loop-sheet polymerization. *JBiolChem* 268, 15333-15335.

Lomas, DA. (2000). Loop-sheet polymerization: the mechanism of α_1-antitrypsin deficiency. *Respir Med* 94, Suppl C, S3-S6.

Lomas, D.A. (2006).The selective advantage of α_1-antitrypsin deficiency. *Am J Respir Crit Care Med* 173, 1072-1077.

Lomas, D.A., Evans, D.L., Finch, J.J. & Carell, R.W. (1992). The mechanism of Z α_1-antitrypsin accumulation in the liver. *Nature* 357, 605-607.

Long, G.L., Chandra, T., Woo, S.L.C., Davie, E.W. & Kurachi, K. (1984). Complete sequence of the cDNA for human alpha-1-antitrypsin and the gene for the S variant. *Biochemistry* 23, 4828-4837.

Lu, Y., Tang, M., Wasserfall, C., Kou, Z., Campbell-Thompson, M., Gardemann, T., Crawford, J., Atkinson, M., & Song, S. (2006). α_1-antitrypsin gene therapy modulates cellular immunity and efficiently prevents type 1 diabetes in nonobese diabetic mice. *Hum Gene Ther* 17, 625-634.

Luisetti, M. & Seersholm, N. (2004). α_1-antitrypsin deficiency. 1: Epidemiology of α_1-antitrypsin deficiency. *Thorax* 59, 164-169.

Mahadeva, R., Dafforn, T.R., Carrell, R.W. & Lomas, D.A. (2002). 6-mer peptide selectively anneals to a pathogenic serpin conformation and blocks polymerization: implications for the prevention of Z α_1-antitrypsin -related cirrhosis. *J Biol Chem* 277, 6771-6774.

Mahadeva, R., Chang, W.S., Dafforn, T.R., Oakley, D.J., Foreman, R.C., Calvin, J., Wight, D.G. & Lomas, D.A. (1999). Heteropolymerization of S, I, and Z α_1-antitrypsin and liver cirrhosis. *J Clin Invest* 103, 999-1006.

Mahadeva, R. & Lomas, D.A. (1998). Alpha$_1$-antitrypsin deficiency, cirrhosis and emphysema. *Thorax* 53, 501-505.

Malerba, M., Ricciardolo, F., Torregiani, C., Radaeli, A., Ceriani, L., Mori, E., Bontempelli, M., Grassi, V & Tantucci, C. (2006). Neutrophilic inflammation and IL-8 levels in induced sputum of alpha-1-antitrypsin PiMZ subjects. *Thorax* 61, 129-133.

Mallya M, Phillips RL, Saldanha SA, Gooptu B, Brown SC, Termine DJ, Shirvani AM, Wu Y, Sifers, R.N., Abagyan, R. & Lomas, D.A. (2007). Small molecules block the polymerization of Z α_1-antitrypsin and increase the clearance of intracellular aggregates. *J Med Chem* 50, 5357-5363.

Mashiba, S., Wada, Y., Takeya, M., Sugiyama, A., Hamakubo, T., Nakamura, A., Noguchi, N., Niki, E., Izumi, A., Kobayashi, M., Uchida, K. & Kodama, T. (2001). In vivo complex formation of oxidized α_1-antitrypsin and LDL. *Arterioscler Thromb Vasc Biol* 21, 1801-1808.

Matheson, N.R., Wong, P.S. & Travis, J. (1979). Enzymatic inactivation of human alpha-1-proteinase inhibitor by neutrophil myeloperoxidase. *Biochem Biophys Res Commun* 88, 402-409.

Mayer, A.S., Stoller, J.K., Vedal, S., Ruttenber, A.J., Strand, M., Sandhaus, R.A. & Newman, L.S. (2006). Risk factors for symptom onset in PI*Z alpha-1antitrypsin deficiency. *Int J Chron Obstruct Pulmon Dis* 1, 485–492.

McElvaney, N.G., Stoller, J.K., Buist, A.S., Prakash, U.B.S., Brantly, M.L., Schluchter, M.D. & Crystal, R.D. (1997). Baseline characteristics of enrollees in the national heart, lung, and blood institute registry of α_1-antitrypsin deficiency. *Chest* 111, 394–403.

Miravitlles, M., Herr, C., Ferrarotti, I., Jardi, R., Rodriguez-Frias, F., Luisetti. M. & Bals. R. (2010). Laboratory testing of individuals with severe α_1-antitrypsin deficiency in three European centres. *Eur Respir J* 35, 960-968.

Mohsenin, V. (1991). Lipid peroxidation and antielastase activity in the lung under oxidant stress: role of antioxidant defenses. *J Appl Physiol* 70, 1456-1462.

Molmenti, E. P., Perlmutter, D. H. & Rubin, D.C. (1993). Cell-specific expression of α_1-antitrypsin in human intestinal epithelium. *J Clin Invest* 92, 2022-2034.

Moraga, F. & Janciauskiene, S. (2000). Activation of primary human monocytes by the oxidized form of α_1-antitrypsin. *J Biol Chem* 275, 7693-7700.

Moraga, F., Lindgren, S. & Janciaskiene, S. (2001). Effects of noninhibitory α_1-antitrypsin on primary human monocyte activation in vitro. *Arch Biochem Biophys* 386: 221-226.

Mornex, J.F., Chytil-Weir, A., Martinet, Y., Courtney, M., LeCocq, J.P. & Crystal, R.G. (1986). Expression of the alpha-1-antitrypsin gene in mononuclear phagocytes of normal and alpha-1-antitrypsin−deficient individuals. *J Clin Invest* 77, 1952-1961.

Mulgrew, A.T., Taggart, C.C., Lawless, M.W., Greene, C.M., Brantly, M.L., O'Neill, S.J. & McElvaney, N.G. (2004). Z α_1-antitrypsin polymerizes in the lung and acts as a neutrophil chemoattractant. *Chest* 125: 1952-1957.

Nukiwa, T., Satoh, K., Brantly, M.L., Ogushi, F., Fells, G.A., Courtney, M. & Crystal, R.G. (1987). Identification of a second mutation in the protein-coding sequence of the Z type alpha 1-antitrypsin gene. *J Biol Chem* 262, 11999-12004.

Oakeshott, J.G, Muir, A., Clark, P., Martin, N.G., Wilson, S.R. & Whitfield, J.B. (1985). Effects of the protease inhibitor (Pi) polymorphism on alpha-1-antitrypsin concentration and elastase inhibitory capacity in human serum. *Ann Hum Biol* 12, 149-160.

Ogushi, F., Hubbard, R.C., Vogelmeier, C., Fells, G.A. & Crystal. R.G. (1991). Risk factors for emphysema. Cigarette smoking is associated with a reduction in the association rate constant of lung α1-antitrypsin for neutrophil elastase. *J Clin Invest* 87, 1060-1065 .

Ogushi, F., Fells, G.A., Hubbard, R.C., Straus, S.D. & Crystal, R.G. (1987). Z-type α1-antitrypsin is less competent then M1-type α1- antitrypsin as an inhibitor of neutropfil elastase. *J Clin Invest* 80, 1366-1374.

Olsen, G.N., Harris, J.O., Castle, J.R., Waldman, R.H. & Karmgard, H.J. (1975). Alpha-1-antitrypsin content in the serum, alveolar macrophages, and alveolar lavage fluid of smoking and nonsmoking normal subjects. *J Clin Invest* 55, 427-30

Owen, M.C., Brennan, S.O., Lewis, J.H. & Carrell, R.W. (1983). Mutation of antitrypsin to antithrombin: α1-antitrypsin Pittsburgh (358 met→arg), a fatal bleeding disorder. *New Eng J Med* 309, 694-698.

Owen, M.C., Carrell, R.W. & Brennan, S.O. (1976).The abnormality of the S variant of human α-1-antitrypsin. *Biochim Biophys Acta* 453, 257-261.

Parfrey, H., Dafforn, T.R., Belorgey, D., Lomas, D.A. & Mahadeva, R. (2004). Inhibiting polymerization: new therapeutic strategies for Z α_1-antitrypsin-related emphysema. *Am J Respir Cell Mol Biol* 31, 133-139.

Parmar, J.S., Mahadeva, R., Reed, B.J., Farahi, N., Cadwallader, K.A., Keogan, M.T., Bilton, D., Chilvers, E.R. & Lomas, D.A. (2002). Polymers of α_1-antitrypsin are chemotactic for human neutrophils. A new paradigm for the pathogenesis of emphysema. *Am J Respir Cell Mol Biol* 26, 723–730.

Perlino, E., Cortese, R. & Ciliberto, G. (1987). The human α_1-antitrypsin gene is transcribed from two different promoters in macrophages and hepatocytes. *EMBO J* 6, 2767-2771.

Petrache, I., Fijalkowska, I., Medler, T.R., Skirball, J., Cruz, P., Zhen, L., Petrache, H.I., Flotte. T.R. & Tuder, R.M. (2006a). α-1 antitrypsin inhibits caspase-3 activity, preventing lung endothelial cell apoptosis. *Am J Pathol* 169, 1155-1166.

Petrache, I., Fijalkowska, I., Zhen, L., Medler, T.R., Brown, E., Cruz, P., Choe, K.H., Taraseviciene-Stewart, L., Scerbavicius, R., Shapiro, L., Zhang, B., Song, S., Hicklin, D., Voelkel, N.F., Flotte, T. & Tuder, R.M. (2006b). A novel anti-apoptotic role for α_1-antitrypsin in the prevention of pulmonary emphysema. *Am J Respir Crit Care Med* 173, 1222-1228.

Pott, G.B., Chan, E.D., Dinarello, C.A. & Shapiro, L. (2009). α-1-Antitrypsin is an endogenous inhibitor of proinflammatory cytokine production in whole blood. *J Leukoc Biol* 85, 886-895.

Prins, J., van der Maijden, B.B., Kraaijenhagen, R.J. & Wielders, J.P.M. (2008). Inherited chronic obstructive pulmonary disease: new selective-sequencing workup for α_1-antitrypsin deficiency identifies 2 previously unidentified Null alleles. *Clin Chem* 54, 101-107.

Pryor, W.A. (1997). Cigarette smoke radicals and the role of free radicals in chemical carcinogenicity. *Environ Health Perspect* 105, 875-882.

Pryor, W.A., Dooley, M.M. & Church, D.F. (1984). Inactivation of human α-1-proteinase inhibitor by gas-phase cigarette smoke. *Biochem Biophys Res Commun* 122, 676- 681.

Rahman, I. (2005). Oxidative stress in pathogenesis of chronic obstructive pulmonary disease: cellular and molecular mechanisms. *Cell Biochem Biophys* 43, 167-188.

Richards, C.D. & Gauldie, B.B. (1991). Cytokine control of acute phase protein expression. *Eur Cytokine Network* 2, 89-98.

Rodriguez, F., Jardí, R., Costa, X., Cotrina, M., Galimany, R., Vidal, R. & Miravitlles, M. (2002). Rapid screening for α_1-antitrypsin deficiency in patients with chronic obstructive pulmonary disease using dried blood specimens. *Am J Respir Crit Care Med* 166, 814-817.

Rouhani, F., Paone, G., Smith, N.K., Krein, P., Barnes, P. & Mark, L. (2000). Lung neutrophil burden correlates with increased pro-inflammatory cytokines and decreased lung function in individuals with α_1-antitrypsin deficiency. *Chest* 117, 250S- 251S.

Sahin, U., Unlü, M., Ozgüner, F., Sütcü, R., Akkaya, A. & Delibas, N. (2001). Lipid peroxidation and glutathione peroxidase activity in chronic obstructive pulmonary disease exacerbation: prognostic value of malondialdehyde. *J Basic Clin Physiol Pharmacol* 12, 59-68.

Satoh, K., Nukiwa, T., Brantly, M., Garver Jr R.I., Hofker, M., Courtney, M. & Crystal, R.G. (1988). Emphysema associated with complete absence of α 1- antitrypsin of a stop codon in an α 1-antitrypsin-coding exon. *Am J Hum Genet* 42, 77-83.

Schroeder, W.T., Miller, M.F., Woo, S.L. & Saunders, G.F. (1985). Chromosomal localization of the human α_1-antitrypsin gene (PI) to 14q31-32. *Am J Hum Genet*, 37, 868-872.

Scott, L.J., Russell, G.I., Nixon, N.B., Dawes, P.T. & Mattey, D.L. (1999). Oxidation of α_1-proteinase inhibitor by the myeloperoxidase-hydrogen peroxidase system promotes binding to immunoglobulin A. *Biochem Biophys Res Commun* 255, 562-567.

Seixas, S., Garcia, O., Trovoada, M.J., Santos, M.T., Amorim, A. & Rocha, J. (2001). Patterns of haplotype diversity within the serpine gene cluster at 14q32.1: insights into the natural history of the α_1-antitrypsin polymorphism. *Hum Genet* 108, 20-30.

Senn, O., Russi, E.W., Schindler, C., Imboden, M., von Eckardstein, A., Brändli, O., Zemp, E., Ackermann-Liebrich, U., Berger, W., Rochat, T., Luisetti, M. & Probst-Hensch, N.M. (2008). Circulating alpha1-antitrypsin in the general population: determinants and association with lung function. *Clin Chem* 54, 1331-1338.

Sharafkhaneh, A., Hanania, N.A. & Kim, V. (2008). Pathogenesis of emphysema: from the bench to the bedside. *Proc Am Thorac Soc* 5, 475-477.

Silverman, E.K., Pierce, J.A., Province, M.A., Rao, D.C. & Campbell, E,J. (1989). Variability of pulmonary function in alpha-1-antitrypsin deficiency: clinical correlates. *Ann Intern Med* 111, 982-991.

Silverman, E.K., Province, M.A., Campbell, E.J., Pierce, J.A. & Rao, D.C. (1990). Biochemical intermediates in alpha 1-antitrypsin deficiency: residual family resemblance for total alpha 1-antitrypsin, oxidized alpha 1-antitrypsin, and immunoglobulin E after adjustment for the effect of the Pi locus. *Genet Epidemiol* 7, 137-149.

Simsek, H., Pinar, A., Altinbas, A., Alp, A., Balaban, Y.H., Buyukasik, Y., Ozcebe, O., Hascelik, G., Gedikoglu, G. & Tatar, G. (2011). Cutoff level to detect heterozygous α_1-antitrypsin deficiency in Turkish population. *J Clin Lab Anal* 25, 296-299.

Snyder, M.S, Katzmann, J.A., Butz, M.L., Yang, P., Dawson, D.B., Halling, K.C., Highsmith, W.E. & Thibodeau, S.N. (2006). Diagnosis of α-1-antitrypsin deficiency: an algorithm of quantification, genotyping, and phenotyping. *Clin Chem* 52, 2236-2242.

Sohrab, S., Petrusca, D.N., Lockett, A.D., Schweitzer, K.S., Rush, N.I., Gu, Y., Kamocki, K., Garrison, J. & Petrache, I. (2009). Mechanism of α-1 antitrypsin endocytosis by lung endothelium. *FASEB J* 23, 3149-3158.

Sørheim, I.C., Bakke, P., Gulsvik, A., Pillai, S.G., Johannessen, A., Gaarder, P.I., Campbell, E.J., Agustí, A., Calverley, P.M., Donner, C.F., Make, B.J., Rennard, S.I., Vestbo, J., Wouters, E.F., Paré, P.D., Levy, R.D., Coxson, H.O., Lomas, D.A., Hersh, C.P. & Silverman, E.K. (2010). α_1-antitrypsin protease inhibitor MZ heterozygosity is asssociated with airflow obstruction in two large cohorts. *Chest* 138, 1125-1132.

Stein, P.D., Leu, J.D., Welch, M.H. & Guenter, C.A. (1971). Pathophysiology of the pulmonary circulation in emphysema associated with α 1 antitrypsin deficiency. *Circulation* 43, 227-239.

Stockley, R.A. & Burnett D. (1979). Alpha-1-antitrypsin and leucocyte elastase in infected and noninfected sputum. *Am Rev Respir Dis* 120, 1081-1086.

Stockley, R.A. (1984). Measurement of soluble proteins in lung secretions. *Thorax* 39, 241–247.

Stoller JK, Smith P, Yang P. & Spray, J. (1994). Physical and social impact of alpha-1 antitrypsin deficiency: results of a mail survey of the readership of a national newsletter. *Cleve Clin J Med* 61, 461-467.

Stoller, J.K., Sandhaus, R.A., Turino, G., Dickson, R., Rodgers, K. & Strange, C. (2005a). Delay in diagnosis of α_1-antitrypsin deficiency: a continuing problem. *Chest* 128, 1989-1994.

Stoller, J.K, Tomashefski, J.Jr, Crystal, R.G., Arroliga, A., Strange, C., Killian, D.N., Schluchter, M.D. & Wiedemann, H.P. (2005b). Mortality in individuals with severe deficiency of α1-antitrypsin: findings from the National Heart, Lung, and Blood Institute Registry. *Chest*, 127, 1196-1204.

Summers, F.A., Morgan, P.E., Davies, M.J. & Hawkins, C.L. (2008). Identification of plasma proteins that are susceptible to thiol oxidation by hypochlorous acid and N-chloramines. *Chem Res Toxicol* 21, 1832-1840.

Sveger, T. (1976). Liver disease in α_1-antitrypsin deficiency detected by screening of 200,000 infants. *N Engl J Med* 294, 1316-1321.

Taggart, C., Cervantes-Laurean, D., Kim, G., McElvaney, N.G., Wehr, N., Moss, J. & Levine, R.L. (2000). Oxidation of either methionine 351 or methionine 358 in α_1-antitrypsin causes loss of anti-neutrophil elastase activity. *J Biol Chem* 275, 27258-27265.

Takahashi, H. & Crystal, R.G. (1990). α1-antitrypsin $\text{Null}_{\text{isola di procida}}$: an α1-antitrypsin deficiency allele caused by deletion of all α1-antitrypsin coding exons. *Am J Hum Genet* 47, 403-413.

Taliercio, R.M., Chatburn, R.L. & Stoller, J.K. (2010). Knowledge of alpha-1 antitrypsin deficiency among internal medicine house officers and respiratory therapists: results of a survey. *Respir Care* 55, 322-327.

Talmud, P.J., Martin, S., Steiner, G., Flavell, D.M., Whitehouse, D.B., Nagl, S., Jackson, R., Taskinen, M.R., Frick, M.H., Nieminen, M.S., Kesaniemi, Y.A., Pasternack, A., Humphries, S.E. & Syvanne, M. (2003). Progression of atherosclerosis is associated with variation in the α_1-antitrypsin gene. *Arterioscler Thromb Vasc Biol* 23, 644–649.

Tanash, H.A., Nilsson, P.M., Nilsson, J.A. & Piitulainen, E. (2008). Clinical course and prognosis of never-smokers with severe alpha-1-antitrypsin deficiency (PiZZ). *Thorax* 63, 1091-1095.

Tanash, H.A, Nilsson, P.M., Nilsson, J.A. & Piitulainen. E. (2010). Survival in severe alpha-1-antitrypsin deficiency (PiZZ). *Respir Res* 11, 44.

Tarjan, E., Magyar, P., Vaczi, Z., Lantos, A. & Vaszar, L. (1994). Longitudinal lung function study in heterozygous PiMZ phenotype subjects. *Eur Respir J* 7, 2199-2204.

Theegarten, D., Teschler, H., Stamatis, G., Konietzko, N. & Morgenroth, K. (1998). Pathologico-anatomical results in surgical lung volume reduction of advanced emphysema. *Pneumologie* 52, 702-706.

Tobin, M.J., Cook, P.J.L. & Hutchinson, D.C.S. (1983). Alpha$_1$-antitrypsin deficiency: the c linical and physiological features of pulmonary emphysema in subjects homozygous for Pi type Z. A survey by the British Thoracic Association. *Br J Dis Chest* 77, 14-27.

Torres-Ramos, Y.D., García-Guillen, M.L., Olivares-Corichi, I.M. & Hicks, J.J. (2009). Correlation of plasma protein carbonyls and C-reactive protein with GOLD stage progression in COPD patients. *Open Respir Med J* 3, 61-66.

Turino, G.M., Barker, A.F., Brantly, M.L., Cohen, A.B., Connelly, R.P., Crystal, R.G., Eden, E., Schluchter, M.D. & Stoller, J.K. (1996).Clinical features of individuals with PI*SZ phenotype of α-1 antitrypsin deficiency. *Am J Respir Crit Care Med* 154, 1718- 1725.

Ueda, U., Mashiba, S. & Uchida, K. (2002). Evaluation of oxidized alpha-1-antitrypsin in blood as an oxidative stress marker using anti-oxidative α1-AT monoclonal antibody. *Clin Chim Acta* 317, 125-131.

Wallaert, B., Gressier, B., Aerts, C., Mizon, C., Voisin, C. & Mizon, J. (1991). Oxidative inactivation of α_1-proteinase inhibitor by alveolar macrophages from healthy smokers requires the presence of myeloperoxidase. *Am J Respir Cell Mol Biol* 5, 437-444.

Vogt, W. (1995). Oxidation of methionyl residues in proteins: tools, targets, and reversal. *Free Radic Biol Med* 18, 93-105.

WHO Meeting on Alpha$_1$-Antitrypsin Deficiency, Geneva, March 18-20, 1996.

Wood, A.M., Harrison, R.M., Semple, S., Ayres, J.G. & Stockley, R.A. (2009). Outdoor air pollution is associated with disease severity in α_1-antitrypsin deficiency. *Eur Respir J* 34, 346-353.

Woolhouse, I.S., Bayley, D.L. & Stockley, R.A. (2002). Sputum chemotactic activity in chronic obstructive pulmonary disease: effect of α_1-antitrypsin deficiency and the role of leukotriene B(4) and interleukin 8. *Thorax* 57, 709-714.

Yang, S.R., Chida, A.S., Bauter, M.R., Shafiq, N., Seweryniak, K., Maggirwar, S.B., Kilty, I. & Rahman I. (2006). Cigarette smoke induces proinflammatory cytokine release by activation of NF-kappaB and posttranslational modifications of histone deacetylase in macrophages. *Am J Physiol Lung Cell Mol Physiol* 291, :L46-L57.

Yoshida, A., Ewing, C., Wessels, M., Lieberman, J. & Gaidulis, L. (1977). Molecular abnormality of PI S variant of human alpha1-antitrypsin. *Am J Hum Genet* 29, 233-239.

Yu, M.H., Lee, K.N. & Kim, J. (1995). The Z type variation of human α_1-antitrypsin causes a protein folding defect. *Nature Structural Biol* 2, 363-367.

Zorzetto, M., Russi, E., Senn, O., Imboden, M., Ferrarotti, I., Tinelli, C., Campo, I., Ottaviani, S., Scabini, R., von Eckardstein, A., Berger, W., Brändli, O., Rochat, T., Luisetti, M. & Probst-Hensch, N. (2008). SERPINA1 gene variants in individuals from the general populationwith reduced α_1-antitrypsin concentrations. *Clin Chem* 54, 1331-1338.

3

Recent Advances in the Research and Development of Alpha-1 Proteinase Inhibitor for Therapeutic Use

Elena Karnaukhova*
Division of Hematology,
Center for Biologics Evaluation and Research
Food and Drug Administration
USA

1. Introduction

Human alpha-1-proteinase inhibitor (α_1-PI) is a well-characterized multifunctional protease inhibitor, the major physiological role of which is inhibition of neutrophil elastase (NE) in the lungs. The importance of α_1-PI is underlined by its deficiency which is characterized by low levels of α_1-PI in the circulation. Under such conditions, lower levels of α_1-PI are transported to tissues, including the fragile alveoli of the lungs. α_1-PI deficiency (with levels of α_1-PI in blood below 11 μM, insufficient for inhibition of proteolytic enzymes in the lungs) is a common genetic condition predisposing α_1-PI-deficient individuals to the development of chronic obstructive pulmonary disease (COPD). Hereditary α_1-PI deficiency is classically associated with the development of premature, ultimately fatal, panacinar emphysema. To slow down the progression of emphysema, several licensed α_1-PI concentrate preparations derived from pooled human plasma are currently available for intravenous augmentation therapy for patients with congenital α_1-PI deficiency and clinically evident emphysema. In addition, and as an alternative to the plasma-derived α_1-PI products, multiple efforts have been made to develop recombinant versions of human α_1-PI over the last three decades. This review describes the recent advances in the research and development of human α_1-PI for therapetic use and covers the following: characterization of human α_1-PI; epidemiology of α_1-PI deficiency and currently licensed treatment; summary of the manufacturing and recent quality improvements of the α_1-PI plasma-derived products; safety and efficacy of α_1-PI intravenous augmentation and alternative routes; development of recombinant versions of human α_1-PI; conditions other than emphysema that are associated with α_1-PI; and some other aspects related to the research and development of α_1-PI for therapeutic use.

---

* The findings and conclusions in this article have not been formally disseminated by the Food and Drug Administration and should not be construed to represent any Agency determination or policy

2. Human α_1-PI and α_1-PI deficiency

2.1 Structure and function of α_1-PI

Human alpha-1-proteinase inhibitor (α_1–PI), also known as alpha-1-antitrypsin, is the most abundant inhibitor of serine proteases in plasma. It is predominantly synthesized in hepatocytes, but is also produced, to a lower extent, by alveolar macrophages, neutrophils, and some other cells (White et al., 1981; Carlson et al., 1988; Paakko et al., 1996). In healthy individuals, the concentration of α_1–PI in blood normally varies from 20 μM to 53 μM (1.04-2.76 g/L) (Brantly et al., 1988; Brantly et al., 1991) with a half-life in the circulation of about 3-5 days (Crystal, 1989; Kalsheker et al., 2002). Though α_1–PI has a wide range of inhibitory activities, its main physiological role is known to be the inhibition of polymorphonuclear leukocyte (neutrophil) elastase (NE) in the lungs (Travis, 1988). In the lower respiratory tract of healthy lungs, α_1–PI provides more than 90% of the anti–neutrophil elastase protection (Crystal, 1991; Crystal et al., 1989). Hereditary α_1–PI deficiency (with levels of α_1–PI in blood below 11 μM, insufficient for inhibition of NE) is classically associated with development of early-onset pulmonary emphysema, a hallmark of α_1–PI deficiency (Crystal et al., 1989; Snider, 1992). Smoking is known to be the biggest risk factor for developing emphysema; in smokers with α_1–PI deficiency a severe lung impairment is usually observed in their fourth decade of life.

α_1-PI is encoded by a single 12.2 kb gene (Pi) located on the long arm of chromosome 14 (Long et al., 1984; Rabin et al., 1986). Over 120 alleles of α_1–PI have been identified with approximately 35 of them being associated with α_1–PI deficiency, including Z-allele, which is the most common cause of the deficiency when inherited in a homozygous fashion. Due to a single mutation in the mobile domain (Glu342Lys), the α_1–PI Z-mutant undergoes aberrant conformational transitions that prompts the protein to aggregate. This results in retention of polymerized α_1–PI Z mutant within hepatocytes, thus inducing disease conditions in the liver and causing α_1–PI deficiency in the circulation (Ekeowa et al., 2011; Lomas, 2005; Volpert et al., 2000). The prevalence of three major α_1–PI variants (PiM, PiS, and PiZ) defines the number of carriers (PiMZ and PiMS) and individuals with deficiency phenotypes (PiZZ, PiSZ, and PiSS). The epidemiology of α_1–PI deficiency and its clinical manifestations, including lung diseases and liver diseases, has been described in detail (Ekeowa et al., 2011; Luisetti & Seersholm, 2004; Needham & Stockley, 2004; Gooptu & Lomas, 2009). Based on the α_1–PI serum concentration, a common classification to define α_1–PI deficiency includes the four major categories: (1) normal (with α_1–PI serum levels not lower than 20 μM); (2) deficient (with α_1–PI concentrations in serum lower than 20 μM); (3) dysfunctional (with normal α_1–PI level, but lost or lower inhibitory activity); and (4) null (with α_1–PI serum concentrations below the detectable level).

α_1–PI is a 52 kDa glycoprotein belonging to the serine protease inhibitor (serpin) superfamily, which in addition to α_1-PI also includes α_1-antichymotrypsin, antithrombin, plasminogen activator inhibitor, C1 esterase inhibitor, and many others (Stein & Carrell, 1995; Silverman et al., 2001). A single polypeptide chain of α_1-PI is comprised of 394 amino acid residues, including one cysteine, 2 tryptophanes, and 9 methionine residues (Carp et al., 1982; Johnson & Travis, 1979). Three N-linked glycans attached to asparagine residues 46, 83, and 247 represent ~12% of α_1–PI by molecular weight (Mega et al., 1980a,b;
Carrell et al., 1981, 1982). The carbohydrate moiety is comprised of biantennary N-glycans, but also triantennary and traces of tetraantennary structures grounded on the mannose fork core and containing N-acetyl glucosamine, galactose, and terminal negatively-charged sialic

(N-acetylneuraminic) acid (Mega et al., 1980b; Travis & Salvesen, 1983; Kolarich et al., 2006a). The glycosylation pattern is a major cause of the iso-electric focusing (IEF) pattern typical for α_1–PI with major isoforms M2, M4, M6, and also M7 and M8 due to the N-terminal truncation (Jeppsson et al., 1985; Kolarich et al., 2006a,b). Some characteristics of human α_1–PI are listed in Table 1. Like the majority of other native glycoproteins, α_1-PI is intrinsically a highly heterogeneous moiety, mainly due to variably trimmed glycosylation and an N-terminal pentapeptide that can be absent (Hercz, 1985; Krasnewich et al., 1995; Vaughan et al., 1982).

Characteristics	Description
Synonyms	alpha-1-proteinase inhibitor, alpha-1-antitrypsin
Common abbreviations	α_1–PI, alpha-1-PI, α_1–AT, alpha-1-AT, A1AT, ATT, AT
Classification	Serine proteinase inhibitor (serpin)
Substrates	Neutrophil elastase, trypsin, chymotrypsin
Molecular weight	52,000 Da (50,300 Da by mass spectrometric analysis)
Glycosylation	Three N-attached carbohydrates (12% w/w)
Polypeptide	Single polypeptide chain of 394 amino acid residues
Heterogeneity	Highly heterogeneous protein
Major isoforms	M2, M4, M6, M7 and M8
Half-life in circulation	3-5 days (for native plasma α_1–PI)
Concentration in blood	Acute-phase plasma protein, concentration normally varies from 20 µM to 53 µM (1.04-2.76 g/L)
Major biological activities	Inhibitory anti-serine proteinase activity Multiple non-inhibitory activities
Aggregation	α_1–PI Z mutant is naturally prone to aggregation α_1–PI S mutant aggregates to a lower degree
Physiologically important phenotypes	PiMM (normal); PiSS, PiSZ & PiZZ (deficiency phenotypes); PiZZ, PiSS & PiNull (the most abnormal)
Diagnostic α_1-PI variants (serum concentrations)	Normal (NLT[a] 20 µM); Deficient (lower than 20 µM; Dysfunctional (NLT 20 µM, inactive); Null (n.d.[b] level)
Diseases related to α_1–PI deficiency and aggregation	Pulmonary and liver diseases Other rare diseases (putative)[c]

[a] NLT, not lower than; [b] n.d., non-detectable; [c] See Table 3

Table 1. Characteristics of human α_1-PI

Figure 1 shows a crystal structure of α_1-PI, typical for serpins, which features 9 α-helices, 3 β-sheets (A, B, and C), and a mobile 15-residue reactive center loop (RCL) exposed for interaction with the target serine protease (Johnson & Travis, 1979; Lomas, 2005). Protease attack of the RCL results in cleavage at Met358-Ser359, formation of a covalent α_1-PI-protease complex with the amino-terminal polypeptide inserted into the A β-sheet, and an overall dramatic conformational change (Huntington et al., 2000; Ludeman et al., 2001; Stratikos & Gettins, 1999; Wilczynska et al., 1997).

Unlike the majority of proteins, α_1–PI is naturally folded in a metastable structure which is essential for its function. This is not the most thermodynamically stable form, and thus, α_1-PI is prone to a variety of conformational transitions and modifications (Lomas, 2005; Lomas et al., 1995). Much like other serpins, α_1-PI can intramolecularly convert into a more stable latent form, which is inactive, but the biological activity can be restored via denaturation and refolding (Lomas et al., 1995; Silverman et al., 2001).

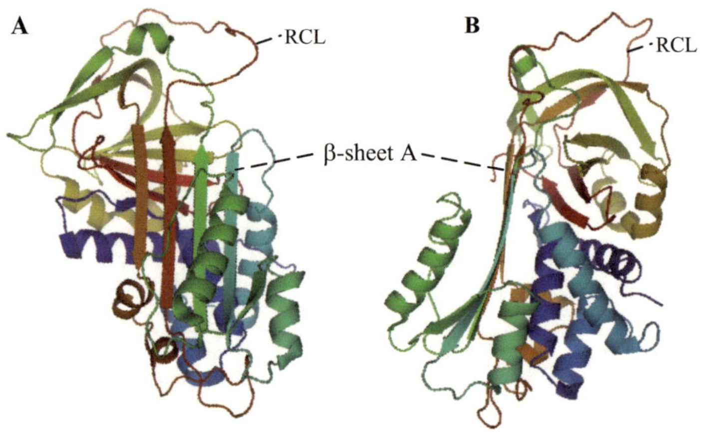

Fig. 1. Crystal structure of α_1-PI (PDB 1HP7) in two projections. (**A**) Front view at the α_1-PI structure in respect to β-sheet A, and (**B**) Side view obtained by 90° clockwise rotation of the molecule. The images were obtained using PyMOL (the PyMOL Molecular Graphics System, Version 1.1r1, Schrödinger, LLC).

In addition to its inhibitory antiprotease function, α_1–PI exhibits a broad spectrum of non-inhibitory activities (Brantly, 2002; Janciauskiene et al., 2011; Nita et al., 2005). Because of the nine methionine residues in α_1–PI molecule, its plausible role as a putative antioxidant has been suggested (*e.g.*, Levine et al., 1999, 2000).

Due to the abundance of α_1–PI in human plasma and its conservative tertiary structure with hydrophobic cavities (Elliott et al., 2000; Lee et al., 2001; Parfrey et al., 2003), α_1–PI has the capacity to bind small hydrophobic molecules. This property has been explored mainly with respect to the peptides and small molecules that may prevent the aggregation of the α_1–PI Z mutant (Mahadeva et al. 2002; Mallya et al., 2007; Chang et al. 2009).

2.2 The α_1-PI deficiency and α_1-PI replacement therapy

There are approximately 60,000-100,000 severely deficient individuals in the United States which define α_1-PI deficiency as a rare disease. However, according to several publications, α_1-PI deficiency is widely under- and mis-diagnosed (*e.g.*, de Serres, 2003; Bals et al., 2007). As reported by the World Health Organization (WHO, 1997), only 4% of the individuals with α_1-PI deficiency cases are identified, and only a portion of them are receiving treatment. Currently licensed treatment of the patients with α_1-PI deficiency and manifestation of pulmonary emphysema involves intravenous infusion of plasma-derived α_1-PI preparations with the recommended dose of 60 mg of active α_1-PI per kg of body weight administered once weekly. To maintain a threshold level of α_1-PI (11μM), α_1–PI-deficient patients should receive augmentation therapy for the duration of their lives, to slow the progression of emphysema. This nadir level has been determined based on α_1-PI levels observed in the plasma of individuals who are heterozygous for Z-mutant α_1−PI and who do not develop emphysema. Evaluation of the efficacy of α_1-PI products used in clinical studies is based on surrogate markers: the infusion of α_1-PI must elevate the circulating serum level of α_1−PI above an epidemiologically established 'protective threshold' and the protein must be detectable in bronchoalveolar lavage fluid (Juvelekian & Stoller, 2004; Sandhaus, 2009). However, the ability of α_1-PI augmentation therapy to reduce the progression of emphysema still remains to be proven. Safety and efficacy of intravenous α_1-PI augmentation are considered in section 3.3.1. For other disease conditions that may possibly benefit from α_1-PI therapy see section 3.3.3.

3. Research and development of α_1-PI for therapeutic use

3.1 Plasma-derived α_1-PI products

3.1.1 Currently approved α_1-PI products

Currently there are six commercial plasma-derived α_1-PI products (Table 2) licensed by the US FDA for intravenous treatment of patients with hereditary α_1-PI deficiency who show evidence of emphysema. Prolastin® (registered trade name of Bayer Corporation since 1987) was the first α_1-PI product to be approved. Since 2005, when Bayer Corporation was acquired by Talecris Biotherapeutics (Research Triangle Park, NC, USA; www.talecris.com), the product has been manufactured by Talecris. Aralast® (initially registered trademark of Alpha Therapeutic Corporation) was approved in 2003, and has been manufactured under the direction of Baxter Healthcare Corporation since then (Baxter, Westlake Village, CA, USA www.baxter.com). Zemaira® (registered trade name of Aventis Behring since 2003), another available product, is now manufactured by CSL Behring LLC (Kankakee, IL, USA; www.cslbehring-us.com). In 2007, the US FDA approved another of Baxter's preparations of α_1-PI concentrate - Aralast NP® - that has the same formulation as its predecessor, but differs from the earlier approved product by having a significantly lower content of C-terminal lysine-truncated α_1-PI (approximately 2% vs. 67%). In 2009, the US FDA approved Prolastin C®, the updated version of the earlier Talecris product that had been on the market for more than two decades. Due to more sophisticated purification and pathogen reduction steps, including two dedicated viral inactivation steps instead of heat treatment, the specific activity of Prolastin C® (above 0.7 mg of functional α_1-PI per mg of total protein) is twice higher than that of Prolastin®, which means that lower volumes and shorter transfusion time are needed. Most recently, in July 2010, the FDA approved Glassia™ (formerly Respira), a product manufactured by Kamada (Weizmann Science Park, Ness Ziona, Israel; www.kamada.com) and commercially launched by Baxter in the United States and some other countries. Glassia™ is another highly purified α_1-PI (with specific activity above 0.7 mg of active α_1-PI per mg of total protein) and the only α_1-PI product that is available in a ready-to-use liquid form with a shelf-life stability of two years under refrigerated conditions.

α_1−PI products are manufactured as part of a complex plasma fractionation scheme which was originally developed for large-scale production of albumin, but now also yields many other plasma therapeutics*. Since products are made from pooled human plasma, they may

* The US FDA product approval information is available at
http://www.fda.gov/BiologicsBloodVaccines/BloodBloodProducts/ApprovedProducts/LicensedProductsBLAs/FractionatedPlasmaProducts/default.htm

Drug product	Manufacturer	Date of licensure	Product form	Major steps of viral inactivation/removal
Prolastin®	Talecris Biotherapeutics	12/2/1987	Lyophilized powder[b]	Depth Filtration Heat Treatment
Aralast®[c]	Baxter Healthcare Co.	3/21/2003	Lyophilized powder	Solvent/Detergent & Nanofiltration
Zemaira®	CSL Behring	7/8/2003	Lyophilized powder	Heat Treatment & Ultrafiltration
Aralast NP®[d]	Baxter Healthcare Co.	5/4/2007	Lyophilized powder	Solvent/Detergent & Nanofiltration
Prolastin C®	Talecris Biotherapeutics	10/16/20099	Lyophilized powder	Solvent/Detergent & Nanofiltration
Glassia™	Kamada	7/1/2010	Ready-to-use liquid	Solvent/Detergent & Nanofiltration

[a] Based on recent publications including (Stockley, 2010; Tonelli & Brantly, 2010)
[b] Reconstitution using Sterile Water for Injection is required
[c] Aralast®, previously known as Respitin, contains approximately 67% of α_1-PI with the truncated C-terminal lysine (Lys394)
[d] Aralast NP® contains approximately 2% of α_1-PI with truncation of C-terminal lysine residue

Table 2. The plasma-derived α_1-PI therapeutic products approved by the US FDA for chronic augmentation and maintenance therapy in adults with congenital α_1-PI deficiency and clinically evident emphysema[a]

carry the risk of transmitting human infectious agents, *e.g.*, some viruses, and theoretically, the Creutzfeldt-Jakob disease (CJD) agent or disease variant agents, as well as emerging or unknown infectious agents. To reduce the potential risk of transmitting infectious agents, the α_1-PI preparations are manufactured using a number of viral inactivation and removal steps. Currently approved α_1−PI products differ in the procedures used for pathogen reduction. For instance, the heat treatment procedure used in manufacturing of Prolastin was one of the reasons for higher content of inactive and aggregated α_1−PI in the product. The manufacturing procedures of the later products (Table 2) include two dedicated steps that are specifically designed for inactivation and removal of viruses (Hotta et al., 2010). Thus, solvent/detergent treatment and nanofiltration are used as the dedicated pathogen reduction steps in the manufacturing of recently approved Prolastin C®, Glassia™ and both Aralast products. Overall, the manufacturing history of plasma-derived α_1-PI therapeutic products reflects a trend of continous improvement of product quality.

3.1.2 Heterogeneity of α_1-PI products

Heterogeneity of α_1-PI therapeutic preparations is a complex phenomenon. First of all, heterogeneous nature of plasma α_1-PI is an intrinsic property of the native glycoproten (see 2.1). Second, the presence of variously processed α_1-PI forms including latent, cleaved, complexed or aggregated α_1-PI species, is barely avoidable. However, it must be kept minimal as the inactive protein species have a direct influence on the product's specific activity. Third, α_1-PI products purified from pooled human plasma contain certain impurities of other plasma proteins, including albumin, haptoglobin, α_1-antichymotrypsin, α_1-lipoprotein, antithrombin III, C1-esterase inhibitor, etc. The human origin of these impurities ensures their tolerability, however, the level of these plasma proteins in α_1-PI concentrate may significantly increase the non-therapeutic protein load in the α_1-PI preparation intended for transfusion. In addition to all that, multistep manufacturing procedures are known to induce various protein alterations, such as aggregation and chemical modifications (*e.g.*, deamidation, cysteinylation, and C-terminal truncation). Some modifications can be observed by IEF and other techniques (Cowden et al., 2005; Kolarich et al., 2006a, 2006b) and reflected in the product specifications. Currently there are no data that would demonstrate whether these alterations affect the *in vivo* activity, safety, efficacy or immunogenicity of α_1-PI therapeutic preparations. In general, commercial plasma-derived α_1-PI products differ in terms of their purity, specific activity, modifications, and excipients (Lomas et al., 1997; Cowden et al., 2005; Stockley, 2010; Tonelli & Brantly, 2010).

3.2 Research and development of the recombinant versions of human α_1-PI

3.2.1 Advances in the development of recombinant α_1-PI

The plasma supply *per se* is a limited source and appears to be insufficient to meet anticipated clinical demand. Moreover, despite effective viral inactivation/removal steps in the manufacturing of plasma proteins (Cai et al., 2005; Hotta et al., 2010), the risk of contamination with new and unknown pathogens may still exist. Therefore, recombinant technology has been widely explored as an alternative approach for the production of human α_1-PI since the pioneering works of the early 1980s (Bollen et al., 1983; Cabezon et al., 1984; Rosenberg et al., 1984). As evident from numerous reports, both from academic research and industry, the human gene for α_1-PI has been expressed in virtually all available hosts (*E. coli*, various yeasts, fungi, insect cells, CHO cells, human neuronal cells, and produced in transgenic plants and animals). For more details on research and development of recombinant α_1-PI (r-α_1-PI) in different systems and advances and limitations of the recombinant approach for production of stable and biologically active α_1-PI, see our comprehensive 2006 review (Karnaukhova et al., 2006). More recently, the human gene for α_1-PI has been expressed in filamentous fungi (Chill et al., 2009; Karnaukhova et al., 2007), transgenic tomato plants (Agarwal et al., 2009), tobacco cell cultures (Huang et al., 2009; Nadai et al., 2009), and human neuronal cell lines (Blanchard et al., 2011). Nevertheless, no r-α_1-PI is available as a licensed therapeutic treatment. In general, the essential criteria for the development of therapeutics for human use are safety, optimal clinical efficacy, and maximum cost-effectiveness. Among many efforts to develop r-α_1-PI of therapeutic quality (see Karnaukhova et al., 2006), there appear to be only two examples of the r-α_1-PIs for which development went far enough to get to clinical trials. The first was r-α_1-PI produced in the yeasts *Saccromyces cerevisiae* and manufactured by Arriva Pharmaceuticals Inc. (Arriva) for several indications. A nebulized formulation of this non-glycosylated r-α_1-PI preparation has been intended for the treatment of respiratory disorders including emphysema and COPD (phase II clinical trials), and asthma (pre-clinical studies) (Brown, 2006a). Although animal studies have been considered to be successful (Pemberton et al., 2006), human trials have not been recommended (see review by Stokley, 2010). A topical gel formulation of r-α_1-PI has been intended for the treatment of dermatitis and other severe dermatological disorders in phase II clinical trials (see Brown, 2006b).

The second example of the advanced development of recombinant human α_1-PI is large scale production performed in transgenic dairy animals (t-α_1-PI): sheep [by PPL Therapeutics (UK) in partnership with Bayer Biologicals (USA), (Dalrymple & Garner, 1998;

Wright et al., 1991)], and goats [by Genzyme Transgenics Corporation (USA), (Ziomek, 1998)]. The transgenic α_1-PI recovered from sheep milk was purified to 99.9% purity. Even so, sheep native α_1-PI and sheep α_1-antichymotrypsin were major impurities, at 6.7-18.7 mg/L and 60.3-75.8 parts per million, respectively. Two sequential clinical studies were performed to evaluate the safety and immunogenicity of aerosolized transgenic human α_1-PI. None of the subjects had an antibody response to human t-α_1-PI (Tebbutt, 2000; Spencer et al., 2005); however, antibody responses were observed to sheep α_1-PI and to sheep α_1-antichymotrypsin (Spencer et al., 2005). Four patients withdrew from the study due to the development of dyspnea and a decline in lung function, and the later product development was terminated.

3.2.2 Pitfalls in the development of r-α_1-PI for therapeutic use

The general regulatory requirements for biologicals intended for therapeutic use, including r-α_1-PI, are purity, safety, and efficacy. In order to be effective, therapeutic proteins have to be stable *in vivo* and *in vitro* (Karnaukhova et al., 2006). Reviewing the work performed over the last two decades to produce stable and biologically active r-α_1-PI of therapeutic quality, one can see basically two major factors that were impeding the progress: (1) impurities that could induce antibody responses and cause adverse reactions in patients, and (2) lower stability than that of plasma counterpart, mainly caused by the lack of glycosylation or non-human type of glycosylation (the latter may also induce immune responses). Although presently the first reason can be technically better solved, removal of trace amounts of non-human native proteins derived from the host, *e.g.*, sheep α_1-PI, from the human r-α_1-PI to exclude further adverse reactions, requires a much higher level of purification than was possible at the time of that development. As for the second reason, indeed, glycosylation is considered to be a cause of rapid clearance of r-α_1-PI from the circulation (Casolaro et al., 1987; Cantin et al., 2002a). Aberrant glycosylation (or lack of glycans) does not neccessarily affect biological activity of the recombinant protein, but it is important for its stability. According to recently published data, glycosylation of α_1-PI does not interfere with the serpin native state flexibility (or instability) essential for its efficient function, though it may confer resistance to degradation by proteases and thus extend its half-life in the circulation (Sarkar & Wintrode, 2011). Extensive work performed over decades for the development of viable r-α_1-PI of therapeutic quality and lessons learned from these experiences truly paved the way for other protein therapeutics. It is worthwhile to mention two serpins produced in transgenic animals that were recently approved. In 2009, the US FDA approved recombinant antithrombin (ATryn®) produced in the milk of transgenic goats (Fyfe & Tait, 2009). In 2010, another serpin, recombinant human C1-esterase inhibitor (Ruconest®) produced in the milk of transgenic rabbits was granted European marketing authorization (Varga & Farkas, 2011). Both pharmaceutical proteins show a faster clearance, yet it may not be an issue depending on the intended use. For instance, Ruconest® was approved for the treatment of acute attacks of hereditary angioedema, and therefore there is no need to maintain its higher level in blood longer than its action is required. Given a shorter *in vivo* half-life of recombinant α_1-PI, it has been considered for other administration routes and applications, such as inhalation for the treatment of emphysematous condition, and topical application for various skin diseases. However, a convincing proof of the recombinant product efficacy and safety in appropriate clinical trials is as problematic as it is for plasma-derived α_1-PI; large clinical trials in the cases of rare diseases are difficult to perform because of small geographically dispersed patient populations. In addition, a limited population means a limited market, which is less attractive for large investments. No doubt, these reasons markedly slow down the development of r-α_1-PI.

3.3 α_1-PI –based therapies

3.3.1 Safety and efficacy of intravenous α_1-PI augmentation

The intravenous augmentation of α_1-PI was shown to be safe and well tolerated over a long history of the replacement therapy. However, its impact on disease progression and mortality still remains to be convincingly proven. α_1-PI augmentation is assumed to slow down the rate of emphysema development and progression and, thus, to improve the life quality and duration of α_1-PI deficient patients, yet the essential proof of efficacy is missing. According to Hubbard & Crystal (1990), only approximately 2-3% of infused α_1−PI actually reaches the lungs; and the effectiveness of α_1-PI replacement therapy has been evaluated mainly on the bases of biochemical (not clinical) criteria (Tonelli & Brantly, 2010). For recently approved α_1-PI products, their pharmacokinetic equivalence and comparable safety profile to Prolastin were demonstrated (*e.g.*, Stocks et al., 2010). α_1-PI therapy is a life-long and very expensive treatment that may cost up to $150,000 (Silverman, 2009) in the United States. Whether this therapy decreases mortality also remains unknown, as there are no reliable data on mortality, as well as morbidity and survival (Gøtzsche & Johansen, 2010a). Some observational studies support the idea that augmentation therapy may help to slow the decline in lung function (Seersholm et al., 1997; Wencker et al., 2001; Kueppers, 2011). But there are also more critical evaluations including the opinion that α_1-PI augmentation therapy cannot be recommended due to lack of evidence of clinical benefit and the cost of treatment (Gøtzsche & Johansen, 2010a, 2010b). It is currently widely admitted that the efficacy of α_1-PI augmentation therapy has never been persuasively demonstrated and must be proven in a proper clinical trial. Due to the widespread and small clusters of patients all over the country, conducting a prospective, randomized, placebo-controlled clinical trial is challenging. In addition, the development of emphysema proceeds slowly, creating the additional difficulties of monitoring lung function decline and mortality data (Hutchinson & Hughes, 1997; Schluchter et al., 2000).

3.3.2 Alternative routes of administration of α_1-PI products

Due to the inconvenience of life-time intravenous augmentation therapy and low levels of α_1−PI reaching lungs, the inhalation of aerosolized α_1-PI has been suggested as a less invasive and more efficient way to deliver large amounts of α_1-PI directly to the lungs where it is most needed (Hubbard et al., 1989; McElvaney et al., 1991; Cockett, 1999). Although strategies for aerosol therapy of α_1-PI deficiency has been proposed two decades ago (Hubbard et al., 1989; Hubbard & Crystal, 1990), there is still no α_1-PI aerosolized treatment approved. Several studies examined efficiency of the α_1-PI inhalation therapy in animals and in humans (Kropp et al., 2001; Siekmeier, 2010). It was demonstrated (Kropp et al., 2001) that significantly more α_1-PI was deposited in the lungs through the inhalational route than via intravenous infusion (14.6% vs. 2%). Although the inhalation route seems attractive, nevertheless, enabling the inhaled material to reach the lung interstitium, the most important to the emphysematous process region, is still problematic. With regards to recombinant versions of α_1-PI, it is generally assumed that products directly delivered to the lungs may not require the same degree of stability as α_1-PI given intravenously. However, as mentioned above, human studies using r-α_1-PI from transgenic sheep were associated with adverse reactions due to impurities derived from the host (Spenser et al., 2005). Thus, higher levels of purification and more clinical studies are required.

3.3.3 Other α_1-PI applications

Currently, α_1-PI therapeutic preparations are licensed exclusively for one indication, *i.e.*, chronic augmentation and maintenance therapy in individuals with emphysema due to congenital α_1-PI deficiency. Previously unrecognized inherited disorder, α_1-PI deficiency was first described in 1963 (Laurell & Eriksson, 1963) based on the serum electrophoretic analysis that revealed five individuals deficient of α_1–fraction; three of those patients had developed emphysematous conditions. Six years later, in 1969, cirrosis associated with α_1-PI deficiency was described (Sharp et al., 1969). These findings initiated a concept of linkage between α_1-PI deficiency and pulmonary and liver diseases. As evident from the available literature, due to the multiple biological activities of α_1-PI, it has been associated with other lung diseases (first of all, cystic fibrosis) and many non-pulmonary diseases (Table 3). Some of these conditions may possibly benefit from α_1-PI augmentation therapy (see recent reviewes by Blanco et al., 2011 and Janciauskiene et al., 2011).

According to Blanco et al. (2011), α_1-PI therapy has proven remarkable efficacy in small cohorts of α_1-PI-deficient patients who also suffer from fibromyalgia, systemic vasculitis, relapsing panniculitis and bronchial asthma. Although the putative benefits of α_1-PI therapy for treatment of additional rare diseases (some are listed in Table 3) requires much more clinical data than are currently available to support clinical efficacy and safety of α_1-PI treatment, in general it indicates a clear potential for additional α_1-PI supply to satisfy the anticipated clinical demand in near future. Because of controversy related to the additional clinical implications of α_1-PI deficiency, more clinical data are needed to verify whether the reported links between α_1-PI deficiency and other rare diseases are real or accidental.

As a potent anti-inflammatory agent, α_1-PI has been investigated in clinical studies for treatment of cystic fibrosis (Jones & Helm, 2009). Whereas patients with emphysematous conditions suffer from the hereditary α_1-PI deficiency and, thus, insufficient levels of the protease inhibitor in the lungs due to impaired α_1-PI synthesis in hepatocytes, patients with cystic fibrosis may have normal synthesis of α_1-PI and suffer from severe pulmonary inflammation due to high excess of NE in the lungs, leading to a progressive loss of lung function (Allen, 1996; Siekmeier, 2010). Therefore, it has been proposed that both groups of patients may benefit from α_1-PI augmentation therapy to prevent the deleterious effect of free protease (Allen, 1996; Birrer, 1995; Birrer et al, 1996) However, intravenous administration of α_1-PI did not result in a suppression of the respiratory neutrophil elastase burden (McElvaney et al, 1991). Several studies have been conducted using inhalation of an aerosolized α_1-PI in cystic fibrosis and α_1-PI deficiency (Hubbard et al., 1989; Griese et al, 2001, 2007; Martin et al, 2006; Brand et al, 2009).

Whereas several studies that investigated the efficacy of treatment with an aerosolized α_1-PI both in patients with cystic fibrosis and in those with α_1-PI deficiency came to positive conclusions regarding deposition of inhaled α_1-PI in the lungs and its anti-elastase activity (see review by Siekmeier, 2010), the conclusion from other studies was that treatment with α_1-PI did not demonstrate any clinical improvements (Martin, 2006). If further clinical studies support the safety and efficacy of an aerosolized α_1-PI, and it is approved for treatment of cystic fibrosis, the demand for therapeutic α_1-PI preparations could be significantly increased.

Disease	References
Vasculitis	Dowd et al., 1995; Esnault, 1997; Griffith et al., 1996
Panniculitis	Chowdhury et al., 2002; Gross et al., 2009; Kjus et al., 2002; Smith et al., 1987; Valverde et al., 2008
Fibromyalgia	Ablin et al., 2009; Blanco et al., 2004; Blanco et al., 2010
Asthma	Blanco et al., 2008; Blanco et al., 2011; Eden et al., 1997
Pancreatitis	Rabassa et al., 1995; Needlham & Stockley, 2004
Renal	Szönyi et al., 2006; Ting et., 2008
Diabetes	Kalis et al., 2010; Lisowska-Myjak et al., 2006;
Cancer	Li et al., 2011; Lindor et al., 2010; Topic et al., 2011
Rheumatoid arthritis	Grimstein et al., 2010; Grimstein et al., 2011
Atherosclerosis	Stakisaitis et al., 2001; Talmud et al., 2003;
Acute anterior uveitis	Fearnley et al., 1988; Saari et al., 1986
Chronic rhinosinusitis	Kilty et al., 2008, 2010; Maune et al., 1995

Table 3. Conditions other than emphysema and liver disease possibly associated with α_1-PI

3.3.4 Research toward the enhancement of α_1-PI-therapies

During last decade various approaches have been considered for the enhancement of α_1-PI-based therapies. For instance, to prolong a short half-life of r-α_1-PI in the circulation, Cantin and co-workers hypothesized that conjugation of r-α_1-PI with polyethylene glycol (PEG) at Cys^{232} could extend the *in vivo* half-life of recombinant protein in blood and lung (Cantin et al., 2002b). According to their data, the site-specific conjugation with either 20 or 40 kD PEG at Cys^{232} of nonglycosylated r-α_1-PI (human) results in an active inhibitor with extended *in vivo* stability. Moreover, 72 h later after airway instillation, the PEG-r-α_1-PI seemed to be significantly better than glycosylated α_1-PI at protecting the lung against elastase-induced lung hemorrhage. As an example of the *in vitro* biochemical evaluation of the concept, α_1−PI has been considered for its affinity to various small ligands and drugs for different reasons. Mainly this approach has been explored with respect to the peptides and small molecules in order to prevent the aggregation of Z mutant (*e.g.*, Mallya et al., 2007; Chang et al. 2009). In the meantime, the protein's potential for binding small ligands of pharmaceutical interest has been proposed as a promising approach that is directed at, and may ultimately enhance, currently existing α_1−PI therapies (Karnaukhova et al., 2010). For instance, α_1−PI's affinity to retinoic acid, which is known for a wide range of physiological activities including alveolar repair and regrowth (Roche clinical studies, see Stockley, 2010; Massaro & Massaro, 1996, 1997) and tissue rejuvenation in various dermatologic diseases, has been convincingly demonstrated in biochemical experiments *in vitro* (Karnaukhova et al., 2010). As α_1−PI augmentation therapy cannot cure, but may only slow down, the progression of emphysema, its complexation with retinoic acid could be more efficient for treatment than α_1−PI alone. It is noteworthy that the interactions of α_1−PI with several other physiologically active ligands (including porphyrins) may reveal additional properties of this multifunctional serpin.

4. Conclusions

Since α_1-PI deficiency was first described by Carl-Bertil Laurell and Sten Eriksson (Laurell & Eriksson, 1963) as a condition that could lead to the development of severe obstructive pulmonary disease, our knowledge about α_1-PI structure-function relationships and clinical manifestations of α_1-PI deficiency has increased tremendously. Moreover, multi-disciplinary research efforts prompted the development of α_1-PI-based augmentation therapy to maintain the inhibitor level above the protective threshold. Since 1987, several α_1-PI products derived from pooled human plasma have been approved and are currently available to slow down the progression of emphysematous conditions in α_1-PI-deficient patients. In addition, due to its multiple physiological activities, α_1-PI has been identified for its putative involvement in several other rare diseases, the treatment of which may possibly benefit from α_1-PI-based therapies. As an alternative to intravenous administration that may improve the efficacy of α_1-PI treatment, the inhalation of aerosolized α_1-PI preparations has been in clinical trials. Recombinant versions of human α_1-PI have been produced in all available hosts and in several transgenic animals. These efforts made a remarkable impact on the research realm of recombinant protein therapeutics, but did not yet bring any viable version of recombinant α_1-PI to the treatment. In regards to therapeutic preparations and their use, there are several questions to be addressed when looking to the future. Keeping in mind the long history of replacement therapy using currently approved plasma-derived α_1-PI products, it is essential that the efficacy of α_1-PI replacement therapy be clearly demonstrated in prospective, randomized, placebo-controlled trials. Will the efficacy of inhalation therapy using aerosolized α_1-PI preparations be proven to be superior to that of the intravenous route? Will the recombinant/transgenic versions of human α_1-PI be optimized to meet the requirements for protein therapeutics? Will other rare diseases currently implicated in association with α_1-PI and α_1-PI deficiency be clearly proven to benefit from α_1-PI treatment? From the standpoint of product quality, safety and efficacy, the current state of research and development of α_1-PI for therapeutic use demonstrates a symbiosis of the recent achievements and controversies, hopefully typical of our progress.

5. References

Ablin, J.N., Bar-Shira, A., Yaron, M. & Orr-Urtreger, A. (2009). Candidate-gene approach in fibromyalgia syndrome: association analysis of the genes encoding substance P receptor, dopamine transporter and alpha1-antitrypsin. *Clin Exp Rheumatol,* Vol. 27, No.5 Suppl 56, (September-October 2009), pp. S33-S38, ISSN 0392-856X

Agarwal, S., Jha, S., Sanyal, I. & Amla, D.V. (2009). Effect of point mutations in translation initiation context on the expression of recombinant human alpha (1)- proteinase inhibitor in transgenic tomato plants. *Plant Cell Rep,* Vol.28, No.12, (December 2009), pp. 1791-1798, ISSN: 0721-7714

Allen, E.D. (1996). Opportunities for the use of aerosolized α_1-antitrypsin for the treatment of cystic fibrosis. *Chest,* Vol.110, Supl.6, (December 1996), pp. 256S-260S, ISSN 0012-3692

Bals, R., Koczulla, R., Kotke, V., Andress, J., et al. (2007). Identification of individuals with alpha-1-antitrypsin deficiency by a targeted screening program. *Respir Med,* Vol. 101, No.8, (August 2007), pp. 1708-1714, ISSN 0954-6111

Birrer, P. (1995). Proteases and antiproteases in cystic fibrosis: pathogenetic considerations and therapeutic strategies. *Respiration* Vol. 62, Suppl.1, pp. 25S–28S, ISSN 0025-7931

Birrer, P., McElvaney, N.G., Rudeberg, A., et al. (1994). Protease-antiprotease imbalance in the lungs of children with cystic fibrosis. *Am J Respir Crit Care Med*, Vol.150, (July 1994), pp. 207–213, ISSN ISSN 1073-449X

Blanchard, V., Liu, X., Eigel, S., Kaup, M., Rieck, S., Janciauskiene, S., Sandig, V., Marx, U., Walden, P., Tauber, R. & Berger, M. (2011). N-Glycosylation and biological activity of recombinant human alpha1-antitrypsin expressed in a novel human neuronal cell line. *Biotechnol Bioeng*, Vol.108, No.9, (September 2011), pp. 2118-2128, ISSN 0006-3592

Blanco. I., Canto, H., de Serres, F.J., Bustillo, E.F. & Rodríguez, M.C. (2004). Alpha-1-antitrypsin replacement therapy efficiently controls fibromyalgia symptoms in two PI ZZ alpha-1-antitrypsin deficiency patients. *J Rheumatol*, Vol.31, No.10, (October 2004), pp. 2082-2085, ISSN 0315-162X

Blanco, I., Canto, H., Flóres, J., Camblor, C., Cárcaba, V., de Serres, F.J., Janciauskiene, S. & Bustillo, E.F. (2008). Long-term augmentation therapy with alpha-1 antitrypsin in an MZ-AAT severe persistent asthma. *Monaldi Arch Chest Dis*, Vol.69, No.4, (December 2008) pp. 178-82, ISSN 1122-0643

Blanco, I., Astudillo, A., Domínguez, F., Janciauskiene, S., Cárcaba, V., Gallo, C., Canto, H., de Serres, F.J. & Bustillo, E.F. (2010). Intravenous infusions of purified alpha 1-antitrypsin effectively controls symptoms and reverts muscle biopsy changes in an MZ-alpha-1 antitripsyn deficiency and fibromyalgia syndrome patient. *J Musculoskel Pain*, Vol.18, No.2, (June 2010), pp. 167-172, ISSN 1058-2452

Blanco, I., Lara, B. & de Serres, F. (2011). Efficacy of alpha1-antitrypsin augmentation therapy in conditions other than pulmonary emphysema. *Orphanet J Rare Dis*, Vol.6, No.14, doi:10.1186/1750-1172-6-14, (April 2011), ISSN 1750-1172

Bollen, A., Herzog, A., Cravador, A., Herion, P. et al. (1983). Cloning and expression in *E. coli* of full length DNA coding for human A_1AT. *DNA* Vol.4, No.4, pp.255-264, ISSN 0198-0238

Brand, P., Schulte, M., Wencker, M., Herpich, C.H., Klein, G., Hanna, K. & Meyer, T. (2009). Lung deposition of inhaled α_1-proteinase inhibitor in cystic fibrosis and α_1-antitrypsin deficiency. *Eur Respir J*, Vol.34, (August 2009), pp. 354-360, ISSN 0903-1936

Brantly, M. (2002). α1−Antitrypsin: Not just an antiprotease: Extending the half-life of a natural anti-inflammatory molecule by conjugation with polyethylene glycol. *Am J Respir Cell Mol Biol*, Vol.27, No.6, (December 2002), 652-654, ISSN 1044-1549

Brantly, M., Nukiwa, Y. & Crystal, R.G. (1988). Molecular basis of α1-antitrypsin deficiency. *Am J Med, Vol.*84, No. 6A, (June 1988), pp. 13-31, ISSN 0002-9343

Brantly, M.L., Wittes, J.T., Vogelmeier, C.F., Hubbard R.C., et al. (1991). Use of highly purified α1-antitrypsin standard to establish ranges for the common normal and deficient α1- antitrypsin phenotypes. *Chest*, Vol.100, No.3, (September 1991), pp. 703-708, ISSN 0012-3692

Brown, W.M. (2006b). rAAt (dermatological) Arriva/ProMetric. *Curr Opin Mol Ther*, Vol.8, No.1, (February 2006), pp. 69-75, ISSN 1464-8431

Brown, W.M. (2006a). rAAt (inhaled) Arriva/Hyland Immuno. *Curr Opin Mol Ther*, Vol.8, No.1, (February 2006), pp. 76-82, ISSN 1464-8431

Cabezon, T., De Wilde, M., Herion, P., Lorian, R. & Bollen, A. (1984). Expression of human α_1-antitrypsin cDNA in the yeast Saccharomyces cerevisiae. *Proc Natl Acad Sci USA,* Vol.81, No.21, (November 1984), pp. 6594–6598, ISSN 0027-8424

Cai, K., Gierman, T.M., Hotta, J., Stenland, C.J., Lee, D.C., Pifat, D.Y. & Petteway, Jr. S.R. (2005). Ensuring the biologic safety of plasma-derived therapeutic proteins. Detection, inactivation and removal of pathogens. *Biodrugs,* Vol.19, No.2, pp. 79-96, ISSN 1173-8804

Cantin, A., Woods, D.E., Cloutier, D., Heroux, J., Dufour, E.K. & Ledoc, R. (2002a). Leukocyte elastase inhibition therapy in cystic fibrosis: role of glycosylation on the distribution of alpha-1-proteinase inhibitor in blood versus lung. *J Aerosol Med,* Vol.15, No.2, (Summer 2002), pp. 141-148, ISSN 0894-2684

Cantin, A.M., Woods, D.E., Cloutier, D., Dufour, E.K. & Leduc, R. (2002b). Polyethylene glycol conjugation at Cys232 prolongs the half life α1 proteinase inhibitor. *Am J Respir Cell Mol Biol,* Vol.27, No.6, (December 2002), pp. 659–665, ISSN 1044-1549

Carlson, J.A., Rogers, B.B., Sifers, R.N., et al. (1988). Multiple tissues express alpha 1-antitrypsin in transgenic mice and man. *J Clin Invest,* Vol.82, No.1 (April 1988), pp. 26–36, ISSN 0021-9738

Carp, H., Miller, F., Hoidal, J.R. & Janoff, A. (1982). Potential mechanism of emphysema: alpha 1-proteinase inhibitor recovered from lungs of cigarette smokers contains oxidized methionine and has decreased elastase inhibitory capacity. *Proc Natl Acad Sci USA,* Vol.79, No.6, (March 1982), pp. 2041-2045, ISSN 0027-8424

Carrell, R.W., Jeppson, J.O., Vaughan, L., Brennan, S.O., Owen, M.C. & Boswell, D.R. (1981). Human α_1-antitrypsin: carbohydrate attachment and sequence homology. *FEBS Lett,* Vol.135, No.2, (December 1981), pp. 301-303, ISSN 0014-5793

Carrell, R.W., Jeppson, J.O., Laurell, C.B., Brennan, S.O., Owen, M.C., Vaughan, L. & Boswell, D.R. (1982). Structure and variation of human α_1-antitrypsin. *Nature* (London), Vol.298, No.5872, (July 1982), pp. 329-334, ISSN 0028-0836

Casolaro, M.A., Fells, G., Wewers, M., et al. (1987). Augmentation of lung antineutrophil elastase capacity with recombinant human alpha-1-antitrypsin. *J Appl Physiol,* Vol.63, No.5, (November 1987), pp. 2015-2023, ISSN 8750-7587

Chang, Y.P., Mahadeva, R., Chang, W.S., Lin, S.C. & Chu, Y.H. (2009). Small-molecule peptides inhibit Z alpha(1)-antitrypsin polymerization. *J Cell Mol Med,* Vol.13, No.8B, (August 2009), pp. 2304-2316, ISSN 1582-1838

Chill, L., Trinh, L., Azadi, P., Ishihara, M., Sonon, R., Karnaukhova, E., Ophir, Y., Golding, B. & Shiloach, J. Production, purification, and characterization of human α_1-proteinase inhibitor from *Aspergillus niger*. *Biotechnol Bioeng,* Vol.102, No.3, (February 2009), pp. 828-844, ISSN 0006-3592

Chowdhury, M.M., Williams, E.J., Morris, J.S., Ferguson, B.J., McGregor, A.D., Hedges, A.R., Stamatakis, J.D. & Pope, F.M. (2002). Severe panniculitis caused by homozygous ZZ alpha1- antitrypsin deficiency treated successfully with human purified enzyme (Prolastin). *Br J Dermatol,* Vol.147, No.6, (December 2002), pp. 1258-1261, ISSN 0007-0963

Cockett, M.I. (1999). Technology evaluation: cystic fibrosis therapy, Genzyme. *Curr Opin Mol Ther* Vol.1, No.2, (April 1999), pp. 279-283, ISSN 1464-8431

Cowden, D.I., Fisher, G.E. & Weeks, R.L. (2005). A pilot study comparing the purity, functionality and isoform composition of alpha-1-proteinase inhibitor (human) products. *Curr Med Research Opinion* Vol.21, No.6 (June 2005), pp. 877-883, ISSN 0300-7995

Crystal, R.G. (1989). The α1-antitrypsin gene and its deficiency states. *Trends Genet,* Vol. 5, No.12, (December 1989), pp. 411-417, ISSN 0168-9525

Crystal, R.G., Brantly, M.L., Hubbard, R.C., Curiel, D.T., States, D.J, & Holmes, M.D. (1989). The alpha 1-antitrypsin gene and its mutations. Clinical consequences and strategies for therapy. *Chest,* Vol.95, No.1, (January 1989), pp. 196-208, ISSN 0012-3692

Crystal, R.G. (1991). α_1-Antitrypsin deficiency: pathogenesis and treatment. *Hospital Practice,* Vol.15, (February 1991), pp. 81-94, ISSN 8750-2836

Dalrymple, M.A. & Garner, I. (1998). Genetically modified livestock for the production of human proteins in milk. *Biotechnol Genet Eng Rev,* Vol.15, pp. 33-49, ISSN 0264-8725

de Serres, F.J. (2003). Alpha-1 Antitrypsin deficiency is not a rare disease but a disease that is rarely diagnosed. *Environ Health Perspect,* Vol.111, No.16, (December 2003), pp. 1851–1854, ISSN 0091-6765

Dowd, S.K., Rodgers, G.C. & Callen, J.P. (1995). Effective treatment with alpha 1-protease inhibitor of chronic cutaneous vasculitis associated with alpha 1-antitrypsin deficiency. *J Am Acad Dermatol,* Vol.33, No.5, Pt. 2, (November 1995), Pt. 2, pp. 913-916, ISSN 0190-9622

Eden, E., Mitchell, D., Mehlman, B. et al. (1997). Atopy, asthma, and emphysema in patients with severe alpha-1-antitrypsin deficiency. *Am J Respir Crit Care Med,* Vol.156, (July 1997), pp. 68-74, ISSN 1073-449X

Ekeowa, U.I., Marciniak, S.J. & Lomas, D.A. (2011). α(1)-antitrypsin deficiency and inflammation. *Expert Rev Clin Immunol,* Vol.7, No.2, (March 2011), pp. 243-252, ISSN 1744-666X

Elliott, P.R., Pei, X.Y., Dafforn, T.R., Lomas, D.A. (2000). Topography of a 2.0 Å structure of a1-antitrypsin reveals targets for rational drug design to prevent conformational disease. *Protein Sci,* Vol.9, No.7, (July 2000), pp. 1274–1281, ISSN 0961-8368

Esnault, V.L. (1997). ANCA-positive vasculitis and alpha 1-antitrypsin deficiency: could free ANCA antigens released by neutrophils mediate vasculitic lesions? *Nephro Dlial Transplant,* Vol.12, (February 1997), pp. 249-251, ISSN 0931-0509

Fearnley, I.R., Spalton, D.J., Ward, A.M., Slavin, B. & Muncey, F. (1988). Alpha 1- antitrypsin phenotypes in acute anterior uveitis. *Br J Ophthalmol,* Vol.72, (August 1988), pp. 636-639, ISSN 0007-1161

Fyfe, A. & Tait, R.C. (2009). Antithrombin-α for the prophylaxis of venous thrombosis in congenital antithrombin deficiency. *Expert Rev Hematol,* Vol.2, No.5, (October 2009), pp. 499-507, ISSN 1747-4086

Gooptu, B. & Lomas, D.A. (2009). Conformational pathology of the serpins: themes, variations, and therapeutic strategies. *Annu Rev Biochem,* Vol.78, (July 2009), pp. 147-76, ISSN 0066-4154

Gøtzsche, P.C. & Johansen, H.K. (2010a). Intravenous alpha-1 antitrypsin augmentation therapy for treating patients with alpha-1 antitrypsin deficiency and lung disease *Cochrane Database of Syst Rev,* Vol. 7, (July 2010), p. CD007851, ISSN 1469-493X

Gøtzsche, P.C. & Johansen, H.K. (2010b). Intravenous alpha-1 antitrypsin augmentation therapy: systematic review. *Dan Med Bull,* Vol. 57, No.9, (September 2010), p. A4175, ISSN 0907-8916

Griese, M., Latzin, P., Kappler, M., Weckerle, K., Heinzlmaier, T., Bernhardt, T. & Hartl, D. (2007). α_1-Antitrypsin inhalation reduces airway inflammation in cystic fibrosis patients. *Eur Respir J*, Vol.29, (February 2007), pp. 240-250, ISSN 0903-1936.

Griese, M., von Bredow, C., Birrer, P., Schams, A. (2001). Inhalation of α_1-protease inhibitor in cystic fibrosis does not affect surfactant convertase and surface activity. *Pulm Pharmacol Ther*, Vol.14, pp. 461-467, ISSN 1094-5539

Griffith, M.E., Lovegrove, J.U., Gaskin, G., Whitehouse, D.B. & Pusey, C.D. (1996). C-antineutrophil cytoplasmic antibody positivity in vasculitis patients is associated with the Z allele of alpha-1-antitrypsin, and the P-antineutrophil cytoplasmic antibody positivity with the S allele. *Nephrol Dial Transplant*, Vol.11, (March 1996), pp. 438-443, ISSN 0931-0509

Grimstein, C., Choi, Y.K., Satoh, M., et al. (2010). Combination of alpha-1 antitrypsin and doxycycline suppresses collagen-induced arthritis. *J Gene Med*, Vol.12, No.1 (January 2010), pp. 35-44, ISSN 1099-498X

Grimstein, C., Choi, Y.K., Wasserfall, C.H., et al. (2011). Alpha-1 antitrypsin protein and gene therapies decrease autoimmunity and delay arthritis development in mouse model. *J Transl Med*, Vol.9, (February 2011), No.21, pp. 1-13, ISSN 1479-5876

Gross, B., Grebe, M., Wencker, M., Stoller, J.K., Bjursten, L.M., Janciauskiene, S. (2009). New findings in PiZZ alpha(1)-antitrypsin deficiency-related panniculitis. Demonstration of skin polymers and high dosing requirements of intravenous augmentation therapy. *Dermatology*, Vol.218, No.4, pp. 370-375, ISSN 1018-8665

Hercz, A. (1985). Proteolytic cleavages in α1-antitrypsin and microheterogeneity. *Biochem Biophys Res Commun*, Vol.128, No.1, (April 1985), pp. 199-203, ISSN 0006-291X

Hotta, J., Chao, S.F., Gall, M., Roth, N.J., Lang, J. & Lee, D. (2010). Effective and robust enveloped virus inactivation by a non-traditional solvent/detergent treatment step. *US Respiratory Disease*, Vol.6, pp. 40–46

Huang, T.K., Plesha, MA., Falk, B.W., Dandekar, A.M. & McDonald, K.A. (2009). Bioreactor strategies for improving production yield and functionality of a recombinant human protein in transgenic tobacco cell cultures. *Biotechnol Bioeng*, (February 2009), Vol.102, No.2, pp. 508-520, ISSN 0006-3592

Hubbard, R.C., Brantly, M.L., Sellers, S.E., et al. (1989). Anti-neutrophil-elastase defenses of the lower respiratory tract in a1-antitrypsin deficiency directly augmented with an aerosol of a1-antitrypsin. *Ann Intern Med*, Vol.111, (August 1989), pp. 206–212, ISSN 0003-4819

Hubbard, R.C. & Crystal, R.G. (1990). Strategies for aerosol therapy of alpha1-antitrypsin deficiency by the aerosol route. *Lung*, Vol.168 (Suppl), pp. 565-578, ISSN 0341-2040

Hutchinson, D.C. & Hughes, M.D. (1997). Alpha-1-antitrypsin replacement therapy: will its efficacy ever be proved? *Eur Respir J*, Vol.10, pp. 2191-2193, ISSN 0903-1936

Huntington, J.A., Read, R.J. & Carrell, R.W. (2000). Structure of a serpin-protease complex shows inhibition by deformation. *Nature*, Vol.407, No.6806, (October 2000), pp. 923–926, ISSN 0028-0836

Janciauskiene, S.M., Bals, R., Koszulla, R., Vogelmeier, C., Köhnlein, T. & Welte, T. (2011). The discovery of α1-antitrypsin and its role in health and disease. *Respir Med*, Vol.105, (August 2011), pp. 1129-1139, ISSN 0954-6111

Jeppsson, J. O., Lilja, H. & Johansson, M. (1985). Isolation and characterization of two minor fractions of alpha 1-antitrypsin by high-performance liquid chromatographic chromatofocusing. *J Chromatogr,* (June 1985), Vol.*327*, pp. 173–177, ISSN 0021-9673

Jones, A.M. & Helm, J.M. (2009). Emerging treatments in cystic fibrosis. *Drugs,* Vol.69. No.14, (October 2009), pp. 1903-1910, ISSN 0012-6667

Johnson, D. & Travis, J. (1979). The oxidative inactivation of human alpha-1-proteinase inhibitor. Further evidence for methionine at the reactive center. *J Biol Chem,* Vol.254, No.10, (May 1979), pp. 4022-4026, ISSN 0021-9258

Juvelekian, G.S. & Stoller, J.K. (2004). Augmentation therapy for α1-antitrypsin deficiency. *Drugs,* Vol.64, No.16, pp. 1743-1756, ISSN 0012-6667

Kalis, M., Kumar, R., Janciauskiene, S., Salehi, A. & Cilio, C.M. (2010). α1-antitrypsin enhances insulin secretion and prevents cytokine-mediated apoptosis in pancreatic β-cells. *Islets,* Vol.2, No.3 (May-June 2010), pp. 185-189, ISSN 1938-2014

Kalsheker, N., Morley, S. & Morgan, K. (2002). Gene regulation of the serine proteinase inhibitors alpha1-antitrypsin and alpha1- antichymotrypsin. *Biochem Soc Trans,* Vol.30, No.2, (April 2002), pp. 93-98, ISSN 0300-5127

Karnaukhova, E. (2010). Interactions of alpha1-proteinase inhibitor with small ligands of therapeutic potential: binding with retinoic acid. *Amino Acids,* Vol.38, No.4, (April 2010), pp. 1011-1020, ISSN 0939-2199

Karnaukhova, E., Ophir, Y., Trinh, L., Dalal, N., Punt, P.J., Golding, B. & Shiloach, J. (2007). Expression of human α_1-proteinase inhibitor in *Aspergillus niger. Microbial Cell Factories,* Vol. 6, No.34, (October 2007), pp. 1-10, ISSN 1475-2859

Karnaukhova, E., Ophir, Y. & Golding, B. (2006). Recombinant human alpha-1 proteinase inhibitor: towards therapeutic use. *Amino Acids,* Vol.30, No.4, (June 2006), pp. 317-332, ISSN 0939-4451

Kjus, T., Lützow-Holm, C., Christensen, O.B. (2002). Treatment of panniculitis associated with alpha-1-antitrypsin deficiency with alpha-1-protease inhibitor. *Br J Dermatol,* Vol.147, No.6, pp. 1258-1261, ISSN 0007-0963

Kilty, S.J. & Desrosiers, M.Y. (2008). Chronic sinusitis and alpha1-antitrypsin deficiency: potential role for protease in rhinosinusitis? *J Otolaryngol Head Neck Surg,* Vol.37, No.6, (December 2008), pp. e179-e182, ISSN 1916-0216

Kilty, S.J., Bossé, Y., Cormier, C., Endam, L.M. & Desrosiers, M.Y. (2010). Polymorphisms in the SERPINA1 (Alpha-1-Antitrypsin) gene are associated with severe chronic rhinosinusitis unresponsive to medical therapy. *Am J Rhinol Allergy,* Vol.24, No.1, (January 2010), pp. e4-e9, ISSN 1945-8924

Kolarich, D., Weber, A., Turecek, P.L., et al. (2006a). Comprehensive glyco-proteomic analysis of human alpha1-antitrypsin and its charge isoforms. *Proteomics,* Vol.6, No.11, (June 2006), pp. 3369-3380, ISSN 1615-9853

Kolarich, D., Turecek, P.L., Weber, A., et al. (2006b). Biochemical, molecular characterization, and glycoproteomic analyses of alpha(1)-proteinase inhibitor products used for replacement therapy. *Transfusion,* Vol.46, No.11, (November 2006), pp. 1959-1977, ISSN 0041-1132

Krasnewich, D.M., Holt, G.D., Brantly, M., Skovby, F., Redwine, J. & Gahl, W.A. (1995). Abnormal synthesis of dolichol-linked oligosaccharides in carbohydrate-deficient glycoprotein syndrome. *Glycobiology,* Vol.5, No.5, (July 1995), pp. 503-510, ISSN 0959-6658

Kropp, J., Wencker, M., Hotze, A., et al. (2001). Inhalation of [^{123}I]α_1-protease inhibitor: toward a new therapeutic concept of α_1-protease inhibitor deficiency? *J Nucl Med,* Vol.42, No.5, (May 2001), pp. 744–751, ISSN 0161-5505

Kueppers, F. (2011). The role of augmentation therapy in alpha-1 antitrypsin deficiency. *Curr Med Res Opin,* Vol.27, No.3, (March 2011), pp. 579-588, ISSN 0300-7995

Laurell, C.B. & Eriksson, S. (1963). The elecrophoreic alpha-1-globulin pattern of serum in alpha1-antitrypsin deficiency. *Scan J Clin Lab Invest,* Vol.15, pp. 132-140, ISSN 0036-5513

Lee, C., Maeng, J.S., Kocher, J.P., Lee, B. & Yu, M.H. (2001). Cavities of a1-antitrypsin that play structural and functional role. *Protein Sci,* Vol.10, No.7, (July 2001), pp. 1446–1453, ISSN 0961-8368

Levine, R.L., Berlett, B.S., Moskovitz, J., Mosoni, L. & Stadtman, E.R. (1999). Methionine residues may protect proteins from critical oxidative damage. *Mech Ageing Dev,* Vol.107, No.3, (March 1999), pp. 323–332, ISSN 0047-6374

Levine, R.L., Moskovitz, J. & Stadtman, E.R. (2000). Oxidation of methionine in proteins: roles in antioxidant defense and cellular regulation. *IUBMB Life,* Vol.50, No.4-5, (October-November 2000), pp. 301- 307, ISSN 1521-6543

Li, Y., Krowka, M.J., Qi, Y., et al. (2011). Alpha1-antitrypsin deficiency carriers, serum alpha 1-antitrypsin concentration, and non-small cell lung cancer survival. *J Thorac Oncol,* Vol.6, No.2, (February 2011), pp. 291-295, ISSN 1556-0864

Lindor, N.M., Yang, P., Evans, I., et al. (2010). Alpha-1-antitrypsin deficiency and smoking as risk factors for mismatch repair deficient colorectal cancer: a study from the colon cancer family registry. *Mol Genet Metab,* Vol.99, (February 2010), pp. 157-159, ISSN 1096-7192

Lisowska-Myjak, B., Pachecka, J., Kaczyńska, B., Miszkurka, G. & Kadziela, K. (2006). Serum protease inhibitor concentrations and total antitrypsin activity in diabetic and non-diabetic children during adolescence. *Acta Diabetol,* Vol. 43, (December 2006), pp. 88-92, ISSN 0940-5429

Lomas, D.A., Elliott, P.R., Chang, W.S.W., Wardell, M.R. & Carrell, R.W. (1995). Preparation and characterization of latent α_1-antitrypsin. *J Biol Chem,* Vol.270, No.10, (March 1995), pp. 5282–5288, ISSN 0021-9258

Lomas, D.A., Elliott, P.R., Carrell, R.W. (1997). Commercial plasma α1-antitrypsin (Prolastin®) contains a conformationally inactive, latent component. *Eur Respir J,* Vol. 10, (March 1997), pp. 672–675, ISSN 0903-1936

Lomas, D. (2005). Molecular mousetraps, α1-antitrypsin deficiency and the serpinopathies. *Clin Med,* Vol.5, No.3, (May-June 2005), pp. 249–57, ISSN 1470-2118

Long, G.L., Chandra, T., Woo, S.L., Davie, E.W. & Kurachi, K. (1984). Complete sequence of the cDNA for human α_1-antitrypsinand the gene for the S variant. *Biochemistry,* Vol.23, No.21, (October 1984), pp. 4828-4837, ISSN 0006-2960

Ludeman, J.P., Whisstock, J.C., Hopkins, P.C.R, Le Bonniec, B.F. & Bottomley, S.P. (2001). Structure of a serpin-enzyme complex probed by cysteine substitutions and fluorescence spectroscopy. *Biophys J,* Vol.80, No.1, (May 2001), pp. 491-497, ISSN 0006-3495

Luisetti, M. & Seersholm, N. (2004). Alpha1-antitrypsin deficiency. 1: epidemiology of alpha1-antitrypsin deficiency. *Thorax,* Vol.59, No.2 (February 2004), pp. 164-169, ISSN 0040-6376

Mahadeva, R., Dafforn, T.R., Carrell, R.W. & Lomas, D.A. (2002). 6-mer peptide selectively anneals to a pathogenic serpin conformation and blocks polymerization. Implications for the prevention of Z alpha(1)-antitrypsin-related cirrhosis. *J Biol Chem,* Vol.277, No.9, (March 2002), pp. 6771–6774, ISSN 0021-9258

Mallya, M., Phillips, R.L., Saldanha, S.A., Gooptu, B., et al. (2007). Small molecules block the polymerization of Z a1-Antitrypsin and increase the clearance of intracellular aggregates. *J Med Chem,* Vol.50, No.22, (November 2007), pp. 5357–5363, ISSN 0022-2623

Massaro, G.D. & Massaro, D. (1996). Postnatal treatment with retinoic acid increases the number of pulmonary alveoli in rats. *Am J Physiol,* Vol.270, No.2 Pt1, (February 1996), pp. L305–L310, ISSN 0002-9513

Massaro, G.D. & Massaro, D. (1997). Retinoic acid treatment abrogates elastase induced pulmonary emphysema in rats. *Nat Med,* Vol.3, No.6, (June 1997), pp. 675–677, ISSN 1078-8956

Martin, S.L., Downey, D., Bilton, D., et al. on behalf of the Recombinant AAT CF Study Team (2006). Safety and efficacy of recombinant α_1-antitrypsin therapy in cystic fibrosis. *Pediatr Pulmonol,* Vol. 41, (February 2006), pp. 177-183, ISSN 8755-6863

Maune, S., Rath, N.F., Görögh, T. & Steinert, R. (1995). Genetic disposition to chronic polypoid sinusitis and alpha 1-proteinase inhibitor deficiency types. *HNO,* Vol.43, (September 1995), pp. 537-539, ISSN 0017-6192

McElvaney, N.G., Hubbard, R.C., Birrer, P., Chernick, M.S., Caplan, D.B., Frank, M.M. & Crystal, R.G. (1991). Aerosol α_1-antitrypsin treatment for cystic fibrosis. *Lancet,* Vol. 337, (February 1991), pp. 392-395, ISSN 0140-6736

Mega, T., Lujan, E. & Yoshida, A. (1980a). Studies on the oligosaccharade chains of human α1-protease inhibitor: I. Isolation of glycopeptides. *J Biol Chem,* Vol.255, No.9, (May 1980), pp. 4053-4056, ISSN 0021-9258

Mega, T., Lujan E. & Yoshida, A. (1980b) Studies on the oligosaccharade chains of human α1-protease inhibitor: II. Structure of oligosaccharides. *J Biol Chem* Vol.255, No.9, (May 1980), pp. 4057-4061, ISSN 0021-9258

Nadai, M., Bally, J., Vitel, M., Job, C., Tissot, G., Botterman, J. & Dubald, M. (2009). High-level expression of active human alpha1-antitrypsin in transgenic tobacco chloroplasts. *Transgenic Res,* Vol.18, No.2, (April 2009), pp. 173-183, ISSN 0962- 8819

Needham, M. & Stockley, R.A. (2004). Alpha 1-antitrypsin deficiency. 3: Clinical manifestations and natural history. *Thorax,* Vol. 59, No.5, (May 2004), 441-445, ISSN 0040-6376

Nita, I., Hollander, C., Westin, U. & Janciauskiene, S.M. (2005). Prolastin, a pharmaceutical preparation of purified human alpha1-antitrypsin, blocks endotoxin-mediated cytokine release. *Respir Res,* Vol.6, No.12, doi:10.1186/1465-9921-6-12; ISSN 1465-9921

Paakko, P., Kirby, M., du Bois, R.M., et al. (1996). Activated neutrophils secrete stored α_1-antitrypsin. *Am J Respir Crit Care Med,* Vol.154, No. 6 Pt1, (December 1996), pp. 1829–1833, ISSN 1073-449X

Parfrey, H., Mahadeva, R., Ravenhill, N.A., et al. (2003). Targeting a surface cavity of alpha 1-antitrypsin to prevent conformational disease. *J Biol Chem,* Vol.278, No.35, (August 2003), pp. 33060–33066, ISSN 0021-9258

Pemberton, P.A., Kobayashi, D., Wilk, B.J., et al. (2006). Inhaled recombinant alpha 1-antitrypsin ameliorates cigarette smoke-induced emphysema in the mouse. *COPD*, Vol.3, No.2, (June 2006), pp. 101-108, ISSN 1541-2555

Rabassa, A.A., Schwartz, M.R. & Ertan, A. (1995). Alpha 1-antitrypsin deficiency and chronic pancreatitis. *Dig Dis Sci*, Vol.40, (September 1995), pp. 1997-2001, ISSN 0163-2116

Rabin, M., Watson, M., Kidd, V., Woo, S.L., Breg, W.R. & Ruddle, F.H. (1986). Regional location of α1-antichymotrypsin and α1-antitrypsin genes on human chromosome 14. *Somatic Cell Mol Gen,* Vol.12, No. (March 1986), pp. 209-214, ISSN 0740-7750

Rosenberg, S., Barr, P.J., Najarian, R.C. & Hallewell, R.A. (1984). Synthesis in yeast of a functional oxidation-resistant mutant of human α_1-antitrypsin. *Nature,* Vol.312, No.5989, (November 1984), pp. 77-80, ISSN 0028-0836

Saari, K.M., Kaarela, K., Korpela, T., Laippala, P., Frants, R.R. & Eriksson, A.W. (1986). Alpha 1-antitrypsin in acute anterior uveitis and rheumatic diseases. *Acta Ophthalmol,* Vol.64, No.5 (October 1986), pp. 522-529, ISSN 0001-639X

Sandhaus, R.A. (2009). Augmentation therapy in alpha-1 antitrypsin deficiency. *COPD*, Vol.6, No.3, (June 2009), pp. 147-148, ISSN 1541-2555

Sarkar, A. & Wintrode, P.L. (2011). Effects of glycosylation on the stability and flexibility of a metastable protein: the human serpin α(1)-antitrypsin. *Int J Mass Spectrom,* Vol. 302, No.1-3, (April 2011), pp. 69-75, ISSN 1387-3806

Seersholm, N., Wencker, M., Banik, N., et al. (1997). Does alpha1-antitrypsin augmentation therapy slow the annual decline in FEV1 in patients with severe hereditary alpha1-antitrypsin deficiency? Wissenschaftliche Arbeitsgemeinschaft zur Therapie von Lungenerkrankungen (WATL) alpha1-AT study group. *Eur Respir J,* Vol.10, (October 1997), pp. 2260–2263, ISSN 0903-1936

Sharp, H.L., Bridges, R.A., Krivit, W. & Freier, E.F. (1969). Cirrhosis associated with alpha-1-antitrypsin deficiency: a previously unrecognized inherited disorder. *J Lab Clin Med,* Vol.73, (June 1969), pp. 934–939, ISSN 0022-2143

Schluchter, M.D., Stoller, J.K., Barker, A.F. et al. (2000). Feasibility of a clinical trial of augmentation therapy for α_1-antitrypsin deficiency. *Am J Respir Crit Care Med,* Vol.161, No.3, (March 2000), pp.796-801, ISSN 1073-449X

Siekmeier, R. (2010). Lung deposition of inhaled alpha-1-proteinase ingibitor (Alpha$_1$-PI) – Problems and experience of Alpha$_1$-PI inhalation therapy in patients with hereditary Alpha$_1$-PI deficiency and cystic fibrosis. *Eur J Med Res,* Vol.15, Suppl. II, (November 2010), pp. 164-174, ISSN 0949-2321

Silverman, G.A., Bird, P.I., Carrell, R.W., et al., (2001). The serpins are an expanding super-family of structurally similar but functionally diverse proteins: evolution, mechanism of inhibition, novel functions, and a revised nomenclature. *J Biol Chem,* Vol.276, No. (September 2001), pp. 33293–33296, ISSN 0021-9258

Silverman, E.K. & Sandhaus, R.A. (2009). Alpha1-antitrypsin deficiency. *New Engl J Med,* Vol. 360, (June 2009), pp. 2749–2757, ISSN 0028-4793

Smith, K.C., Pittelkow, M.R. & Su, W.P. (1987). Panniculitis associated with severe alpha 1-antitrypsin deficiency. Treatment and review of the literature. *Arch Dermatol,* Vol.123, No.12, (December 1987), pp. 1655-1661, ISSN 0003-987X

Snider, G.L. (1992). Emphysema: the first two centuries and beyond: a historical overview, with suggestions for future research. *Am Rev Respir Dis,* Vol.146, No.5 Pt 1, (December 1992), pp. 1334-44 & No.6, pp. 1615-22, ISSN 0003-0805

Spencer, L.T., Humphries, J.E. & Brantly, M.L. (2005). Transgenic Human Alpha 1-Antitrypsin Study Group. Antibody response to aerosolized transgenic human alpha1-antitrypsin. *N Engl J Med,* Vol.352, No.19, (May 2005), pp. 2030-2031, ISSN 0028-4793

Stakisaitis, D., Basys, V. & Benetis, R. (2001). Does alpha-1-proteinase inhibitor play a protective role in coronary atherosclerosis? *Med Sci Monit,* Vol.4, No.4, (Jul-Aug, 2001), pp. 701-11, ISSN 1234-1010

Stein, P.E. & Carrell, R.W. (1995). What do dysfunctional serpins tell us about molecular mobility and disease? *Nat Struct Biol,* Vol.2, No.2, (February 1995), pp. 96-113, ISSN 1072-8368

Stockley, R.A. (2010). Emerging drugs for alpha-1-antitrypsin deficiency. *Expert Opin Emerg Drugs,* Vol.15, No.4, (December 2010), pp. 685-694, ISSN 1472-8214

Stocks, J.M., Brantly, M.L., Wang-Smith, L., et al. (2010). Pharmacokinetic comparability of Prolastin®-C to Prolastin® in $alpha_1$-antitrypsin deficiency: a randomized study. *BMC Clin Pharmacol,* Vol.10, No.13, (September 2010), doi:10.1186/1472-6904-10- 13, ISSN 1472-6904

Stratikos, E. & Gettins P.G.W. (1999). Formation of the covalent serpin-proteinase complex involves translocation of the proteinase by more than 70Å and full insertion of the reactive centre loop into β-sheet A. *Proc Natl Acad Sci USA,* Vol.96, No.9, (April 1999), pp. 4808–4813, ISSN 0027-8424

Szönyi, L., Dobos, M., Vásárhelyi, B., et al. (2006). Prevalence of alpha1-antitrypsin phenotypes in patients with IgA nephropathy. *Clin Nephrol,* Vol.62, pp. 418-422

Talmud, P.J., Martin, S., Steiner, G., et al. (2003). Progression of atherosclerosis is associated with variation in the alpha1-antitrypsin gene. *Arterioscler Thromb Vasc Biol,* Vol.23, No.4, (April 2003), pp. 644-649, ISSN: 1524-4636

Tebbutt, S.J. (2000). Technology evaluation: transgenic alpha-1-antitrypsin (AAT), PPL therapeutics. *Curr Opin Mol Ther,* Vol.2, No.2, (April 2000), pp. 199-204, ISSN 1464-8431

Ting, S.M., Toth, T. & Caskey, F. (2008). Alpha1-antitrypsin (A1AT) deficiency presenting with IgA nephropathy and nephritic syndrome: is renal involvement caused by A1AT deposition? *Clin Nephrol,* Vol. 70, (August 2008), pp. 159-162, ISSN 0301-0430

Tonelli, A.R. & Brantly, M.L. (2010). Augmentation therapy in alpha-1 antitrypsin deficiency: advances and controversies. *Ther Adv Respir Dis,* Vol.4, No.5, (October 2010), pp. 289-312, ISSN 1753-4658

Topic, A., Ljujic, M., Nikolic, A., Petrovic-Stanoevic, N., et al. (2011). Alpha-1-antitrypsin phenotypes and neutrophil elastase gene promoter polymorphisms in lung cancer. *Pathol Oncol Res,* Vol.17, No.1, (March 2011), pp. 75-80, ISSN 1219-4956

Travis, J. (1988). Structure, function, and control of neutrophil proteinases. *Am J Med,* Vol. 84, No.6A, (June 1988), pp. 37-42, ISSN 0002-9343

Travis, J. & Salvesen, G.S. (1983). Human plasma proteinase inhibitors. *Annu Rev Biochem,* Vol.52, No. (1983), pp. 655–709, ISSN 0066-4154

Valverde, R., Rosales, B., Ortiz-de Frutos, F.J., Rodriguez-Peralto, J.L., Ortiz-Romero, P.L. (2008). Alpha-1-antitrypsin deficiency panniculitis. *Dermatol Clin,* Vol.26, (October 2008), pp. 447-451 , ISSN 0733-8635

Varga, L. & Farkas, H. (2011). rhC1INH: a new drug for the treatment of attacks in hereditary angioedema caused by C1-inhibitor deficiency. *Expert Rev Clin Immunol,* Vol.7, No.2, (March 2011), pp. 143-153, ISSN 1744-666X

Vaughan, L., Lorier, M.A. & Carrell, R.W. (1982). α1-Antitrypsin microheterogeneity: isolation and physiological significance of isoforms. *Biochem Biophys Acta,* Vol.701, No.3, (March 1982), pp. 339-345, ISSN 0006-3002

Volpert, D., Molleston, J.P.& Perlmutter, D.H. (2000). Alpha1-antitrypsin deficiency-associated liver disease progresses slowly in some children. *J Pediatr Gastroenterol Nutr*, Vol.31, No.3, (September 2000), pp. 258–63, ISSN 0277-2116

Wencker, M., Fuhrmann, B., Banik, N. & Konietzko, N. (2001). Longitudinal follow-up of patients with alpha1-protease inhibitor deficiency before and during IV alpha1-protease inhibitor, *Chest,* Vol.119, No.3, (March 2001), pp. 737–744, ISSN 0012- 3692

White, R., Lee, D., Habicht, G.S. & Janoff, A. (1981). Secretion of alpha-1-proteinase inhibitor by cultured rat alveolar macrophages. *Am Rev Respir Dis,* Vol.123, No.4, Pt 1, (April 1981), pp. 447–449, ISSN 0003-0805

WHO (1997). World Health Organization, Human Genetics Programme. Alpha-1-antitrypsin deficiency. Report of WHO meeting held in Geneva on 18-20 March 1996, *Bull World Health Organ*, Vol.75, No.5, pp. 397-415

Wilczynska, M., Fa, M., Karolin, J., Ohlsson, P.I., Johansson, L.B. & Ny, T. (1997). Structural insights into serpin-protease complexes reveal the inhibitory mechanism of serpins. *Nat Struct Biol,* Vol.4, No.5, (May 1997), pp. 354–357, ISSN 1072-8368

Wright, G., Carver, A., Cottom, D., Reeves, D., Scott A., Simons, P., Wilmut, I., Gamer, J. & Colman, A. (1991). High level of expression of active human alpha-1-antitrypsin in the milk of transgenic sheep. *Bio/Technology,* Vo.9, No.9, (September 1991), pp. 830−834, ISSN 0733-222X

Ziomek, C.A. (1998). Commercialization of proteins produced in the mammary gland. *Theriogenology,* Vol.49, No.1, (January 1998), pp. 139-144, ISSN 0093-691X

4

Mechanisms Promoting Chronic Lung Diseases: Will Targeting Stromal Cells Cure COPD and IPF?

Lynne A. Murray[1] and Cory M. Hogaboam[2]
[1]*Respiratory, Inflammation and Autoimmunity, MedImmune Ltd, Cambridge,*
[2]*Department of Pathology, University of Michigan Medical School, Ann Arbor, MI,*
[1]*UK*
[2]*USA*

1. Introduction

Tissue remodeling is a common pathology in many diseases. The reparative processes of wound healing result in an increase in extracellular matrix (ECM) generation, serving to restore barrier protection and normal tissue architecture. However in the lung, increased formation of ECM results in decreased lung compliance and impaired gas exchange. The chronic lung diseases COPD (chronic obstructive pulmonary disease) and IPF (idiopathic pulmonary fibrosis) both exhibit increased extracellular matrix (ECM) deposition within the lung due to increased stromal cell number and activation. The chronic nature of the disease is hypothesized to correlate with the extent of scarring and remodeling, with greater evidence being available for COPD rather than IPF. The potential underlying causes of both diseases are numerous, including direct insults to the lung such as cigarette smoke or exhaust particles; as well as underlying autoimmune conditions such as scleroderma or collagen vascular disease. Moreover, a correlation between COPD and smoking is well established; however, any causes for IPF, apart from a familial link, are currently not understood. To date there are no approved anti-fibrotic therapies that target the underlying remodeling in either disease. In order to treat this pathology, understanding the mechanisms promoting continual ECM deposition may elucidate novel therapeutic approaches that could provide clinical benefit to patients suffering from these debilitating diseases. This Chapter will focus on the cellular mechanisms and interactions within the fibrotic lung including resident fibroblast-epithelial cells as well as the cross-talk between fibroblasts and recruited bone marrow derived cells such as fibrocytes and monocytes. Also, the soluble mediators that have been associated with disease and how these can directly and indirectly modulate stromal cell activation will be discussed.

2. COPD and IPF disease pathogenesis

One of the common features between COPD and IPF is the heterogeneous pathology observed in the lung at the macroscopic level in both disease settings. Both diseases exhibit patchy areas of pathology, consisting of ECM proteins or inflammatory infiltrates, with fibrotic regions being juxtaposed to regions of normal alveolar tissue or areas with interstitial leukocyte accumulation. Grossly, COPD contains regions dense in bronchiolar inflammation and consolidated lung tissue, as well as emphysematous areas, due to alveolar destruction [1,2]. In IPF, salient hallmarks of disease included profound collagen deposition, as well as regions of honeycombed lung due to a collapse of alveolar walls [3]. COPD has been clinically separated into distinct GOLD (Global initiative for chronic Obstructive Lung Disease) Stages based primarily on a key parameter of lung function, Forced Expiratory Volume in one second (FEV_1). Here, patients with more significant impairment in FEV_1 have a higher GOLD Stage status. Supporting these changes in lung function analysis of the underlying pathologies of patients within each GOLD Stage has also highlighted that, as the disease progresses, there is an increase in airway wall thickness [4]. Even though the GOLD staging system is universally recognized, there are efforts underway to also separate COPD patients in to fast decliners and slow decliners based on lung function parameters. Extensive work is currently underway to try and stage IPF in an equivalent manner. In this disease, retrospective analysis of patient survival has indicated that there is both a rapidly progressing phenotype and a more slowly progressing phenotype of IPF patients. In the 'rapid' IPF progressors, approximately 50% of patients will die within 6-8 months, whereas this is greatly extended in slow progressors [5,6].

Chronic remodeling is a common feature between IPF and COPD. In order to understand the mechanisms underlying the maintenance, progression and staging of disease, this Book Chapter will focus on the similarities and differences between stromal cells in these patients. We will focus on the phenotypic differences in fibroblasts and myofibroblasts as well as how these cell types interact within the lung (Fig. 1). We will also describe some of the key families of mediators that are found to be elevated in disease and how their mechanism may be directly promoting chronic lung disease. Lastly, we will discuss the potential therapeutic approaches to targeting stromal cells clinically.

3. Profibrotic role of fibroblasts

Fibroblasts play a myriad of important roles in normal tissue function. In the lung they coordinate organogenesis and budding of the lung from the foregut through intimate bi-directional communication with adjacent epithelial cells. Myofibroblasts are "smooth muscle-like cells" that are morphologically similar to fibroblasts, but also express alpha-smooth muscle actin (α-SMA) [7]. Fibroblasts and myofibroblasts are also key cells in the production and homeostatic maintenance of the ECM of the tissue or organ in which they reside. They are metabolically active cells, capable of synthesizing and secreting ECM components such as collagens and proteoglycans. Fibroblasts continually synthesize ECM proteins although the amount they secrete is tightly regulated, with up to 90% of all procollagen molecules being degraded intracellularly prior to secretion, depending on tissue and age. Further, fibroblasts generate both matrix metalloproteinases (MMPs) and tissue inhibitors of metalloproteinases, thus controlling homeostatic tissue architecture.

Myofibroblasts were first described by Gabbiani and colleagues as cells central to wound healing [8]. The actin filaments result in myofibroblasts having contractile properties, which, at sites of wound healing serve to close the wound. However, the presence of contractile myofibroblasts in the interstitium of the lung may cause a retraction of parenchymal tissue resulting in alveolar collapse giving the characteristic honeycombing as observed in the lungs of IPF patients, or add to the increase in alveolar size, which is characteristic of COPD [9].

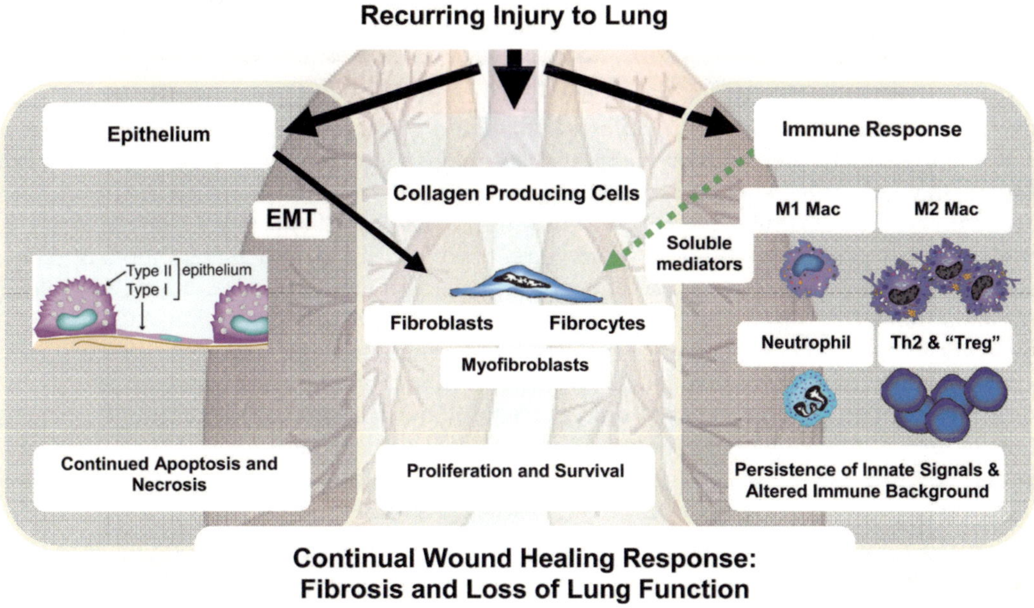

Fig. 1. *Cellular Pathways in Lung Fibrosis: Multi-Faceted Aberrant Response*
Chronic lung remodelling is hypothesized to occur following repeated trauma or injury to the lung. Multiple cellular pathways and interactions which can all promote ECM deposition have been described in lung fibrosis which promote fibroblast and myofibroblast activation, proliferation and survival. Following injury to the epithelium, apoptotic and necrotic signals stimulate collagen producing cells. These resident epithelial cells can also differentiate into a collagen-producing phenotype during EMT. The immune response in the lung is also altered in chronic lung diseases, with pro-fibrotic M2 macrophages and type 2 T cells predominating. These cells generate soluble mediators such as TGFβ, CCL2 and IL13 which directly activates collagen producing cells.
Key: EMT: epithelial to mesenchymal transition; Mac: Macrophage; Treg: regulatory T cell

Under normal conditions, myofibroblasts sequentially perpetuate and then dampen inflammation via the secretion of chemokines, cytokines, arachidonic acid metabolites and protease inhibitors. When activated, they express cell surface adhesion molecules allowing specific interactions with immune and inflammatory cells, including lymphocytes, mast cells and neutrophils. If these processes become dysregulated, fibrosis may ensue with catastrophic consequences for lung function.

Most insight into the potential role of fibroblasts at driving pulmonary remodeling, as well as phenotypic differences in fibroblasts found in fibrotic regions versus those located in normal tissue has been garnered from *in vitro* studies using fibroblasts isolated from IPF lungs and animal models. Fibroblasts isolated from fibrotic environments are phenotypically different than non-fibrotic fibroblasts [10-12]. Fibroblasts from a profibrotic environment exhibit altered responsiveness to growth factors, express enhanced receptor levels for chemokines, which has also been observed in murine models of pulmonary remodeling. These studies suggest a distinct heterogeneity in fibroblast function and phenotype in the fibrotic lung.

We and other investigators have reported that fibroblasts derived from IPF lungs proliferate faster than cells derived from normal lung tissue. In contrast, others have shown that the growth rate of IPF fibroblasts was significantly slower than normal fibroblasts. This discrepancy may be due to the site in the lung from which fibroblasts are harvested, since the magnitude of inflammation and fibrosis are heterogeneous in distribution. Thus, areas of active fibrosis may yield hyperproliferative fibroblasts compared to areas of established fibrosis in which cells may be hypoproliferative.

To begin to address this diversity, recent studies have used microarray technologies to profile global gene expression in pulmonary fibrosis in man and mouse models. These studies have showed expression of almost 500 genes are increased more than two- fold in fibrotic lungs, including many genes related to cytoskeletal reorganization, ECM, cellular metabolism and protein biosynthesis, signaling, proliferation and survival [13,14]. There was excellent concordance between gene expression in human and experimental models, giving us some confidence in the value of our efforts to model human disease. Studies examining human lung fibroblast global gene expression in response to TGFβ1 have shown almost 150 genes upregulated, representing several functional categories described above. This included 80 genes that were not previously known to be TGFβ -responsive.

The progression and severity of many lung diseases, most notably IPF, are tightly associated with regions of fibroblast accumulation and proliferation, to the extent that these regions have become a reliable indicator of survival. The increased number of (myo)fibroblasts seen in these diseases, implies that they are either hyper-proliferative and/or resistant to apoptosis. However, most studies suggest that these cells proliferate faster than normal [10,15,16]

4. Sources and fates of fibroblasts and myofibroblasts

As remodeling of the lung is associated with accumulation and activation of fibroblasts and myofibroblasts, the derivation of both cell types is currently under examination. Reports indicate that there may be multiple pathways through which fibroblasts and myofibroblasts are derived [17]. Fibroblasts isolated from human or murine fibrotic tissue exhibit enhanced basal proliferation. Therefore an increase in the fibroblast pool could be due to local proliferation. Myofibroblasts express a panel of markers and these markers have been correlated with site of derivation. For example, myofibroblasts found in the peripheral and subpleural regions of fibrosis express α-SMA, vimentin and desmin, whereas cells found in other regions of the lung do not express desmin [18].

4.1 Epithelial to mesenchymal transition

Another potential source of fibroblasts is by a process called epithelial to mesenchymal transition (EMT). EMT is a dynamic process by which epithelial cells undergo phenotypic transition to fully differentiated motile mesenchymal cells, such as fibroblasts and myofibroblasts. This process occurs normally during early fetal development where there is seamless plasticity between epithelial and mesenchymal cells [19]. Furthermore, this phenomenon is well accepted in cancer as a key mechanism that supports tumor metastases [20]. However, the process of EMT in development and cancer differ greatly in that, unlike developmental EMT, the tumorigenic EMT process is poorly regulated [21]. During the process of EMT, the downregulation of epithelial and tight junction proteins is associated with a concomitant increase in mesenchymal cell markers [22,23]. In chronic lung diseases, the dual expression of epithelial and mesenchymal markers in the same cells has led investigators to postulate that EMT is a mechanism resulting in more ECM-generating mesenchymal cells in the lung [24,25]. The differentiation of airway epithelial cells has been previously described, for example, type I pneumocytes transitioning into goblet cells [26-29]. However, the switching of an epithelial cell into a phenotype that moves beyond the original cell's embryonic lineage, has only recently been suggested to be a causative factor in fibrosis [23,30,31].

The initial events of EMT include the loss of cell polarity and the induction of matrix metalloproteinases (MMPs) that promote basement membrane degradation and cell detachment. The cells also undergo cytoskeletal changes, as well as altered expression of surface molecules which allow for the migration and transition of these cells to a mesenchymal phenotype [32,33]. The majority of the work evaluating EMT has been performed *in vitro;* however the full extent of this pathogenic pathway *in vivo* is currently being evaluated. In animal models of kidney fibrosis, it has been estimated that up to 20% of the fibroblasts found in the fibrotic lesions were derived from the epithelium through EMT [30,34-37].

The idea of EMT promoting the fibrosis observed in COPD and IPF is rapidly beginning to evolve [29]. Several recent studies have also shown that EMT occurs in lung epithelial cells both *in vitro* and *in vivo,* supporting the concept of EMT contributing to the fibrosis observed in IPF [29,38,39]. Moreover, we have recently published an alteration in the microRNA regulation of genes associated with EMT in IPF[40]. The potential of EMT promoting COPD requires further investigation. Nevertheless, there is an emerging link between COPD and lung cancer, thus increasing the likelihood of EMT being present in the COPD lung. The link between smoking, lung cancer and COPD is also apparent, in that smoking is a risk factor for COPD and also for lung cancer [41,42]. An underlying response to cigarette smoke is generating an altered inflammatory environment in the lung [43], which can then be susceptible to either COPD or lung cancer development [44]. Therefore, future work correlating the timecourse of EMT induction with COPD and IPF disease staging will be insightful to determine the extent of contribution mediated by this process.

4.2 Circulating progenitor mesenchymal cells

Along with the epithelium, studies have also highlighted a role for bone marrow-derived circulating progenitor mesenchymal cells, or fibrocytes, in promoting lung fibrosis by differentiating into fibroblasts or myofibroblasts [45,46,47] (Fig. 1). Fibrocytes have been observed at sites of active fibrosis and increased numbers of these cells in the circulation correlate with mortality in IPF [5]. They are induced by pro-fibrotic mediators such as TGFβ1 and Th2 cytokines [48]; and the cell markers include leukocyte markers (CD45, CD34), mesenchymal markers (collagen I, fibronectin) and chemokine receptors (CCR3, CCR5, CCR7 and CXCR4) [49]. Human and mouse studies have demonstrated that fibrocytes from peripheral blood migrate to skin wound chambers [49-51] and bronchial mucosa after antigen challenge [52]. Furthermore, these cells have been reported in disease states with fibrotic pathologies including hypertrophic scars, asthma and IPF [52-55].

Fibrocytes are pleiotropic and may contribute to fibrogenesis by directly producing collagen, as well as inflammatory cytokines, hematopoietic growth factors, and chemokines [54-58] (Fig. 2). In a study performed in collaboration between AstraZeneca and Malmö University Hospital, increased fibrocyte numbers were observed in the circulation of COPD patients, where patients with mild COPD had the most elevated number of fibrocytes in comparison to moderate COPD, severe COPD or healthy patients [59]. Although there was no correlation of fibrocyte number with any lung function parameter, inhaled glucocorticosteroid use

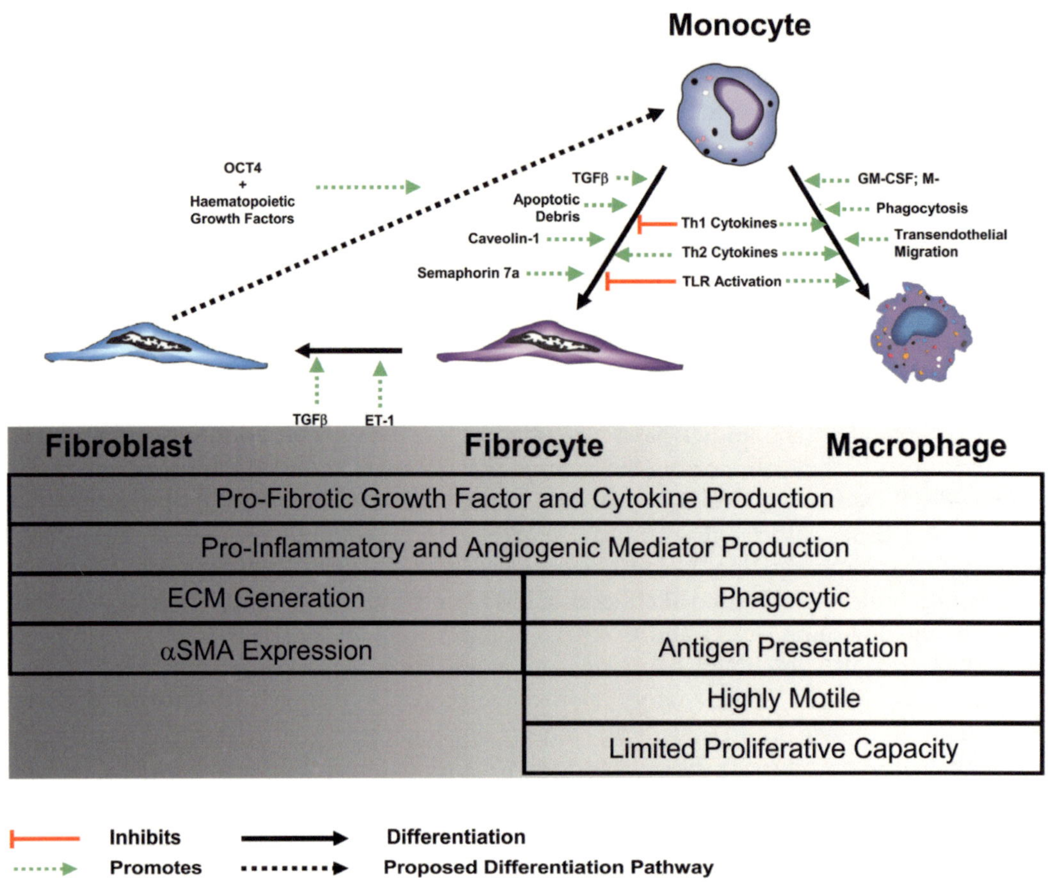

Fig. 2. Overlapping Differentiation Pathways and Functions of Fibroblasts, Fibrocytes and Macrophages

Fibroblasts, fibrocytes and macrophages share many *in vitro* and *in vivo* functions such as mediator production, host defence and extracellular matrix deposition. Monocytes can differentiate into fibrocytes or macrophages depending on the environment and the nature of the stimulus. *In vitro* studies have highlighted a role for various mediators such as cytokines, TLR signals, cellular debris and cell function at promoting differentiation. However, it is likely a combination of these pathways *in situ* which dictates the fate of the monocyte. Fibrocytes have been shown to differentiate into fibroblasts, in part through losing CD45 expression but retaining collagen I expression. Moreover in vitro, fibrocytes stimulated with TGFβ or ET-1 can promote fibrocyte to fibroblast differentiation. Recent evidence has indicated that fibroblasts can differentiate into haematopoietic cells when stimulated with appropriate growth factors.

Key: TGFβ: transforming growth factor β; GM-CSF: granulocyte macrophage colony-stimulating factor; M-CSF: macrophage colony-stimulating factor; TLR: toll-like receptors; ET-1: endothelin-1; OCT4: octamer-binding transcription factor 4); ECM: extracellular matrix; αSMA: α-smooth muscle actin.

significantly inhibited circulating fibrocyte numbers, corroborating the pro-inflammatory association of fibrocytes [59]. While it was originally thought that fibrocytes promote fibrosis through production of ECM components, it is becoming increasingly hypothesized that their primary role in tissue remodelling may be through secretion of soluble factors.

Fibrocytes have pleuripotent potential to differentiate into other cell lineages, as has been demonstrated with fibrocyte-derived adipocytes [60]. Furthermore, the extreme plasticity of these cells *in vitro*, makes both the derivation and characterization of these cells difficult. Exposure of fibrocytes to TGFβ1 *in vitro* results in the cells transitioning into a myofibroblast phenotype that expresses both fibronectin and type III collagen [52]. Using an adoptive transfer model of bone marrow cells from green fluorescent protein (GFP) transgenic mice into mice challenged with intratracheal bleomycin to initiate lung injury, recruited GFP+ fibrocytes were shown to differentiate into fibroblasts while resident lung fibroblasts differentiated into myofibroblasts [56].

At sites of normal wound healing, once sufficient ECM has been deposited, fibroblasts and myofibroblasts undergo apoptosis [61,62]. This serves to limit the excessive deposition of ECM and also dampen the pro-inflammatory and pro-fibrotic milieu. However, myofibroblasts persist in fibrotic conditions. Moreover, IPF fibroblasts are relatively resistant to apoptosis *in vitro*, with IPF cells inducing a different pattern of pro-apoptotic enzymes in response to Fas-L stimulation compared to normal fibroblasts [63].

A recently described study showed an alternate potential fate of fibroblasts in that they can de-differentiation or transition into haematopoietic cells[64]. Here the investigators showed that, in the presence of haematopoietic transcription factors, fibroblasts can convert into haematopoietic progenitor cells, indicating a stem-like potential of cells that have traditionally thought to be resident to the lung [64]. Therefore, expanding our understanding on the pathways that control fibroblast to myofibroblast fate, as well as fibroblast to non-fibroblast cell fate, particularly in disease, will greatly expand our understanding of disease.

5. Fibroblast cell: Cell interactions

In the lung, fibroblasts are found in the greatest number in the subepithelial layer of the conducting airways and the interstitium of the lung parenchyma (Fig. 1). Here they are in a prime location to interact with the epithelial and endothelial cells, as well as leukocytes in the airspaces, interstitium and vasculature. One of the key inflammatory cells that is found in the lung, and one that is becoming more associated with the maintenance and progression of fibrosis, is the alternatively activated (M2) macrophage. The M2 macrophage is the predominant macrophage found in the lungs of IPF patients [65]. Moreover, M2 macrophages have been associated with COPD [66,67]. In healthy tissue, alveolar macrophages are known to remove apoptotic and necrotic debris and pathogens via phagocytosis in a non-phlogistic mechanism, in that downstream inflammation is limited and the inflammatory process is attenuated [68].

In chronic lung disease, the predominant M2 macrophage phenotype is inefficient at clearing debris. M2 macrophages are defective in phagocytosis and do not dampen the inflammatory response [69]. These macrophages are capable of synthesizing pro-fibrotic mediators, which supports their role in wound healing, yet this cell type is inefficient at supporting host defense [69]. This may explain why COPD and IPF patients are susceptible to repeated bouts of pulmonary infections or exacerbation of disease. These cells express elevated levels of scavenger receptors such as macrophage scavenger receptor (MSR) and mannose receptor C (MRC/ CD206) [69,70]. Assessing circulating primary cells from IPF patients, we have determined an elevation of CD163+CD14+ cells and M2-associated soluble mediators in the circulation, which was more pronounced in progressive IPF patients, suggestive of an overall elevated M2 background in these patients [71]. We have also shown that peripheral blood monocytes from patients with scleroderma-related lung disease display a pro-fibrotic phenotype, characterized by increased CD163 expression and CCL18 production [72]. Interestingly, macrophages in the lungs of COPD patients, as well as smokers with or without COPD, also demonstrate a skewing towards an M2 phenotype, with a deactivated M1 phenotype [73,74]. Moreover *in vitro*, cigarette smoke induces a M2-type phenotype and this result was also seen in an *in vivo* cigarette smoke model in mice [73]. *In vitro*, macrophage polarization to an M2 phenotype has only been shown robustly with mouse cells. Here the differentiation of a monocyte to an M2 phenotype requires a cocktail of cytokines including IL13 and CCL17/TARC[75]. Therefore the Th2 cytokine profile observed in remodeled lungs contributes to the appearance of M2 macrophages.

Studies of bleomycin-induced fibrosis have assessed either M2 macrophage or fibrocyte number [71,76]. It is increasingly recognized that there is some overlap between these cell subsets in terms of both function and markers [76]. However, although both fibrocytes and M2 macrophages can be derived from monocytes, they are not completely redundant in function. Recently, using a lung-specific TGFβ1 over-expression model of lung fibrosis, we determined that depletion of lung monocyte/macrophages using liposomal clodronate reduced collagen accumulation, but this had no effect on the TGFβ-induced fibrocyte recruitment [77]. Therefore, for novel therapeutic approaches such as cell depletion or specific targeting, the M2 macrophage may be a more compelling target for chronic lung remodeling.

In COPD, alveolar macrophages have been hypothesized to have reduced anti-inflammatory properties, as well as a reduced capacity to turn over matrix [78]. However a recent study looking at macrophage number, MMP expression and emphysema determined a correlation between a greater infiltration of macrophage to the lung and emphysema in COPD patients [79]. *Ex vivo*, cigarette smoke induces a wide array of changes in the inflammatory profile and the host defence potential of COPD alveolar macrophages [80]. Moreover, microarray analysis indicated a correlation between alveolar macrophage gene expression, circulating monocyte gene expression and lung function [81]. The investigators hypothesized that there is a "COPD-related gene expression pattern" as many genes differentially expressed in COPD alveolar macrophages were also expressed in COPD circulating monocytes [81].

6. Activators of fibroblasts/ mesenchymal cells

Fibroblasts are activated by numerous signals including: mechanical forces such as those imposed during bronchoconstriction; matrix interactions; hypoxia and resultant changes in pH levels; and soluble mediators (Fig. 1). The large variety of soluble mediators capable of activating mesenchymal cells are produced by many different cell types found in fibrotic regions. Furthermore, proteases of the coagulation cascade and other serum factors also promote fibroblast proliferation, collagen synthesis, migration and differentiation.

6.1 Growth factors

Growth factors are the most recognized mediators that activate mesenchymal cells. Transforming growth factor β (TGFβ) is one of the most potent profibrotic mediators *in vitro* and is a central driver in the remodeling process. TGFβ1 regulates numerous biologic

activities such as proliferation, apoptosis, and differentiation [82,83]. TGFβ1 is upregulated in the lungs of IPF patients and patients with other chronic lung diseases [84-89]. Interestingly, expression of TGFβ1 is nearly absent in the bronchial epithelial cells but is highly expressed in inflammatory cells beneath the basement membrane where subepithelial fibrosis predominates [90]. In COPD, TGFβ has also been reported to be produced by circulating and interstitial T cells and monocytes [91]. Polymorphisms in the promoter region of TGFβ1 have been reported in COPD patients [92]. However, TGFβ SNPs have been associated with protection in COPD [93] or have been linked to COPD but not related to worsening of disease [94].
Transient overexpression of TGFβ1, or pulmonary delivery of this cytokine to mouse lungs, induces a pronounced interstitial fibrosis mediated by excess ECM generation and deposition, as well as the presence of myofibroblasts[95]. Using a transgenic mouse model of SMAD-3 deficiency, TGFβ/SMAD-3 signaling has been shown to be required for alveolar integrity and ECM homeostasis and that this pathway is involved in pathogenic mechanisms mediating both tissue destruction and fibrogenesis.
Due to TGFβ1 being such a potent growth factor, the release and activation of this growth factor is tightly regulated. TGFβ is released in a latent complex, associated with LAP (latency activated peptide) and LTBP. There are several mechanisms by which TGFβ is then activated and these include integrin-mediated cell cytoskeletal rearrangement in the case of integrin αvβ6[96]; cell membrane MMP recruitment for enzymatic cleavage in the case of integrin αvβ8[97] and other protease-related mechanisms exhibited by components of the coagulation cascade[98] (discussed later). The integrin αvβ6 is upregulated in IPF[99] and neutralization of this integrin *in vivo* reduces fibrosis in various experimental models [99-101].
There are also endogenous inhibitors of TGFβ, the largest being the BMP (bone morphogenic protein) family. The BMP family is structurally and functionally related to the TGFβ superfamily [102]. BMPs inhibit TGFβ signaling through either inhibiting Smad 2/3 phosphorylation or competing for Smad 4 or both [103,104]. Recombinant BMP7 has been shown to inhibit TGFβ-induced EMT *in vitro,* as well as reducing renal fibrosis [105]. However, we have shown that BMP7 had no anti-fibrotic effect in models of lung fibrosis, nor were there effects on lung epithelial cells *in vitro* [106].

6.2 Th2-associated mediators

Interleukin 13 (IL13) and IL4 are two pleiotropic, Th2-associated cytokines, with numerous distinct and overlapping functions. They share overlapping roles due to the shared IL13Rα1 receptor subunit. However they also have unique subunits that confer the distinct functions. IL13 activates epithelial cells and goblet cells causing mucous production, goblet cell hyperplasia and EMT [107,108]. Various animal models of pulmonary fibrosis have indicated a more pro-fibrotic role for IL13 than IL4. Indeed it has been hypothesized that IL4 is involved in the initiation of fibrosis whereas IL13 is central to the maintenance of the fibrotic response.
We have published that IL-13 is elevated in the lungs of IPF patients [71] and this protein is associated with fibrotic pathologies and aberrant remodeling at various tissue sites [65,109]. There is also elevated expression of the two IL13 receptor subunits IL13Rα1 and IL13Rα2 which are prominant on fibroblasts [110,111]. More recently we have shown that IPF fibroblasts are hyper-responsive to IL13 in comparison to non-fibrotic fibroblasts[58]. It was originally hypothesized that IL13Rα2 is a decoy receptor as it has a short cytoplasmic tail and although it is the higher affinity receptor subunit, it is found at high levels in a soluble form, but only

in murine models of fibrosis[112] and not in humans[113]. However, recent data has suggested that signaling of IL13 through IL13Rα2 is pro-fibrotic, resulting in TGFβ1 production [114]. Lung-specific over-expression of IL13 in mice results in remodeling and emphysema [115]. Moreover, various MMPs and cathepsins that are associated with COPD[1] are also induced in the IL13-transgenic lung [116]. However robust detection of IL13 has not been consistently reported. IL13 producing macrophages and NKT cells have been detected in the COPD lung [117]. Also, the presence of the cytokine and IL13 positive cells have been shown in the bronchial epithelium of smokers with chronic bronchitis [118]. In contrast, decreased IL13 has been measured in emphysema compared to non-emphysematous lungs [119]. An inverse correlation between plasma IL13 and the lung diffusion capacity for carbon monoxide (DLCO) parameter, used to determine the efficiency of gas exchange in COPD has been reported [120].
Another Th2-associated mediator that is being actively researched in fibrosis is the chemokine CCL18/ PARC. In IPF, CCL18 has been associated with poor outcome, namely, patients with CCL18 levels greater than 150ng/ml in the circulation will typically have more progressive disease, compared to those with CCL18 levels below 150ng/ml [6]. CCL18 expression is also a marker for M2 macrophages [121], therefore linking the profibrotic cell phenotype with IPF progression. In the recent ECLISPE study, elevated CCL18 levels in COPD patients has been associated with increased chance of COPD exacerbation [122]. This association of CCL18 with COPD exacerbations was in stark contrast to TNFα, IL6 or CXCL8/ IL8 levels, or the number of pack years of smoking [122]. These observations may change the understanding of the pleiotropic nature of the underlying mechanisms for COPD, as CCL18 is not associated with smoking or with neutrophil accumulation and activation.

6.3 Coagulation cascade

Thrombin is a serine protease generated during activation of the coagulation pathway [123]. Thrombin has been implicated in a number of pulmonary fibrotic diseases such as acute lung injury (ALI) [124,125] acute respiratory distress syndrome (ARDS) [126], interstitial lung disease (ILD) [127,128] and IPF [127,129-132] and IPF BAL fluid thrombin has been shown to promote fibroblast proliferation [131]. In COPD, elevated procoagulant activity has been observed in the serum of patients with moderate to severe disease [133]. Animal models of fibrosis have strengthened the connection between thrombin and fibrosis. Increased thrombin is found in the lungs of mice challenged with bleomycin and pharmacological inhibition of thrombin significantly reduced the collagen deposition [130].
At the cellular level, thrombin has numerous biologic effects that are in addition to its role as a coagulation pathway proteinase. It has been shown to promote inflammation and fibrosis through inducing chemokine and growth factor production from fibroblasts. Many of the cell-based activities of thrombin are mediated through a family of receptors termed proteinase-activated receptors (PARs). PARs are G-protein coupled receptors (GPCR), with 4 known subtypes identified to date. A defining feature of these receptors is that they are activated by proteases that cleave a portion of the extracellular amino terminus to unmask a new N-terminal sequence, which then functions as a tethered ligand that autoactivates the receptor. PAR-1-deficient mice are protected from bleomycin induced lung fibrosis [134]. Further, PAR-2-deficient mice had decreased eotaxin/CCL11 and reduced eosinophilia in the lungs following antigen challenge in an allergen sensitization and challenge model of asthma [135,136]. Furthermore, thrombin and other PAR1 agonists promote the integrin-mediated activation latent TGFβ in a model of acute lung injury [98] . Thus, the local activation of TGFβ at sites of fibrosis may be enhanced by the coagulation cascade in both IPF and COPD.

6.4 Pentraxins

Pentraxins comprise a highly conserved superfamily of cyclic pentameric proteins. These proteins interact with numerous ligands, including selected pathogens and apoptotic cells[137], and are recognized by macrophages via mannose 6P and Fc gamma (γ) receptors, ultimately leading to complement activation, pathogen recognition, and apoptotic cell clearance [138-140]. Pentraxins are subdivided into the short pentraxins that include C-reactive protein (CRP) and serum amyloid P component (SAP, PTX2), and the long pentraxin 3 (PTX3) [141,142]. SAP appears to be uniquely involved in the resolution or repair phase of tissue injury via its modulator effects on resident and bone marrow derived collagen producing cells [76,143]. SAP binds to Fcγ receptors[144] and the anti-fibrotic activities of SAP have been shown to be mediated through Fcγ receptors[143] which affect peripheral blood monocyte differentiation and activation states.

SAP promotes the differentiation of M1 classically activated macrophages in a tuberculosis model of lung infection [145]. We have recently demonstrated that SAP has prominent immunomodulatory effects on mouse macrophages, thereby providing a mechanism for its ability to prevent the development and reverse established experimental fungal airway disease [75]. Moreover, human SAP has been shown to potently inhibit the differentiation of monocytes into fibrocytes[146] and it has consequently been used therapeutically in animal models to inhibit lung fibrosis and fibrosis in a number of organ sites. In addition, SAP causes an inhibition of the differentiation of peripheral blood mononuclear cells into $CD45^+$/collagen I^+ cells called fibrocytes[76,146,147], as well as reducing M2 macrophage number [75,77].

6.5 Matrix Metalloproteinases and Chitinases

Active remodeling of the ECM is dependent on the coordinated activities of proteases and protease inhibitors [148,149]. Fibroblasts generate metalloproteinases (MMPs), which are elevated in asthma and COPD (reviewed in [150]). MMPs are a family of proteins that exert proteolytic activities on various proteins including ECM components and are thus central to ECM formation and organization [150]. Tissue inhibitors of metalloproteinases (TIMP)s are endogenous inhibitors of MMPs that bind to the catalytic site on these proteinases [151]. In IPF, MMP1, 2 and 9 were co-localized to the epithelium surrounding fibrotic lesions, whereas increased TIMP2 was also observed suggesting that the MMP activity may be inhibited and that the fibrotic region not degraded [152].

Another family of enzymes associated with fibrosis and remodeling is the chitinase family. Chitinases are proteolytic enzymes that bind, but do not cleave chitin [153]. Chitin is the main component of the insect exoskeleton, thought to be absent in human tissue. However, these proteins are postulated to play important, yet currently undefined roles in biology. The prototypic chitinase-like protein is derived from the chitinase 3 like 1 (*Ch3l1*) gene, called YKL40 in humans and BRP39 in mice. YKL40/BRP39 is a circulating regulator of apoptosis, and shown to have a role in M2 macrophage activation, TGFβ1 induction and tissue fibrosis [154]. An early report in asthmatics indicated that YKL40 is elevated in the circulation and is associated with asthma severity [155]. Chitinolytic activity has also been demonstrated in COPD patients [156,157], as well as in models of cigarette smoke induced emphysema [157]. Interestingly, BRP39 gene deficient mice have increased epithelial cell apoptosis and alveolar destruction in response to cigarette smoke, but worsened pathology in hyperoxia-induced lung injury which is a more acute ARDS-like model [157,158]. Increased YKL40 has also been detected in the lungs and circulation of IPF patients, with levels correlating with survival [159,160]. Thus, there is clear disease association with chitinase activity, however because of discrepancies in the different animal models, whether these chitinases are promoting disease or uniquely serve as a marker of disease activity still requires further elucidation.

7. Therapeutic options for targeting pro-fibrotic cells

IPF is a disease that is driven by continual parenchymal ECM deposition, which reduces lung compliance and effective gas exchange. The fibrosis observed in the lungs of COPD patients predominates around small airways[4,161] and may not be the main driving factor causing the loss in lung function and death. Emphysema and lung tissue destruction is often observed in COPD patients and honeycombing is a salient feature in IPF patient lungs [162]. Overall this suggests an imbalance in repair processes within the lung and targeting the underlying pro-fibrotic mechanisms may impact COPD and IPF in a positive way. In IPF, the capacity of the lungs (FVC, forced vital capacity); as well as the efficiency of gas exchange (DLCO) may improve with a reduction in fibrosis. Both of these parameters are used clinically in IPF patients to measure lung function and monitor disease progression[162]. In COPD, anti-fibrotic strategies directed at the same cells and/or mediators may attenuate the obstructive nature in the airways and this may be the most discernible improvement in lung function. This would translate to an improvement in forced expiratory volume in a short time frame (FEV_1). Again, FEV_1 is commonly used in COPD patient management and is used to segregate patients into the various GOLD stages of disease[4].

As has been highlighted in this Chapter, monocytes and mesenchymal cells express a variety of receptor that can promote recruitment, proliferation or activation, as well as differentiation into other phenotypes (Fig. 2). In experimental mouse models of lung fibrosis, blocking fibrocyte recruitment through chemokine ligand/ receptor blockade significantly attenuated ECM deposition [54-56,163]. However, these chemokine receptors are not uniquely expressed on fibrocytes[164], so the anti-fibrotic effects observed following blockade of these G-protein coupled receptors might extend beyond impaired fibrocyte recruitment. Also, we have demonstrated that depletion of lung monocyte/ macrophages inhibits TGFβ-induced lung fibrosis, but has no effect on lung fibrocyte number, suggesting a redundant role for fibrocyte recruitment in promoting TGFβ-induced lung fibrosis [77].

One other mechanism to consider in any therapeutic approach in pulmonary fibrosis is fibrocyte activation. A prototypic activator of fibrocytes, fibroblasts and myofibroblasts is TGFβ. Adenoviral-mediated over-expression of TGFβ in the lungs of mice or rats, or lung-specific transgenic over-expression in mice induces significant lung pathology[95,165,166]. In the lung specific TGFβ over expression, active TGFβ is expressed by airway epithelial cells. At early timepoints following over-expression, apoptosis is observed, following by interstitial leukocyte accumulation and then increased collagen deposition, predominating around the airways and then gradually increasing in the parenchyma[77,165,167]. At later stages of lung-specific TGFβ over-expression, alveolar collapse is observed[77] whereas adenoviral TGFβ expression results in a prolonged, severe fibrosis[95]. These apparent chronic differences may be due to the initial extent of acute lung injury immediately following TGFβ over-expression, in that transgenic mediated TGFβ induces extensive apoptosis, whereby blocking apoptosis inhibits subsequent fibrosis[165]. Blockade of TGFβ in experimental models of lung fibrosis through either antibody neutralization, receptor inhibition of TGFβ activation has been shown to attenuate lung remodelling [99,100,168-170]. However, TGFβ1 gene deficient mice die within 3-4 weeks of age and demonstrate significant autoimmune pathologies, potentially due to the lack of immunoregulation in the absence of TGFβ [171,172].

Therefore direct neutralization of this target might have significant safety concerns in IPF or COPD patients.

Other factors that work in concert with TGF-β include IL4 and IL13. In order to examine the role of IL4- and IL13-responsive cells in pulmonary fibrosis, we have conducted preclinical studies using IL13 conjugated to a Pseudomonas exotoxin, IL13-PE[173], which targets cells expressing the type 2 IL4 receptor and IL13Rα2. This protein-toxin conjugate selectively targets IPF fibroblasts because they express these receptor subunits, resulting in specific cell death. Moreover, *in vivo* use in a murine model of bleomycin-induced lung fibrosis showed that selective targeting of fibroblasts at the end stages or maintenance phase of fibrosis, attenuated remodelling. In contrast, IL13-PE delivered to the lung during the onset or initiation of disease had no therapeutic benefit[173]. This suggests that targeting these cells in established disease may allow for the resolution of lung pathology that is observed in chronic lung disease patients.

Taken together, targeting stromal cells to dampen the extent of activation and the amount of ECM deposition, regardless of disease, or region within the lung may have an impact in lung function that can either halt disease progression or promote resolution and restoration of lung function.

8. Acknowledgements

We also thank Dr. Judith Connett for her critical reading of the manuscript.

9. References

[1] Gosselink, J.V., *et al.* Differential expression of tissue repair genes in the pathogenesis of chronic obstructive pulmonary disease. *American journal of respiratory and critical care medicine* 181, 1329-1335.

[2] Hogg, J.C., McDonough, J.E., Gosselink, J.V. & Hayashi, S. What drives the peripheral lung-remodeling process in chronic obstructive pulmonary disease? *Proceedings of the American Thoracic Society* 6, 668-672 (2009).

[3] Gross, T.J. & Hunninghake, G.W. Idiopathic pulmonary fibrosis. *N Engl J Med* 345, 517-525 (2001).

[4] Hogg, J.C., *et al.* The nature of small-airway obstruction in chronic obstructive pulmonary disease. *N Engl J Med* 350, 2645-2653 (2004).

[5] Moeller, A., *et al.* Circulating fibrocytes are an indicator of poor prognosis in idiopathic pulmonary fibrosis. *American journal of respiratory and critical care medicine* 179, 588 594 (2009).

[6] Prasse, A., *et al.* CCL18 as an indicator of pulmonary fibrotic activity in idiopathic interstitial pneumonias and systemic sclerosis. *Arthritis and rheumatism* 56, 1685-1693 (2007).

[7] Ohta, K., Mortenson, R.L., Clark, R.A., Hirose, N. & King, T.E., Jr. Immunohistochemical identification and characterization of smooth muscle-like cells in idiopathic pulmonary fibrosis. *Am J Respir Crit Care Med* 152, 1659-1665 (1995).

[8] Gabbiani, G. & Badonnel, M.C. Contractile events during inflammation. *Agents Actions* 6, 277-280 (1976).

[9] Dacic, S. & Yousem, S.A. Histologic classification of idiopathic chronic interstitial pneumonias. *Am J Respir Cell Mol Biol* 29, S5-9 (2003).

[10] Moodley, Y.P., *et al.* Fibroblasts isolated from normal lungs and those with idiopathic pulmonary fibrosis differ in interleukin-6/gp130-mediated cell signaling and proliferation. *Am J Pathol* 163, 345-354 (2003).
[11] Scaffidi, A.K., *et al.* Oncostatin M stimulates proliferation, induces collagen production and inhibits apoptosis of human lung fibroblasts. *Br J Pharmacol* 136, 793-801 (2002).
[12] McAnulty, R.J. Fibroblasts and myofibroblasts: their source, function and role in disease. *The international journal of biochemistry & cell biology* 39, 666-671 (2007).
[13] Selman, M., Pardo, A. & Kaminski, N. Idiopathic pulmonary fibrosis: aberrant recapitulation of developmental programs? *PLoS medicine* 5, e62 (2008).
[14] Selman, M., *et al.* Accelerated variant of idiopathic pulmonary fibrosis: clinical behavior and gene expression pattern. *PloS one* 2, e482 (2007).
[15] Jacoby, D.B., Gleich, G.J. & Fryer, A.D. Human eosinophil major basic protein is an endogenous allosteric antagonist at the inhibitory muscarinic M2 receptor. *J Clin Invest* 91, 1314-1318 (1993).
[16] Ramos, C., *et al.* Fibroblasts from idiopathic pulmonary fibrosis and normal lungs differ in growth rate, apoptosis, and tissue inhibitor of metalloproteinases expression. *Am J Respir Cell Mol Biol* 24, 591-598 (2001).
[17] Hinz, B., *et al.* The myofibroblast: one function, multiple origins. *Am J Pathol* 170, 1807-1816 (2007).
[18] Zhang, K., Rekhter, M.D., Gordon, D. & Phan, S.H. Myofibroblasts and their role in lung collagen gene expression during pulmonary fibrosis. A combined immunohistochemical and in situ hybridization study. *Am J Pathol* 145, 114-125 (1994).
[19] Thiery, J.P. Epithelial-mesenchymal transitions in development and pathologies. *Current opinion in cell biology* 15, 740-746 (2003).
[20] Kalluri, R. & Weinberg, R.A. The basics of epithelial-mesenchymal transition. *The Journal of clinical investigation* 119, 1420-1428 (2009).
[21] Dasari, V., Gallup, M., Lemjabbar, H., Maltseva, I. & McNamara, N. Epithelial-mesenchymal transition in lung cancer: is tobacco the "smoking gun"? *Am J Respir Cell Mol Biol* 35, 3-9 (2006).
[22] Willis, B.C. & Borok, Z. TGF-{beta}-induced EMT: mechanisms and implications for fibrotic lung disease. *Am J Physiol Lung Cell Mol Physiol* (2007).
[23] Valcourt, U., Kowanetz, M., Niimi, H., Heldin, C.H. & Moustakas, A. TGF-beta and the Smad signaling pathway support transcriptomic reprogramming during epithelial-mesenchymal cell transition. *Mol Biol Cell* 16, 1987-2002 (2005).
[24] Zavadil, J. & Bottinger, E.P. TGF-beta and epithelial-to-mesenchymal transitions. *Oncogene* 24, 5764-5774 (2005).
[25] Zavadil, J., Cermak, L., Soto-Nieves, N. & Bottinger, E.P. Integration of TGF-beta/Smad and Jagged1/Notch signalling in epithelial-to-mesenchymal transition. *Embo J* 23, 1155-1165 (2004).
[26] Borok, Z., *et al.* Modulation of t1alpha expression with alveolar epithelial cell phenotype in vitro. *Am J Physiol* 275, L155-164 (1998).
[27] Danto, S.I., Shannon, J.M., Borok, Z., Zabski, S.M. & Crandall, E.D. Reversible transdifferentiation of alveolar epithelial cells. *Am J Respir Cell Mol Biol* 12, 497-502 (1995).

[28] Torday, J.S., Torres, E. & Rehan, V.K. The role of fibroblast transdifferentiation in lung epithelial cell proliferation, differentiation, and repair in vitro. *Pediatr Pathol Mol Med* 22, 189-207 (2003).
[29] Kim, K.K., *et al.* Alveolar epithelial cell mesenchymal transition develops in vivo during pulmonary fibrosis and is regulated by the extracellular matrix. *Proc Natl Acad Sci U S A* 103, 13180-13185 (2006).
[30] Kalluri, R. & Neilson, E.G. Epithelial-mesenchymal transition and its implications for fibrosis. *J Clin Invest* 112, 1776-1784 (2003).
[31] Selgas, R., Jimenez-Heffernan, J. & Lopez-Cabrera, M. On the epithelial-mesenchymal transition of mesothelial cells. *Kidney Int* 66, 866-867; author reply 867 (2004).
[32] Grunert, S., Jechlinger, M. & Beug, H. Diverse cellular and molecular mechanisms contribute to epithelial plasticity and metastasis. *Nat Rev Mol Cell Biol* 4, 657-665 (2003).
[33] Iwano, M., *et al.* Evidence that fibroblasts derive from epithelium during tissue fibrosis. *J Clin Invest* 110, 341-350 (2002).
[34] Okada, H., Danoff, T.M., Kalluri, R. & Neilson, E.G. Early role of Fsp1 in epithelial-mesenchymal transformation. *Am J Physiol* 273, F563-574 (1997).
[35] Iwano, M., *et al.* Evidence that fibroblasts derive from epithelium during tissue fibrosis. *J Clin Invest* 110, 341-350. (2002).
[36] Kalluri, R. & Neilson, E.G. Epithelial-mesenchymal transition and its implications for fibrosis. *J. Clin. Invest.* 112, 1776-1784 (2003).
[37] Saika, S., *et al.* Smad3 Signaling Is Required for Epithelial-Mesenchymal Transition of Lens Epithelium after Injury. *Am J Pathol* 164, 651-663 (2004).
[38] Kasai, H., Allen, J.T., Mason, R.M., Kamimura, T. & Zhang, Z. TGF-beta1 induces human alveolar epithelial to mesenchymal cell transition (EMT). *Respir Res* 6, 56 (2005).
[39] Willis, B.C., *et al.* Induction of epithelial-mesenchymal transition in alveolar epithelial cells by transforming growth factor-beta1: potential role in idiopathic pulmonary fibrosis. *The American journal of pathology* 166, 1321-1332 (2005).
[40] Oak, S.R., *et al.* A micro RNA processing defect in rapidly progressing idiopathic pulmonary fibrosis. *PloS one* 6, e21253.
[41] Youlden, D.R., Cramb, S.M. & Baade, P.D. The International Epidemiology of Lung Cancer: geographical distribution and secular trends. *J Thorac Oncol* 3, 819-831 (2008).
[42] Proctor, R.N. Tobacco and the global lung cancer epidemic. *Nat Rev Cancer* 1, 82-86 (2001).
[43] Cosio, M.G., Saetta, M. & Agusti, A. Immunologic aspects of chronic obstructive pulmonary disease. *N Engl J Med* 360, 2445-2454 (2009).
[44] Walser, T., *et al.* Smoking and lung cancer: the role of inflammation. *Proceedings of the American Thoracic Society* 5, 811-815 (2008).
[45] Quan, T.E., Cowper, S.E. & Bucala, R. The role of circulating fibrocytes in fibrosis. *Curr Rheumatol Rep* 8, 145-150 (2006).
[46] Quan, T.E., Cowper, S., Wu, S.P., Bockenstedt, L.K. & Bucala, R. Circulating fibrocytes: collagen-secreting cells of the peripheral blood. *Int J Biochem Cell Biol* 36, 598-606 (2004).
[47] Lama, V.N. & Phan, S.H. The extrapulmonary origin of fibroblasts: stem/progenitor cells and beyond. *Proceedings of the American Thoracic Society* 3, 373-376 (2006).

[48] Shao, D.D., Suresh, R., Vakil, V., Gomer, R.H. & Pilling, D. Pivotal Advance: Th-1 cytokines inhibit, and Th-2 cytokines promote fibrocyte differentiation. *J Leukoc Biol* 83, 1323-1333 (2008).

[49] Abe, R., Donnelly, S.C., Peng, T., Bucala, R. & Metz, C.N. Peripheral blood fibrocytes: differentiation pathway and migration to wound sites. *J Immunol* 166, 7556-7562 (2001).

[50] Bucala, R., Spiegel, L.A., Chesney, J., Hogan, M. & Cerami, A. Circulating fibrocytes define a new leukocyte subpopulation that mediates tissue repair. *Mol Med* 1, 71-81 (1994).

[51] Chesney, J., Metz, C., Stavitsky, A.B., Bacher, M. & Bucala, R. Regulated production of type I collagen and inflammatory cytokines by peripheral blood fibrocytes. *J Immunol* 160, 419-425 (1998).

[52] Schmidt, M., Sun, G., Stacey, M.A., Mori, L. & Mattoli, S. Identification of circulating fibrocytes as precursors of bronchial myofibroblasts in asthma. *J Immunol* 171, 380-389 (2003).

[53] Abe, S., *et al.* Cells derived from the circulation contribute to the repair of lung injury. *Am J Respir Crit Care Med* 170, 1158-1163 (2004).

[54] Moore, B.B., *et al.* CCR2-mediated recruitment of fibrocytes to the alveolar space after fibrotic injury. *Am J Pathol* 166, 675-684 (2005).

[55] Moore, B.B., *et al.* The role of CCL12 in the recruitment of fibrocytes and lung fibrosis. *Am J Respir Cell Mol Biol* 35, 175-181 (2006).

[56] Hashimoto, N., Jin, H., Liu, T., Chensue, S.W. & Phan, S.H. Bone marrow-derived progenitor cells in pulmonary fibrosis. *J Clin Invest* 113, 243-252 (2004).

[57] Phillips, R.J., *et al.* Circulating fibrocytes traffic to the lungs in response to CXCL12 and mediate fibrosis. *J Clin Invest* 114, 438-446 (2004).

[58] Murray, L.A., *et al.* Hyper-responsiveness of IPF/UIP fibroblasts: interplay between TGFbeta1, IL-13 and CCL2. *The international journal of biochemistry & cell biology* 40, 2174-2182 (2008).

[59] Weislander, E., *et al.* Increased circulating levels of fibroscytes in COPD - a sign of ongoing lung repair? *American journal of respiratory and critical care medicine* 179, A1992 (2010).

[60] Hong, K.M., Burdick, M.D., Phillips, R.J., Heber, D. & Strieter, R.M. Characterization of human fibrocytes as circulating adipocyte progenitors and the formation of human adipose tissue in SCID mice. *Faseb J* 19, 2029-2031 (2005).

[61] Desmouliere, A., Redard, M., Darby, I. & Gabbiani, G. Apoptosis mediates the decrease in cellularity during the transition between granulation tissue and scar. *Am J Pathol* 146, 56-66 (1995).

[62] Darby, I., Skalli, O. & Gabbiani, G. Alpha-smooth muscle actin is transiently expressed by myofibroblasts during experimental wound healing. *Lab Invest* 63, 21-29 (1990).

[63] Moodley, Y.P., *et al.* Comparison of the morphological and biochemical changes in normal human lung fibroblasts and fibroblasts derived from lungs of patients with idiopathic pulmonary fibrosis during FasL-induced apoptosis. *The Journal of pathology* 202, 486-495 (2004).

[64] Szabo, E., *et al.* Direct conversion of human fibroblasts to multilineage blood progenitors. *Nature* 468, 521-526.

[65] Hancock, A., Armstrong, L., Gama, R. & Millar, A. Production of interleukin 13 by alveolar macrophages from normal and fibrotic lung. *Am J Respir Cell Mol Biol* 18, 60-65 (1998).
[66] Zhou, Y., Murthy, J.N., Zeng, D., Belardinelli, L. & Blackburn, M.R. Alterations in adenosine metabolism and signaling in patients with chronic obstructive pulmonary disease and idiopathic pulmonary fibrosis. *PloS one* 5, e9224.
[67] Barnes, P.J. Alveolar macrophages as orchestrators of COPD. *Copd* 1, 59-70 (2004).
[68] Savill, J. Apoptosis in resolution of inflammation. *J Leukoc Biol* 61, 375-380 (1997).
[69] Gordon, S. Alternative activation of macrophages. *Nat Rev Immunol* 3, 23-35 (2003).
[70] Tiemessen, M.M., *et al.* CD4+CD25+Foxp3+ regulatory T cells induce alternative activation of human monocytes/macrophages. *Proc Natl Acad Sci U S A* 104, 19446-19451 (2007).
[71] Murray, L.A., *et al.* Serum amyloid P therapeutically attenuates murine bleomycin-induced pulmonary fibrosis via its effects on macrophages. *PloS one* 5, e9683.
[72] Mathai, S.K., *et al.* Circulating monocytes from systemic sclerosis patients with interstitial lung disease show an enhanced profibrotic phenotype. *Laboratory investigation; a journal of technical methods and pathology* 90, 812-823.
[73] Hodge, S., *et al.* Cigarette Smoke-induced Changes to Alveolar Macrophage Phenotype and Function is Improved by Treatment with Procysteine. *Am J Respir Cell Mol Biol.*
[74] Shaykhiev, R., *et al.* Smoking-dependent reprogramming of alveolar macrophage polarization: implication for pathogenesis of chronic obstructive pulmonary disease. *J Immunol* 183, 2867-2883 (2009).
[75] Moreira, A.P., *et al.* Serum amyloid P attenuates M2 macrophage activation and protects against fungal spore-induced allergic airway disease. *The Journal of allergy and clinical immunology* 126, 712-721 e717.
[76] Pilling, D., *et al.* Reduction of bleomycin-induced pulmonary fibrosis by serum amyloid P. *J Immunol* 179, 4035-4044 (2007).
[77] Murray, L.A., *et al.* TGF-beta driven lung fibrosis is macrophage dependent and blocked by Serum amyloid P. *The international journal of biochemistry & cell biology* 43, 154-162.
[78] Pons, A.R., *et al.* Decreased macrophage release of TGF-beta and TIMP-1 in chronic obstructive pulmonary disease. *Eur Respir J* 26, 60-66 (2005).
[79] Haq, I., Lowrey, G.E., Kalsheker, N. & Johnson, S.R. Matrix metalloproteinase-12 (MMP-12) SNP affects MMP activity, lung macrophage infiltration and protects against emphysema in COPD. *Thorax.*
[80] Kent, L., *et al.* Cigarette smoke extract induced cytokine and chemokine gene expression changes in COPD macrophages. *Cytokine* 42, 205-216 (2008).
[81] Poliska, S., *et al.* Chronic obstructive pulmonary disease-specific gene expression signatures of alveolar macrophages as well as peripheral blood monocytes overlap and correlate with lung function. *Respiration; international review of thoracic diseases* 81, 499-510.
[82] Pinkas, J. & Teicher, B.A. TGF-beta in cancer and as a therapeutic target. *Biochem Pharmacol* 72, 523-529 (2006).
[83] Sanders, Y.Y., Kumbla, P. & Hagood, J.S. Enhanced Myofibroblastic Differentiation and Survival in Thy-1(-) Lung Fibroblasts. *Am J Respir Cell Mol Biol* (2006).

[84] Coker, R.K., *et al.* Diverse cellular TGF-beta 1 and TGF-beta 3 gene expression in normal human and murine lung. *Eur Respir J* 9, 2501-2507 (1996).

[85] Khalil, N., O'Connor, R.N., Flanders, K.C. & Unruh, H. TGF-beta 1, but not TGF-beta 2 or TGF-beta 3, is differentially present in epithelial cells of advanced pulmonary fibrosis: an immunohistochemical study. *Am J Respir Cell Mol Biol* 14, 131-138 (1996).

[86] Khalil, N., *et al.* Increased production and immunohistochemical localization of transforming growth factor-beta in idiopathic pulmonary fibrosis. *Am J Respir Cell Mol Biol* 5, 155-162 (1991).

[87] Yoshida, K. & Gage, F.H. Cooperative regulation of nerve growth factor synthesis and secretion in fibroblasts and astrocytes by fibroblast growth factor and other cytokines. *Brain Res* 569, 14-25 (1992).

[88] Okumura, K.K., *et al.* Cortisol and TGF-beta inhibit secretion of platelet-activating factor-acetylhydrolase in a monocyte-macrophage model system [corrected]. *Mol Hum Reprod* 3, 927-932 (1997).

[89] Vignola, A.M., *et al.* Transforming growth factor-beta expression in mucosal biopsies in asthma and chronic bronchitis. *Am J Respir Crit Care Med* 156, 591-599 (1997).

[90] Magnan, A., *et al.* Altered compartmentalization of transforming growth factor-beta in asthmatic airways. *Clin Exp Allergy* 27, 389-395 (1997).

[91] Hodge, S.J., Hodge, G.L., Reynolds, P.N., Scicchitano, R. & Holmes, M. Increased production of TGF-beta and apoptosis of T lymphocytes isolated from peripheral blood in COPD. *American journal of physiology* 285, L492-499 (2003).

[92] Su, Z.G., Wen, F.Q., Feng, Y.L., Xiao, M. & Wu, X.L. Transforming growth factor-beta1 gene polymorphisms associated with chronic obstructive pulmonary disease in Chinese population. *Acta pharmacologica Sinica* 26, 714-720 (2005).

[93] Wu, L., *et al.* Transforming growth factor-beta1 genotype and susceptibility to chronic obstructive pulmonary disease. *Thorax* 59, 126-129 (2004).

[94] van Diemen, C.C., *et al.* Decorin and TGF-beta1 polymorphisms and development of COPD in a general population. *Respiratory research* 7, 89 (2006).

[95] Sime, P.J., Xing, Z., Graham, F.L., Csaky, K.G. & Gauldie, J. Adenovector-mediated gene transfer of active transforming growth factor-beta1 induces prolonged severe fibrosis in rat lung. *The Journal of clinical investigation* 100, 768-776 (1997).

[96] Munger, J.S., *et al.* The integrin alpha v beta 6 binds and activates latent TGF beta 1: a mechanism for regulating pulmonary inflammation and fibrosis. *Cell* 96, 319-328 (1999).

[97] Mu, D., *et al.* The integrin alpha(v)beta8 mediates epithelial homeostasis through MT1-MMP-dependent activation of TGF-beta1. *J Cell Biol* 157, 493-507 (2002).

[98] Jenkins, R.G., *et al.* Ligation of protease-activated receptor 1 enhances alpha(v)beta6 integrin-dependent TGF-beta activation and promotes acute lung injury. *The Journal of clinical investigation* 116, 1606-1614 (2006).

[99] Horan, G.S., *et al.* Partial inhibition of integrin alpha(v)beta6 prevents pulmonary fibrosis without exacerbating inflammation. *American journal of respiratory and critical care medicine* 177, 56-65 (2008).

[100] Puthawala, K., *et al.* Inhibition of integrin alpha(v)beta6, an activator of latent transforming growth factor-beta, prevents radiation-induced lung fibrosis. *American journal of respiratory and critical care medicine* 177, 82-90 (2008).

[101] Hahm, K., *et al.* Alphav beta6 integrin regulates renal fibrosis and inflammation in Alport mouse. *The American journal of pathology* 170, 110-125 (2007).
[102] Eickelberg, O. & Morty, R.E. Transforming growth factor beta/bone morphogenic protein signaling in pulmonary arterial hypertension: remodeling revisited. *Trends in cardiovascular medicine* 17, 263-269 (2007).
[103] Massague, J. How cells read TGF-beta signals. *Nat Rev Mol Cell Biol* 1, 169-178 (2000).
[104] Wrana, J.L. Regulation of Smad activity. *Cell* 100, 189-192 (2000).
[105] Kalluri, R. & Zeisberg, M. Exploring the connection between chronic renal fibrosis and bone morphogenic protein-7. *Histol Histopathol* 18, 217-224 (2003).
[106] Murray, L.A., *et al.* BMP-7 does not protect against bleomycin-induced lung or skin fibrosis. *PloS one* 3, e4039 (2008).
[107] Yasuo, M., *et al.* Relationship between calcium-activated chloride channel 1 and MUC5AC in goblet cell hyperplasia induced by interleukin-13 in human bronchial epithelial cells. *Respiration* 73, 347-359 (2006).
[108] Atherton, H.C., Jones, G. & Danahay, H. IL-13-induced changes in the goblet cell density of human bronchial epithelial cell cultures: MAP kinase and phosphatidylinositol 3-kinase regulation. *Am J Physiol Lung Cell Mol Physiol* 285, L730-739 (2003).
[109] Wynn, T.A. Fibrotic disease and the T(H)1/T(H)2 paradigm. *Nat Rev Immunol* 4, 583-594 (2004).
[110] Jakubzick, C., *et al.* Human pulmonary fibroblasts exhibit altered interleukin-4 and interleukin-13 receptor subunit expression in idiopathic interstitial pneumonia. *Am J Pathol* 164, 1989-2001 (2004).
[111] Jakubzick, C., *et al.* Augmented pulmonary IL-4 and IL-13 receptor subunit expression in idiopathic interstitial pneumonia. *J Clin Pathol* 57, 477-486 (2004).
[112] Chiaramonte, M.G., *et al.* Regulation and function of the interleukin 13 receptor alpha 2 during a T helper cell type 2-dominant immune response. *The Journal of experimental medicine* 197, 687-701 (2003).
[113] O'Toole, M., Legault, H., Ramsey, R., Wynn, T.A. & Kasaian, M.T. A novel and sensitive ELISA reveals that the soluble form of IL-13R-alpha2 is not expressed in plasma of healthy or asthmatic subjects. *Clin Exp Allergy* 38, 594-601 (2008).
[114] Fichtner-Feigl, S., Strober, W., Kawakami, K., Puri, R.K. & Kitani, A. IL-13 signaling through the IL-13alpha2 receptor is involved in induction of TGF-beta1 production and fibrosis. *Nat Med* 12, 99-106 (2006).
[115] Lee, C.G., *et al.* Interleukin-13 induces tissue fibrosis by selectively stimulating and activating transforming growth factor beta(1). *The Journal of experimental medicine* 194, 809-821 (2001).
[116] Zhu, Z., *et al.* IL-13-induced chemokine responses in the lung: role of CCR2 in the pathogenesis of IL-13-induced inflammation and remodeling. *J Immunol* 168, 2953-2962 (2002).
[117] Kim, E.Y., *et al.* Persistent activation of an innate immune response translates respiratory viral infection into chronic lung disease. *Nat Med* 14, 633-640 (2008).
[118] Miotto, D., *et al.* Interleukin-13 and -4 expression in the central airways of smokers with chronic bronchitis. *Eur Respir J* 22, 602-608 (2003).
[119] Boutten, A., *et al.* Decreased expression of interleukin 13 in human lung emphysema. *Thorax* 59, 850-854 (2004).

[120] Lee, J.S., *et al.* Inverse association of plasma IL-13 and inflammatory chemokines with lung function impairment in stable COPD: a cross-sectional cohort study. *Respir Res* 8, 64 (2007).
[121] Prasse, A., *et al.* A vicious circle of alveolar macrophages and fibroblasts perpetuates pulmonary fibrosis via CCL18. *American journal of respiratory and critical care medicine* 173, 781-792 (2006).
[122] Hurst, J.R., *et al.* Susceptibility to exacerbation in chronic obstructive pulmonary disease. *N Engl J Med* 363, 1128-1138.
[123] Overduin, M. & de Beer, T. The plot thickens: how thrombin modulates blood clotting. *Nat Struct Biol* 7, 267-269 (2000).
[124] Kipnis, E., *et al.* Massive alveolar thrombin activation in Pseudomonas aeruginosa-induced acute lung injury. *Shock* 21, 444-451 (2004).
[125] Schmidt, B., *et al.* Thrombin inhibitors reduce intrapulmonary accumulation of fibrinogen and procoagulant activity of bronchoalveolar lavage fluid during acute lung injury induced by pulmonary overdistention in newborn piglets. *Pediatr Res* 39, 798-804 (1996).
[126] Burchardi, H., *et al.* Adult respiratory distress syndrome (ARDS): experimental models with elastase and thrombin infusion in pigs. *Adv Exp Med Biol* 167, 319-333 (1984).
[127] Kimura, M., *et al.* The significance of cathepsins, thrombin and aminopeptidase in diffuse interstitial lung diseases. *J Med Invest* 52, 93-100 (2005).
[128] Fujimoto, H., *et al.* Thrombin-activatable fibrinolysis inhibitor and protein C inhibitor in interstitial lung disease. *Am J Respir Crit Care Med* 167, 1687-1694 (2003).
[129] Ludwicka-Bradley, A., Bogatkevich, G. & Silver, R.M. Thrombin-mediated cellular events in pulmonary fibrosis associated with systemic sclerosis (scleroderma). *Clin Exp Rheumatol* 22, S38-46 (2004).
[130] Howell, D.C., Laurent, G.J. & Chambers, R.C. Role of thrombin and its major cellular receptor, protease-activated receptor-1, in pulmonary fibrosis. *Biochem Soc Trans* 30, 211-216 (2002).
[131] Hernandez-Rodriguez, N.A., *et al.* Role of thrombin in pulmonary fibrosis. *Lancet* 346, 1071-1073 (1995).
[132] Ohba, T., *et al.* Scleroderma bronchoalveolar lavage fluid contains thrombin, a mediator of human lung fibroblast proliferation via induction of platelet-derived growth factor alpha-receptor. *Am J Respir Cell Mol Biol* 10, 405-412 (1994).
[133] Vaidyula, V.R., Criner, G.J., Grabianowski, C. & Rao, A.K. Circulating tissue factor procoagulant activity is elevated in stable moderate to severe chronic obstructive pulmonary disease. *Thrombosis research* 124, 259-261 (2009).
[134] Howell, D.C., *et al.* Absence of proteinase-activated receptor-1 signaling affords protection from bleomycin-induced lung inflammation and fibrosis. *Am J Pathol* 166, 1353-1365 (2005).
[135] Takizawa, T., *et al.* Abrogation of bronchial eosinophilic inflammation and attenuated eotaxin content in protease-activated receptor 2-deficient mice. *J Pharmacol Sci* 98, 99-102 (2005).
[136] Schmidlin, F., *et al.* Protease-activated receptor 2 mediates eosinophil infiltration and hyperreactivity in allergic inflammation of the airway. *J Immunol* 169, 5315-5321 (2002).

[137] Manfredi, A.A., Rovere-Querini, P., Bottazzi, B., Garlanda, C. & Mantovani, A. Pentraxins, humoral innate immunity and tissue injury. *Current opinion in immunology* 20, 538-544 (2008).
[138] Siripont, J., Tebo, J.M. & Mortensen, R.F. Receptor-mediated binding of the acute-phase reactant mouse serum amyloid P-component (SAP) to macrophages. *Cellular immunology* 117, 239-252 (1988).
[139] Mantovani, A., Garlanda, C., Doni, A. & Bottazzi, B. Pentraxins in innate immunity: from C-reactive protein to the long pentraxin PTX3. *Journal of clinical immunology* 28, 1-13 (2008).
[140] Lu, J., *et al.* Structural recognition and functional activation of FcgammaR by innate pentraxins. *Nature* 456, 989-992 (2008).
[141] Garlanda, C., *et al.* Non-redundant role of the long pentraxin PTX3 in anti-fungal innate immune response. *Nature* 420, 182-186 (2002).
[142] Hirschfield, G.M. & Pepys, M.B. C-reactive protein and cardiovascular disease: new insights from an old molecule. *Qjm* 96, 793-807 (2003).
[143] Haudek, S.B., *et al.* Fc receptor engagement mediates differentiation of cardiac fibroblast precursor cells. *Proc Natl Acad Sci U S A* 105, 10179-10184 (2008).
[144] Lu, J., *et al.* Structural recognition and functional activation of FcgammaR by innate pentraxins. *Nature* (2008).
[145] Singh, P.P. & Kaur, S. Serum amyloid P-component in murine tuberculosis: induction kinetics and intramacrophage Mycobacterium tuberculosis growth inhibition in vitro. *Microbes and infection / Institut Pasteur* 8, 541-551 (2006).
[146] Pilling, D., Buckley, C.D., Salmon, M. & Gomer, R.H. Inhibition of fibrocyte differentiation by serum amyloid P. *J Immunol.* 171, 5537-5546. (2003).
[147] Haudek, S.B., *et al.* Bone marrow-derived fibroblast precursors mediate ischemic cardiomyopathy in mice. *Proc Natl Acad Sci U S A* 103, 18284-18289 (2006).
[148] Matrisian, L.M. The matrix-degrading metalloproteinases. *Bioessays* 14, 455-463 (1992).
[149] O'Connor, C.M. & FitzGerald, M.X. Matrix metalloproteases and lung disease. *Thorax* 49, 602-609 (1994).
[150] Demedts, I.K., Brusselle, G.G., Bracke, K.R., Vermaelen, K.Y. & Pauwels, R.A. Matrix metalloproteinases in asthma and COPD. *Curr Opin Pharmacol* 5, 257-263 (2005).
[151] Visse, R. & Nagase, H. Matrix metalloproteinases and tissue inhibitors of metalloproteinases: structure, function, and biochemistry. *Circ Res* 92, 827-839 (2003).
[152] Fukuda, Y., Ishizaki, M., Kudoh, S., Kitaichi, M. & Yamanaka, N. Localization of matrix metalloproteinases-1, -2, and -9 and tissue inhibitor of metalloproteinase-2 in interstitial lung diseases. *Lab Invest* 78, 687-698 (1998).
[153] Lee, C.G., *et al.* Role of Chitin, Chitinase/Chitinase-Like Proteins in Inflammation, Tissue Remodeling, and Injury. *Annual review of physiology*.
[154] Lee, C.G., *et al.* Role of breast regression protein 39 (BRP-39)/chitinase 3-like-1 in Th2 and IL-13-induced tissue responses and apoptosis. *The Journal of experimental medicine* 206, 1149-1166 (2009).
[155] Chupp, G.L., *et al.* A chitinase-like protein in the lung and circulation of patients with severe asthma. *N Engl J Med* 357, 2016-2027 (2007).
[156] Letuve, S., *et al.* Lung chitinolytic activity and chitotriosidase are elevated in chronic obstructive pulmonary disease and contribute to lung inflammation. *Am J Pathol* 176, 638-649.

[157] Matsuura, H., *et al.* Role of Breast Regression Protein (BRP)-39 in the Pathogenesis of Cigarette Smoke-Induced Inflammation and Emphysema. *Am J Respir Cell Mol Biol.*

[158] Sohn, M.H., *et al.* The chitinase-like proteins breast regression protein-39 and YKL-40 regulate hyperoxia-induced acute lung injury. *American journal of respiratory and critical care medicine* 182, 918-928.

[159] Korthagen, N.M., *et al.* Serum and BALF YKL-40 levels are predictors of survival in idiopathic pulmonary fibrosis. *Respir Med* 105, 106-113.

[160] Furuhashi, K., *et al.* Increased expression of YKL-40, a chitinase-like protein, in serum and lung of patients with idiopathic pulmonary fibrosis. *Respiratory medicine* 104, 1204-1210.

[161] Hogg, J. Peripheral lung remodelling in asthma and chronic obstructive pulmonary disease. *Eur Respir J* 24, 893-894 (2004).

[162] Raghu, G., *et al.* An official ATS/ERS/JRS/ALAT statement: idiopathic pulmonary fibrosis: evidence-based guidelines for diagnosis and management. *American journal of respiratory and critical care medicine* 183, 788-824.

[163] Phillips, R.J., *et al.* Circulating fibrocytes traffic to the lungs in response to CXCL12 and mediate fibrosis. *J Clin Invest.* 114, 438-446. (2004).

[164] Murphy, P.M., *et al.* International union of pharmacology. XXII. Nomenclature for chemokine receptors. *Pharmacological reviews* 52, 145-176 (2000).

[165] Lee, C.G., *et al.* Early growth response gene 1-mediated apoptosis is essential for transforming growth factor beta1-induced pulmonary fibrosis. *The Journal of experimental medicine* 200, 377-389 (2004).

[166] Gauldie, J., Sime, P.J., Xing, Z., Marr, B. & Tremblay, G.M. Transforming growth factor-beta gene transfer to the lung induces myofibroblast presence and pulmonary fibrosis. *Current topics in pathology* 93, 35-45 (1999).

[167] Lee, C.G., Kang, H.R., Homer, R.J., Chupp, G. & Elias, J.A. Transgenic modeling of transforming growth factor-beta(1): role of apoptosis in fibrosis and alveolar remodeling. *Proceedings of the American Thoracic Society* 3, 418-423 (2006).

[168] Li, M., *et al.* Epithelium-specific deletion of TGF-beta receptor type II protects mice from bleomycin-induced pulmonary fibrosis. *The Journal of clinical investigation* 121, 277-287.

[169] Higashiyama, H., *et al.* Inhibition of activin receptor-like kinase 5 attenuates bleomycin-induced pulmonary fibrosis. *Experimental and molecular pathology* 83, 39-46 (2007).

[170] Yamada, M., *et al.* Gene transfer of soluble transforming growth factor type II receptor by in vivo electroporation attenuates lung injury and fibrosis. *Journal of clinical pathology* 60, 916-920 (2007).

[171] Shull, M.M., *et al.* Targeted disruption of the mouse transforming growth factor-beta 1 gene results in multifocal inflammatory disease. *Nature* 359, 693-699 (1992).

[172] Kulkarni, A.B., *et al.* Transforming growth factor beta 1 null mutation in mice causes excessive inflammatory response and early death. *Proceedings of the National Academy of Sciences of the United States of America* 90, 770-774 (1993).

[173] Jakubzick, C., *et al.* Therapeutic Attenuation of Pulmonary Fibrosis Via Targeting of IL-4- and IL-13-Responsive Cells *J Immunol* 171, 2684-2693 (2003).

Part 2

Neoplasia

5

Cancer Stem Cells (CSCs) in Lung Cancer

Hiroyuki Sakashita, Yuki Sumi and Naohiko Inase
Department of Integrated Pulmonology,
Graduate School of Medical and Dental Science,
Tokyo Medical and Dental University
Japan

1. Introduction

The cancer stem cell model for tumor progression is the first model of its type to suggest that only one subpopulation of cancer cells is capable of proliferating indefinitely. These cells resemble normal stem cells in their capacity for self-renewal and multi-potential differentiation, and can both initiate and maintain tumors. The prevailing names for these cells are "cancer stem cells (CSCs)" and "cancer initiating cells (CICs)." The CSC model implies a hierarchical organization within the tumor in which a limited number of CSCs represents the apex of the hierarchy. CSCs are chemo-resistant, radio-resistant, and quiescent, and have been shown to cause both metastasis and relapse.

CSCs were first described in patients with acute myeloid leukemia (AML) by Dick et al. (Lapidot et al., 1994). As to be expected from leukemia stem cells, these CSCs exhibited the properties of self-renewal, proliferation and multipotency. The frequency of these leukemia-initiating cells in the peripheral blood of those AML patients was one engraftment unit in 250,000 cells. Dick et al. identified the leukemia-initiating cells as $CD34^{+}CD38^{-}$.

In the years since, CSCs have been identified in cancers of the breast(Al-Hajj et al., 2003), brain (Singh et al., 2003) and prostate, pancreas and lung (Eramo et al., 2008). In this chapter we review CSCs in lung cancer.

2. Overview of CSCs in lung cancer

2.1 Concept of CSCs

Two major models have been described for tumor propagation: the clonal evolution model, which involves a stochastic component, and the CSC model, which is defined as hierarchical. According to the clonal evolution model, a neoplasm arises from a single cell of origin, whereupon an acquired genetic variability within the original clone allows a sequential selection to more aggressive clones, thereby allowing the tumor to progress. According to the CSC model, tumor cells are heterogeneous, and only the CSC subset has the ability to proliferate extensively and form new tumors (Wicha et al., 2006). Yet neither model alone can adequately explain the complex biology of tumor progression, resistance, and metastasis. Fig. 1 describes a new CSC hypothesis model that encompasses both the CSC hierarchical and clonal evolution components, a model in which pre-existing CSCs can transform into secondary CSCs (Takebe & Ivy, 2003).

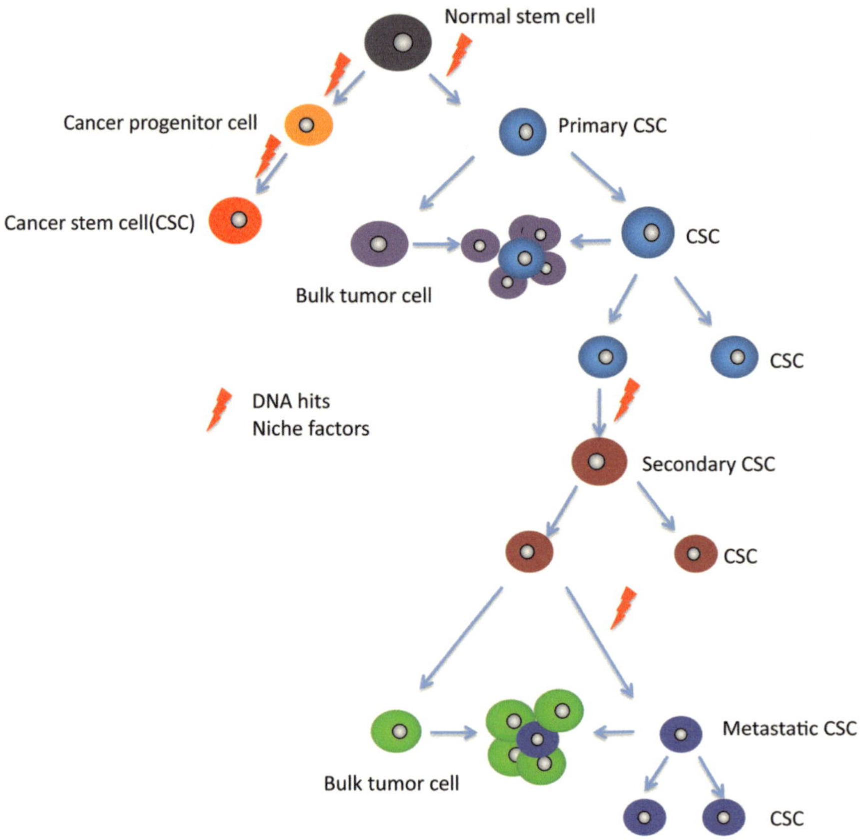

Fig. 1. CSC development.

A combination of DNA hits and niche microenvironmental factors can transform normal stem cells into primary CSCs or more differentiated cancer progenitor cells. Primary tumors are formed mostly from bulk tumor cells together with a small percentage of CSCs. The accumulation of additional DNA hits plus an altered niche microenvironment may drive primary CSCs to evolve into a genetically distinct population of secondary CSCs. Metastatic CSCs have the potential to proliferate and form metastatic tumors at distant sites composed mostly of bulk tumor cells together with a minority of metastatic CSCs (Takebe & Ivy, 2003).

2.2 Origins of CSCs

It remains uncertain whether CSCs originate from normal (somatic) stem cells that acquire oncogenic mutations or from non-stem cells of more differentiated forms that dedifferentiate and acquire stem-cell-like properties through mutation and reprogramming. CSCs can convert into differentiated cells, (Fig. 2) and evidence has suggested that these differentiated cells can acquire stem-cell-like properties via exogenous circumstances (including the niche), with plasticity. (Fig. 2) Cancer stem cells, for example, might be supplied from cancer cells of a non-metastatic epithelial form through a process referred to as "epithelial–mesenchymal transition" (EMT). Besides tissue stem cells, bone marrow-derived cells (BMDCs) may also represent a potential source of malignancy (Fig. 2). Houghton et al.

showed that chronic infection of C57BL/6 mice with Helicobacter, a known carcinogen, repopulated the stomach with BMDCs (Houghton et al., 2004). Not long after, these cells progressed through metaplasia and dysplasia to intraepithelial cancer. These findings have broad implications for the multistep model of cancer progression, as they suggest that epithelial cancers can originate from bone-marrow-derived sources. The BMDCs may also be the precursors to CSCs in lung cancer.

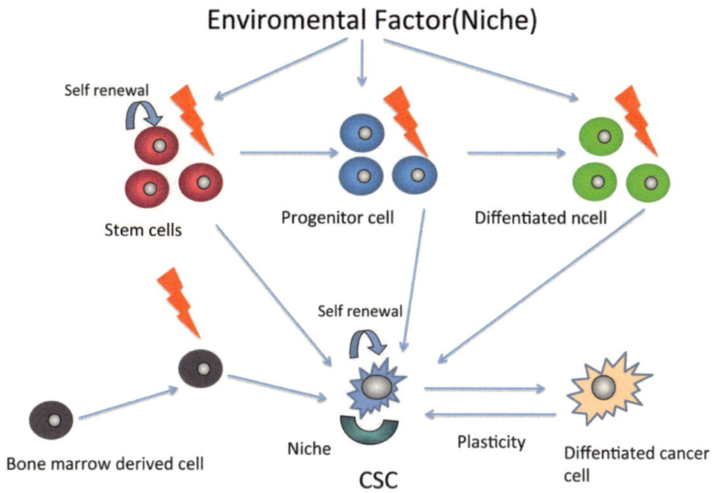

Fig. 2. Origins of CSCs

2.3 How CSCs can be identified?

Cancer stem cells are difficult to isolate in solid cancers, though several possible methodologies for attempting isolation are available. The process can be attempted with a surface marker (CD44 or CD133), or with non-adherent cells cultured in a specific condition (sphere-forming), or with side population (SP) cells identified by efflux of dye and an intracellular enzyme activity (aldehyde dehydrogenase, ALDH). As yet, there is no apparent consensus about the 'best marker' by which to identify CSCs. The gold standard assay *in vivo*, the assessment that isolates what most closely fits the definition of CSCs, may be serial transplantation in animal models.

2.3.1 Surface marker

CD44 or CD133 have served as CSC markers in many solid cancers. In a lung cancer study by Eramo et al., some tumors contained a rare population of $CD133^+$ cancer stem-like cells that could both self-renew and generate an unlimited progeny of non-tumorigenic cells (Eramo et al., 2008). Eramo's group found that the tumorigenic cells in small cell lung cancer (SCLC) and non-small cell lung cancer (NSCLC) consisted of rare populations of undifferentiated cells expressing CD133, an antigen present in the cell membrane of normal and cancer-primitive cells of the hematopoietic, neural, endothelial and epithelial lineages. In their cultures, lung cancer $CD133^+$ cells were able to grow indefinitely as 'tumor spheres.' Meanwhile, Bertolini et al. independently reported similar findings using $CD133^+$ cells isolated from 60 samples of human lung cancer (Bertolini et al., 2009). In their experiments, a $CD133^+$ population was increased in primary NSCLC compared with normal lung tissue.

Importantly, the expression of CD133 in tumors was linked to shorter progression-free survival of NSCLC patients treated with platinum-based regimens. The proliferative potential, invasiveness, and chemoresistance of $CD133^+$ cells isolated from human lung tumors are reported to depend on the expression of Oct-4 (Chen et al., 2008), a protein important in embryonic stem cell development. Lung cancer $CD133^+$ cells have higher Oct-4 expression, can self-renew, and robustly resist both chemotherapy agents and radiotherapy. Leung et al. found that stem cell-like properties are enriched in $CD44^+$ subpopulations of some lung cancer cell lines, while most cancer cell lines showed no significant CD133 expression (Leung et al., 2010).

Urokinase plasminogen activator (uPA) and its receptor (uPAR/CD87) are major regulators of extracellular matrix degradation. Both take part in cell migration and invasion under physiological and pathological conditions. uPAR/CD87 was identified as one of the candidate CSC markers in SCLC (Gutova et al., 2007). $uPAR^+$ cells exhibited multi-drug resistance, high clonogenic activity, and co-expression of the putative cancer stem cell markers CD44 and MDR1 in all of the SCLC cell lines examined.

2.3.2 Sphere formation in culture

Primary cancer cells can be propagated in spheroid cultures (Reynolds & Weiss, 1992), and doing so may allow extensive CSC characterization *in vitro*. The cells are grown *in vitro* as tumor spheres under nonadherent conditions using a serum-free medium supplemented with growth factors. Once cultured by this technique, they exhibit high clonogenic potential and readily renew themselves, generate differentiated progeny, and generate tumors *in vivo* (Singh et al., 2003; Ricci-Vitiani et al., 2007). From the major subtypes of lung cancer, 'tumor spheres' were found to possess CSC properties, both *in vitro* (expression of the CSC marker CD133, unlimited proliferative potential, extended abilities to self-renew and differentiate) and *in vivo* (high tumorigenic potential, capacity to recapitulate tumor heterogeneity and mimic the histology of the specific tumor subtype from which CSCs were derived). Lung cancer 'spheres' are also extremely resistant to most conventional drugs currently used to treat lung cancer patients. This spheroid culture method serves adequately in isolating CSCs from clinical samples.

2.3.3 Side population (SP) on flow cytometry

SP cells are a subpopulation of cells rich in stem-cell-like characteristics. This subpopulation was first identified by flow-cytometer-based cell sorting defined by Hoechst 33342 dye exclusion (Goodell et al., 1996). Hoechst low cells are described as side population (SP) cells by virtue of their typical profiles in Hoechst red versus Hoechst blue bivariate fluorescent-activated cell sorting dot plots. This test is based on ABCG2 transporter, the second member of the G subfamily of ATP binding cassette (ABC) transporters. ABCG2 is one of the most important multidrug-resistance transporters, and its substrates include Hoeschst 33342 (Ding et al., 1996). SP cells were isolated from several solid cancers and certified to have stemness. Regarding the lung, SP cells isolated from six lung cancer cell lines exhibited higher invasiveness, higher resistance to chemotherapeutic drugs, and higher tumorigenicity *in vivo* compared with non-SP cells (Ho et al., 2007). Most of the SP fraction appeared to be in the G(0) quiescent state. Several SCLC cell lines examined by Salcido et al. contained a consistent SP fraction comprising $<1\%$ of the bulk population. SP cells had higher proliferative capacity *in vitro*, were able to efficiently self-renew, and exhibited reduced cell surface expression of differentiation markers. These cells also over-expressed many genes associated with cancer stem cells, drug resistance, and angiogenesis (Salcido et al., 2010).

2.3.4 ALDH activity

Aldehyde dehydrogenase (ALDH) is a detoxifying enzyme known for its role in the oxidation of intracellular aldehydes and for its contribution to the oxidation of retinol to retinoic acid in early stem cell differentiation (Jiang et al., 2009). Class 1 of the ALDH family (ALDH1) is the predominant ALDH isoform in mammals, and ALDH1 activity might serve as a common marker for both normal and malignant stem cell populations. Jiang et al. used the Aldefluor assay and fluorescence-activated cell sorting (FACS) analysis to isolate ALDH1-positive cells from human lung cancer cell lines. The ALDH1-positive cancer cells they isolated exhibited several of the important CSC properties: self-renewal, differentiation, multidrug resistance and expression of stem cell marker *in vitro*; tumor initiation and occurrence of a heterogeneous population of cancer cells *in vivo*. Jiang et al. also found that relatively high ALDH1 protein levels were positively associated with the stage and grade of the tumors, and inversely related to patient survival.

2.3.5 Surface marker may vary even when the cells originate from the same tumor subtype

The marked heterogeneity within CSC sub-populations underlines the need to find more specific single markers or to define new marker combinations for the prospective isolation of CSCs in solid tumors. CD133 is generally considered a stem cell marker, but $CD133^-$ tumors also contain cells with CSC activity. Independent studies have shown that $CD133^-$ glioblastoma cells can establish tumors in recipient mice with efficiencies comparable to those of $CD133^+$ cells (Beier et al., 2007). In a study by Meng et al., $CD133^+$ and $CD133^-$ subpopulations in lung cancer cells exhibited similar levels of colony formation, self-renewal, proliferation, differentiation, and invasion, as well as similar resistance to chemotherapy drugs (Meng et al., 2009). As such, these $CD133^+$ and $CD133^-$ subpopulations can be assumed to have contained similar numbers of cancer stem cells. In some cases, CD133 is undetectable among lung cancer samples. In a study by Tirino et al., for example, $CD133^+$ was found in only 72% of 89 fresh specimens (Tirino et al., 2009). As to be expected from heterogeneous populations, the CSC phenotype is less than uniform, even when the cells originate from the same tumor subtype. Primary tumors with different genotypes at just one locus can have tumor propagating cell populations with distinct markers. Fig. 3 (Curtis et al., 2010)

Transgenic mice carrying mutant Kras (left), mutant Kras with p53 deficiency (center), and mutant EGFR (right) all develop lung adenocarcinomas that harbor similar proportions of cells expressing the mouse stem cell marker Sca-1 (blue cells). The tumor-propagating capacity of $Sca\text{-}1^+$ and $Sca\text{-}1^-$ cells from each primary tumor genotype was tested by implanting small numbers of sorted cells into the lungs of recipient mice. When isolated from primary Kras tumors, both $Sca\text{-}1^+$ and $Sca\text{-}1^-$ cells generated secondary tumors that recapitulated the Sca-1 cell heterogeneity found in the primary tumor (left). Yet in tumors with the mutant Kras and p53 deficiency, $Sca\text{-}1^+$ cells were better able to form secondary tumors (represented as larger tumors) than $Sca\text{-}1^-$ cells (center). Further, the secondary tumors derived from $Sca\text{-}1^+$ cells harbored $Sca\text{-}1^+$ cells in a proportion comparable to the

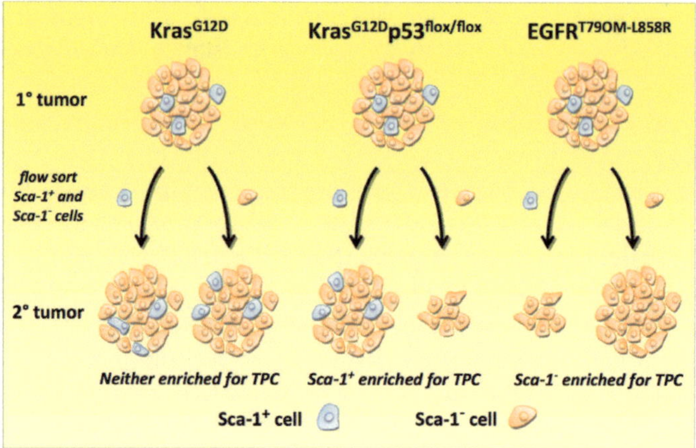

Fig. 3. Tumor Propagating Capacity of Sca-1+ Lung Cancer Cells

primary tumor, whereas the few small tumors derived from Sca-1- cells had no detectable Sca-1+ population. These data suggest that the Sca-1+ cells in this tumor genotype are enriched in lung cancer stem cells. The opposite appears to be true in mutant EGFR adenocarcinomas, in which Sca-1- cells exhibited a greater capacity for generating secondary tumors (right). The distribution of Sca-1+ cells in secondary mutant EGFR tumors remains undetermined. Adapted with permission from Sullivan JP, Minna JD. Tumor oncogenotypes and lung cancer stem cell identity. Cell Stem Cell. 2010 Jul 2;7(1):2-4.

2.4 Serial transplantation is the gold standard to validate CSCs

Serial transplantation in animal models has been the gold standard to certify stemness, but animal models fail to mimic the human tumor microenvironment as closely as desired. This can be overcome, however, by orthotopic transplantation of candidate cancer-initiating cells back into their normal microenvironment. When working with putative lung cancer-initiating cells, this can be achieved by intratracheal delivery into the lung cavity using a methodology employed for the delivery of an adeno-Cre virus in sporadic murine models of human lung cancer (Meuwissen et al., 2001, 2003). In serial transplantation in animal models, the presence of residual immune effector cells in recipient mice may influence the efficiency of human cell engraftment in NOD/SCID mice. Shultz et al. showed that NOD-*scid IL2Rγnull* (NSG) mice engrafted with human hemopoietic stem cells generate a 6-fold higher percentage of human CD45+ cells in host bone marrow compared to similarly treated NOD-*scid* mice (Shultz et al., 2005).

2.5 How do we overcome obstacles of researching CSCs?

It would be impossible to extensively investigate CSCs without expanding the cell populations *in vitro*. Given the low frequency of lung CSCs within primary tumor tissues, we have difficulty in finding agents which can kill CSCs with strong selective toxicity. There are two methods to surmount this obstacle.

2.5.1 Sphere formation is the best way to obtain CSCs from patients

This experimental strategy is the best approach so far developed to obtain the unlimited expansion of a tumorigenic lung cancer cell population from primary patients. As such, it serves as a powerful enabler for extensive studies on these cells. Yet CSC spheres are difficult to establish from epithelial tumors, particularly in the case of lung cancer. Indeed, only a few specialized laboratories in the world are able to use CSC spheroids from primary tumors. And as another potential limiting factor, CSCs constitute 5 - 30% of the cells in an average tumor sphere (Eramo et al., 2008).

2.5.2 Inducing CSCs by EMT

Another potential solution is the generation of 'induced' CSCs (iCSC). The induction of an epithelial-mesenchymal transition (EMT) in normal or neoplastic mammary epithelial cell populations has been shown to enrich the cells with stem-like properties. Gupta et al. demonstrated that normal and cancer cell populations experimentally induced into an EMT also exhibited an increased resistance to chemotherapy drug treatment. When cancer cell populations are induced to pass through an EMT, the proportion of CSCs could increase (Gupta et al., 2009).

2.6 Lung stem cells and lung cancer stem cells

The lung is a complex organ made up of regionally and functionally distinct cell phenotypes. A diverse class of lung stem cells drives the development and turnover of these populations. The epithelium of the adult airways consists of three distinct compartments arranged along a proximal-distal axis. One factor impeding efforts to demonstrate the existence of adult lung stem cells has been the slow turnover rates in the adult epithelium. Yet in spite of this factor, findings from new studies on pollutant- and pathogen-induced injuries leading to massive lung cell proliferation suggest that adult stem cells are present in each of the epithelial compartments. These different tumor subclasses may arise from distinct cells of origin localized within a defined regional compartment/microenvironment. (Fig. 4)

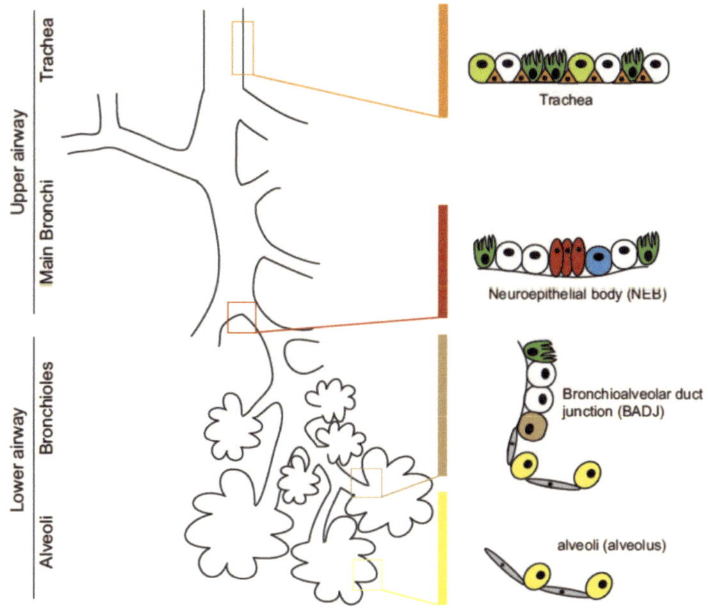

Fig. 4. Airway stem cell microenvironments and associated human carcinomas.

A schematic diagram of the mouse lung highlighting the spatially distinct cellular environments shown to harbour airway stem/progenitor cells. Candidate epithelial niches (depicted on the right hand side) have been identified and found to exist in spatially defined regions: the tracheal submucosal gland ducts, neuroendocrine bodies (NEB) of the bronchi/bronchioles, and the broncholalveolar duct junction (BADJ). Adapted with permission from Sutherland KD, Berns A. Cell of origin of lung cancer. Mol Oncol. 2010 Oct;4(5):398.

2.6.1 Adenocarcinoma

The distal airways are composed of respiratory bronchioles and alveoli lined with cuboidal epithelium. The bronchioalveolar duct junction (BADJ) has been identified as a microenvironment harboring airway stem cells (Giangreco et al., 2002). With regard to tumorigenicity, Jackson et al. reported that lung tumors were suggested to initiate by oncogenic K-Ras activation appeared to be derived from targeted cells located in the BAD (Fig. 5A) (Jackson et al., 2001). Kim et al. have isolated bronchioalveolar stem cells (BASCs), a regional pulmonary stem cell population, in BADJ, and have identified the candidate origins of CSCs in lung adenocarcinomas (Kim et al., 2005). The BASCs in their experiments resisted bronchiolar and alveolar damage and proliferated during epithelial cell renewal *in vivo*. The BASCs also exhibited self-renewal capability and multipotent properties in clonal assays, and expanded in response to oncogenic K-ras in culture and developed to the lung tumor precursors *in vivo*.

2.6.2 Squamaous carcinoma

The histopathology and gene expression patterns of mouse lung SCC-like lesions frequently resemble those of tracheal basal cell progenitors. This presents the appealing prospect that these are the target cells of origin in this subclass of lung cancer (Fig. 5C). Keratin (K) 5/14-expressing basal cells are located at the submucosal gland duct junctions or intracartilaginous boundaries and are capable of self-renewal, proliferation, and multipotency (Borthwick et al., 2001; Hong et al., 2004a, 2004b; Rawlins et al., 2008; Rock et al., 2009). As such, K 5/14-expressing cells are the putative major airway stem cells. But the clear relationship between basal progenitors and lung SCC has not been established yet.

2.6.3 Small cell carcinoma

The specific cell population that gives rise, upon genetic alteration, to SCLC remains to be identified. Human and mouse SCLC predominately localize to the midlevel bronchioles and typically express a range of neuroendocrine markers, including calcitonin-gene related peptide (CGRP) and other neuropeptides normally expressed within pulmonary neuroendocrine cells (PNECs) (Meuwissen et al., 2003). Some investigators have hypothesized, based on these observations, that a rare population of PNECs are the progenitors of SCLC. (Fig. 5B) In the mouse lung, microenvironments found in close proximity to neuroepithelial bodies (NEB) have been shown to maintain putative stem cell populations containing both PNECs and variant CCSP-expressing (vCE) cells (Reynolds et al., 2000a). These may be the CSCs of small cell carcinoma.

2.6.4 Human lung stem cells

Kajstura et al. recently identified a set of potential stem cells in the human lung (Kajstura et al., 2011). These cells were self renewing, clonogenic and multipotent *in vitro*. And when

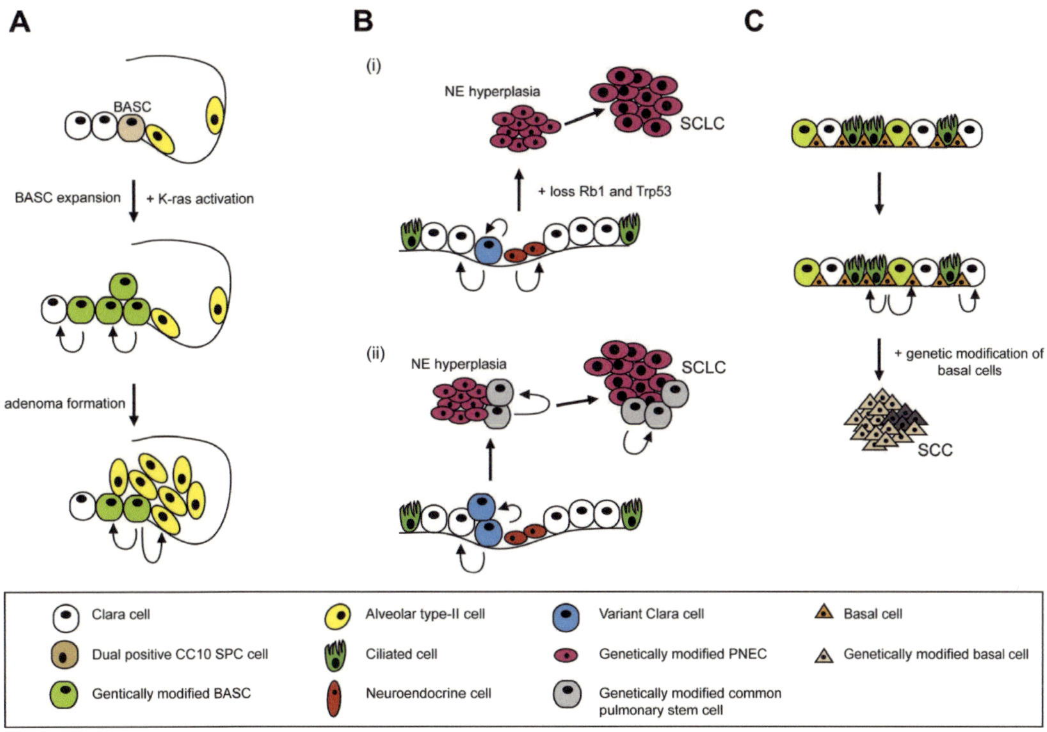

Fig. 5. Schematic overview of the putative role of normal tissue stem/progenitor cells in lung cancer.
(A) BADJ contains a rare cell population that expresses both Clara-specific and alveolar-specific markers. These cells are BASCs. K-Ras activation enhances the proliferation of BASCs. (B) Two hypotheses on the origin of lung NE tumors. NEBs in the epithelial lining of the bronchi harbor PNECs associated with vCEs. The first hypothesis proposes that (i) NE tumors arise from these PNECs. The second hypothesis proposes (ii) that NE hyperplasia and SCLC arise from a less-differentiated progenitor-like cell (for example vCE). (C) Given the basal-like phenotype of SCC, one could hypothesize that squamous cell tumors arise from these basal stem cells. Adapted with permission from Sutherland KD, Berns A. Cell of origin of lung cancer. Mol Oncol. 2010 Oct;4(5):397-403.

injected into a mouse model of lung injury, they regenerated bronchioles, alveoli, smooth muscle, pulmonary vessels and many other lung components. The experiments were performed using c-kit as a stem cell marker. These results are exciting, though rigorous validation will be required. CSCs of the human lung with the potential to differentiate into NSCLCs and SCLCs may originate from not only regional lung stem cells, but also multipotent stem cells.

2.6.5 Analysis of important molecules and pathways of CSCs in the mouse model

Several papers have reported analyses of important molecules related with CSCs in mouse models.

2.6.5.1 Bmi1

Bmi1 is requisite for K-ras–induced tumorigenesis in the mouse model (Dovey et al., 2008). Loss of Bmi1 in K-ras transgenic mice decreased the prevalence and progression of lung tumors and impaired BADJ stem cell proliferation and self-renewal *in vivo* and *in vitro*.

2.6.5.2 PI3K/PTEN/Akt

The phosphoinositide 3-kinases (PI3K)/phosphatase and tensin homolog (PTEN)/protein kinase B (Akt) pathway is requisite for normal stem cell function. The tumor suppressor PTEN encodes a lipid phosphatase that negatively regulates the PI3K /Akt cell survival pathway. In NSCLC, loss of PTEN protein expression occurs frequently (Marsit et al., 2005).

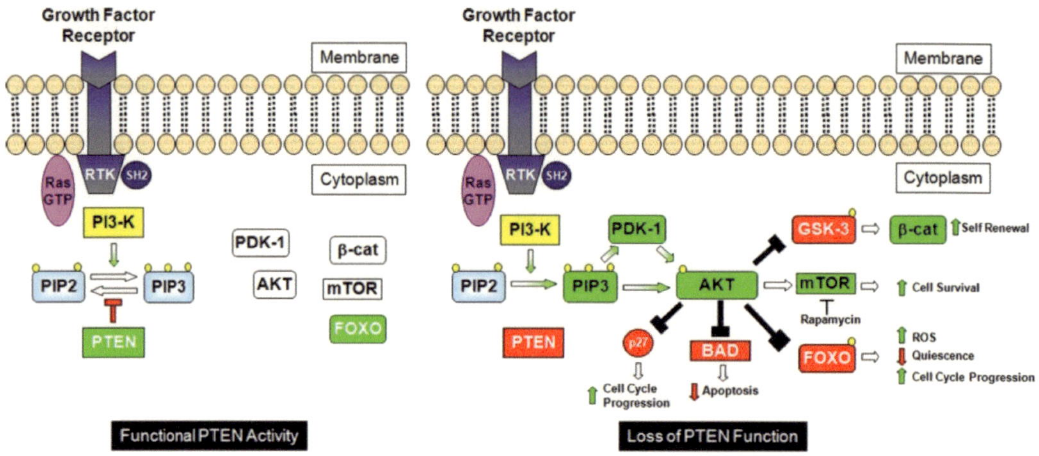

Fig. 6. Loss of PTEN function results in accumulation of PIP3, which activates a cascade of signaling molecules.
AKT activation inhibits pro-apoptotic factors and stimulates cell cycle progression. The loss of PTEN function leads to increased cell survival and proliferation. RTK, receptor tyrosine kinase. Adapted with permission from Hill R, Wu H. PTEN, stem cells, and cancer stem cells. J Biol Chem. 2009 May 1;284(18):11755-9.

Recent work has linked the PI3K/PTEN/Akt pathway to lung cancer stem cells and to the suppression of K-ras mutations. (Fig. 6) Spontaneous lung adenocarcinomas develop in transgenic mice with an inducible loss of PTEN expression in bronchioalveolar cells (Yanagi et al., 2007). Interestingly, a loss of PTEN expression resulted in K-ras mutations in 33% of mice and developed spontaneous adenocarcinomas. A loss of PTEN expression and PI3K activation may elicit increases in BADJ stem cells, side-population (SP) cells, and the frequency of K-ras mutations, and thereby initiate the development of lung adenocarcinoma over time.

2.6.5.3 Hedgehog

The Hedgehog (Hh) signaling pathway acts as an important regulator of stem cell fates during embryonic development and has been linked to SCLC (Watkins et al., 2003a, 2003b). The observation that intraepithelial Hh signaling is increased after naphthalene-induced airway injury suggests that progenitor cells activate Hh signaling in response to injury. Increased Hh signaling is also observed in the lungs of PTEN-deficient mice that develop spontaneous lung adenocarcinomas in conjunction with BADJ stem cell expansion, and thus may play a causal role in this process (Yanagi et al., 2007).

2.6.5.4 Wnt

The Wnt developmental pathway is an another critical regulator of embryonic lung stem cells (Reynolds et al., 2008; Zhang et al., 2008). In adult mice, conditional deletion of p38+, a known downstream target of noncanonical Wnt signaling (Ma & Wang, 2007), leads to an expansion of $CCSP^{+}SP\text{-}C^{+}$ stem cells, hyperproliferation, and increased sensitization to K-ras–induced tumorigenesis (Ventura et al., 2007).

2.7 Therapeutic strategy against CSCs

CSCs are thought to be responsible for disease relapse or metastasis, and also for resistance to radiation or conventional chemotherapy. CSCs showed increased quiescence *in vivo* and *in vitro*, which suggests that they may respond poorly to conventional treatments designed to mainly kill the proliferating cells or terminally differentiated cells forming the bulk of tumors (Guan et al., 2003). Several therapies against CSCs have been considered, but none have been fully developed for lung cancer CSCs. The remainder of this chapter will discuss strategies for targeting CSCs in various organs.

2.7.1 Targeting the key molecule (stem cell marker), key gene & key signaling pathways

Given that CSCs share many of the same features as normal stem cells, there is a potential risk of killing normal stem cells while targeting CSCs. It thus becomes important to further characterize the similarities and differences between these two types of stem cells. New therapeutic approaches to selectively target CSC-specific markers, genes, and pathways are needed.

2.7.1.1 Antibody-based treatment against surface markers

One recently introduced therapeutic approach for human AML employs an activating mAb directed to the adhesion molecule CD44, a known CSC marker of AML (Jin et al., 2006). The *in vivo* administration of this Ab to NOD/SCID mice transplanted with human AML markedly reduced leukemic repopulation. Mechanistically, CD44-specific Ab treatment induced differentiation to a more mature cancer cell progeny that were unable to establish robust leukemia upon xenotransplantation. For solid tumors, CD13, a CSC marker of hepatocellular carcinoma, is expected to become a target of CSC therapy (Haraguchi et al., 2010).

2.7.1.2 Inhibition of essential pathways in the CSCs function

The eventual goal is to generate targeted therapeutics that inhibit essential pathways in the CSC fraction. It will probably be complicated to target these pathways, as the same pathways are also pivotal in normal stem cell function. The Wnt pathway, hedgehog pathway, and notch pathway are all reportedly essential for maintaining stemness. The blocking of these pathways thus holds promise as a therapeutic approach. Many reports and target drugs have been published and developed in pursuit of such a therapy, but only few of these reports have touched upon lung cancer CSCs. The hedgehog pathway may play an important role in lung CSCs, as the pharmacological inhibition of this pathway reduced the growth of lung tumor cells in xenograft models (Watkins et al., 2003a). Suppression of the

Notch pathway by treatment with either a γ-secretase inhibitor or stable expression of shRNA against NOTCH3 significantly decreased $ALDH^+$ lung cancer cells, and commensurate reductions in tumor cell proliferation and clonogenicity were observed (Sullivan et al., 2010). Notch signaling thus appears to take part in lung cancer stem cell maintenance.

2.7.1.3 Blocking of the stemness gene

$CD133^+$ cells in lung cancer exhibit higher Oct-4 expression. Oct-4 plays a crucial role in maintaining the self-renewing, cancer stem-like, and chemoradioresistant properties of $CD133^+$ cells. Knock-down of Oct-4 expression can significantly inhibit the abilities of tumor invasion and colony formation, increase apoptotic activities, and enhance the treatment effect of chemoradiotherapy (Chen et al., 2008). The downregulation of transcription factor SOX in lung CSCs reportedly suppresses growth and metastasis (Xiang et al., 2011), and the blocking of the SCF/c-kit signaling pathway inhibits CSC proliferation and survival after chemotherapy exposure in human lung cancer cell lines (Levina et al., 2010). Cisplatin treatment eliminated most of the tumor cells, but unlike the blocking of c-kit, it was unsuccessful in eliminating CSCs. A combination treatment with cisplatin and c-kit blocking prevented the growth of both tumor cell subpopulations.

2.7.2 Regulation of micro RNA

Micro RNAs can affect the signaling pathways that influence stem cell self-renewal. A lack of let-7 is required for self renewal *in vitro* and for tumorigenicity *in vivo*. In other words, an overexpression of let-7a reduces self renewal and proliferative capacity and converts highly malignant and metastasizing CSCs into less malignant cells (Yu et al., 2007).

2.7.3 Induction of diffentiation of CSCs

Differentiation therapy aims at converting tumorigenic CSCs in their non-tumorigenic progeny. Treatment with bone morphogenic protein 4 (BMP4) reduced the tumor-initiating cell pool in a glioma model and markedly slowed down tumor growth *in vivo* without toxic side effects (Piccirillo et al., 2006).

2.7.4 Altering the CSCs' environment (niche)

The stem cell niche plays an important role in maintaining CSCs and apparently enhances the therapy resistance of CSCs by sheltering the cells from diverse insults (Folkins et al., 2007). Perivascular, hypoxic, premetastatic and stromal myofibroblast niches have all been reported. The perivascular niche in brain tumors has been shown to contribute directly to the generation of CSCs and tumor growth. Anti-angiogenic therapy using vascular endothelial growth factor inhibitors not only depleted tumor vascularization, but also ablated CSCs in the xenograft (Calabrese et al., 2007). While some stem cells are perivascular, others may occupy hypoxic niches and be regulated by O_2 gradients (Parmar et al., 2007). However, the underlying mechanisms are still unclear. O_2 availability may have a direct role in stem cell regulation through the HIF-1α modulation of Wnt/β-catenin signaling (Mazumdar et al., 2010). These niches are expected to become targets of CSC therapy. In experiments with colon adenocarcinomas, Vermeulen et al. found that hepatocyte growth factor and other myofibroblast-secreted factors activate CSC clonogenicity (Vermeulen et al., 2010). More significantly, myofibroblast-secreted factors restored the CSC phenotype in more differentiated tumor cells both *in vitro* and *in vivo*. Vermeulen's group therefore propose that the stemness of colon cancer cells is in part orchestrated by the microenvironment.

2.7.5 Activation of reactive oxygen species (ROS)

CSCs have the ability to keep ROS levels low. Subsets of CSCs in some tumors contain lower ROS levels and enhanced ROS defenses compared to their non-tumorigenic progeny. This may contribute to tumor radioresistance. Overcoming low ROS levels within CSCs may be a useful method for improving local and systemic oncologic therapies (Diehn et al., 2009). Haraguchi et al. found that CD13 is a marker for semiquiescent CSCs in human liver cancer cell lines and clinical samples. Mechanistically, CD13 reduced ROS-induced DNA damage after genotoxic chemo/radiation stress and protected cells from apoptosis. In mouse xenograft models, a combination of a CD13 inhibitor and the genotoxic chemotherapeutic fluorouracil (5-FU) drastically reduced tumor volume compared with either agent alone. Thus, the combination of a CD13 inhibitor with a ROS-inducing chemo/radiation therapy may improve the treatment of liver cancer (Haraguchi et al., 2010). CD44 is an adhesion molecule expressed in cancer stem-like cells in gastric cancer. Ishimoto et al. showed that a CD44 variant (CD44v) interacts with xCT, a glutamate-cystine transporter, and controls the intracellular level of reduced glutathione (GSH) (Ishimoto et al., 2011). Human gastrointestinal cancer cells with strong CD44 expression showed an enhanced capacity for GSH synthesis and defense against ROS. Ablation of CD44 induced a loss of xCT from the cell surface and suppressed tumor growth in a transgenic mouse model of gastric cancer. The activation of ROS may be viable as another target therapy for CSCs.

2.7.6 Overcoming of chemoresistance and radioresistance in CSCs

Reversing chemoresistance in CSC populations can be achieved through a specific blockade of multidrug resistance ABC transporters (Frank et al., 2005). Enhanced drug efflux mediated by ABCB1 P-glycoprotein and related ATP-binding cassette transporters is one of several mechanisms of multidrug resistance thought to impair chemotherapeutic success in human cancers. In CD133$^+$ CSC in malignant melanoma, ABCB5, a novel human ABC transporter, mediates melanoma resistance to the chemotherapeutic agent doxorubicin, and this effect is reversible by both mAb-mediated inhibition of ABCB5-dependent drug efflux. In addition, ABCB5 gene silencing substantially increases the sensitivity of human melanoma cells to the anticancer chemotherapeutics 5-fluorouracil (5-FU) and camptothecin (Huang et al., 2004). CSC-targeted therapeutic approaches might also include strategies directed at reversal of radioresistance. Bao et al. reported that CD133$^+$ human glioma CSCs contributed to tumor radioresistance by preferentially activating the DNA damage checkpoint response and enhancing the DNA repair capacity (Bao et al., 2006). An inhibition of the Chk1 and Chk2 checkpoint kinases reversed the radioresistance of CD133$^+$ glioma CSCs in their experiments.

2.7.7 Supressing EMT and inducing MET

EMT in carcinoma seems to be associated with the acquisition of a CSC phenotype endowed with a more invasive and metastatic phenotype. As such, a new drug to suppress EMT is expected as a target therapy for CSCs. Metastatic progression might involve the dissemination of CSCs at tumor margins that have undergone EMT. Thus, the mesenchymal-epithelial transition (MET) seems to hold promise as a therapy. Gupta et al. identified small molecules (salinomycin) that specifically inhibit cancer stem cell proliferation through the induction of MET (Gupta et al., 2009).

3. Conclusion

Though targeted therapies have been developed, we have witnessed only limited improvement in the prognosis of lung cancer patients. Ultimately, patient cure will require the eradication of all cells within a cancer. From this standpoint, combination therapies targeting both CSCs and bulk cancer populations hold promise. In the coming years we must clarify the origin of CSCs, find more specific CSC markers, elucidate the CSC niche, and develop more effective innovative agents against resistant tumorigenic lung CSCs. CSCs may vary in different lung cancers, so personalized CSC therapy may be needed.

4. References

Al-Hajj, M., Wicha, MS. & Benito-Hernandez, A. (2003), Prospective identification of tumorigenic breast cancer cells. *Proc Natl Acad Sci U S A, 100,* 7, (Apr 1), pp. 3983-8,ISSN 0027-8424

Beier, D., Hau, P. & Proescholdt, M. (2007), CD133(+) and CD133(-) glioblastoma-derived cancer stem cells show differential growth characteristics and molecular profiles. *Cancer Res,* 67, 9, (May 1), pp. 4010-5, ISSN 0008-5472

Bertolini, G., Roz, L. & Perego, P. (2009), Highly tumorigenic lung cancer CD133+ cells display stem-like features and are spared by cisplatin treatment. *Proc Natl Acad Sci U S A,* 106, 38, (Sep 22), pp. 16281-6,ISSN 0027-8424

Borthwick, DW., Shahbazian, M. & Krantz, QT. (2001), Evidence for stem-cell niches in the tracheal epithelium. *Am J Respir Cell Mol Biol,* 24, 6, (Jun),pp. 662-70, ISSN 1044-1549

Calabrese, C., Poppleton, H. & Kocak M. (2007), A perivascular niche for brain tumor stem cells. *Cancer Cell,* 11, 1, (Jan), pp. 69-82, ISSN 1535-6108

Campbell, LL. & Polyak, K. (2007), Breast tumor heterogeneity: cancer stem cells or clonal evolution? *Cell Cycle,* 6, 19, (Oct 1), pp. 2332-8, ISSN 1551-4005

Chen, YC., Hsu, HS. & Chen, YW. (2008), Oct-4 expression maintained cancer stem-like properties in lung cancer-derived CD133-positive cells. *PLoS One,* 3, 7, e2637, ISSN 1932-6203

Chen YC, Hsu HS, Curtis, SJ., Sinkevicius, KW. &Li, D. (2010), Primary tumor genotype is an important determinant in identification of lung cancer propagating cells. *Cell Stem Cell,* 7, 1, (Jul 2), pp. 127-33

Diehn, M., Cho, RW. & Lobo, NA. (2009), Association of reactive oxygen species levels and radioresistance in cancer stem cells. *Nature,* 458, 7239, (Apr 9), pp. 780-3, ISSN 0028-0836

Ding, XW. ,Wu, JH. & Jiang, CP. (2010), ABCG2: a potential marker of stem cells and novel target in stem cell and cancer therapy. *Life Sci,* 86, 17-18, (Apr 24), pp. 631-7, ISSN 0024-3205

Dovey, JS., Zacharek, SJ. &Kim, CF. (2008), Bmi1 is critical for lung tumorigenesis and bronchioalveolar stem cell expansion. *Proc Natl Acad Sci U S A,* 105, 33, (Aug 19), pp. 11857-62, ISSN 0027-8424

Eramo, A., Lotti, F. & Sette, G. (2008), Identification and expansion of the tumorigenic lung cancer stem cell population. *Cell Death Differ,* 15, 3, (Mar), pp. 504-14, ISSN 1350-9047

Folkins, C., Man, S. &Xu, P. (2007), Anticancer therapies combining antiangiogenic and tumor cell cytotoxic effects reduce the tumor stem-like cell fraction in glioma xenograft tumors. *Cancer Res,* 67, 8, (Apr 15), pp. 3560-4, ISSN 0008-5472

Frank, NY., Margaryan, A. & Huang, Y. (2005), ABCB5-mediated doxorubicin transport and chemoresistance in human malignant melanoma. *Cancer Res,* 65, 10, (May 15), pp. 4320-33, ISSN 0008-5472

Gutova, M., Najbauer, J., Gevorgyan, A., Metz, MZ., Weng, Y., Shih, CC,,& Aboody, KS. (2007). Identification of uPAR-positive chemoresistant cells in small cell lung cancer. *PLoS One,* 2, 2, (Feb 2007), pp. e243., Available from www.ncbi.nlm.nih.gov/pmc/articles/PMC1800348/pdf/pone.0000243.pdf

Giangreco, A., Reynolds, SD. & Stripp, BR. (2002), Terminal bronchioles harbor a unique airway stem cell population that localizes to the bronchoalveolar duct junction. *Am J Pathol,* 161, 1, (Jul), pp. 173-82, ISSN 0002-9440

Giangreco, A., Groot, KR. & Janes, SM. (2007), Lung cancer and lung stem cells: strange bedfellows? *Am J Respir Crit Care Med,* 175, 6, (Mar 15), pp. 547-53, ISSN 1073-449X

Goodell, MA., Brose, K. & Paradis, G. (1996), Isolation and functional properties of murine hematopoietic stem cells that are replicating in vivo. *J Exp Med,* 183, 4, (Apr 1), pp. 1797-806, ISSN 0022-1007

Guan, Y., Gerhard, B. & Hogge, DE. (2003), Detection, isolation, and stimulation of quiescent primitive leukemic progenitor cells from patients with acute myeloid leukemia (AML). *Blood,* 101, 8, (Apr 15), pp. 3142-9, ISSN 0006-4971

Gupta, PB., Onder, TT. & Jiang, G. (2009), Identification of selective inhibitors of cancer stem cells by high-throughput screening. *Cell,* 138, 4, (Aug 21), pp. 645-59, ISSN 0092-8674

Haraguchi, N., Ishii, H. & Mimori, K. (2010), CD13 is a therapeutic target in human liver cancer stem cells. *J Clin Invest,* 120, 9, (Sep 1), pp. 3326-39, ISSN 0021-9738

Ho, MM., Ng, AV. &Lam, S. (2007), Side population in human lung cancer cell lines and tumors is enriched with stem-like cancer cells. *Cancer Res,* 67, 10, (May 15), pp. 4827-33, ISSN 0008-5472

Hong, KU., Reynolds, SD. &Watkins, S. (2004), Basal cells are a multipotent progenitor capable of renewing the bronchial epithelium. *Am J Pathol,* 164, 2, (Feb), pp. 577-88, ISSN 0002-9440

Hong, KU., Reynolds, SD. & Watkins, S. (2004), In vivo differentiation potential of tracheal basal cells: evidence for multipotent and unipotent subpopulations. *Am J Physiol Lung Cell Mol Physiol,* 286, 4, (Apr), pp. L643-9, ISSN 1040-0605

Houghton, J., Stoicov, C. & Nomura, S. (2004), Gastric cancer originating from bone marrow-derived cells. *Science,* 306, 5701, (Nov 26), pp. 1568-71, ISSN 0036-8075

Huang, Y., Anderle, P. & Bussey, KJ. (2004), Membrane transporters and channels: role of the transportome in cancer chemosensitivity and chemoresistance. *Cancer Res,* 64, 12, (Jun 15), pp. 4294-301, ISSN 0008-5472

Ishimoto, T., Nagano, O. & Yae, T. (2011), CD44 variant regulates redox status in cancer cells by stabilizing the xCT subunit of system xc(-) and thereby promotes tumor growth. *Cancer Cell,* 19, 3, (Mar 8), pp. 387-400, ISSN 1535-6108

Ishizawa, K., Rasheed, ZA. & Karisch, R. (2010), Tumor-initiating cells are rare in many human tumors. *Cell Stem Cell,* 7, 3, (Sep 3), pp. 279-82

Jackson, EL., Willis, N. &Mercer, K. (2001), Analysis of lung tumor initiation and progression using conditional expression of oncogenic K-ras. *Genes Dev,* 15, 24, (Dec 15), pp. 3243-8, ISSN 0890-9369

Jiang, F., Qiu, Q. & Khanna, A. (2009), Aldehyde dehydrogenase 1 is a tumor stem cell-associated marker in lung cancer. *Mol Cancer Res,* 7, 3, (Mar), pp. 330-8, ISSN 1541-7786

Jin, L., Hope, KJ. & Zhai, Q. (2006), Targeting of CD44 eradicates human acute myeloid leukemic stem cells. *Nat Med,* 12, 10, (Oct), pp. 1167-74, ISSN 1078-8956

Kajstura, J., Rota, M. & Hall, SR. (2011), Evidence for human lung stem cells. *N Engl J Med,* 364, 19, (May 12), pp. 1795-806, ISSN 0028-4793

Kim, CF., Jackson, EL. & Woolfenden, AE. (2005), Identification of bronchioalveolar stem cells in normal lung and lung cancer. *Cell,* 121, 6, (Jun 17) , pp. 823-35, ISSN 0092-8674

Lapidot, T., Sirard, C. & Vormoor, J. (1994), A cell initiating human acute myeloid leukaemia after transplantation into SCID mice. *Nature,* 367, 6464, (Feb 17) ,pp. 645-8, ISSN 0028-0836

Leung, EL., Fiscus, RR. & Tung, JW. (2010), Non-small cell lung cancer cells expressing CD44 are enriched for stem cell-like properties. *PLoS One,* 5, 11, e14062, ISSN 1932-6203

Levina, V., Marrangoni, A. & Wang, T. (2010), Elimination of human lung cancer stem cells through targeting of the stem cell factor-c-kit autocrine signaling loop. *Cancer Res,* 70, 1, (Jan 1), pp. 338-46, ISSN 0008-5472

Ma, L. & Wang, HY. (2007), Mitogen-activated protein kinase p38 regulates the Wnt/cyclic GMP/Ca2+ non-canonical pathway. *J Biol Chem,* 282, 39, (Sep 28), pp. 28980-90, ISSN 0021-9258

Marsit, CJ., Zheng, S. & Aldape, K. (2005), PTEN expression in non-small-cell lung cancer: evaluating its relation to tumor characteristics, allelic loss, and epigenetic alteration. *Hum Pathol,* 36, 7, (Jul), pp. 768-76, ISSN 0046-8177

Mazumdar, J., O'Brien, WT. & Johnson, RS. (2010), O2 regulates stem cells through Wnt/beta-catenin signalling. *Nat Cell Biol,* 12, 10, (Oct), pp. 1007-13, ISSN 1465-7392

Meng, X., Li, M. & Wang, X. (2009), Both CD133+ and CD133- subpopulations of A549 and H446 cells contain cancer-initiating cells. *Cancer Sci,* 100, 6, (Jun), pp. 1040-6, ISSN 1347-9032

Meuwissen, R., Linn, SC. & Linnoila, RI. (2003), Induction of small cell lung cancer by somatic inactivation of both Trp53 and Rb1 in a conditional mouse model. *Cancer Cell,* 4, 3, (Sep), pp. 181-9, ISSN1535-6108

Meuwissen, R., Linn, SC. & van der Valk, M. (2001), Mouse model for lung tumorigenesis through Cre/lox controlled sporadic activation of the K-Ras oncogene. *Oncogene,* 20, 45, (Oct 4), pp. 6551-8, ISSN 0950-9232

Parmar, K., Mauch, P. & Vergilio, JA. (2007), Distribution of hematopoietic stem cells in the bone marrow according to regional hypoxia. *Proc Natl Acad Sci U S A,* 104, 13, (Mar 27), pp. 5431-6, ISSN 0027-8424

Pece, S., Tosoni, D. & Confalonieri, S. (2010), Biological and molecular heterogeneity of breast cancers correlates with their cancer stem cell content. *Cell,* 140, 1, (Jan 8), pp. 62-73, ISSN 0092-8674

Piccirillo, SG., Reynolds, BA. & Zanetti, N. (2006), Bone morphogenetic proteins inhibit the tumorigenic potential of human brain tumour-initiating cells. *Nature,* 444, 7120, (Dec 7), pp. 761-5, ISSN 0028-0836

Rawlins, EL., Okubo, T. & Que, J. (2008), Epithelial stem/progenitor cells in lung postnatal growth, maintenance, and repair. *Cold Spring Harb Symp Quant Biol,* 73, 291-5, ISSN 0091-7451

Reynolds, BA. & Weiss, S. (1992), Generation of neurons and astrocytes from isolated cells of the adult mammalian central nervous system. *Science,* 255, 5052, (Mar 27), pp. 1707-10, ISSN 0036-8075

Reynolds, SD., Giangreco, A. & Power, JH. (2000), Neuroepithelial bodies of pulmonary airways serve as a reservoir of progenitor cells capable of epithelial regeneration. *Am J Pathol,* 156, 1, (Jan), pp. 269-78, ISSN 0002-9440

Reynolds, SD., Hong, KU. & Giangreco, A. (2000), Conditional clara cell ablation reveals a self-renewing progenitor function of pulmonary neuroendocrine cells. *Am J Physiol Lung Cell Mol Physiol,* 278, 6, (Jun), pp. L1256-63, ISSN 1040-0605

Reynolds, SD., Zemke, AC. & Giangreco, A. (2008), Conditional stabilization of beta-catenin expands the pool of lung stem cells. *Stem Cells,* 26, 5, (May), pp. 1337-46, ISSN 1066-5099

Ricci-Vitiani, L., Lombardi, DG. & Pilozzi, E. (2007), Identification and expansion of human colon-cancer-initiating cells. *Nature,* 445, 7123, (Jan 4), pp. 111-5, ISSN 0028-0836

Rock, JR., Onaitis, MW. & Rawlins, EL. (2009), Basal cells as stem cells of the mouse trachea and human airway epithelium. *Proc Natl Acad Sci U S A,* 106, 31, (Aug 4), pp. 12771-5,ISSN 0027-8424

Salcido, CD., Larochelle, A. & Taylor, BJ. (2010), Molecular characterisation of side population cells with cancer stem cell like characteristics in small-cell lung cancer. *Br J Cancer,* 102, 11, (May 25), pp. 1636-44, ISSN 0007-0920

Shultz, LD., Lyons, BL. & Burzenski, LM. (2005), Human lymphoid and myeloid cell development in NOD/LtSz-scid IL2R gamma null mice engrafted with mobilized human hemopoietic stem cells. *J Immunol,* 174, 10, (May 15), pp. 6477-89, ISSN 0022-1767

Singh, SK., Clarke, ID. & Terasaki, M. (2003), Identification of a cancer stem cell in human brain tumors. *Cancer Res,* 63, 18, (Sep 15), pp. 5821-8, ISSN 0008-5472

Sullivan, JP., Spinola, M. & Dodge, M. (2010), Aldehyde dehydrogenase activity selects for lung adenocarcinoma stem cells dependent on notch signaling. *Cancer Res,* 70, 23, (Dec 1), pp. 9937-48, ISSN 0008-5472

Takebe, N. & Ivy, SP. (2010), Controversies in cancer stem cells: targeting embryonic signaling pathways. *Clin Cancer Res,* 16, 12, (Jun 15), pp. 3106-12, ISSN 1078-0432

Tirino, V., Camerlingo, R. & Franco, R. (2009), The role of CD133 in the identification and characterisation of tumour-initiating cells in non-small-cell lung cancer. *Eur J Cardiothorac Surg,* 36, 3, (Sep), pp. 446-53, ISSN 1010-7940

Ventura, JJ., Tenbaum, S. & Perdiguero, E. (2007), p38alpha MAP kinase is essential in lung stem and progenitor cell proliferation and differentiation. *Nat Genet,* 39, 6, (Jun), pp. 750-8, ISSN 1061-4036

Vermeulen, L., De Sousa, EMF. & van der Heijden, M. (2010), Wnt activity defines colon cancer stem cells and is regulated by the microenvironment. *Nat Cell Biol,* 12, 5, (May), pp. 468-76, ISSN 1465-7392

Watkins, DN., Berman, DM. & Baylin, SB. (2003), Hedgehog signaling: progenitor phenotype in small-cell lung cancer. *Cell Cycle,* 2, 3, (May-Jun), pp. 196-8, ISSN 1551-4005

Watkins, DN., Berman, DM. & Burkholder, SG. (2003), Hedgehog signalling within airway epithelial progenitors and in small-cell lung cancer. *Nature,* 422, 6929, (Mar 20), pp. 313-7, ISSN 0028-0836

Wicha, MS., Liu, S. & Dontu, G. (2006), Cancer stem cells: an old idea--a paradigm shift. *Cancer Res,* 66, 4, (Feb 15), pp. 1883-90; discussion 95-6, ISSN 0008-5472

Xiang, R., Liao, D. & Cheng, T. (2011), Downregulation of transcription factor SOX2 in cancer stem cells suppresses growth and metastasis of lung cancer. *Br J Cancer,* 104, 12, (Jun 7), pp. 1931, ISSN 0007-0920

Yanagi, S., Kishimoto, H. & Kawahara, K. (2007), Pten controls lung morphogenesis, bronchioalveolar stem cells, and onset of lung adenocarcinomas in mice. *J Clin Invest,* 117, 10, (Oct), pp. 2929-40, ISSN 0021-9738

Yu, F., Yao, H. & Zhu, P. (2007), let-7 regulates self renewal and tumorigenicity of breast cancer cells. *Cell,* 131, 6, (Dec 14), pp. 1109-23, ISSN 0092-8674

Zhang, Y., Goss, AM. & Cohen, ED. (2008), A Gata6-Wnt pathway required for epithelial stem cell development and airway regeneration. *Nat Genet,* 40, 7, (Jul), pp. 862-70, ISSN 1061-4036

6

Oncogenes and Tumor Suppressor Genes in Small Cell Lung Carcinoma

Pankaj Taneja[1,2], Robert D. Kendig[1,2], Sinan Zhu[1,3], Dejan Maglic[1,2,3], Elizabeth A. Fry[1,2] and Kazushi Inoue[1,2,3,*]
[1]The Departments of Pathology,
[2]Cancer Biology,
[3]Graduate Program in Molecular Medicine,
Wake Forest University Health Sciences,
Medical Center Boulevard, Winston-Salem
USA

1. Introduction

Small cell lung cancer (SCLC) makes up almost 15% of all cases of lung cancer and occurs almost exclusively in individuals with a history of smoking (Blackhall & Faivre-Finn, 2011; Meyerson et al., 2004; Tamasi and Muller, 2011; Walenkamp et al., 2009). However, SCLCs differ significantly from NSCLCs in specific genetic alterations that occur. Moreover, smoking-damaged bronchial epithelia accompanying SCLCs appears to have undergone significantly more acquired genetic damage than is frequently found in NSCLCs. Two subtypes of SCLC exist: homogeneous small cell carcinoma and combined SCLC (mixture of any non-small cell type) (Meyerson et al., 2004; Tamasi and Muller, 2011). SCLC in its advanced stage has an aggressive clinical course and is commonly accompanied by paraneoplastic syndromes. Autocrine growth factors, such as neuroendocrine regulatory peptides (e.g. bombesin/gastrin-releasing peptide), are prominent in SCLC.
SCLC is categorized as limited stage disease (LS) when confined to the ipsilateral hemithorax and within a single radiation port, while extensive stage disease (ES) includes metastatic disease outside the ipsilateral hemithorax (Blackhall & Faivre-Finn, 2011; Meyerson et al., 2004; Tamasi and Muller, 2011; Walenkamp et al., 2009). SCLC is sensitive to chemotherapy; response rates to front-line agents are often in the range of 60%, with approximately 10% of patients achieving a complete response, even in the setting of metastatic disease (Brambilla et al., 2009 Jemal et al., 2006). Despite this, the relapse rates are quite high and survival with currently available salvage therapy is quite modest. With current therapy, patients with LS-SCLC have a median survival of 17 months and a 5-year overall survival rate of 12% , while patients with ES-SCLC have a median survival of 8.9 months, and a 5-year survival rate of approximately 2%. (Brambilla et al., 2009 Jemal et al., 2006; Tamasi and Muller, 2011). This article will review the molecular targeted agents, the genetic abnormalities, and therapeutic efficacy in SCLC.

---

* Corresponding Author

2. *Trp53* gene

The *p53* gene located on chromosome 17p13.1 encodes a nuclear protein that acts as a transcription factor and causes cell cycle arrest or apoptosis. Mutations of this gene lead to the loss of tumor suppressor function, thereby promoting cellular proliferation. The majority of the mutations seen in lung cancers are G to T transversions on the non-transcribed strand, suggesting mutagenesis secondary to tobacco smoke. Wild-type p53 protein is present in very low levels in normal cells, whereas mutant p53 is present in much greater quantities in tumor cells due to its prolonged half-life. In fact, 40–70% of SCLC express abnormal p53 protein (Wistuba et al., 2001). Inactivating mutations of *p53*, seen in approximately 90% of SCLC, are typically missense mutations in the DNA binding domain and, to a lesser degree, homozygous deletions (Demirhan et al., 2010). Preclinical studies have shown that a vaccine composed of dendritic cells transduced with a human wild-type *P53* containing recombinant adenovirus (DC-Ad-p53) causes an antitumor response (Ishihda et al., 1999). The differential expression of the mutant *P53* gene between normal and tumor cells could provide a basis for vaccine therapy.

Antonia et al. (2006) treated 29 patients with relapsed/refractory ES-SCLC with a vaccine consisting of dendritic cells transduced with the full-length wild-type *P53* gene delivered via an adenoviral vector. Only one patient showed a clinical response to the vaccine therapy. Interestingly, there was a high rate of objective clinical responses to chemotherapy (61.9%) that immediately followed vaccination. This clinical response to subsequent chemotherapy was closely associated with induction of immunologic response to vaccination. Hence, it is likely that vaccine therapy could serve as an adjunct to chemotherapy, rather than a primary treatment modality. Using this rationale, a current phase I/II trial is evaluating an autologous dendritic cell-adenovirus p53 vaccine following standard platinum-etoposide chemotherapy in patients with ES- SCLC (Horn et al., 2011). Another approach towards vaccination therapy is to target the ganglioside GD3, a cell surface glycosphingolipid antigen that is typically expressed on cells of neuroectodermal origin and a subset of T-lymphocytes (Grant et al., 1999). Studies using SCLC cell lines suggest that these cell lines express significant levels of GD3. The anti-idiotypic antibody BEC-2, which mimics the structure of the GD3 ganglioside, showed promising results in a pilot study (Grant et al., 1999). Based on these results, the European Organization for Research and Treatment of Cancer (EORTC) performed a randomized phase III study in 515 patients with LS-SCLC who were randomized to receive BEC-2 or not as a maintenance treatment following standard induction chemotherapy (Giaccone et al., 2005). Although there was no improvement in overall survival, progression-free survival, or quality of life in the vaccination arm, there was a trend toward prolonged survival in patients who had a humoral response. The authors concluded that vaccination strategies may be warranted with vaccines that were better able to induce a humoral immune response.

Yang et al. (2011) evaluated the role of genetic *P53* polymorphism in radiation-induced pneumonitis (RP), a common dose-limiting toxicity of radiotherapy. In a cohort comprised of 253 (188 NSCLC and 65 SCLC) lung cancer patients receiving thoracic irradiation, the *P53* 72Arg/Arg genotype was associated with increased radiation-induced pneumonitis risk compared with the 72Pro/Pro genotype. Furthermore, the *P53* Arg72Pro and ATM-111G>A polymorphisms displayed an additive effect in intensifying the risk of developing RP. The cross-validation test showed that 63.2% of RP cases could be identified by *P53* and *ATM* genotypes. Thus, genotyping *P53* and *ATM* polymorphisms might help proactively identify patients susceptible to developing RP when receiving radiotherapy. A recent report by Garcia and co-workers (2010) describe the association of SCLC with ovarian metastases. A 54-year-old woman with SCLC presented with a left ovarian mass, 4.8 cm in diameter, the microscopic appearance of which was identical to the previous bronchoscopic biopsy. Molecular analysis of *P53* demonstrated an identical point mutation (S215) in both tumor sites. Moreover, a *P53* DNA polymorphism (P52R) was identified in normal tissue, but present in homozygosity in both tumor sites.

3. Retinoblastoma (*RB*) gene

The *RB* gene, located on chromosome 13q14.11, has been implicated in the regulation of cell cycle progression, particularly the G1 to S-phase transition, in part, through inactivation of members of the E2F transcription factor family (Modi et al., 2000; Schaffer et al., 2010; Wikman et al., 2006). Hypophosphorylated RB is the growth suppressing form that controls the transcription factors E2F1, E2F2 and E2F3, which are necessary for the G1/S transition. (Modi et al., 2000; Wikman et al., 2006). When bound to hypophosphorylated RB, E2F is in its inactive form, causing cell arrest in the G1 phase. The cyclin D1/CDK4 complex phosphorylates RB, which in turn releases E2F, allowing its activation and promoting entry into S phase. During S phase, cyclin E and CDK2 assert control over the phosphorylation of RB (Wikman et al., 2006; Xue et al., 2003). Inactivation of pRB by gross structural alterations or point mutations in the *RB-1* gene has been described in >90% of all SCLC (Wikman et al., 2006; Xue et al., 2003). The types of mutations that occur in the *RB* gene include deletions, nonsense mutations and splicing abnormalities. Phosphorylated RB suppresses apoptosis by repressing other pro-apoptotic target genes, including apoptotic protease activating factor-1 (Apaf-1) and caspases.

There have been numerous reports of RB protein expression in lung cancer (Wikman & Kettunen, 2006). Similar to human tumor entities in general, different lung cancer types show extensively varying expression patterns: SCLC and large cell neuroendocrine carcinomas (LCNEC) are mostly characterized by loss of RB expression (~90%). Conversely, altered expression of RB is rare (~25%) in squamous cell carcinoma (SCC) and adenocarcinoma (AC), which comprise most cases of NSCLC (Leversha et al., 2003; Gouyer et al., 1998). Rather, NSCLC is attributed to $p16^{INK4a}$ loss or CCND1 overexpression (Schauer et al., 1994). Interestingly, a few cases of SCLC display $p16^{INK4a}$ alterations, but retain normal RB. Preinvasive bronchial lesions and carcinoid tumors also rarely exhibit abnormal RB expression. It is thought that SCLC and other neuroendocrine lung tumors originate from the progenitor neural crest that is similar to the origin of RB.

RB is altered by mutations (20–30%) or small deletions and chromosomal loss (80–90%) in SCLC (Mori et al., 1990; Kashii et al., 1994). Even though 58% of neuroendocrine lung tumors show low or absent mRNA levels, no hypermethylation has been observed in these tumors. In NSCLC, some reports have detected no *RB* DNA alterations, whereas others, somewhat controversially, have found frequent loss of heterozygosity (LOH) (up to 75%) and mutations (33%) of *RB* in SCC (Gouyer et al., 1998; Leversha et al., 2003). DNA Alterations of *RB* have rarely bee described in AC (Sachse et al., 1994). In summary, complete loss of *RB* or a mutant form of *RB* are present in greater than 90% of SCLC cases (Modi et al., 2000). As all normal cells express functional RB, drugs that target cells with inactived or deleted *RB* would be appropriate candidates for testing in patients with SCLC. Such drugs include heat shock protein-90 (Hsp90) inhibitors (Rodina et al., 2007).

4. *BCL2* gene

BCL2 is an oncogene that plays a major role in suppressing apoptosis and thus in treatment resistance (Ilievska et al., 2008; Tudor et al., 2000). Therefore, suppression of BCL2 may increase therapeutic efficacy (Ilievska et al., 2008; Lawson et al., 2010; Ziegler et al., 1997). Since BCL2 is expressed in the vast majority of SCLC cases, it represents a potential therapeutic target in this disease. G3139 (oblimersen) is an 18-base antisense phosphorothioate oligonucleotide complementary to the *BCL2* mRNA in the region encoding the first six amino acids (Reed et al., 1990). Preclinical and clinical studies have demonstrated that intravenous administration of G3139 reduces BCL2 protein production (Waters et al., 2000). The combination of oblimersen and paclitaxel was evaluated in a phase II trial of 12 patients with chemo-refractory SCLC (Rudin et al., 2002). There were no objective responses, but four patients had stable disease. The low yield of this small study was attributed to the relatively low doses of both agents; the dose of oblimersen chosen may have been insufficient to suppress expression of the target gene *BCL2*, while paclitaxel had to be given at a dose clearly below that routinely used. Also, since inhibition of BCL2 expression may increase therapeutic efficacy of cytotoxic agents, this strategy may be more beneficial in patients who responded positively to chemotherapy. In order to test this hypothesis, Rudin et al. (2004) combined oblimersen with etoposide and carboplatin in 16 patients with newly diagnosed extensive stage SCLC. This combination yielded promising results with reasonable toxicity and is currently being studied in a randomized phase III trial to define an exact role for this molecule. Additionally, a small molecule BCL2 inhibitor, AT101, is currently being evaluated in combination with topotecan in patients with relapsed/refractory SCLC. ABT-263 has also been identified as a Bcl-2 inhibitor in numerous SCLC and leukemia/lymphoma cell lines *in vitro* and *in vivo* (Tahir et al., 2010). In another study, Knoefel et al. (2011) studied the single-nucleotide polymorphism C-938A to assess the potential impact as a genetic marker for response to chemotherapy and outcome prediction in 188 Caucasian SCLC patients. Patients carrying the *BCL2-938CC* genotype showed significantly worse time to progression and overall survival than those with the *BCL2-938AA* genotype. This genetic marker might particularly impact on treatment strategies using *BCL2* antisense approaches.

5. *MYC* genes

c-MYC, N-MYC and *L-MYC* are proto-oncogenes that code for proteins involved in the regulation of proliferation, differentiation, and apoptosis (Komiya et al., 2011; Paulson et al., 2009; Xion et al., 2011). Amplification of the *c-MYC* oncogene has been observed in various human malignancies (Komiya et al., 2011). Studies in small cell lung cancer have suggested that although amplification of the *MYC* family genes is seen in only about 10% of patients with newly diagnosed SCLC, this proportion increases following treatment (Komiya et al., 2011; Paulson et al., 2009; Xion et al., 2011 ; Barr et al., 1998), suggesting that MYC expression increases with resistance of SCLC to therapy. Other studies have suggested that higher levels of expression of the *MYC* gene family may play a significant role in the carcinogenesis of SCLC (Kumimoto et al., 2002). Protein overexpression is seen with *MYC* activation by gene amplification or transcriptional dysregulation (Komiya et al., 2011). In addition, amplification of these genes may have a predictive value, since tumors with *N-MYC* amplification have been associated with poor response to chemotherapy, rapid tumor growth, and short survival (Komiya et al., 2011).

6. c-KIT receptor

c-Kit is a tyrosine kinase receptor that, when activated by its ligand stem cell factor (SCF), enhances the growth and survival of hematopoietic cells (Reber et al., 2006; Schneider et al., 2010). Preclinical studies have demonstrated the expression of c-KIT and SCF on almost 70% of SCLC cell lines (Reber et al., 2006), suggesting a possible role in the autocrine/paracrine stimulation of tumor growth. Almost a third of patients with ES-SCLC show evidence of c-kit overexpression by immunohistochemistry (IHC) (Potti et al., 2003; 2005). In a phase II study of imatinib in SCLC, Johnson et al. (2003) enrolled 19 patients with extensive disease who were either treatment-naïve or had a chemo-sensitive relapse. No activity for imatinib was reported, with only one patient showing disease stabilization. A major drawback of this study was that 79% of the enrolled patients lacked c-KIT expression. In an attempt to improve on these findings, the Cancer and Leukemia Group B (CALGB) refined the study design and conducted a similar trial (Dy et al., 2005) in patients with c-KIT overexpression. Despite this, the results were similar to those seen in the previous study, with no observed responses and only one patient with stable disease for 31 weeks. In a third study, imatinib was used as maintenance therapy following cisplatin and irinotecan in patients with ES-SCLC and c-KIT overexpression in tumor tissue (Schneider et al., 2010). Patients who received imatinib did not have any improvement in the progression-free survival, and thus, this strategy did not warrant further investigation. One of the reasons for the inactivity of imatinib in SCLC may be that the putative cells of origin of SCLC are not developmentally dependent on c-KIT (Heinrich et al., 2002), as opposed to hematopoietic stem cells. Another reason could be the absence of activating mutations in patients with SCLC in c-*KIT* exon 11 that predict for imatinib activity in gastrointestinal stromal tumors (Burger et al., 2003).

7. Vascular endothelial growth factor (VEGF) and basic fibroblast growth factor (bFGF)

The vascular endothelial growth factor (VEGF) family is comprised of VEGF-A, VEGF-B, VEGF-C, VEGF-D and VEGF-E growth factors and their three VEGF receptors (VEGFR 1-3) (Tanno et al., 2004; Wójcik et. al., 2010). The VEGF signaling pathway leads to increased proliferation, migration, and invasion of endothelial cells, thus mediating tumor angiogenesis (Tanno et al., 2004; Sattler & Salgia, 2003). VEGF is a key factor in the development of new blood vessels that increases the permeability of microvessels (Thomas et al., 2003). High levels of VEGF have been reported in patients with SCLC, which are associated with tumor stage, disease progression, resistance to chemotherapy and poorer outcomes (Fischer et al., 2007). Studies affecting angiogenesis in SCLC have involved: (1) External inhibitors of angiogenesis, chiefly targeting VEGF and its receptor, (2) Endogenous inhibitors such as interferons, and, (3) Miscellaneous agents, e.g., thalidomide. SCLCs express VEGFR1-3 and VEGFR-2, which are actively involved in tumor growth and invasion (Tanno et al., 2004). The VEGF/VEGFR autocrine signaling pathway mediates proliferation and metastasis, which can be inhibited with the use of monoclonal antibodies against VEGFR-2 and VEGFR-3 in SCLC (Tanno et al., 2004). SU6668, which inhibits VEGFR, c-KIT and FGFR, blocks proliferation and angiogenesis in human lung tumor xenografts (Laird et al., 2000). In a study of 87 patients with SCLC who underwent primary resection followed by adjuvant therapy, microvessel count and expression of VEGF significantly affected survival, thereby establishing a role for angiogenesis in SCLC (Lucchi et al., 2002). Another

preclinical trial demonstrated that ZD6474, a VEGFR-2 and EGFR kinase inhibitor, successfully interfered with VEGF signaling and angiogenesis, leading to decreased proliferation and increased apoptosis in SCLC xenographs. Bevacizumab is a recombinant humanized monoclonal antibody against VEGF that has been approved by the US Food and Drug Administration (FDA) for the treatment of metastatic colon cancer and NSCLC. Preliminary reports of bevacizumab following carboplatin and irinotecan treatment in patients with LS-SCLC have demonstrated response rates, 1- and 2-year survival rates and a safety profile comparable to standard therapy (Raefsky et al., 2005). However, whether the addition of bevacizumab increases progression-free and overall survival is currently unclear and needs to be studied in a randomized phase III trial. VEGF-tyrosine kinase (VEGF-TK) inhibitors have been shown to inhibit downstream signaling pathways that are activated following ligand binding to the VEGF receptor. Multiple agents with VEGF-TK inhibitory activity are being tested for their utility in therapy of various malignancies. A number of small molecules that inhibit VEGFTKs are currently in development, including ZD6474, PTK787/ ZKI222584 (vatalanib), AZD2171, BAY 43-9006 (sorafenib), SU11248 (sunitinib), and AMG706 (Herbst et al., 2005; Morabito et al., 2009). Trials incorporating SU11248 (sunitinib), a multi-targeted TK inhibitor, are being planned in SCLC.
The interferons are a family of naturally-occurring cytokines that have anticancer activity through immunomodulatory and antiangiogenic properties (Blackhall & Shepherd, 2004). Interferons affect endothelial cells by blocking production of basic fibroblast growth factor (bFGF). Patients who achieved a response to chemotherapy were randomized to either interferon maintenance or placebo in different randomized trials. In each of those trials, administration of interferon was associated with considerable toxicity, although two studies showed a trend towards improved survival with interferon treatment (Lebeau et al., 1999). Current trials are investigating the role of interferon either as a vaccine or in combination with cytotoxic chemotherapy in SCLC. Initial reports of maintenance therapy with thalidomide following induction with platinum - etoposide in patients with ES-SCLC have been promising (Conney et al., 2005; Ustuner et al., 2008). This approach needs evaluation in the future.

8. Epidermal growth factor receptor (EGFR)

Although EGFR expression has been reported to be low in SCLC, gefitinib, an oral EGFR tyrosine kinase inhibitor, has been shown to inhibit EGFR signaling in SCLC cell lines (Schmid et al., 2010; Tanno et al., 2004). Anecdotal evidence has suggested tumor regression in patients with advanced stage SCLC following treatment with gefitinib (Araki et al., 2005; Okamoto et al., 2006). This suggests a potential role for gefitinib and other agents targeting the EGFR pathway in this disease. Sequist et al. (2011) performed systematic genetic and histological analyses of tumor biopsies from 37 patients with drug-resistant NSCLCs carrying EGFR mutations. All drug-resistant tumors retained their original activating EGFR mutations, and some acquired known mechanisms of resistance including, the EGFR T790M mutation or *MET* gene amplification. Furthermore, some resistant cancers showed unexpected genetic changes, such as EGFR amplification and mutations in the *PIK3CA* gene, whereas others underwent a pronounced epithelial-to-mesenchymal transition. Surprisingly, five resistant tumors (14%) transformed from NSCLC into SCLC, and were sensitive to standard SCLC treatments. Serial biopsies in three patients revealed that genetic mechanisms of resistance were lost in the absence of the continued selective pressure of EGFR inhibitor treatment, and were sensitive to a second round of treatment with EGFR

inhibitors (Sequist et al., 2011). Collectively, these results deepen our understanding of resistance to EGFR inhibitors and underscore the importance of repeatedly assessing cancers throughout the course of the disease.
HER2/neu expression in SCLC has been less well studied. Studies have demonstrated overexpression of HER2/neu by immunohistochemistry in approximately 13–30% of patients with advanced stage SCLC (Micke et al., 2001; Potti et al., 2002, 2003). These studies also found that HER2/neu expression was associated with a poor prognosis for patients with advanced disease. Based on these findings, the anti-HER2/neu monoclonal antibody trastuzumab may be useful as a therapeutic agent in SCLC.

9. Matrix metalloproteinase (MMP) inhibitors

Matrix metalloproteinases are involved in extracellular matrix (ECM) degradation (Stetler-Stevenson et al., 1993), a key process in metastasis. Use of protease inhibitors to limit extracellular matrix proteolysis by cancer cells, thereby interfering with tumor cell invasion, would thus be an attractive therapeutic target. In a retrospective analysis, elevated MMP expression was identified as a negative predictor of survival in SCLC (Michael et al., 1999). 60 to 70% of tumor cells stained positive by IHC for MMP-1 and -9, while positive signals for MMP-11, -13, and -14 were observed in 70 to 100% of tumor cells. Expression of MMP-11 and MMP-14 was determined to be an independent negative prognostic factor for Marimastat, a synthetic, orally administrated, broad spectrum MMPI with activity against collagenases, gelatinases, and stromolysins (Brown & Giavazzi 1995). The National Cancer Institute of Canada-Clinical Trials Group (NCIC-CTG) and EORTC conducted a randomized placebo-controlled trial of marimastat following induction chemotherapy in 532 patients with sensitive SCLC (Shepherd et al., 2002). The addition of marimastat after induction chemotherapy did not result in improved survival and also had a negative impact on quality of life. These disappointing results may be due to patient selection, as MMP expression was not studied in these patients. The proteinases MMP11 and MMP14 were expressed, a more selective MMPI-targeting these two proteins would arguably be more beneficial. In another study, Jumper et al. (2004) evaluated the relationship between circulating MMP-9 and tissue inhibitor of matrix metalloproteinase (TIMP-1). Thirty one male and female patients with either stage III or IV NSCLC and 17 with either stage III or IV SCLC were compared to 117 age-matched non-smoking controls of both sexes. Prior to any treatment of the patient, a baseline serum sample was obtained from each of the patients for the determination of circulating MMP-9 and TIMP-1. The results indicate that both MMP-9 and TIMP-1 were elevated in the serum of patients with SCLC or NSCLC when compared to the controls. However, the mean values for both MMP-9 and TIMP-1 in the two tumors did not differ. The natural physiological relationship between MMP-9 and the inhibitor TIMP-1 was lost in both SCLC and NSCLC, indicative of abnormal alterations by the tumor. This study suggests that advanced lung cancer alters the normal circulatory pattern of MMP-9 and TIMP-1 a finding that could aid in the understanding of tumor invasion and/or metastasis.

10. Sonic hedgehog pathway

The hedgehog (HH) signaling pathway is important during embryonic development and may be involved in development and progression of several human malignancies (Datta &

Datta, 2006; Watkins & Peacock, 2004). *In vitro* studies have demonstrated extensive activation of this pathway in a subset of SCLC cell lines (Watkins et al., 2003). The Hedgehog (Hh) pathway is essential in early lung formation and development through epithelial-mesenchymal interactions (Peacock & Watkins, 2008; Watkins et al., 2003). The signaling cascade is initiated by Hh binding to the Patched-1 receptor (Ptch-1), a twelve transmembrane protein. In the absence of Hh ligand, Ptch-1 constitutively inhibits the seven transmembrane protein Smoothened (Smo), and renders the pathway inactive. However, binding of Hh ligand to Ptch-1 causes the inhibition of Smo to be relieved, which then activates a protein complex and downstream transcription of Hh targets in the nucleus, including Gli-1 and Ptch-1. Present at low levels in the basal layer of bronchial epithelium in the adult, active Hedgehog signaling results in expansion of an intraepithelial cell population during airway regeneration induced by naphthalene injury. In SCLC, there is ligand-dependent activation of the Hedgehog pathway in a juxtacrine fashion, with adjacent cells expressing Sonic hedgehog (Peacock & Watkins, 2008; Watkins et al., 2003). Further, *in vitro* and *in vivo* studies have demonstrated that SCLC can be inhibited by the steroidal alkaloid Hedgehog antagonist, cyclopamine (Watkins et al., 2003; Vestergaard et al., 2006). These data support the presence of a progenitor cell in SCLC that remains chemotherapy-resistant and relies on the Hedgehog developmental pathway, which can be targeted. Gene expression analysis on members of this pathway showed that although the key transcription factor of this pathway, GL1, was only weakly expressed in cell lines, it was expressed on most SCLC tumors studied, thereby suggesting an important role for this pathway for tumor growth *in vivo* (Vestergaard et al., 2006). Thus, the data support the idea that the HH pathway may be an ideal therapeutic target in SCLC. Agents that inhibit this pathway, cyclopamine and its analog KAAD cyclopamine, will soon be in clinical trials.

11. mTOR pathway

Mammalian target of rapamycin (mTOR), a downstream mediator in the PI3K/Akt signaling pathway, plays a critical role in the regulation of cell proliferation, survival, mobility and angiogenesis (Schmid et al., 2010). Inhibition of this pathway leads to inhibition of downstream signaling elements, thereby resulting in cell cycle arrest in the G1 phase (Chan 2004). Temsirolimus (CCI-779), an inhibitor of mTOR, is being investigated in a phase II trial in patients with ES-SCLC in remission following platinum-based chemotherapy. Genome-wide gene expression profiling revealed that mutant NRF2 affects diverse molecular pathways including the mTOR pathway. Mutant NRF2 upregulates RagD, a small G-protein activator of the mTOR pathway, which was also overexpressed in primary lung cancer (Shibata et al., 2010). Preliminary results show a prolongation of progression-free survival, thereby suggesting significant activity for this agent in SCLC (Pandya et al., 2005). Another agent from this class, everolimus (RAD-001), is currently being tested in a phase II trial for patients with relapsed SCLC (Schmid et al., 2010).

12. CD56 (NCAM)

The neural cell adhesion molecule (NCAM, CD56) is associated with the immunoglobulin family and modulates neuroendocrine cell growth, migration, and differentiation (Jensen & Berthold, 2007; Kim and Kwon, 2010). CD56 is an isoform encoded by the NCAM gene. NCAM is found in almost 100% of SCLC and is also expressed on natural killer cells, neuroendocrine glands, cardiomyocytes, and in the central and peripheral nervous system (Kim and Kwon, 2010). Since malignant cells can be influenced by NCAM signaling, it has been investigated as a target for anti-cancer therapy (Jensen & Berthold, 2007). N901 is an anti-CD56 monoclonal antibody covalently linked to a blocked ricin molecule binds to SCLC tumors and cell lines (Lynch, 1993). Initial studies showed promising activity, but were hampered by the immune response that developed against the murine monoclonal antibody and the ricin molecule, leading to potentially fatal side effects (Fidias et al., 2002). In order to overcome this, a humanized version of this antibody covalently bound to the maytasinoid (microtubule- depolymerizing compound) effector molecule DM-1 has now been made available (BB-10901 or huN901-DM1). Initial studies of this compound have shown evidence of efficacy and safety (Fossella et al., 2005) and a phase II trial is currently underway.

13. Chromosomal alterations

In SCLC and other epithelial tumors, multiple chromosomal aberrations are found, reflecting genomic instability (Balsara& Testa, 2002; Sato et al., 2007.). Loss of the short arm of chromosome 3 has been consistently seen in SCLC (Balsara & Testa, 2002). The deletion of 3p leads to inactivation of three putative tumor-suppressor genes. The majority of SCLCs have deletions affecting multiple chromosomal sites, with recurrent losses at 3p, 5q, 13q and 17p, which are loci with tumor suppressor genes including p53 (Balsara& Testa, 2002). Comparative genomic hybridization analyses have revealed that a large number of SCLCs harbor gains of 1p, 2p, 3q, 5p, 8q and 19p, regions which encode well-known oncogenes, such as *MYC* and *KRAS*. SCLC cell lines found to have amplifications of 1p, 2p and 3q, and deletion of 18q display a more aggressive phenotype of the disease (Balsara & Testa, 2002). Allele loss on chromosome 3p occurs with a frequency greater than 90% in SCLC and is believed to be an early event found in lung carcinogenesis (Sato et al., 2007). The loss of the fragile histidine triad *(FHIT)* gene results in the accumulation of diadenosine tetraphosphate, stimulating DNA synthesis and proliferation (Sozzi et al., 1996). This gene has been localized to 3p14.2 and is believed to be an important tumor suppressor gene involved in the pathogenesis of lung cancer (Sozzi et al., 1996; Wistuba et al., 2001). The second tumor suppressor gene is believed to be *RASSF1A,* which is located within a 120 kilobase region of chromosome 3p21.3 which also contains the *FUS1, SEMA3B* and *SEMA3F* loci. *RASSF1A* encodes a protein similar to RAS effector proteins and is inactivated by tumor-acquired promoter hypermethylation in 90-100% of SCLC samples (Burbee et al., 2001; Dammann et al., 2000). ASSF1 is involved in cell cycle pathways, apoptosis and microtubule stability (Agathanggelou et al., 2005).

FUS1 is a novel tumor suppressor gene identified in the human chromosome 3p21.3 region where allele losses and genetic alterations occur early and frequently for many human cancers. Expression of FUS1 protein is absent or reduced in the majority of lung cancers and premalignant lung lesions. Specificially, expression of the FUS1 protein is lost in 100% of SCLC cases. Interestingly, restoration of wild-type FUS1 function in 3p21.3-deficient non-small cell lung carcinoma cells significantly inhibited tumor cell growth by induction of apoptosis and alteration of cell cycle kinetics (Ji & Ross, 2008). They report that FUS1 induces apoptosis through the activation of the intrinsic mitochondrial-dependent and Apaf-1-associated pathways and inhibits the function of protein tyrosine kinases including EGFR, PDGFR, AKT, c-Abl, and c-Kit. Moreover, intravenous administration of a nanoparticle encapsulated FUS1 expression plasmid effectively delivered FUS1 to distant

tumor sites and mediated an antitumor effect in orthotopic human lung cancer xenograft models (Ji & Ross, 2008). This approach is the rationale for an ongoing FUS1-nanoparticle-mediated gene delivery clinical trial for the treatment of lung cancer.
Deletion of a third gene, *TGFBR2*, located at 3p21.3.22, that encodes the transforming growth factor β (TGF-β) type II receptor, has also been described in SCLC (Hougaard et al., 1999). This nonsense mutation results in the synthesis of a truncated receptor and has been linked to exposure to benzo[a]-pyrene, a component of cigarette smoke. The gene coding for Retinoic Acid Receptor Beta *(RAR-β)* is located on chromosome 3p24 (Mattei et al., 1991). Retinoic acid plays an important role in lung development and differentiation, acting primarily via nuclear receptors. Loss of heterozygosity of *RAR-B2* and *RAR-B4* isoforms is seen in almost all cases of SCLC. Methylation of the promoter region of these two isoforms may be responsible for the silencing of their expression in SCLC (Virmani et al., 2000).

14. Telomerase

Telomeres are genetic elements present at the ends of linear chromosomes that play an important role in stabilizing chromosomes from degradation and cell death (Counter et al., 1992; Hyer & Silvestri, 2000). Telomerase is a ribonucleoenzyme that compensates for telomere shortening during cell division by synthesizing hexameric TTAGGG repeats at the end of the chromosomes. The functional unit of this enzyme consists of an RNA component hTR, and a catalytic component hTERT. Repression of telomerase in the somatic tissues of humans seems to have evolved as a powerful protective barrier against carcinogenesis (Newbold, 2002). Studies in patients with neuroendocrine lung tumors have demonstrated upregulation of the RNA component of telomerase in 98% of human SCLC (Sarvesvaran et al., 1999). Similar studies assessing telomerase activity in small cell lung cancer showed increased activity in all specimens analyzed (Hiyama et al., 1995). Zaffaroni et al. (2003) studied telomerase activity by the telomeric repeat amplification protocol (TRAP) assay in 38 neuroendocrine (NE) lung tumors. A positive TRAP signal was observed in 14 of 15 (93%) SCLCs, 7 of 8 (87%) large-cell NE carcinomas, and only 1 of 15 (7%) typical carcinoid tumors. When telomerase activity was correlated with the gene product-based immunophenotypic profile of individual tumors, the absence of telomerase activity was associated with a lack of BCL-2, P53, c-KIT, and CDK4 expression and presence of RB. Such a phenotype was appreciable in most of the carcinoid tumors. Conversely, telomerase-positive tumors generally showed an immunophenotype consistent with gene product alterations (including high expression of BCL-2, P53, and c-KIT, and loss of RB) and were characterized by a high proliferative index. These data support the previously reported evidence for two genetically unrelated groups of NE lung tumors that have distinct phenotypic profiles (Zaffaroni et al., 2003).

15. Knockout Mouse Models for SCLC

Contrary to NSCLC, neuroendocrine carcinomas are virtually never found in spontaneous or chemically induced murine lung cancer. One reason for this could be that in these murine models, a combination of both *p53* and *Rb* mutations is almost never found, unlike most human SCLCs. To address this issue, a Cre/lox based deletion of both conditional alleles for *Rb* and *p53* was performed by intratracheal instillation with Adeno-Cre (Meuwissen et al., 2003). After 3 months, foci of neuroendocrine hyperplasia developed through the proximal as well as distal bronchi. After a further 3 months, these early lesions progressed into massive lung tumors with histological features typical of SCLC. Interestingly, some early type lesions remained even in the presence of extensive SCLC. Consequently, it was of importance to determine if the early neuroendocrine lesions are indeed precursors for SCLC and, if so, which additional epigenetic events are then needed for progression. Immunohistological characterization of the full-blown tumors revealed that they indeed shared neuroendocrine features with human SCLC. As in human SCLC all neuroendocrine differentiation markers, such as calcitonin gene-related protein (CGRP), neuron-specific enolase, synaptophysin, neural cell adhesion molecule, and achaete-scute homolog-1 (ASH-1) were not expressed. Furthermore, the murine SCLC readily metastasized towards similar organs as found with human SCLC (Meuwissen et al., 2003). All primary SCLC, as well as their metastases, had all *Rb* and *p53* alleles inactivated. Tumors that retained one WT *Rb* allele were all invariably adenocarcinomas without any neuroendocrine features. Therefore, the status of *Rb* most likely determines if tumors occur with mixed SCLC and NSCLC phenotypes, as has been observed in some patients (Brambilla et al., 2000). No lung tumors were found in *Rb*$^{F/F}$ mice, which suggested that loss of *Rb* alone is not enough to initiate lung tumorigenesis (Meuwissen et al., 2003) and the additional loss of *p53* is needed.

Not only does *Rb* loss require additional genetic events to initiate lung tumorigenesis, the nature of these complementary lesions also determines which type of lung cancer will develop. For instance, *RB* inactivation and *KRas* mutations are almost never found together in the same human lung cancer. Moreover, the overall mutation rate of *RB* in human NSCLC is very low (Wistuba & Gazdar, 2003). As noted, Adeno-Cre dependent activation of *Kras* in a broad range of lung epithelial cells leads exclusively to the onset of NSCLC. However, when *LSLKrasG12D* transgenes were combined with *Rb*$^{F/F}$ and Rb family *p130*$^{F/F}$ alleles for Adeno-Cre-dependent lung tumor induction, much more advanced adenocarcinomas of *Kras*^{G12D}; *Rb*$^{-/-}$; *p130*$^{-/-}$ genotypes resulted compared to single *Kras*^{G12D} (Ho et al., 2009). Loss of both *Rb* and *p130*, albeit to a lesser extent, contributed to *Kras* dependent NSCLC. Clearly, in this genetic context Kras^{G12D} overrules any effect of *Rb* loss on neuroendocrine differentiation.

Another intriguing observation came from *CC10-rtTA; tetO7-Cre; Rb*$^{F/F}$ mice administered doxycycline during early embryogenesis, causing a complete *Rb* ablation in all bronchial Clara cells. However, only increased hypercellular neuroendocrine lesions were detected in these mice, and no effect on Clara cell homeostasis could be observed. Alternatively, when all three Rb family proteins (Rb, p107 and p130) were inactivated by a truncated SV40 large T-antigen oncoprotein (T121) in *CC10-T121* mice, severe bronchial hyperplasia with complete dedifferentiation of all Clara cells occurred. These results suggest that Rb might be specifically required for determining neuroendocrine cell fate, but only in a strict cellular and genetic context. The combined evidence from mouse models indicate it is unlikely that NSCLC and SCLC develop from similar target cells. It would be more plausible that separate, non-identical target cells can develop into different lung cancers, although each still depends on specific major genetic pathways.

Apart from the somatic *Rb*$^{F/F}$; *p53*$^{F/F}$ model for SCLC, two other lung cancer models have also been associated with pulmonary neuroendocrine tumors. One model made use of bitransgenic *CC10-hASH1; CC10-SV40 large T* system in which progressive neuroendocrine dysplasia and aggressive lung adenocarcinoma developed with both focal neuroendocrine differentiation (through expression of pro-neural ASH-1 transcription factor) and CC10 expression (Linnoila et al., 2000). These adenocarcinomas closely resembled human NSCLC with neuroendocrine differentiation (Linnoila et al., 1994). In the other model, the cyclin dependent kinase inhibitor *p18*^{Ink4c} and *Men1*, a tumor suppressor gene deleted in human multiple endocrine neoplasia, were both inactivated. To determine how *p18* and *p27* genetically interact with Men1, Pei et al. (2007) characterized *p18-Men1* and *p27-Men1* double mutant mice and showed that p18, but not p27, functionally collaborates with Men1 in suppressing lung tumorigenesis. Lung tumors developed in both *Men1*$^{+/-}$ and *p18*$^{-/-}$; *Men1*$^{+/-}$ mice at a high penetrance and contained both neuroendocrine and non-neuroendocrine cells. The remaining wild-type *Men1* allele was lost in most lung tumors from *Men1*$^{+/-}$ mice, but was retained in most tumors from *p18*$^{-/-}$;*Men1*$^{+/-}$ mice, showing a functional collaboration between p18 and Men1 in lung tumor suppression (Pei et al., 2007). Phosphorylation of Rb protein at both Cdk2 and Cdk4/Cdk6 sites were significantly increased in normal bronchial epithelia and tumor cells derived from *p18*$^{-/-}$;*Men1*$^{+/-}$ mice compared to those from single *p18*$^{-/-}$ or *Men1*$^{+/-}$ mice. Lung tumors developed in *p18*$^{-/-}$;*Men1*$^{+/-}$ mice were multifocal, more heterogeneous, and highly invasive compared to those in either *p18*$^{-/-}$ or *Men1*$^{+/-}$ mice. These results revealed a previously unrecognized function of p18 in lung tumor suppression through collaboration with Men1 to control lung stem cell proliferation. To investigate the cellular origin(s) of this cancer, Sutherland et al. (2011) assessed the effect of *Trp53* and *Rb1* inactivation in distinct cell types in the adult lung using adenoviral vectors that target Cre recombinase to Clara, neuroendocrine (NE), and alveolar type 2 (SPC-expressing) cells. Using these cell type-restricted Adeno-Cre viruses, loss of *Trp53* and *Rb1* efficiently transformed NE and SPC-expressing cells, leading to SCLC, albeit SPC-expressing cells were transformed less efficiently (Sutherland et al., 2011). In contrast, Clara cells were largely resistant to transformation. Their results indicate that although NE cells serve as the predominant cell of origin of SCLC, a subset of SPC-expressing cells are also endowed with this ability.

Increasingly, it is realized that during tumorigenesis a variety of cells are recruited into the tumor to provide a range of functions that are associated with tumor progression (Calbo et al., 2011). Karnoub and colleagues (2007) showed that mesenchymal stem cells recruited into the stroma of breast cancer promote metastasis through CCL5-mediated paracrine signaling, thereby emphasizing the relevance of the interactions between tumor cells and the surrounding microenvironment. Using the mouse model for simultaneous *Rb* and *p53* inactivation, Calbo et al. (2011) established primary cultures from 21 murine NSCLCs. They found mouse SCLC primary cultures attached to the dishes in 9 of 21 cases, consistent with cell culture derived from human SCLC. They seeded single-cell suspensions from 15 mouse SCLC cultures in soft agar-containing medium, and isolated individual colonies and expanded separately. Most of the obtained clones grew as suspending aggregates of very small cells. These cells expressed neuroendocrine protein markers such as synaptophysin, achaete-scute complex homolog 1, and neural cell adhesion molecule. They also obtained clones grew as a cellular monolayer composed of larger cells with visible cytoplasm and spindle-like membrane extensions, spreading on the substrate (mesenchymal cells). This is consistent with human SCLC that are often composed of phenotypically different cells with either a neuroendocrine or a mesenchymal marker profile. Importantly, these two types of cells had a common origin because they shared specific genomic aberrations as demonstrated by SKY analysis. Calbo et al. also showed that the transition from neuroendocrine to mesenchymal phenotype could be achieved by the ectopic expression of oncogenic Ras^{V12} in the former (Calbo et al., 2011). When engrafted as a mixed population, the mesenchymal cells endowed the neuroendocrine cells with metastatic capacity, illustrating the potential relevance of tumor cell heterogeneity in dictating tumor properties (Calbo et al., 2011). In short, they showed a specific type of tumor heterogeneity of SCLC, in which the interaction between clonally derived but diversified subclones alters the behavior of the tumor as a whole (Calbo et al., 2011). One outcome was a substantially increased metastatic potential, a feature with important clinical ramifications in human SCLC. Tumor cell behavior then not only depended on the interactions with stromal cells, but was also influenced by interactions with tumor cell variants that fulfill a distinct role in the tumor tissue. This study provides a unique system, whereby the mesenchymal compartment of the tumor was generated from a separate subclone of SCLC during the tumorigenic process, providing the tumor cell population as a whole with new capabilities such as metastatic potential.

16. Xenograft models for SCLC

For the past three decades, the mainstay of preclinical cancer therapeutic research has been the use of human cancer cells lines cultured *in vitro* and of xenografts derived from these cell lines grown *in vivo* in immunodeficient mice. However, neither model consistently predicted the efficacy in clinical trials, resulting in two major barriers to the successful translation of new cancer therapeutics. First, resources are expended on drug development based on these models that ultimately fail in clinical trials. Second, many potentially useful therapies that might be beneficial in humans are discarded because the animal models fail to demonstrate efficacy in conventional cell culture and xenograft models. Emerging evidence suggests that the process of establishing conventional cell lines from human cancers results in distinct and irreversible loss of important biological properties. These include (*a*) gain or loss of gene amplification, (*b*) the ability to migrate and metastasize, (*c*) the maintenance of a distinct stem cell population, and (*d*) the preservation of dependency on embryonic signaling pathways. These properties are not restored when these conventional cell lines are grown as heterotopic or orthotopic xenografts.

Because SCLC is usually diagnosed by endobronchial biopsy or fine-needle aspiration cytology, substantial quantities of fresh or frozen tissues are typically lacking in most tumor banks. For this reason, most SCLC researches rely on conventional cell lines, which are often chemoresistant because they were derived from patients who had received cytotoxic chemotherapy (Phelps et al., 1996). In addition, all of these cell lines have experimental limitations and lack the three-dimensional tumor-stromal interactions, which seem to significantly affect the response of these cells to chemotherapy (Hodkinson et al., 2007). To establish better models for the study of SCLC, Daniel et al. (2009) generated and characterized a series of primary xenograft models derived from chemo-naive patients to more accurately model SCLC in mice. In parallel, cell lines grown in conventional tissue culture conditions were derived from each xenograft line, passaged for 6 months, and then reimplanted to generate secondary xenografts. When compared with normal lung, primary tumors, xenografts, and cell lines displayed a gene expression signature specific for SCLC (Daniel et al., 2009). Comparison of gene expression within the xenograft model identified a group of tumor-specific genes expressed in primary SCLC and xenografts that was lost during the transition to SCLC cell lines; these genes were not regained when the tumors were re-established as secondary xenografts. Such changes in gene expression may be a common feature of many cancer cell culture systems, with functional implications for the use of such models for preclinical drug development.

Bcl-2 is a central regulator of cell survival that is overexpressed in most SCLC tumors and contributes to both malignant transformation and therapeutic resistance. Hann et al. (2008) compared primary SCLC xenografts prepared from *de novo* human tumors with standard cell line–based xenografts to evaluate a novel and highly potent small molecule inhibitor of Bcl-2, ABT-737. ABT-737 induced dramatic regressions in tumors derived from some SCLC cell lines. In contrast, only one of three primary xenograft SCLC tumors showed significant growth inhibition with ABT-737. Explanations for this apparent difference may include relatively low expression of Bcl-2 in the primary xenografts or inherent differences in the model systems. The addition of etoposide to ABT-737 in the primary xenografts resulted in significantly decreased tumor growth, underscoring the clinical potential of ABT-737 in combination therapy. To identify factors that may contribute to resistance to ABT-737 and related inhibitors, they isolated resistant derivatives of an initially sensitive cell line–based xenograft. Acquired resistance in this model was associated with decreases in the expression of the primary target Bcl-2, of proapoptotic partners of Bcl-2 (Bax and Bim), and of Bcl-2:Bim heterodimers. Expression profiling revealed 85 candidate genes demonstrating consistent changes in gene expression with acquired resistance. These data have specific implications for the clinical development of Bcl-2 inhibitors for SCLC and broader implications for the testing of novel anticancer strategies in relevant preclinical models.

17. Conclusions

There are many distinct genetic pathways present in SCLC, leading to its unique biology and clinical features. A better understanding of these basic molecular and cellular changes will allow for the development of novel therapeutic strategies. Multiple molecularly targeted agents are actively being studied pre-clinically and clinically, with the hope of ultimately improving survival of patients with SCLC. Development of targeted therapy in small cell lung cancer has significantly lagged behind that of non-small cell lung cancer. Etoposide and cisplatin remain the mainstays of first-line SCLC treatment. Although the decreasing prevalence of smoking in industrialized countries will lead to decreased incidence of SCLC, the burden of disease is shifting to developing countries. Further investment in research for this disease is, therefore, warranted. Many phase 1 and 2 studies of drugs with potential activity in SCLC and phase 2 and 3 trials to improve radiotherapy are underway. Inclusion of patients with SCLC in such trials should be encouraged, especially otherwise healthy patients with relapsing or refractory SCLC, for whom treatment options are limited. A new, effective, and active combination for extensive-stage SCLC would be quickly moved up as a treatment priority.

SCLC remains a therapeutic challenge despite high initial responses to chemotherapy and radiotherapy. The fact that several promising molecularly targeted agents have not shown adequate activity in clinical trials does not mean the end of novel targeted therapies for SCLC. Nevertheless, a better understanding of SCLC biology and better preclinical models of SCLC are needed to improve available therapies.

The mouse model presented in the study by Meuwissen et al. clearly showed that somatic inactivation of both *Rb1* and *Trp53* alleles in lung epithelial cells readily leads to formation of small cell NE tumors. Their histopathologic characteristics and metastasizing capacity were strikingly similar to human SCLCs. Their mouse model will prove a valuable tool for (1) comparing genotype-phenotype similarities between human SCLC and MSCLC, (2) the identification of precursor lesions, and (3) additional factors involved in tumor progression, and (4) ultimately, testing of targeted, novel tumor intervention strategies and chemoprevention.

The identification of specific cell type(s) from which SCLC originates is critical in the development of methods for early diagnosis and treatment. By using cell type-restricted Adeno-Cre vectors in directing *Trp53* and *Rb1* loss to distinct cell populations in the adult mouse lung, Sutherland et al. showed that NE cells are the predominant cells of origin of SCLC. Their study provides additional tools to address questions related to the cell of origin of lung cancer, and highlights the importance of specifically targeting NE cells for the treatment of SCLC. Their strategy to manipulate specific adult lung cell populations in a controlled manner by cell type-restricted somatic gene transfer vectors could help to answer the question of whether distinct lung pathologies have a unique cell of origin, and whether this cell of origin is a determining factor in the drug resistance profile of the various tumor subtypes.

The work of Calbo et al. showed a specific type of tumor heterogeneity, in which the interaction between clonally derived but diversified subclones alters the behavior of the tumor as a whole. One outcome was substantially increased metastasis, a feature with important clinical ramifications. Thus, tumor cell behavior not only depends on the interactions with stromal cells, but also interactions with tumor cell variants that fulfill a distinct role in the tumor tissue. Enhanced metastatic capacity serves as an illustrative example of crosstalk between specialized tumor cell clones. Disrupting the paracrine signaling involved in this interaction is worth further exploring as a strategy to mitigate tumor progression in SCLC.

18. Acknowledgements

We thank K. Klein for editing. K. Inoue is supported by NIH/NCI 5R01CA106314, ACS RSG-07-207-01-MGO, a Director's Challenge pilot award (Comprehensive Cancer Center of WFU), and an intramural pilot grant award from Wake Forest University School of Medicine. P. Taneja has been supported by the Susan G. Komen Foundation postdoctoral fellowship KG080179. D. Maglic has been supported by DOD predoctoral fellowship BC100907.

19. References

19.1,2 Introduction and Trp53

Antonia SJ, Mirza N, Fricke I, Chiappori A, Thompson P, Williams N, Bepler G, Simon G, Janssen W, Lee JH, Menander K, Chada S, Gabrilovich DI. (2006). Combination of p53 cancer vaccine with chemotherapy in patients with extensive stage small cell lung cancer. *Clin Cancer Res* 12:878–87.

Blackhall F, Faivre-Finn C. (2011). Treatment of limited small cell lung cancer: an old or new challenge. *Curr Opin Oncol* 23(2):158-62. Review.

Brambilla E, Gazdar A. (2009). Pathogenesis of lung cancer signalling pathways: roadmap for therapies. *Eur Respir J* 33(6):1485-97.

Demirhan O, Taştemir D, Hastürk S, Kuleci S, Hanta I. (2010). Alterations in p16 and p53 genes and chromosomal findings in patients with lung cancer: fluorescence in situ hybridization and cytogenetic studies. *Cancer Epidemiol* 34:472-7.

Garcia V, Velasco A, Gatius S, Gonzalez FJ, Matias-Guiu X. (2010). Pulmonary small cell carcinoma metastatic to the ovary: a clinicopathologic study of one case with emphasis on the importance of p53 analysis in diagnosis. *Gynecol Obstet Invest* 70:87-90.

Giaccone G, Debruyne C, Felip E, Chapman PB, Grant SC, Millward M, Thiberville L, D'Addario G, Coens C, Rome LS, Zatloukal P, Masso O, Legrand C. (2005). Phase III study of adjuvant vaccination with Bec2/bacille Calmette-Guerin in responding patients with limited-disease small-cell lung cancer (European Organisation for Research and Treatment of Cancer 08971-08971B; Silva Study). *J Clin Oncol* 23:6854–64.

Grant SC, Kris MG, Houghton AN, Chapman PB. (1999). Long survival of patients with small cell lung cancer after adjuvant treatment with the anti-idiotypic antibody BEC2 plus Bacillus Calmette-Guerin. *Clin Cancer Res* 5:1319–23.

Horn L, Castellanos EL, Johnson DH. (2011). Update on new drugs in small cell lung cancer. *Expert Opin Investig Drugs* 20(4):441-5. Review.

Ishida, T.; Chada, S; Stipanov, M.; Nadaf S, Ciernik, FI.; Gabrilovich D. (1999). Dendritic cells transduced with wild-type p53 gene elicit potent anti-tumour immune responses. *Clin Exp Immunol* 117:244-51.

Jemal A, Siegel R, Ward E, Murray T, Xu J, Smigal C, Thun MJ. (2006). Cancer statistics, 2006. *CA Cancer J Clin* 56:106–30.

Meyerson M, Franklin WA, Kelley MJ. (2004). Molecular classification and molecular genetics of human lung cancers. *Semin Oncol* 31: 4–19.

Tamási L, Müller V. (2011). Symptoms and diagnostics of lung neuroendocrine tumors. *Orv Hetil* 152(10):366-70. Review

Walenkamp AM, Sonke GS, Sleijfer DT. (2009). Clinical and therapeutic aspects of extrapulmonary small cell carcinoma. *Cancer Treat Rev* 35(3):228-36.

Wistuba, II.; Gazdar, AF. & Minna JD. (2001). Molecular genetics of small cell lung carcinoma. *Semin Oncol* 28; 3-13

Yang M, Zhang L, Bi N, Ji W, Tan W, Zhao L, Yu D, Wu C, Wang L, Lin D. 2011. Association of P53 and ATM polymorphisms with risk of radiation-induced pneumonitis in lung cancer patients treated with radiotherapy. *Int J Radiat Oncol Biol Phys* 79(5):1402-7

19.3 RB

Dosaka-Akita H, Cagle PT, Hiroumi H, Fujita M, Yamashita M, Sharma A, Kawakami Y, Benedict WF. (2000). Differential retinoblastoma and p16(INK4A) protein expression in neuroendocrine tumors of the lung. *Cancer* 88(3):550-6.

Gouyer V, Gazzeri S, Bolon I *et al.* (1998). Mechanism of retinoblastoma gene inactivation in the spectrum of neuroendocrine lung tumors. *Am J Respir Cell Mol Biol* 182(2):188-96.

Gugger M, Burckhardt E, Kappeler A, Hirsiger H, Laissue JA, Mazzucchelli L. (2002). Quantitative expansion of structural genomic alterations in the spectrum of neuroendocrine lung carcinomas. *J Pathol* 196(4):408-15.

Kashii T, Mizushima Y, Monno S, Nakagawa K, Kobayashi M. (1994). Gene analysis of K-, H-ras, p53, and retinoblastoma susceptibility genes in human lung cancer cell lines by the polymerase chain reaction/single-strand conformation polymorphism method. *J Cancer Res Clin Oncol* 120(3):143-8.

Kitamura H, Yazawa T, Sato H, Okudela K, Shimoyamada H. (2009). Small cell lung cancer: significance of RB alterations and TTF-1 expression in its carcinogenesis, phenotype, and biology. *Endocr Pathol* 20(2):101-7. Review.

Leversha MA, Fielding P, Watson S, Gosney JR, Field JK. (2003). Expression of p53, pRB, and p16 in lung tumours: a validation study on tissue microarrays. *J Pathol* 200(5):610-9.

Modi S, Kubo A, Oie H, Coxon AB, Rehmatulla A, Kaye FJ. (2000). Protein expression of the RB-related gene family and SV40 large T antigen in mesothelioma and lung cancer. *Oncogene* 19:4632-9.

Mori N, Yokota J, Akiyama T, Sameshima Y, Okamoto A, Mizoguchi H, Toyoshima K, Sugimura T, Terada M. (1990). Variable mutations of the RB gene in small-cell lung carcinoma. *Oncogene* 5(11), 1713–7.

Rodina A, Vilenchik M, Moulick K, Aguirre J, Kim J, Chiang A, et al. (2007). Selective compounds define Hsp90 as a major inhibitor of apoptosis in small-cell lung cancer. *Nat Chem Biol* 3:498-507.

Sachse R, Murakami Y, Shiraishi M, Hayashi K, Sekiya T. (1994). DNA aberrations at the retinoblastoma gene locus in human squamous cell carcinomas of the lung. *Oncogene* 9(1), 39–47.

Schaffer BE, Park KS, Yiu G, Conklin JF, Lin C, Burkhart DL, Karnezis AN, Sweet-Cordero EA, Sage J. (2010). Loss of p130 accelerates tumor development in a mouse model for human small-cell lung carcinoma. *Cancer Res* 70(10):3877-83.

Schauer I, Siriwardana S, Langan T, Sclafani R. (1994). Cyclin D1 overexpression vs. retinoblastomainactivation: implications for growth control evasion in non-small cell and small cell lung cancer. *Proc Natl Acad Sci USA* 91(16), 7827–31.

Wikman H, Kettunen E. (2006). Regulation of the G1/S phase of the cell cycle and alterations in the RB pathway in human lung cancer. Expert Rev Anticancer Ther. 6(4):515-30. Review.

Xue Jun H, Gemma A, Hosoya Y, Matsuda K, Nara M, Hosomi Y, Okano T, Kurimoto F, Seike M, Takenaka K, Yoshimura A, Toyota M, Kudoh S. (2003). Reduced transcription of the RB2/p130 gene in human lung cancer. *Mol Carcinog* 38(3):124-9.

19.4 BCL2

Knoefel LF, Werle-Schneider G, Dally H, Müller PJ, Edler L, Bartsch H, Tuengerthal S, Heussel CP, Reinmuth N, Thomas M, Risch A. (2011). Polymorphisms in the apoptotic pathway gene BCL-2 and survival in small cell lung cancer. *J Thorac Oncol* 6(1):183-9.

Lawson MH, Cummings NM, Rassl DM, Vowler SL, Wickens M, Howat WJ, Brenton JD, Murphy G, Rintoul RC. (2010). Bcl-2 and β1-integrin predict survival in a tissue microarray of small cell lung cancer. *Br J Cancer* 103(11):1710-5.

Tudor G, Aguilera A, Halverson DO, Laing ND, Sausville EA. (2000). Susceptibility to drug-induced apoptosis correlates with differential modulation of Bad, Bcl-2 and Bcl-xL protein levels. *Cell Death Differ* 7:574–86.

Reed JC, Stein C, Subasinghe C, Haldar S, Croce CM, Yum S, Cohen J. (1990). Antisense-mediated inhibition of BCL2 protooncogene expression and leukemic cell growth and survival: comparisons of phosphodiester and phosphorothioate oligodeoxynucleotides. *Cancer Res* 50:6565–70.

Rudin CM, Otterson GA, Mauer AM, Villalona-Calero MA, Tomek R, Prange B, George CM, Szeto L, Vokes EE. (2002). A pilot trial of G3139, a bcl-2 antisense oligonucleotide, and paclitaxel in patients with chemorefractory small-cell lung cancer. *Ann Oncol* 13:539–45.

Rudin CM, Kozloff M, Hoffman PC, Edelman MJ, Karnauskas R, Tomek R, Szeto L, Vokes EE. (2004). Phase I study of G3139, a bcl-2 antisense oligonucleotide, combined with carboplatin and etoposide in patients with small-cell lung cancer. *J Clin Oncol* 22:1110–7.

Tahir SK, Wass J, Joseph MK, Devanarayan V, Hessler P, Zhang H, Elmore SW, Kroeger PE, Tse C, Rosenberg SH, Anderson MG. (2010). Identification of expression signatures predictive of sensitivity to the Bcl-2 family member inhibitor ABT-263 in small cell lung carcinoma and leukemia/lymphoma cell lines. *Mol Cancer Ther* 9(3):545-57.

Waters JS, Webb A, Cunningham D, Clarke PA, Raynaud F, di Stefano F, Cotter FE. (2000). Phase I clinical and pharmacokinetic study of bcl-2 antisense oligonucleotide therapy in patients with non-Hodgkin's lymphoma. *J Clin Oncol* 18:1812–23.

19.5 MYC

Barr LF, Campbell SE, Bochner BS, Dang CV. (1998). Association of the decreased expression of alpha3beta1 integrin with the altered cell: environmental interactions and enhanced soft agar cloning ability of c-myc-overexpressing small cell lung cancer cells. *Cancer Res* 58(23):5537-45.

Paulson KG, Lemos BD, Feng B, Jaimes N, Peñas PF, Bi X, Maher E, Cohen L, Leonard JH, Granter SR, Chin L, Nghiem P. (2009). Array-CGH reveals recurrent genomic changes in Merkel cell carcinoma including amplification of L-Myc. *J Invest Dermatol* 129(6):1547-55.

Xiong F, Wu C, Chang J, Yu D, Xu B, Yuan P, Zhai K, Xu J, Tan W, Lin D. (2011). Genetic variation in an MiRNA-1827 binding site in MYCL1 alters susceptibility to small cell lung cancer *Cancer Res* 2011, Jun 15.

19.6 c-Kit

Burger H, den Bakker MA, Stoter G, Verweij J, Nooter K. (2003). Lack of c-kit exon 11 activating mutations in c-KIT/CD117- positive SCLC tumour specimens. *Eur J Cancer* 39:793–9.

Dy GK, Miller AA, Mandrekar SJ, Aubry MC, Langdon RM, Jr., Morton RF, Schild SE, Jett JR, Adjei AA. (2005). A phase II trial of imatinib (ST1571) in patients with c-kit expressing relapsed small-cell lung cancer: a CALGB and NCCTG study. *Ann Oncol* 16:1811–6.

Heinrich MC, Blanke CD, Druker BJ, Corless CL. (2002). Inhibition of KIT tyrosine kinase activity: a novel molecular approach to the treatment of KIT-positive malignancies. *J Clin Oncol* 20:1692–703.

Johnson BE, Fischer T, Fischer B, Dunlop D, Rischin D, Silberman S, Kowalski MO, Sayles D, Dimitrijevic S, Fletcher C, Hornick J, Salgia R, Le Chevalier T. (2003). Phase II study of imatinib in patients with small cell lung cancer. *Clin Cancer Res* 9:5880–7.

Reber L, Da Silva CA, Frossard N. (2006). Stem cell factor and its receptor c-kit as targets for inflammatory diseases. Eur J Pharmacol 533:327–40.

Schneider BJ, Kalemkerian GP, Ramnath N, Kraut MJ, Wozniak AJ, Worden FP, Ruckdeschel JC, Zhang X, Chen W, Gadgeel SM. (2010). Phase II trial of imatinib maintenance therapy after irinotecan and cisplatin in patients with c-Kit-positive, extensive-stage small-cell lung cancer. *Clin Lung Cancer* 11(4):223-7.

Potti A, Moazzam N, Ramar K, Hanekom DS, Kargas S, Koch M. (2003). CD117 (c-kit) overexpression in patients with extensivestage small-cell lung carcinoma. *Ann Oncol* 14:894–7.

Potti A, Ganti AK, Tuchman SA, Sholes K, Langness E, Koka V, Koch M. (2005). HER-2/neu and CD117 (c-kit) overexpression in patients with pesticide exposure and extensive stage small cell lung carcinoma (ESSCLC). *J Carcinog* 4:8.

19.7 VEGF

Bogos K, Renyi-Vamos F, Dobos J, Kenessey I, Tovari J, Timar J, Strausz J, Ostoros G, Klepetko W, Ankersmit HJ, Lang G, Hoda MA, Nierlich P, Dome B. (2009). High VEGFR-3-positive circulating lymphatic/vascular endothelial progenitor cell level is associated with poor prognosis in human small cell lung cancer. *Clin Cancer Res* 15(5):1741-6.

Blackhall FH, Shepherd FA. (2004). Angiogenesis inhibitors in the treatment of small cell and non-small cell lung cancer. *Hematol Oncol Clin North Am* 18:1121–41.

Cooney MM, Subbiah S, Chapman R, Ness A, Rutherford K, Warren G, Saltzman J, Mekhail T, Levitan N, Dowlati A. (2005). Phase II trial of maintenance daily oral thalidomide in patients with extensive-stage small cell lung cancer (ES-SCLC) in remission. *J Clin Oncol* (Meeting Abstracts) 23:7166.

Fischer B, Marinov M, Arcaro A. (2007). Targeting receptor tyrosine kinase signalling in small cell lung cancer (SCLC): what have we learned so far? *Cancer Treat Rev* 33:391-406.

Laird AD, Vajkoczy P, Shawver LK, Thurnher A, Liang C, Mohammadi M, Schlessinger J, Ullrich A, Hubbard SR, Blake RA, Fong TA, Strawn LM, Sun L, Tang C, Hawtin R, Tang F, Shenoy N, Hirth KP, McMahon G, Cherrington. (2000). SU6668 is a potent antiangiogenic and antitumor agent that induces regression of established tumors. *Cancer Res* 60:4152-60.

Herbst RS, Onn A, Sandler A. (2005). Angiogenesis and lung cancer: prognostic and therapeutic implications. *J Clin Oncol* 23:3243–56.

Lebeau B, Salmoniere P, Ozenne G, Blanchon F, Leclerc P, Coetmeur D. (1999). Alpha interferon as maintenance therapy for small cell lung cancer (SCLC). *Proc Am Soc Clin Oncol* 18:475a.

Lucchi M, Mussi A, Fontanini G, Faviana P, Ribechini A, Angeletti CA. (2002). Small cell lung carcinoma (SCLC): the angiogenic phenomenon. *Eur J Cardio-thorac Surg* 21:1105–10.

Morabito A, Piccirillo MC, Falasconi F, De Feo G, Del Giudice A, Bryce J, Di Maio M, De Maio E, Normanno N, Perrone F. (2009). Vandetanib (ZD6474), a dual inhibitor of vascular endothelial growth factor receptor (VEGFR) and epidermal growth factor receptor (EGFR) tyrosine kinases: current status and future directions. *Oncologist* 14(4):378-90.

Raefsky EL, Spigel DR, Greco FA, Yardley DA, Bradof JE, Woytowitz DV, Schreeder MT, Liggett WH, Zubkus JD, Petrone D, Hainsworth JD. (2005). Irinotecan (I), carboplatin (C), and radiotherapy (RT) followed by bevacizumab (B) in the treatment of limited-stage small cell lung cancer (SCLC): A phase II trial of the Minnie Pearl Cancer Research Network. *ASCO Meeting Abstracts* 23:7050.

Sattler M, Salgia R. (2003). Molecular and cellular biology of small cell lung cancer. *Semin Oncol* 30:57-71.

Tanno S, Ohsaki Y, Nakanishi K, Toyoshima E, Kikuchi K. (2004). Human small cell lung cancer cells express functional VEGF receptors, VEGFR-2 and VEGFR-3. *Lung Cancer* 46:11-9.

Thomas A, Morgan B, Drevs J, Unger C, Wiedenmann B, Vanhoefer U, Laurent D, Dugan M, Steward W (2003) Vascular endothelial growth factor receptor tyrosine kinase inhibitors: PTK787/ZK 222584. *Semin Oncol* 30:32–8.

Ustuner Z, Saip P, Yasasever V, Vural B, Yazar A, Bal C, Ozturk B, Ozbek U, Topuz E. (2008). Prognostic and predictive value of vascular endothelial growth factor and its soluble receptors, VEGFR-1 and VEGFR-2 levels in the sera of small cell lung cancer patients. *Med Oncol* 25(4):394-9.

Wójcik E, Jakubowicz J, Skotnicki P, Sas-Korczyńska B, Kulpa JK. (2010). IL-6 and VEGF in small cell lung cancer patients. *Anticancer Res* 30(5):1773-8.

19.8 EGFR

Araki J, Okamoto I, Suto R, Ichikawa Y, Sasaki J. (2005). Efficacy of the tyrosine kinase inhibitor gefitinib in a patient withn metastatic small cell lung cancer. *Lung Cancer* 48:141–4.

Micke P, Hengstler JG, Ros R, Bittinger F, Metz T, Gebhard S, Beeh KM, Oesch F, Buhl R. (2001). c-erbB-2 expression in small cell lung cancer is associated with poor prognosis. *Int J Cancer* 92:474–9.

Okamoto I, Araki J, Suto R, Shimada M, Nakagawa K, Fukuoka M. (2006). EGFR mutation in gefitinib-responsive small-cell lung cancer. *Ann Oncol* 17:1028–9.

Potti A, Ganti AK, Sholes K, Langness E, Koka V, Horvarth L, Koch M. (2003). Effect of pesticide exposure on HER-2/neu overexpression seen in patients with extensive stage small cell lung carcinoma. *Clin Cancer Res* 9:4872–6.

Potti A, Willardson J, Forseen C, Kishor Ganti A, Koch M, Hebert B, Levitt R, Mehdi SA. (2002). Predictive role of HER-2/ neu overexpression and clinical features at initial presentation in patients with extensive stage small cell lung carcinoma. Lung *Cancer* 36:257–61.

Schmid K, Bago-Horvath Z, Berger W, Haitel A, Cejka D, Werzowa J, Filipits M, Herberger B, Hayden H, Sieghart W. (2010). Dual inhibition of EGFR and mTOR pathways in small cell lung cancer. *Br J Cancer* 103(5):622-8.

Sequist LV, Waltman BA, Dias-Santagata D, Digumarthy S, Turke AB, Fidias P, Bergethon K, Shaw AT, Gettinger S, Cosper AK, Akhavanfard S, Heist RS, Temel J, Christensen JG, Wain JC, Lynch TJ, Vernovsky K, Mark EJ, Lanuti M, Iafrate AJ, Mino-Kenudson M, Engelman JA. (2011). Genotypic and histological evolution of lung cancers acquiring resistance to EGFR inhibitors. *Sci Transl Med* 3(75):75ra26.

Tanno S, Ohsaki Y, Nakanishi K, Toyoshima E, Kikuchi K. (2004). Small cell lung cancer cells express EGFR and tyrosine phosphorylation of EGFR is inhibited by gefitinib ("Iressa", ZD1839). *Oncol Rep* 12:1053–7.

19.9 Matrix Metalloproteinase

Brown PD, Giavazzi R. (1995). Matrix metalloproteinase inhibition:a review of anti-tumour activity. *Ann Oncol* 6:967–74.

Jumper C, Cobos E, Lox C. (2004). Determination of the serum matrix metalloproteinase-9 (MMP-9) and tissue inhibitor of matrix metalloproteinase-1 (TIMP-1) in patients with either advanced small-cell lung cancer or non-small-cell lung cancer prior to treatment. Respir Med. 98:173-7.

Komiya K, Sueoka-Aragane N, Sato A, Hisatomi T, Sakuragi T, Mitsuoka M, Sato T, Hayashi S, Izumi H, Tsuneoka M, Sueoka E. (2010). Expression of Mina53, a novel c-Myc target gene, is a favorable prognostic marker in early stage lung cancer. *Lung Cancer* 69:232-8.

Kumimoto H, Hamajima N, Nishimoto Y, Matsuo K, Shinoda M, Hatooka S, Ishizaki K. (2002). L-myc genotype is associated with different susceptibility to lung cancer in smokers. *Jpn J Cancer Res* 93:1-5.

Michael M, Babic B, Khokha R, Tsao M, Ho J, Pintilie M, Leco K, Chamberlain D, Shepherd FA. (1999). Expression and prognostic significance of metalloproteinases and their tissue inhibitors in patients with small-cell lung cancer. *J Clin Oncol* 17:1802–8.

Shepherd FA, Giaccone G, Seymour L, Debruyne C, Bezjak A, Hirsh V, Smylie M, Rubin S, Martins H, Lamont A, Krzakowski M, Sadura A, Zee B. (2002). Prospective, randomized, doubleblind, placebo-controlled trial of marimastat after response to firstl inechemotherapy in patients with small-cell lung cancer: a trial of the National Cancer Institute of Canada-Clinical Trials Group and the European Organization for Research and Treatment of Cancer. *J Clin Oncol* 20:4434–9.

Stetler-Stevenson WG, Aznavoorian S, Liotta LA. (1993). Tumor cell interactions with the extracellular matrix during invasion and metastasis. *Annu Rev Cell Biol* 9:541–73.

19.10 Sonic Hedghog pathway

Datta S, Datta MW. (2006). Sonic hedgehog signaling in advanced prostate cancer. *Cell Mol Life Sci* 63(4):435-48.

Berman DM, Burkholder SG, Wang B, Beachy PA, Baylin SB. (2003). Hedgehog signalling within airway epithelial progenitors and in small-cell lung cancer. *Nature* 422:313–7.

Peacock CD, Watkins DN. (2008). Cancer stem cells and the ontogeny of lung cancer. *J Clin Oncol* 26:2883-9.

Vestergaard J, Pedersen MW, Pedersen N, Ensinger C, Tumer Z, Tommerup N, Poulsen HS, Larsen LA. (2006). Hedgehog signaling in small-cell lung cancer: frequent in vivo but a rare event in vitro. *Lung Cancer* 52:281–90.

Watkins DN, Peacock CD. (2004). Hedgehog signalling in foregut malignancy. *Biochem Pharmacol* 68:1055–60.

19.11 mTOR pathway

Chan S. (2004). Targeting the mammalian target of rapamycin (mTOR): a new approach to treating cancer. *Br J Cancer* 91:1420–24.

Lohar MV, Mundada R, Bhonde M, Padgaonkar A, Deore V, Yewalkar N, Bhatia D, Rathos M, Joshi K, Vishwakarma RA, Kumar S. (2008). Design and synthesis of novel furoquinoline based inhibitors of multiple targets in the PI3K/Akt-mTOR pathway. *Bioorg Med Chem Lett* 18(12):3603-6.

Oh SH, Jin Q, Kim ES, Khuri FR, Lee HY. (2008). Insulin-like growth factor-I receptor signaling pathway induces resistance to the apoptotic activities of SCH66336 (lonafarnib) through Akt/mammalian target of rapamycin-mediated increases in survivin expression. *Clin Cancer Res* 14(5):1581-9.

Pandya KJ, Levy DE, Hidalgo M, Cohen RB, Lee MW, Schiller JH, Johnson DH. (2005). A randomized, phase II ECOG trial of two dose levels of temsirolimus (CCI-779) in patients with extensive stage small cell lung cancer in remission after induction chemotherapy. A preliminary report. *J Clin Oncol* (Meeting Abstracts) 23:7005.

Shibata T, Saito S, Kokubu A, Suzuki T, Yamamoto M, Hirohashi S. (2010). Global downstream pathway analysis reveals a dependence of oncogenic NF-E2-related factor 2 mutation on the mTOR growth signaling pathway. *Cancer Res* 70(22):9095-105.

Schmid K, Bago-Horvath Z, Berger W, Haitel A, Cejka D, Werzowa J, Filipits M, Herberger B, Hayden H, Sieghart W. (2010). Dual inhibition of EGFR and mTOR pathways in small cell lung cancer. *Br J Cancer* 103(5):622-8.

19.12 CD56 (NCAM)

Fidias P, Grossbard M, Lynch TJ Jr. (2002.) A phase II study of the immunotoxin N901-blocked ricin in small-cell lung cancer. *Clin Lung Cancer* 3:219–22.

J Fossella F, McCann J, Tolcher A, Xie H, Hwang LL, Carr C, Berg K, Fram R. (2005). Phase II trial of BB-10901 (huN901-DM1) given weekly for four consecutive weeks every 6 weeks in patients with relapsed SCLC and CD56-positive small cell carcinoma. *J Clin Oncol* (Meeting Abstracts) 23:7159.

ensen M, Berthold F. (2007). Targeting the neural cell adhesion molecule in cancer. *Cancer Lett* 258:9-21.

Kim DH, Kwon MS. (2010). Role of fine needle aspiration cytology, cell block preparation and CD63, P63 and CD56 immunostaining in classifying the specific tumor type of the lung. *Acta Cytol* 54(1):55-9.

Lynch TJ Jr. (1993). Immunotoxin therapy of small cell lung cancer. N901-blocked ricin for relapsed small-cell lung cancer. *Chest* 103:436S–439S.

19.13 Chromosomal alterations

Agathanggelou A, Cooper WN, Latif F. (2005). Role of the Ras-association domain family 1 tumor suppressor gene in human cancers. *Cancer Res* 65:3497-508.

Balsara BR, Testa JR. (2002). Chromosomal imbalances in human lung cancer. *Oncogene* 21:6877-83.

Burbee DG, Forgacs E, Zochbauer-Muller S, Shivakumar L, Fong K, Gao B, Randle D, Kondo M, Virmani A, Bader S, Sekido Y, Latif F, Milchgrub S, Toyooka S, Gazdar AF, Lerman MI, Zabarovsky E, White M, Minna JD. (2001). Epigenetic inactivation of RASSF1A in lung and breast cancers and malignant phenotype suppression. *J Natl Cancer Inst* 93:691–9.

Dammann R, Li C, Yoon JH, Chin PL, Bates S, Pfeifer GP. (2000). Epigenetic inactivation of a RAS association domain family protein from the lung tumour suppressor locus 3p21.3. *Nat Genet* 25:315–9.
Hougaard S, Norgaard P, Abrahamsen N, Moses HL, Spang- Thomsen M, Skovgaard Poulsen H. (1999). Inactivation of the transforming growth factor beta type II receptor in human small cell lung cancer cell lines. *Br J Cancer* 79:1005–11.
Ji L, Roth JA. (2008). Tumor suppressor FUS1 signaling pathway. *J Thorac Oncol* 3(4):327-30.
Mattei MG, Riviere M, Krust A, Ingvarsson S, Vennstrom B, Islam MQ, Levan G, Kautner P, Zelent A, Chambon P et al. (1991). Chromosomal assignment of retinoic acid receptor (RAR) genes in the human, mouse, and rat genomes. *Genomics* 10:1061–9.
Sato M, Shames DS, Gazdar AF, Minna JD. (2007). A translational view of the molecular pathogenesis of lung cancer. *J Thorac Oncol* 2:327-43.
Sozzi G, Veronese ML, Negrini M, Baffa R, Cotticelli MG, Inoue H, Tornielli S, Pilotti S, De Gregorio L, Pastorino U, Pierotti MA, Ohta M, Huebner K, Croce CM. (1996). The FHIT gene 3p14.2 is abnormal in lung cancer. *Cell* 85:17–26.
Virmani AK, Rathi A, Zochbauer-Muller S, Sacchi N, Fukuyama Y, Bryant D, Maitra A, Heda S, Fong KM, Thunnissen F, Minna JD, Gazdar AF. (2000). Promoter methylation and silencing of the retinoic acid receptor-beta gene in lung carcinomas. *J Natl Cancer Inst* 92:1303–7.
Wistuba, II, Gazdar AF, Minna JD. (2001). Molecular genetics of small cell lung carcinoma. *Semin Oncol* 28:3–13.

19.14 Telomerase

Counter CM, Avilion AA, LeFeuvre CE, Stewart NG, Greider CW, Harley CB, Bacchetti S. (1992). Telomere shortening associated with chromosome instability is arrested in immortal cells which express telomerase activity. *EMBO J* 11:1921-9.
Hiyama K, Hiyama E, Ishioka S, Yamakido M, Inai K, Gazdar AF, Piatyszek MA, Shay JW. (1995). Telomerase activity in small-cell and non-small cell lung cancers. *J Natl Cancer Inst* 87:895–902.
Hyer JD, Silvestri G. (2000). Diagnosis and staging of lung cancer. 21:95-106.
Newbold RF. (2002). The significance of telomerase activation and cellular immortalization in human cancer. *Mutagenesis* 17:539–50.
Sarvesvaran J, Going JJ, Milroy R, Kaye SB, Keith WN. (1999). Is small cell lung cancer the perfect target for anti-telomerase treatment? *Carcinogenesis* 20:1649–51.
Zaffaroni N, De Polo D, Villa R, Della Porta C, Collini P, Fabbri A, Pilotti S, Daidone MG. (2003). Differential expression of telomerase activity in neuroendocrine lung tumours: correlation with gene product immunophenotyping. *J Pathol* 201(1):127-33.

19.15 Knockout mouse models

Brambilla E, Lantuejoul S, Sturm N. (2000). Divergent differentiation in neuroendocrine lung tumors. *Semin Diagn Pathol* 17: 138–48.
Calbo J, van Montfort E, Proost N, van Drunen E, Beverloo HB, Meuwissen R, Berns A. (2011). A functional role for tumor cell heterogeneity in a mouse model of small cell lung cancer. *Cancer Cell* 19(2):244-56.

Ho VM, Schaffer BE, Karnezis AN, Park KS, Sage J. (2009). The retinoblastoma gene Rb and its family member p130 suppress lung adenocarcinoma induced by oncogenic K-Ras. *Oncogene* 28:1393–9.

Karnoub AE, Dash AB, Vo AP, Sullivan A, Brooks MW, Bell GW, Richardson AL, Polyak K, Tubo R, Weinberg RA. (2007). Mesenchymal stem cells within tumour stroma promote breast cancer metastasis. *Nature* 449(7162):557-63.

Linnoila RI, Piantadosi S, Ruckdeschel JC. (1994). Impact of neuroendocrine differentiation in non-small cell lung cancer. The LCSG experience. *Chest* 106: Suppl. 6, 367S–371S.

Linnoila RI, Zhao B, DeMayo JL, Nelkin BD, Baylin SB, DeMayo FJ, Ball DW. (2000). Constitutive achaete-scute homologue-1 promotes airway dysplasia and lung neuroendocrine tumors in transgenic mice. *Cancer Res* 60: 4005–9.

Meuwissen R, Linn SC, Linnoila RI, Zevenhoven J, Mooi WJ, Berns A. (2003). Induction of small cell lung cancer by somatic inactivation of both Trp53 and Rb1 in a conditional mouse model. *Cancer Cell*; 4: 181–9.

Pei XH, Bai F, Smith MD, Xiong Y. (2007). p18Ink4c collaborates with Men1 to constrain lung stem cell expansion and suppress non-smallcell lung cancers. *Cancer Res* 67: 3162–70.

Sutherland KD, Proost N, Brouns I, Adriaensen D, Song JY, Berns A. (2011).Cell of origin of small cell lung cancer: inactivation of Trp53 and rb1 in distinct cell types of adult mouse lung. *Cancer Cell* 19(6):754-64.

Wistuba II, Gazdar AF. (2003). Characteristic genetic alterations in lung cancer. *Methods Mol Med* 74:3–28.

19.16 Mouse xenograft models

Daniel VC, Marchionni L, Hierman JS, Rhodes JT, Devereux WL, Rudin CM, Yung R, Parmigiani G, Dorsch M, Peacock CD, Watkins DN. (2009). A primary xenograft model of small-cell lung cancer reveals irreversible changes in gene expression imposed by culture in vitro. Cancer Res. 69(8):3364-73.

Hann CL, Daniel VC, Sugar EA, Dobromilskaya I, Murphy SC, Cope L, Lin X, Hierman JS, Wilburn DL, Watkins DN, Rudin CM. (2008). Therapeutic efficacy of ABT-737, a selective inhibitor of BCL-2, in small cell lung cancer. *Cancer Res* 68(7):2321-8.

Hodkinson PS, Mackinnon AC, Sethi T. (2007). Extracellular matrix regulation of drug resistance in small-cell lung cancer. *Int J Radiat Biol* 83: 733–4

Phelps RM, Johnson BE, Ihde DC, Gazdar AF, Carbone DP, McClintock PR, Linnoila RI, Matthews MJ, Bunn PA Jr, Carney D, Minna JD, Mulshine JL. (1996). NCI-Navy Medical Oncology Branch cell line data base. *J Cell Biochem* 24: 32–91.

7

Centrosome Abnormality and Human Lung Cancer

Kazuya Shinmura and Haruhiko Sugimura
Hamamatsu University School of Medicine
Japan

1. Introduction

The centrosome, which functions as a major microtubule-organizing center (MTOC), is composed of a pair of centrioles and surrounding protein aggregates called pericentriolar material (PCM); at any given time during the cell cycle, each cell contains one or two centrosomes (Fukasawa, 2007). Centrosomes play a crucial role in the formation of bipolar mitotic spindles, which are essential for accurate chromosome segregation (Zyss & Gergely, 2009). Numerical and functional abnormalities of centrosomes result in an increase in aberrant mitotic spindle formation, merotelic kinetochore-microtubule attachment errors, lagging chromosome formation, and chromosome segregation errors, all of which are thought to be possible causes of chromosome instability (Ganem et al., 2009; Nigg & Raff, 2009). Centrosome abnormalities and chromosome instability are characteristics of human lung cancer (Masuda and Takahashi, 2002; Koutsami et al., 2006; Jung et al., 2007; Shinmura et al., 2008), and abnormalities in genes responsible for centrosome regulation have been reported in lung cancer (Fukasawa, 2007; Lee et al., 2010). In this Review, the status of centrosome abnormalities in lung cancer, the mechanisms responsible for inducing centrosome abnormalities, and the relationship between centrosome abnormalities and chromosome instability are summarized.

2. Centrosome abnormalities in human lung cancer: Mechanisms causing centrosome abnormalities and chromosome instability

The presence of two centrosomes at mitosis is an important factor in the formation of bipolar mitotic spindles. Therefore, the numerical integrity of centrosomes is carefully controlled in human cells, and abrogation of this control results in centrosome amplification. First, we describe the normal centrosome duplication cycle, followed by three reports on centrosome abnormalities in lung cancer. Next, we describe investigations of the mechanism responsible for inducing centrosome amplification. Finally, we summarize the possible reasons why centrosome abnormalities cause chromosome instability.

2.1 Centrosome duplication cycle in human cells

Centrioles are cylindrical structures (-0.2 μm in diameter and 0.2-0.5 μm in length) and are composed of nine triplet microtubule arrays organized around a central cartwheel. Centrioles contain several tubulin isoforms and non-tubulin proteins such as CETN2, CP110,

SAS-6, and SAS-4 (Bettencourt-Dias & Glover, 2009). In animal cells, a pair of centrioles is embedded in a cloud of electron dense material known as PCM, and both structures constitute a larger structure named the centrosome, which serves as the main MTOC during both interphase and mitotic phase (Vorobjev & Nadezhdina, 1987). Centrosome duplication occurs once per cell cycle and is subject to strict control within cells. To organize a bipolar mitotic spindle, a centrosome is duplicated in S phase, additional PCM proteins are recruited during centrosome maturation in G2, and the two centrosomes separate at mitotic entry (Figure 1). The primary function of PCM is microtubule nucleation. The assembly of microtubules is initiated on a γ-tubulin ring complex (γTuRC), composed by γ-tubulin and additional subunits known as γ-tubulin complex proteins (Teixidó-Travesa et al., 2010).

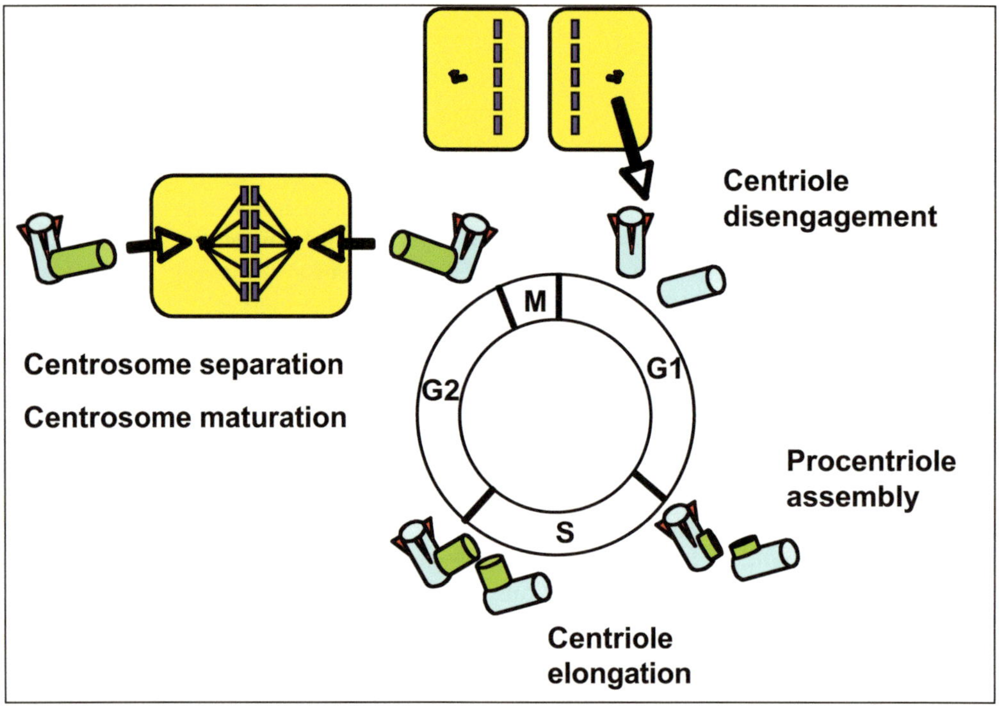

Fig. 1. Centrosome duplication cycle.

The centrioles duplicate once per cell cycle. The formation of the daughter centriole on each mother centriole occurs during the late G1 and S phases of the cell cycle. The daughter and mother centrioles are tightly associated in an orthogonal manner until the end of mitosis, and centriole disengagement occurs during mitotic exit. The initiation of centriole duplication requires the activity of several proteins, such as Cdk2-cyclin E and PLK4 kinases. The procentriole starts to assemble, and elongation depends on several proteins including centrin, CEP135, and γ-tubulin. During G2 phase, additional PCM proteins are recruited, and centrosome maturation requires the activity of Aurora A and PLK1 kinases. During late G2, the daughter centriole of the parental pair acquires subdistal appendages. Then, the two duplicated centrosomes separate and move to opposite end of the cell (centrosome separation). Finally, the two centrosomes form the poles of the bipolar mitotic spindle.

2.2 Centrosome abnormalities in lung cancer

Centrosome amplification has been reported in a variety of human primary cancers (e.g., breast cancer, lung cancer, bladder cancer, pancreatic cancer, and prostatic cancer) (Pihan et al., 1998; Sato et al., 1999; Pihan et al., 2001; Kawamura et al., 2004; Zyss & Gergely, 2009). With regard to primary lung cancer, Koutsami et al. (2006) examined 68 primary non-small cell lung carcinomas (NSCLCs) for the presence or absence of centrosome amplification using an immunofluorescence analysis with a monoclonal antibody for γ-tubulin, a centrosome marker; they showed that 36 (53%) of the 68 NSCLCs exhibited centrosome amplification. Centrosome amplification was not associated with clinicopathological markers such as stage, tumor grade, and histological subtype, but was associated with aneuploidy. Jung et al. (2007) examined 175 NSCLCs for centrosome abnormalities using an immunofluorescence analysis with an anti-γ-tubulin antibody; they showed that 50 (29%) of the 175 NSCLCs exhibited a centrosome abnormality. Aneuploidy, p16 expression, and the loss of pRB expression were significantly associated with centrosome abnormalities. Shinmura et al. (2008) examined 182 primary lung carcinomas for the presence or absence of centrosome amplification using an immunohistochemical analysis with an anti-γ-tubulin antibody and showed that 67 (37%) of the 182 cancers exhibited centrosome amplification. Thus, centrosome amplification is a common abnormality seen in human primary lung cancers.

2.3 Mechanisms inducing centrosome abnormalities

An immunofluorescence analysis using an antibody for centrosome or centriole markers in cultured cell lines can be used to determine the status of the centrosome number in the cells. The involvement of many kinds of agents and genes in centrosome regulation has been examined using such analyses. Here, these analyses are divided into those using lung cells and those using cells derived from other organs.

2.3.1 Mechanisms identified by using the lung cells

Holmes et al. (2006) showed that chronic exposure to lead chromate causes centrosome abnormalities and aneuploidy using WTHBF-6 cells, a cell line derived from normal human bronchial fibroblasts. Hexavalent chromium compounds [Cr(VI)] are human lung carcinogens (Le´onard & Lauwerys, 1980), and "particulate" Cr(VI) compounds are one of the most potent forms. They reported centrosome amplification in interphase and mitotic cells in response to treatment with lead chromate as a model particulate Cr(VI) compound. They suggested that one possible mechanism for lead chromate induced carcinogenesis is through centrosome dysfunction, leading to the induction of aneuploidy. The same group (Holmes et al., 2010) also showed that chronic exposure to zinc chromate, another particulate Cr(VI) compound, induces centrosome amplification and spindle checkpoint bypass using human lung fibroblasts.

Arsenic is another environmental toxicant, and the biological effects of arsenic have been studied. Liao et al. (2007) showed that arsenic promotes centrosome abnormalities and cell colony formation in p53 compromised human lung cells. They used H1355 (a lung adenocarcinoma cell line with a p53 mutation), BEAS-2B (immortalized lung epithelial cells with functional p53) and pifithrin-α-treated BEAS-2B (p53-inhibited cells) and reported an increase in centrosome abnormalities in both arsenite-treated p53 compromised cell lines, compared with that in arsenite-treated BEAS-2B cells. Their findings provided evidence of the carcinogenic promotional role of arsenic, especially in the presence of p53 abnormalities. The group also showed that arsenite promoted centrosome abnormalities in the presence of a p53-compromised status induced by 4-(methylnitrosamino)-1-(3-pyridyl)-1-butanone (nicotine-derived nitrosamine ketone, NNK) using BEAS-2B cells (Liao et al., 2010). Their findings provided evidence of an interaction between arsenite and cigarette smoking.

Benzo[*a*]pyrene diol epoxide (B[*a*]PDE), the ultimate carcinogenic metabolite of benzo[*a*]pyrene, has been implicated in the mutagenesis of the *p53* gene, which is involved in smoking-associated lung cancer. Shinmura et al. (2008) showed that the exposure of *p53*-deficient H1299 lung cancer cells to B[*a*]PDE resulted in S-phase arrest, leading to abnormal centrosome amplification. They also revealed that the centrosome amplification could be primarily attributed to excessive centrosome duplication, rather than to centriole splitting, and the forced expression of POLK DNA polymerase, which has the ability to bypass B[*a*]PDE–guanine lesions in an error-free manner, suppressing B[*a*]PDE-induced centrosome amplification. The B[*a*]PDE exposure also led to chromosome instability, which was likely to have resulted from centrosome amplification. Thus, they concluded that B[*a*]PDE contributes to neoplasia by inducing centrosome amplification and consequent chromosome destabilization in addition to its mutagenic activity.

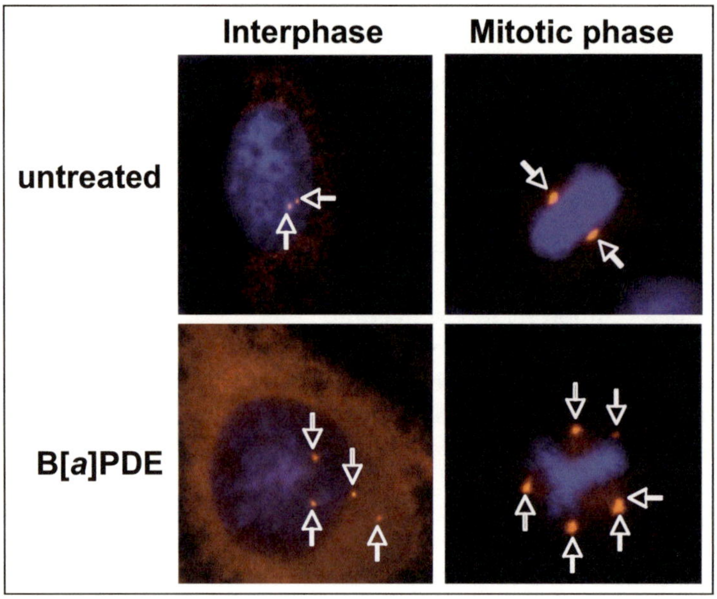

Fig. 2. Induction of centrosome amplification in *p53*-deficient H1299 lung cancer cells by exposure to benzo[*a*]pyrene diol epoxide (B[*a*]PDE).

H1299 cells were exposed to 0.6 μM B[*a*]PDE for 72 hr and then immunostained with mouse anti-γ-tubulin monoclonal antibody (GTU-88; Sigma-Aldrich, St. Louis, MO, USA). Alexa Fluor 546 (red)-conjugated anti-IgG antibody (Molecular Probes, Eugene, OR, USA) was used to detect the antibody–antigen complexes. The nuclei were stained with 4',6-diamidino-2-phenylindol (DAPI, blue). An increase in the number of centrosomes, i.e., centrosome amplification, was observed in both interphase cells and mitotic phase cells. The arrows indicate the positions of centrosomes.

The lung is easily subjected to many kinds of environmental agents, some of which may be derived from cigarette smoking or occupational exposure. As described in the above three paragraphs, some environmental carcinogens induce centrosome amplification. Other environmental carcinogens attacking DNA may also induce centrosome amplification, since cell cycle arrest has been shown to occur during centrosome amplification. Further precise analyses of environmental agent-related centrosome amplification are needed to understand the relationship between environmental carcinogens and lung cancer more clearly.

The S-phase kinase-interacting protein-2 (SKP2) plays a key role in the progression of cells from a quiescent to proliferative state, and the SKP2 protein is overexpressed in lung cancer. Jiang et al. (2005) showed that the RNA silencing of SKP2 inhibits proliferation and centrosome amplification using the lung cancer cell lines A549 and H1792. Their results suggest that SKP2 plays an oncogenic role in lung cancer and has a centrosome regulating function.

NORE1 (RASSF5) is a member of the *RASSF* gene family, and NORE1A is the longest and major splice isoform of the *NORE1* gene (Nakamura et al., 2005). Its product, NORE1A, is a nucleocytoplasmic shuttling protein and has a growth-suppressive function (Moshnikova et al., 2006). Shinmura et al. (2011) showed that NORE1A suppresses the centrosome amplification induced by hydroxyurea using a *p53*-deficient H1299 lung cancer cell line, and NORE1A expression was down-regulated in NSCLC. Both of these findings imply that NORE1A has a key preventative role against the carcinogenesis of NSCLC.

2.3.2 Mechanisms identified using cells derived from other organs

CDK2–cyclin E, a known inducer of S-phase entry (Heichman, 1994), has an important role in the regulation of centrosome duplication (Hinchcliffe et al., 1999; Matsumoto et al., 1999). The activation of CDK2–cyclin E during late-G1 phase coordinates the initiation of centrosome and DNA duplication. Several CDK2–cyclin E targets, including nucleophosmin (NPM) (Okuda et al., 2000), have been identified. NPM binds and modulates the activities of multiple proteins including tumor suppressor proteins (e.g., p53) and some oncogenic proteins (e.g., ROCK2) (Colombo et al., 2002; Ma et al., 2006b). The reduced as well as increased expression of NPM can lead to the oncogenic transformation of cells. Actually, NPM is frequently mutated, lost or overexpressed in cancers (Grisendi et al., 2006), and both the overexpression and the depletion of NPM in cultured cells can lead to neoplastic transformation (Kondo et al., 1997; Grisendi et al., 2005). NPM localizes between the paired centrioles of the unduplicated centrosome, probably functioning in centriole pairing (Shinmura et al., 2005). When NPM is phosphorylated by CDK2–cyclin E, most of the NPM dissociates from the centrosomes, leading to the centrosome duplication. In this context, NPM negatively controls centrosome duplication; indeed, the depletion of NPM leads to centrosome amplification (Grisendi et al., 2005; Wang et al., 2005). NPM was reported to have the ability to control centrosome duplication in association with ROCK2 (Ma et al., 2006b), a member of the Rho-associated, coiled-coil containing protein kinase family that is frequently overexpressed in cancer (Nishimura et al., 2003). After NPM phosphorylation by CDK2–cyclin E, the binding between NPM and ROCK2 increases and ROCK2 is activated at centrosomes, leading to centrosome duplication (Ma et al., 2006b). In ROCK2 activation, the binding of Rho small GTPase to the auto-inhibitory region is also required (Kanai et al., 2010). Among three isoforms of Rho, both RhoA and RhoC, but not RhoB, promoted centrosome duplication and centrosome amplification.

Another target of CDK2–cyclin E in centrosome regulation is MPS1, a spindle checkpoint kinase that is localized at the centrosome (Fisk et al., 2003). MPS1 is stabilized and activated by CDK2–cyclin E phosphorylation and involved in centrosome duplication. Mortalin, a member of the heat-shock protein 70 molecular chaperone family, is localized at the centrosome and physically interacts with and is phosphorylated by MPS1. The phosphorylation of mortalin activates MPS1 in a positive-feedback manner, and this phenomenon is important for MPS1-related centrosome duplication (Kanai et al., 2007). Mortalin is frequently upregulated in cancers (Wadhwa et al., 2006).

CDK2 forms a complex with cyclin A in addition to cyclin E, and CDK2–cyclin A has been implicated in the regulation of centrosome duplication (Meraldi et al., 1999). CDK2–cyclin A and CDK2–cyclin E share some substrates (Tokuyama et al., 2001). The CDK2–cyclin A complex is active in S and G2 phases during the cell cycle, and CDK2–cyclin A may have a crucial role in centrosome over-duplication and/or amplification (Hanashiro et al., 2008). As another type of CDK-cyclin complex, the overactivation of CDK4/6–cyclin D has been shown to induce centrosome amplification (Nelsen et al., 2005). The major target of CDK4/6–cyclin D is the RB tumor-suppressor protein (Duensing et al., 2000). The conditional loss of *Rb* in mice results in centrosome amplification (Balsitis et al., 2003; Iovino et al., 2006).

CDK2 activity is also negatively controlled by the CDK inhibitor p21, one of the major transactivation targets of the p53 tumor-suppressor protein (Bálint & Vousden, 2001). p53 is involved in the regulation of centrosome duplication, which was first demonstrated in cells and tissues from *p53*-deficient mice (Fukasawa et al., 1996; Fukasawa et al., 1997). When cells are exposed to DNA-synthesis inhibitors such as hydroxyurea, centrosomes undergo reduplication without DNA synthesis, resulting in centrosome amplification (Balczon et al., 1995). Centrosome reduplication occurs efficiently when *p53* is mutated or lost (Tarapore et al., 2001a). In normal cells, p53 is stabilized under cellular stresses by the inhibition of MDM2, leading to the upregulation of p21, which blocks the initiation of centrosome reduplication through the inhibition of cyclin–CDK2 complexes (Bálint & Vousden, 2001). On the other hand, p21 is not upregulated in cells lacking *p53*, allowing the activation of CDK2, which in turn triggers centrosome reduplication.

Besides the p53–p21 pathway, p53 has the ability to control centrosome duplication. p53 is localized at centrosomes (Blair Zajdel & Blair, 1988; Brown et al., 1994; Tarapore et al., 2001b; Tritarelli et al., 2004; Ma et al., 2006a; Shinmura et al., 2007) and appears to control centrosome duplication independently of its transactivation function. Even if p53 is a mutant without transactivation function, p53 retains the ability to localize to centrosomes and partially suppresses centrosome duplication (Shinmura et al., 2007). However, the mechanism underlying this role of p53 is currently unknown.

The proteins that control p53 stability are also involved in the regulation of centrosome duplication. The ectopic expression of human papilloma virus (HPV) E6 protein, which promotes the degradation of p53, induces centrosome amplification (Duensing et al., 2000). MDM2 is an E3 ubiquitin ligase that promotes the degradation of p53 and is often overexpressed in cancers (Manfredi, 2010). The forced expression of MDM2 in cells containing wild-type p53 efficiently leads to centrosome amplification (Carroll et al., 1999). Aurora A kinase (AURKA) phosphorylates p53 at Ser315, resulting in MDM2-mediated p53 destabilization (Katayama et al., 2004), and the forced expression of Aurora A induces centrosome amplification (Zhou et al., 1998).

Polo-like kinase 1 (PLK1) is a key regulator of centrosome maturation (Barr et al., 2004; Bettencourt-Dias and Glover, 2007). Its deregulation is linked to centrosome abnormalities and oncogenesis (Zyss and Gergely, 2009). PLK1 belongs to the mammalian PLK family, which is comprised of five members (PLK1 - PLK4 and PLK5P) (Lens et al., 2010). PLK1 is involved in a variety of mitotic events, including centrosome maturation and separation, G2/M transition, mitotic spindle formation, chromosome segregation, and cytokinesis, and several kinds of PLK1 substrates are known (Barr et al., 2004; Petronczki et al., 2008). PLK1 targets multiple centrosomal proteins (e.g., γ-tubulin) to fulfill the mitotic function of centrosomes. Ninein-like protein (NLP) interacts with γTuRC during interphase, and participates in the establishment of the cytoplasmic microtubule network (Casenghi et al., 2003; Rapley et al., 2005). At the onset of mitosis, the cooperation of PLK1 and NLP promotes the centrosomal localization of γ-tubulin and other mitosis specific PCM components, resulting in a higher microtubule nucleation capacity of the mitotic centrosome (Casenghi et al., 2003; Rapley et al., 2005). The phosphorylation of NEDD1 by PLK1 is required for the targeting of γTuRC to the centrosome (Zhang et al., 2009). In mitosis, centrosomes must withstand the pulling forces exerted by chromosome-attached microtubules. To withstand such forces, PLK1 also plays a role in maintaining the structural integrity of the centrosome during mitosis (Oshimori et al., 2006). Kizuna is localized at the centrosomes and is phosphorylated by PLK1 during mitosis. The reduced expression of kizuna results in centrosome fragmentation and the dispersion of PCM, leading to the formation of aberrant mitotic spindles and chromosome segregation errors.

Another PLK, PLK4, is involved in recruiting the structural components required for the formation of procentrioles at the proximal side of the older centriole, in cooperation with CDK2-cyclin E (Habedanck et al., 2004). The upregulation of PLK4 expression is a strong stimulus for centriole multiplication (Kleylein-Sohn et al., 2007). The timely degradation of PLK4 by the SCF slimb ubiquitin ligase is important for the restriction of procentriole formation (Cunha-Ferreira et al., 2009). The SCF component CUL1 also functions as a centrosomal suppressor of centriole multiplication by regulating the PLK4 protein level (Korzeniewski et al., 2009). PLK4 kinase activity also regulates its own stability (Holland et al., 2010; Guderian et al., 2010). CEP152 interacts with PLK4 and CPAP and controls centrosome duplication in human cells (Dzhindzhev et al., 2010). PLK4 is transcriptionally regulated by p53 (Li et al., 2005). Clinically, the expression of PLK4 is upregulated in colon cancer (Macmillan et al., 2001), while the expression of PLK4 is downregulated in hepatocellular carcinoma because of promoter hypermethylation and the loss of heterozygosity (LOH) (Pellegrino et al., 2010; Rosario et al., 2010)

The role of the morgana/chp-1 in centrosome regulation has been reported by Ferretti et al. (2010). Mutations in morgana result in centrosome amplification. Morgana forms a complex with Hsp90, ROCK1 and ROCK2, and directly binds to ROCK2. Morgana downregulation promotes the interaction between ROCK2 and NPM, leading to an increase in ROCK2 activity, which in turn results in centrosome amplification. Morgana is downregulated in a large fraction of lung and breast cancers. They suggested that morgana plays a role in preventing centrosome amplification and tumorigenesis.

NLP, a previously described substrate of PLK1 (Casenghi et al., 2003), is a BRCA1-associated centrosomal protein that is involved in microtubule nucleation and spindle formation (Jin et al., 2009). NLP is overexpressed as a result of *NLP* gene amplification in lung cancer, and NLP overexpression causes centrosome amplification (Shao et al., 2010).

The *BRCA1* gene is responsible for susceptibility to familial breast/ovarian cancer and participates in diverse cellular functions (Venkitaraman, 2002). The BRCA1 is localized at the centrosomes (Hsu & White, 1998; Okada & Ouchi, 2003) and is involved in the regulation of centrosome duplication (Xu et al., 1999). BRCA1 is associated with BARD1, and this association mediates the ubiquitylation of γ-tubulin, which is important for maintaining the numeral integrity of centrosomes. The *BRCA2* gene is another causative gene of familial breast/ovarian cancer and its protein product functions in homologous recombination (HR) repair (Venkitaraman, 2002). The loss of *BRCA2* results in centrosome amplification (Tutt et al., 1999), implying a relationship between a defect in DNA repair and the abnormal amplification of the centrosomes. HR repair is mediated by several proteins including RAD51, and the downregulation of RAD51 leads to centrosome amplification (Bertrand et al., 2003). The reduced expression or loss of XRCC2, XRCC3, and RAD51B-D, which are other HR components, induces centrosome amplification and chromosome instability (Griffin et al., 2000; Smiraldo et al., 2005; Date et al., 2006; Renglin Lindh et al., 2007; Cappelli et al., 2011).

Centrosome amplification induced by DNA damage occurs during a prolonged G2 phase (Dodson et al., 2004). A centrosome-autonomous signal that involves centriole disengagement causes centrosome amplification in G2 phase after DNA damage (Inanç et al., 2010), suggesting that genotoxic stress can decouple the centrosome cycle and chromosome cycle.

The active nucleocytoplasmic transport of proteins is mediated by the nuclear localization signal (NLS) and nuclear export signal (NES) (Turner & Sullivan, 2008). NLS-containing proteins are transported from the cytoplasm to the nucleus, whereas NES-containing proteins are exported from the nucleus to the cytoplasm by XPO1, the human homolog of yeast Crm1. The inhibition of XPO1 causes centrosome amplification via the disruption of the nucleocytoplasmic transport of NPM (Forgues et al., 2003; Shinmura et al., 2005; Wang et al., 2005). XPO1 is involved in the centrosomal localization of various proteins (Han et al., 2008). Importin β and RANBP1 are other proteins involved in nucleocytoplasmic transport, and these proteins also have the ability to regulate centrosomes (Di Fiore et al., 2003; Ciciarello et al., 2004).

SGOL1 interacts with protein phosphatase 2A, is localized in the centromere, and prevents the cohesin complex from precocious cleavage at the centromere via the dephosphorylation of SA2, one of the cohesin subunits (Kitajima et al., 2006; Riedel et al., 2006). Clinically, SGOL1 expression is downregulated in colorectal cancer, and SGOL1-knockdown leads to centrosome amplification and chromosome instability in a colon cancer cell line (Iwaizumi et al., 2009; Dai et al., 2009). A SGOL1-P1 transcript containing an exon-skip of exon 3, resulting in the formation of a premature stop codon, is expressed in colorectal cancer, and the overexpression of SGOL1-P1 in a colon cancer cell line resulted in an increased number of cells with aberrant chromosome alignment, precociously separated chromatids, delayed mitotic progression, and centrosome amplification (Kahyo et al., 2011). Furthermore, the overexpression of SGOL1-P1 inhibited the localization of endogenous SGOL1 and cohesin subunit RAD21/SCC1 to the centromere, suggesting that SGOL1-P1 may function as a negative factor to native SGOL1 (Kahyo et al., 2011).

2.4 Relationship between centrosome abnormalities and chromosome instability

Chromosome instability is defined as a persistently high rate of the gain and loss of whole chromosomes (Thompson et al., 2010). Chromosome instability is a major source of aneuploidy (Lengauer et al., 1997; Rajagopalan and Lengauer, 2004), and chromosome instability is thought to be involved not only in cancer initiation, where aneuploidy may have a causal role, but also in cancer development, where increased rates of chromosome missegregation may enable the clonal expansion of cells with a greater malignant potential (Rajagopalan & Lengauer, 2004; Weaver et al., 2007; Gao et al., 2007; Ganem et al., 2009). Defects in chromosome cohesion, weakened spindle assembly checkpoint (SAC) signalling, impaired microtubule-kinetochore attachment, defects in cell cycle regulation, and centrosome abnormalities can cause chromosome instability (Lingle et al., 1998; Draviam et al., 2004; Thompson & Compton, 2008; Weaver & Cleveland, 2008; Thompson et al., 2010). Regarding centrosome abnormalities, two mechanisms underlying chromosome instability have been proposed. The first mechanism is that centrosome amplification generates chromosome instability by promoting multipolar anaphase, which is an abnormal division that produces more than three aneuploid daughter cells (Nigg, 2002). The other mechanism is that centrosome amplification generates chromosome instability by promoting merotelic kinetochore–microtubule attachments (Ganem et al., 2009; Silkworth et al., 2009). Merotely is a type of error in which single kinetochores attach to microtubules emanating from different poles (Salmon et al., 2005; Cimini, 2008) and is common in cells showing chromosome instability (Thompson & Compton, 2008). Cells with centrosome amplification often coalesce the extra centrosomes during mitosis to ensure that anaphase occurs with a bipolar spindle (Quintyne et al., 2005). The extra centrosomes induce transient multipolar spindle intermediates prior to the coalescence of the centrosomes into bipolar spindles; this event increases the incidence of merotelic kinetochore–microtubule attachments and elevates the chromosome missegregation rates (Ganem et al., 2009; Silkworth et al., 2009). Ganem et al. (2009) showed that the presence of extra centrosomes is correlated with an increase in lagging chromosomes (Figure 3), promoting chromosome missegregation through excessive merotely induced by transient multipolar spindle intermediates. Since merotelic attachments are poorly sensed by the SAC (Salmon et al., 2005; Cimini, 2008), the merotelic attachments arising from centrosome amplification are not fully repaired and give rise to lagging chromosomes during anaphase, possibly leading to missegregation events.

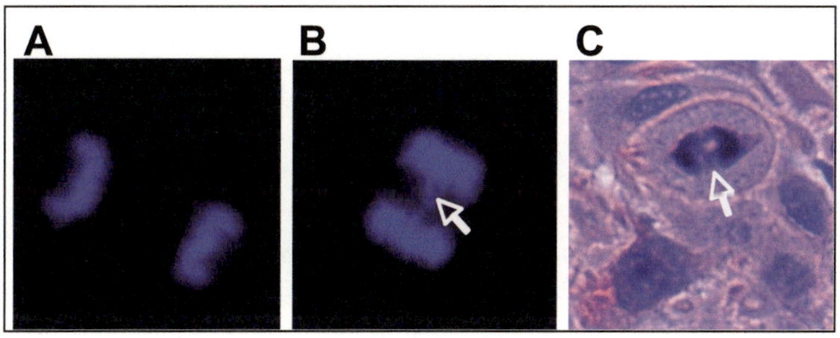

Fig. 3. Lagging chromosomes in human cancer cells.

(A, B) Lagging chromosome formation detected in a B[*a*]PDE-treated H1299 lung cancer cell line. (A) Normal segregation; (B) an anaphase cell showing lagging chromosome formation. The nuclei were stained with DAPI (blue). (C) Lagging chromosomes are shown in a hematoxylin-and-eosin-stained section of a squamous cell carcinoma of the lung. In (B) and (C), the arrows indicate lagging chromosomes.

3. Conclusion

The progress in our understanding of the relationship between centrosome abnormalities and cancer during the past 15 years has been enormous. We have learned that centrosome abnormalities are common among diverse human cancers including lung cancer. Many molecules are involved in the control of the numeral and/or functional integrity of centrosomes, and the abrogation of these mechanisms results in centrosome abnormalities, which promote chromosome instability. From a therapeutic standpoint, anti-cancer drugs targeting the centrosome have now been developed (Mazzorana et al., 2011). Future studies using a genome-wide approach and new scientific technologies will further increase our knowledge of the role of the centrosome in human cells, and such knowledge will likely help to establish effective cancer therapies.

4. Acknowledgment

This work was supported by grants from the MHLW (21-1), the JSPS (22590356), the MEXT (20014007 and 221S0001), and the Smoking Research Foundation.

5. References

Balczon, R., Bao, L., Zimmer, W.E., Brown, K., Zinkowski, R.P., & Brinkley, B.R. (1995). Dissociation of centrosome replication events from cycles of DNA synthesis and mitotic division in hydroxyurea-arrested Chinese hamster ovary cells. *Journal of Cell Biology,* Vol.130, No.1, (July), pp. 105-115, ISSN 0021-9525

Bálint, E.E. & Vousden, K.H. (2001). Activation and activities of the p53 tumour suppressor protein. *British Journal of Cancer,* Vol.85, No.12, (December 14), pp. 1813-1823, ISSN 0007-0920

Balsitis, S.J., Sage, J., Duensing, S., Münger, K., Jacks, T., & Lambert, P.F. (2003). Recapitulation of the effects of the human papillomavirus type 16 E7 oncogene on mouse epithelium by somatic Rb deletion and detection of pRb-independent effects of E7 in vivo. *Molecular and Cellular Biology,* Vol.23, No.24, (December), pp. 9094-9103, ISSN 0270-7306

Barr, F.A., Sillјé, H.H., & Nigg, E.A. (2004). Polo-like kinases and the orchestration of cell division. *Nature Reviews Molecular Cell Biology,* Vol.5, No.6, (June), pp. 429-440, ISSN 1471-0072

Bertrand, P., Lambert, S., Joubert, C., & Lopez, B.S. (2003). Overexpression of mammalian Rad51 does not stimulate tumorigenesis while a dominant-negative Rad51 affects centrosome fragmentation, ploidy and stimulates tumorigenesis, in p53-defective CHO cells. *Oncogene,* Vol.22, No.48, (October 23), pp. 7587-7592, ISSN 0950-9232

Bettencourt-Dias, M. & Glover, D.M. (2007). Centrosome biogenesis and function: centrosomics brings new understanding. *Nature Reviews Molecular Cell Biology,* Vol.8, No.6, (June), pp. 451-463, ISSN 1471-0072

Bettencourt-Dias, M. & Glover, D.M. (2009). SnapShot: centriole biogenesis. *Cell,* Vol.136, No.1, (January 9), pp. 188-188.e1, ISSN 0092-8674

Blair Zajdel, M.E. & Blair, G.E. (1988). The intracellular distribution of the transformation-associated protein p53 in adenovirus-transformed rodent cells. *Oncogene,* Vol.2, No.6, (June), pp. 579-584, ISSN 0950-9232

Brown, C.R., Doxsey, S.J., White, E., & Welch, W.J. (1994). Both viral (adenovirus E1B) and cellular (hsp 70, p53) components interact with centrosomes. *Journal of Cellular Physiology,* Vol.160, No.1, (July), pp. 47-60, ISSN 0021-9541

Cappelli, E., Townsend, S., Griffin, C., & Thacker, J. (2011). Homologous recombination proteins are associated with centrosomes and are required for mitotic stability. *Experimental Cell Research,* Vol.317, No.8, (May 1), pp. 1203-1213, ISSN 0014-4827

Carroll, P.E., Okuda, M., Horn, H.F., et al. (1999). Centrosome hyperamplification in human cancer: chromosome instability induced by p53 mutation and/or Mdm2 overexpression. *Oncogene,* Vol.18, No.11, (March 18), pp. 1935-1944, ISSN 0950-9232

Casenghi, M., Meraldi, P., Weinhart, U., Duncan, P.I., Körner, R., & Nigg, E.A. (2003). Polo-like kinase 1 regulates Nlp, a centrosome protein involved in microtubule nucleation. *Developmental Cell,* Vol.5, No.1, (July), pp. 113-125, ISSN 1534-5807

Ciciarello, M., Mangiacasale, R., Thibier, C., et al. (2004). Importin beta is transported to spindle poles during mitosis and regulates Ran-dependent spindle assembly factors in mammalian cells. *Journal of Cell Science,* Vol.117, No.26, (December 15), pp. 6511-6522, ISSN 0021-9533

Cimini, D. (2008). Merotelic kinetochore orientation, aneuploidy, and cancer. *Biochimica et Biophysica Acta-Reviews on Cancer,* Vol.1786, No.1, (September), pp. 32-40, ISSN 0304-419X

Colombo, E., Marine, J.C., Danovi, D., Falini, B., & Pelicci, P.G. (2002). Nucleophosmin regulates the stability and transcriptional activity of p53. *Nature Cell Biology,* Vol.4, No.7, (July), pp. 529-533, ISSN 1465-7392

Cunha-Ferreira, I., Rodrigues-Martins, A., Bento, I., et al. (2009). The SCF/Slimb ubiquitin ligase limits centrosome amplification through degradation of SAK/PLK4. *Current Biology,* Vol.19, No.1, (January 13), pp. 43-49, ISSN 0960-9822

Dai, J., Kateneva, A.V., & Higgins, J.M. (2009). Studies of haspin-depleted cells reveal that spindle-pole integrity in mitosis requires chromosome cohesion. *Journal of Cell Science,* Vol.122, No.22, (November 15), pp. 4168-4176, ISSN 0021-9533

Date, O., Katsura, M., Ishida, M., et al. (2006). Haploinsufficiency of RAD51B causes centrosome fragmentation and aneuploidy in human cells. *Cancer Research,* Vol.66, No.12, (June 15), pp. 6018-6024, ISSN 0008-5472

Di Fiore, B., Ciciarello, M., Mangiacasale, R., et al. (2003). Mammalian RanBP1 regulates centrosome cohesion during mitosis. *Journal of Cell Science,* Vol.116, No.16, (August 15), pp. 3399-3411, ISSN 0021-9533

Dodson, H., Bourke, E., Jeffers, L.J., et al. (2004). Centrosome amplification induced by DNA damage occurs during a prolonged G2 phase and involves ATM. *EMBO Journal,* Vol.23, No.19, (October 1), pp. 3864-3873, ISSN 0261-4189

Draviam, V.M., Xie, S., & Sorger, P.K. (2004). Chromosome segregation and genomic stability. *Current Opinion in Genetics & Development,* Vol.14, No.2, (April), pp. 120-125, ISSN 0959-437X

Duensing, S., Lee, L.Y., Duensing, A., et al. (2000). The human papillomavirus type 16 E6 and E7 oncoproteins cooperate to induce mitotic defects and genomic instability by uncoupling centrosome duplication from the cell division cycle. *Proceedings of the National Academy of Sciences of the United States of America,* Vol.97, No.18, (August 29), pp. 10002-10007, ISSN 0027-8424

Dzhindzhev, N.S., Yu, Q.D., Weiskopf, K., et al. (2010). Asterless is a scaffold for the onset of centriole assembly. *Nature,* Vol.467, No.7316, (October 7), pp. 714-718, ISSN 0028-0836

Ferretti, R., Palumbo, V., Di Savino, A., et al. (2010). Morgana/chp-1, a ROCK inhibitor involved in centrosome duplication and tumorigenesis. *Developmental Cell,* Vol.18, No.3, (March 16), pp. 486-495, ISSN 1534-5807

Fisk, H.A., Mattison, C.P., & Winey, M. (2003). Human Mps1 protein kinase is required for centrosome duplication and normal mitotic progression. *Proceedings of the National Academy of Sciences of the United States of America,* Vol.100, No.25, (December 9), pp. 14875-14880, ISSN 0027-8424

Forgues, M., Difilippantonio, M.J., Linke, S.P., et al. (2003). Involvement of Crm1 in hepatitis B virus X protein-induced aberrant centriole replication and abnormal mitotic spindles. *Molecular and Cellular Biology,* Vol.23, No.15, (August), pp. 5282-5292, ISSN 0270-7306

Fukasawa, K., Choi, T., Kuriyama, R., Rulong, S., & Vande Woude, G.F. (1996). Abnormal centrosome amplification in the absence of p53. *Science,* Vol.271, No.5256, (March 22), pp. 1744-1747, ISSN 0036-8075

Fukasawa, K., Wiener, F., Vande Woude, G.F., & Mai, S. (1997). Genomic instability and apoptosis are frequent in p53 deficient young mice. *Oncogene,* Vol.15, No.11, (September), pp. 1295-1302, ISSN 0950-9232

Fukasawa, K. (2007). Oncogenes and tumour suppressors take on centrosomes. *Nature Reviews Cancer,* Vol.7, No.12, (December), pp. 911-924, ISSN 1474-175X

Ganem, N.J., Godinho, S.A., & Pellman, D. (2009). A mechanism linking extra centrosomes to chromosomal instability. *Nature,* Vol.460, No.7252, (July 9), pp. 278-282, ISSN 0028-0836

Gao, C., Furge, K., Koeman, J., et al. (2007). Chromosome instability, chromosome transcriptome, and clonal evolution of tumor cell populations. *Proceedings of the National Academy of Sciences of the United States of America,* Vol.104, No.21, (May 22), pp. 8995-9000, ISSN 0027-8424

Griffin, C.S., Simpson, P.J., Wilson, C.R., & Thacker, J. (2000). Mammalian recombination-repair genes XRCC2 and XRCC3 promote correct chromosome segregation. *Nature Cell Biology,* Vol.2, No.10, (October), pp. 757-761, ISSN 1465-7392

Grisendi, S., Bernardi, R., Rossi, M., et al. (2005). Role of nucleophosmin in embryonic development and tumorigenesis. *Nature,* Vol. 437, No. 7055, (September 1), pp. 147-153, ISSN 0028-0836

Grisendi, S., Mecucci, C., Falini, B., & Pandolfi, P.P. (2006). Nucleophosmin and cancer. *Nature Reviews Cancer,* Vol.6, No.7, (July), pp. 493-505, ISSN 1474-175X

Guderian, G., Westendorf, J., Uldschmid, A., & Nigg, E.A. (2010). Plk4 trans-autophosphorylation regulates centriole number by controlling betaTrCP-mediated degradation. *Journal of Cell Science,* Vol.123, No.13, (July 1), pp. 2163-2169, ISSN 0021-9533

Habedanck, R., Stierhof, Y.D., Wilkinson, C.J., & Nigg, E.A. (2005). The Polo kinase Plk4 functions in centriole duplication. *Nature Cell Biology,* Vol.7, No.11, (November), pp. 1140-1146, ISSN 1465-7392

Han, X., Saito, H., Miki, Y., & Nakanishi, A. (2008). A CRM1-mediated nuclear export signal governs cytoplasmic localization of BRCA2 and is essential for centrosomal localization of BRCA2. *Oncogene,* Vol.27, No.21, (May 8), pp. 2969-2977, ISSN 0950-9232

Hanashiro, K., Kanai, M., Geng, Y., Sicinski, P., & Fukasawa, K. (2008). Roles of cyclins A and E in induction of centrosome amplification in p53-compromised cells. *Oncogene,* Vol.27, No.40, (September 11), pp. 5288-5302, ISSN 0950-9232

Heichman, K.A. & Roberts, J.M. (1994). Rules to replicate by. *Cell,* Vol.79, No.4, (November 18), pp. 557-562, ISSN 0092-8674

Hinchcliffe, E.H., Li, C., Thompson, E.A., Maller, J.L., & Sluder, G. (1999). Requirement of Cdk2-cyclin E activity for repeated centrosome reproduction in Xenopus egg extracts. *Science,* Vol.283, No.5403, (February 5), pp. 851-854, ISSN 0036-8075

Holland, A.J., Lan, W., Niessen, S., Hoover, H., & Cleveland, D.W. (2010). Polo-like kinase 4 kinase activity limits centrosome overduplication by autoregulating its own stability. *Journal of Cell Biology,* Vol.188, No.2, (January 25), pp. 191-198, ISSN 0021-9525

Holmes, A.L., Wise, S.S., Sandwick, S.J., et al. (2006). Chronic exposure to lead chromate causes centrosome abnormalities and aneuploidy in human lung cells. *Cancer Research,* Vol.66, No.8, (April 15), pp. 4041-4048, ISSN 0008-5472

Holmes, A.L., Wise, S.S., Pelsue, S.C., et al. (2010). Chronic exposure to zinc chromate induces centrosome amplification and spindle assembly checkpoint bypass in human lung fibroblasts. *Chemical Research in Toxicology,* Vol.23, No.2, (February 15), pp. 386-395, ISSN 0893-228X

Hsu, L.C. & White, R.L. (1998). BRCA1 is associated with the centrosome during mitosis. *Proceedings of the National Academy of Sciences of the United States of America,* Vol.95, No.22, (October 27), pp. 12983-12988, ISSN 0027-8424

Inanç, B., Dodson, H., & Morrison, C.G. (2010). A centrosome-autonomous signal that involves centriole disengagement permits centrosome duplication in G2 phase after DNA damage. *Molecular Biology of the Cell,* Vol.21, No.22, (November 15), pp. 3866-3877, ISSN 1059-1524

Iovino, F., Lentini, L., Amato, A., & Di Leonardo, A. (2006). RB acute loss induces centrosome amplification and aneuploidy in murine primary fibroblasts. *Molecular Cancer,* Vol.5, (September 20), pp. 38, ISSN 1476-4598

Iwaizumi, M., Shinmura, K., Mori, H., et al. (2009). Human Sgo1 downregulation leads to chromosomal instability in colorectal cancer. *Gut,* Vol.58, No.2, (February), pp. 249-260, ISSN 0017-5749

Jiang, F., Caraway, N.P., Li, R., & Katz, R.L. (2005). RNA silencing of S-phase kinase-interacting protein 2 inhibits proliferation and centrosome amplification in lung cancer cells. *Oncogene,* Vol.24, No.21, (May 12), pp. 3409-3418, ISSN 0950-9232

Jin, S., Gao, H., Mazzacurati, L., et al. (2009). BRCA1 interaction of centrosomal protein Nlp is required for successful mitotic progression. *Journal of Biological Chemistry,* Vol.284, No.34, (August 21), pp. 22970-22977, ISSN 0021-9258

Jung, C.K., Jung, J.H., Lee, K.Y., et al. (2007). Centrosome abnormalities in non-small cell lung cancer: correlations with DNA aneuploidy and expression of cell cycle regulatory proteins. *Pathology Research and Practice,* Vol.203, No.12, pp. 839-847, ISSN 0344-0338

Kahyo, T., Iwaizumi, M., Shinmura, K., et al. (2011). A novel tumor-derived SGOL1 variant causes abnormal mitosis and unstable chromatid cohesion. *Oncogene,* Vol.30, No.44, (November 3), pp.4453-4463, ISSN 0950-9232

Kanai, M., Ma, Z., Izumi, H., et al. (2007). Physical and functional interaction between mortalin and Mps1 kinase. *Genes to Cells,* Vol.12, No.6, (June), pp. 797-810, ISSN 1356-9597

Kanai, M., Crowe, M.S., Zheng, Y., Vande Woude, G.F., & Fukasawa, K. (2010). RhoA and RhoC are both required for the ROCK II-dependent promotion of centrosome duplication. *Oncogene,* Vol.29, No.45, (November 11), pp. 6040-6050, ISSN 0950-9232

Katayama, H., Sasai, K., Kawai, H., et al. (2004). Phosphorylation by aurora kinase A induces Mdm2-mediated destabilization and inhibition of p53. *Nature Genetics,* Vol.36, No.1, (January), pp. 55-62, ISSN 1061-4036

Kawamura, K., Izumi, H., Ma, Z., et al. (2004). Induction of centrosome amplification and chromosome instability in human bladder cancer cells by p53 mutation and cyclin E overexpression. *Cancer Research,* Vol.64, No.14, (July 15), pp. 4800-4809, ISSN 0008-5472

Kitajima, T.S., Sakuno, T., Ishiguro, K., et al. (2006). Shugoshin collaborates with protein phosphatase 2A to protect cohesin. *Nature,* Vol.441, No.7089, (May 4), pp. 46-52, ISSN 0028-0836

Kleylein-Sohn, J., Westendorf, J., Le Clech, M., Habedanck, R., Stierhof, Y.D., & Nigg, E.A. (2007). Plk4-induced centriole biogenesis in human cells. *Developmental Cell,* Vol.13, No.2, (August), pp. 190-202, ISSN 1534-5807

Kondo, T., Minamino, N., Nagamura-Inoue, T., Matsumoto, M., Taniguchi, T., & Tanaka, N. (1997). Identification and characterization of nucleophosmin/B23/numatrin which binds the anti-oncogenic transcription factor IRF-1 and manifests oncogenic activity. *Oncogene,* Vol.15, No.11, (September), pp. 1275-1281, ISSN 0950-9232

Korzeniewski, N., Zheng, L., Cuevas, R., et al. (2009). Cullin 1 functions as a centrosomal suppressor of centriole multiplication by regulating polo-like kinase 4 protein levels. *Cancer Research,* Vol.69, No.16, (August 15), pp. 6668-6675, ISSN 0008-5472

Koutsami, M.K., Tsantoulis, P.K., Kouloukoussa, M., et al. (2006). Centrosome abnormalities are frequently observed in non-small-cell lung cancer and are associated with aneuploidy and cyclin E overexpression. *Journal of Pathology,* Vol.209, No.4, (August), pp. 512-521, ISSN 0022-3417

Lee, W., Jiang, Z., Liu, J., et al. (2010). The mutation spectrum revealed by paired genome sequences from a lung cancer patient. *Nature,* Vol.465, No.7297, (May 27), pp. 473-477, ISSN 0028-0836

Lengauer, C., Kinzler, K.W., & Vogelstein, B. (1997). Genetic instability in colorectal cancers. *Nature,* Vol.386, No.6625, (April 10), pp. 623-627, ISSN 0028-0836

Lens, S.M., Voest, E.E., & Medema, R.H. (2010). Shared and separate functions of polo-like kinases and aurora kinases in cancer. *Nature Reviews Cancer,* Vol.10, No.12, (December), pp. 825-841, ISSN 1474-175X

Le´onard, A. & Lauwerys, R.R. (1980). Carcinogenicity and mutagenicity of chromium. *Mutation Research-Reviews in Mutation Research,* Vol.76, pp. 227-239. ISSN 1383-5742

Li, J., Tan, M., Li, L., Pamarthy, D., Lawrence, T.S., & Sun, Y. (2005). SAK, a new polo-like kinase, is transcriptionally repressed by p53 and induces apoptosis upon RNAi silencing. *Neoplasia,* Vol.7, No.4, (April), pp. 312-323, ISSN 1522-8002

Liao, W.T., Lin, P., Cheng, T.S., Yu, H.S., & Chang, L.W. (2007). Arsenic promotes centrosome abnormalities and cell colony formation in p53 compromised human lung cells. *Toxicology and Applied Pharmacology,* Vol.225, No.2, (December 1), pp. 162-170, ISSN 0041-008X

Liao, W.T., Yu, H.S., Lin, P., & Chang, L.W. (2010). Arsenite promotes centrosome abnormalities under a p53 compromised status induced by 4-(methylnitrosamino)-1-(3-pyridyl)-1-butanone (NNK). *Toxicology and Applied Pharmacology,* Vol.243, No.1, (February 15), pp. 55-62, ISSN 0041-008X

Lingle, W.L., Barrett, S.L., Negron, V.C., et al. (2002). Centrosome amplification drives chromosomal instability in breast tumor development. *Proceedings of the National Academy of Sciences of the United States of America,* Vol.99, No.4, (February 19), pp. 1978-1983, ISSN 0027-8424

Ma, Z., Izumi, H., Kanai, M., Kabuyama, Y., Ahn, N.G., & Fukasawa, K. (2006a). Mortalin controls centrosome duplication via modulating centrosomal localization of p53. *Oncogene,* Vol.25, No.39, (August 31), pp. 5377-5390, ISSN 0950-9232

Ma, Z., Kanai, M., Kawamura, K., Kaibuchi, K., Ye, K., & Fukasawa, K. (2006b). Interaction between ROCK II and nucleophosmin/B23 in the regulation of centrosome duplication. *Molecular and Cellular Biology,* Vol.26, No.23, (December), pp. 9016-9034, ISSN 0270-7306

Macmillan, J.C., Hudson, J.W., Bull, S., Dennis, J.W., & Swallow, C.J. (2001). Comparative expression of the mitotic regulators SAK and PLK in colorectal cancer. *Annals of Surgical Oncology,* Vol.8, No.9, (October), pp. 729-740, ISSN 1068-9265

Manfredi, J.J. (2010). The Mdm2-p53 relationship evolves: Mdm2 swings both ways as an oncogene and a tumor suppressor. *Genes & Development,* Vol.24, No.15, (August 1), pp. 1580-1589, ISSN 0890-9369

Masuda, A. & Takahashi, T. (2002). Chromosome instability in human lung cancers: possible underlying mechanisms and potential consequences in the pathogenesis. *Oncogene,* Vol.21, No.45, (October 7), pp. 6884-6897, ISSN 0950-9232

Matsumoto, Y., Hayashi, K., & Nishida, E. (1999). Cyclin-dependent kinase 2 (Cdk2) is required for centrosome duplication in mammalian cells. *Current Biology,* Vol.9, No.8, (April 22), pp. 429-432, ISSN 0960-9822

Mazzorana, M., Montoya, G., & Mortuza, G.B. (2011). The centrosome: a target for cancer therapy. *Current Cancer Drug Targets,* Vol.11, No.5, (June 1), pp. 600-612, ISSN 1568-0096

Meraldi, P., Lukas, J., Fry, A.M., Bartek, J., & Nigg, E.A. (1999). Centrosome duplication in mammalian somatic cells requires E2F and Cdk2-cyclin A. *Nature Cell Biology,* Vol.1, No.2, (June), pp. 88-93, ISSN 1465-7392

Moshnikova, A., Frye, J., Shay, J.W., Minna, J.D., & Khokhlatchev, A.V. (2006). The growth and tumor suppressor NORE1A is a cytoskeletal protein that suppresses growth by inhibition of the ERK pathway. *Journal of Biological Chemistry,* Vol.281, No.12, (March 24), pp. 8143-8152, ISSN 1059-1524

Nakamura, N., Carney, J.A., Jin, L., et al. (2005). RASSF1A and NORE1A methylation and BRAFV600E mutations in thyroid tumors. *Laboratory Investigation,* Vol.85, No.9, (September), pp. 1065-1075, ISSN 0023-6837

Nelsen, C.J., Kuriyama, R., Hirsch, B., et al. (2005). Short term cyclin D1 overexpression induces centrosome amplification, mitotic spindle abnormalities, and aneuploidy. *Journal of Biological Chemistry,* Vol.280, No.1, (January 7), pp. 768-776, ISSN 0021-9258

Nigg, E.A. (2002). Centrosome aberrations: cause or consequence of cancer progression? *Nature Reviews Cancer,* Vol.2, No.11, (November), pp. 815-825, ISSN 1474-175X

Nigg, E.A. & Raff, J.W. (2009). Centrioles, centrosomes, and cilia in health and disease. *Cell,* Vol.139, No.4, (November 13), pp. 663-678, ISSN 0092-8674

Nishimura, Y., Itoh, K., Yoshioka, K., Tokuda, K., & Himeno, M. (2003). Overexpression of ROCK in human breast cancer cells: evidence that ROCK activity mediates intracellular membrane traffic of lysosomes. *Pathology & Oncology Research,* Vol.9, No.2, pp. 83-95, ISSN 1219-4956

Okada, S. & Ouchi, T. (2003). Cell cycle differences in DNA damage-induced BRCA1 phosphorylation affect its subcellular localization. *Journal of Biological Chemistry,* Vol.278, No.3, (January 17), pp. 2015-2020, ISSN 0021-9258

Okuda, M., Horn, H.F., Tarapore, P., et al. (2000). Nucleophosmin/B23 is a target of CDK2/cyclin E in centrosome duplication. *Cell,* Vol.103, No.1, (September 29), pp. 127-140, ISSN 0092-8674

Oshimori, N., Ohsugi, M., & Yamamoto, T. (2006). The Plk1 target Kizuna stabilizes mitotic centrosomes to ensure spindle bipolarity. *Nature Cell Biology,* Vol.8, No.10, (October), pp. 1095-1101, ISSN 1465-7392

Pellegrino, R., Calvisi, D.F., Ladu, S., et al. (2010). Oncogenic and tumor suppressive roles of polo-like kinases in human hepatocellular carcinoma. *Hepatology,* Vol.51, No.3, (March), pp. 857-868, ISSN 0270-9139

Petronczki, M., Lénárt, P., & Peters, J.M. (2008). Polo on the Rise-from Mitotic Entry to Cytokinesis with Plk1. *Developmental Cell,* Vol.14, No.5, (May), pp. 646-659, ISSN 1534-5807

Pihan, G.A., Purohit, A., Wallace, J., et al. (1998). Centrosome defects and genetic instability in malignant tumors. *Cancer Research,* Vol.58, No.17, (September 1), pp. 3974-3985, ISSN 0008-5472

Pihan, G.A., Purohit, A., Wallace, J., Malhotra, R., Liotta, L., & Doxsey, S.J. (2001). Centrosome defects can account for cellular and genetic changes that characterize prostate cancer progression. *Cancer Research,* Vol.61, No.5, (March 1), pp. 2212-2219, ISSN 0008-5472

Quintyne, N.J., Reing, J.E., Hoffelder, D.R., Gollin, S.M., & Saunders, W.S. (2005). Spindle multipolarity is prevented by centrosomal clustering. *Science,* Vol.307, No.5706, (January 7), pp. 127-129, ISSN 0036-8075

Rajagopalan, H. & Lengauer, C. (2004). Aneuploidy and cancer. *Nature,* Vol.432, No. 7015, (November 18), pp. 338-341, ISSN 0028-0836

Rapley, J., Baxter, J.E., Blot, J., et al. (2005). Coordinate regulation of the mother centriole component nlp by nek2 and plk1 protein kinases. *Molecular and Cellular Biology,* Vol.25, No.4, (February), pp. 1309-1324, ISSN 0270-7306

Renglin Lindh, A., Schultz, N., Saleh-Gohari, N., & Helleday, T. (2007). RAD51C (RAD51L2) is involved in maintaining centrosome number in mitosis. *Cytogenetic and Genome Research,* Vol.116, No.1-2, pp. 38-45, ISSN 1424-8581

Riedel, C.G., Katis, V.L., Katou, Y., et al. (2006). Protein phosphatase 2A protects centromeric sister chromatid cohesion during meiosis I. *Nature,* Vol.441, No. 7089, (May 4), pp. 53-61, ISSN 0028-0836

Rosario, C.O., Ko, M.A., Haffani, Y.Z., et al. (2010). Plk4 is required for cytokinesis and maintenance of chromosomal stability. *Proceedings of the National Academy of Sciences of the United States of America,* Vol.107, No.15, (April 13), pp. 6888-6893, ISSN 0027-8424

Salmon, E.D., Cimini, D., Cameron, L.A., & DeLuca, J.G. (2005). Merotelic kinetochores in mammalian tissue cells. *Philosophical Transactions of the Royal Society of London. Series B, Biological Sciences,* Vol.360, No.1455, (March 29), pp. 553-568, ISSN 0080-4622

Sato, N., Mizumoto, K., Nakamura, M., et al. (1999). Centrosome abnormalities in pancreatic ductal carcinoma. *Clinical Cancer Research,* Vol.5, No.5, (May), pp. 963-970, ISSN 1078-0432

Shao, S., Liu, R., Wang, Y., et al. (2010). Centrosomal Nlp is an oncogenic protein that is gene-amplified in human tumors and causes spontaneous tumorigenesis in transgenic mice. *Journal of Clinical Investigation,* Vol.120, No.2, (February 1), pp. 498-507, ISSN 0021-9738

Shinmura, K., Tarapore, P., Tokuyama, Y., George, K.R., & Fukasawa, K. (2005). Characterization of centrosomal association of nucleophosmin/B23 linked to Crm1 activity. *FEBS Letters,* Vol.579, No.29, (December 5), pp. 6621-6634, ISSN 0014-5793

Shinmura, K., Bennett, R.A., Tarapore, P., & Fukasawa, K. (2007). Direct evidence for the role of centrosomally localized p53 in the regulation of centrosome duplication. *Oncogene,* Vol.26, No.20, (May 3), pp. 2939-2944, ISSN 0950-9232

Shinmura, K., Iwaizumi, M., Igarashi, H., et al. (2008). Induction of centrosome amplification and chromosome instability in p53-deficient lung cancer cells exposed to benzo[a]pyrene diol epoxide (B[a]PDE). *Journal of Pathology,* Vol.216, No.3, (November), pp. 365-374, ISSN 0022-3417

Shinmura, K., Tao, H., Nagura, K., et al. (2011). Suppression of hydroxyurea-induced centrosome amplification by NORE1A and down-regulation of NORE1A mRNA expression in non-small cell lung carcinoma. *Lung Cancer,* Vol.71, No.1, (January), pp. 19-27, ISSN 0169-5002

Silkworth, W.T., Nardi, I.K., Scholl, L.M., & Cimini, D. (2009). Multipolar spindle pole coalescence is a major source of kinetochore mis-attachment and chromosome mis-segregation in cancer cells. *PLoS One,* Vol.4, No.8, (August 10), pp. e6564, ISSN 1932-6203

Smiraldo, P.G., Gruver, A.M., Osborn, J.C., & Pittman, D.L. (2005). Extensive chromosomal instability in Rad51d-deficient mouse cells. *Cancer Research,* Vol.65, No.6, (March 15), pp. 2089-2096, ISSN 0008-5472

Tarapore, P., Horn, H.F., Tokuyama, Y., & Fukasawa, K. (2001a). Direct regulation of the centrosome duplication cycle by the p53-p21Waf1/Cip1 pathway. *Oncogene,* Vol.20, No.25, (May 31), pp. 3173-3184, ISSN 0950-9232

Tarapore, P., Tokuyama, Y., Horn, H.F., & Fukasawa, K. (2001b). Difference in the centrosome duplication regulatory activity among p53 'hot spot' mutants: potential role of Ser 315 phosphorylation-dependent centrosome binding of p53. *Oncogene,* Vol.20, No.47, (October 18), pp. 6851-6863, ISSN 0950-9232

Teixidó-Travesa, N., Villén, J., Lacasa, C., et al. (2010). The gammaTuRC revisited: a comparative analysis of interphase and mitotic human gammaTuRC redefines the set of core components and identifies the novel subunit GCP8. *Molecular Biology of the Cell,* Vol.21, No.22, (November 15), pp. 3963-3972, ISSN 1059-1524

Thompson, S.L. & Compton, D.A. (2008). Examining the link between chromosomal instability and aneuploidy in human cells. *Journal of Cell Biology,* Vol.180, No.4, (February 25), pp. 665-672, ISSN 0021-9525

Thompson, S.L., Bakhoum, S.F., & Compton, D.A. (2010). Mechanisms of chromosomal instability. *Current Biology,* Vol.20, No.6, (March 23), pp. R285-R295, ISSN 0960-9822

Tokuyama, Y., Horn, H.F., Kawamura, K., Tarapore, P., & Fukasawa, K. (2001). Specific phosphorylation of nucleophosmin on Thr(199) by cyclin-dependent kinase 2-cyclin E and its role in centrosome duplication. *Journal of Biological Chemistry,* Vol.276, No.24, (June 15), pp. 21529-21537, ISSN 0021-9258

Tritarelli, A., Oricchio, E., Ciciarello, M., et al. (2004). p53 localization at centrosomes during mitosis and postmitotic checkpoint are ATM-dependent and require serine 15 phosphorylation. *Molecular Biology of the Cell,* Vol.15, No.8, (August), pp. 3751-3757, ISSN 1059-1524

Turner, J.G. & Sullivan, D.M. (2008). CRM1-mediated nuclear export of proteins and drug resistance in cancer. *Current Medicinal Chemistry,* Vol.15, No.26, pp. 2648-2655, ISSN 0929-8673

Tutt, A., Gabriel, A., Bertwistle, D., et al. (1999). Absence of Brca2 causes genome instability by chromosome breakage and loss associated with centrosome amplification. *Current Biology,* Vol.9, No.19, (October 7), pp. 1107-1110, ISSN 0960-9822

Venkitaraman, A.R. (2002). Cancer susceptibility and the functions of BRCA1 and BRCA2. *Cell,* Vol.108, No.2, (January 25), pp. 171-182, ISSN 0092-8674

Vorobjev, I.A. & Nadezhdina, E.S. (1987). The centrosome and its role in the organization of microtubules. *International Review of Cytology-A Survey of Cell Biology,* Vol.106, pp. 227-293, ISSN 0074-7696

Wadhwa, R., Takano, S., Kaur, K., et al. (2006). Upregulation of mortalin/mthsp70/Grp75 contributes to human carcinogenesis. *International Journal of Cancer,* Vol.118, No.12, (June 15), pp. 2973-2980, ISSN 0020-7136

Wang, W., Budhu, A., Forgues, M., & Wang, X.W. (2005). Temporal and spatial control of nucleophosmin by the Ran-Crm1 complex in centrosome duplication. *Nature Cell Biology,* Vol.7, No.8, (August), pp. 823-830, ISSN 1465-7392

Weaver, B.A., Silk, A.D., Montagna, C., Verdier-Pinard, P., & Cleveland, D.W. (2007). Aneuploidy acts both oncogenically and as a tumor suppressor. *Cancer Cell,* Vol.11, No.1, (January), pp. 25-36, ISSN 1535-6108

Weaver, B.A. & Cleveland, D.W. (2008). The aneuploidy paradox in cell growth and tumorigenesis. Cancer Cell, Vol.14, No.6, (December 9), pp. 431-433, ISSN 1535-6108

Xu, X., Weaver, Z., Linke, S.P., et al. (1999). Centrosome amplification and a defective G2-M cell cycle checkpoint induce genetic instability in BRCA1 exon 11 isoform-deficient cells. *Molecular Cell,* Vol.3, No.3, (March), pp. 389-395, ISSN 1097-2765

Zhang, X., Chen, Q., Feng, J., et al. (2009). Sequential phosphorylation of Nedd1 by Cdk1 and Plk1 is required for targeting of the gammaTuRC to the centrosome. *Journal of Cell Science,* Vol.122, No.13, (July 1), pp. 2240-2251, ISSN 0021-9533

Zhou, H., Kuang, J., Zhong, L., et al. (1998). Tumour amplified kinase STK15/BTAK induces centrosome amplification, aneuploidy and transformation. *Nature Genetics,* Vol.20, No.2, (October), pp. 189-193, ISSN 1061-4036

Zyss, D. & Gergely, F. (2009). Centrosome function in cancer: guilty or innocent? *Trends in Cell Biology,* Vol.19, No.7, (July), pp. 334-346, ISSN 0962-8924

8

Defective Expression and DNA Variants of TGFBR2 in Chinese Small Cell Lung Carcinoma

ZhenHong Zhao[1], Jibin Xu[2], Jun Xie[2], Yang Bao[2,3], Xiaotian Wang[1], Lei Wang[2], Junjie Wu[4], Li Jin[1], Zhiyun Xu[2*] and Jiucun Wang[1,*]
[1]MOE Key Laboratory of Contemporary Anthropology and State Key Laboratory of Genetic Engineering, School of Life Sciences, Fudan University, Shanghai,
[2]Department of Cardiac and Thoracic Surgery, Changhai Hospital, Shanghai,
[3]Yangzhou No.1 People's Hospital, Jiangsu Province,
[4]Department of Pneumology, Changhai Hospital, Shanghai,
China

1. Introduction

Lung cancer is one of the most commonly diagnosed malignant tumors, and has the highest death rate of all cancer types. Both the incidence rate and death rate of lung cancer have increased rapidly worldwide during the last 50 years. Lung cancer has now become the leading cause of cancer death in males, and the second most common cause of cancer death in females, after breast cancer. According to data provided by the International Agency for Research on Cancer, about 1.6 million new lung cancer patients were confirmed in 2008, accounting for 13% of the total cancer cases, while about 1.4 million patients died, amounting to 18% of the total deaths caused by cancer worldwide (Jemal et al., 2011).

Lung cancer can be divided according to histological subtype into non-small cell lung cancer (NSCLC) and small cell lung cancer (SCLC), with the latter accounting for about 14% of new lung cancer cases in the USA and Europe in 2004 (Jemal et al., 2004). The clinical and histological features of SCLC were first recognized by Barnard in 1926 as being distinct from those of other types of lung cancer (Barnard, 1926). SCLC cells develop from lung Kulchitsky cells, and SCLC can be further subdivided into three different types: oat-cell type, intermediate-cell type and mixed-cell type (Travis, 1999). Smoking is the key risk factor for SCLC, and more than 95% of patients develop SCLC as a result of tobacco smoking. Smoking more cigarettes and prolonging the duration of smoking can both increase the risk of developing SCLC (Brownson et al., 1992), while stopping smoking reduces its risk, compared to persistent smokers (Khuder and Mutgi, 2001; Jackman and Johnson, 2005). SCLC is very aggressive and the median survival time without treatment is less than 4 months. Chemotherapy and radiotherapy represent the two major treatments for SCLC. According to the standards developed by the Veterans Administration Lung Cancer Study Group, SCLC can be divided into two stages: a limited stage and an extensive stage (Simon, 2003). Cancer cells in limited-stage SCLC are restricted to the ipsilateral hemithorax

* Corresponding Author

and can be treated by both chemotherapy and radiation therapy. About 20% of patients are cured after treatment, and the median survival time is about 18 months. Patients with extensive-stage SCLC have a high response rate to chemotherapy, which is the primary treatment for this disease, but the median survival time is only about 9 months because most patients relapse and the results of salvage therapy are poor (Janne et al., 2002; Demedts et al., 2010).

Transforming growth factor-beta (TGF-β) belongs to a large superfamily of cell cytokines, and is an important component of several cellular metabolic pathways. TGF-β signaling pathways regulate many aspects of cellular function, such as cellular proliferation, differentiation, migration, apoptosis, adhesion, angiogenesis, immune surveillance and survival (Jakowlew, 2006). TGF-β plays a very complex dual role in cancer development, progress and metastasis (Akhurst & Derynck, 2001; Elliott & Blobe, 2005). TGF-β inhibits primary tumor development and growth by inducing cell cycle arrest and apoptosis as a tumor suppressor during the early phase of tumorigenesis (Arteaga, et al. 1993), but also promotes tumor invasion and metastasis by inducing the epithelial-mesenchymal transition in some epithelial cells, indicating that TGF-β can also act as a tumor promoter in the late stage of cancer (Miyazono, 2009).

There are two types of TGF-β signaling pathways; Smad-dependent and Smad-independent pathways. In Smad-dependent TGF-β signaling pathways, autocrine or exogenous TGF-β binds to the TGFBR2 and TGFBR1 membrane receptors. TGFBR2 then phosphorylates TGFBR1, which activates receptor-regulated Smads (also known as R-Smads). The R-Smads usually comprise Smad2 and Smad3. Activated Smad2 and Smad3 form complexes with Smad4, the common-partner Smad (co-Smad) in mammals. The subsequent R-Smad-co-Smad complexes shuttle between the nucleus and cytoplasm, and interact with various transcription factors and transcriptional co-activators such as AP-1, Sp1, p300, and SMIF to regulate the transcription of target genes (Derynck & Zhang, 2003). The phosphorylation of R-Smads can be blocked by inhibitory Smad, which starts the ubiquitination and degradation of the R-Smad-co-Smad complexes, thus inhibiting signal transduction (Itoh & ten Dijke, 2007). This TGF-β signal transduction pathway mainly regulates cell metabolism through this network involving cell cycle capture and apoptosis. In addition to Smad-mediated signaling pathways, TGF-β also activates other pathways, including Erk, JNK and p38 MAPK kinase pathways, via Smad-independent mechanisms (Moustakas & Heldin, 2007).

Both Smad-dependent and -independent TGF-β signaling pathways start by binding TGF-β to its transmembrane receptor TGFBR2, which then activates the downstream signal transduction. However, TGFBR2 expression is often reduced or even blocked in tumor cells (Levy & Hill, 2006). In bladder cancer, deficient TGFBR2 expression leads to loss of the growth inhibition function of TGF-β, and loss of expression of TGFBR2 has been shown to correlate with tumor grade (Tokunaga, et al., 1999). Other studies also found that inactivation of TGFBR2 played a central role in the development and progression of human gastric cancer, and TGFBR2 expression has shown a strong association with the degree of malignancy in gastric cancer (Chang, et al., 1997). The expression of TGFBR2 was also reduced in breast cancer (Gobbi, et al. 2000). Although the reasons for defective TGFBR2 expression are still unknown, loss of or reduced expression of TGFBR2 may be caused by histone deacetylation in lung cancer cell lines (Osada et al., 2001).

TGFBR2 mutations have also been observed in tumor cells. A DNA variant with a frameshift mutation in the poly$(A)_{10}$ repeat, resulting in microsatellite instability (MSI), has been detected in the coding region of the TGFBR2 gene in several types of tumors, including colon cancer, gastric cancer, and gliomas (Markowitz et al. 1995; Pinto et al., 1997; Izumoto et al. 1997). This frameshift could affect gene function and be related to cancer development. This MSI also been detected in both NSCLC and SCLC (Kim et al., 2000; Tani et al., 1997), though the mutation rate seems to be much lower than that of deficient TGFBR2 expression rate in lung cancer. A previous study identified a novel microdeletion (c.492_507del) in giant cell carcinoma (GCC) and large cell carcinoma (LCC) patients, compared to other NSCLC subtypes. This 16-bp microdeletion introduced a premature stop codon at positions 590–592 of the cDNA, resulting in a truncated TGFBR2 protein with a mutated transmembrane domain and loss of a kinase domain. Although the mutated TGFBR2 played an important role in the abrogation of TGF-β signal transduction in LCC cells (Wang et al., 2007), it was not correlated with the reduced TGFBR2 expression seen in NSCLC (Xu et al., 2007).

However, TGFBR2 has rarely been studied in Chinese SCLC samples and its role in TGF-β insensitivity in this population thus remains unknown. The present study therefore examined the levels of TGFBR2 expression in 27 pairs of formalin-fixed, paraffin-embedded SCLC tumors and compared them with NSCLC samples. The entire cDNA region and promoter of the gene was then sequenced to identify the causal variants in the TGFBR2 gene that accounted for its defective expression.

2. Materials and methods

2.1 Specimens

Twenty-seven formalin-fixed, paraffin-embedded SCLC samples and their corresponding normal tissues were collected by the Laboratory of the Department of Thoracic Surgery, Changhai Hospital between 2000 and 2007. All the patients had undergone pulmonary resection for primary SCLC at Changhai Hospital and had provided informed consent, and none had received preoperative radiotherapy or chemotherapy. The demographic and clinical features of these SCLC cases are summarized in Table 1. This research was conducted with the official approval of the academic advisory board of the Institute of Genetics, Fudan University, Shanghai, P. R. China.

An additional 65 formalin-fixed, paraffin-embedded NSCLC samples and their corresponding normal tissues were collected between 2005 and 2007, as a control group to compare with SCLC (Table 2). These tissues were also provided by the Laboratory of the Department of Thoracic Surgery, Changhai Hospital after obtaining the patients' consent. None of these patients had received radiotherapy or chemotherapy prior to surgery.

2.2 Immunohistochemistry

Expression of TGFBR2 was detected by immunohistochemistry assay using a monoclonal antibody against the extracellular domain of TGFBR2 (R & D Systems, Minneapolis, MN) via two-step immunohistochemical staining using the EnVision system (DAKO Cytomation, Denmark), as described in our previous report (26). In brief, after the paraffin sections were deparaffinized and hydrated, serial 4-μm thick sections were placed into 3% hydrogen peroxide solution for 10 min to block endogenous peroxidase activity. For antigen retrieval, the sections were treated with boiling 0.01 mol/L citrate buffer (pH 6.0) for 25 min and then incubated with 10% fetal calf serum for 20 min at room temperature. After the blocking serum was removed, the sections were incubated with the primary antibody (1:50) at room temperature for 1 h, followed by rinsing three times with phosphate-buffered saline (PBS).

Patient No.	Age	Gender	Type	Subtype	TNM	Stage	Smoking Status	Family History	TGFBR2 expression		
							Pack*Year		Normal	Tumor	
S1	32	Male	SCLC	Limited	T2N1MO	II a	No	No	9	9	Pr
S2	65	Male	SCLC	Limited	T2N1MO	II a	720	No	9	9	Pr
S3	46	Female	SCLC	Limited	T2N2MO	IIIa	No	No	9	6	Re
S4	52	Female	SCLC	Limited	T2N1MO	II a	No	No	9	9	Pr
S5	64	Male	SCLC	Limited	T2N1MO	II a	Little	No	9	6	Re
S6	45	Male	SCLC	Extensive	T4N3MO	IIIb	600	No	9	3	Re
S7	46	Male	SCLC	Limited	T2N2MO	IIIa	200	No	9	3	Re
S8	63	Male	SCLC	Limited	T2N1MO	II a	600	No	9	3	Re
S9	47	Male	SCLC	Extensive	T4N2MO	IIIb	600	No	9	9	Pr
S10	69	Male	SCLC	Limited	T1N0M0	I a	600	No	9	6	Re
S11	57	Female	SCLC	Limited	T2N1MO	II a	No	No	9	9	Pr
S12	48	Male	SCLC	Limited	T3N3M0	IIIb	300	No	9	6	Re
S13	57	Male	SCLC	Limited	T3N2M0	IIIa	No	No	9	6	Re
S14	62	Male	SCLC	Limited	T2N1M0	II a	500	No	9	4	Re
S15	46	Male	SCLC	Limited	T2N2MO	IIIa	520	No	9	6	Re
S16	57	Female	SCLC	Limited	T1N2M0	IIIa	600	No	9	6	Re
S17	63	Male	SCLC	Limited	T2N1MO	II a	600	No	9	9	Pr
S18	37	Female	SCLC	Limited	T2N2MO	IIIa	No	No	9	9	Pr
S19	52	Male	SCLC	Extensive	T4N0M1	IV	No	No	9	9	Pr
S20	77	Male	SCLC	Limited	T2N1MO	II a	1200	No	9	3	Re
S21	60	Female	SCLC	Limited	T2NIM0	II a	Unknown	No	9	9	Pr
S22	50	Male	SCLC	Limited	T2N2MO	IIIa	300	No	9	6	Re
S23	55	Male	SCLC	Extensive	T4N0M0	IIIa	600	Yes	9	6	Re
S24	71	Male	SCLC	Limited	T1N0M0	I a	1600	No	9	9	Pr
S25	43	Male	SCLC	Limited	T3N0M0	II b	400	No	9	6	Re
S26	63	Male	SCLC	Limited	T1N2M0	IIIa	No	No	9	0	Re
S27	71	Male	SCLC	Limited	T2N2MO	IIIa	Unknown	No	9	6	Re

Re: reduced TGFBR2 expression in tumor tissues, Loss: loss of TGFBR2 expression, Pr: preserved TGFBR2 expression.
The staining score of each tissue is the product of the proportion of positive staining cells and intensity scores.

Table 1. Clinical features and TGFBR2 expression of the 27 SCLC patients

Type	Total	TGFBR2 expression	
		Pr	Re
AdC	33	21	12
SqC	27	18	9
Ad-SqC	3	2	1
Atypical Carcinoid	1	1	
Low Differentiation Sarcoma	1		1
Grand Total	65	42	23

Re: reduced TGFBR2 expression in tumor tissues, Pr: preserved TGFBR2 expression.

Table 2. Clinical features and TGFBR2 expression in NSCLC samples

The sections were then incubated with a working solution of horseradish peroxidase-labeled goat anti-mouse immunoglobulin, as provided in the EnVision kit, for 30 min. Finally, the peroxidase activity was developed with 3,3-diaminobenzidine tetrahydrochloride and hydrogen peroxide. Because NSCLC develops from bronchial epithelium precursors, human normal bronchial epithelium was used as a positive control. A negative control for each specimen was provided by treating the sections with PBS instead of the primary antibody.

2.3 Interpretation of the staining and data evaluation

All sections were examined by standard light microscopy and scored semi-quantitatively on the basis of the percentage of immunoreactive cells and on the intensity of the staining reaction. The samples were initially classified into one of four grades, according to staining intensity: 0 (negative staining, equivalent to the negative control), 1 (weak staining), 2 (medium staining) and 3 (strong staining). The percentages of positively-stained cells were assigned as 0 for 0–25%, 1 for 26–50%, 2 for 51–75% and 3 for 76–100%, respectively. The final score was determined as the product of the proportion and intensity scores, and ranged from 0–9. Samples were considered to be negatively stained if the final score was 0, and positively stained if the final score was 1–9. Moreover, cancer samples were classified as preserved- or reduced-type in terms of TGFBR2 expression, depending on whether the final score was the same as or less than that of its corresponding normal lung tissue.

2.4 DNA Extraction and mutation analysis

Target cells from formalin-fixed, paraffin-embedded tissue sections were microdissected and scraped into microtubes. After deparaffinization with xylene and washing in ethanol, DNA was extracted by standard proteinase K digestion and phenol-chloroform extraction (Sambrook & Maniatis, 1989).

The presence of the 16-bp microdeletion in exon 4, which was previously detected in LCC and GCC, was examined in all SCLC tissues using the following forward and reverse primers to amplify the fragments of 117/101 bp, representing the wild/mutant alleles: 5'-caccagcaatcctgacttgttg-3' and 5'-cggttaacgcggtagcagtag-3'. The MSI in exon 3 was detected by the STR method using an ABI 3100 Sequencer and the following forward and reverse primers were used to amplify the exon 3 fragment (normally 242 bp) of the TGFBR2 gene: 5′-tccaatgaatctcttcactc-3′ and 5′-cccacacccttaagagaaga-3′. c.1167 C>T in exon 4 of TGFBR2 was detected by direct sequencing using an ABI 3100 Sequencer and the following forward and reverse primers to amplify the exon 4 fragment (242 bp) of the TGFBR2 gene: 5′-

cccaagatgcccatcgtg-3′ and 5′-tcccaggctcaaggtaaagg-3′. The other primers used for promoter and exon sequencing are listed in Table 3.

Fragments	Region	Direction	Sequence (5' - 3')
TGFBR2 promoter	Promoter part1	Forward	aactacaaaacatgtacaccagg
TGFBR2 promoter		Reverse	ttctttaggtcgaagtctagagg
TGFBR2 promoter	Promoter part2	Forward	atgcagaatctctgcctgcctc
TGFBR2 promoter		Reverse	cgagagctttggccgacttt
TGFBR2 promoter	Promoter part3	Forward	gtaaatacttggagcgaggaactc
TGFBR2 promoter		Reverse	ttctgaacgtgcggtgggat
TGFBR2 exon	exon 1	Forward	tcggtctatgacgagcag
TGFBR2 exon		Reverse	gggaccccaggaagaccc
TGFBR2 exon	exon 2	Forward	gggctggtatcaagttcatttg
TGFBR2 exon		Reverse	ggagacagagatacactgactgtg
TGFBR2 exon	exon 3	Forward	tccaatgaatctcttcactc
TGFBR2 exon		Reverse	cccacacccttaagagaaga
TGFBR2 exon	exon 4-1	Forward	ccaactccttctctccttgttttg
TGFBR2 exon		Reverse	tccaagaggcatactcctcatagg
TGFBR2 exon	exon 4-2	Forward	gtcgctttgctgaggtctataagg
TGFBR2 exon		Reverse	ccaggctcaaggtaaaggggatctagca
TGFBR2 exon	exon 5	Forward	ggcagctggaattaaatgatgggc
TGFBR2 exon		Reverse	tgctcgaagcaacacatg
TGFBR2 exon	exon 6	Forward	tttcctttgggctgcacatg
TGFBR2 exon		Reverse	cctaagaggcaacttggttgaatc
TGFBR2 exon	exon 7	Forward	ccaactcatggtgtccctttg
TGFBR2 exon		Reverse	tctttggacatgcccagcctg
TGFBR2 MSI	Exon 3	Forward	Fam-tccaatgaatctcttcactc
TGFBR2 MSI		Reverse	cccacacccttaagagaaga
TGFBR2 LOH	Exon 4	Forward	cccaagatgcccatcgtg
TGFBR2 LOH		Reverse	tcccaggctcaaggtaaagg

Table 3. Primers used in the study

2.5 Statistical analysis

Data were analyzed using χ^2 tests, corrected χ^2 tests, or Fisher's exact tests. A P value of less than 0.05 was considered statistically significant.

3. Results

3.1 TGFBR2 expression was more often reduced in SCLC than in NSCLC

TGFBR2 expression was assessed using immunohistochemistry. Normal human lung tissues and normal human bronchial epithelium were used as positive controls. Over 75% of cells in these tissues exhibited consistently strong staining, both showing staining scores of 3 × 3 = 9, indicating normal TGFBR2 expression (Figure 1). Immunostaining of TGFBR2 was performed in 27 SCLC tumor tissue samples and their corresponding normal tissues. All the normal tissues showed strong staining in over 75% cells with staining scores of 9. One SCLC sample showed negative TGFBR2 expression (score of 0), while the remaining 26 were TGFBR2-positive. Furthermore, 16 of the total 27 SCLC tumor samples showed reduced TGFBR2 expression (score of 1–6) and 10 showed preserved expression (Table 1).

None of the 65 NSCLC samples showed negative TGFBR2 expression (staining score of 0). In addition, only 35.4% (23/65) of all NSCLC tumor tissues showed reduced (score of 1–6) TGFBR2 expression and 64.6% (42/65) of tumors had preserved expression (score of 9) (Table 2). When adenocarcinoma and squamous cell carcinoma tissues were analyzed separately, the frequencies of preserved type were also higher (63.6% (21/33) and 66.7% (18/27) respectively) than those of reduced type (36.4% (12/33) and 33.4% (9/27) respectively). In contrast, the frequency of preserved type in SCLCs (47%, 10/27) was much lower than that of reduced type (63%, 17/27), indicating that reduced TGFBR2 expression was more frequent in SCLC cells (Table 1 & 2).

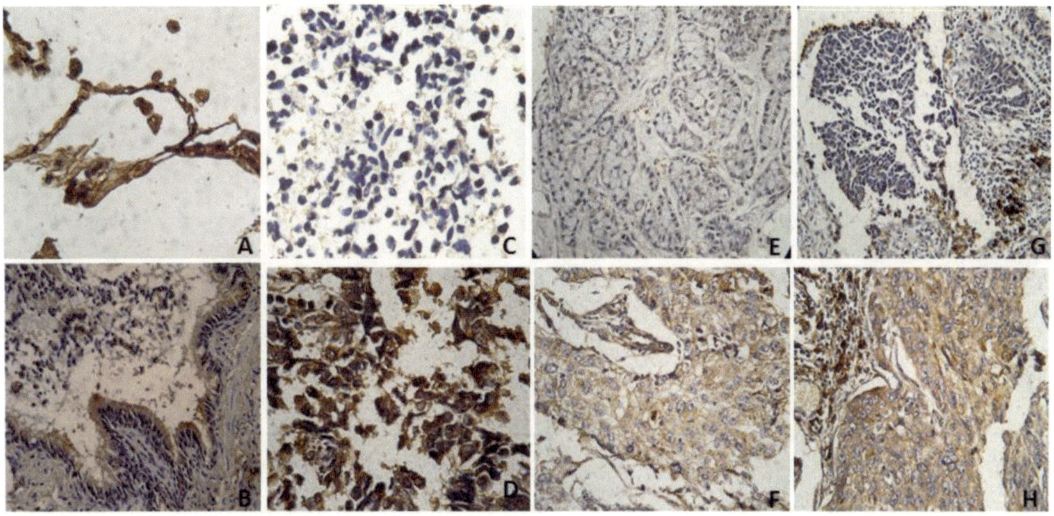

Fig. 1. Expression of TGFBR2 in lung cancer by immunohistochemical analysis (×400).
A. The expression of normal lung epithelium;
B. The expression of normal bronchus epithelium;
C. Reduced expression of SCLC;
D. Preserved expression of SCLC;
E. Reduced expression of AdC;
F. Preserved expression of AdC;
G. Reduced expression of SCC;
H. Preserved expression of SCC.

3.2 No significant relationship was found between TGFBR2 expression and clinical features in SCLC patients

The associations between TGFBR2 expression and other clinical features were analyzed. No significant associations were found between TGFBR2 expression and gender (P = 1.00), age (P = 0.14), tumor size (P = 1.00), nodal involvement (P = 1.00), metastasis (P = 1.00) or stage (P = 0.12) (Table 4).

	Cases	Gender		TGFBR2 expression		Age	P-value
		M	F	Re	Pr		
Age							
≤60	16 (59.26%)	11	5	10	6	32-57	P=1.0000
>60	11 (40.74%)	10	1	7	4	61-77	
Gender							
Male	21 (77.78%)	21	0	15	6		P=0.1358
Female	6 (22.22%)	0	6	2	4		
Tumor Size							
T1	4	3	1	3	1		P=1.0000
T2	16	11	5	14	9	T≥2	
T3	3	3	0				
T4	4	4	0				
Nodal involvement							
N0	5	5	0	3	2		P=1.0000
N1	10	8	2	14	8	N≥1	
N2	10	8	2				
N3	2	2	0				
Metastasis							
M0	26	20	6	16	10		P=1.0000
M1	1	1	0	1	0		
Stage							
I	2	2	0	1	1		P=0.1164
II	11	8	3	5	6		
III	13	10	3	11	2		
IV	1	1	0	0	1		

Table 4. Association between TGFBR2 expression and clinical features of 27 SCLC patients

3.3 TGFBR2 expression is related to tumor types

The relationship between TGFBR2 expression and histological type was analyzed. Samples were categorized as SCLC or NSCLC subtypes because they developed from different lung cells. As shown in Table 5, a significant association between TGFBR2 expression and histological type was identified (P = 0.0151), indicating the existence of a significant difference in TGFBR2 expression levels between SCLC and NSCLC subtypes (Table 5).

For further statistical analysis, NSCLC cases were divided into AdC, SqC, Ad-SqC and other subtypes. Because of the sample sizes, comparisons were only made between SCLC and AdC, and between SCLC and SqC. The results demonstrated significant differences in TGFBR2 expression between SCLC and AdC, and between SCLC and SqC (P = 0.0402 and 0.0293, respectively) (Table 5).

3.4 Mutations in exon 4 of TGFBR2

In a previous study, we identified a microdeletion (c.492_507del) in patients with GCC and LCC. We therefore investigated the occurrence of this microdeletion in SCLC in the present study. Genomic DNA was extracted from 21 pairs of formalin-fixed, paraffin-embedded SCLC tissues and their corresponding normal tissues. The coding and promoter regions of

Item	n	Reduced	Preserved	P-value
(1)				
SCLC	27	17 (63.0%)	10 (37.0%)	0.0151
NSCLC	65	23 (35.4%)	42 (64.6%)	
(2)				
SCLC	27	17 (63.0%)	10 (37.0%)	0.0402
AdC	33	12 (36.4%)	21 (63.6%)	
(3)				
SCLC	27	17 (63.0%)	10 (37.0%)	0.0293
SqC	27	9 (33.3%)	18 (66.7%)	

Table 5. TGFBR2 expression in different subtypes of tumor

TGFBR2 were sequenced. The DNA from the other six pairs of tissues was degraded and was unsuitable for amplification. No microdeletion was observed in any of the tested SCLC samples.

However, another novel variant in exon 4 of TGFBR2 was identified in 11 of 21 SCLC tumor samples. This variant at c.1167 in the TGFBR2 coding region was T/T homozygous in eight out of 11 cases, and C/T heterozygous in the other three cases, compared with C/C homozygous in normal individuals. The corresponding normal samples for these were C/T heterozygous. In the other 10 pairs of samples, however, the site was C/C homozygous. These results suggest that loss of heterozygosity (LOH) occurred in the eight tumors whose alleles became T/T homozygous from C/T heterozygous (Figure 2 and Table 6).

Interestingly, this change was a synonymous mutation that did not alter the amino acid sequence. We investigated its effect on the expression of TGFBR2, and found that TGFBR2 expression was reduced in nearly all T carriers (81.8%), compared with that in normal tissues, while only 60% of CC carriers had reduced TGFBR2 expression (Table 6).

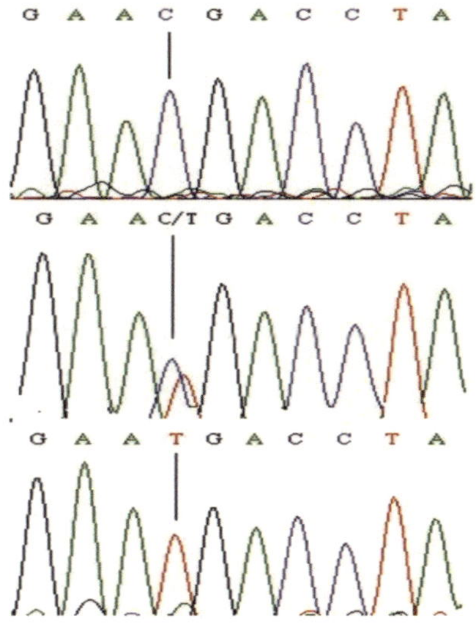

Fig. 2. LOH in SCLC.
A. CC sequence in normal lung tissue from SCLC patients;
B. TC sequence in normal lung tissue from SCLC patients;
C. TT sequence in tumor tissue from SCLC patients.

Patient No.	Tissue	LOH	TGFBR2 expression
S1	+	TT	Pr
	-	CT	
S3	+	CC	Re
	-	CC	
S5	+	CC	Re
	-	CC	
S6	+	TT	Re
	-	CT	
S7	+	CC	Re
	-	CC	
S8	+	TT	Re
	-	CT	
S9	+	CC	Pr
	-	CC	
S11	+	CC	Pr
	-	CC	
S12	+	TT	Re
	-	CT	
S13	+	TT	Re
	-	CT	
S15	+	CT	Re
	-	CT	
S16	+	CC	Re
	-	CC	
S18	+	CC	Pr
	-	CC	
S19	+	TT	Pr
	-	CT	
S20	+	CT	Re
	-	CT	
S21	+	CC	Pr
	-	CC	
S22	+	CT	Re
	-	CT	
S23	+	TT	Re
	-	CT	
S25	+	CC	Re
	-	CC	
S26	+	TT	Re
	-	CT	
S27	+	CC	Re
	-	CC	

+: tumor tissues; -: normal lung tissue of patients;
Re: reduced TGFBR2 expression in tumor tissues, Pr: preserved TGFBR2 expression.

Table 6. Relationship between LOH in exon 4 and TGFBR2 expression

3.5 MSI in TGFBR2 in SCLC

Poly$(A)_{10}/(A)_9$ heterozygosity in exon 3 of TGFBR2, representing MSI, was detected in 60% of SCLC samples (9 out of 15), as shown in Table 7. However, no association between MSI and TGFBR2 expression was found ($P = 0.264$).

Patient No.	Tissue	MSI	TGF-BRII expression
S1	+	poly $(A)_{10}$	Preserved
	-	poly $(A)_{10}$	
S2	+	poly $(A)_{10}$	Preserved
	-	poly $(A)_{10}$	
S3	+	poly $(A)_{10}/(A)_9$	Reduced
	-	poly $(A)_{10}/(A)_9$	
S5	+	poly $(A)_{10}/(A)_9$	Reduced
	-	poly $(A)_{10}/(A)_9$	
S6	+	poly $(A)_{10}/(A)_9$	Reduced
	-	poly $(A)_{10}/(A)_9$	
S9	+	poly $(A)_{10}/(A)_9$	Preserved
	-	poly $(A)_{10}$	
S13	+	poly $(A)_{10}/(A)_9$	Reduced
	-	poly $(A)_{10}$	
S16	+	poly $(A)_{10}/(A)_9$	Reduced
	-	poly $(A)_{10}/(A)_9$	
S19	+	poly $(A)_{10}/(A)_9$	Preserved
	-	poly $(A)_{10}$	
S21	+	poly $(A)_{10}$	Preserved
	-	poly $(A)_{10}$	
S22	+	poly $(A)_{10}$	Reduced
	-	poly $(A)_{10}$	
S23	+	poly $(A)_{10}/(A)_9$	Reduced
	-	poly $(A)_{10}/(A)_9$	
S25	+	poly $(A)_{10}$	Reduced
	-	poly $(A)_{10}$	
S26	+	poly $(A)_{10}/(A)_9$	Reduced
	-	poly $(A)_{10}/(A)_9$	
S28	+	poly $(A)_{10}$	Reduced
	-	poly $(A)_{10}$	
S29	+	poly $(A)_{10}$	Reduced
	-	poly $(A)_{10}$	
S30	+	poly $(A)_{10}$	Reduced
	-	poly $(A)_{10}$	

+: tumor tissues; -: normal lung tissue of patients;
Re: reduced TGFBR2 expression in tumor tissues, Pr: preserved TGFBR2 expression.

Table 7. MSI detection and relation with TGFBR2 expression

4. Discussion

Tumor cells are often able to escape from TGF-β-signaling-induced cell cycle capture and apoptosis. TGF-β has a dual function in tumor development (Akhurst & Derynck, 2001; Elliott & Blobe, 2005); it acts as a tumor suppressor during the initial stages of tumor development (Arteaga, et al. 1993), but promotes tumor progression during the later stages (Miyazono, 2009). High levels of TGF-β expression in tumor cells can induce tumor evolution by stimulating angiogenesis and through other potential immunosuppressive effects, as well as by directly affecting tumor cell invasion and metastasis (Pardali & Moustakas, 2007). These direct effects can be achieved via Smad-dependent pathways, or may be mediated by interference with these pathways (Derynck & Zhang, 2003). Changes in the TGF-β signaling pathway may lead to abnormal signal transduction and cause dysregulated cell growth and differentiation. The first step in any mechanism involves binding of autocrine or paracrine TGF-β to the TGFBR2 receptor on the cell membrane, before activation of various downstream receptors can occur. TGFBR2 thus plays a key role in TGF-β signaling pathways, and its expression is reduced or blocked in many tumors (Chang et al., 1997; Tokunaga et al., 1999; Gobbi et al. 2000;Levy & Hill, 2006), resulting in partial or complete disruption of the TGF-β pathway.

Previous studies demonstrated that TGFBR2 expression in NSCLC differed between LCC and AdC, SqC or non-LCC cases, but the role of defective TGFBR2 expression in the initiation and/or development of SCLC (Xu et al., 2007), and its expression status in SCLC remain largely unknown. Furthermore, SCLC is phenotypically distinct from and much more malignant than NSCLC. We therefore compared TGFBR2 expression between SCLC and NSCLC. Immunohistochemical staining with TGFBR2 antibody revealed significant differences in the incidence of reduced expression in SCLC (63.0% of cases) versus AdC (36.4% of cases, $P = 0.0402$) and SqC (33.3% of cases, $P = 0.0293$), or SCLC versus NSCLC (35% of cases, $P = 0.0151$). These differences in expression levels between SCLC and NSCLC were consistent with the histopathologic classification of these tumors, suggesting that defective TGFBR2 expression might contribute to the initiation and/or development of SCLC.

To determine the reason for the reduced expression of TGFBR2, we examined the mutation status of c.492 507del in exon 4, but found no changes in this sequence in SCLC tumor samples. We subsequently determined the MSI status in exon 3, and identified a DNA variant with a frameshift mutation in the TGFBR2 poly$(A)_{10}$ repeat (which causes MSI) in the coding region of the TGFBR2 gene. A total of 60.0% of SCLC were poly$(A)_{10}/(A)_9$ heterozygous, but no association was found between the MSI and TGFBR2 expression. However, no MSI was identified in our previous study of NSCLC, suggesting that the MSI in SCLC is at least partly associated with its carcinogenesis. We also sequenced all seven exons and the promoter region of the TGFBR2 gene and identified a novel LOH at c.1167 in 38.1% (8/21) of SCLC tissues. Further analysis showed that most of the mutant T-allele carriers (81.8%) had reduced TGFBR2 expression in tumor tissues, compared with only 60% of C-allele carriers. These results suggest that the change from wild type to mutant type might contribute, at least in part, to the defective expression of TGFBR2 in SCLC patients, though further studies are needed to clarify the mechanisms responsible.

5. Conclusion

The present study identified reduced TGFBR2 gene expression levels in formalin-fixed, paraffin-embedded sections from most SCLC tumors examined, suggesting that this might contribute to the initiation and/or development of SCLC. Sequencing analysis also indicated that change of the wild-type C-allele to the mutant T-allele at c.1167 might contribute to the defective expression of TGFBR2 in SCLC patients. Another DNA variant with a frameshift mutation in the TGFBR2 poly$(A)_{10}$ repeat, leading to MSI, was found in the coding region of the TGFBR2 gene, but this was not associated with TGFBR2 expression.

These results suggest that defective expression of TGFBR2 might inactivate TGF-β signal transduction, leading to the loss of growth inhibition and acceleration of tumor formation, and that a C>T substitution at c.1167 might be partially responsible for this reduced expression of TGFBR2 in SCLC.

6. Acknowledgement

This study was supported by grants from the National Science Foundation of China, grant number 30971594 to JC Wang and grant number 30890034 to L Jin.

7. References

Akhurst RJ, Derynck R: TGF-beta signaling in cancer--a double-edged sword.Trends Cell Biol 2001, 11:S44-51.

Arteaga, C.L., et al., Anti-transforming growth-factor (TGF)-beta antibodies inhibit breast-cancer cell tumorigenecity and increase mouse spleen mature-killer-cell activity-implications for a possible role of tumor-cell host TGF-beta interactions in human breast-cancer progression. Journal of Clinical Investigation, 1993. 92(6): p. 2569-2576.

Barnard, W.G., The nature of the "oat-celled sarcoma" of the mediastinum. Journal of Pathology and Bacteriology, 1926. 29(3): p. 241-244.

Brownson, R.C., J.C. Chang, and J.R. Davis, Gender and Histologic type variations in smoking-related risk of lung-cancer. Epidemiology, 1992. 3(1): p. 61-64.

Chang, J., et al., Expression of transforming growth factor beta type II receptor reduces tumorigenicity in human gastric cancer cells. Cancer Research, 1997. 57(14): p. 2856-2859.

deJonge, R.R., et al., Frequent inactivation of the transforming growth factor beta type II receptor in small-cell lung carcinoma cells. Oncology Research, 1997. 9(2): p. 89-98.

Demedts, I.K., K.Y. Vermaelen, and J.P. van Meerbeeck, Treatment of extensive-stage small cell lung carcinoma: current status and future prospects. European Respiratory Journal, 2010. 35(1): p. 202-215.

Derynck, R. and Y.E. Zhang, Smad-dependent and Smad-independent pathways in TGF-beta family signalling. Nature, 2003. 425(6958): p. 577-584.

Elliott, R.L. and G.C. Blobe, Role of transforming growth factor beta in human cancer. Journal of Clinical Oncology, 2005. 23(9): p. 2078-2093.

Gobbi, H., et al., Loss of expression of transforming growth factor beta type II receptor correlates with high tumour grade in human breast in-situ and invasive carcinomas. Histopathology, 2000. 36(2): p. 168-177.

Itoh S, ten Dijke P. Negative regulation of TGF-β receptor/Smad signal transduction, Curr Opin Cell Biol, 2007, 19(2):176-184

Izumoto, S., et al., Microsatellite instability and mutated type II transforming growth factor-beta receptor gene in gliomas. Cancer Letters, 1997. 112(2): p. 251-256.

Jackman, D.M. and B.E. Johnson, Small-cell lung cancer. Lancet, 2005. 366(9494): p. 1385-1396.

Jakowlew, S.B., Transforming growth factor-beta in cancer and metastasis. Cancer and Metastasis Reviews, 2006. 25(3): p. 435-457.

Janne, P.A., et al., Twenty-five years of clinical research for patients with limited-stage small cell lung carcinoma in North America - Meaningful improvements in survival. Cancer, 2002. 95(7): p. 1528-1538.

Jemal, A., et al., Cancer statistics, 2004. Ca-a Cancer Journal for Clinicians, 2004. 54(1): p. 8-29.

Jemal, A., et al., Global Cancer Statistics. Ca-a Cancer Journal for Clinicians, 2011. 61(2): p. 69-90.

Khuder, S.A. and A.B. Mutgi, Effect of smoking cessation on major histologic types of lung cancer. Chest, 2001. 120(5): p. 1577-1583.

Kim, W.S., et al., Microsatellite instability(MSI) in non-small cell lung cancer(NSCLC) is highly associated with transforming growth factor-beta type II receptor(TGF-beta RII) frameshift mutation. Anticancer Research, 2000. 20(3A): p. 1499-1502.

Kim, W.S., et al., Reduced transforming growth factor-beta type II receptor (TGF-beta RII) expression in adenocarcinoma of the lung. Anticancer Research, 1999. 19(1A): p. 301-306.

Levy, L. and C.S. Hill, Alterations in components of the TGF-beta superfamily signaling pathways in human cancer. Cytokine & Growth Factor Reviews, 2006. 17(1-2): p. 41-58.

Markowitz, S., et al., Inactivation of the type-II TGF-beta receptor in colon-cancer cells with microsatellite instability. Science, 1995. 268(5215): p. 1336-1338.

Miyazono, K., Transforming growth factor-beta signaling in epithelial-mesenchymal transition and progression of cancer. Proceedings of the Japan Academy Series B-Physical and Biological Sciences, 2009. 85(8): p. 314-323.

Moustakas, A. and C.-H. Heldin, Signaling networks guiding epithelial-mesenchymal transitions during embryogenesis and cancer progression. Cancer Science, 2007. 98(10): p. 1512-1520.

Nagatake, M., et al., Somatic in vivo alterations of the DPC4 gene at 18q21 in human lung cancers. Cancer Research, 1996. 56(12): p. 2718-2720.

Osada, H., et al., Heterogeneous transforming growth factor (TGF)-beta unresponsiveness and loss of TGF-beta receptor type II expression caused by histone deacetylation in lung cancer cell lines. Cancer Research, 2001. 61(22): p. 8331-8339.

Pardali K, Moustakas A: Actions of TGF-beta as tumor suppressor and pro-metastatic factor in human cancer. Biochim Biophys Acta 2007, 1775:21-62.

Pinto, M., et al., Promoter methylation of TGF beta receptor I and mutation of TGF beta receptor II are frequent events in MSI sporadic gastric carcinomas. Journal of Pathology, 2003. 200(1): p. 32-38.

Sambrook J, F.E., Maniatis T., Molecular cloning: A laboratory manual 2nd ed. Molecular cloning: A laboratory manual. 1989, New York: Cold Spring Harbor Laboratory.

Simon, G.R. and H. Wagner, Small cell lung cancer. Chest, 2003. 123(1): p. 259S-271S.

Tani, M., et al., Infrequent mutations of the transforming growth factor beta-type II receptor gene at chromosome 3p22 in human lung cancers with chromosome 3p deletions. Carcinogenesis, 1997. 18(5): p. 1119-1121.

Tokunaga, H., et al., Decreased expression of transforming growth factor beta receptor type I is associated with poor prognosis in bladder transitional cell carcinoma patients. Clinical Cancer Research, 1999. 5(9): p. 2520-2525.

Travis WD, C.T., Corrin B, Shimosato Y, Brambilla E. Epithelial tumours. In: Travis WD, CV, Corrin B, et al., Histological typing of lung and pleural tumours, 3rd edn. Washington DC: Armed Forces Institute of Pathology. 1999, Washington DC: Armed Forces Institute of Pathology. 25-47.

Uchida, K., et al., Somatic in vivo alterations of the JV18-1 gene at 18q21 in human lung cancers. Cancer Research, 1996. 56(24): p. 5583-5585.

Wang, J.-C., et al., Novel microdeletion in the transforming growth factor beta Type II receptor gene is associated with giant and large cell variants of nonsmall cell lung carcinoma. Genes Chromosomes & Cancer, 2007. 46(2): p. 192-201.

Xu, J. B., et al., Defective expression of transforming growth factor P type II receptor (TGFBR2) in the large cell variant of non-small cell lung carcinoma. Lung Cancer, 2007. 58(1): p. 36-43.

9

Neuroendocrine Tumours of the Lung

Guadalupe Aparicio Gallego[1], Vanessa Medina Villaamil[1], Ana Capdevila Puerta[2], Enrique Grande Pulido[3] and L.M. Antón Aparicio[4,5]
[1]*Biomedical Research Institute, A Coruña University Hospital, A Coruña,*
[2]*Anatomic Pathology Service, A Coruña University Hospital, A Coruña,*
[3]*Medical Oncology Service, Ramon y Cajal University Hospital, Madrid,*
[4]*Medical Oncology Service, A Coruña University Hospital, A Coruña*
[5]*Medicine Department, University of A Coruña, A Coruña*
Spain

1. Introduction

Lung cancer arises from neoplastic changes of the epithelial cells in the lung. However, it is not known whether all or only a subset of these lung epithelial cells is susceptible to malignant transformation. Specifically, a major question is whether the changes need to take place in lung epithelial cells involving stem-cell–like properties. Lung cancer is a clinically, biologically, histologically, molecularly, and genetically heterogeneous disease. The underlying causes of this heterogeneity are unknown and could reflect changes occurring in cells with various potential for differentiation or represent different molecular changes occurring in the same lung epithelial target cells. Transformation from a normal to malignant lung cancer phenotype is thought to arise in a multistep fashion, through a series of genetic versus epigenetic alterations, ultimately evolving into an invasive cancer by clonal expansion. These progressive pathological changes in the bronchial epithelium occur primarily as one of three distinct morphological forms: squamous dysplasia, atypical adenomatous hyperplasia, and diffuse idiopathic pulmonary neuroendocrine cell hyperplasia. Bronchial squamous dysplasia and carcinoma in situ (CIS) are the recognised preneoplastic lesions for squamous cell carcinoma (SCC); atypical adenomatous hyperplasia (AAH), a putative preneoplastic lesion, for a subset of adenocarcinomas (ADC); and diffuse idiopathic pulmonary neuroendocrine cell hyperplasia (DIPNECH) for neuroendocrine lung carcinomas. Pulmonary neuroendocrine tumours comprise approximately 2% of all lung malignancies. According to the most recent World Health Organization classification, pulmonary neuroendocrine tumours are histologically divided into a three-tier, four-category system including low-grade (typical carcinoid), intermediate-grade (atypical carcinoid), and high-grade (small cell carcinoma and large cell neuroendocrine carcinoma) tumours. Nearly all lung cancers exhibit the morphological and molecular features of epithelial cells and are accordingly classified as carcinomas. The cells of origin of virtually all lung cancers reside in the epithelial lining of the airways. As more is learned about the origin of neuroendocrine lung tumours, it is also increasingly clear that the biology of neuroendocrine lung tumours arising in the central airways (i.e., SCLC) is distinct from that of peripheral airway lesions. The purpose of this chapter is not so much to recapitulate the details of the neuroendocrine lung tumour classification but rather to provide an understanding of the main categories of lung carcinoma, to highlight potential pitfalls in the histopathological diagnosis of lung cancer, to summarise current information on molecular properties and cellular origins of individual neuroendocrine lung tumour subtypes, and to relate pathologies to biological behaviours.

2. Neuroendocrine system of the lung

The endocrine cells within the gut epithelium (foregut, midgut, and hindgut) constitute the largest population of hormone producing cells in the body. So far, approximately 10 different neuroendocrine lineages have been identified, and most of them show a specific rostro-caudal distribution. Pulmonary neuroendocrine cells (PNECs) are part of the diffuse neuroendocrine system (DNES) distributed throughout the body. The PNEC system (solitary PNECs and neuroepithelial bodies, or NEBs) consists of a distinct population of airway epithelial cells displaying endocrine and paracrine secretory mechanisms. Pulmonary neuroendocrine cells were readily demonstrated and uniformly distributed in normal adult human lungs. Overall, as identified by neurone specific enolase immunoreactivity, there were 10.5 neuroendocrine cells per 10 cm of epithelial length and 4 per 10,000 epithelial cells; they extended from the trachea to the alveolar ducts but none was seen in the alveoli (72% were in bronchi, 24% in bronchioles, and 4% in alveolar ducts). Of the cells identified by gastrin-releasing peptide immunoreactivity, there were 6.9 neuroendocrine cells per 10 cm of epithelial length and 2.4 per 10,000 epithelial cells. Of the cells identified by calcitonin immunoreactivity, there were 3.5 neuroendocrine cells per 10 cm of epithelial length and 1.3 per 10,000 epithelial cells. Minor cells contained serotonin (all in the terminal bronchioles), and in a small minority no peptide or amine was detected. It is currently thought that PNECs, like their counterparts in the gastrointestinal tract, are derived from multipotent epithelial progenitors, and that all epithelial cells arise from a single stem cell. All pulmonary epithelial cells including PNECs and non-NE airway epithelial cells are likely to be derived from a single stem cell. Epithelial lung stem cells, as in many organs, are often confined to discretely localised niches that are protected from environmental insults. In the lung, PNECs are associated with the stem cell niches in both the proximal and distal airways. One of the lung stem-cell niches is located in the trachea that reveals two stem-cell niches: gland ducts in the proximal compartment and select foci near the cartilage-intercartilage junction in the distal trachea. Other intrapulmonary stem cell niches include NEBs located at the airway bifurcation. Another stem cell niche is at the bronchoalveolar junctions, although PNECs may play a diminished role at this location. Among many functions assigned to them, there is a possible dual role: the regulation of lung maturation/growth and chemoreception. First, during the early stages of lung organogenesis, PNECs acting via their amine and peptide products may function as local modulators of lung growth and differentiation. Second, later in foetal life and in postnatal stages, PNECs and in particular innervated NEBs could play a role as airway chemoreceptors. The diffuse neuroendocrine system (DNES) of the lung involves neuroendocrine cells that have been shown to express a functional oxygen sensing mechanism. Aggregates of neuroendocrine cells, called neuroepithelial bodies (NEBs), are diffusely spread in the epithelium at all levels of the intrapulmonary airways, preferentially located at the airway bifurcation of the lungs. Neuroendocrine cells are selectively contacted by different nerve fibres. NEBs are contacted by at least three different nerve-fibre populations: vagal sensory calbidin D28k, calcitonin gene related peptide (CGRP)/substance P (SP) innervation, and intrinsic pulmonary nitrergic neurons.

2.1 Neuroendocrine epithelial cells

Neuroendocrine epithelial cells (NEC) of the respiratory system tend to occur either as single cells that are sparsely distributed throughout the epithelium of the tracheobronchial tract or in small, well-defined clusters that are supported by nonciliated bronchiolar (Clara) cells. The latter are referred to as neuroepithelial bodies (NEBs) and are located only in the epithelium of the intrapulmonary airways, often at or near a bronchiolar bifurcation. The solitary pulmonary NEC cells of most of the investigated species are fusiform or flask-shaped, resting on the basement membrane with an apical process pointing toward the airway lumen. Adult human NEC cells generally lack luminal contact. Although there are some differences between solitary NEC cells and NEBs, a large body of evidence points to their being a member of the amine precursor uptake and decarboxylation (APUD) cell series or of the paraneuron family. The endocrine system of the lung consists of at least two different cell categories. These categories exhibit similar main characteristics. They contain a biogenic amine and neuropeptide mediators, and their cytoplasm harbours neurosecretory-like granules. Regarding morphological features and location, these cells presumably have a receptor secretory function. Consequently, these classes of endocrine cells can be designated as paraneurons. Solitary NEC cells were found to be distributed over almost the entire respiratory system, while NEBs seemed to be restricted to the epithelium of the intrapulmonary airways. Neuroepithelial bodies generally consist of nonciliated, cylindrical cells with a palisade-like arrangement between the airway surface and the underlying connective tissue, although they may also appear as stratified cells. Most of the luminal side of the NEBs is covered by the supporting Clara cells. The NEBs are strategically located on the surface of the airway bifurcations. They, in fact, contain the serotonin-bioactive amine and neuropeptides, leading to the speculation of these cells as a homogeneous or heterogeneous class. They also exert control on pulmonary vessels and airway tone. The NEC cell may function as the transducer of the stimulus or the sensory nerve ending, the activity of the latter being modulated by the release of bioactive substances from NEC cells. Investigations have indicated the influence of NEC cells on epithelial cell differentiation, mucous secretion, and proliferation of local endoderm in developing airways.

2.2 Pulmonary neuroendocrine cells

Pulmonary neuroendocrine cells (PNECs) are commonly organised into innervated clusters, called NEBs, which have been proposed to serve various functions, including the regulation of embryonic lung growth and maturation through the elaboration of a variety of potent neuropeptides. Several studies have suggested that PNECs are quiescent cells with limited self-renewal capacity. However, it was recently demonstrated that PNECs have a self-renewal capacity and can be activated to undergo multiple rounds of proliferation after TA (Clara) cell depletion. It has been suggested that PNEC-derived paracrine factors might play a role in the regulation of epithelial cell differentiation and proliferation during foetal lung development and possibly in the normal or injured adult lung. Cell proliferation has also been shown to contribute to the maintenance of PNE cells in the normal lung as well as in hyperplasia of this population in various disease states. PNE cells are known to act as a progenitor cell for the establishment of NEB hyperplasia and represent one of two proliferative populations within hyperplastic NEBs of the naphthalene-injured lung. Participation of non-PNE progenitor cells in this process has also been demonstrated and may contribute to the intermediate phase of NEB hyperplasia. These data suggest that multiple cell types contribute to the maintenance and expansion of the NEB-associated PNE population and that progenitor selection may be a dynamic feature of NEB hyperplasia. Findings from various studies have established PNE cells as a progenitor population that is sufficient for the development of both NEB hypertrophy and hyperplasia. Although NEB dysplasia is correlated with preneoplastic conditions and PNE cells are thought to serve as a precursor for the development of small cell lung carcinoma, mechanisms regulating the expansion of the PNE cell population are not well understood. Based on studies performed in animal models, it has been suggested that NEB-associated progenitor cells that are phenotypically distinct from PNE cells contribute to PNE cell hyperplasia. However, when considering mechanisms that may account for PNE cell hyperplasia, the finding that multiple cell types proliferate in the NEB microenvironment raises the possibility that a non-PNE cell progenitor may yield progeny cells with the capacity to undergo PNE cell differentiation.

2.3 Neuroepithelial bodies

Neuroendocrine bodies were illustrated in 1949 in the description of neuroendocrine cells in the bronchiolar mucosa. Neuroendocrine bodies consist of a cluster of 4 to 10 neuroendocrine cells. On well-oriented sections, they can extend from the subepithelial basement membrane to the airway lumens. They are found not only in the epithelium of bronchi and bronchioles, but also in alveoli. The neuroepithelial body (NEB) is a highly dynamic structure that responds to chronic airway injury through hyperplasia of the associated PNEC. NEB-associated epithelial cells share many morphological and biochemical characteristics with cells that are distributed throughout the airway. Pulmonary NEBs are prime candidates to serve as sensory end organs in the lung. NEBs consist of highly organised clusters of specialised cells with neuroendocrine characteristics, arranged into organoids that are dispersed throughout the epithelium at all levels of the intrapulmonary airways. Structurally, NEB cells harbour cytoplasmic neurosecretory granules that are known to contain monoamine, peptide, and purine transmitters. Neuroendocrine cells are able to synthesise and release ATP, monoamine, and peptide transmitters, resulting in autocrine, paracrine, or endocrine effects. Morphologically, NEBs resemble other known chemoreceptors, such as taste buds and carotid bodies, and are thought to represent "chemosensors" among other possible functions. Hypoxic conditions appear to depolarise NEB cells via a potassium channel-mediated mechanism. In particular, the extensively innervated aggregates of the neuroendocrine cells, called neuroepithelial bodies (NEBs), are diffusely spread in the epithelium at all levels of the intrapulmonary airways but are preferentially located at the airway bifurcation points in the lungs. Proportionally, most NEBs are found in the bronchioles and in the terminal respiratory bronchioles. The NEB microenvironment may represent an analogous structure within the conducting airway epithelium for maintenance of an airway stem-cell pool. It may influence the phenotype of the CE cells, blocking the differentiation from Clara to ciliated cells and preserving a population of regenerative cells that can contribute to epithelial renewal after exposure to Clara cell toxicants. Regeneration of the chronically injured airway epithelium is associated with alterations in the number and cellularity of the NEBs as well as the enrichment of nascent epithelial cell populations of epithelial cells that are candidate stem cells. The NEB microenvironment is multifunctional, serving to maintain slow-cycling epithelial cells in the steady state epithelium and to stimulate the proliferation of TA cells either after airway injury or during airway development. Many studies have presented extensive evidence that NEBs in the lungs may be selectively contacted by at least 5 distinct nerve-fibre populations that are both sensory and motor in nature. In addition, they have different origins, indicating that NEBs should be regarded as very complex airway receptors that may be capable of accommodating various chemo- and mechano-sensory modalities.

2.3.1 Functions

It has been estimated that NEBs represent <1% of the epithelial cells in human lungs.
Some of the supposed functions of NEB in mammalian lungs include the following: 1) the ability of NEB to function as transducers (hypoxia); 2) modulation of bronchomotor tone via targeting bronchial smooth muscle and the associated nerves located directly beneath NEB; 3) promotion and regulation of the growth of developing airways by stimulating the proliferation of local endoderm; 4) release of amine and peptide modulators; and 5) neonatal respiratory adaptation. The lung bud epithelium grows into the adjacent mesenchyme and stars branching to form the future bronchial tree. The various stages are divided into the embryonic, pseudoglandular, canalicular, saccullar and alveolar/microvascular periods. Pulmonary neuroendocrine cells are the first specialised epithelial cell type to appear in lung development. In humans, ultrastructurally distinct primitive PNECs (pre-NE cells), which contain serotonin and neuro-specific enolase (NSE), can be detected in the beginning of the pseudoglandular period. Solitary and clustered PNECs contain bombesin, the major neuropeptide in human lungs, which appears in the early weeks of gestation. As the distal segments of the developing airways elongate, a process referred to as the canalicular period, PNECs differentiate first, followed by ciliated and secretory (Clara) cells. Parallel with the increasing number of peripheral airways, the number of PNECs also increases. In the developing bronchioles, small NEBs composed of 3-5 bombesin and serotonin-immunoreactive cells appear at the airway branching points, and rare nerve endings have been demonstrated to be in contact with NEBs already in the human foetal lung. Proposed roles for PNECs in foetal and newborn lung development include the regulation of branching morphogenesis as well as cellular growth and maturation.

2.3.2 Airway oxygen sensors

Since 1930, evidence has accumulated to suggest that NEBs may function as hypoxia-sensitive airway sensors. NEB cells express membrane-bound O_2 sensors and are the transducers of the hypoxic stimulus. NEB cells respond to acute hypoxia, but apparently not to hypercapnia with the degranulation of dense core vesicles and release of 5-hydroxytryptamine (5-HT). Morphologic and experimental studies to support NEB functions as hypoxia-sensitive airway chemoreceptors modulated by the central nervous system include the following: a) preferential location of NEB at airway branching points; b) apical microvilli in contact with the airway lumen; c) cytoplasmic neurosecretory granules containing monoamine and neuropeptides; d) afferent sensory innervation derived from the vagus nerve; and e) proximity to blood capillaries. NEBs are predominantly innervated by sensory nerve fibres derived from cell bodies in the nodose ganglion of the vagus nerve.

Morphological data support the role of NEBs as hypoxia-sensitive airway sensor systems. Studies on the effects of chronic hypoxia have shown induced cellular hyperplasia and hypertrophy in the peripheral chemoreceptors; chronic normobaric hypoxia showed a significant increase in the number of solitary pulmonary neuroendocrine cells (PNECs) as well as the enlargement of NEBs. NEB cells possess an oxygen-binding protein, cytochrome *b*, an NADPH oxidase located in the cellular membranes that acts as the O_2 receptor both during normoxia and hypoxia.

3. Pathology of neuroendocrine tumours of the lung

The neuroendocrine cell system is divided into cell types that form glands and diffusely distributed cells. This second group is collectively known as the diffuse neuroendocrine system (DNES), and its representatives are found in the lung, gastrointestinal tract, or urogenital tract. Neuroendocrine tumours of the lung arise from bronchial mucosal cells known as Kulchitsky cells, which are part of the DNES. The classification of lung neuroendocrine malignancies has been an evolving process (Table 1).

WHO/IASLC histological classification
Preinvasive Lesions
Diffuse idiopathic pulmonary neuroendocrine cell hyperplasia (DIPNECH)
Large Cells carcinoma (Variants)
Large cell neuroendocrine carcinoma (LCNEC)
Combined large cell neuroendocrine carcinoma (C-LCNEC)
Carcinoid tumour
Typical carcinoid (TC)
Atypical carcinoid (AC)
Small cell carcinoma
Combined small cell carcinoma
Non-small Cell Lung Carcinoma with Neuroendocrine Differentiation (NSCLC-NED)

WHO: World Health Organization; IASLC: International Association for the Study of Lung Cancer
*From Travis WD, Colby TV, Corrin B, et al in collaboration with pathologists from 14 countries. Histological typing of lung and pleural tumors. 3rd ed. Berlin: Springer Verlag, 1999, with permission.

Table 1. Lung tumours with neuroendocrine morphology include the low-grade typical carcinoid (TC), intermediate-grade atypical carcinoid (AC), and the high-grade LCNEC and SCLC.

These classifications date back to 1972, when atypical carcinoids were initially defined according to histological criteria, including the number of mitoses per high-power field (hpf), the presence of necrosis, increased cellularity with disorganisation, nuclear pleomorphism, hyperchromatism, and an abnormal nuclear to cytoplasmic ratio (Table 2).
In 1991, a new classification proposed 4 categories of neuroendocrine lung tumours that included the following: typical carcinoid (TC), which is a low-grade malignancy; atypical carcinoid (AC), which is a medium-grade malignancy; large-cell neuroendocrine carcinoma (LCNEC), which is a high-grade malignancy; and small-cell lung cancer (SCLC), which is also a high-grade malignancy. The 2004 WHO categorisation of tumours with neuroendocrine features included the classic carcinoid low-grade TC and intermediate-grade AC, as well as the high-grade malignancies LCNEC and SCLC.

Tumor	Mitoses	Nuclear chromatin	N/C ratio	Nucleoli	Necrosis	Shape
TC	<2/10 HPF	Finely granular	Moderate	Occasional	None	Round, oval
AC	2-10/10 HPF	Finely granular, occasional atypia	Moderate	Common	+(focal)	Round,oval
SCLC	≥11/10 HPF Median 80/10	Finely granular	High	Absent or inconspicuous	+(large zones)	Round, oval,spindle
LCNEC	>11/10 HPF Median 70/10	Vesicular or coarsely granular	Low	Very common	+(large zones)	Round, oval polygonal

N/C: nuclear/cytoplasmic; HPF: high power fields; LCNEC: large cell neuroendocrine carcinoma; SCLC: small cell lung carcinoma

Table 2. Histopathological Classification of Neuroendocrine Tumours of Lung

3.1 Tumourlets

Carcinoid tumours that grow in the peripheral lung and are smaller than 5 mm are referred to as tumourlets. By definition, tumourlets are comprised of increased numbers of individual cells, small group cells, or nodular aggregates of cells that are confined to the bronchial/bronchiolar epithelium (with larger lesions bulging into the lumen but not breaking the subepithelial basement membrane).

3.2 Diffuse Idiopathic Pulmonary Neuroendocrine Cell Hyperplasia

Diffuse idiopathic pulmonary neuroendocrine cell hyperplasia (DIPNECH) is a rare condition in which neuroendocrine cells proliferate throughout the peripheral airways in the form of neuroendocrine cell hyperplasia, tumourlets, and sometimes carcinoid tumours. In DIPNECH, neuroendocrine cell hyperplasia and tumourlets are thought to be a primary proliferation in contrast to the much more common situation where these lesions are seen as a reactive secondary lesion in the setting of airway inflammation and/or fibrosis. This condition is regarded as a precursor to carcinoid tumours because a subset of these patients experience one or more carcinoid tumours. More aggressive forms of lung carcinoma, including SCLC, have not been associated with DIPNECH.

3.3 Carcinoid tumours

Pulmonary or bronchial carcinoid tumours account for over 25% of all carcinoid tumours and for 1%-2% of all pulmonary neoplasms. Approximately 10%-20% of pulmonary carcinoids are typical carcinoids; the remaining 80%-90% are atypical carcinoids. Most of these tumours occur centrally and involve the main, lobar, or segmental airways. Sometimes they are located distal to the segmental bronchi; such tumours are the so-called peripheral carcinoids. Atypical carcinoids have been reported to be larger than typical carcinoids, with mean diameters of 3.6 cm and 2.3 cm, respectively. Moreover, atypical carcinoids are more likely to occur in the periphery of the lung than are typical carcinoids. It was generally accepted that a carcinoid tumour was a very slow-growing and benign neoplasm with no potential for invasiveness and no tendency to give rise to metastases. Carcinoid tumours have subsequently been reported in a wide range of organs, but they most commonly involve the lungs and the gastrointestinal tract. The histopathologic features that distinguish atypical carcinoids from typical carcinoids are as follows: increased mitotic activity; greater cytological pleomorphism and higher nuclear to cytoplasmic ratios; increased cellularity and architectural irregularities, and more areas of tumour necrosis. In terms of histological features, typical carcinoids show no evidence of necrosis and fewer than 2 mitoses per 10 high-power fields (or 2 mm^2) of viable tumour, whereas atypical carcinoids do have areas of necrosis and 2-10 mitoses per 10 high-power fields.

3.4 Large-Cell Neuroendocrine Carcinoma

Large-cell neuroendocrine carcinoma (LCNEC) was proposed as the fourth category of pulmonary neuroendocrine tumours due to its distinct clinical and pathologic findings versus the typical carcinoid, atypical carcinoid, and SCLC. LCNEC is defined as a poorly differentiated and high-grade neuroendocrine tumour that morphologically is between an atypical carcinoid and SCLC. According to the WHO suggestions, the morphologic features of LCNEC represent a spectrum between those of atypical carcinoid and those of SCLC. In 70%-80% of cases, LCNEC appears as a peripheral mass or nodule, whereas 25% manifests as a central mass. Histopathologic diagnosis criteria for LCNEC are as follows: neuroendocrine morphologic features; a high mitotic rate (>10 per 10 high-power fields); necrosis (often large zones); cytologic features different from those of SCLC; and positive immunohistochemical staining for one or more neuroendocrine markers including chromogranin A, synaptophysin , and neural cell adhesion molecular (NCAM/CD56).

3.5 Small-cell lung carcinoma

SCLC accounts for approximately 20% of all bronchogenic carcinomas. Approximately 90%-95% of SCLCs occur centrally, apparently arising in a lobar or main bronchus. In 5%-10% of cases, SCLC manifests as a peripheral nodule. These tumour cells are usually small with a round or fusiform shape and have high cellularity with a very high mitotic rate. SCLCs are highly proliferative and rarely are the mitotic rates less than 10 mitoses per 10 high-power fields. As such, virtually every high-power field contains one or more mitoses. The architecture of the tumour clusters is poorly preserved, with large areas of necrosis separating small islands of viable tumour. A distinguishing feature of SCLC is its expression of neuroendocrine markers including neuron specific enolase (NSE), synaptophysin, neural cell adhesion molecule (NCAM/CD56), and Leu-7 (CD57).

4. The neuroendocrine differentiation in lung tumours

4.1 Non-small cell lung cancer (NSCLC)

The hypothesis that tumours with neuroendocrine properties should be grouped into a single category is not universally accepted for several reasons. First, a large proportion of lung carcinomas have mixed non-neuroendocrine and neuroendocrine properties. This is particularly evident in molecular profiling studies where otherwise unremarkable adenocarcinomas have been shown to express clusters of genes that are thought to reflect neuroendocrine differentiation. Second, many of the markers that are regarded as neuroendocrine markers are expressed in a variety of cells in addition to neuroendocrine cells. Third, neuroendocrine markers are expressed during the embryonic development of the lung.

4.1.1 Adenocarcinoma (ACA)

Pathology reports frequently mention the presence of NE immunophenotype or NE differentiation in NSCLC. Travis et al. have provided a new classification of the pulmonary NE proliferations and neoplasms of the lung, as part of the WHO classification of lung cancers. In this classification, NSCLC with NE differentiation (NSCLC-ND) detected only by immunostaining via electron microscopy is presented as a distinct entity in which no histological features of NE differentiation are appreciated on routine hematoxylin and eosin (HE). NSCLC represents a histologically heterogeneous group of tumours with variable clinical behaviours. Evidence for NE differentiation in non-small cell lung carcinomas (NSCLCs) is, at present, based on histochemical, ultrastructural, and immunohistochemical data. The existence of nonsmall cell lung carcinoma with neuroendocrine differentiation as a distinct entity, as well as its relevance for prognostic and treatment purpose, is controversial. A minority of NSCLCs (10-30%) show NE differentiation, and in contrast to large cell NE carcinoma, they show no evidence of this differentiation on routine light microscopic examination. Previous studies have identified NE differentiation in NSCLC in 10 to 70% of cases. Positivity for all 3 NE (Ch, SNP, and CD56) markers was not seen. The co-expression of SNP and Ch, the two most commonly used NE markers, accounted for only 0.2% (ACA) of the NSCLC. SNP staining was observed in a significant minority of NSCLC (7.5%), whereas Ch, the most specific NE marker, was very uncommon (0.4%) (Table3).

NSCLC Cell Type	Chromogranin (Ch)	Synaptophysin (SNP)	N-CAM (CD56)
Adenocarcinoma	0.4%	11.2%	5.1%
Squamous cell carcinoma	0.4%	4.3%	12.4%
Non-small cell carcinoma	0%	12%	7.4%
Large cell carcinoma	0%	9.3%	6.2%
Others	0%	0%	0%

Table 3. Immunoreactivity for Neuroendocrine Markers in Different Subtypes of NSCLC

As has been suggested, the derivation of all lung tumours from a common endodermal stem cell, along with the adoption of amine precursor uptake and decarboxylation properties by this endodermal stem cell, explains divergent differentiation in NE lung tumours and the occurrence of NE subsets in NSCLC.

4.1.2 Large cell carcinoma (LCC)

Large cell carcinomas of the lung are classified into four types based on light microscopic evidence of neuroendocrine morphology. Immunohistochemical or electron microscopic assessments of neuroendocrine differentiation are categorised as follows: (1) large cell neuroendocrine carcinoma exhibits both neuroendocrine morphology and evidence of neuroendocrine differentiation; (2) large cell carcinoma with neuroendocrine differentiation exhibits neuroendocrine markers but lacks neuroendocrine morphology; (3) large cell carcinoma with neuroendocrine morphology exhibits neuroendocrine markers; and (4) classic large cell carcinoma exhibits neither neuroendocrine morphology nor differentiation. Neuroendocrine markers in NSCLC are expressed not only in large cell carcinoma but also in adenocarcinomas.

4.2 NETs of the lung with NE differentiation

Lung tumours with neuroendocrine morphology include the low-grade typical carcinoid (TC), intermediate-grade atypical carcinoid (AC), and the high-grade LCNEC and SCLC. Neuroendocrine differentiation may be detected by immunohistochemical or ultrastructural studies in 10% to 20% of histologically ordinary NSCLCs such as squamous cell carcinomas, adenocarcinomas, or large cell carcinomas.

4.2.1 Small cell lung carcinoma (SCLC)

SCLC tumors are considered poorly differentiated NE cancers in contrast to typical and atypical bronchial carcinoid tumors. In addition to SCLC, approximately 20-30% of NSCLC tumors express some degree of NE differentiation, predominatly in adenocarcinomas and large cell cancers. SCLC exhibits characteristic molecular abnormalities which partially overlap with those of NSCLC including frequent inactivation of the Rb-p16INK4A-related G1 checkpoint pathway, loss of p53, and frequent abnormalities in chromosome

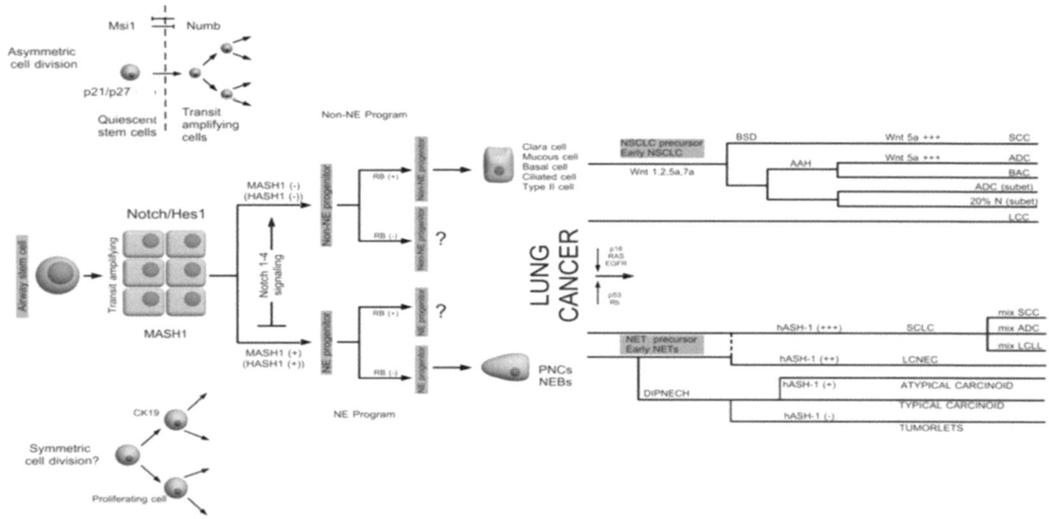

Fig. 1. Hypothetical carcinogenetic pathway in lung cancer: The specification of distinct cell fates is often achieved through the activation of specific intercellular signaling pathways by growth factors whose expression must be spatially and temporally controlled to ensure accurate response. Typically, a target cell expresses an excess of receptors such that the availability of its ligands is rate-limiting for pathway activation. Overall, for a signal to elicit the desired response, the intensity and duration of ligand expression must be sufficient to meet its threshold concentration, and yet the signal response must be restricted to prevent excessive signaling. Excessive activation of a signaling pathway can have broad deleterious effects, thus prompting a requirement for antagonistic regulation. Abbreviations: AAA (Atypical Adenomatous Hyperplasia), ADC (Adenocarcinoma), BAC (Bronchioalveolar Carcinoma), BSD (Basal Squamous Dysplasia), DIPNECH (Diffuse Idiopathic Pulmonary Neuroendocrine Cell Hyperplasia), LCC (Large Cell Carcinoma), LCNEC (Large Cell Neuroendocrine Carcinoma), NEBs (Neuroepithelial Bodies), PNCs (Pulmonary Neuroendocrine Cells), SCC (Squamous Cell Carcinoma), SCLC (Small Cell Lung Carcinoma).

3p-assocaited tumor suppressor activity. In addition to these changes, SCLCs frequently overexpress myc genes, especially c-Myc, often via gene amplification events. Of all the genetic changes in SCLC, Rb gene mutations are utterly characteristic. Functioning RB protein is lacking in greater than 90% of SCLC and NSCLC with NE features.

4.2.2 Large cell neuroendocrine carcinoma (LCNEC)

The term combined LCNEC is used for those tumours associated with other histologic types of NSCLC. Most often this represents a component of adenocarcinoma. LCNEC must be distinguished from adenocarcinoma, SCLC, large cell carcinoma, and large cell carcinoma with neuroendocrine differentiation (LCC-ND).

5. Embryological pathways in lung tumours

5.1 Notch

The three main functions of Notch signalling in self-renewing tissues include stem-cell maintenance, binary cell-fate decisions, and induction of differentiation. A critical aspect of Notch function in both development and post-natal life is the maintenance of stem cell viability and asymmetric cell division. Intrinsic to this process is an unequal distribution of Notch signals in the daughter cells, with the Notch-active cell maintaining its stem cell

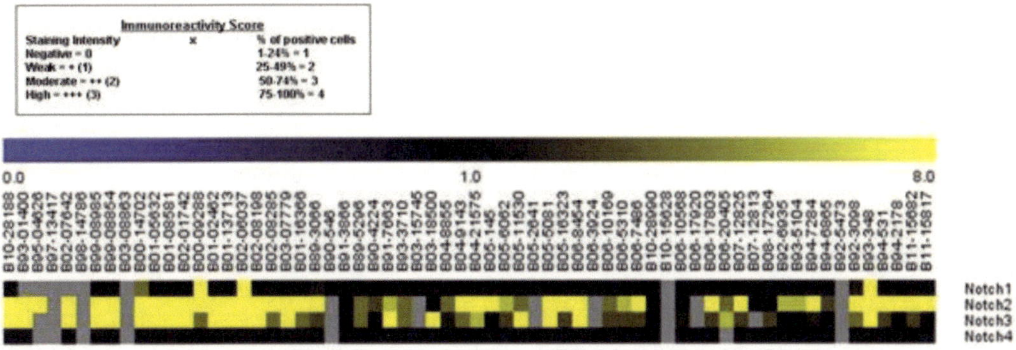

Fig. 2. Heat map for Notch1-4 expression in a serie of 64 carcinoids studied by tissue array technology in our lab gave the next information: The mean of expression for Notch1 is 2.33 and the mode 0. 76.6% of the samples showed no expression for this marker, 4.7% showed weak expression, 1.6% moderate expression; 4.7% of the samples showed strong reactivity for Notch1 in more than 75 % of tumour cells in the core biopsy arrayed, 12.5% of the samples did not show enough tissue for testing. The average expression for Notch2 is 8.56 and the mode 12. 7. 8% of the samples showed no expression for this marker, 4.7% showed weak expression, 17.2% moderate expression, 54.7% of the samples showed intense staining for Notch2 in almost all tumour cells present in the sample, 15.6% of the samples did not show enough tissue for testing. The average Notch3 expression is 6.3, and mode of 8. 10.9% of the samples showed no expression for this marker, and 25% showed weak expression, 14% moderate expression, 31.3% of the samples showed intense staining for Notch3 in almost all tumour cells present in the sample 18.8% of the samples did not show enough tissue for testing. Finally, for Notch4 we did not find reactivity in any of the 87, 5% samples with enough tissue for its evaluation.

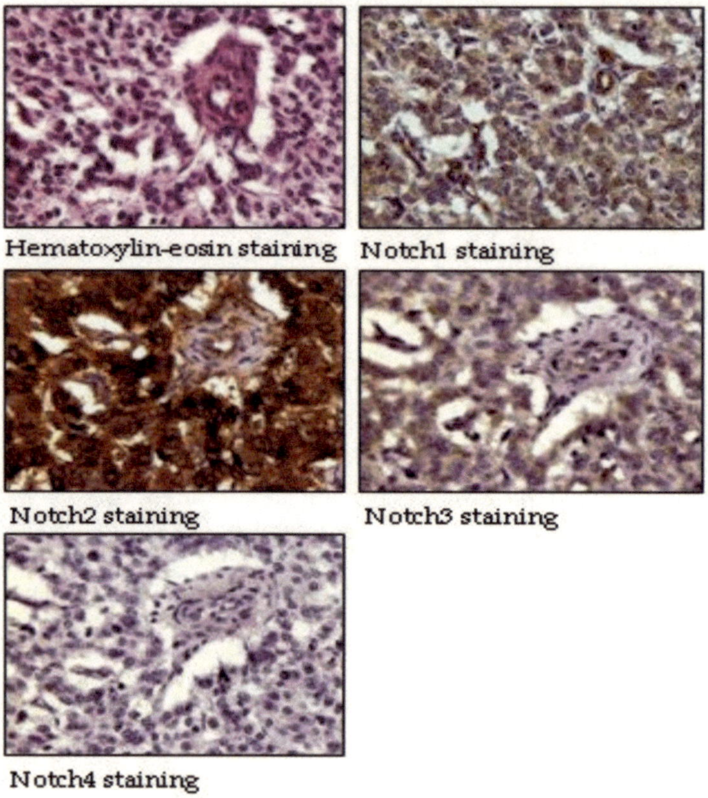

Fig. 3. Immunohistochemical findings for Notch1-4 in carcinoids tumors.

character and with transit-amplifying cells typically losing Notch activity. Interestingly, Notch function in lung cancer exhibits properties suggesting both tumour promotion and inhibition, depending on the tumour cell type. A prominent function of Notch signalling is to inhibit the transcriptional activities of the widely expressed E2A proteins. Notch signalling rapidly induces degradation and inactivation of E proteins and tissue-specific bHLH proteins such as hASH1. This inhibition may occur as a consequence of forming inhibitory complexes of E2A proteins with the Hes/HERP/HEY proteins, as well as the promotion of E2A protein ubiquitinylation and degradation by Notch. Notch1 and Notch2 proteins are frequently expressed in non-small-cell lung cancer (NSCLC), while Notch3 mRNA expression was detected in one-third of all NSCLC cell lines. NSCLC, which includes adenocarcinoma, squamous cell carcinoma, large cell undifferentiated carcinoma, and bronchoalveolar cell carcinoma, was initially shown to express significant levels of the Hes1 protein. In addition, there is an inverse correlation in these cell lines between the expressions of hASH1/ASCL1 and of the Hes1 protein. In contrast to NSCLC, where Notch is suspected to have a growth promoting function, SCLC appears to be growth inhibited, at least by the high level over-expression of activated Notch1 and Notch2. Notch1 is rarely detectable or inactive in SCLC, whereas a subset of SCLC exhibit Notch2. Notch3 mRNA expression was not detected in the SCLC cell lines. Expression of Notch3 has been reported to be common in NSCLC but not in SCLC. Significantly, Notch signaling has recently been shown to be induced by the ras pathway, which is active in a large fraction of NSCLC, but only rarely in SCLC. Notch in the SCLC cells lead to a significant increase in Hes1 and a marked down-regulation of the neurally related transcription factors hASH1 and Hes6. The loss of hASH1 may be critical in mediating the growth inhibitory effect of Notch1 in SCLC, although a role for other as yet unidentified targets cannot be excluded Activated Notch1 and Notch2, but not Hes1, caused a potent G1 arrest in the SCLC cells, accompanied by the marked up-regulation of $p21^{wasl/cip1}$, overall abundance of p53, and a Rb mutant typifying the majority of SCLC

5.2 Hedgehog signalling in lung cancer

The hedgehog (Hh) signalling network functions in cell-cell communication and regulates pattern formation, proliferation, cell fate, and the stem/progenitor cell maintenance and self-renewal in many organs. A greatly simplified version of "canonical" hedgehog signalling in mammals typically involves two types of cells, a signalling cell expressing a member of the Hedgehog family of secreted ligands (*Sonic Hedgehog* (Shh), *Indian Hedgehog* (Ihh), or *Desert Hedgehog* (Dhh)) and a responding cell expressing one or more *Patched* family hedgehog receptors (*Patched-1* (PTCH2)). In the Hh pathway, increased signalling results in activation of the GLI oncogenes (GLI1, GLI2, and GLI3) that can regulate gene transcription. The Hh signalling pathway was originally shown to have persistent activation in SCLC with high expression of Shh, PTCK, and GLI1, but an important role in NSCLC, was also demonstrated.

5.3 BMPs and BMPRs

The BMPs comprise a branch of the TGF-β superfamily that also plays a key role in development. Several BMP ligands and BMPRs including BMP3, 4 and 7 as well as type I BMPR are expressed during embryonic lung development. BMP4 mRNA is localized at high levels in the epithelium of distal tips of terminal buds, with lower levels in the adjacent mesenchyme. These loci of BMP expression overlap with the expression domains of some other important morphogenetic signaling molecules including HNF-3β, Wnt-2, Shh and FGF-10. Also, since BMPs and Shh are co-expressed in the same domains, and since Decapentaplegic, the Drosophila BMP homologue, is regulated by the Hedgehog signaling pathway, it seems possible that BMP-Shh interactions may prove to play key roles in lung morphogenesis. Recently published data on fibroblast growth factor interactions suggest that Shh, TGF-β1 and BMP4 all counteract the bud-promoting effects of FGF-10.

5.4 Wnt pathway in lung cancer

Wnt signaling has many functions in animal development including its development role in empbryogenesis and in the adult lung. More specifically, studies of knockout mice demonstrated the importance of Wnt-2, Wnt-5a, and Wnt-7b in lung maturation. In addition to its role in stem cell self-renewal, tissue regeneration, and lung development, Wnt signaling is also intimately involved in tumorigenesis and cancer progression. For example, the organs where Wnt signaling influences stem cell self-renewal are the same organs where those Wnt-pathway-dependent cancers originate. Numerous reportes have demonstrated aberrant Wnt activation in lung cancer. Overexpression of Wnt-1 has been demonstrated in NSCLC cell lines and primary cancer tissues. This activation can be caused by mutations and/or deregulation of many different Wnt signaling components. Mutations in Wnt pathway components are rarely found in lung cancer. Also overexpression of Wnt-2 in NSCLC has been demonstrated. The human Wnt-2 gene, located on chromosome 7q31.3, is highly expressed in fetal lung. The link between Wnt-2 and tumorigenesis was first proposed after data indicated that Wnt-2 was amplified in human cancers. Indeed, in patients with NSCLC found that Wnt-5a expression is squamous cell carcinoma was significantly higher than that in adenocarcinoma. Recently there has been a suggested role for Wnt-7 in lung cancer. It has been reported that expression of Wnt-7a is downregulated in most lung cancer cell lines and tumor samples.

5.5 bHLH

Helix-loop-helix proteins are a diverse family of transcriptional regulators involved in fetal development and cancer. The 125 recognized human HLH proteins can be subdivided into 45 families, almost all of which have Drosophila representatives as well. These families include achaete-scute homologs, E proteins, Atonal, NeuroD, neurogenin, ID proteins, HES, and Hes-related proteins, and others. bHLH genes control cell differentiation in various tissues and are categorised into two distinct groups, activator genes and repressor genes. In mammals, bHLH genes such as mammalian achaete-scute complex homolog-1 (MASH1) and mammalian atonal homolog (MATH)-1 are expressed in neural precursor cells, and they up-regulate late-expressing bHLH genes such as NeuroD to direct terminal differentiation. On the other hand, HES1, one of the hairy and enhancer of split (HES) homologues, represses neuronal differentiation by the suppression of proneural bHLH factors. Repressive bHLH factors such as HES1 are regulated by the Notch pathway. The Notch ligands activate the Notch receptors, and the activated intracellular domain of the Notch receptors interacts with the DNA-binding protein RBP-Jk to activate the expression of repressive bHLHs such as HES1 and HES5, which, in turn, suppress the expression of activator bHLHs such as MASH1 and NeuroD. Immunohistochemical studies have revealed that Notch1, Notch3, Jagged1, and Jagged2 were expressed in neuroendocrine cells of the airway epithelium, while Dll1 was detected in the pulmonary neuroendocrine cells. Thus, the differentiation of the lung epithelial cells depends on a bHLH factor network, and the Notch pathway may be involved in determining the cell differentiation fate in the airway epithelium.

5.5.1 Achaete-scute homolog (ASH-1)

Mash1 (termed Hash1 in humans) plays a critical role in development of the central and autonomic nervous systems and in tissues of the so-called diffuse NE system including the adrenal medullary chromaffin cells, thyroid parafollicular C-cells, and pulmonary NE cells. MASH1 is important in the development of the diffuse neuroendocrine system, including pulmonary neuroendocrine cells. During neurogenesis, MASH1 expression is confined to mitotically active precursors where it is involved in the early stages of lineage commitment; in more mature neurons the expression is extinguished. MASH1 and mammalian atonal homolog-1 (Math1) up-regulate NeuroD in neural precursor cells to direct terminal differentiation, whereas HES1 represses neuronal differentiation by the suppression of pro-neural factors such as MASH1. In the developing mouse lung, Mash1 first becomes detectable at approximately E13.5 in neuroepitelial bodies (NEB´S), clusters of NE cells frequently located at branchpoints of large and medium-sized airways. Mash 1 expression in mouse lung peaks near birth and the declines in adulthood, following the peak and decline of lung NE cells. One target of achaete-scute proteins is the cell surface ligand delta, which leads to activation of the Notch pathway in adjoining cells and repression of the neuronal fate. In human lung tumours, the expression of hASH1 mRNA was significantly higher in

SCLC (75%) than in LCNEC (50%); conversely, HES1 mRNA was lower in SCLC (59%) than in LCNEC (87%). These findings reveal that SCLC more strongly expresses the neuroendocrine phenotype, while LCNEC shows characteristics that are more similar to the epithelium phenotype, suggesting that the biological characteristics of these two tumours are different. On the contrary, non-neuroendocrine carcinoma cells do not express hASH1 but show high HES1 expression. In NSCLC (squamous cell carcinoma vs. adenocarcinoma), the expression of hASH1 mRNA was lower, (0% vs. 15%, respectively), whereas HES1 mRNA was higher (10% vs. 100%, respectively). Neuroendocrine pulmonary carcinomas express MASH1 but not HES1, whereas adenocarcinoma and squamous cell carcinoma express HES1. Surprisingly, Merkel cell carcinoma, the cutaneous counterpart of small cell carcinoma MASH1, was completely negative in 100% of the cases.

5.5.2 Hairy and Enhancer-of-split (HES)

Hes1, a key effector of the Notch signalling pathway, is expressed broadly in non-neuroendocrine cells in the airway epithelium. In the developing lung, Notch1 and HES1 are strongly expressed in the non-neuroendocrine airway epithelial cells, whereas MASH1 is restricted to the clustered pulmonary neuroendocrine cells. HES1 directly represses hASH1 expression by binding to a class C site in the ASH1 promoter. Today, the published results suggest that the differentiation of neuroendocrine cells in normal lungs is affected by the absence of the MASH1 gene. Elements of the Notch signalling pathway, especially that of HES1, appear to be critical negative regulators of achaete-scute homolog 1 expression in normal lungs and in lung cancer. For example, HES1 transgenic knockout mice exhibit substantial hyperplasia and premature differentiation of lung NE cells associated with an increase in MASH1-expressing pulmonary epithelium. It has been shown that the over-expression of HES1 in SCLC cells leads to the repression of hASH1 expression via a transcriptional mechanism.

5.5.3 Retinoblastoma (Rb)

The RB gene is a prototypical tumour suppressor gene, and the loss of RB function is believed to be a key event in the initiation or progression of several human malignancies. Most RB gene alterations result in the loss of RB protein expression or in a truncated RB protein, which does not enter the nucleus. Thus, heterogeneous positive nuclear RB immunostaining is, in general, indicative of normal RB function, whereas negative intranuclear RB immunostaining in all tumour cells reflects aberrant RB protein expression. Typical and atypical carcinoids manifest a heterogeneous RB-positive staining pattern. Atypical carcinoids in general show an increase in the number of tumour cells with nuclear staining compared to typical carcinoids. In contrast, small-cell and large-cell neuroendocrine carcinomas fail to show RB staining in any tumour nuclei, indicating the loss of RB function. From these results, it can be concluded that a progressively higher degree of malignancy from typical carcinoids to atypical carcinoids to small-cell carcinomas is paralleled by the loss of neuroendocrine markers, increased proliferative markers, increased frequency of p53 immunostaining, and decreased frequency of RB immunostaining.

5.5.4 p53

Although p53 alterations have been previously studied in pulmonary neuroendocrine tumours, either these studies have used immunochemistry alone rather than genotypic analysis or they have examined a limited spectrum of pulmonary neuroendocrine neoplasias. The distribution of p53 immunohistochemical staining has 4 patterns: negative in typical carcinoids (TCs), 50% of ACs, 20% LCNECs, and 12% SCLCs; less than 10% but more than 5-10 HPF (focal) in a subset (30%) of aggressive adenocarcinomas; and 50-100% of tumour cells (diffuse), exclusively seen in LCNECs and SCLCs. Three patterns of immunohistochemical staining intensities of the p53 protein were seen: negative; weak or mild; and moderate to marked staining. Similar to other cancers, multiple genetic events contribute to the development of neuroendocrine lung tumours. This has already been demonstrated in SCLCs, which are known to exhibit alterations in their oncogenes such as *c-myc* and in tumour suppressor genes such as p53 and Rb. In addition, it has been shown that alterations in oncogenes such as H-ras, c-myc, and c-raf-1 can modulate the expression of neuroendocrine antigens in lung cancer cell lines. Thus, evidence is accumulating that the expression of neuroendocrine differentiation in pulmonary neuroendocrine tumours is fundamentally controlled by multiple genetic determinants.

6. Conclusions

Although incidence of newly diagnosed patients with carcinoid tumors of the lung is low, the long survival for those with low and intermediate differentiation grade, and the deeper knowledge we now have on molecular processes that governs tumors growth make these tumors a challenging field in Oncology. Systemic treatment for metastatic carcinoid tumors of the lung has not change significantly in the last two decades, and this fact leads to a poor improvement in overall survival, contrary to what has happened in other solid tumors. Nowadays, most of researchers in neuroendocrine field consider that every single neuroendocrine tumors has its own features depending on the organ where it seats, the capacity to produce and secrete active hormones to blood stream, and the proliferation rate. Novel agents like antiangiogenic tyroisine kinase inhibitors, mTOR inhibitors or oral chemotherapeutic agents like temozolomide and capecitabine have been used to treat metastatic neuroendocrine tumors of the lung without a clear activity. Unfortunately, these clinical trials with new agents were not driven to lung tumors but to other neuroendocrine tumors of the gastrointestinal tract. Therefore, other pathways are needed to be investigated. A non insignificant number of recent publications are correlating embryological pathways with carcinoid tumors of the lung development. In this sense, some elements of the Notch signalling pathway, especially HES1, appear to be critical negative regulators of hASH-1 expression in normal lungs and in lung cancer. This fact may influence in carcinoid tumor development at this place. New compounds under clinical development targeting embryological pathways like Notch, Hedgehog or Wnt pathways may have a future impact in the treatment of disseminated carcinoids of the lung. The more we are able to select patients molecularly the greater the chance of success in future clinical trials conducted in this setting. However, none of this would be meaningless if the histological diagnosis is not accurate. There is a need to leverage the knowledge in the scientific community of the variety of neuroendocrine-derived tumors that may arise in the lung. The teamwork between pulmonologists, thoracic surgeons, pathologists, molecular biologists, oncologists, and radiotherapists is mandatory to offer to our patients the best treatment approach at the right time for their diseases.

7. References

7.1 Neuroendocrine system of the lung

Dimaline RN, Struthers J. Expression and regulation of a vesicular monoamine transporter (VMAT2) in rat stomach a putative histamine transporter. J Physiol. 1996; 490: 249-56.

Erickson JD, Schafer MK, Bonner TI, et al. Distinct pharmacological properties and distribution in neurons and endocrine cells of two isoforms of the human vesicular monoamine transporter. Proc Natl Acad Sci USA. 1996; 93: 5166-71.

Feyrter F. Über diffuse endocrine ephiteliale Organe. Liepzig Zentr Inn Mediz. 1938; 29: 545-71.

Feyrter F. Über die peripheren endockrinen (parakrinen) Druesen des Menschen. 1993; Maudrich. Vienna.

Jin L, Hemperly JJ, Lloyd RV. Expression of neural cell adhesion molecule in normal and neoplastic human neuroendocrine tissues. Am J Pathol. 1991; 138: 961-9.

Komminoth P, Roth J, Lacke PM, et al. Polysialic of the neural cell adhesion molecule distinguishes small cell lung carcinoma from carcinoids. Am J Pathol. 1991; 139: 297-304.

Lantuejoul S, Moro D, Michalides RJ, et al. Neural cell adhesion molecules (NCAM) and NCAM-PSA expression in neuroendocrine lung tumors. Am J Surg Pathol. 1998; 22: 1267-76.

Lloyd RV, Wilson BS. Specific endocrine tissue marker defined by a monoclonal antibody. Science. 1983; 222: 628-30.

Masson P. Carcinoid (argentaffin-cell tumors) and nerve hyperplasia of the appendicular mucosa. Am J Pathol. 1928; 4: 181-212.

Pearse AG. The cytochemistry and ultrastrusture of polypeptide hormone-producing cells of the APUD series and the embryologic, physiologic and pathologic implications of the concept. J Histochem Cytochem 1969;17:303-313

Rode J, Dhillon AP, Doran JF, et al. PGP 9.5, a new marker for human neuroendocrine tumours. Histopathology. 1985; 9: 147-58.

Wiedenmann B, Franke WW, Kuhn C, et al. Synaptophysin: a marker protein for neuroendocrine cells and neoplasms. Proc Natl Acad Sci USA. 1986; 83: 3500-4.

Wilkinson KD, Lee KM, Desphande S, et al. The neuron-specific protein PGP 9.5 is a ubiquitin carboxyl-terminal hrydrolase. Science. 1989; 246: 670-3.

7.2 Neuroendocrine epithelial cells

DiAugustine RP, Sonstegard KS. Neuroendocrinelike (small granule) epithelial cell of the lung. Environ Health Perspect. 1984; 55: 271-95.

Fujita T. concept of paraneurons. Arch Histol Jpn. 1977; 40 suppl: 1-2

Fujita T. Present status of paraneuron concept. Arch Histol Cytol. 1989; 52 suppl: 1-8.

Hoyt RF Jr, McNelly NA, Sorokin SP. Dynamics of neuroenpithelial body (NEB) formation in developing hamster lung: light microscopic autoradiography after 3H-thymidine labelling in vivo. Anat Rec. 1990; 227: 340-50

Hoyt RF Jr, McNelly NA, McDowell EM, Sorokin SP. Neuroepithelial bodies stimulate proliferation of airway epithelium in fetal hamster lung. Am J Physiol. 1991; 260: L234-L240

Linnoila RI, Nettesheim P, Di Augustine RP. Lung endocrine-like cells in hamsters treated with diethylnitrosamine: alterations in vivo and in cell cultire. Proc Natl Acad Sci USA. 1981; 78: 5170-4

MacDowell EM, Sorokin SP, hoyt RF Jr, Trump BF. An unusual bronchial carcinoid tumor: light and electron microscopy. Hum Pathol. 1981; 12 : 338-48.

Pearse AGE. The cytochemistry and ultrastructure of polypeptide hormone-producing cells of the APUD series and the embryologic, physiologic and pathologic implications of the concept. J Histochem Cytochem. 1969; 17: 303-13.

Polark JM, Bloom SR. Regulatory peptides. Localization and measurement. In: Becker KL, Gazdar AF, eds. The endocrine lung in health and disease. Philadephia: Saunders; 198. P. 300-27.

Scheuermann DW. Morphology and cytchemistry of the endocrine epithelial system in the lung. Int Rev Cytol. 1987; 106: 35-88.

Simon J-P, Aunis D. Biochemistry of the chromogranin A protein family. Biochem J. 1989; 262: 1-13.

7.3 Neuroendocrine epithelial cells & pulmonary neuroendocrine cells

DiAugustine RP, Sonstegard KS. Neuroendocrinelike (small granule) epithelial cell of the lung. Environ Health Perspect. 1984; 55: 271-95.

Fujita T. concept of paraneurons. Arch Histol Jpn. 1977; 40 suppl: 1-2

Fujita T. Present status of paraneuron concept. Arch Histol Cytol. 1989; 52 suppl: 1-8.

Hoyt RF Jr, McNelly NA, Sorokin SP. Dynamics of neuroenpithelial body (NEB) formation in developing hamster lung: light microscopic autoradiography after 3H-thymidine labelling in vivo. Anat Rec. 1990; 227: 340-50

Hoyt RF Jr, McNelly NA, McDowell EM, Sorokin SP. Neuroepithelial bodies stimulate proliferation of airway epithelium in fetal hamster lung. Am J Physiol. 1991; 260: L234-L240

Linnoila RI, Nettesheim P, Di Augustine RP. Lung endocrine-like cells in hamsters treated with diethylnitrosamine: alterations in vivo and in cell cultire. Proc Natl Acad Sci USA. 1981; 78: 5170-4

McDowell EM, Sorokin SP, Hoyt RF J, Trump BF. An unuasual bronchial carcinoid tumor: light and electron microscopy. Hum Pathol. 1981; 12: 338-48.

Pearse AGE. The cytochemistry and ultrastructure of polypeptide hormone-producing cells of the APUD series and the embryologic, physiologic and pathologic implications of the concept. J Histochem Cytochem. 1969; 17: 303-13.

Polark JM, Bloom SR. Regulatory peptides. Localization and measurement. In: Becker KL, Gazdar AF, eds. The endocrine lung in health and disease. Philadephia: Saunders; 198. P. 300-27.

Scheuermann DW. Morphology and cytchemistry of the endocrine epithelial system in the lung. Int Rev Cytol. 1987; 106: 35-88.

Simon J-P, Aunis D. Biochemistry of the chromogranin A protein family. Biochem J. 1989; 262: 1-13.

7.4 Neuroepithelial body structure

Adriaensen D, Timmermans JT, Brouns I, et al. Pulmonary intraepithelial vagal nodose afferent nerve terminals are confined to neuroenpithelial bodies: an anterograde tracing and confocal microscopy study in adult rats. Tissue Res. 1998; 293: 395-405.

Adriaensen D, Sheurman DW. Neuroendocrine cells and nerves of the lung. Anat Rev. 1993; 236: 70-85.

Adriaensen D, Brouns I, Van Genechten J, and Timmermans JP. Functional morphology of pulmonary neuroepithgelial bpodies: extremely complex aairway receptors. Anat Rec 2003;270A:25-40

Barth PJ, Wolf M, Ramaswamy A. Dristribution and number of Clara cells in the normal and disturbed development of the human fetal lung. Pediatr Pathol. 1994; 14: 637-51.

Brouns I, Adriaensen D, Burnstock G, Timmermans JP. Intraepithelial vagal sensory nerve terminals in rat pulmonary neuroepithelial bodies express P2X3 receptors. Am J Respir Cell Mol Biol. 2000; 23: 52-61.

Brouns I, Van Genechten J, Sheuermann D, et al. Neuroepithelial bodies: a morphologic substrate for the link between neuronal nitric oxide and sensitivily to airway hypoxia? J Comp Neurol. 2002; 449: 343-54.

Brouns I, Van Genechten J, Hayashi H, Gajda M, Gomi T, Burnstock G, Timmermans JP, and Adriaensen D. Dual sensory innervation of pulmonary neuroepithelial bodies. Am J Respir Cell Mol Biol2003;28:275-285

Cho T, Chan W, Cutz E. Distribution and frequency of neuroephitelial bodies in post-natal rabbit lung: quantitative study with monoclonal antibody against serotonin. Cell Tissue Res. 1989; 255: 353-62.

Cutz E, Gillan JE, Perrin DG. Pulmonary neuroendocrine cell system: an overview of cell biology. In pulmonary Disease. Perspect Pdiatr Pathol. F.B. Askin FB, Langston C, Rosemberg HS, Bertnstein J (eds). Basel, Karger. 1995; 18: 32-70.

Frölich F. Die ´Helle Zelle´der Bronchialschleimhaut und ihre Beziehungen zum problem der Chemoreceptoren. Frankfurter Z Pathol. 1949; 60: 517-59.

Gould Ve, Linnoila RI, Memoli VA, Warren WH. Neuroendocrine components of the bronchiopulmonary tract: hyperplasias, dysplasias, and neoplasms. Lab invest 1983; 49: 519-37.

Haller CJ. A Scanning and transmission electron microscopic study of the development of the surface structure of neuroepithelial bodies in the mouse lung. Micron. 1994; 25: 527-38.

Hartness ME, Lewis A, Searle GJ, et al. Combinedantisense and pharmacological approaches implicate hTASK as a airway o2 sensing K+ channel. J Biol Chem. 2001; 276: 26499-508.

Hong KV, Reynolds SD, Giangreco A, et al Clara cell secretory protein-expressing cells of the neuroepithelial body microenvironment include a label-retaining subset and are critical for eithelial renewal after progenitor depletion. Am J Respir Cell Mol Biol 2001;24:671-681

Hoyt RF Jr, Sorokin SP, McDowell EM, McNelly NA. Neuroepithelial bodies and growth of the airway epithelium in developing hamster lung. Anat. Rec. 1993; 236: 15-22.

Hoyt RF Jr, McNelly NA, McDowell EM, Sorokin SP. Neuroepithelial bodies stimulate proliferation of airway epithelium in fetal hamster lung. Am J Physiol. 1991; 260: L234-L240

Kemp PJ, Searle GJ, Hartness ME, et al. Acute oxygen sensing in cellular models:relevance to the physiology of pulmonary neuroepithelial and carotid bodies. Anat Rec 2003;270A:41-50

Khoor A, Gray ME, Singh G, Stahiman MT. Oncologeny of Clara cell-specific protein and its mRNA: their association with neuroepithelial bodies in human fetal lung and in bronchiopulmonary dysplasia. J Histochem Cytochem. 1996; 44: 1429-38.
Lauweryns JM, Goddeeris P. Neuroepithelial bodies in the human child and adult lung. Am Rev Respir Dis. 1975; 111: 469-76.
Lauweryns JM, Cokelaere M, Theunynck P. Neuroepithelial bodies in the respiratory mucosa of various mammals: a light optical, histochemical and ultrastructural investigation. Z. ZelforshMidrosk Anat. 1972; 135; 569-92.
Linnoila RI. Effects of diethylnitrosamine on lung neuroendocrine cells. Exp Lung Res 1982; 3: 225-36.
Magdaline SM, Barrish F, Fingold MJ, DeMayo FJ. Investigating stem cells in the lung Adv Pediatr. 1998; 45: 363-97.
Reynolds SD, Giangreco A, Power JH et al. Neuroepithelial bodies of pulmonary airways serve as a reservoir of progenitor cells capable of epithelial regeneration. Am J Pathol 2000; 156: 269-278
Rocall M, Springall DR, Maggioni M, et al. Early changes in the calcitonin generelated peptide (CGRP) content of pulmonary endocrine cells concomitant with vascular remodelling in the hypoxic rat. Am J respire Cell Mol Biol. 1993; 9: 467-74.
Sorokin SP, Hoyt F. Neuroepithelial bodies and solitary small-granule cells. In Lung cell Biology. D. Massaro, editor. Marcel Dekker. New York; 1989. P. 191-344.
Spindel ER. Roles of bombesin-like peptides in lung development and lung injury. Am J Respir Cell Mol Biol. 1996; 14: 407-8.
Stevens TP, McBride JT, Peake JL, et al. Cell proliferation contributes to PNEC hyperplasia after acute airway injury. Am J Physiol Lung cell Mol Physiol. 1997; 272: L486-L493.
Sunday ME, Willet CG, Patidar K, Graham SA. Modulation of oncogene and tumor suppressor gene expression in ahamster model of chronic lung injury with varying degrees of pulmonary neuroendocrine cell hyperplasia. Lab Invest. 1994; 70: 875-88.
Van Lommel A, Bolle T, Fannes W, et al. The pulmonary reuroiendocrine system:the past decade. Arch Histol Cytol 1999;62:1-16
Van Lommel A and Lauwerys JM. Neuroepithelial bodies in the Fawn Hooded rat lung: morphological and neuroanatomical evidence for a sensory innervation. J Anat. 1993; 183: 553-66.
Van Genechten J, Brouns I, Burnstock G, et al. Quantification of neuroepithelial bodies and their innervation in Fawn-Hooded and Wistar rat lungs. Am. J. Resp Cell Mol Biol. 2004; 30: 20-30.

7.5 Stem cells and neuroephitelial bodies

Bishop AE. Pulmonary epithelial stem cells. Cell Prolif. 2003; 37: 89-96.
Boers JE, Ambergen AW, Thunnissen FB. Number and proliferation of clara cells in normal human airway epithelium. Am J Respir Crit Care Med. 1999; 159: 1585.
Emura E. Stem cells of the respiratory tract. Paed Respir Rev. 2002; 3: 36.
Gosbey JR. Pulmonary neuroendocrine cell system in pediatric and adult lung disease. Microsc Res Techn. 1997; 37: 107.
Inayama Y, Hook GE, Brody AR, et al. The differentiation potential of tracheal basal cells. Lab Invest. 1988; 58: 706.

Linnoila RI, Mulshine JL, Steinberg SM, et al. Neuroendocrine differentiation in endocrine and nonendocrine lung carcinomas. Am J Clin Pathol. 1988; 90: 641-52.

Linnoila RI. Effects of diethylnitrosamine on lung neuroendocrine cells. Exp Lung Res 1982; 3: 225-36.

Liu JY, Nettesheim P, Randall SH. Growth and differentiation of tracheal epithelial progenitor cells. Am J Physiol. 1994; 266: 96.

McDowell EM, Trump BF. Pulmonary small cell carcinoma showing tripartite differentiation in individual cells. Hum Pathol. 1981; 12: 296-94.

Nettesheim P, jetten AM, Inayama Y, et al. Pathways of differentiation of airway epithelial cells. Environ. Health Perspect. 1990; 85: 317.

Reynolds SD, Giangreco A, Power JH et al. Neuroepithelial bodies of pulmonary airways serve as a reservoir of progenitor cells capable of epithelial regeneration. Am J Pathol 2000; 156: 269-278

Reynolds SD, Hong KU, Giangreco A, et al. Conditional Clara cells ablation reveals a self-renewing progenitor function of pulmonary neuroendocrine cells. Am J Physiol Lung Cell Mol Physiol 2000;278:L1256-L1263

Sell S, Pierce G. Biology of disease: Maturation arrest of stem cell differentiation is a common pathway for the cellular origin of teratorcarcinomas and epithelial cancers. Lab Invest. 1994; 70: 6-22.

Sunday ME, Willet CG, Patidar K, Graham SA. Modulation of oncogene and tumor suppressor gene expression in ahamster model of chronic lung injury with varying degrees of pulmonary neuroendocrine cell hyperplasia. Lab Invest. 1994; 70: 875-88.

Sunday ME, Willet CG. Induction and spontaneous regression of intense pulmonary neuroendocrine cell differentiation in a model of preneoplastic lung injury. Cancer Res. 1992; 52: 2677s

Taipale J, Beachy PA. The hedgehog and Wnt signalling pathways in cancer. Nature. 2001; 441: 349-54.

Travis WD, Colby TV, Corrin B, et al. Histological Typing of Lung and pleural tumors (Springer, Berlin) 1999.

Watkins DN, Berman DM, Burkholder SG, et al. Hedgehog signalling Within Airway epithelial progenitors and in small cell lung cancer. Nature 2003; 422: 313-7.

7.6 Pathology of neuroendocrine tumours of the lung

Aguayo SM, Millar YE, Waldron JA Jr ewt al. Brief report:idiopathic diffuse hyperplasia of pulmonary neuroendocrine cells and airways disease. N Engl J med 1992;327:1285-1288

Arrigoni MG, Woolner LB, Bernatz PE. Atypical carcinoid tumors of the lung. J Thorac Cardiovasc Surg 192;64:413-421

Aubry MC, Thomas CF Jr, Jett JR, Swensen SJ, Myers JL. Significance of multiple carcinoid tumors and tumorlets in surgical lung specimens: analysis of 20 patientys. Chest 2007;131:1635-1643

Beasley MB, Brambilla E, Travis WD. The 2004 World Health Organization classification of lung tumors. Semin Roentgenol 2005;40:90-97

Brambilla E, Travis WD, Colby TV, Corrin B, Shimosato Y. The new World Health Organization classification of lung tumors. Eur Respir J 2001;18:1059-1068

Cerilli LA, Ritter JH, Mills SE, Wick MR. Neuroendocrine neoplasms of the lung. Am J Clin Pathol 2001;116:S65-S96

Cutz E. Neuroendocrine cells of the lung. An overview of morphologic characteristics and development. Exp Lung Res 1982;3:185-208

Cutz E, Gillan JE, Perrin DG. Pulmonary neuroendocrine cell system: an overview of cell biology and pathology with emphasis on pediatric lung disease. In:Askin FB, Langston C, Rosemberg HS, Bertnstein J (eds). Pulmonary Disease. Karger:Basel, 1995

Churg A, Warnock ML. Pulmonary tumorlet. A form of peripheral carcinoid. Cancer 1976;37:1469-1477

Fink G, Krelbaium T, Yellin A, et al. Pulmonary carcinod presentation, diagnosis, and outcome in 142 cases in Israel and review of 640 cases from the literature. Chest 2001;119:1647-1651

Franklin WA. Diagnosis of lung cancer:pathology of invasive and preinvasive neoplasia. Chest 200;117:80S-89S

Hage R, de la Riviere AB, Seldenrijk CA, van den Bosch JM. Update in pulmonary carcinoid tumors: a review article. Ann Surg Oncol 2003;10:697-704

Hiroshima K, Iyoda A, Shida T, et al. Distinction of pulmonaru large cell neuroendocrine carcinoma from small cell lung carcinoma :a morphological, immunohistrochemical, and molecular analysis. Mod Pathol 2006 ;19 :1358-1368

Jiang SX, kameya T, Shoji M, Dobashi Y, Shinada J, Yoshimura H. Large cell neuroendocrine carcinoma of the lung: a histologic and immunohistochemical study of 22 cases. Am J Surg Oathol 1998;22:5265-537

Jung KJ, Lee KS, Han J, et al. Large cell neuroendocrine carcinoma of the lung: clinical, CT, and pathologic findings in 11 patients. J Thorac Imaging 2001;16:156-162

Kaufmann O, Georgi T, Dietel M. Utility of 123C3 monoclonal antibody against CD56 (NCAM) for the diagnosis of small cell carcinomas on paraffin sections. Hum Pathol 1997;28:1373-1378

Kloppel G. Tumour biology and histopathology of neuroendocrine tumours. Best Patct Res Clin Endocrinol Metab 2007;21:15-31

Kulke MH, Mayer RJ. Carcinoid tumors. N Engl J Med 1999;340:858-869

Lantuejoul S, Moro D, Michalides RJ, et al. Neural cell adhesion molecules (NCAM) and NCAM-PSA expression in neuroendocrine lung tumors. Am J Surg Pathol 1998;22:1267-1276

Mazieres J, daste G, Molinier L, et al. Large cell neuroendocrine carcinoma of the lung: pathological study and clinmcial outcome of 18 resected cases. Lung Cancer 2002;37:287-292

Modlin IM, Sandor A. An analysis of 8305 cases of carcinod tumors. Cancer 1997;79:813-829

Modlin IM, Lye KD, Kidd M. A 5-decade analysis of 13,715 carcinoid tumors. Cancer 2003;97:934-959

Muller NL, Miller RR. Neuroendocrine carcinomas of the lung. Semin Roentgenal 1990;25:96-104

Nowell PC. The clonal evolution of tumor cell populations. Science 1976;194:23-28

Nylen ES, Becker KL. The diffuse neuroendocrine system. In:Becker KL.(ed). Principles and Practice of Endocrinology and Metabolim, 3rd edn. Lippincott Williams and Wilkins:Philadelphia, 2001

Oberg K. Carcinoid tumors: current concepts in diagnosis and treatment. Oncologits 1998;3:339-345

Oshiro Y, Kusumoto M, matsuno Y, et al. CT findings of surgically resected large cell neuroendocrine carcinoma of the lung in 38 patients. AJR Am J Roentgenol 2004;182:87-91

Quoix E, Fraser R, Wolkove N, Finkelstein H, Kreisman H. Small cell lung cancer presenting as a soilitary pulmonary nodule. Cancer 1990;66:577-582

Rosado de CXhristenson ML, Abbott GF, Kirejcyk WM, Galvin JR, Travis WD. Thoracic carcinoids:radiologic-pathologic correlation. RadioGraphics 1999;19:707-736

Skuladottir H, Hirsch FR, Hansen HH, et al. Pulmoanry neuroendocrine tumors: incidence and prognosis of histological subtypes. A population-based study in Denmark. Lung Cancer 2002;37:127-135

Takei H, Asamura H, Maeshima A, et al. Large cell neuroendocrine carcinoma of the lung: a clinicopathologic study of eight-seven caees. J Thorac cardiovasc Surg 2002;124:285-292

Travis WD, Linnoila RI, Tsokos MG, et al. Neuroendocrine tumors of the lung with proposed criteria for large-cell neuroendocrine carcinoma. An ultrastructural, immunohistochemical, and flow cytometric study of 35 cases. Am J Surg Pathol 1991;15:529-553

Travis WD, Rush W, Flieder DB, et al. Survival analysis of 200 pulmonary neuroendocrine tumors with clarification of criteria for atypical carcinoid and its separation from typical carcinod. Am J Surg Pathol 1998;22:934-944

Travis WD, Brambilla E, Muller-Hermelink H, harris C. World Health Organization Classification of Tumors. Pathology and Genetics of Tumors of the Lung, Plaura, Thymus and Heart. Lyon, France. IARC Press; 2004

Vadasz P, Palffy G, Egervary M, Schaff Z. Diagnosis and treatment of bronchial carcinoid tumors:clinical and pathological review of 120 operated patients. Eur J Cardiothorac Surg 1993;7:8-11

Van Lommel A, Bolle T, Fannes W, et al. The pulmonary neuroendocrine system:the past decade. Arch Histol Cytol 1999;62:1-16

Van Lommel A. Pulmonary neuroendocrine cells (PNEC) and neuroepithelial bodies (NEB):chemoreceptors and regulators of lung development. Paediatric Respir Rev 2001;2:171-176

Warren WH, Could VE. Neuroendocrine tumors of the bronchopulmonary tract: a reappraisal of their classification after 20 years. Surg Clin Noth Am 2002;82:525-540

Wistuba II, gazdar AF. Lung cancer preneoplasia. Annu rev Oathol 2006;1:331-348

Yabuuchi H, Murayama S, Sakai S, et al. Resected peripheral small cell carcinoma of the lung:computed tomographic-histologic correlation. J Thorac Imaging 1999;14:105-108

7.7 The neuroendocrine differentiation in lung tumours

Abbott G, Papotti M, Viberti L, et al. Chromogranin A gene expression in non-small cell lung carcinomas. J Pathol. 1998; 186: 151-156.

Baldi A, Groger AM, Esposito V, et al. Neuroendocrine differentiation in non-small cell lung carcinomas. In Vivo. 2000; 14: 109-114.

Bhattacharjee A, Richards WG, Stauton J, et al. Classification of human lung carcinomas by mRNA expression profiling reveals distinct adenocarcinoma subclasses. PNAS USA 2001;98:13790-13795.
Beer DG, kardia SL, Huang CC, et al. Gene-expression profiles predict survival of patients with lung adenocarcinoma. Nat Med 2002;8:816-824.
Bobrow LG, Happerfield L, Patel K. The expression of small cell lung cancer related antigens in foetal lung and kidney. Br J Cancer 1991; 14:56-58.
Brambilla E, Lantuejoul S, Sturm N. Divergent differentiation in neuroendocrine lung tumors. Semin Diagn Pathol. 2000; 17: 138-148.
Carles J, Rosell R, Ariza A, et al. Neuroendocrine differentiation as a prognostic factor in non-small cell lung cancer. Lung Cancer. 1993; 10: 209-219.
Freeman M, Gurdon JB. Regulatory principles of developmental signaling . Annu Rev Cell Dev Biol 2002;18:515-539
Garber MF, Troyanskaya OG, Schluens K, et al. Diversity of gene expression in adenocarcinoma of the lung. PNAS USA 2001;98:13784-13789
Graziano SL, Tatum AH, Newman NB, et al. The prognostic significance of neuroendocrine markers and carcinoembryonic antigen in patients with resected stage I and II non-small cell lung cancer. Cancer Res. 1994; 54: 2908-2913.
Iyoda A, Hiroshima K, Toyozaki T, et al. Clinical characterization of pulmonary large cell neuroendocrine carcinoma and large cell carcinoma with neuroendocrine morphology. Cancer 2001; 91: 1992-2000.
Linnoila RI, Mulshine JL, Steinberg SM, et al. Neuroendocrine differentiation in endocrine and nonendocrine lung carcinomas. Am J Clin Pathol. 1998; 90: 641-652.
Skov BG, Sorensen JB, Hirsch FR, et al. Prognostic impact of histologic demonstration of chromogranin A and neuron specific enolase in pulmonary adenocarcinoma. Ann Oncol. 1991; 2: 355-360.
Travis WD, Linnoila RI, Tsokos MG, et al. Neuroendocrine tumors of the lung with proposed criteria for large-cell neuroendocrine carcinoma. An ultrastructural, immunohistochemical, and flow cytometric study of 35 cases. Am J Surg Pathol. 1991; 15: 529-553.
World Health Organization. Epithelial tumours. In: Histological typing of lung and pleural tumours. 3rd ed. Berlin: Spring-Verlag, 1999:25-47.
World Health Organization. International Histological Classification of Tumours. Histological Typing of Lung and Pleural Tumours. 3rd ed. Geneva: WHO; 1999.
Yesner R. Heterogeneity of so-called neuroendocrine lung tumors. Exp Mol pasthol 2001; 70:179-182

7.8 Embryological signalling pathways in lung tumours

Adhikary S, Eilers M. Transcriptional regulation and transformation by Myc proteins. Nat Rev Mol Cell Biol 2005; 6:635-645.
Apelqvist A, Li H, Sommer L, Beatus P, Anderson DJ, Honjo T, Hrabe de Angelis M, Lendahl U, Edlund H. Notch signaling controls pancreatic cells differentiation. Nature 1999; 400: 877-881.
Artavansis-Tsakonas S, Rand MD, Lake RJ. Notch signalling: cell fate control and signal integation in development. Science 284:770-776, 1999.

Barbareschi M, Girlando S, Mauri FA, et al. Tumor supressor gene product, proliferation and differentiation markers in lung neuroendocrine neoplasms. J Pathol 1992, 166: 343-350.

Bellusci S, Furuta Y, Rush MG, Henderson R, Winnier G, Hogan B. Involvement of Sonic Hedgehog (Shh) in mouse embryonic lung growth and morphogenesis. Development 1997; 124: 53-63.

Bellusci S, Furuta Y, Rush MG, Henderson R, Winnier G, Hogan BL. Involvement of Sonic hedgehog (Shh) in mouse embryonic lung growth and morphogenesis, Development 1997; 124: 53-63.

Bellusci S, Grindley J, Emoto H, Itoh N, Hogan BL. Fibroblast growth factor 10 (FGF10) and branching morphogenesis in the embryonic mouse lung. Development 1997; 124: 4867-4878.

Bellusci S, Henderson R, Winnier G, Oikawa T, Hogan B. Evidence from normal expression and targeted misexpression that bone morphogenetic protein-4 (Bmp-4) plays a role in mouse embryonic lung morphogenesis. Development 1996; 122: 1693-1702.

Borges MW, Linnoila RI, van de Velde HJ, Chen H, et al. An achaete-scute homologue essential for neuroendocrine differentiation in the lung. Nature 1997; 386:852-855

Bray S. Notch signaling in Drosophila: three ways to use a pathway. Semin Cell Dev 1998;9:591-597.

Broers JL, Viallet J, Jensen SM, et al. Expression of c-myc in progenitor cells of the bronchopulmonary epithelium and in a large number of non-small cell lung cancers. Am J Respir Cell Mol Biol 1993; 9:33-43.

Cagle PT, El-Naggar AK, Xu HJ, et al. Differential retinoblastoma protein expression in neuroendocrine tumors of the lung. Ann J Pathol 1997, 150:393-400.

Calvo R et al. Altered HOX and WNT7A expression in human lung cancer. Proc Natl Acad Sci USA. 2000; 97: 12776-12781.

Chen H, Thiagalingam A, Chopra H, Borges MW, Feder JN, Nelkin BD, et al. Conservation of the Drosophila lateral inhibition pathway in human lung cancer: a hairy-related protein (HES-1) directly represses achaete-scute homolog-1 expression. PNAS USA 1997; 94:5355-5360

Chen H, Thiagalingan A, Chopra H, Borges MW, et al. Conservation of the Drosophila lateral ionhibition pathway in human lung cancer: a hairy-related protein (HES-1) directly represses achaete-scute homologue-1 expression. PNAS USA 1997; 94:5355-5360

Clarke RB, Anderson E, Howell A, Potten CS. Regulation of human breast epithelial stem cells. Cell Prolif 2003; 36:45-58

Dang TP, Eichenberg S, Gonzalez A, et al. Cosntitutive activation of Notch3 inhibits terminal differentiation in lungs of transgenic mice. Oncogene 2003; 22:1988-1997

Dang TP, Gazdar AF, Virmani AK, Sepetavec T, Hande KR, Minna JD, Roberts JR, Carbone DP. Chromosome 19 translocation, overexpression of Notch3, and human lung cancer. J Natl. Cancer Inst. 2000; 92: 1355-1357.

Dang TP, gazdar AF, Virmani AK, Sepetavec T, Hande KR, Minna JD, et al. Chromosome 19 translocation, overexpression of Notch3, and human lung cancer. J Natl cancer Inst 2000; 92:1355-1357

Daniel VC, Peacock CD, Watkins DN. Developmental signaling pathways in lung cancer. Respirology 2006; 11:234-240

Eberhard DA, Johnson BE, Amler LC, et al. Mutations in the epidermal growth factor receptor and in KRAS are predictive and prognostic indicators in patients with non-small-cell lung cancer treated with chemotherapy alone and in combination with erlotininb. J Clin Oncol 2005; 23:5900-5909

Fitzgerald K, Harrington A, Leder P. Ras pathway signals are required for notch-mediated oncogenesis. Oncogene 19:4191-4198

Fong KM, Sekido Y, Minna JD. Molecular patogénesis of lung cancer. J Throac Cardiovasc Surg 1999; 118:1136-1152

Franklin WA, Veve R, Hirsch FR, et al. Epidermal growth factor receptor family in lung cancer and premalignancy. Semin Oncol 2002; 29:3-14

Fujino S, Enokibori T, Tezuka N, et al. A Comparison of epidermal growth factor receptor levels and other prognostic parameters in non-small cell lung cancer. Eur J Cancer 1996; 32A:2070-2074

Fukui T, Kondo M, Ito G, et al. Transcriptional silencing of secreted frizzled related protein 1 (SFRP1) by promoter hypermethylation in non-samll-cell lung cancer. Oncogene 2005; 24:6323-63327

Gouyer V, Gazzeri S, Brambilla E, et al. Loss of heterozygosity at the RB locus correlates with loss of RB protein in primary malignant neuro-endocrine lung carcinomas. Int J Cancer 1994, 58:818-824.

Gray GE , Mann RS, Mitsiadis E, Henrique D, Carnagin ML, Banks A, et al. Human ligands of the Notch receptor. Am J Pathol 1999; 154:785-794

Haruki K, Kawaguchi KS, Eichenberg S, et al. Dominant-negative Notch3 receptor inhibits mitogen-activated protein kinase pathway and the growth of human lung cancers. Cancer Res 2005; 65:3555-3561

He B et al. A monoclonal antibody against Wnt-1 induces apoptosis in human cancer cells. Neoplasia 2004; 6: 7-14.

He B, You L, Uematsu K, et al. A monoclonal antibody against Wnt-1 induces apoptosis in human cancer cells. Neoplasia 2004; 6:7-14

Huang CL et al. Wnt5a expression is associated with the tumor proliferation and the stromal vascular endothelial growth factor - an expression in non-small-cell lung cancer. J Clin Oncol 2005; 23: 8765-8773.

Ito T, Udaka N, Yazawa T, Okudela K, et al. Basic herlix-loop-helix transcription factors regulate the neuroendocrine differentiation of fetal mouse pulmonary epithelium. Development 2000; 127:3913-3921

Jan YN, Jan LY. Genetic control of cell fate specification in Drosophila peripheral nervous system. Annu Rev Genet 28:373-393, 1994.

Jensen J, Pedersen EE, Galante P, Hald J, Heller RS, Ishibashi M, Kageyama R, Guillemot F, Serup P, Madsen OD. Control of endodermal endocrine development by Hes-1. Nat. Genet. 2000; 24: 36-44.

Jiang SX, Kameya T, Asamura H, Umezawa A, et al. hASH1 expression is closely correlated with endocrine phenotype and differentiation extent uin pulmonary neuroendocrine tumors. Modern Pathol 2004; 17:222-229

Kageyama R, Nakanishi S. Helix-loop-helix factors in growth and differentiation of the vertebrate nervous system. Curr Opin Genet Dev 7:659-665, 1997.

Katoh M. Differential regulation of Wnt2 and Wnt2B expression in human cancer. Int J Mol Med 2001; 8: 657-660.

Kegeyama R, Nakanish S. Helix-loop-helix factors in growth and differentiation of the vertebrate nervous system. Curr Opin Genet Dev 1997; 7:659-665

Kunnimalaiyaan M, Chen H. Tumor suppressor role of Notch-1 signaling in neuroendocrine tumors. The Oncologist 2007; 12:535-542

Lai SL, Brauch H, Knutsen T, et al. Molecular genetic characterization of neuroendocrine lung cancer cell lines. Antcancer Res 1995, 15:225-232.

Lebeche D, Malpel S, Cardoso WV. Fibroblast growth factor interactions in the developing lung. Mech. Dev. 1999; 86: 125-136.

Li C, et al. Wnt5a participates in distal lung morphogenesis. Dev Biol 2002: 248: 68-81.

Mazieres J, He B, You L, et al. Wnt inhibitory factor-1 is silenced by promoter hypermethylation in human lung cancer. Cancer Res 2004; 64:4717-4720

Miki M, Ball DW, Linnoila I. Insights into the achaete-scute homoog-1 gene (hASH1) in normal and neoplatic human lung. Lung Cancer 2011;

Miyamoto Y, Maitra A, Ghosh B, Zechner U, Argani P, Iacobuzio-Donahue CA, et al. Notch mediates TGF alpha-induced changes in epithelial differentiation during pancreatic tumorigenesis. Cancer Cell 2003; 3:565-576

Nasgashio R, Sato Y, Matsumoto T, Kageyama T, et al. The balance between the expression of hASH1 and HES1 differs between large cell neuroencodrine carcinoma and small cell carcinoma of the lung. Lung Cancer 2011;

Nau MM, Brooks BJ Jr, Carney DN, et al. Human small-cell lung cancers show amplification and expression of the M-Myc gene. PNAS USA 1986; 83:1092-1096

Nie L, Xu M, Vladimirova A, Sun XH. Notch-induce E2A ubiquitination and degradation are controlled by MAP kinase activities. EMBO J 2003;22:5780-5782

Normanno N, Bianco C, Strizzi L, et al. The ErbB receptors and their ligands in cancer: an overview. Curr Drug Targets 2005;6:243-257

Pao W, Wang TY, Riely GJ, et al. KRAS mutations and primary resistance of lung adenocarcinomas to genitinif or erlotinib. PLoS Med 2005;2:E17

Price JV, Savenye ED, Lum D, amnd Breitkrwutz A. Genetics 1997; 147:1139-1153

Przygodzki RM, Finkelstein SD, Langer JC, et al. Analysis of p53, K-ras2, and C-raf-1 in pulmonary neuroendocrine tumors: correlation with histological subtype and clinical outcome. Am J Pathol 1996, 148:1531-1541.

Radtke F, raj K. The role of Notch in tumorigenesis: oncogene or tumor suppressor. Nature rev Cancer 2003; 3:756-767

Ralston J, Chiriboga, Nonaka D. MASH1: a useful marker in differentiating pulmonary small cell carcinoma from Merkel cell carcinoma. Modern Pathol 2008; 21:1357-1362

Riely GJ, Kris MG, Rosenbaum D, et al. Frequency and distinctive sapectrum of KRAS mutations in never smokers with lung adenocarcioma. Clin Cancer Res 2008; 14:5731-5734

Rodenhuis S, Slebos RJ, Clinical significance of ras oncogene activation in human lung cancer. Cancer Res 1992; 52:S2665-S2669

Rubin LL, de Sauvage FJ. Targeting the Hedgehog pathway in cancer. Nat rev Drug Discov 2006;5:1026-1033

Rusch V, Baselga J, Cordon-Cardo C, et al. Differential expression of epidermal growth factor and its ligands in primary non-small cell lung cancers and adjacent benign lung. . Cancer Res; 53:2379-2385

Sasai Y, Kageyama R, Tagawa Y, Shiemoto R, et al. Two mammalian helix-loop-helix factors structurally related to *Drosophila hairy* and *Enhancer of split*. Genes Dev 6:2620-2634, 1992.

Shu W et al. Wnt7b regulates mesenchymal proliferation and vascular development in the lung. Development 2002; 129: 4831-4842.

Sriuranpong V, Borges MW, Ravi RK, Arnold DR, Nelkin BD, Baylin SB, et al. Notch signaling induces cell cycle arrest in small cell lung cancer cells. Cancer Res 2001; 61:3200-3205

Sriuranpong V, Borges MW, Strock CL, Nakakura EK, Watkins DN, Blaumuller CM, et al. Notch signaling induces rapid degradation of achaete-scute homolog.1. Mol Cell Biol 2002; 22:3129-3139

7.10 The neuroendocrine pathway of differentiation

Uematsu K, He B, You L, et al. Activation of the Wnt pathway in non small cell lung cancer: evidence of dishevelled oversexpression. Oncogene 2003; 22:7218-7221

Wang XY, el Dakir H, Naizhen X, et al. Achaete-scute-homolog-1 limnked to remodeling and preneoplasia of pulmonary epithelium. Lab Invest 2007; 87:527-539

Watkins DN, Berman DM, Burkjholder SG, et al. Hedgehog signalling within airway epithelial progenitors and in small-cell lung cancer. Nature 2003; 422:313-317

Weidenfeld J et al. The WNT7b promoter is regulated by TTF-1, GATA6, and Foxa2 in lung epithelium. J Biol Chem 2002; 277: 21061-21070.

Weijzen S, Rizzo P, Braid M, Vaishnav R, Jonkheer SM, Zlobin A, et al. Activation of Notch-1 signaling maintains the neoplastic phenotype in human Ras-tansformed cells. Nat med 2002; 8:979-986

Winn Ra et al. Restoration of Wnt-7a expression reverses non-small cell lung cancer cellular transformation through frizzled-9-mediated growth inhibition and promotion of cell differentiation. J Biol Chem 2005; 280: 19625-19634.

Winn RA, Van Scoyk M, Hammond M, et al. Antitumorigenic efefct of Wnt 7a and Fzl 9 in non-small cell lung cancer cells is mediated through ERK-5-dependent activation of peroxisome proliferator-activated receptor gamma. J Biol Chem 2006; 281:26943-26950

Wissman C, Wild PJ, Kaiser S, et al. WIF1, a component of the Wnt pathway, is down-regulated in prostate, breast, lung and bladder cancer. J Pathol 2003; 201:204-212

Yamaguchi T et al. A Wnt5a pathway underlies outgrowth of multiple structures in the vertebrate embryo. Development 1999; 126: 1211-1223.

Yoshida M C et al. Human HST1 (HSTF1) gene maps to chromosome band 11q13 and coamplifies with the INT2 gen in human cancer. Proc Natl Acad Sci USA 1998; 85: 4861-4864.

You L et al. Inhibition of Wnt-2-mediated signaling induces programmed cell death in non small cell lung cancer cells. Oncogene 2004; 23: 6170-6174.

You L, He B, Xu Z, et al. Inhibition of Wnt-2-mediated signaling inducew programmed cell death in non-small-cell lung cancer cells. Oncogene 2004; 23:6170-6174

Zayzafoon M, Abdulkadir SA, McDonald JM. Nocth signaling and ERK activation are important for the osteomimetic properties of prostate cancer bone metastatic cell lines. J Biol Chem 2004; 279:3662-3670

10

Chemotherapy for Large Cell Neuroendocrine Carcinoma of the Lung: Should It Be Treated with the Same Strategy as Small Cell Lung Carcinoma?

Katsuhiko Naoki, Kenzo Soejima, Takashi Sato, Shinnosuke Ikemura, Hideki Terai, Ryosuke Satomi, Sohei Nakayama, Satoshi Yoda and Koichiro Asano

Keio Cancer Center / Division of Respiratory Medicine, Department of Internal Medicine, School of Medicine, Keio University, Tokyo / Yuai Clinic, Yokohama Japan

1. Introduction

Lung cancer is leading cause of cancer death in many advanced countries and one of the challenging malignancies because of poor prognosis. Lung cancer is traditionally divided into two major categories, so called small cell lung carcinoma (SCLC) and non-small cell lung carcinoma (NSCLC) because of distinctive prognostic and treatment strategies between them. On the other hand, there is a spectrum of tumors called pulmonary neuroendocrine (NE) tumors that are thought to originate from neuroendocrine cells in the pulmonary and bronchial epithelium. Until recently, pulmonary NE tumors were classified into three categories, i.e., typical carcinoid (TC), atypical carcinoid (AC), and SCLC. Large cell neuroendocrine carcinoma (LCNEC) of the lung was officially identified by Travis et al. in 1991 as a fourth category, a unique higher grade NSCLC existing between TC and SCLC (Travis et al., 1991). It is often difficult to diagnose LCNEC with small biopsy specimens because accurate diagnosis needs morphological and immunohistochemical information. Although earlier reports mainly focused on prognosis after surgical procedures, several recent studies reported on the efficacy of chemotherapy for advanced LCNEC. Because of the limited numbers of cases (in surgical series, LCNEC represents ~3% of lung cancers), large scale prospective studies have not been reported. Standard treatment for LCNEC, especially if advanced, is not established although LCNEC is included in NSCLC in the treatment algorithm in many guidelines. However, accumulating data including recent retrospective studies have suggested that there is similarity in the prognosis and treatment response between LCNEC and SCLC.

In this review, we will focus on the treatment of advanced LCNEC for the better selection of chemotherapeutic regimens for the patients with this relatively rare lung cancer.

2. Large cell neuroendocrine carcinoma of the lung

LCNEC is classified as a variant of large cell carcinoma in NSCLC whilst LCNEC has neuroendocrine characteristics similar to SCLC such as morphology and the immunohistochemical staining pattern. This discrepancy raises the question as to what the best therapeutic modality is, that is, should we treat LCNEC as NSCLC or SCLC?

	Typical Carcinoid	Atypical Carcinoid	LCNEC	Small cell carcinoma
Morphology	carcinoid	carcinoid	neuroendocrine	neuroendocrine
Mitosis	<2 / 2mm^2 (10HPF)	<2-10 / 2mm^2 (10HPF)	high: >11 / 2mm2 (10HPF)	high: >11 / 2mm2 (10HPF)
Necrosis	abscent	present (focal punctate)	present (extensive)	present (extensive)
Cytologic features			NSCLC (large cell, low N/C)	small cell, scant cytoplasm
Immunohistochemistry			positive for NE markers	positive for NE markers

Abbreviations: LCNEC, large cell neuroendocrine carcinoma;
HPF, high power field;
NSCLC, non-small cell lung carcinoma;
N/C, nuclear-cytoplasmic ratio;
NE, neuroendocrine

Table 1. Tumors with neuroendocrine morphology (Travis 2010, Gollard et al., 2010)

Recently, Varlotto et al. reported survival analysis of resected cases with LCNEC and SCLC (Varlotto et al., 2011). They compared overall survival (OS) and lung cancer-specific survival (LCSS) of patients with LCNEC and SCLC or other large cell lung carcinomas (OLCs) using the US National Cancer Institute database (SEER program). Although, the survival rates tended to be better in LCNEC and OLCs compared to SCLC, multivariate analysis showed no statistical differences (4-year OS rates are 41 % in LCNEC, 42% in OLC, and 32% in SCLC; 4-year LCSS rates are 57 % in LCNEC, 54% in OLC, and 42% in SCLC). The SEER database does not include chemotherapy information, so that we do not know the impact of chemotherapy on survival. Other reports also noted that survival in the early stage LCNEC is similar to SCLC (Asamura et al., 2006, Sun et al., 2009) and not better than NSCLC (Iyoda et al., 2007).

3. Chemotherapy for advanced LCNEC

LCNEC is classified in the category of NSCLC pathologically (Brambilla et al., 2001), so that the guideline recommended treatment of advanced LCNEC as NSCLC (NCCN guideline™ 2011), and many trials have included this disease as a NSCLC. However, recent accumulating data have brought new insights regarding possibly better results with SCLC regimens.

From the published literature, we found four major studies showing the treatment results with chemotherapy for advanced LCNEC (Igawa et al., 2010, Fujiwara et al., 2007, Yamazaki et al., 2005, Rossi et al., 2005) (Table 2). All studies were retrospective and a total of 83 patients were treated with first line systemic chemotherapy. Chemotherapy regimens can be classified into two groups: SCLC-based regimens (total n=44; platinum and etoposide n=27, platinum and irinotecan (CPT-11) n=16, CPT-11 only n=1) and NSCLC-based regimens (total n=39; platinum and paclitaxel (PTX) n=11, platinum and gemcitabine n=10, cisplatin with vindesine and mitomycin n=6, cisplatin and vindesine n=4, other platinum doublet n=2, other single agent n=6).

Report				OS	1yr survival	Chemotherapy	Pt	RR
Igawa	2010	Lung Cancer	n=14	10M	34%	total	n=14	50%
						CDDP+CPT11	n=7	57%
						CBDCA+VP16	n=2	50%
						CPT11	n=1	0%
						CBDCA+PTX	n=1	100%
						CDDP+PTX	n=1	100%
						VNR	n=1	0%
						DTX	n=1	0%
Fujiwara	2007	Jpn J Clin Oncol	n=22	10.3M	43.3%	total	n=22	59%
						Platinum+CPT11	n=9	56%
						Platinum+VP16	n=4	25%
						Platinum+PTX	n=6	67%
						PTX	n=1	100%
						CDDP+VNR	n=1	100%
						CDDP+DTX	n=1	100%
Yamazaki	2005	Lung Cancer	n=20	7.9M	35%	total	n=20	50%
						CDDP+VP16	n=9	56%
						MVP	n=6	33%
						CDDP+VDS	n=4	75%
						CDDP	n=1	0%
Rossi	2005	Lung Cancer	n=27	no data	no data	total	n=27	29%
						Platinum+VP16	n=12	50%
						CDDP+GEM	n=10	0%
						CBDCA+PTX	n=3	0%
						GEM	n=2	0%

Abbreviations: OS, overall survival;
Pt, patient number;
RR response rate;
PTX, paclitaxel;
VNR, vinorelbine;
DTX, docetaxel;
MVP, mitomycin + vindesine + cisplatin;
VDS, vindesine;
GEM, gemcitabine.

Table 2. Previous report regarding 1st line chemotherapy for advanced large cell neuroendocrine cell carcinoma (LCNEC)

The response rate (RR) was 47.7% (21/44) for SCLC-based regimens and 35.9% (14/39) for NSCLC-based regimens (Table 3). In particular, a platinum doublet yielded a RR of 56.3% (9/16) with platinum and CPT-11, 44.4% (12/27) with platinum and etoposide, 54.5% (6/11) with platinum and PTX, 16.7% (2/12) with platinum and other third generation agents.

Rossi et al. (2005) showed a significant survival benefit with a SCLC-based regimen compared with a NSCLC regimen (OS of 51 months (M) vs 21M). This result is far better than other reports (OS 7.9M-10.3M, 1-year survival rate 35-47.6%), suggesting that the result was from combined effects of surgery and chemotherapy.

	Chemotherapy	Pt	RR
SCLC based	total	n=44	48%
	Platinum+VP16	n=27	44%
	Platinum+CPT11	n=16	56%
	CPT11	n=1	0%
NSCLC based	total	n=39	36%
	Platinum+PTX	n=11	55%
	PTX	n=1	100%
	CDDP+VNR	n=1	100%
	VNR	n=1	0%
	CDDP+DTX	n=1	100%
	DTX	n=1	0%
	CDDP+GEM	n=10	0%
	GEM	n=2	0%
	MVP	n=6	33%
	CDDP+VDS	n=4	75%
	CDDP	n=1	0%

(Abbreviations are the same as in Table 1)

Table 3. Summary of previous reports regarding 1st line chemotherapy for advanced large cell neuroendocrine cell carcinoma (LCNEC)

As for second line treatment, there is no report other than a recent publication with amrubicin treatment (Yoshida et al., 2011). Amrubicin has efficacy for both SCLC and NSCLC, and has been used commonly in Japan in a second line setting with SCLC. Promising results for SCLC have also been recently reported from the USA (Ettinger et al., 2010, Jotte et al., 2011).

Currently there are a few prospective clinical trials for LCNEC in the 1st line settings (ClinicalTrials.gov and UMIN-CTR Clinical Trial, accessed 2nd Aug, 2011). One is not yet open but is an interesting phase II study with RAD001 + carboplatin/paclitaxel for advanced LCNEC. The other is an ongoing phase II study with cisplatin + irinotecan for advanced LCNEC.

The former study with RAD001 is an interesting study utilizing an mTOR inhibitor which inhibits one of the signaling pathways, i.e. the PI3K-mTOR pathway, that lies downstream of receptor tyrosine kinases (RTKs) such as EGFR and c-MET. EGFR is one of the most

Disease	Report	Study	Pt	RR	PFS	OS
LCNEC	Yoshida, 2011	retrospective	n=18	27.7%	3.1M	5.1M
SCLC (sensitive)	Jotte, 2011	prospective	n=50	44%	4.5M	9.2M
SCLC (refractory)	Ettinger, 2010	prospective	n=75	21.3%	3.2M	6.0M
SCLC (sensitive)	Inoue, 2008	prospective	n=9	53%	3.9M	9.9M
SCLC (refractory)			n=2	17%	2.6M	5.3M
SCLC (sensitive)	Onoda, 2006	prospective	n=44	52%	10.3M	11.6M
SCLC (refractory)			n=16	50%	2.6M	4.4M

Table 4. Efficacy of Amrubicin in the 2nd line treatment for LCNEC and SCLC

important RTKs in NSCLC (Paez et al., 2004), and moreover c-MET is reported to be an important RTK in SCLC as well as NSCLC (Nakachi et al., 2010, Rossi et al., 2005, Schmid et al., 2010). RAD001 has limited but apparent antitumor activity against pretreated SCLC as a single agent (Tarhini et al., 2010). According to these results, targeting signaling pathways with cytotoxic agent might be the next challenge for SCLC and LCNEC. Because many of the current effort in NSCLC is searching for driver mutations (Paez et al., 2004, Naoki et al., 2002), such an effort is also important in SCLC and LCNEC.

4. Conclusion

Although there is an issue regarding accurate diagnosis with small biopsy specimens, accumulating retrospective data suggest that patients with advanced LCNEC will benefit from systemic chemotherapy.

The current recommendation for the treatment of advanced LCNEC is similar to that of SCLC, i.e. platinum based combination chemotherapy, mainly with etoposide or CPT-11 and possibly with PTX. Further prospective data is needed to elucidate the best combination therapy.

5. References

Asamura H, Kameya T, Matsuno Y, Noguchi M, Tada H, Ishikawa Y, Yokose T, Jiang SX, Inoue T, Nakagawa K, Tajima K, & Nagai K. Neuroendocrine neoplasms of the lung: a prognostic spectrum. *J Clin Oncol* 2006 Jan 1;24(1):70-6, ISSN 0732-183X

Brambilla E, Travis WD, Colby TV, Corrin B, & Shimosato Y. The new World Health Organization classification of lung tumours. *Eur Respir J* 2001 Dec;18(6):1059-68, ISSN:0903-1936

Clinical Trials.gov, 2011 Aug,
http://clinicaltrials.gov/

Ettinger DS, Jotte R, Lorigan P, Gupta V, Garbo L, Alemany C, Conkling P, Spigel DR, Dudek AZ, Shah C, Salgia R, McNally R, Renschler MF, & Oliver JW. Phase II study of amrubicin as second-line therapy in patients with platinum-refractory small-cell lung cancer. *J Clin Oncol* 2010 May 20;28(15):2598-603, ISSN 0732-183X

Fujiwara Y, Sekine I, Tsuta K, Ohe Y, Kunitoh H, Yamamoto N, Nokihara H, Yamada K, & Tamura T. Effect of platinum combined with irinotecan or paclitaxel against large cell neuroendocrine carcinoma of the lung. *Jpn J Clin Oncol* 2007 Jul;37(7):482-6, ISSN 0368-2811

Gollard R, Jhatakia S, Elliott M, & Kosty M. Large cell/neuroendocrine carcinoma. *Lung Cancer* 2010 Jul;69(1):13-8, ISSN 0169-5002

Igawa S, Watanabe R, Ito I, Murakami H, Takahashi T, Nakamura Y, Tsuya A, Kaira K, Naito T, Endo M, Yamamoto N, & Kameya T. Comparison of chemotherapy for unresectable pulmonary high-grade non-small cell neuroendocrine carcinoma and small-cell lung cancer. *Lung Cancer* 2010 Jun;68(3):438-45, ISSN 0169-5002

Inoue A, Sugawara S, Yamazaki K, Maemondo M, Suzuki T, Gomi K, Takanashi S, Inoue C, Inage M, Yokouchi H, Watanabe H, Tsukamoto T, Saijo Y, Ishimoto O, Hommura F, & Nukiwa T. Randomized phase II trial comparing amrubicin with topotecan in patients with previously treated small-cell lung cancer: North Japan Lung Cancer Study Group Trial 0402. *J Clin Oncol* 2008 Nov 20;26(33):5401-6, ISSN 0732-183X

Iyoda A, Hiroshima K, Nakatani Y, & Fujisawa T. Pulmonary large cell neuroendocrine carcinoma: its place in the spectrum of pulmonary carcinoma. *Ann Thorac Surg* 2007 Aug;84(2):702-7, ISSN 0003-4975

Jotte R, Conkling P, Reynolds C, Galsky MD, Klein L, Fitzgibbons JF, McNally R, Renschler MF, & Oliver JW. Randomized phase II trial of single-agent amrubicin or topotecan as second-line treatment in patients with small-cell lung cancer sensitive to first-line platinum-based chemotherapy. *J Clin Oncol*. 2011 Jan 20;29(3):287-93, ISSN 0732-183X

Nakachi I, Naoki K, Soejima K, Kawada I, Watanabe H, Yasuda H, Nakayama S, Yoda S, Satomi R, Ikemura S, Terai H, Sato T, & Ishizaka A. The combination of multiple receptor tyrosine kinase inhibitor and mammalian target of rapamycin inhibitor overcomes erlotinib resistance in lung cancer cell lines through c-Met inhibition. *Mol Cancer Res* 2010 Aug;8(8):1142-51, ISSN:1541-7786

Naoki K, Chen TH, Richards WG, Sugarbaker DJ, Meyerson M. Missense mutations of the BRAF gene in human lung adenocarcinoma. *Cancer Res* 2002 Dec 1;62(23):7001-3, ISSN:0008-5472

Non-Small Cell Lung Cancer, *NCCN Guidelines™*, 2011 Aug,
http://www.nccn.org/professionals/physician_gls/pdf/nscl.pdf

Onoda S, Masuda N, Seto T, Eguchi K, Takiguchi Y, Isobe H, Okamoto H, Ogura T, Yokoyama A, Seki N, Asaka-Amano Y, Harada M, Tagawa A, Kunikane H, Yokoba M, Uematsu K, Kuriyama T, Kuroiwa Y, & Watanabe K; Thoracic Oncology

Research Group Study 0301. Phase II trial of amrubicin for treatment of refractory or relapsed small-cell lung cancer: Thoracic Oncology Research Group Study 0301. *J Clin Oncol* 2006 Dec 1;24(34):5448-53, ISSN 0732-183X

Paez JG, Jänne PA, Lee JC, Tracy S, Greulich H, Gabriel S, Herman P, Kaye FJ, Lindeman N, Boggon TJ, Naoki K, Sasaki H, Fujii Y, Eck MJ, Sellers WR, Johnson BE, & Meyerson M. EGFR mutations in lung cancer: correlation with clinical response to gefitinib therapy. *Science* 2004 Jun 4;304(5676):1497-500, ISSN:0036-8075

Rekhtman N. Neuroendocrine tumors of the lung: an update. *Arch Pathol Lab Med* 2010 Nov;134(11):1628-38, ISSN 0003-9985

Rossi G, Cavazza A, Marchioni A, Longo L, Migaldi M, Sartori G, Bigiani N, Schirosi L, Casali C, Morandi U, Facciolongo N, Maiorana A, Bavieri M, Fabbri LM, & Brambilla E. Role of chemotherapy and the receptor tyrosine kinases KIT, PDGFRalpha, PDGFRbeta, and Met in large-cell neuroendocrine carcinoma of the lung. *J Clin Oncol* 2005 Dec 1;23(34):8774-85, ISSN 0732-183X

Schmid K, Bago-Horvath Z, Berger W, Haitel A, Cejka D, Werzowa J, Filipits M, Herberger B, Hayden H, & Sieghart W. Dual inhibition of EGFR and mTOR pathways in small cell lung cancer. *Br J Cancer* 2010 Aug 24;103(5):622-8, ISSN:0007-0920

Sun L, Sakurai S, Sano T, Hironaka M, Kawashima O, & Nakajima T. High-grade neuroendocrine carcinoma of the lung: comparative clinicopathological study of large cell neuroendocrine carcinoma and small cell lung carcinoma. *Pathol Int* 2009 Aug; 59(8):522-9, ISSN 1320-5463

Tarhini A, Kotsakis A, Gooding W, Shuai Y, Petro D, Friedland D, Belani CP, Dacic S, & Argiris A. Phase II study of everolimus (RAD001) in previously treated small cell lung cancer. *Clin Cancer Res* 2010 Dec 1;16(23):5900-7, ISSN:1078-0432

Travis WD, Linnoila RI, Tsokos MG, Hitchcock CL, Cutler GB Jr, Nieman L, Chrousos G, Pass H, & Doppman J. Neuroendocrine tumors of the lung with proposed criteria for large-cell neuroendocrine carcinoma. An ultrastructural, immunohistochemical, and flow cytometric study of 35 cases. *Am J Surg Pathol* 1991 Jun;15(6):529-53, ISSN 0147-5185

Travis WD. Advances in neuroendocrine lung tumors. *Ann Oncol* 2010 Oct;21 Suppl 7:vii65-71, ISSN 0923-7534

UMIN-CTR Clinical Trial, 2011 Aug,
http://www.umin.ac.jp/ctr/

Varlotto JM, Medford-Davis LN, Recht A, Flickinger JC, Schaefer E, Zander DS, & DeCamp MM. Should large cell neuroendocrine lung carcinoma be classified and treated as a small cell lung cancer or with other large cell carcinomas? *J Thorac Oncol* 2011 Jun;6(6):1050-8, ISSN 1556-0864

Yamazaki S, Sekine I, Matsuno Y, Takei H, Yamamoto N, Kunitoh H, Ohe Y, Tamura T, Kodama T, Asamura H, Tsuchiya R, & Saijo N. Clinical responses of large cell neuroendocrine carcinoma of the lung to cisplatin-based chemotherapy. *Lung Cancer* 2005 Aug;49(2):217-23, ISSN 0169-5002

Yoshida H, Sekine I, Tsuta K, Horinouchi H, Nokihara H, Yamamoto N, Kubota K, & Tamura T. Amrubicin Monotherapy for Patients with Previously Treated Advanced Large-cell Neuroendocrine Carcinoma of the Lung. *Jpn J Clin Oncol* 2011 Jul;41(7):897-901, ISSN 0368-2811

11

Radiation Therapy in Management of Small-Cell Lung Cancer

Erkan Topkan and Cem Parlak
Baskent University Adana Medical Faculty, Department of Radiation Oncology Turkey

1. Introduction

Worldwide, lung carcinoma (LC) is the commonest and deadliest form of cancer in men and women, exceeding the mortality of prostate, breast, and colorectal cancers combined (Jemal et al., 2009). Irrespective of histologic subtype, more than 90% of all LC is strongly associated with cigarette smoking (Alavanja et al., 2002), and the risk significantly increases with the number of cigarettes smoked per day, degree of inhalation, age at initiation, and life-long cumulative exposure (Tyczynski et al., 2003). Although survival at 5-year is less than 15%, yet, there exists no single proven chemopreventive measure reducing the risk of LC development, except for cessation of cigarette smoking.

Histologically, non-small cell LC (NSCLC) and small-cell LC (SCLC) are the two commonest types of LC, constituting 85-90% and 10-15% of all cases, respectively (Rosenzweig et al., 2010). SCLC (previously called oat cell carcinoma) is relatively less common than NSCLC; however, because of a more aggressive growth pattern and clinical course, its treatment is more challenging. Although there is no significant difference in outcome by histologic subtype, the World Health Organization classification subdivides SCLC into three cell types; pure or classic, variant cell, and mixed (Brambilla et al., 2001). SCLC displays a high propensity to metastasize, and usually a remarkable but temporary responsiveness to chemotherapy and radiotherapy (RT). Although some may be cured, most patients succumb to disease because of rapid development of drug resistance and resultant disease progression. Median survival for metastatic SCLC is only 10 months, which is interestingly very similar to patients with relatively much more drug resistant NSCLC of similar stage (Chute et al., 1997). Despite great improvements in imaging, pathology, genetics, chemotherapy, and RT techniques, this did not translate into the clinical outcomes, thus, the current overall survival rate for SCLC patients is not different than that was 20 years before (Chute et al., 1997).

This chapter has been designated to focus specifically on treatment of SCLC patients, with specific emphasises on the technical basis and outcomes of current RT and concurrent chemoradiotherapy (C-CRT). Therefore, readers interested in more comprehensive information about the epidemiology, etiology, preventive measures, pathologic and genetic basis and surgical treatment of SCLC are referred to excellent reviews available in this book.

2. Staging

Management of SCLC begins with the accurate staging of the disease. Historically, using the Veteran's Administration Lung Study Group (VALG) criteria (Zelen, 1973), staging of SCLC was simplified to include two stages: limited stage SCLC (LS-SCLC), and extensive stage SCLC (ES-SCLC). LS-SCLC is defined as the disease confined to the ipsilateral hemithorax which can be safely encompassed within a tolerable single radiation port. Involvement of ipsilateral supraclavicular lymph node region is also included in limited-stage disease. In contrast; patients with ES-SCLC have disease that is beyond the ipsilateral hemithorax. Besides the hematogenous spread, involvement of contralateral supraclavicular lymph node region and/or presence of malignant pleural- and/or pericardial effusion are included in extensive-stage disease. Only less than one third of SCLC patients present with limited-stage disease, while remaining two thirds have extensive-stage disease, and are treated with palliative chemotherapy.

The revised American Joint Committee on Cancer (AJCC) staging system implemented the TNM staging for NSCLC, but its use for SCLC was also recommended in sixth and seventh editions (Edge, 2010; Greene, 2002). Recent study by Vallieres et al., constituting of 349 patients with resected SCLC confirmed the utility of TNM-based pathologic staging in terms of survival outcomes. But, because of being restricted to only 5% SCLC patients presenting with an operable disease at presentation, TNM-based staging has not been routinely adopted two tired VALG staging system (LS-SCLC and ES-SCLC) in this group of patients (Vallieres et al., 2009).

3. Prognostic factors

Despite paramount improvements in imaging and treatment modalities, prognosis of patients with SCLC is still unacceptably poor with median survival ranges of only 15-20 months for LS-SCLC and 8-13 months for ES-SCLC (Lally et al, 2007). Furthermore, 5-year survivors are reported to be only in the respective ranges of 10-13% and 1-2%, emphasizing the futility of the condition (Lassen, 1995; Tai, 2003). A number of factors have been assigned to carry prognostic importance for patients with SCLC but the most important tumor related factor is the VALG stage (LS-SCLC versus ES-SCLC). In LS-SCLC, early stage disease that corresponds to TNM stage 1 carries the best prognosis specifically in the absence of elevated serum lactate dehydrogenase levels (Byhardt, 1986; Lassen, 1995). Similar to other tumor sites, weight loss and poor performance status are significant predictors of unfavorable outcome (Paesmans et al., 2000). Likewise, men fare poorer than women (Lally et al, 2007). In ES-SCLC, the number of organ sites and site of involvement are also strongly associated with prognosis (Albain et al, 1991). Compared to other sites, involvement of bone marrow, liver, or central nervous system signify unfavorable disease course.

Compared to NSCLC, SCLC is more frequently associated with paraneoplastic syndromes either via antibody-mediated tissue destruction or via ectopic hormone production (Lally et al, 2007). Although, some debate exists, unlike antibody-mediated paraneoplastic syndromes, ectopic hormone production is generally accepted as a predictor of poor outcome. Favorable prognosis linked to antibody-mediated paraneoplastic syndromes may be related with presence of a fully competent immune system, indicating the need for exploration of immunotherapy adjunct to standard treatment approaches in this patients group.

4. Treatment for limited-stage small cell lung carcinoma

4.1 Chemotherapy

In LS-NSCLC, chemotherapy trials conducted in the 1970s improved survival from weeks to months. Over the following three decades, several studies have shown that combination chemotherapy regimens were clearly more efficacious than single agent regimens. Response rates of 70%-85%, with complete response of 20%-30%, are encouraging but virtually almost every patient relapses (Lally et al, 2007). Results of randomized investigations and meta-analysis for the most active regimen indicated the superiority of etoposide plus cisplatin (EP) combination over the other tested combinations (Fukuoka, 1991; Pujol, 2000; Roth, 1992; Sundstrom, 2002). Therefore, the EP combination has become the standard care chemotherapy combination in United States and Europe since 1980s. Although cisplatin is the backbone of chemotherapy, carboplatin may be substituted for cisplatin in older patients or in those with renal insufficiency without an apparent efficacy loss (Okamoto et al., 2005).

Chemotherapy combinations constituting a variety of newer agents, like irinotecan, have been tested in an effort to improve current outcomes in LS-SCLC. However, these agents do not appear to be more active than older counterparts. Irinotecan, which was the most promising of them, has been tested in three randomized phase 3 trials (Hanna, 2006; Lara, 2009; Noda, 2002). The first trial by Noda et al. demonstrated the superiority of cisplatin plus irinotecan (IP) over the standard EP combination in a Japanese Clinical Oncology Group (JCOG) trial (Noda et al., 2002). However, two subsequent trials launched in United States could not validate these results (Hanna, 2006; Lara, 2009). In both trials response and survival rates in patients treated with investigational IP were found to be equivalent to standard EP. The potential benefit of adding a third agent to standard EP has also been extensively investigated. Higher response rates at a cost of significantly increased toxicity were achieved, with no notable improvement in median survival duration over EP alone (Loehrer, 1995; Mavroudis, 2001; Niell, 2005; Pujol, 2001).

Based on these results, the current standard for the first line chemotherapy in this group of patients is 4 to 6 cycles of EP combination, and further treatment with either maintenance therapy or four cycles of topotecan following standard EP regimen has not been proved to improve outcomes (Schiller, 2001; Sculier, 1998).

4.2 Thoracic radiotherapy

Before the introduction of chemotherapy in the 1970s, thoracic radiotherapy (TRT) was the mainstay of treatment for LS-SCLC. However, management of LS-SCLC with chemotherapy alone results in unacceptable rates of intrathoracic failures, ranging from 75 to90% (Faivre-Finn et al. 2005). In this setting, integration of TRT to chemotherapy reduces these failures up to 30 to 60%. Impact of such a decrease in intrathoracic failures has been extensively investigated by two meta-analyses (Pignon, 1992; Warde & Payne, 1992). In the first one, Warde and Payne (Warde & Payne, 1992) analyzed 11 randomized studies including 1911 patients, and reported a significantly longer overall survival with the combination of TRT and chemotherapy than with chemotherapy alone, with an absolute benefit of 5.4% at 2-year ($p<0.001$). In the other meta-analysis, Pignon et al. (Pignon et al., 1992) included 13 trials consisting of 2103 LS-SCLC patients. Combination of TRT and chemotherapy again resulted in an absolute survival advantage of 5.4% at 3-year compared to chemotherapy alone ($p=0.001$). Based on the results of these two meta-analyses combination of TRT and chemotherapy became the established standard of care in LS-SCLC.

TRT delivered both sequentially and concurrently with chemotherapy has been intensively assessed. Although sequential treatment approach has the theoretical benefits by chance of irradiating smaller target volumes with resultant reduced toxicity rates, the associated longer overall treatment time potentially increases the risk of accelerated tumor repopulation and development of treatment-resistant clones. In this context, concurrent use of chemotherapy and TRT does not only reduce the risk for accelerated repopulation but also offers a chance for better locoregional control by utilizing the radiosensitizing efficacy of chemotherapeutic agents. Nevertheless, despite such potential benefits, because of increased risk for higher rates of acute toxicity with concurrent chemoradiotherapy, sequential use of chemotherapy and TRT may be more feasible in elderly patients or those with larger tumors.

Data on the optimum radiotherapy dose and fractionation come mostly from retrospective and phase 2 prospective studies. The results from non-randomized studies indicate a notable increase in local control when the dose of TRT is increased from 35 to 40 Gy, and a slightly further gain with 50 Gy. Laboratory studies have suggested that typical SCLC cell lines have radiation survival curves with little shoulders indicating that accelerated fractionation schemes would, therefore, be advantageous (van Meerbeeck et al., 2011). In 1999, two different cooperative groups randomized patients to once-a-day versus twice-a-day TRT with concurrent chemotherapy, as depicted in Table 1 (Bonner, 1999; Turrisi, 1999). In the study by Bonner et al., authors reported the North Central Cancer Treatment Group (NCCTG) experience, and concluded that there was no difference in survival with twice-daily TRT versus once daily counterpart (Bonner et al., 1999). However, this study has been criticized because of using split-course RT schedule which is currently an established factor to increase the chance for accelerated repopulation, and therefore, affect treatment outcomes in an unfavorable fashion. In the landmark study by Turissi et al. (Int-0096), authors reported the long-term outcomes of 358 patients enrolled onto the cooperative group study of Eastern Cooperative Oncology Group/ Radiation Therapy Oncology Group (ECOG/RTOG) with the diagnosis of LS-SCLC. Results of this study demonstrated that twice-daily 45 Gy (1.5 Gy BID) and concurrent CRT was significantly superior over conventionally fractionated TRT scheme (Turrisi et al., 1999). Based on the results of this latter study, the current standard of care for medically fit LS-SCLC became the 45 Gy (1.5 Gy BID) TRT and concurrent EP. Nonetheless, because of the higher frequency of dose limiting ≥ Grade 3 esophagitis in twice-daily TRT scheme, 54 Gy (1.8 Gy per fraction) in 30 days and concurrent EP is also a common and acceptable treatment scheme.

Carcinoma and Leukemia Group B (CALGB) conducted two phase 2 trials to investigate the potential benefit of a higher dose of 70 Gy given in 35 fractions within 7 weeks (Bogart, 2004; Miller, 2007). In the first study, median survival, 2-year survival rate, and ≥ Grade 3 esophagitis rate were 22 months, 48%, and 21%, respectively (Bogart et al., 2004). In the second study respective rates were 20 months, 35%, and 30% (Miller et al., 2007). Based on the promising results of these two trials, two ongoing randomized Phase 3 trials were conducted to compare standard Turissi protocol with escalated doses of conventionally fractionated TRT. Results of these two landmark trials summarized in Table 2, will address the question whether the higher doses delivered by once daily scheme in 7-week, could compensate for the longer interval between the initiation of treatment and the end of TRT, in the expense of increased risk for accelerated tumor cell repopulation.

In treatment of LS-SCLC, another issue of interest is whether TRT should be administered early or late during the chemotherapy course. This question has been addressed by a number of trials with no firm conclusions (Gregor, 1997; Jeremic, 1997; Murray, 1993; Perry,

	ECOG/RTOG		P	NCCTG		P
Study Arms	Chemo + TRT	Chemo + twice daily TRT		Chemo + TRT	Chemo + twice daily TRT	
Number	176	182	-	133	130	-
Total cycles of CTX	4	4	-	6	6	-
Cycles of concurrent CTX	2	2	-	2	2	-
Median survival (mo)	18.6	20.3	0.04	21	21	0.49
2-year survival (%)	42	44		47	45	
3-year survival (%)	-	-		34	29	
5-year survival (%)	16	26		-	-	
≥Grad 3 Esophagitis	33 (16%)	67 (32%)	<0.001	7 (5.3%)	16 (12.3%)	0.05
≥Grad 3 Pulmonary toxicity	8 (4%)	14 (5%)	0.97	6 (4.5%)	8 (6.2%)	>0.05

Table 1. Limited-stage small cell lung cancer with daily versus twice-daily TRT

Study	CTX	Standard arm	Experimental arm	Primary endpoint	Expected enrollment
CONVERT	4xEP	45 Gy/30 fx, 3 week, BID, starting at second course	66 Gy/33 fx, 6.6 week, once-daily, starting at second course	Overall survival	532
RTOG0538/ CALGB30610	4xEP	45 Gy/30 fx, 3 week, BID, starting at first or second course	A: 70 Gy/35 fx, 7 week, once-daily B: 61.2 Gy/34 fx, 5 week, BID, starting at first course	Overall survival	712

Table 2. Benchmark ongoing trials of chemoradiotherapy for limited-stage small-cell lung carcinoma

1987; Skarlos, 2001; Takada, 2002; Work, 1997). In the landmark phase 3 ECOG/RTOG trial reported by Turissi et al., the shortening of total irradiation period from 5 weeks to 3 weeks was associated with an absolute 10% (16% versus 26%) increase in 5-year survival (Turrisi et al., 1999). Results of three other trials revealed a significantly superior survival advantage for early TRT over late TRT, confirming the findings of intergroup trial (Jeremic, 1997; Murray, 1993; Takada, 2002). The impact of timing of TRT relative to chemotherapy has also been addressed by various meta-analyses. De Ruysscher and colleagues conducted a meta-analysis of phase III trials combining TRT and platinum-based chemotherapy, and concluded that the most important predictor of 5-year survival was the interim between the start of any treatment until the end of RT (SER), with shorter SERs (<30 days) being associated with the highest 5-year survival rates (>20%) (De Ruysscher et al., 2006). With a subsequent meta-analysis, Pijls-Johannesma and colleagues evaluated the impact of timing of TRT by comparing early versus late TRT, by defining early TRT as within 30 days of beginning chemotherapy. In presence of platinum-based chemotherapy, the 2- and 5-year survival rates were favoring early TRT, and this difference was significant only if the TRT was administered in a treatment period of less than 30 days. In this study, patient compliance was found to be of paramount importance, indicating the importance of patient selection in clinical trials (Pijls-Johannesma et al., 2007). In a relatively older meta-analysis by Fried et al., late TRT was defined as beginning 9 weeks after the initiation of chemotherapy or after the completion of third cycle of chemotherapy. Similar to other subsequent meta-analyses, this meta-analysis also demonstrated a statistically significant benefit of early TRT over late TRT in terms of 2-year overall survival. On subset analysis of studies that used hyperfractionated TRT, treatment with early versus late TRT revealed a survival benefit, but not when once-daily TRT was employed. Likewise, the survival benefit for early versus late TRT was observed uniquely in studies using platinum-based chemotherapy, which was not notable in studies using non-platinum-based chemotherapy (Fried et al., 2004). Results of the available studies and meta-analyses suggested an interaction between TRT and chemotherapy and, accelerated tumor cell repopulation was postulated to be triggered by the first dose of any effective cytotoxic agent (De Ruysscher et al., 2006). Therefore, to obtain the highest chance for local/regional control, the last clonogenic tumor cell should be killed by the end of TRT (van Meerbeeck et al., 2011). Hence, long-term survival decreases with increasing time between the initiations of any treatment and the completion of TRT.

In summary, current evidence recommends the early administration of 45 Gy (1.5 Gy, BID) with concurrent EP at systemic doses in medically fit LS-SCLC patients.

4.4 Radiotherapy techniques and treatment fields

Treatment for lung tumors, including SCLC, is complex. In order to ensure safe and effective RT, several issues must be considered: (a) accurate target volume delineation; (b) proximity of dose limiting normal structures (lung, spinal cord, esophagus, heart, brachial plexus, and liver); (c) anatomic slope of the chest surface; (d) inhomogenities resulting from the presence of nonuniform tissues on the way of RT; (e) frequent need for irregular field dose calculations; (f) respiratory motion of the targeted tumor and normal tissues such as lung, heart and liver, depending on the location of the primary tumor and involved lymphatic region(s).

The ultimate goal of any RT application is to deliver the prescribed dose homogenously (not cooler than 95% and not hotter than 107%) to the planned target volume and keep the dose to non-tumorous normal tissues as minimum as possible respecting their tissue architecture (serial versus parallel) and their radiation tolerance limits. In this setting, with the aid of imaging with anatomic computerized tomography (CT), functional 18-F-fluorodeoxyglucose positron emission tomography (PET), preferably fusion of both) and the use of 3–dimensional conformal RT, and novel 4-dimensional image-guided RT (IGRT), it is easier than before to achieve these goals. Additionally, the dose-volume histograms (DVH) created for each patient makes it possible to anticipate the potential early and late toxicity risks based on the organ of interest measures and, therefore, modify the treatment plans as necessitated.

There is considerable debate on the size of the RT portals of SCLC. Historically, RT portals were large, encompassing the primary tumor as well as both hilar, entire mediastinal and both supraclavicular lymph node regions with generous margins. This was believed to be necessary to ensure adequate coverage of gross disease prior to the routine use of CT- based RT planning. Although such large field plans may guarantee the irradiation of target volumes, they are also associated with increased acute and late toxicity rates and unplanned

treatment delays, which may negatively impact both quality of life measures and local/regional control rates and related survival outcomes. This issue is specifically argued when TRT is delayed after the completion of induction chemotherapy. Although some authors advocate generous portals encompassing the pre-chemotherapy volumes as stated above, others argue that only limited portals encompassing the pre-chemotherapy primary tumor and high-risk nodal areas with a 1-cm margin are adequate, since effective chemotherapy has the theoretical chance to cope with subclinical or microscopic disease eliminating the need for generous portals. This latter approach has the additional potential for decreased treatment related toxicity specifically when TRT is administered concurrently with chemotherapy. Treatment directed at pre- versus post-chemotherapy volumes is also an ongoing issue of conflict. The unique randomized trial that addressed this issue is the one conducted by the South West Oncology Group (SWOG). In this study, patients achieving a partial response after chemotherapy were randomized to pre- versus post-chemotherapy volume irradiation arms. Outcomes of this benchmark study did not indicate any superiority for pre-chemotherapy volume irradiation arm over post-chemotherapy irradiation counterpart, in terms of neither local/regional nor survival rates (Kies et al., 1987). This issue has latter been investigated by Liengswangwong et al. in a retrospective analysis. The authors were unable to find a benefit favoring pre-chemotherapy large-field TRT over post-chemotherapy limited-field TRT (Liengswangwong et al., 1994).
In NSCLC, elective irradiation of hilar and/or mediastinal lymphatic regions has gradually been replaced by treatment limited to nodes identified by CT or FDG -PET as being involved. For SCLC, evidence is scarce to support this approach. In a prospective study by De Ruysscher et al., authors limited the RT fields to only CT-positive mediastinal lymph nodes in a cohort of 27 patients with LS-SCLC. The authors reported an isolated regional recurrence rate of 11%, which was higher than similar studies using elective mediastinal irradiation. However, because of small sample size, no definitive conclusions can be drawn from this study (De Ruysscher et al., 2006). In a larger phase 2 study including 60 LS-SCLC patients, van Loon et al., irradiated only the lymph nodes that appeared to be involved on FDG-PET, and reported an isolated nodal failure rate of 3%, which awaits to be confirmed by further studies with larger cohorts (van Loon et al., 2010). A typical 3-D conformal RT plan used in our institution and associated DVH is shown in Figure 1.

4.5 Prophylactic cranial irradiation

Approximately 10-14% of SCLC patients have detectable brain metastases (BM) at the time of initial diagnosis (Hardy et al., 1990). During the course of disease, the incidence of BM increases up to more than 50%, which is far beyond in postmortem examinations (Hirsch, 1983; Nicholson, 2002). The incidence of BM is directly proportional with the survival time, indicating a potential for further increase with implementation of more effective treatment protocols (Komaki, 1981; van Oosterhout, 1996). Compared to patients with LS-SCLC, the risk for BM occurrence is higher for patients with ES-SCLC reaching 69% at 2- years of diagnosis (van Oosterhout, 1996; Yang GY & Matthews, 2000).
Impact of BM on socioeconomic issues and quality of life is significantly worse than the impact of failure at other metastatic sites. Patients with BM are often obliged to spend significant time hospitalized, and suffer loss of independence (Felletti et al., 1985). Despite cranial irradiation and/or chemotherapy, the treatment of clinically established BM is partially satisfactory with intracranial disease control rates of about 50% and overall survival of 4 to 6 months (Carmichael, 1988; Lucas, 1986; Postmus, 1989).

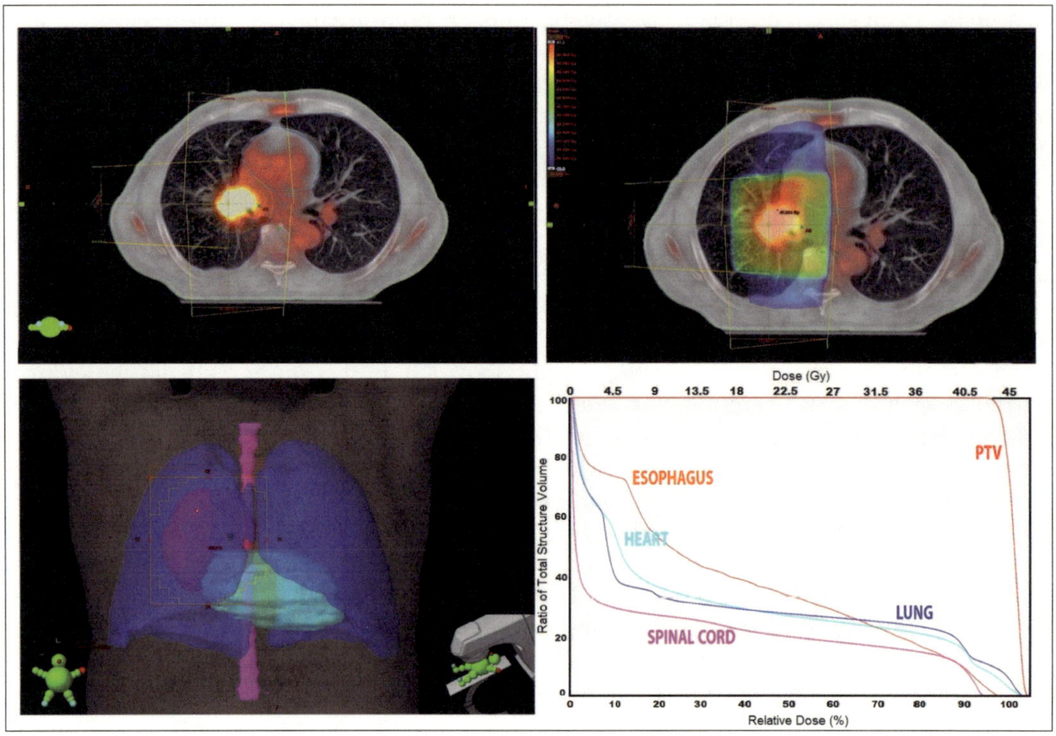

Fig. 1. An example of typical 3-D conformal RT plan and associated DVH.

Several randomized trials have been conducted to investigate the utility of prophylactic cranial irradiation (PCI) in prevention of BM development in patients with LS-SCLC. Logically, in patients with extracranial disease under control, PCI may eliminate the intracranial microscopic tumor cell deposits with relatively low radiation doses and, therefore, may increase the long-term survival. Results of two randomized controlled trials from France (PCI85) and United Kingdom (UK02) demonstrated a trend for better survival with PCI but neither could reach statistical significance (Arriagada, 1995; Gregor, 1997). Up till now, no individual randomized trial has conclusively demonstrated a survival benefit for PCI, which may be related with their deficiency in provision of sufficient power to detect moderate differences in survival.

To conduct a meta-analysis of trials using PCI and to make recommendations for clinical practice, the PCI Overview Collaborative Group was established. The meta-analysis reported by Auperin et al. in 1999 included individual data from patients enrolled on seven prospective randomized PCI trials. Trials eligible in the meta-analysis were limited to those, in which patients had been treated with systemic chemotherapy with/without TRT to a complete clinical response, and no known BM. PCI treatments were generally between 24 to 40 Gy, administered in 2-3 Gy per day. Results of this meta-analysis, for the first time, demonstrated a statistically significant survival advantage favoring PCI over non-PCI arm. The relative risk for death in the treatment group, as compared to control group, was 0.84 (95 CI, 0.73-0.97; P= 0.01), which corresponds to a 5.4% higher rate of survival at 3 years (20.7% versus 15.3%), and the survival advantage persisted over time. As a percent gain over control, this represents a 35% increase in the proportion of surviving patients. There was also significant difference in disease-free survival at 3 years from 13.3% in the non-PCI group to 22.1% in the PCI group ($p<0.0001$). PCI was additionally associated with a 25.3% absolute decrease in the cumulative incidence of BM at 3 years, from 58.6% to 33.3% ($p<0.0001$) (Auperin et al., 1999). Results of this comprehensive meta-analysis have recently been confirmed by the review of data from Surveillance Epidemiology and End Results (SEER) reported by Patel et al. Of 7995 LS-SCLC patients included, 670 received PCI. Better overall and cause-specific survival were observed in patients treated with PCI, and corresponding 2- and 5-year survival rates were 23% and 11% without PCI and 425% and 19% with PCI (Patel et al., 2009).

Based on the results of meta-analysis by Auperin et al., PCI became the standard of care in patients with LS-SCLC demonstrating complete response following systemic and/or local/regional treatment (Auperin et al., 1999). However, an important concern about the use of PCI is the need for determination of an established non-toxic but effective fractionation scheme and total dose. Available data have shown that lower doses of PCI may be less effective in preventing CNS failures (Auperin, 1999; Gregor, 1997). Recently, Le Pechoux et al. published the results of benchmark international PCI trial evaluating radiation dose for PCI in LS-SCLC. The study randomized 720 LS-SCLC patients from 157 centers to one of two PCI arms: Arm-1 included patients receiving standard-dose PCI to 25 Gy in 2.5 Gy per fraction, and Arm 2 included patients receiving higher dose PCI to 36 Gy delivered in 2 Gy once daily or 1.5 Gy twice daily. No significant difference of BM incidence was reported between two study arms, but there was a significantly higher rate of cancer-related mortality in the higher dose arm as a result of unexplained finding of more deaths from extracranial disease progression (Le Pechoux et al., 2009). Based on the results of this study, 25 Gy delivered at 2.5 Gy per fraction per day remains the standard of care for PCI in LS-SCLC patients.

5. Treatment for extensive-stage small cell lung carcinoma

5.1 Radiotherapy

Combination chemotherapy is the mainstay in the management of ES-SCLC, but as intrathoracic disease control may be a significant challenge to overcome in a significant proportion of patients, role of consolidative TRT has been addressed in several trials. Jeremic et al. randomized patients with ES-SCLC, who responded completely at extrathoracic sites and at least partially at thorax, to consolidation TRT versus observation arms after 3 cycles of systemic chemotherapy. In experimental arm, TRT was administered in an accelerated hyperfractionated scheme of 54 Gy given in 1.5 Gy twice daily fractions concurrently with EP chemotherapy. The median and a 5-year overall survival in the TRT arm and no TRT arm were 17 versus 11 month and 9.1% versus 3.7%, respectively (Jeremic et al, 1999). However, the results of ongoing studies addressing the question of TRT both in Netherlands and in Canada should be awaited before its routine recommendation for patients with ES-SCLC.

5.2 Prophylactic cranial irradiation

Although the beneficial effects of PCI on prevention of BM occurrence and on augmentation of overall and disease-free survival have been well established in LS-SCLC patients, this issue had remained to be answered in ES-SCLC until the publication of the results of recent EORTC trial. In this benchmark study, patients with ES-SCLC who had a response to chemotherapy were randomized to PCI versus observation arms. The cumulative risk of symptomatic BM at 1-year and the 1-year survival rate were 14.6% versus 40.4% ($p<0.001$), and 27.1% versus 13.3% (p=0.003), both favoring the PCI arm (Slotman et al., 2007). Following this study, similar to LS-SCLC, PCI became the standard of care in ES-SCLC patients except for those experience disease progression during chemotherapy.

6. Treatment related toxicity

Acute side effects of CRT often begin during the second or third weeks of treatment. Cessation of the tobacco abuse should be the first step in the management of SCLC patients to increase the efficacy of intended CRT as well as to decrease the incidence and severity of the treatment related side effects. Dermatitis may be seen but severe cases are rare. Prevention of trauma is the key for prevention of severe and difficult to treat dermatitis development. Aloe vera gel and perfume-free ointments can be safely used in mild to moderate dermatitis. Acute esophagitis is usually the dose limiting toxicity of mediastinal irradiation, which rarely progress to severe late esophagitis. In patients with mild to moderate swallowing difficulty, semisolid nutrition and liquid form analgesics may be beneficial. Although confirmation with randomized controlled Phase 3 trials are needed, based on the results of two recent retrospective series by Algara et al. and Topkan et al., prophylactic use of glutamine may be beneficial in preventing and reducing the severity of acute esophagitis (Algara, 2007; Topkan, 2009). Nonproductive dry cough may be seen if trachea and/or major bronchi is/are involved in the high dose radiation portals.

After the completion of TRT, radiation pneumonitis (RP) may be seen at 2 to 4 weeks. RP is a form of radiation-induced lung disease, mimicking bacterial pneumonia. Symptoms usually include non-productive dry cough, dyspnea, chest pain, palpitations, malaise, and occasionally fever. Rales can be noted on auscultation. Plain X-rays and CT are beneficial in demonstrating the extent of perivascular haziness and alveolar filling densities primarily within the radiation portal. Treatment of RP includes use of 60 mg/day prednisone for two weeks followed by gradual tapering at following 3 to 12 weeks. There is no evidence supporting the use of prophylactic use of glucocorticoids or antibiotics in preventing or reducing the severity of RP.

Late toxicities involve chronic esophagitis, pericarditis, myocarditis, pancarditis, spinal cord injury, radiation induced lung fibrosis, and secondary cancers. Incidence and severity of all these late toxicities depend on the total dose and dose per fraction, fractionation scheme, interim between subsequent fractions, volume of non-target organ exposed to specified doses of RT, and concurrent use of chemotherapy. Currently, excluding the symptomatic management measures, the best treatment method is prevention of toxicity in the presence of agents with at best limited healing efficacy. To achieve this, tolerance doses must be strictly respected. Specific for radiation-induced lung fibrosis, which may potentially be fatal, a recent study demonstrated promising efficacy of pentoxyfilline and alpha-tocopherol combination in reduction of fibrotic lung area up to 50% at median 24 months of drug use.

At long-term, potential neurocognitive toxicity of PCI is of great concern, since sequalae like severe memory loss, intellectual impairment or even dementia, ataxia, or seizures have been reported in retrospective studies with small size and questionable methodology. For example, neurocognitive assessments prior to chemotherapy and/or PCI are lacking despite the fact that almost 50% of SCLC patients have neurologic and neurocognitive impairments prior to onset of PCI (Arriagada, 1995; Gregor, 1997; Grosshans, 2008; Komaki, 1995). Neurocognitive impairment risk has been reported to strongly associate with daily fraction sizes of >3 Gy (Paumier & A Le Péchoux, 2010). In one study, Shaw et al. found that the risk for neurocognitive impairment following PCI was 2% and 10% at 2- and 5-year follow-ups, respectively. Furthermore, the authors reported that all toxicities were seen with regimens using daily fraction sizes of >3 Gy (Shaw et al., 1994). Notably, two randomized studies with neurocognitive assessments in patients randomized to PCI versus non-PCI did not demonstrate any deterioration in neurologic functions at 30 months, and quality of life measures at baseline, at 6 and 12 months (Arriagada, 1995; Gregor, 1997). However, these findings do not mean that PCI has no potential toxicity and should be administered to every patient with the diagnosis SCLC, rather they impact the importance of patient selection based on neurocognitive tests for safer PCI applications.

7. Treatment algorithm for LS-SCLC and ES-SCLC

Our current instutitional treatment algorithm for LS-SCLC and ES-SCLC patients is as depicted in Figure 2.

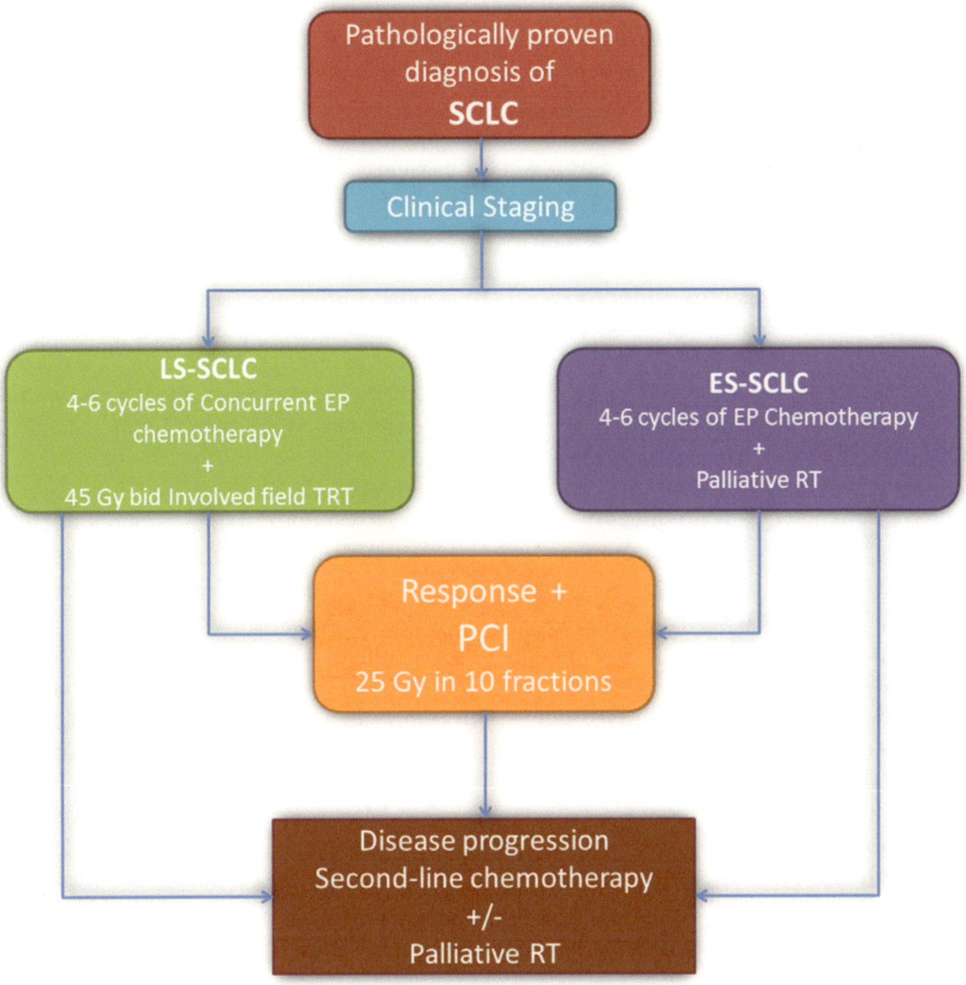

Fig. 2. Management Algorithm for LS-SCLC and ES-SCLC

8. Conclusion

Significant progress has been made in diagnosis and treatment of SCLC in the last 25 years, but, with an overall median survival time of 18 to 20 months, even in patients with limited-stage disease, it is still not possible to consider SCLC in the category of curable cancers. Despite this disappointing figure, mandating further research on this highly fatal disease, all improvements in LS-SCLC have been achieved by concurrent use chemotherapy and TRT (as early as possible), chemotherapy and PCI. For medically fit patients with ES-SCLC, combination chemotherapy followed by PCI (in non-progressive cases) is the standard of care, and further consolidation with TRT is currently under investigation. It is of paramount importance that patients with ES-SCLC be given the chance to participate in future trials for identification of a new and effective treatment combination, which may potentially offer a longer survival.

9. References

Alavanja, M.C. (2002). Biologic damage resulting from exposure to tobacco smoke and from radon: Implication for preventive interventions. *Oncogene*, Vol.21, No.48, (October 2002), pp.7365-7375.

Albain, K.S., Crowley, J.J., & Livingston, R.B. Long-term survival and toxicity in small cell lung cancer. Expanded Southwest Oncology Group experience. (1991). *Chest*, Vol.99, No.6, (June 1991), pp.1425-32.

Algara, M., Rodriguez, N., Vinals, P., Lacruz, M., Foro, P., Reig, A., Quera, J., Lozano, J., Fernandez-Velilla, E., Membrive, I., Dengra, J., & Sanz, X. (2007). Prevention of radiochemotherapy-induced esophagitis with glutamine: results of a pilot study. *Int J Radiat Oncol Biol Phys*, Vol.69, No.2, (October 2007), pp.342-349.

Arriagada, R., Le Chevalier, T., Borie, F., Riviere, A., Chomy, P., Monnet, I., Tardivon, A., Viader, F., Tarayre, M., & Benhamou, S. (1995). Prophylactic cranial irradiation for patients with small-cell lung cancer in complete remission. *J Natl Cancer Inst*, Vol.87, No.3, (February 1995), pp.183-190.

Auperin, A., Arriagada, R., Pignon, J.P., Le Pechoux, C., Gregor, A., Stephens, R.J., Kristjansen, P.E., Johnson, B.E., Ueoka, H., Wagner, H., & Aisner, J. (1999). Prophylactic cranial irradiation for patients with small-cell lung cancer in complete remission. Prophylactic Cranial Irradiation Overview Collaborative Group. *N Engl J Med*, Vol.341, No.7, (August 1999), pp.476-484.

Bogart, J.A., Herndon, J.E., Lyss, A.P., Watson, D., Miller, A.A., Lee, M.E., Turrisi, A.T., & Green, M.R. (2004). 70 Gy thoracic radiotherapy is feasible concurrent with chemotherapy for limited-stage small-cell lung cancer: analysis of Cancer and Leukemia Group B study 39808. *Int J Radiat Oncol Biol Phys*, Vol.59, No.2, (June 2004), pp.460-468.

Bonner, J.A., Sloan, J.A., Shanahan, T.G., Brooks, B.J., Marks, R.S., Krook, J.E., Gerstner, J.B., Maksymiuk, A., Levitt, R., Mailliard, J.A., Tazelaar, H.D., Hillman, S., & Jett, J.R. (1999). Phase III comparison of twice-daily split-course irradiation versus once-daily irradiation for patients with limited stage small-cell lung carcinoma. *J Clin Oncol*, Vol.17, No.9, (September 1999), pp.2681-2691.

Brambilla, E., Travis, W.D., Colby, T.V., Corrin, B., & Shimosato, Y. (2001). The new World Health Organization classification of lung tumors. Eur Respir J, Vol.18, No.6, pp.1059-68.

Byhardt, R.W., Hartz, A., Libnoch, J.A., Hansen, R., & Cox JD. (1986). Prognostic influence of TNM staging and LDH levels in small cell carcinoma of the lung (SCCL). *Int J Radiat Oncol Biol Phys,* Vol.12, No.5, (May 1986), pp.771-777.

Carmichael, J., Crane, J.M., Bunn, P.A., Glatstein, E., & Ihde, D.C. (1988). Results of therapeutic cranial irradiation in small cell lung cancer. *Int J Radiat Oncol Biol Phys,* Vol.14, No.3, (March 1988) pp.455-459.

Chute, J.P., Venzon, D.J., Hankins, B.S., Okunieff, P., Frame, J.N., Ihde, D.C., & Johnson, B.E. (1997). Outcome of patients with small-cell lung cancer during 20 years of clinical research at the US National Cancer Institute. *Mayo Clin Proc* Vol.72, No.10, (October 1997), pp.901-912.

De Ruysscher, D., Pijls-Johannesma, M., Bentzen, S.M., Minken, A., Wanders, R., Lutgens, L., Hochstenbag, M., Boersma, L., Wouters, B., Lammering, G., Vansteenkiste, J., & Lambin, P. (2006).Time between the first day of chemotherapy and the last day of chest radiation is the most important predictor of survival in limited-disease small-cell lung cancer. *J Clin Oncol,* Vol.24, No.7, (March 2006), pp.1057-1063.

De Ruysscher, D., Bremer, R.H., Koppe, F., Wanders, S., van Haren, E., Hochstenbag, M., Geeraedts, W., Pitz, C., Simons, J., ten Velde, G., Dohmen, J., Snoep, G., Boersma, L., Verschueren, T., van Baardwijk, A., Dehing, C., Pijls, M., Minken, A., & Lambin, P. (2006). Omission of elective node irradiation on basis of CT-scans in patients with limited disease small cell lung cancer: a phase II trial. *Radiother Oncol,* Vol.80, No.3, (September 2006), pp.307-312.

Edge, S.B., Byrd, D.R., Compton, C.C., Fritz, A.G., Greene, F.L., & Trotti, A. (2010). *AJCC Cancer Staging Manual, 7th ed.,*ISBN: 0387884408, Springer, New York.

Faivre-Finn, C., Lorigan, P., West, C., & Thatcher, N. (2005). Thoracic radiation therapy for limited-stage small-cell lung cancer: unanswered questions. *Clin Lung Cancer,* Vol.7, No.1, (July 2005), pp.23-29.

Felletti, R., Souhami, R.L., Spiro, S.G., Geddes, D.M., Tobias, J.S., Mantell, B.S., Harper, P.G., & Trask, C. (1985). Social consequences of brain or liver relapse in small cell carcinoma of the bronchus. *Radiother Oncol,* Vol.4, No.4, (December 1985), pp.335-339.

Fried, D.B., Morris, D.E., Poole, C., Rosenman, J.G., Halle, J.S., Detterbeck, F.C., Hensing, T.A., & Socinski, M.A. (2004) Systematic review evaluating the timing of thoracic radiation therapy in combined modality therapy for limited-stage small-cell lung cancer. *J Clin Oncol,* Vol.22, No.23, (December 2004), pp.4837-4845.

Fukuoka, M., Furuse, K., Saijo, N., Nishiwaki, Y., Ikegami, H., Tamura, T., Shimoyama, M., & Suemasu, K. (1991). Randomized trial of cyclophosphamide, doxorubicin, and vincristine versus cisplatin and etoposide versus alternation of these regimens in small-cell lung cancer. *J Natl Cancer Inst,* Vol. 83, No.12, pp.855-861.

Greene, F.L., Page, D.L., Fleeming, I.D., Fritz, A., Balch, C.M., Haller, D.G., & Marrow M. (2002). *AJCC Cancer Staging Manual, 6th ed.* ISBN: 0387952713, Springer, New York.

Gregor, A., Drings, P., Burghouts, J., Postmus, P.E., Morgan, D., Sahmoud, T., Kirkpatrick, A., Dalesio, O., & Giaccone, G. (1997). Randomized trial of alternating versus sequential radiotherapy/chemotherapy in limited-disease patients with small-cell lung cancer: a

European Organization for Research and Treatment of Cancer Lung Cancer Cooperative Group Study. *J Clin Oncol*, Vol.15, No.8, (August 1997), pp.2840-2849.

Gregor, A., Cull, A., Stephens, R.J., Kirkpatrick, J.A., Yarnold, J.R., Girling, D.J., Macbeth, F.R., Stout, R., & Machin, D. (1997). Prophylactic cranial irradiation is indicated following complete response to induction therapy in small cell lung cancer: results of a multicentre randomised trial. United Kingdom Coordinating Committee for Cancer Research (UKCCCR) and the European Organization for Research and Treatment of Cancer (EORTC). *Eur J Cancer*, Vol.33, No.11, (October 1997), pp.1752-1758.

Grosshans, D.R., Meyers, C.A., Allen, P.K., Davenport, S.D., & Komaki, R. (2008). Neurocognitive function in patients with small cell lung cancer: effect of prophylactic cranial irradiation. *Cancer*, Vol.112, No.3, (February 2008), pp.589-595.

Hanna, N., Bunn, P.A., Langer, C., Einhorn, L., Guthrie, T., Beck, T., Ansari, R., Ellis, P., Byrne, M., Morrison, M., Hariharan, S., Wang, B., & Sandler, A. (2006). Randomized phase III trial comparing irinotecan/cisplatin with etoposide/cisplatin in patients with previously untreated extensive-stage disease small-cell lung cancer. *J Clin Oncol*, Vol.24, (May 2006), No.13, pp.2038-2043.

Hardy, J., Smith, I., Cherryman, G., Vincent, M., Judson, I., Perren, T., & Williams, M. (1990). The value of computed tomographic (CT) scan surveillance in the detection and management of brain metastases in patients with small cell lung cancer. *Br J Cancer*. Vol.62, No.4, (October 1990), pp.684-686.

Hirsch, F.R., Paulson, O.B., Hansen, H.H., & Larsen, S.O. (1983). Intracranial metastases in small cell carcinoma of the lung. Prognostic aspects. *Cancer*. Vol.51, No.3, (February 1983), pp.529-533.

Jemal, A., Siegel, R., Ward, E., Hao, Y., Xu, J., & Thun, M.J. (2009). Cancer statistics, 2009. *CA Cancer J Clin*, Vol.59, No.4, (July 2009), pp.225-249.

Jeremic, B., Shibamoto, Y., Acimovic, L., & Milisavljevic, S. Initial versus delayed accelerated hyperfractionated radiation therapy and concurrent chemotherapy in limited small-cell lung cancer: a randomized study. *J Clin Oncol*, Vol.15, No.3, (March 1997), pp.893-900.

Jeremic, B., Shibamoto, Y., Nikolic, N., Milicic, B., Milisavljevic, S., Dagovic, A., Aleksandrovic, J., & Radosavljevic-Asic G. (1999). Role of radiation therapy in the combined-modality treatment of patients with extensive disease small-cell lung cancer: A randomized study. *J Clin Oncol*, Vol.17, No.7, (July 1999), pp.2092-2099.

Kies, M.S., Mira, J.G., Crowley, J.J., Chen, T.T., Pazdur, R., Grozea, P.N., Rivkin, S.E., Coltman, C.A., Ward, J.H., & Livingston, R.B. (1987). Multimodal therapy for limited small-cell lung cancer: a randomized study of induction combination chemotherapy with or without thoracic radiation in complete responders; and with wide-field versus reduced-field radiation in partial responders: a Southwest Oncology Group Study. *J Clin Oncol*, Vol.5, No.4, (April 1987), pp.592-600.

Komaki, R., Cox, J.D., & Whitson, W. (1981). Risk of brain metastasis from small cell carcinoma of the lung related to length of survival and prophylactic irradiation. *Cancer Treat Rep*,Vol.65, No.9, (September 1981), pp.811-814.

Komaki, R., Meyers, C.A., Shin, D.M., Garden, A.S., Byrne, K., Nickens, J.A., & Cox, J.D. Evaluation of cognitive function in patients with limited small cell lung cancer prior to and shortly following prophylactic cranial irradiation. *Int J Radiat Oncol Biol Phys*, Vol.33, No.1, (1995 August), pp.179-182.

Lally, B.E., Urbanic, J.J., Blackstock, A.W., Miller, A.A., & Perry, M.C. (2007) Small cell lung cancer: Have we made any progress over the last 25 years? *Oncologist*, Vol.12, No.9, (May 2007) pp.1096-1104.

Lara, P.N., Natale, R., Crowley, J., Lenz, H.J., Redman, M.W., Carleton, J.E., Jett, J., Langer, C.J., Kuebler, J.P., Dakhil, S.R., Chansky, K., & Gandara, D.R. (2009). Phase III trial of irinotecan/cisplatin compared with etoposide/cisplatin in extensive-stage small-cell lung cancer: clinical and pharmacogenomic results from SWOG S0124. J Clin Oncol, Vol.27, No.15, (May 2009), pp.2530-2535.

Lassen, U., Osterlind, K., Hansen, M., Dombernowsky, P., Bergman, B., & Hansen, H.H. (1995). Long-term survival in small-cell lung cancer: posttreatment characteristics in patients surviving 5 to 18+ years--an analysis of 1,714 consecutive patients. *J Clin Oncol*, Vol.13, No.5, (May 1995), pp.1215-1220.

Le Pechoux, C., Dunant, A., Senan, S., Wolfson, A., Quoix, E., Faivre-Finn, C., Ciuleanu, T., Arriagada, R., Jones, R., Wanders, R., Lerouge, D., & Laplanche, A. (2009). Prophylactic Cranial Irradiation (PCI) Collaborative Group. Standard-dose versus higher-dose prophylactic cranial irradiation (PCI) in patients with limited-stage small-cell lung cancer in complete remission after chemotherapy and thoracic radiotherapy (PCI 99-01, EORTC 22003-08004, RTOG 0212, and IFCT 99-01): a randomised clinical trial. *Lancet Oncol*, Vol.10, No.5, (May 2009), pp.467-474.

Liengswangwong, V., Bonner, J.A., Shaw, E.G., Foote, R.L., Frytak, S., Eagan, R.T., Jett, J.R., Richardson, R.L., Creagan, E.T., & Su, J.Q. (1994). Limited-stage small-cell lung cancer: patterns of intrathoracic recurrence and the implications for thoracic radiotherapy. *J Clin Oncol*, Vol.12, No.3, (March 1994), pp.496-502.

Loehrer, P.J., Ansari, R., Gonin, R., Monaco, F., Fisher, W., Sandler, A., & Einhorn, L.H. Cisplatin plus etoposide with and without ifosfamide in extensive small-cell lung cancer: a Hoosier Oncology Group study. *J Clin Oncol*, Vol.13, No.10, (October 1995), pp.2594-2599.

Lucas, C.F., Robinson, B., Hoskin, P.J., Yarnold, J.R., Smith, I.E., & Ford, H.T. Morbidity of cranial relapse in small cell lung cancer and the impact of radiation therapy. *Cancer Treat Rep*, Vol.70, No.5, (May 1986), pp.565-570.

Mavroudis, D., Papadakis, E., Veslemes, M., Tsiafaki, X., Stavrakakis, J., Kouroussis, C., Kakolyris, S., Bania, E., Jordanoglou, J., Agelidou, M., Vlachonicolis, J., & Georgoulias, V. (2001). A multicenter randomized clinical trial comparing paclitaxel-cisplatin-etoposide versus cisplatin-etoposide as first-line treatment in patients with small-cell lung cancer. *Ann Oncol*. Vol.12, No.4, (April 2001), pp.463-470.

Miller, A.A., Wang, X.F., Bogart, J.A., Hodgson, L.D., Rocha Lima, C.M., Radford, J.E., Vokes, E.E., & Green, M.R. (2007). Phase II trial of paclitaxel-topotecan-etoposide followed by consolidation chemoradiotherapy for limited-stage small cell lung cancer: CALGB 30002. *J Thorac Oncol*, Vol.2, No.7, (July 2007), pp.645-51.

Murray, N., Coy, P., Pater, J.L., Hodson, .I, Arnold, A., Zee, B.C., Payne, D., Kostashuk, E.C., Evans, W.K., & Dixon, P. (1993). Importance of timing for thoracic irradiation in the combined modality treatment of limited-stage small-cell lung cancer. The National Cancer Institute of Canada Clinical Trials Group. *J Clin Oncol*. Vol.11, No.2, (February 1993), pp.336-344.

Nicholson, S.A., Beasley, M.B., Brambilla, E., Hasleton, P.S., Colby, T.V., Sheppard, M.N., Falk, R., & Travis, W.D. (2002). Small cell lung carcinoma (SCLC): a clinicopathologic study of 100 cases with surgical specimens. *Am J Surg Pathol.* Vol.26, No.9, (September 2002), pp.1184-1197.

Niell, H.B., Herndon, J.E., Miller, A.A., Watson, D.M., Sandler, A.B., Kelly, K., Marks, R.S., Perry, M.C., Ansari, R.H., Otterson, G., Ellerton, J., Vokes, E.E., & Green, M.R. (2005). Randomized phase III intergroup trial of etoposide and cisplatin with or without paclitaxel and granulocyte colony-stimulating factor in patients with extensive-stage small-cell lung cancer: Cancer and Leukemia Group B Trial 9732. *J Clin Oncol*, Vol.23, (Jun 2005), No.16, pp.3752-3759.

Noda, K., Nishiwaki, Y., Kawahara, M., Negoro, S., Sugiura, T., Yokoyama, A., Fukuoka, M., Mori, K., Watanabe, K., Tamura, T., Yamamoto, S., & Saijo, N. (2002). Irinotecan plus cisplatin compared with etoposide plus cisplatin for extensive small-cell lung cancer. N Engl J Med, Vol.346, No.2, (January 2002), pp.85-91.

Okamoto, H., Watanabe, K., Kunikane, H., Yokoyama, A., Kudoh, S., Ishizuka, N., Fukuda, H., Tamura, T., & Saijo, N. (2005). Randomized phase III trial of carboplatin(C) plus etoposide (E) vs. split doses of cisplatin (P) plus etoposide (E) in elderly or poor-risk patients with extensive disease small cell lung cancer (ED-SCLC): JCOG9702. J Clin Oncol, Vol.23, (May 2005), Suppl.16, Abstract.7010.

Paesmans, M., Sculier, J.P., Lecomte, J., Thiriaux, J., Libert, P., Sergysels, R., Bureau, G., Dabouis, G., Van Cutsem, O., Mommen, P., Ninane, V., & Klastersky, J. (2000). Prognostic factors for patients with small cell lung carcinoma: analysis of a series of 763 patients included in 4 consecutive prospective trials with a minimum follow-up of 5 years. *Cancer*. Vol.89, No.3, (August 2000), pp.523-33.

Patel, S., Macdonald, O.K., & Suntharalingam, M. (2009). Evaluation of the use of prophylactic cranial irradiation in small cell lung cancer. *Cancer*, Vol.115, No.4, (February 2009), pp.842-50.

Paumier, A., & Le Pechoux, C. (2010). Radiotherapy in small-cell lung cancer: where should it go? Lung Cancer, Vol.69, No.2, (August 2010), pp.133-40.

Perry MC, Eaton WL, Propert KJ, Ware JH, Zimmer B, Chahinian AP, Skarin A, Carey RW, Kreisman H, Faulkner C, et al. Chemotherapy with or without radiation therapy in limited small-cell carcinoma of the lung. N Engl J Med. 1987 Apr 9;316(15):912-8.

Pignon, J.P., Arriagada, R., Ihde, D.C., Johnson, D.H., Perry, M.C., Souhami, R.L., Brodin, O., Joss, R.A., Kies, M.S., & Lebeau, B. (1992) A meta-analysis of thoracic radiotherapy for small-cell lung cancer. *N Engl J Med*, Vol.327, No.23, (December 1992), pp.1618-1624.

Pijls-Johannesma, M., De Ruysscher, D., Vansteenkiste, J., Kester, A., Rutten, I., & Lambin P. (2007). Timing of chest radiotherapy in patients with limited stage small cell lung cancer: a systematic review and meta-analysis of randomised controlled trials. *Cancer Treat Rev*, Vol.33, No.5, (August 2007), pp.461-73.

Postmus, P.E., Sleijfer, D.T., & Haaxma-Reiche, H. (1989). Chemotherapy for central nervous system metastases from small cell lung cancer: a review. *Lung Cancer,*Vol.5, pp.254-263.

Pujol, J.L., Carestia, L., & Daures JP. (2000). Is there a case for cisplatin in the treatment of small-cell lung cancer? A meta-analysis of randomized trials of a cisplatin-containing regimen versus a regimen without this alkylating agent. *Br J Cancer*, Vol.83, No.1, (July 2000), pp.8-15.

Pujol, J.L., Daures, J.P., Riviere, A., Quoix, E., Westeel, V., Quantin, X., Breton, J.L., Lemari, E., Poudenx, M., Milleron, B., Moro, D., Debieuvre, D., & Le Chevalier, T. Etoposide plus cisplatin with or without the combination of 4'-epidoxorubicin plus cyclophosphamide in treatment of extensive small-cell lung cancer: a French Federation of Cancer Institutes multicenter phase III randomized study. *J Natl Cancer Inst*, Vol.93, No.4, (February 2001), pp.300-308.

Rosenzweig, K.E., Chen, C.P., Yom, S.S., & Krug, L.M. (2010). Tumors of the Lung, Pleura, and Mediastinum, In: *Leibel And Phillips Textbook Of Radiation Oncology*, Richard T. Hoppe, Theodore Locke Phillips, & Mack Roach III, (Ed.), pp. 737-771, Saunders, ISBN: 978-1-4160-5897-7, Philadelphia.

Roth, B.J., Johnson, D.H., Einhorn, L.H., Schacter, L.P., Cherng, N.C., Cohen, H.J., Crawford, J., Randolph, J.A., Goodlow, J.L., & Broun, G.O. (1992). Randomized study of cyclophosphamide, doxorubicin, and vincristine versus etoposide and cisplatin versus alternation of these two regimens in extensive small-cell lung cancer: a phase III trial of the Southeastern Cancer Study Group. *J Clin Oncol*, Vol.10, No.2, (February 1992), pp.282-291.

Schiller, J.H., Adak, S., Cella, D., DeVore, R.F., & Johnson, D.H. (2001). Topotecan versus observation after cisplatin plus etoposide in extensive-stage small-cell lung cancer: E7593--a phase III trial of the Eastern Cooperative Oncology Group. *J Clin Oncol*,Vol.19, No.8, (April 2001), pp.2114-2122.

Sculier, J.P., Berghmans, T., Castaigne, C., Luce, S., Sotiriou, C., Vermylen, P., & Paesmans, M. Maintenance chemotherapy for small cell lung cancer: a critical review of the literature. *Lung Cancer*, Vol.19, No.2, (February 1998), pp.141-51.

Shaw, E.G., Su, J.Q., Eagan, R.T., Jett, J.R., Maksymiuk, A.W., & Deigert, F.A. (1994) Prophylactic cranial irradiation in complete responders with small-cell lung cancer: analysis of the Mayo Clinic and North Central Cancer Treatment Group data bases. *J Clin Oncol*, Vol.12, No.11, (November 1994), pp.2327-2332.

Skarlos, D.V., Samantas, E., Briassoulis, E., Panoussaki, E., Pavlidis, N., Kalofonos, H.P., Kardamakis, D., Tsiakopoulos, E., Kosmidis, P., Tsavdaridis, D., Tzitzikas, J., Tsekeris, P., Kouvatseas, G., Zamboglou, N., & Fountzilas, G. (2001). Randomized comparison of early versus late hyperfractionated thoracic irradiation concurrently with chemotherapy in limited disease small-cell lung cancer: a randomized phase II study of the Hellenic Cooperative Oncology Group (HeCOG). *Ann Oncol*, Vol.12, No.9, (September 2001), pp.1231-1238.

Slotman, B., Faivre-Finn, C., Kramer, G., Rankin, E., Snee, M., Hatton, M., Postmus, P., Collette, L., Musat, E., & Senan, S. (2007). EORTC Radiation Oncology Group and Lung Cancer Group. Prophylactic cranial irradiation in extensive small-cell lung cancer. *N Engl J Med* Vol.357, No.7, (August 2007), pp.664-672.

Sundstrom, S., Bremnes, R.M., Kaasa, S., Aasebo, U., Hatlevoll, R., Dahle, R., Boye, N., Wang, M., Vigander, T., Vilsvik, J., Skovlund, E., Hannisdal, E., Aamdal, S., & Sundstrom. (2002). Cisplatin and etoposide regimen is superior to cyclophosphamide, epirubicin, and vincristine regimen in small-cell lung cancer: results from a randomized phase III trial with 5 years' follow-up. *J Clin Oncol*, Vol.20, No.24, (December 2002), pp.4665-4672.

Tai, P., Tonita, J., Yu, E., & Skarsgard, D. (2003). Twenty-year follow-up study of long-term survival of limited-stage small-cell lung cancer and overview of prognostic and treatment factors. *Int J Radiat Oncol Biol Phys,* Vol.56, No.3, (July 2003), pp.626-633.

Takada, M., Fukuoka, M., Kawahara, M., Sugiura, T., Yokoyama, A., Yokota, S., Nishiwaki, Y., Watanabe, K., Noda, K., Tamura, T., Fukuda, H., & Saijo, N. Phase III study of concurrent versus sequential thoracic radiotherapy in combination with cisplatin and etoposide for limited-stage small-cell lung cancer: results of the Japan Clinical Oncology Group Study 9104. *J Clin Oncol,* Vol.20, No.14, (July 2002), pp.3054-3060.

Tyczynski, J.E., Bray, F., & Parkin D.M. (2003). Lung cancer in Europe in 2000: epidemiology, prevention, and early detection. Lancet Oncol, Vol.4, No.1, (January 2000), pp.45-55.

Topkan, E., Yavuz, M.N., Onal. C., & Yavuz, A.A. (2009). Prevention of acute radiation-induced esophagitis with glutamine in non-small cell lung cancer patients treated with radiotherapy: evaluation of clinical and dosimetric parameters. *Lung Cancer,* Vol.63, No.3, (March 2009), pp.393-399.

Turrisi, A.T., Kim, K., Blum, R., Sause, W.T., Livingston, R.B., Komaki, R., Wagner, H., Aisner, S., & Johnson, D.H. (1999). Twice-daily compared with once-daily thoracic radiotherapy in limited small-cell lung cancer treated concurrently with cisplatin and etoposide. *N Engl J Med,* Vol.340, Vol.4, (January 1999), pp.265-271.

Vallieres, E., Shepherd, F.A., Crowley, J., Van Houtte, P., Postmus, P.E., Carney, D., Chansky, K., Shaikh, Z., & Goldstraw, P. (2009). The IASLC Lung Cancer Staging Project: proposals regarding the relevance of TNM in the pathologic staging of small cell lung cancer in the forthcoming (seventh) edition of the TNM classification for lung cancer. *J Thorac Oncol,* Vol.4, No.9, (September 2009), pp.1049-1059.

van Loon, J., De Ruysscher, D., Wanders, R., Boersma, L., Simons, J., Oellers, M., Dingemans, A.M., Hochstenbag, M., Bootsma, G., Geraedts, W., Pitz, C., Teule, J., Rhami, A., Thimister, W., Snoep, G., Dehing-Oberije, C., & Lambin, P. (2010). Selective nodal irradiation on basis of (18)FDG-PET scans in limited-disease small-cell lung cancer: a prospective study. *Int J Radiat Oncol Biol Phys,* Vol.77, No.2, (June 2010), pp.329-336.

van Meerbeeck JP, Fennell DA, De Ruysscher DK. Small-cell lung cancer. Lancet. 2011 May 10. [Epub ahead of print]

van Oosterhout AG, van de Pol M, ten Velde GP, Twijnstra A. Neurologic disorders in 203 consecutive patients with small cell lung cancer. Results of a longitudinal study. Cancer. 1996 Apr 15;77(8):1434-41.

Yang GY, Matthews RH. Prophylactic cranial irradiation in small-cell lung cancer. Oncologist. 2000;5(4):293-8.

Warde P, Payne D. Does thoracic irradiation improve survival and local control in limited-stage small-cell carcinoma of the lung? A meta-analysis. J Clin Oncol. 1992 Jun;10(6):890-5.

Work E, Nielsen OS, Bentzen SM, Fode K, Palshof T. Randomized study of initial versus late chest irradiation combined with chemotherapy in limited-stage small-cell lung cancer. Aarhus Lung Cancer Group. J Clin Oncol. 1997 Sep;15(9):3030-7.

Zelen, M. (1973). Keynote address on biostatistics and data retrieval. Cancer Chemother Rep 3, Vol.4, No.2, pp.31-42.

12

Lung Parenchyma Sparing Resection for Pulmonary Malignancies

Arpad Pereszlenyi
Department of Thoracic Surgery,
Vivantes Klinikum Neukölln, Berlin,
Germany

1. Introduction

It is well-known that the incidence of lung malignancies increases. The increase of primary lung cancer is especially alarming. But the lung is also a target organ for other secondary malignancies, such as metastases of different origins. For the primary lung cancer, the therapy of choice is its radical resection (together with systematic lymphadenectomy). For pulmonary metastases, less radical resections are necessary. Both could be challenging for thoracic surgeons in case of limited lung function and in the case of multiple bilateral lung nodules – metastases. Furthermore, the newly detected lung tumor is in most cases diagnosed in elderly, active smokers with a limited lung function and significant comorbidity. Therefore, the above-mentioned planned radical resection in these "limited" patients is not possible. Thoracic surgeons face apparently a dead-lock situation having to operate radically and sparing enough functional lung parenchyma at the same time.
This paper is dedicated to the topic of lung parenchyma sparing resection. It's first part describes a laser resection of multiple lung lesions – metastases. The laser segmental lung resection and the sleeve bronchoplastic (angioplastic) resection are introduced in it's second and third part, respectively.

2. Laser resection for lung metastases

2.1 History

Already in 1786, John Hunter reported the first case report in history of pulmonary metastases. The primary cancer was a malignant tumor of the femur and the patient died of widespread pulmonary metastazing only 7 weeks after the leg was amputated (Allen et al., 1993; Van Schil et al. 2008). In 1927, the first surgeon who performed a lung resection of pulmonary metastasis was Jan Divis from Prague (Divis, 1927). Barney and Churchill could note the real success after the surgery, removing a lung metastasis by a lobectomy. The renal-cell carcinoma was removed by nephrectomy, subsequently. The patient survived for over 20 years without any signs of recurrence (Barney & Churchill, 1939).
Finally, a retrospective analysis of 205 patients after resection of pulmonary metastases should be mentioned. This report was published by Thomford in 1965 with a 5 Years-Survival-Rate (Y-S) of 30.3% (Thomford 1965).

2.2 Introducing the laser in thoracic surgery

In 1985, after establishing a 1064 nm Nd:YAG laser for standard endobronchial interventions (Häusinger et al, 1984), LoCicero reopened the debate on the use of lasers in open thoracic surgery as well (LoCicero, 1985, 1989). However, since his CO_2 laser was a pure absorption or cutting laser, it proved inadequate for lung surgery and thus could not establish itself in this medical discipline. As a result, a number of medical centers in the United States, Japan and Europe began experimenting with 1064 nm Nd:YAG lasers, using bare fibers and sapphire tips to perform superficial resections (Branscheid, 1992; Kodama 1991, 1992; Lo Cicero 1985, 1989; Mineo, 1998; Moghissi, 1988; Rolle, 1988). As it follows, all of these teams achieved only low patient-loads and published no further results, mainly because the technical difficulties posed by the available 1064 nm lasers could not be overcome without further basic research. Table 1.

The new era began by introducing the 1318 nm wavelength Nd:YAG laser system of 40 W power output. This high performance Nd: YAG laser system consisted of the thin flexible quartz fibres (400 µm) with low water content and of a four lens focusing handpiece. This new laser system was exclusively used in all patients undergoing a lung parenchyma sparing resection in our study. The next Section presents the description of this laser system.

Author	Article	Laser	Wave Length (nm)	Laser Application
LoCicero	1985 Ann Thorac Surg	CO_2		Hemostasis, Sealing of Air Leaks
Rolle	1988 Laser in Med and Surg	Nd:YAG	1064/1318	Experimental/clinical n=47 Wedge and Segmental Resections
Moghissi	1988 J Thoracic Cardiovasc Surg	Nd:YAG	1064	Local Excision, "Coin Lesions"
LoCicero	1989 J Thoracic Cardiovasc Surg	Nd:YAG	1064	Laser assisted pulmonary resections
Kodama	1991 J Thoracic Cardiovasc Surg	Nd:YAG	1064	Resection of Lung Metastases n=25
Branscheid	1992 Eur J Cardiothorac Surg	Nd:YAG	1064	Resection of Lung Metastases n=14 Laser only n=51 comb. with with Lobectomy
Kodama	1992 Kyobu Geka	Nd:YAG	1064	Resection of Lung Metastases n=25 Segmental Resection (NSCLC) n=25
Mineo	1988 Chest	Nd:YAG	1064	Resection of Lung Metastases n=23
Rolle	2006 J Thorac Cardiovasc Surg	Nd:YAG	1318	Lobe-Sparing Resection of Multiple Pulmonary Metastases n=328

Table 1. Literature Survey: Nd:YAG/CO2 Laser resection in thoracic surgery.

2.2.1 Scientific background, description of 1318 Nd:YAG Laser

Due to its parenchymal tissue having a typical water content of 80% but a very low tissue density (just a fifth of the liver parenchyma), a very low heat capacity and a variable air content, the lung is an ideal organ for phototermal laser applications. Therefore, resecting lung parenchyma requires a laser with a powerful coagulation capability in addition to excellent cutting properties, given the high vessel density. After all, the surgeon must always expect fistulae and increasing bronchopulmonary leaks, particularly when dissecting lung parenchyma, the more so the deeper one works down in central direction. The absorption behavior of different lasers in water differs a lot (Bayly, 1963; Bramson, 1968; Dinstl, 1981).

The 1318 nm wavelength Nd:YAG laser significantly differs from the standard (1064 nm) wavelength by its ten times higher absorption in water but still offers sufficient laser light scatter, due its proximity to the beginning infrared spectrum, to satisfy the vital coagulation requirement as well. In fact the 1318 nm wavelength provided the intended combination effect - cutting capability plus coagulation capability - so perfectly as it could not be achieved with the 1064 nm wavelength (Rolle, 1988, 1989). As a welcome side-effect, we also found strong lung tissue shrinkage, which provides two additional advantages: mechanical reinforcement of the coagulation effect, and fistula sealing far into the central lobe region. In fact, the surfaces coagulated and sealed off through defocused irradiation with the 1318 nm laser withstand artificial ventilation pressures of up to 25 cm H_20.

As for the founding and developing of the above mentioned laser system, the name of Professor Axel Rolle has to be mentioned in this place (Rolle, 1988, 1989, 1999).

The following design features were incorporated to develop a 1318 nm commercial design Trumph (formerly Hüttinger Medizintechnik, Umkirch, Germany) and Martin companies. The second wavelength is first generated by adapted reflection of the laser mirrors. High beam quality allows coupling into thin (less than 0.6 mm) optical quartz fibers with minimum losses. For flexible transmission to the area of application, special water-free quartz fibers are required as laser light absorption in water is 10 times higher at the 1318-nm wavelength (Bayly, et al., 1963; Stokes et al., 1981).

A four-lens focusing handpiece was developed to concentrate the laser light and allow manual manipulation of the beam onto lung tissue to keep the working-point focus in the tissue at 4 mm while avoiding heat generation in the focusing handpiece. The extremely high laser power density of 24kW/cm^2 allows fast and precise cutting with simultaneous coagulation and sealing of lung tissue. A high performance smoke evacuation system eliminates the vaporization fumes, which are unavoidable during parenchyma dissection with this laser (Fig.1).

2.3 Surgical technique

Laser metastasectomy is performed via an anterolateral thoracotomy (staged 3 to 4 weeks, if bilateral) after fulfilling the standard indication criteria for pulmonary metastasectomy (histologically confirmed primary tumor after its radical resection or its fully controlled stage). Preoperative evaluations are the same as a for routine thoracic intervention; including a history and physical examination, chest computed tomography (CT), pulmonary function tests, and a bone scan. If the signs or symptoms are suggestive, a head CT is also obtained. Patients with identified extrapulmonary metastases are excluded from surgery.

The technique, indication and possibility to save lobes are demonstrated on a case report. A 59-years-old female patient with a history of radically resected colorectal carcinoma

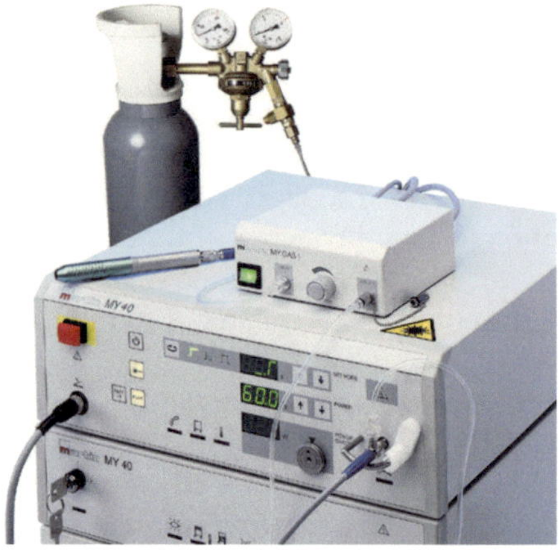

Fig. 1. Components of modern Laser equipment for the application on lung tissue (1318 nm wavelength, 40 W power output, beam quality, energy efficiency, high performance smoke evacuation system, 0.4 mm diameter of fibre, focusing handpiece, flexible quartz fibres /low water content/).

(Adenocarcinoma of rectosigmoid pT4 pN1 pM1 (Liver), G3, Status post hemihepatectomy, chemotherapy and radiation) was referred to our Institute. A significant progress of (isolated) lung metastases was reported. The chest CT demonstrates the situation after the successful laser resection of pulmonary metastases on the right side and just before the procedure on left (Fig. 2).

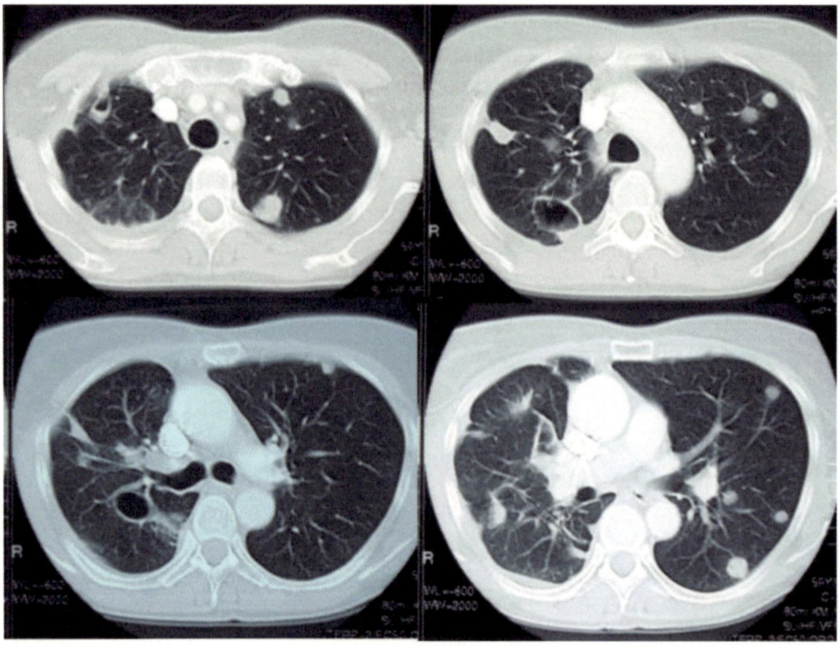

Fig. 2. Case Report 1: The Chest CT demonstrates the situation after the successful laser resection of pulmonary metastases on the right side and just before the procedure on left.

The new 1318 nm Nd:YAG laser system offers a unique opportunity to perform the procedure in a parenchyma-saving and lobe-sparing way. Therefore, the bilateral laser procedure was performed. The intraoperative situation can be seen on the series of photographs: the pulmonary artery is mobilized on a vessel loop; the upper vein lies next to the central, 30 mm great metastasis (Fig. 3). The laser resection of this metastasis was than performed. The next figure (Fig. 4) shows the situation immediately after the laser resection. The intraoperative situation - its close relation to segmental pulmonary vein - can be easily recognized. Exposed bronchial branches and segmental vessels at the segmental level were over-sewn and ligated with absorbable suture (4-0/ 3-0). The lung architecture and orientation was reconstructed following each nodular resection by reapproximating the visceral pleura with a running absorbable suture (4-0 Vicryl) (Fig. 5). This technique avoided a distortion of the lung tissue to allow consistent orientation and palpation of the initially noted lung nodules. At the end of the procedure, the resected lung was re-insuflated by a standard way in accordance with the routine thoracic surgical practice.

By performing the metastasectomy the above-described way, it was possible to save the patient's lobes and to operate on both lungs by a laser parenchyma sparing manner. The patient, now one year after the procedure, is in good condition with a full physical activity, living free of metastases.

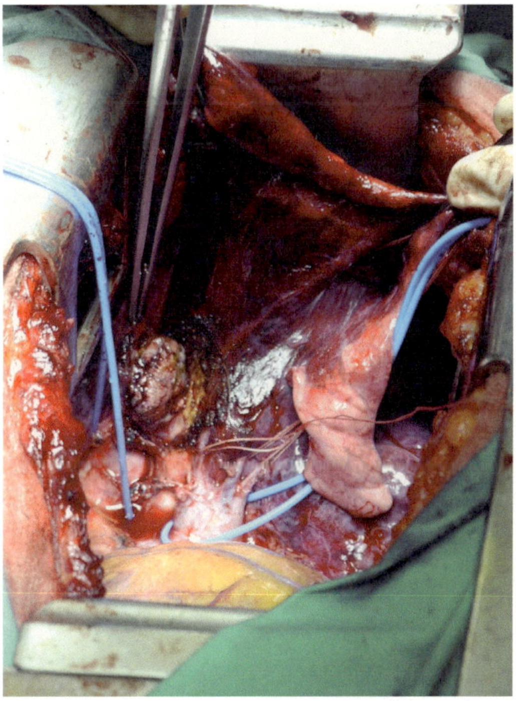

Fig. 3. Intraoperative view: Laser resection of 30 mm central metastasis localized in left upper lobe centrally to pulmonary artery. Intraoperative situation: pulmonary artery and the upper vein are mobilized on vessel loop (blue).

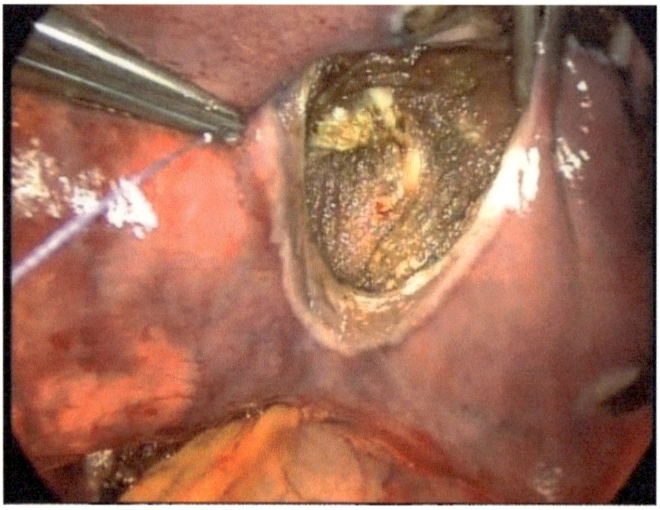

Fig. 4. The intraoperative situation – its close relation to segmental pulmonary vein - can be easily recognized. Exposed bronchial branches and segmental vessels at the segmental level were over-sewn and ligated with absorbable suture (4-0/ 3-0).

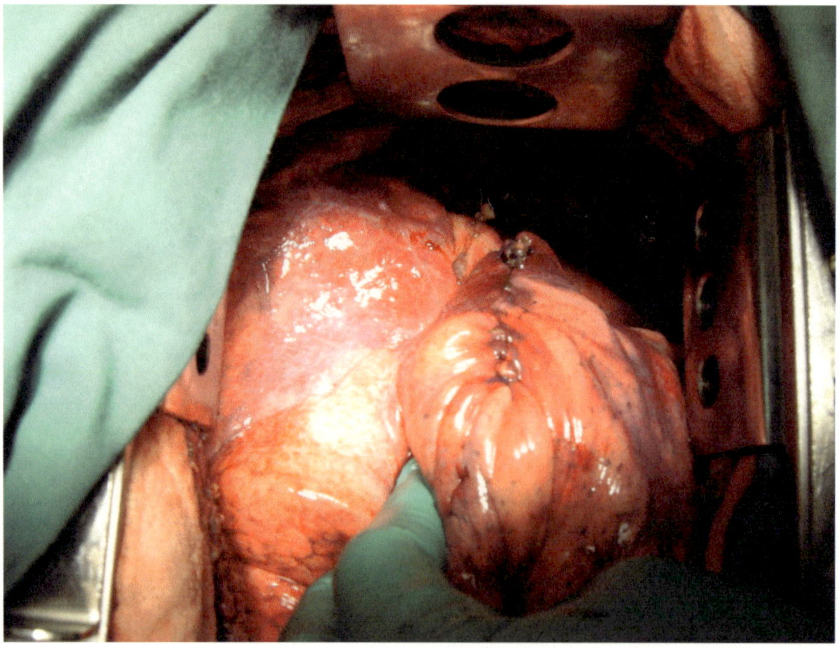

Fig. 5. Intraoperative view: Reconfiguration of the left upper lobe with continuous suture of the pleura visceralis.

2.4 Results

From January 1996 to May 2004, lung laser resections were performed in 328 patients. There were 164 males and 164 females and the main indications for laser lung resections included lung metastases of the following primaries: renal carcinoma in 112 cases, colorectal in 91 and breast cancer in 35 cases. In the remaining 90 cases laser resection was performed for metastases of lung cancer (n=12), malignant melanoma (n=1), sarcomas (n=15), head and neck carcinoma (n=12) and for metastases of other less frequent ones (n=27). These results were already reported and published elsewhere (Rolle et al., 2006).

This retrospective study analyzes the second largest indication group of colorectal carcinoma lung metastases (Pereszlenyi et al., 2006a, 2006b). 46 females and 45 males with median age of 64 yrs, ranged from 43 to 80 years were included. The number of complete removed metastases was 629, ranged 1-56; median 7 per patient. All laser resections were performed by the Nd:YAG laser system of 1318 nm wavelength with its lung parenchyma saving effect. The complete resection (R0) was achieved in 78 patients, incomplete (R1/2) in 13 patients.

There was no perioperative mortality. Follow-up was completed for all patients and ranged from 1-30 Mo with a median of 20 months. 1 Year-Survival (Y-S) for complete (R0) resection was 82%, 2 Y-S was 68%, 3 Y-S 42% and 5 Y-S was 22% (Fig. 6). For incomplete (R1/2) resection (n=13): 1 Year-Survival was 85%, 2 Y-S was 54%, 3 Y-S 46%, 4 Y-S 9% and 5 Y-S was 0 (Fig. 6).

Despite of that the 7 Metastases pro patient was removed and 19% of lymphatic-nodes involvement, the radical resection (R0) could be achieved. In 13 patients was the resection incomplete (R1/R2). For the R0 versus R1/2 see the Figure 6. The survival with and without lymphatic-node-involvement (N1-hilum, N2-mediastinum) after the radical resection (R0N0 versus R0N1/2) is demonstrated in Figure 7.

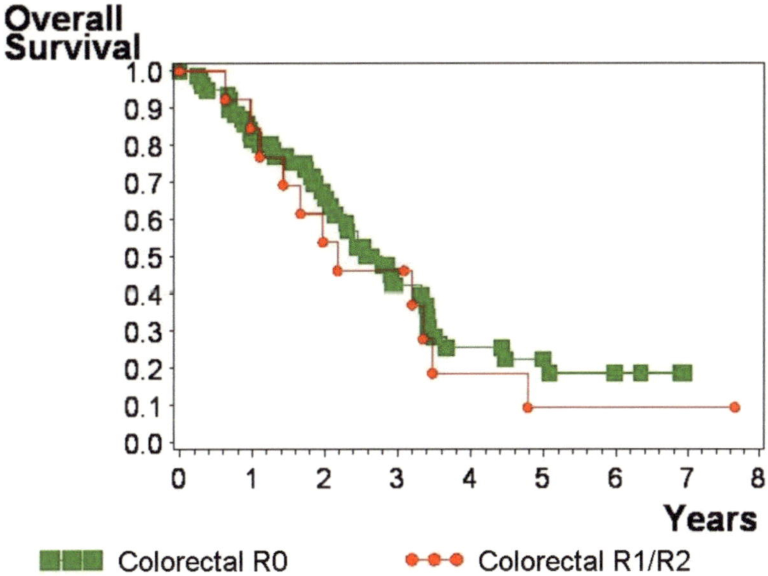

Fig. 6. Kaplan-Meier curve showing survival according to resection (Bullets = complete R0, squares = incomplete R1/R2 resections).

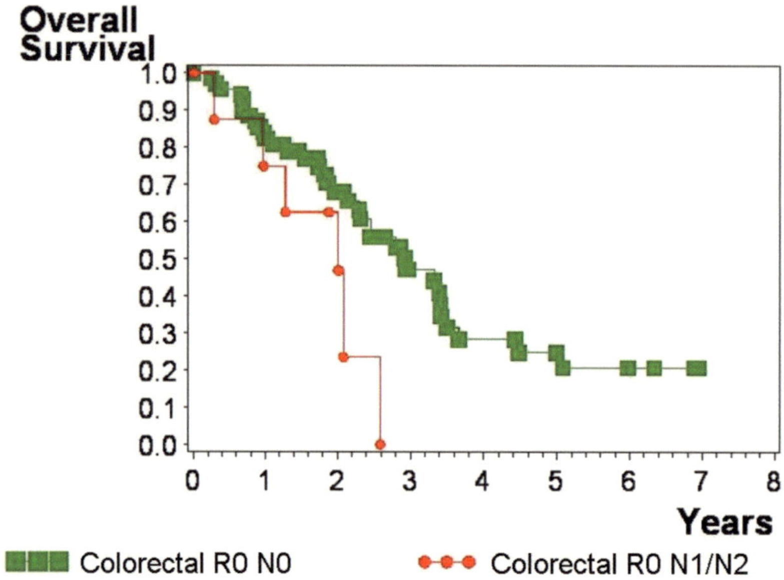

Fig. 7. Kaplan-Meier curve showing survival according to lymphnode-involvement (Bullets = complete without LN-involvement R0N0, squares = complete with LN1/N2-involvement R0 N1/N2).

3. Laser segmental lung resection

The technique of conventional lung segment resection, so called segmentectomy, is well known from the pioneer age of the thoracic surgery (pneumoftiseology) when the apical sublobar lung resections were performed for lung tuberculosis. Nowadays, those resections are not so widely spread due to their "not enough radicalism" for lung cancer cases.

However, as it is already stated in the Introduction, these resections will gain more and more importance due to their lung parenchyma-sparing effect and the improving results on early postoperative morbidity and mortality (Keenan et al., 2004; Harada et al., 2005).

In this place, it should be emphasized that the segmental resection is also an anatomical lung resection as the lobectomy. It respects the anatomical structure of the lung with its bronchial and vascular composites together with its lymphatic flows.

A significant role in the technique of the segmental resection belongs to the laser system. Its cutting effect enables the thoracic surgeon to perform this kind of resection exactly within the anatomical boarders of the pulmonary segment. Therefore it is feasible also for segments where the "classical" segment resections can only hardly be obtained, e.g. segment III, IX, X etc.

3.1 Surgical technique

Laser segmentectomy is performed via an anterolateral muscle-sparing thoracotomy after fulfilling the standard indication criteria for a lung cancer resection (histologically confirmed lung tumor in its functional and oncologic operable stage). Preoperative evaluations are the same as for a routine thoracic intervention; including a history and physical examination, chest computed tomography (CT), pulmonary function tests, and a PET scan. If there are positive mediastinal lymphatic nodes proved by the test, a video-mediastinoscopy in order to clarify the N2/N3 status is added prior to the resection.

Next, a case report presents the technique of laser segmental lung resection. A 66-years-old male patient with histological confirmed Adenocarcinoma of the right upper lobe was evaluated for a lung resection. Because of the patient's significant comorbidity (ischemic heart disease, arterial hypertension, diabetes mellitus) and poor lung function (COPD, active smoker with history of 30 Pack/Years, FEV1 55%), the limited lung resection - Laser resection of the Segment 1 - was performed.
For the patient's preoperative images see Figure 8.

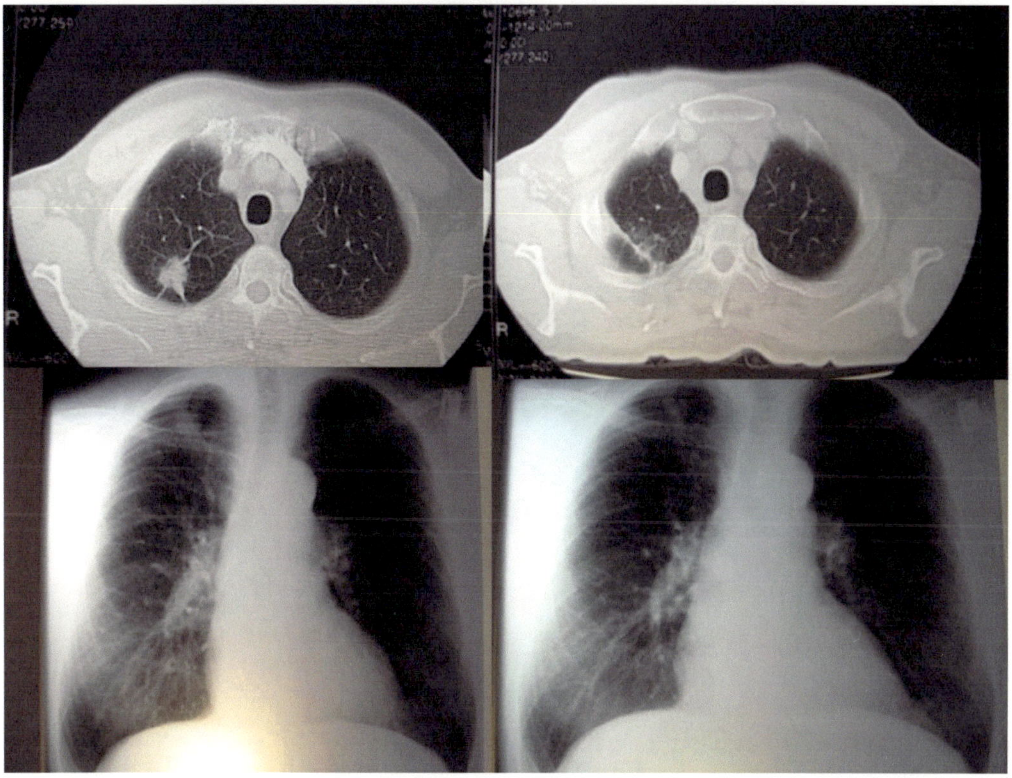

Fig. 8. Chest CT and X-ray pictures of Case 2. The perioperative images are on the left and the postoperative images are on the right side.

After the mobilization of the lung hilus, the segmental vessels and bronchus were mobilized on vessel loops. Fig.9. After this step, the lung parenchyma resection was performed by the laser system within the anatomical boarders of the Segment 1. Fig.10. The visceralisation (reapproximating the visceral pleura with a running absorbable suture /4-0 Vicryl/) in order to restore the architecture of the upper lobe followed. As it was already described above, this technique avoided a distortion of the lung tissue to allow consistent orientation and palpation of the lung parenchyma. At the end of the procedure, the resected lung was re-insuflated by a standard way in accordance with the routine thoracic surgical practice. Radical lymphadenectomy is routinely added to this procedure (Pereszlenyi et al., 2006).
The patient is now 3 years after the procedure, without any signs of tumor recurrence. The histological examination of the resected specimen has proved an Adenocarcinoma of the lung 3 cm of diameter, radically (R0) removed via the laser resection of the Segment 1. For postoperative CT scans see Figure 8.

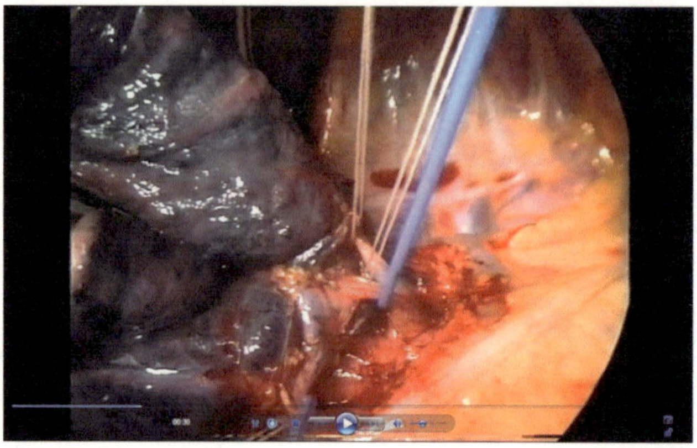

Fig. 9. Right lung hilus is mobilized; truncus anterior on the blue vessel loop with its segmental artery branches A1, A3.

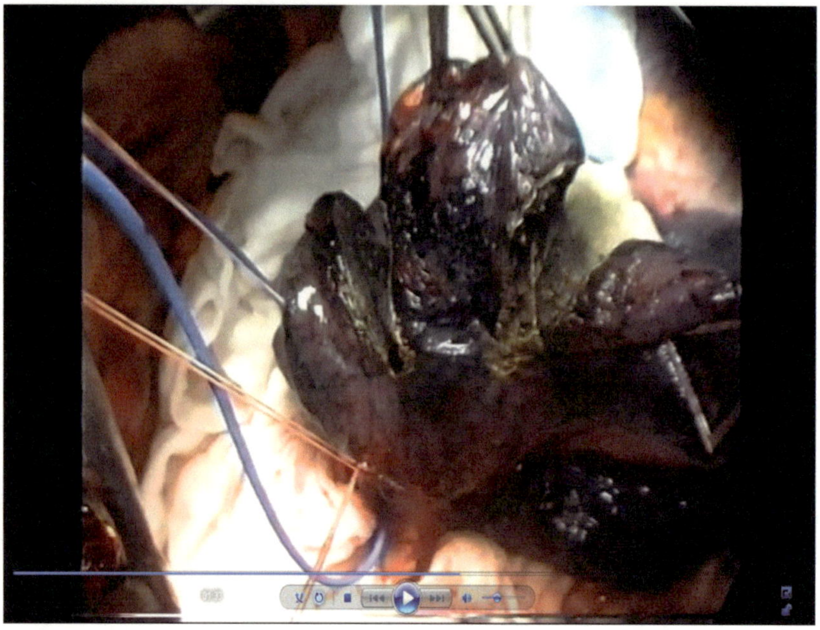

Fig. 10. Laser segmental resection within the anatomical boarders of the Segment 1.

3.2 Results

From January 1996 to December 2001, laser segmental lung resections were performed in 53 patients (Pereszlenyi et al., 2006). The results after these resections were compared to standard lobectomies /n=154/ for non-small cell lung cancer (NSCLC). The data of this comparison are presented in the Table 2.

As it follows, the 1, 3, 5 Year-Survival (Y-S) is comparable in both groups, there is no statistical significance /p=0.696/ in terms of tumor recurrence rate (26.4% versus 29.2%). The postoperative mortality rate (11.3%) after laser lung segmental resection is explained by the significant comorbidity, limited lung function in elderly patients in whom this kind of lung parenchyma sparing resection was performed. Tab.2.

To conclude, we are convinced that radical surgical resection is still the therapy of choice in NSCLC treatment. However, laser segmental lung resection represents an optimal treatment eventuality especially for those high risk patients in whom the standard resection - lobectomy is not feasible or performable.
Our study demonstrates the possibility and justification of this treatment modality with comparable results after the standard ones (Harada et al., 2005).

	n	Mean Age/yrs (Range)	Intraoperative mortality	Postoperative mortality	1,3,5 Years Survival	Tumor Recurrence Rate
Laser Segmental Resection	53	67.5 (49.5-82.7)	0	11.3%	95% 82% 65%	26.4%
Lobectomy	154	62.5 (28.3-77.6)	0	1.9%	92% 71% 58%	29.2%

Table 2. Laser segmental lung resection versus standard lobectomy for primary lung cancer (n=207). Selection criteria for laser segmental resection: high risk patients (elderly patient, poor performance status, FEV1<65%, significant comorbidity) and peripheral tumors of ≤ 4cm diameter.

4. Sleeve bronchoplastic lung resection

Last but not least, the sleeve lobectomy should be mentioned. Centrally localized lung tumors can be resected by a lobectomy extended into a resection of central part of the invaded bronchus. The shape of such resected bronchus has a form of a sleeve. That's where the term "sleeve" lobectomy originates. There are numerous published studies showing the clear benefit for this type of lung resections. The most important advantage includes the avoidance of a major lung resection, e.g. pneumonectomy by performing a sleeve lobectomy. Its technique is well known, but in case of constructing so called "Neo-carina" followed by its re-implantation to the main stem bronchus can be very challenging also for experienced surgeons. Fig.11.

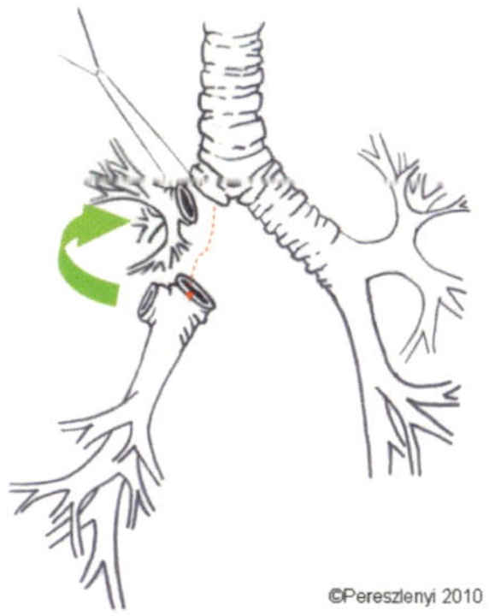

Fig. 11. Sleeve middle and lower (bi-)lobectomy: Re-implantation the upper lobe bronchus into main-stem bronchus right (or into distal trachea with construction of the "neo-carina") after resection the tumor within the bilobectomy. Scheme.

In case of multiple lung lesions, the laser system plays a significant role. The centrally located endobronchial tumor is removed by a sleeve lobectomy, and any smaller peripheral lesions (satellites) are resected by laser. Fig.12. The technique of the laser resection is presented in detail in the first part of this chapter. Fig. 13.

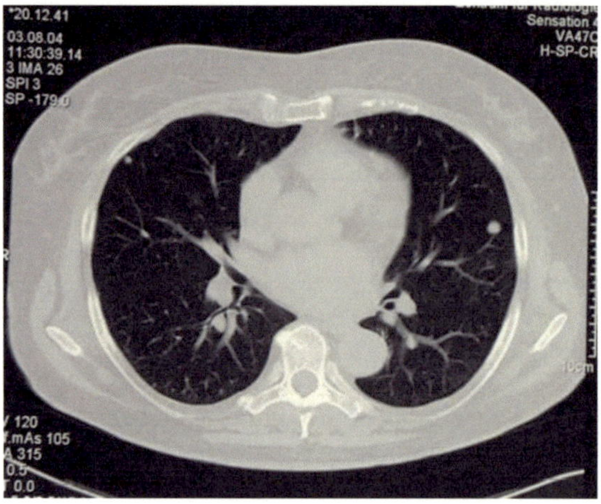

Fig. 12. Case Report 3: Chest CT shows the central lung tumor in the right lower lobe and two small satellites in the periphery of the lung.

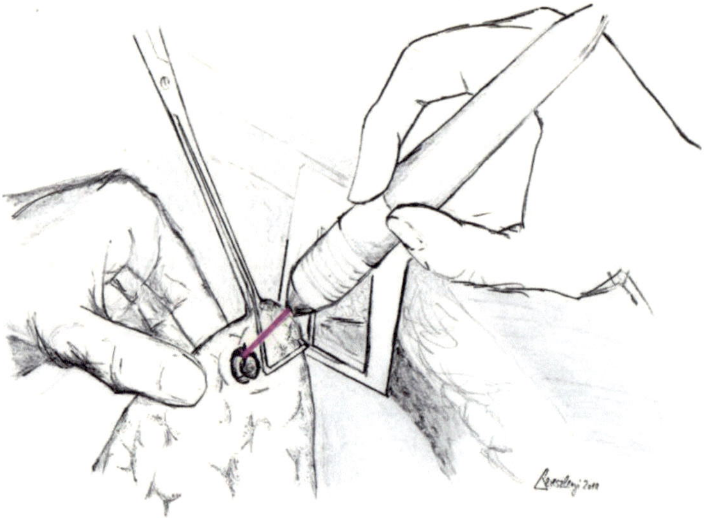

Fig. 13. Scheme of laser resection of small peripheral nodule located in the middle lobe after sleeve lower lobe resection for a large central located endobronchial tumor.

4.1 Surgical technique, patients and methods

Between January 2005 and January 2011, 58 patients (42 males, 16 females, mean age 61 yrs range 24 – 83) underwent sleeve lobectomy (SL) in our Institute. The indications for SL were: non-small cell lung carcinoma (NSCLC) in 47 /Fig.14/, and pulmonary metastases in 11 patients. Fig.15. As the metastatic pulmonary lesions were multiple, the Laser Resection (LR) of these satellites was added to the SL procedure. The main indication for laser resection were metastases of renal-cell (n=4) and colorectal-carcinoma (n=3). Fig.15. The most detected histologic type of NSCLC was squamous-cell carcinoma (n=22), followed by adenocarcinoma (n=14). The laser resection (combined by SL) was performed after fulfilling the standard criteria for metastasectomy: primary tumors were radically removed and there were no evidence of any distant extrathoracic metastases. In four NSCLC patients the arterial sleeve was added to the left upper bronchial SL. Lymphadenectomy was routinely added to the both parenchyma-saving procedures.

The Tumor Stage is shown in the Figure 16 according to the newest, revised TNM Classification from 2009 (Goldstraw et al., 2007).

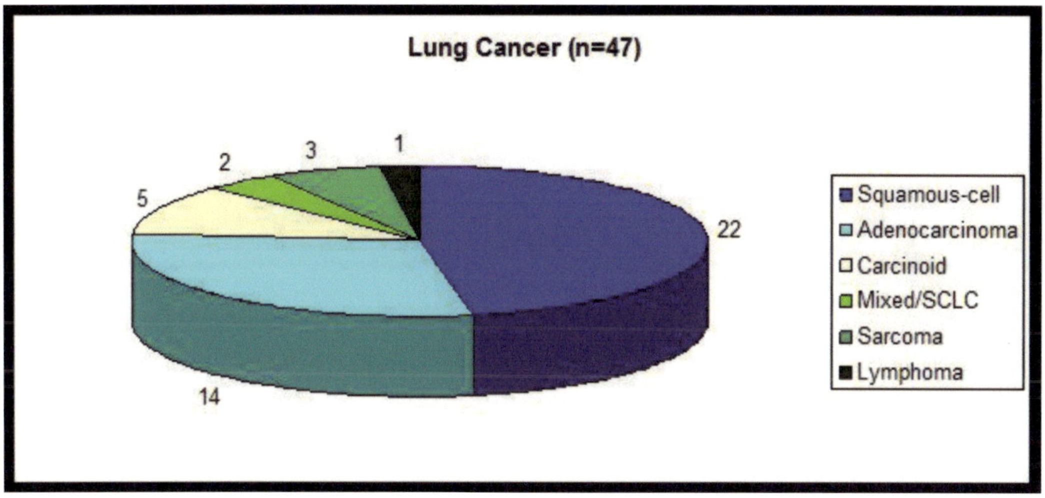

Fig. 14. Tumor histology distribution (NSCLC; n=47).

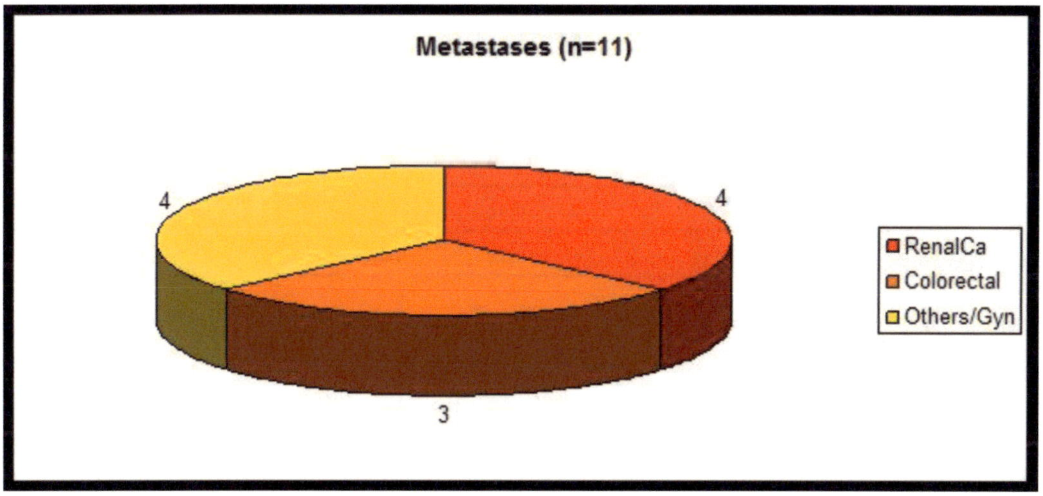

Fig. 15. Tumor histology distribution (Lung Metastases; n=11).

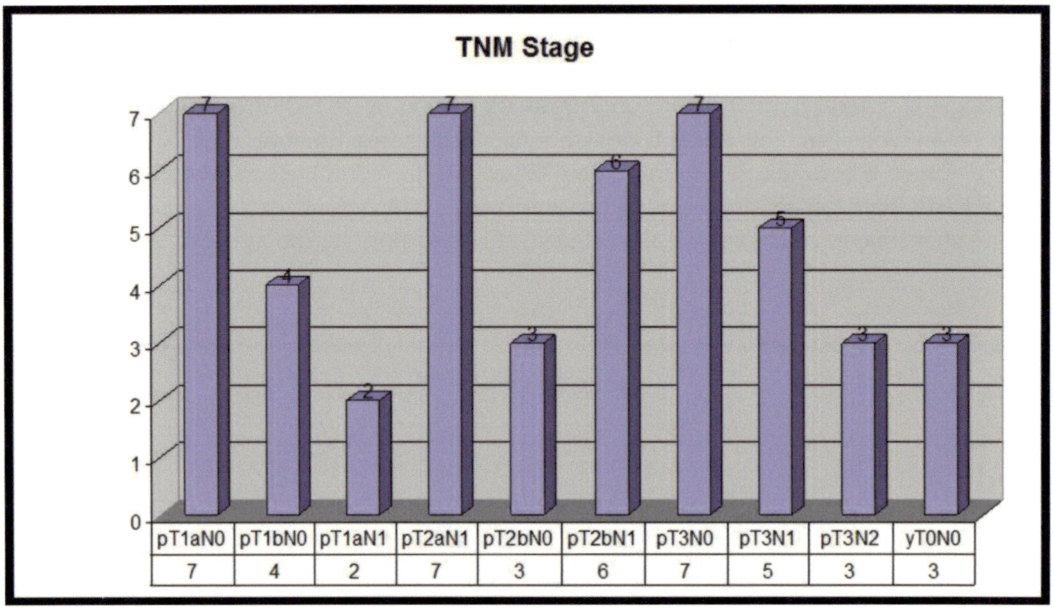

Fig. 16. Tumor Stage according to TNM Classification 2009 (n=47). yT0N0 - As the result of the successful neoadjuvant treatment, the tumor is not detectable in the resected lung specimen.

The location of the tumors and types of sleeve resections are shown in Table 3. Almost 40% of the patients underwent right sleeve upper lobe resection.

Side and Type of Procedure	**Number of Patients (%)**
Right Lung	
Upper Lobe	23 (39)
Middle Lobe	1 (2)
Middle and Lower Lobe	1 (2)
Lower Lobe	14 (24)
Left Lung	
Upper Lobe	12 (21)
Lower Lobe	7 (12)

Table 3. The location of tumors and types of sleeve resections (n=58).

Following the double-lumen tube intubation and the standard anterolateral, muscle-sparing thoracotomy, we proceed with the resection. A bronchial anastomosis is performed by interrupted monofilament absorbable suture of PDS 3-0 or 4-0. The vascular anastomosis was performed by running suture of the non-absorbable material of Prolene 5-0 (or 4-0) in four NSCLC patients after the left upper sleeve lobectomy was finished.

Mediastinal (hilar) lymphadenectomy is routinely performed as well as an intraoperative frozen section analysis of the resected bronchus (and vessel). After the reconstruction of the bronchus, a routine fiber bronchoscopy is always performed by the first surgeon. In our series, we didn't cover the bronchial anastomosis by any autologeous flap or any other materials.

4.2 Results

A negative bronchial (vascular) margin was achieved in all. No 30-days postoperative mortality occurred. Follow-up (completed for all patients with median of 12 Mo) showed no anastomotic complications, no local recurrence on the bronchial (arterial) anastomosis. Survival was analyzed according to Kaplan-Meier method with the estimated 1, 2, 4 years overall survival. Fig. 17.

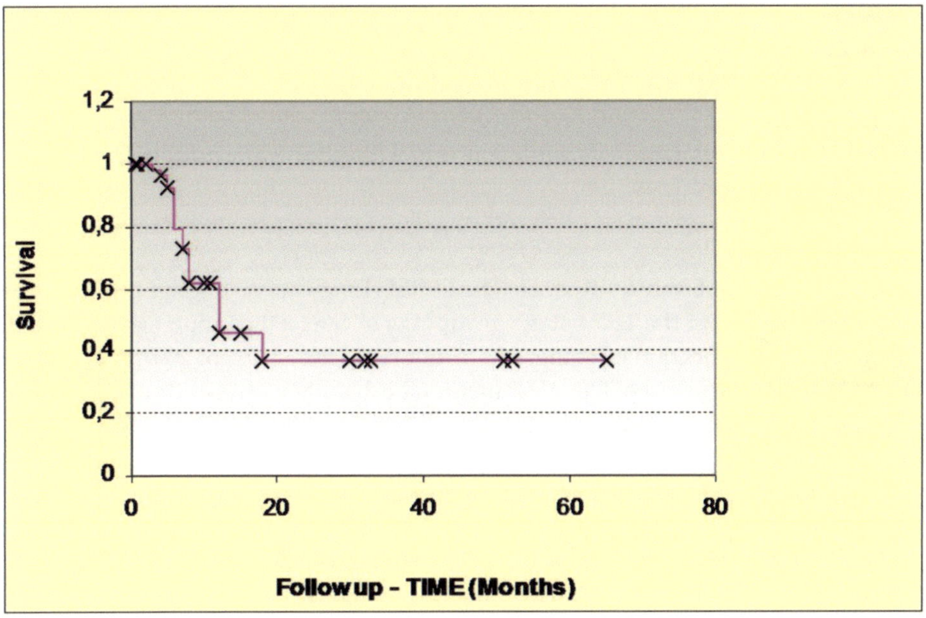

Fig. 17. Kaplan-Meier curve showing Survival at 20, 40, 60 Months.

In accordance with the reported results from the literature we can also conclude, the bronchial and vascular sleeve lobectomy can be performed safely, and is a good alternative solution to avoid pneumonectomy (Konstantinou et al., 2009; Ludwig et al., 2005).

As shown in our study, selected patients with central lung metastases can be also included for this procedure after fulfilling the standard criteria for pulmonary metastasectomy. The central role for these kinds of procedures belongs to the laser lung-parenchyma-saving

resection. In our study all laser resections were performed by a 1318-nm Nd:YAG laser system of 40 W power output.
Laser resection may expand the scope of surgical treatment for pulmonary metastases, allowing a more complete resection. The indications for laser resection may expand to include patients who are not considered ideal candidates for lung metastasectomy because of poor residual lung function or multifocal pulmonary disease. The 1318-nm Nd:YAG laser for the resection of pulmonary metastases demonstrates a significant influence on the conservation of tissue during metastasectomy and appears to minimize complications.

5. References

Allen E, Turk JL, Murley R. The case book of John Hunter FRS. London: Royal Society of Medicine Services; 1993.

Barney JD, Churchill ET. Adenocarcinoma of the kidney with metastasis to the lung cured by nephrectomy and lobectomy. J Urol 1939;42:269-76.

Bayly IG, Kartha VB, Stevens WH. The absorption spectra of liquid phase H_2O, HDO, and D_20 from 0.7 micron to 10 micron. Infrared Physics 1963;3:211-23.

Bramson M. Infrared Radiation. A handbook for applications. Plenum Press, New York, 1968.

Branscheid D, Krysa S, Wollkopf G, Bulzebruck H, Probst G, Horn M, Schirren J, Vogt-Moykopf I. Does ND-YAG laser extend the indicatons for resection of pulmonary metastases? Eur J Cardiothorac Surg 1992;6:590-7.

Dinstl K, Fischer PL. Der Laser. Grundlagen und klinische Anwendung. Springer, Berlin, Heidelberg, New York, 1981.

Divis J. Ein Beitrag zur operativen Behandlung der Lungengeschwülste. Acta Chir Scand 1927;62:329-41.

Goldstraw P, Crowley J, Chansky K, et al. The IASLC lung cancer staging project: proposals for the revision of the TNM stage groupings in the forthcoming (seventh) edition of the TNM classification of malignant tumours. J Thorac Oncol 2007;2:706 –714.

Harada H, Okada M, Sakamoto T et al. Functional advantage after radical segmentectomy versus lobectomy for lung cancer. Ann Thorac Surg 2005;80:2041-2045.

Häussinger K, Held E, Huber R: Endobronchial laser therapy, differential therapeutic use, and clinical value. Klin Wochenschr 1984;62:74-80.

Keenan RJ, Landreneau RJ, Maley RH Jr et al. Segmental resection spares pulmonary function in patients with stage I lung cancer. Ann Thorac Surg 2004;78:228-233.

Kodama K, Doi O, Higashiyama M, Tatsuta M, Iwanaga T. Surgical management of lung metastases. Usefulness of resection with the neodymium:yttrium-aluminium-garnet laser with median sternotomy. J Thorac Cardiovasc Surg 1991;101:901-8.

Kodama K, Doi O, Higashiyama M, Yokoouchi H. Usefulness of Nd:YAG laser for the excision of multiple lung metastases and segmentectomy for primary lung cancer. Kyobu Geka 1992;45:51-5.

Konstantinou M, Potaris K, Sakellaridis T, Chamalakis G. Sleeve lobectomy for patients with non small-cell lung cancer: a simplified approach. Eur J Cardiothorac Surg 2009;36:1045-1051.

LoCicero J, Hartz RS, Frederiksen JW, Michaelis LL. Laser assisted parenchyma-sparing pulmonary resection. J Thorac Cardiovasc Surg 1989;97:732-6.

LoCicero J, Hartz RS, Frederiksen JW, Michaelis LL. New applications of the laser in pulmonary surgery. Hemostasis and sealing of air leaks. Ann Thoracic Surg 1985;40:546-50.

Ludwig C, Stoelben E, Olschewski M, Hasse J. Comparison of morbidity. 30-day mortality and long-term survival after pneumonectomy and sleeve lobectomy for non-small cell carcinoma. Ann Thorac Surg 2005;79:968-73.

Mineo TC, Ambrogi V, Pompeo E, Nofroni I. The value of the Nd:YAG laser for the surgery of lung metastases in a randomized trial. Chest 1998;113:1402-7.

Moghissi K. Experience in non-contact Nd:YAG laser in pulmonary surgery. Eur J Cardiothorac Surg 1988;2:87-94.

Pereszlenyi A, Bis B, Baier B, Schilling A, Rudek B, Rolle A. Metastasized colorectal carcinoma - is there a place for a lung laser metastasectomy? An Oncol 2006;17(Suppl 6): vi 84.

Pereszlenyi A, Rolle A, Huscher S, Bis B, Baier B, Rudek B: Laser segmental lung resection for stage I non-small cell lung cancer (VIDEO). 11th International Thoracic Surgery Congress - 23rd Annual Meeting - Austrian Society of Surgical Oncology (ACO-ASSO), St. Wolfgang, Austria, October 5-7, 2006.

Pereszlenyi A, Rolle A, Huscher S, Koch R, Rudek B: Laser segmental lung resection versus lobectomy for stage I non-small cell lung cancer - a prospective single institution study. Eur. Surg. 2006,Vol.38,Supplement Nr.210:55.

Pereszlenyi A, Schilling A, Rudek B, Baier B, Rolle A. Ergebnisse nach Laserresektion metastasierender Lungenmetastasen von kolorektalem Karzinom. 146. Jahrestagung der West- und Norddeutschen Gesellschaft für Chirurgie. Hamburg, 31.11.-03.12.2006.

Rolle A, Eulerich E. Extensive multiple and lobe-sparing pulmonary resections with the Nd:YAG laser and a new wavelength of 1318 nm. Acta Chirurgica Hungarica 1999;38(1):115-7.

Rolle A, Pereszlenyi A, Koch R, Richard M, Baier B. Is surgery for multiple lung metastases reasonable? A total of 328 consecutive patients with multiple-laser metastasectomies with a new 1318-nm Nd:YAG laser. J Thorac Cardiovasc Surg. 2006;131:1236-41.

Rolle A, Thetter O, Häussinger K, Hallfeldt KKJ, Schmölder A. Einsatz des Neodym YAG Lasers in der Thoraxchirurgie. Herz Gefäss Thorax Chir 1989;3:85-91.

Rolle A, Unsöld E, Ruprecht L, Permanetter W, Frank F. Morphologic aspects of Nd:YAG laser application (wavelengths 1064 nm and 1318 nm) on lung tissue. Laser Med Surg 1988;4:10-14.

Stokes LF, Auth DC, Tanaka D, Gray JL, Gulasik C. Biomedical utility of 1320 nm Nd:YAG laser radiation. IEEE Trans Biomed Eng 1981;28:297-9.

Thomford NR, Woolner LD, Clagett OT. The surgical treatment of metastatic tumors in the lungs. J Thorac Cardiovasc Surg. 1965;49:357-63.

Van Schil PE, Hendriks JM, Van Putte BP, Stockman BA, Lauwers PR, Ten Broecke PW, Grootenboers MJ, Schramel FM: Isolated lung perfusion and realted techniques for the treatment of pulmonary metastases. Eur J Cardiothorac Surg 2008;33: 486-495.

13

Surgery in Small-Cell Lung Cancer: Past, Present and Future

Cristian Rapicetta[1], Sara Tenconi[1], Tommaso Ricchetti[1], Sally Maramotti[2] and Massimiliano Paci[1]
[1]*Thoracic Surgery Unit, Cardio-Thoracic-Vascular and Critical Care Department*
[2]*Laboratory of Molecular Biology, Department of Oncology*
Arcispedale Santa Maria Nuova - IRCCS, Reggio nell'Emilia
Italy

1. Introduction

Small-Cell Lung Carcinoma (SCLC) represents about 15% of all lung cancers diagnosed worldwide. Although its incidence is diminished in the last decades, SCLC continues to represent an almost fatal disease due to its propensity to local relapse and distant metastasis, despite initial responsiveness to therapies. Biological behaviour of SCLC has therefore lead to consider it as a systemic disease *per se* not amenable of surgical resection: the Veterans Administration Lung Study Group (VALSG) two-stage classification was in fact based on field irradiation criteria and has been applied to SCLC for long-time.

The introduction of TNM staging system, the common recurrences of local disease despite initial complete response after chemo-radiation therapy, the lack of a valid maintenance therapy after remission or a second-line therapy after relapse renewed interest in surgery in a multimodal treatment setting. However, the second prospective randomized trial in 1994, did not confirm any significant advantage of surgery compared to chemo-radiation therapy and several retrospective studies published in the same years failed to provide strong evidences of surgery's benefits. Lack of homogeneity in design of clinical trials, which are mostly dated, patients selection and other confounding factors made results of meta-analysis too much inconsistent to be added to guidelines; for these reasons, nowadays, surgery is recommended only in small peripheral nodules without nodal involvement (proven by invasive preoperative staging).

Advances in comprehension of biological pathways underlying carcinogenesis in SCLC are the next steps that could deeply modify the approach to disease (patients selection and prognostic stratification, chemosensitivity and treatment modality) beyond the mere histology. Molecular profile should lead to identify subsets of tumours with more favourable prognosis, especially in terms of systemic control of disease, which is actually a major issue in SCLC; these subsets could be overlapped to NSCLC regarding to natural history of disease, making their treatment similar, including indication to surgery.

The aim of this review is to analyze literature to deduce which has been, is actually and could be the role of surgery on overall survival and pattern of recurrence of patients affected by SCLC.

2. Clinical background

2.1 Epidemiology

Small-cell Lung Carcinoma (SCLC) accounts for approximately for 13-15%% of all newly diagnosed cases of lung cancer worldwide (in United States, more than 220.000 new cases lung carcinoma were diagnosed in 2010, with about 160.000 cancer-related deaths [American Cancer Society, 2010].

More than 90% of patients with SCLC are elderly, current or past heavy smokers, and risk rises with increasing duration and intensity of smoking [Devesa et al., 2005]; rare cases have been reported in people who never smoked [Antony et al., 2010].

Incidence of SCLC is decreasing compared to that of adenocarcinoma [Govindan, 2006]; this reflects the decreased prevalence of smoking in industrialised countries. However, the burden of disease is shifting to developing countries (Asia and Eastern Europe), where, on the contrary, an increase of incidence is expected in next years. Further investment in research against SCLC is therefore warranted.

A revision in the WHO classification of lung cancers might also have contributed to incidence falling of SCLC, as some borderline cases previously described as mixed subtypes are now classified as NSCLC [Travis et al., 2004].

Median survival of untreated patients ranges from 2 to 4 months from diagnosis: historical data of untreated patients come from an old study of VALSG (Veterans Association of Lung Study Group) comparing cyclophosphamide to placebo. In IASLC (International Association for Study of Lung Cancer) database for staging project (the largest series of SCLCs reported), 5-year survival rates were 38/21% for clinical stages IA/IB and 38/18% for clinical stages IIA/IIB, respectively. Considering only resected, fully staged patients, 5-years survival rates were 53/44% for p-stages IA/IB and 43/35% in p-stages IIA/IIB, respectively.

2.2 Clinical presentation

Two thirds of SCLCs present as peribronchial lesions with infiltration of bronchial submucosa. Extensive mediastinal lymph node metastases are a common finding at diagnosis; sometimes mediastinal involvement presents as "bulky" disease, causing superior vena cava syndrome. Only in 4-12% of cases SCLC presents as a peripheral "coin lesion" [Quoix et al., 1990].

Clinical presentation of SCLC is strictly related to stage and presence of paraneoplastic syndrome. Common symptoms are cough, wheeze, dyspnoea, haemoptysis for hilar localization. Symptoms may reflect direct involvement of chest wall, superior vena cava, oesophagus, recurrent nerve (pain, mediastinal syndrome, dysphagia, dysphonia) or the site of metastasis (brain, liver, adrenal glands, bone and bone marrow). SCLC is more frequently associated to paraneoplastic syndromes than NSCLC [Gandhi et al., 2006]. The most common are syndrome of inappropriate antidiuresis (15-40% of SCLC patients) and Cushing's syndrome (2-5% of SCLC patients), that can be responsible of infective complications during chemotherapy. Sometimes SCLC presents with dermatological abnormalities as acquired tylosis, trip palms, erythema gyratum repens [Master et al., 2010]. Occasionally SCLC is associated to dermatomyositis, hyperglycemia or hypoglicemia, hypercalcemia and gynecomastia. Neurological syndromes, that may precede diagnosis of SCLC by several months, are caused by cross-reaction of auto-antibodies and T-lymphocytes specific for common tumour epitopes and nervous components [Darnell et al., 2003]. Antibodies directed against the P/Q- type voltage-gated calcium channel in the presynaptic nerve terminal (expressed by 3% of SCLC) are responsible of Lambert-Eaton syndrome [Payne et al., 2010], that should be differentiated from miastenia gravis, rarely associated to SCLC. Similarly, paraneoplastic encephalomyelitis and paraneoplastic sensory neuropathy have been associated with antibodies directed against Hu proteins, a family of DNA-binding proteins (<1% of SCLC patients) [Gultekin et al., 2000]; neurological symptoms are not always reversible with therapy.

2.3 Diagnosis

Although diagnosis of SCLC could be suspected on the basis of clinical and radiological findings, histo-patological diagnosis is required prior to establish the proper treatment.

SCLC represents the extreme of spectrum of neuro-endocrine lung carcinomas and is defined as pure SCLC or combined SCLC if the non small-cell component accounts for at least 10%of burden disease.

While pre-invasive and in situ lesions are frequently found in NSCLC, they are uncommon in SCLC [Kumar et al., 2005].

Samples can be obtained by bronchoscopy biopsy or fine-needle aspiration from primary tumour, lymph nodes or other metastatic sites. Since tumour shows propensity to spread through tunica submucosa, superficial bronchoscopic biopsy or brush may be falsely negatives. Colliquative necrosis can sometimes hamper diagnosis, especially for cytological samples; however there is a good interobserver agreement among pathologists for differential diagnosis with NSCLC. Immunohistochemistry is used in difficult cases: less than 10% of SCLC tumours are negative for all neuroendocrine markers (chromogranin, synaptophysin, and CD56. Positivity for TTF-1 and cytokeratins helps to distinguish them from lymphomas and other small-cell tumours [van Meerbeeck et al., 2011]

2.4 Staging

Historically, SCLC had been classified according to the Veterans Administration Lung Study Group (VALSG). In 1957 the VALSG created a dichotomous staging system that took into account the aggressive behaviour of SCLC and the standard of care at that time. This classification underlined the highest importance of radiation therapy and allowed a better selection of patients for this kind of treatment.

The Limited Disease (LD) was characterized by a tumour volume encompassed in one radiation portal (30% of cases): all that was not comprised in one radiation portal was classified as extensive stage (ED), including malignant pleural effusion and haematogenous metastases. [Zelen et al., 1973]. In 1989 the International Association for the Study of Lung Cancer modified the VALSG staging including all non-metastatic patients in the limited stage [Stahel et al., 1991] (Tab.1).

More recently, in 2007, the IASLC based on a retrospective analysis of survival of 8088 patients with SCLC recommended the TNM classification system also for SCLC [Shepherd et al., 2007]. This suggestion comes from the evidence of significantly worse survival of patients with limited-stage disease and N2-N3 lymph node involvement, than for those with N0-N1 lymph node involvement. Patients with pleural effusion without extrathoracic metastasis showed a survival intermediate between stage III and stage IV. In the TNM classification patients with cytology-negative pleural effusion are classified as having stage III disease. This classification is used less frequently in clinical practice because it relies on surgical confirmation for its accuracy and patients with SCLC seldom present at a stage for which surgery is appropriate (in IASLC database only 349 patients out of 12.620 affected by SCLC were resected, representing only 2,8%).

VALSG staging	TNM staging
Limited Disease: disease encompassed within a tolerable radiation therapy portal • Tumour confined to one hemithorax • Involvement of ipsilateral and contralateral mediastinal nodes • Involvement of ipsilateral supraclavicular nodes • Ipsilateral pleural effusion	From IA to IIIB
Extensive Disease: any other	IV

Table 1. Comparison between VALSG and TNM staging

Considering the therapeutic options (chemotherapy and radiotherapy) representing, to date, the standard of care, it could be argued that the more precise staging of SCLC using the TNM system does not provide extra benefits to select the treatment modality. However TNM has been shown to be prognostic of outcome [Micke et al., 2002], and a more precise definition of nodal involvement may be relevant for radiation treatment. Moreover, surgery for limited disease (T1-2, N0, M0) is nowadays considered a valid therapeutic option [Varlotto et al., 2011]. For these reasons clinicians and cancer registrars recommend to classify SCLC with the TNM staging system [Shepherd et al., 2007]. This recommendation is particularly strong for those trials in LD addressing thoracic and prophylactic cranial irradiation questions and those that include a surgical treatment arm [Vallieres et al., 2009]. In the future a better definition of N stage is needed and prognostic difference in patients with or without cytology-positive pleural and/or pericardial effusions must be addressed.

To assess the extent of disease, which remains the main prognostic factor, several staging tests are available; their execution sequence should be guided by the patient's signs and symptoms at presentation and the availability of the diagnostic tests. Staging should be accurate and fast, considering the rapid growth of SCLC. Staging work-up should include full medical history, physical examination, chest X-ray, hematology and chemistry panels including differential blood count, liver and renal function tests, lactate dehydrogenase (LDH) and sodium levels (hyponatremia, due to ectopic production of antidiuretic hormone or atrial natriuretic peptide, is observed in up to 15% of patients), pulmonary function tests, and contrast-enhanced CT of the chest and upper abdomen. SCLC displays the propensity for early distant metastases to liver, bones, adrenal glands, and above all brain. Therefore, in patients with suspect for distant metastases, additional tests may include bone scintigraphy, CT scan with intravenous contrast or MRI of the brain, and bone marrow aspiration and biopsy. Bone marrow is involved in 15 to 30 percent of patients at presentation, but it represents rarely a solitary site of metastatic disease (2 to 6%). Bone-marrow infiltration should be suspected in presence of an isolated rise in lactate dehydrogenase (LDH) concentration or blood counts indicating otherwise unexplained anemia or a leucoerythroblastic response or if bone scan is positive [Campling et al., 1986]. CT or MRI of the brain are recommended if chemo-radiation with curative intent is under consideration. In one report, the prevalence of brain metastases was 10% with CT and 24% with MRI. In this series all CT-detected brain metastases were symptomatic, whereas 11% of those detected by MRI were asymptomatic [Seute et al., 2008]. Chest CT scan, abdominal CT scan, brain MRI and bone scintigraphy are mandatory in the evaluation of patients amenable to surgery [Koletsis et al., 2009]. Fluorodeoxyglucose (FDG) uptake is usually high in SCLC, leading to a sensitivity of nearly 100% but its routine use in SCLC remains controversial [Thomson et al., 2011]. PET is, anyway, useful to plan radiotherapy in some countries [Van Loon et al., 2010]. Pathological confirmation is still required for PET-detected lesions that could result in upstaging, in particular if radical resection could be offered. The role of combined fluorodeoxyglucose PET (FDG-PET) and CT scanning is yet to be completely defined but, if available, it may be useful to improve the accuracy of staging by the detection of mediastinal nodal and occult distant metastatic spread. In patients who present with pleural effusion, in the absence of extrathoracic disease, cytopathologic confirmation of tumour involvement is needed.

With improvements in staging through the use of PET/CT and magnetic resonance imaging (MRI), more patients are found to have ES-SCLC: the ratio of LS-SCLC to ES-SCLC was formerly 1:1 and is now 1:3 as more subtle lesions, such as silent adrenal and brain metastases, are identified.

If extensive disease is detected by one test, further staging can be omitted, although bone scintigraphy may be used to identify symptomatic lesions amenable of palliation radiotherapy and brain CT/MRI could be performed or repeated in patients who respond to treatment in order to plan a brain irradiation of symptomatic lesions or to plan PCI in absence of metastasis (since PCI has been extended to ED-SCLC responsive to primary treatments)

2.5 Prognosis

Stage is the major prognostic factor of survival but some other prognostic factors have been identified: performance status, weight loss, sex and some laboratory tests (CEA, LDH, NSE, hypoalbuminemia, elevated alkaline phosphatase). No histological or molecular features have been validated yet. Several algorithms have been elaborated for predicting survival but the reliability for individual patients remains poor. Paraneoplastic syndromes are more frequently found in patients with limited-stage SCLC and they are considered positive prognostic factors.

3. Historical background of SCLC

SCLC was firstly recognized by Barnard in 1926, who noted that "oat-cell sarcomas of the mediastinum" were metastatic carcinomas of the lung instead.

In the 85 years of SCLC life, some milestones should be reminded:

1959: Pathogists recognized SCLC as a separate entity among carcinomas of the lung and Azzopardi defined six features of cells at light microscopic examination [Azzopardi, 1959]

1963: VALSG introduced the 2-stage system for SCLC

1969: British Medical Research Council reported better survival of radiotherapy arm versus surgical arm in the first clinical randomized trial on SCLC [Miller et al., 1969]. Cyclophosphamide showed to be effective against lung cancer [Green et al., 1969]

1979: Medical Research Council showed advantage in survival with combination of chemotherapy (cyclophosphamide) and radiation therapy compared with radiation alone in LD-SCLC [Medical Research Council Lung Cancer Working Party, 1979]

1982: Shields re-evaluated surgery as initial treatment in SCLC after introduction of TNM staging system [Shields, 1982]
1987: Adding RT to chemotherapy improved survival in LD-SCLC [Perry et al., 1987]
1989: The International Association for Study of Lung Cancer (IASLC) was revised for the first time by its introduction the Veterans Administration Lung Study Group staging system [Stahel, 1989]
1994: Lung Cancer Study Group published results of the first (and unique, so far) perspective randomized trial in LD-SCLC comparing surgery to RT after induction chemotherapy: Authors concluded that surgery offered no advantage in terms of either survival or local control of disease.
1995-1999: Prophylactic Cranial Irradiation (PCI) showed to improve overall and disease-free survival in selected patients (responders to first-line treatments) [Aupérin et al., 1999]
1999: studies of dose fractionation of RT demonstrated that twice-daily administration was superior compared to once-daily in terms of local control and overall survival [Turrisi et al., 1999]
Combining this dates we can schematically recognize three periods.

3.1 The "Surgical Era" (early 1900-1960s)

The dramatic increase of tobacco consumption in early 900's produced a sharp increase of incidence of SCLC; on the other hand, prevalence of pulmonary tuberculosis and chest wounds during World Wars promoted advances in thoracic surgery and lung resections. Surgery was considered the standard of care for Small-Cell as well as Non small-cell lung cancer. However high rates of recurrence (both local and distant), even after apparently complete resection, were observed. Results published by British Medical Council Group in first clinical prospective trial randomizing patients affected by SCLC to either surgery or thoracic radiation therapy reported the slight advantage in survival of RT arm. This was enough to abandon surgery at least for primary therapy for SCLC. Dichotomous staging by Veterans Administration Lung Cancer Study Group (1968) reflected and anticipated the centrality of RT as primary treatment for local control of disease

3.2 The "advent of Chemotherapy" (1960s-1980s)

Few years later report of British Medical Council, the pathology study conducted by Matthews in autopsies of patients deceased within 30 days of attempted curative resection showed that SCLC had, in almost all patients, microscopic but widely metastatic disease [Matthews et al., 1973]. This enforced the importance of accurate staging of disease and promoted the need of systemic control of disease. The chemosensitivity of SCLC was first recognized in 1940s when nitrogen mustard (methyl-bis-B-Chloro-ethyl amine hydrochloride) demonstrated capability of inducing tumour regression in more than 50% of patients. Despite a large amount of active drugs towards SCLC, it was perceived quite early that single-agent regimens were associated to frail remissions and high rates of precocious recurrences. In 1970s combination chemotherapy, mainly based on cyclophosphamide showed dramatic responses, even in very incapacitated patients, although long term disease-free survival remained disappointing and natural history of disease did not seem to change. Chemotherapy became the standard of care also in limited disease when Medical Research Council demonstrated the advantage of a combination of cyclophosphamide and radiation compared with radiation alone. During the 1970s thoracic radiation was relegated to an adjuvant, "consolidative" role in LD-SCLC.

3.3 Evolution of combined modality treatment (1980s-today)

The last period could be considered as "quiescent": no tools against disease proved to be revolutionary and efforts were made towards integration of multimodal approach. Paradigms and flow charts of treatment did not reflect the chronological sequence of most important studies but rather controlled studies and consensus expressed by expertise panels of Authors. Etoposide and platinum became from 1980s the first-line treatment. An important study from National Cancer Institute (NCI) in 1976 firstly tested a very aggressive protocol involving simultaneous irradiation of brain, primary tumour and mediastinum and concomitant CAV chemotherapy (cyclophosphamide/doxorubicine/vincristine). Despite unacceptable toxicity (radiation pneumonitis in 38%, mielodepression with fatal sepsis in 24%), this regimen showed the best results, never reached before (nearly 100% complete remissions, 80% of long term survival) [Greco et al., 1979]. This work firstly recognized the importance of tumour repopulation by clones of cells whose resistance was allowed by sequentiality of treatments. Efforts were made in order to minimize tissue interaction without compromising delivery of both radiation and chemo-therapy: timing of radiation therapy [Perry et al., 1987] and dose fractioning [Turrisi et al. 1999] were largely studied by various Authors.

In this period surgery revived with first report from Shields and coll. who concluded that primary surgery and adjuvant chemotherapy could be offered to patients with SCLC in early stages (i.e. T1N0). A large number of subsequent studies (discussed in the chapter) reported favourable long-term survival after surgery with improved local control of disease: one of the most remarkable experience was that of Toronto Group [Shepherd, 1983].

Undoubtedly, advances in both imaging and invasive staging tools (spiral CT, PET/CT, FNA-EBUS) lead to a more precise stratification of disease, allowing selection of patients in really "limited" disease amenable for radical resection. Application of TNM staging as used for NSCLC eliminated one of the barriers that divided SCLC and NSCLC and contributed to better define prognosis of patients previously classified as having Limited Disease (an heterogeneous stage ranging from isolated coin lesion to extensive hilar mass with supraclavicular node metastasis).

Times were mature for another clinical perspective randomized trial involving surgery: it was started by Lung Cancer Study Group in 1983 and ended in 1994. Results again excluded a benefit of surgery even on a multimodal approach, but did not prevent further Authors to report their retrospective experiences on surgically resected SCLC, criticizing at the same time this study.

Main changes of treatment modalities in SCLC are summarized in Fig. 1

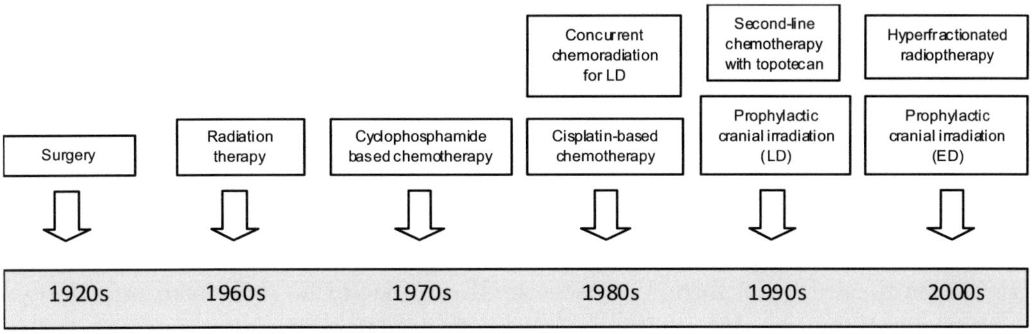

Fig. 1. Evolution of treatment modalities through decades

4. Current guidelines for treatment (NCCN/ACCP)

It should be noted that guidelines for the treatment of SCLC are based on review of a literature that lacks of big randomized prospective trials and is heterogeneous regarding to kind of treatment, timing, endpoints and selection of patients.
The National Comprehensive Cancer Network (NCCN) has recently developed a review of its guidelines, declaring that every recommendation for SCLC has to be considered category 2A, because they are "based upon lower-level evidence" but "uniform NCCN consensus that the intervention is appropriate" (see Table 2). [NCCN Clinical Practice Guidelines in Oncology]

Category 1	The recommendation is based on high-level evidence (e.g., randomized trials) and there is uniform NCCN consensus
Category 2A	The recommendation is based on lower-level evidence and there is uniform NCCN consensus
Category 2B	The recommendation is based on lower-level evidence and there is nonuniform NCCN consensus (but no major disagreement).
Category 3	The recommendation is based on any level of evidence but reflects major disagreement

Table 2. NCCN category of recommendation.

The American College of Chest Physicians (ACCP) in 2007 produced a systematic literature review resulting in evidence–based guidelines, graded upon the "ACCP grading system for guideline recommendations"
Both documents debate on diagnostic and therapeutic options for SCLC and are quite similar in recommendations, except for the use of PET (not yet standardized in 2007 ACCP guidelines) and for the choice of staging system (NCCN recommending the use of the new TNM instead of Veterans Administration Lung Study Group classification).
Guidelines for treatment have a key point in the use of platinum-based chemotherapy plus radiotherapy for all fit patients (Performance Status 0-2) with limited stage disease, followed by Prophylactic Cranial Irradiation (PCI); topics of discussion are timing of radiotherapy (concurrent versus sequential, early versus late), volume, dose and fractionation of radiations, treatment of unfit-elderly patients, maintenance and second line chemotherapy and surgery.
Cisplatin has to be preferred to Carboplatin in combination with Etoposide in first line treatment; in phase III randomized trials, Irinotecan was substituted for Etoposide in combination with Carboplatin in advanced disease with mild improve in survival and thus being added to guidelines as an option for patients with extensive-stage disease. In these patients, where the treatment of choice is chemotherapy alone with initial response of about 60-70% but median survival of 9-11 months due to early relapse, maintenance or consolidation chemotherapy beyond 4 to 6 cycles is currently not recommended outside clinical trials (grade of recommendation IB); likewise, the introduction of a third agent (alkylating agent with or without anthracycline) showed minor advantage in duration of response without improving survival and carried greater cumulative toxicity. The use of cytochine or anti-angiogenetic agents (i.e. Bevacizumab) is not currently recommended in first line treatment, even though randomized phase III trials are currently running.
Second line treatment is generally a single agent therapy, administered with an interval of at least 3 month since initial therapy (otherwise disease has to be considered refractory or resistant) and should be given until 2 cycles beyond best response, progression of disease, development of major toxicity.

The addition of thoracic radiotherapy has improved survival in patients with limited stage disease (grade of recommendation 1A); staging of SCLC actually involves relationship between extension of disease and radiation port field. As far as timing is concerned, early (within 30 days to 9 weeks since the beginning of chemotherapy) concurrent chemo-radiotherapy is recommended for patients with limited-stage disease (grade of recommendation 1A). Hyper-fractionation of radiation dose has not yet being correctly compared to once-daily administration in available trials, according to NCCN review of literature.

PCI given after completion of chemotherapy in a low dose per fraction causes less neurological toxicity and prevent the emergence of brain metastasis, both in limited and extensive stage disease; it is recommended for fit patients who achieve a complete or partial response to initial treatment (Grade of recommendation 1B).

Radiotherapy is also recommended in relapse for palliation of symptoms.

The European Society of Medical Oncology (ESMO) in the 1st consensus conference in lung cancer stated guidelines for diagnosis, treatment and follow up of SCLC, underlying the absence of randomized trials comparing surgery with concurrent chemo-radiotherapy. Nevertheless, with grade of recommendation III D, surgical resection may be considered for very limited disease (T1-2, N0), only after histological confirmation of N parameters by mediastinoscopy, followed by PCI.

ACCP guidelines stress the importance of invasive mediastinal staging, with grade of recommendation 1A. NCCN guidelines specify that lobectomy has to be preferred if resection is performed and that adjuvant chemotherapy alone is recommended for patients without nodal metastasis, while mediastinal RT has to be added in case of nodal involvement (Fig. 2)

5. Studies regarding surgery in SCLC

Except from those by British Medical Council and Lung Cancer Study Group, all studies focused on surgery in SCLC are retrospective or prospective non-randomized, so conclusions should be interpreted cautiously.

However, also those phase III trials have been criticised on several points.

The British Medical Council study, dated 1963, did not include patients with peripheral lung lesions, since preoperative evaluation and diagnosis were made using rigid bronchoscopy available at that time; secondly, rate of complete (R0) resection was low (approximately 50%) compared to resections for NSCLC; finally, staging was performed without modern tools, like contrast CT-scan or PET, nor histological confirmation by mediastinoscopy was obtained. So it is likely that a remarkable number of patients with occult intrathoracic and extrathoracic disease was included in the study and randomized to surgery, compromising the long term survival results.

Twenty years later, after advent of chemotherapy as standard primary treatment, times were mature for another randomized trials, set up by Lung Cancer Study Group in 1983. Eligibility criteria include LD stage, according to VALSG staging: this means that also patients with clinical evident mediastinal adenopaties were included in the study. Conversely, patients with peripheral nodules and normal bronchoscopy were specifically excluded from the study. Induction therapy was quite heterogeneous (anthracycline based regimen) and only 144 of 340 patients (42%) accrued in the trial were randomized (68 to surgery arm and 76 to radiotherapy arm). Six patients randomized to surgery refused

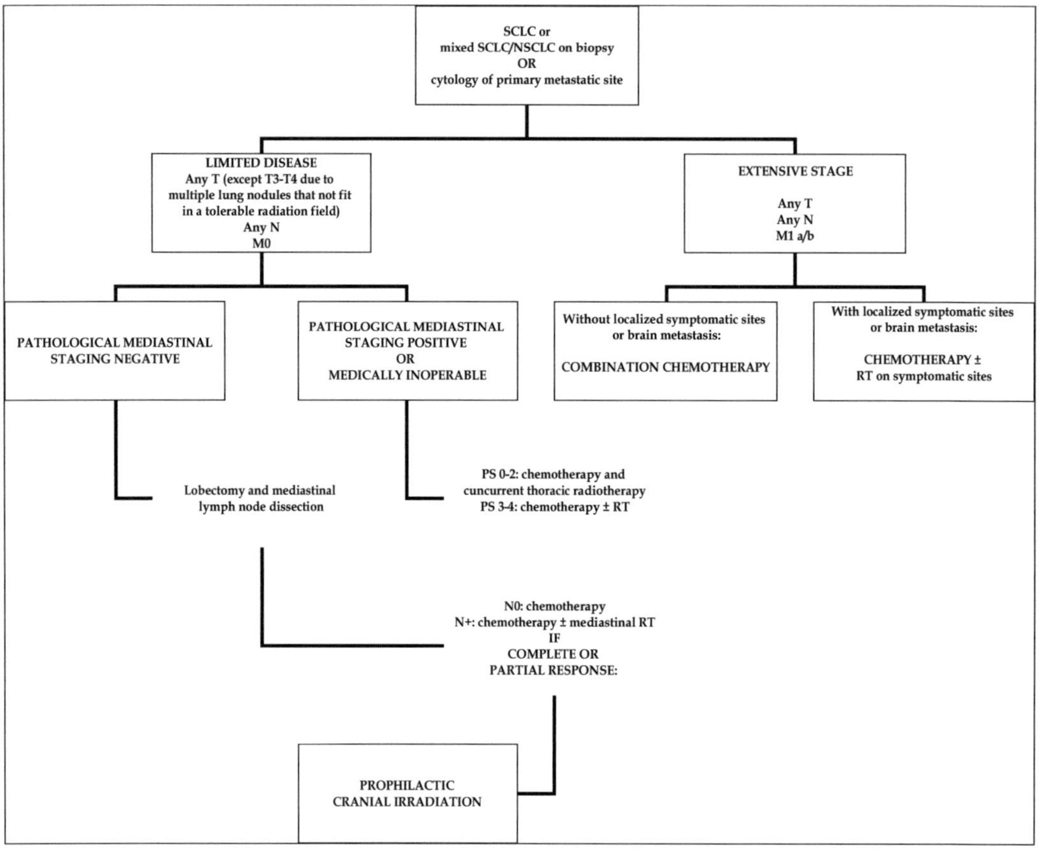

Fig. 2. NCCN clinical practice guidelines

thoracotomy and, on the contrary, eight patients requested surgical intervention and received off-randomization surgery, representing a significant cross-over (10%) between the two arms. Moreover, few other data should be pointed out: only 65% of patients responded to induction chemotherapy, in 17% of patients assigned to surgery only exploratory thoracotomy was performed and, above all, the high proportion of patients included with bulky N2 or N3 nodal metastasis (who unlikely achieved a complete mediastinal downstaging). Interestingly N status and post-treatment clinical stage did not influence resectability (a result correlated with clinical understaging).

The conclusion of the study was that surgery did not add any benefit neither in terms of survival nor of pattern of recurrence.

The same results were anticipated in a retrospective study of 1985 based on 33 operated patients compared to 46 patients who fulfilled criteria of operability and resectability but were treated with non-surgical management. However microscopic or macroscopic residual disease was left in half of patients, suggesting that clinical staging was not so accurate in predicting resectability of disease [Østerlind, 1985]

Considering these weak points, rejection of surgery did not discourage several Authors, which continued to report good results with surgery combined to either induction or adjuvant chemotherapy and radiotherapy in some cases.

Rostad et al. analyzed 2442 patients with SCLC in a national survey in Norway, 38 of which were surgically resected (25 received adjuvant therapies). For stage I addition of surgery to conventional treatments (chemo-radiation) improved 5-year survival rate from 11.3% to 44.9%, so Authors concluded that patients with resectable disease in stage I should be referred to surgery [Rostad, 2004].

The same conclusion is reported by Leo and Pastorino in their review [Leo & Pastorino, 2003] for T1-2N0M0 patients which can be treated by surgery and adjuvant chemotherapy, while patients in stage II-III should undergo surgery only in the context of clinical trials.

Rea et al. reported a 32% overall survival in 104 patients with SCLC surgically resected, despite a remarkable percentage of stage III (43.3%), which resulted as a major negative prognostic factors [Rea, 1998]

Brock et al reviewed their institutional experience of 1415 SCLC among whom 82 (6%) underwent surgery with curative intent from 1976 to 2002 [Brock, 2005]. Surgery was accompanied by induction or adjuvant chemotherapy in 77% of patients. Authors found a 5-year survival of 85.7% for stage I SCLC (similar to that historically expected for completely resected stage I NSCLC without adjuvant chemotherapy). Favourable prognostic factors were early stage, lobectomy as surgical procedure, female gender and date of intervention after 1987 (a surrogate marker for availability of platinum based chemotherapy). Pattern of recurrence was not reported in this study, however Authors concluded that lobectomy plus platinum based chemotherapy is a feasible option yielding excellent results in T1-T2N0-M0 SCLC.

High 5 years survival rate was reported also by Tsuchiya in a retrospective series of patients treated with a similar protocol [Tsuchiya, 2005]. Interestingly, Authors reported only 10% of local failure after surgery, which is lower than commonly reported after chemo-radiation therapies alone.

Badzio and coll. in a retrospective series of patients treated with surgery or non-surgical management reported a significative improvement in survival in surgical resected patients (22 months Vs 11, P<0.001) [Badzio, 2004]. The control group of patients treated with chemo-radiotherapy was built using pair-matched case-control according to main prognostic factors, stage and resectability; moreover diagnosis of surgical treated patients was established only postoperatively, thus minimizing some bias related to selection of patients.

In 2006 the Bronchogenic Carcinoma Cooperative Group of the Spanish Society of Pneumology and Thoracic Surgery (GCCB-S) presented a multicenter study on 47 patients with SCLC out a total of 2994 lung cancers resected [Gomez de Antonio, 2006]. Thirty-three % of patients had incomplete resection suggesting that the criteria for surgery were not predictable enough for resectability. The routine use of mediastinoscopy (performed only in 19% of cases) might have identified some of the patients whose clinical staging was underestimated and which added to low rate of respectability. Moreover a low proportion of patients received adjuvant treatments. These factors accounts for an overall survival which does not exceed that reported in literature for patients with possibly more advanced stage managed with chemo-radiotherapy.

Recently, Schreiber and coll. analyzed patients included in the Surveillance, Epidemiology and End Results registry (SEER), which is the cancer registry representative of United States [Schreiber, 2010]. Among 14.179 patients affected by SCLC coded as localized (T1-2Nx-0) or regional disease (T3-4Nx-0), 863 (6%) had undergone surgical resection, making them one of the larger population based cohort ever reported in literature. Overall 5-year survival rates were 26.3 Vs 9.3% (P=0.01) in favour of surgery with median survival of 22 Vs 12 months, respectively. Advantage of surgery to survival was much more substantial in N0 patients (median survival 40 Vs 15 months), which on the other hand did show benefit from addition of PORT (Post-Operative Radiation Therapy). These data seem to suggest that radical surgery alone could be adequate for local control of disease and, conversely PORT may be detrimental for survival. Another retrospective analysis of SEER database conducted in 2010 and focused only on stage I confirmed reasonable outcome in patients who underwent lobectomy without PORT [Yu et al., 2010]. Unfortunately both studies, although based on large population, lack of data concerning chemotherapy, margins of resection, pathologic confirmation of diagnosis and performance status (not recorded in SEER database).

Study	**Number of patients**	**Treatment Modality**	**Local recurrence**	**5-year survival**
Fujimori, 1997	22	PE x 2/4 → S	5%	Cumulative: 66.7% (3-year) Stage I-II: 73.3% (3-year) Stage IIIA: 42.9%
Lucchi, 1997	127	S (15) S → CT (RT) (92) CT → S → CT (15)	4.1% (10.6% local+distant)	Cumulative: 22.6% 47% in stage I 0% in N2 patients 0% with surgery alone
Eberhardt, 2003	46	Stage I-IIA: PE x 4 → S Stage IIB-IIIA: PE x 3 → CTRx (HfRTx) → S	0%	Cumulative: 39%
Badzio, 2004	134	S → CT (67) CTRx (67)	5% 15%	Cumulative: 27% (4% CTRx) Stage IA: 59%
Rostad, 2004	38	S S → adjuvant	n/a	Stage I: 44.9%
Brock, 2005	82	(CT) → S → (CT)		Stage I: 58% Stage II: 18% Stage III: 23% Stage IV: 0%
Tsuchiya, 2005	62	S → PE x 4	10%	Stage IA/IB: 73/67% Stage II: 38% Stage III: 39%
Granetzny, 2006	95	S → CTRx (Stage I) CT → S → CTRx (Stage III)	n/a	Median survival (months) 31.3 (Stage I) 31.7 (Stage III – downstaged) 12.4 (Stage III – not downstaged)
Gomez De Antonio, 2006	47	CT → S (3) S → CT (30) S (14)	n/a	Cumulative: 26% R0 resection: 31% Stage I: 36%
Schreiber, 2009	863	S S → RT CT data n/a		Cumulative: 34.6% Stage I: 44.8% Stage II-III: 26.3%

S: surgery, CT: chemotherapy, CTRx: chemoradiation therapy, PE: Platinum-Etoposide, HfRTx: Hyperfractioned Radiation therapy

Table 3. Some of the recent trials supporting the role of surgery

A current year report on a small series of patients (28) underlines the low rate of local failure (3/28) after surgery compared to distant (especially brain) metastasis, which confirms the role of PCI [Ogawa et al. 2011]

5.1 Rationale of surgery in SCLC

As pointed out by Anraku and Waddell [Anraku, 2006] in their review, rationale of surgery can be can summarized in the following clinical presentations.

- **Small peripheral coin lesions**: typical or atypical carcinoids may be misdiagnosed as SCLC since their diagnosis is often made on cytological samples obtained by either trans-thoracic fine needle biopsy or trans-bronchial biopsy by bronchoscopy
- **Combined histology tumours**: definitive histology of tumours initially diagnosed as pure SCLC reveals a Non Small-Cell component in 11-25% [Asamura, 2006]. Percentages are higher in surgical reports possibly due to the fact that combined SCLC tends to arise peripherally and resection is feasible more frequently and because a larger amount of tissue for individuation of both components is available with surgical specimen [Mangum, 1989]. Although prognosis is mainly determined by the aggressiveness of Small-Cell component, the Non Small-Cell one may fail to chemoradiation protocols commonly used against SCLC being responsible of weak responses or early relapses.
- **Early stages (T1-2N0M0)** benefit of surgical resection in terms of improved local control of disease: first site of recurrence (which occurs in approximately 50% of cases after concurrent chemo-radiation protocols [Turrisi, 1999]) is the tumour bed site followed by hilar/mediastinal lymph nodes, even in patients who achieve complete pathological remission [Elliott, 1987]. Adjuvant radical resection (i.e. with R0 margins) after induction chemoradiotherapy has shown local control of disease in almost all cases and this is reflected in a slight advantage in long-term survival [Eberhardt, 2003]. Table with local recurrences and survival
- If general criteria for operability and resectability are met, **adjuvant "salvage" surgery** is preferable in cases of a chemotherapy resistant tumour or early local relapse (usually: 3 months) after an initial response, compared to second-line therapies which are often uneffective against SCLC. In their report, the Toronto Group identified a small subset of patients without node metastasis that benefit from salvage surgery). A second biopsy, if feasible, is worthy to be considered before surgery [Shepherd, 1991] to demonstrate a NSCLC component.
- **New metachronous tumours** appearing two years after a SCLC successfully treated patients could be second primary NSCLC and after a complete re-staging should be surgically resected even if histology can not be obtained preoperatively [Anraku, 2006]

5.2 Patient selection criteria and choice of surgical procedure

If a diagnosis is obtained preoperatively, pathologists should exclude any possible coexisting NSCLC component. Even more than in NSCLC, accurate staging is crucial before planning surgery in fit patients, as discussed before. Toronto Group demonstrated better 5-year survival (18% vs 6%) in patients without mediastinal nodes involvement preoperatively [Shepherd, 1991]; in a recent phase II trial on surgery after induction chemotherapy only patients who achieved complete nodal downstaging had a fair survival. Mediastinoscopy and eventually re-mediastinoscopy after primary treatment is therefore

recommended to detect nodal involvement which is microscopic and subclinical in a considerable percentage of patients. This matter accounts for discordance between clinical and pathological staging in SCLC.
If a SCLC is diagnosed in operative theatre at frozen section of specimens, radical resection (preferably lobectomy) is recommended if intraoperative histological examination of mediastinal lymph nodes does not reveal metastasis; however, surgery can be proposed to patients with mediastinal nodes micrometastasis if they can easily tolerate the procedure. Sublobar resections are recommended in less fit patients or in presence of nodal involvement.

6. Targeting the complex biology of SCLC

First cytogenetic studies, dated 1982, found that a deletion on chromosome 3p was present in 95% of SCLC [Whang, 1982]. This chromosomal region contains tumour-suppressor genes relevant to the pathogenesis of the tumour e.g. RARβ [Naylor 1987, Kok 1987] and FITH [Franklin, 2010]. The 3p loss alone is not specific of SCLC, since it is frequent encountered also in other tumours. Thanks to the high-throughput technology as comparative genomic hybridization (CGH) and gene expression arrays, researchers discovered that in 90% of SCLC samples, the most frequent sites of chromosome loss are 3p, 5q and 13q, the last determining the loss of retinoblastoma gene (RB1) [Ried, 1994]. Mutation studies on biology of SCLC showed that this type of tumour has frequent mutation in the gene encoding for p53 protein (TP53) [Hanahan, 200] but rarely presents mutation in the tyrosine-kinase signalling gene including KRAS and EGFR [Franklin, 2010], which are actually the most known pathways with larger number of active drugs (mainly tested in lung adenocarcinomas).
Targeted cancer therapies are drugs or antibodies that block the growth and the spread of cancer by interfering with specific molecules involved in tumour growth and progression. These therapies are being studied for use alone, in combination with other targeted therapies, and in combination with other cancer treatments, such as chemotherapy. By blocking signals that make cancer cell grow and replicate, targeted cancer therapies can help to stop cancer progression and may induce cancer cell death through apoptosis.
To give an example the PI3K/AKT/mTOR intracellular pathway is chronically activated in SCLC through inactivating mutations in PTEN gene and this activation pathway correlates with sensitivity to Everolimus in vitro [Marinov, 2009]. Furthermore, the amplification of BCL-2 genes seems to be correlate with the sensitivity to the highly potent small-molecule called ABT-737 suggesting that patients with bcl-2 protein over expression, may have some benefits from bcl-2 inhibitors [Olejniczak, 2007]. In SCLC cell lines, microRNA and gene-expression signatures of chemo-resistance have been described [Guo, 2010] and several inhibitors of growth factor pathways implicated in SCLC are in clinical development (NCT00896752); the compound PD173074 induces apoptosis in vitro and in vivo in SCLC by inhibition of FGF2 signalling [Pardo, 2009].
The targeting of specific molecules has been already studied in several trials, even though with limited success. One of the emerging need in clinical research dealing with SCLC is inadequacy of preclinical models of disease used to date. Cancer-cell-line-based xenograft models employed as standard testing ground especially for drugs have revealed as a surrogate of disease. In vitro activity level is then weakly predictable of clinical efficacy thus explaining the high rates of failure of new drugs tested in clinical studies. Human cancers

cells, compared to cancer-cell cultures, grow up in hypoxic and nutrient-poor complex environments which promotes continue selection of more aggressive cell-clones. This explains the reason why cell-line-based SCLC xenografts tend to grow as relatively indolent tumours, while corresponding human disease is characterized by aggressive clinical and biological behaviour.

Moreover, as for standard chemotherapy, the use of a single molecular target drug in such complex malignancy as SCLC, is wrong. The inhibition of multiple targets or the combination with standard chemotherapic agents are likely to have greater potential. The customizing of therapy with novel agent to individual patient's characteristics is becoming the most beneficial approach to treatment of SCLC. In addition to new agents, biomarkers of chemosensitivity need be identified to efficaciously assess single agents for relapse after first-line therapy or as a maintenance therapy in placebo-controlled, randomised designs. Several studies have identified genes or proteins in lung cancer whose expression levels are associated with response to antitumor drugs. The breast cancer resistant protein (BCRP), is one of the ABC transporters reported to be associated with resistance to anticancer drugs like doxorubicin, irinotecan, mitoxantrone, and its expression was found to be associated with a poor clinical outcome in SCLC patients undergoing chemotherapy [Kim, 2009]. Chiappori et al. reported that RRM1 and Topo2 alpha proteins expression are biomarkers of chemotherapeutic efficacy in SCLC [Chiappori, 2010] and, recently, Usuda et al. demonstrated that the expression levels of Klotho protein was correlated with the prognosis following resection in SCLC patients [Usuda, 2011]. These results are encouraging; however, this findings need to be incorporated into common signatures for individual therapies and further tested in prospective clinical trials. Of course, biostatistical concerns still exist for predicting response to drugs as for predicting patient prognosis.

7. Conclusions

Although the incidence of SCLC has been steadily decreasing over time, it continues to represent a relevant problem of public health due to its aggressive clinical behaviour and the lack of effective therapies; it is considered one of the most elusive cancers. Twenty-five years ago it was considered to be the next malignancy added to the list of curable cancers, because of the effectiveness of several chemotherapeutic agents and radiation therapy, and the discover of central nervous system sanctuary, which would require distinct treatment.

Conversely, despite active and ongoing research involving novel approaches to treat SCLC, few discovers had a successful translation in clinical practice over the past 25 years, with cumulative improvement of only 15% in survival which remains dismal and moreover seems to have now reached a plateau.

7.1 Current evidences

Over the last 25 years, few landmarks in therapy have been provided by clinical trials focused on LS-SCLC. Minimal progress was noted in ES-SCLC.

Main strategies that demonstrated able to add small but significant improvements in survival can be summarized in the followings:

- **Advantage of addition of radiotherapy to chemotherapy**: The defining report, Cancer and Leukemia Group B (CALGB) 8083 [14], published in the New England Journal of Medicine, showed, for patients with LS-SCLC, a local control, failure-free survival, and overall survival benefit with the addition of thoracic radiation to chemotherapy using a cyclophosphamide and doxorubicin-based regimen. At 2 years, only 13% of patients who received chemotherapy alone maintained local control, compared with 54% of patients receiving chest radiotherapy. Although the likelihood of relapse in the chest may be reduced by up to 50% when thoracic irradiation is administered after chemotherapy, 20–36% of patients will have local recurrence even after combined modality treatment [12,13]. An analysis of the site of first relapse demonstrated that, even for patients who have achieved clinical complete response, the primary tumour bed and hilar or mediastinal lymph node areas are the most frequent single sites of failure [Elliott, 1987]. Failure to achieve control at the primary site remains the most important obstacle to cure in patients with limited SCLC [Shepherd, 1991].

- **superiority of twice-daily radiation therapy over daily fractionation**: hyperfractioning radiation therapy was defined and experimented in order to respond to the need of improve local control of disease, which remains a serious issue in non-surgical managed patients
- **advantage of prophylactic central nervous system radiation** (PCI) in all responding patients (also with ES-SCLC)

7.2 Take home messages

There are other recommendations without strong evidence, but for which there is general agreement:

- **Resection is a reasonable option as initial treatments for early stages T1-2N0-M0 patients**: if preoperative diagnosis of SCLC has been obtained, nodal or distant metastasis must be excluded using by either non invasive or invasive staging, avoiding futile thoracotomies. Induction chemo-radiotherapy did not demonstrated superior to adjuvant setting. In any other stage of presentation, surgery is contemplated only in clinical trials.
- **Clinical understaging is frequent in SCLC** (concordance with pathological stage is only 58% in IASLC database) and common criteria of resectability often fails to predict complete resections in SCLC, due to propensity to spread through peribronchial lymphatic vessels to regional lymph-nodes. Introduction and more liberal use of EUS in flexible bronchoscopy or mediastinoscopy may help to rule out patients with micrometastasis not amenable of surgical resection
- **Surgery improves local control of disease** if radical resection is achieved. Local failure rates vary in literature from 0 to 15%, which is considerably lesser than 35-50% reported for chemo-therapy with twice-daily radiation therapy (the standard of care, to date) [Pijls-Johannesma et al., 2007; Turrisi et al., 1999]. In resected specimens after concurrent CT with HfRTx, Eberhardt found persistence of vital disease at the primary site [Eberhardt & Korfee, 2003]. However, there is no evidence, to date, that this translates in an improvement of overall and disease-free survival, which could eventually derive from progresses in systemic treatments.

7.3 Challenge to systemic disease

Since the overwhelming majority of patients with LD-SCLC have subclinical metastatic foci at the time of diagnosis, chemotherapy is an essential part of multimodal treatment to control systemic disease.

Cytotoxic drugs active in SCLC discovered in the early 1980s remains a standard of care at present. Advances in supportive care and technical advances in radiation therapy have allowed the application of therapies with less toxicity and well tolerated by most patients. Fall in treatment-related deaths implies an improvement on survival (compared to history of 20-yrs ago) which is actually difficult to be discriminated by the true prolongation of survival due to change in natural history of disease.

At now, most of ongoing clinical trials deal with various combination of active cytotoxic agents, but it has become evident that only small improvements in survival should be expected by such protocols. The issue is not spectrum of active drugs, as is the case in melanoma, for example but rather the rapid development of drug resistance and the failure of second-line therapy, especially in case of no response to primary treatment or early relapse of disease (< 3 months). Therefore clinical research on SCLC is shifting towards target-therapy, although most efforts have been and are still spent on lung adenocarcinoma, because its arise in incidence makes it more attractive in terms of cost/effectiveness of research.

Another issue in SCLC-related researches is paradoxically the introduction of fine-needle aspiration techniques rather than biopsy for histologic diagnosis: this has dramatically diminished the material available for studying compared with other lung cancers and other epithelial tumors.

7.4 Current perspectives: "Time to fish or cut bait"

"Immortalization" of old randomized trials which refused surgery in multimodal treatment of SCLC in others era is no more acceptable today. A different staging system, lack or routine diagnostic tools and some evident weak points make these milestones anachronistic at now.

However, due to small number of cases and bias in selection of patients, retrospective series starts to carry a small usefulness in adding greater evidence in any type of treatment not contemplated in current guidelines. Meta-analyses too seem not to be reliable on studies that encompass sometimes two or three decades: lack of homogeneity between cohorts characteristics, staging system, diagnostic tools and type of treatments administered are a major issue to significance of results reported.

As brilliantly stated from Shepherd in comment to another retrospective trial on SEER database [Yu, 2010] "it is time to fish or cut bait": thoracic oncologists have to seriously face the question of role of surgery in multimodal approach to SCLC,: if they decide to fish, a large multi-center, international prospective randomized trial seem the only feasible option to achieve powerful statistical results [Shepherd, 2010]. Trial should accrue a large number of patients in a limited period of time with strict eligibility criteria in order to ensure as more homogeneity as possible among centres regarding patients selection, staging criteria and treatment modalities. In the forthcoming seventh edition of the TNM staging system, the IASLC has recommended to apply TNM stratification to SCLC in future clinical trials on LD-SCLC. At least one of the arm should be treated with chemo-radiation therapy followed by PCI, which represents actually the standard of care.

The small number of patients eligible for surgical trials makes accrual extremely slow, so that 3 trials started before 2003 have not been published yet (Essen Thoracic Oncology Group, West Japan Thoracic Oncology group, German Multicenter Randomised Trial).

Meanwhile advances in comprehension of molecular biology of SCLC will perhaps improve systemic control of disease, supporting and not excluding the role of surgery as the most powerful tool of cytoreduction local strategy even in more locally advanced disease in order to eliminate potential residual clones of resistant cells. It seems in fact still REMOTE the possibility discover of definitive systemic therapy capable of achieve complete local and distant, permanent remission of disease

8. Acknowledgment

Many thanks to Dr. Giorgio Sgarbi, Chief of Thoracic Surgery Unit, Dr. Salvatore De Franco, Clinical Director of IRCCS and "Associazione Vittorio Lodini per la ricerca in chirurgia" for supporting our research activity.
Many thanks to Ms Giulia Mazzi for her English revision.

9. References

American Cancer Society. (2010) Cancer Facts and Figures 2010. Atlanta

Anraku, M. & Waddell, TK. (2006) Surgery for small-cell lung cancer. *Semin Thorac Cardiovasc Surg*, Vol. 18, No. 3, pp. 211-216

Antony, GK., Bertino, E., Franklin, M. et al. (2010) Small cell lung cancer in never smokers. Report of 2 cases. *J Thorac Oncol*, Vol. 5, pp. 747-748

Asamura, H., Kameya, T., Matsuno, Y. et al. (2006) Neuroendocrine neoplasms of the lung: a prognostic spectrum. *J Clin Oncol*, Vol. 24, No. 1, (Jan 2006), pp. 70-76

Aupérin A., Arriagada R., Pignon JP. et al. (1999) Prophylactic cranial irradiation for patients with small-cell lung cancer in complete remission. Prophylactic Cranial Irradiation Overview Collaborative Group. *N Engl J Med*, Vol. 341, No. 7, (Aug 1999), pp. 476-84

Azzopardi, JG. (1959) Oat-cell carcinoma of the bronchus. *J Pathol Bacteriol*, (1959), Vol. 78, (Oct 1959), pp.513-519

Badzio, A., Kurowskib, K., Karnicka-Mlodkowska, H. et al. (2004) A retrospective comparative study of surgery followed by chemotherapy vs. non-surgical management in limited-disease small cell lung cancer. *Eur J Cardiothorac Surg*, Vol. 26, No 1, pp.183-188

Brock, M.V., Hooker, G.M., Shyphard, J.E. at al. (2005) Surgical resection of limited disease SCLC in the era of platinum chemotherapy: its time has come. *J Thorac Cardiovasc Surg*, Vol. 129, pp. 64-72

Campling, B., Quirt, I., DeBoer, G. et al. (1986) Is bone marrow examination in small-cell lung cancer rally necessary? *Ann Intern Med*, Vol. 105, pp. 508-512, ISSN

Chiappori, A.A., Zheng, Z., Chen, T. et al. (2010) Features of potentially predictive biomarkers of chemotherapeutic efficacy in small cell lung cancer. *J Thorac Oncol*, Vol. 5, pp. 484–490

Darnell, R.B. & Posner, J.B. (2003) Paraneoplastic syndromes involving the nervous system. *N Engl J Med*, Vol. 349, pp. 1543-1554

Devesa, S.S., Bray F, Vizcaino, A.P. & Parkin, D.M. (2005) International lung cancer trends by histologic type: male, female differences diminishing and adenocarcinoma rising. *Int J Cancer* , Vol. 117, pp. 249-299

Eberhardt, W., Korfee, S. (2003) New approaches for small-cell lung cancer: local treatments. *Cancer Control*, Vol. 10, No. 4, (Jul-Aug 2003) pp. 289-296

Elliot, J.A., Osterlind, K., Hirsch, F.R., et al. (1987) Metastatic patterns in small- cell lung cancer: correlation of autopsy finding with clinical parameters in 537 patients. *J Clin Oncol*, Vol. 5, pp. 246–254

Franklin, W.F., Noguchi, M. & Gonzalez, A. (2010) Molecular and cellular pathology of lung cancer. In: *Principles and practice of lung cancer*, Pass HI, Carbone DP, Johnson DH, Minna JD, Scagliotti GV, Turrisi AT pp. 287-324, Lippincott Williams & Wilkins, Philadelphia

Gandhi, L. & Johnson, B.E. (2006) Paraneoplastic syndromes associated with small cell lung cancer. *J Natl Compr Canc Netw*, Vol. 4, pp 631-638

Gomez de Antonio, D., Alfageme, F., Gamez, P. et al. (2006) Results of surgery in small cell carcinoma of the lung. *Lung Cancer*, Vol. 52, pp. 299-304

Govindan, R., Page, N., Morgensztern, D. et al. (2006) Changing epidemiology of small cell lung cancer in the United States over the last 30 years: analysis of the surveillance, epidemiologic and end results database. *J Clin Oncol*, Vol. 24, pp. 4539-4544

Green, R.A., Humphrey, E., Close, H. & Patno, M.E. (1969) Alkylating agents in bronchogenic carcinoma. *Am J Med*, Vol. 46, No. 4, (Apr 1969), pp. 516-25

Guo, L. et al. (2010) Gene expression profiling of drug-resistant small cell lung cancer cells by combining microRNA and cDNA expression analysis. *Eur J Cancer*, Vol. 46, pp. 1692–1702

Gultekin, S.H., Rosenfeld, M.R., Voltz, R. et al. (2000) Paraneoplastic limbic encephalitis: neurological symptoms, immunological findings and tumour association in 50 patients. *Brain*, Vol. 123, pp. 1481-1494

Hanahan, D. & Weinberg, R.A. (2000) The hallmarks of cancer. *Cell*, Vol. 100, pp. 57–70

Yokomizo, A. et al. (1998) PTEN/MMAC1 mutations identified in small cell, but not in non-small cell lung cancers. *Oncogene*, Vol. 17, pp. 475–479

Kim, Y.H., Ishii, G., Goto, K. et al. (2009) Expression of breast cancer resistant protein is associated with a poor clinical outcome in patients with small cell lung cancer. *Lung Cancer*, Vol. 65, pp. 105–11

Kok, K. et al. (1987) Deletion of a DNA sequence at the chromosomal region 3p21 in all major types of lung cancer. *Nature*, Vol. 330, pp. 578–581

Koletsis, E.N., Prokakis, C., Kranikolas, M., et al. (2009) Current role of surgery in small cell lung carcinoma. *J Cardiothorac Surg*, Vol. 4, pp. 30

Kumar, V., Abbas, A. & Fausto, N. (2005) *Robbins and Cotran Pathologic Basis of Disease.* (7th edition) Elsevier Inc, Philadelphia

Leo, F. & Pastorino, U. (2003) Surgery in small cell lung carcinoma: where is the rationale? *Semin Surg Oncol* Vol. 21, pp. 176-181

Mangum, M.D., Greco, F.A., Hainsworth, J.D. et al. (1989) Combined small-cell and non-small-cell lung cancer. *J Clin Oncol*, Vol.7, No. 5, (May 1989) pp. 607-612

Marinov, M. et al. (2009) AKT/mTOR pathway activation and BCL 2 family proteins modulate the sensitivity of human small cell lung cancer cells to RAD001. *Clin. Cancer Res*, Vol. 15, pp. 1277–1287

Master, G.A. Clinical presentiation of small cell lung cancer. (2010) In: *Principles and practice of lung cancer*. Pass HI, Carbone DP, Johnson DH, Minna JD, Scagliotti GV, Turrisi AT, pp. 341-351, Lippincott Williams & Wilkins, Philadelphia

Matthews, M.J., Kanhouwa, S., Pickren, J. & Robinette, D. (1973) Frequency of residual and metastatic tumor in patients undergoing curative surgical resection for lung cancer. *Cancer Chemother Rep*, Vol. 4, No. 2, (Mar 1973), pp. 63-67

Medical Research Council Lung Cancer Working Party. (1979) Radiotherapy alone or with chemotherapy in the treatment of small-cell carcinoma of the lung. *Br J Cancer*, Vol. 40, No. 1(Jul 1979), 1-10

Micke, P., Faldum, A., Metz, T., et al. (2002) Staging small cell lung cancer: Veterans Administration Lung Cancer Study Group versus International Association for the Study of Lung Cancer-what limits limited disease? *Lung cancer*, Vol. 37, No. 3, pp. 271-276

Miller, A.B., Fox, W. & Tall, R. (1969) Five-year follow-up of the Medical Research Council comparative trial of surgery and radiotherapy for the primary treatment of small-celled or oat-celled carcinoma of the bronchus. *Lancet*, Vol. 6, No. 2, (sept 1969), pp.501-505

Naylor, S.L., Johnson. B.E., Minna, J.D. & Sakaguchi, A.Y. (1987) Loss of heterozygosity of chromosome 3p markers in small-cell lung cancer. *Nature*, Vol. 329, pp. 451–454

Ogawa, S., Horio, Y., Yatabe, Y. et al. (2010) Patterns of recurrence and outcome in patients with surgically resected small cell lung cancer. *Int J Clin Oncol.* DOI 10.1007/s10147-011-0277-4

Olejniczak, E.T. et al. (2007) Integrative genomic analysis of small-cell lung carcinoma reveals correlates of sensitivity to bcl 2 antagonists and uncovers novel chromosomal gains. *Mol Cancer Res*, Vol. 5, pp. 331–339

Østerlind, K., Hansen, M. & Hansen, H. (1985) Treatment policy of surgery in small cell carcinoma of the lung: retrospective analysis of a series of 874 consecutive patients. *Thorax,* Vol. 40, pp. 272-277

Payne, M., Bradboury, P., Lang, B. et al. (2010) Prospective study into incidence of Lambert-Eaton myasthenic syndrome in small cell lung cancer. *J Thorac Oncol*, Vol. 5, No. 1, pp. 34-38

Pardo, O.E., Latigo, J., Jeffery, R.E., et al. (2009) The fibroblast growth factor receptor inhibitor PD173074 blocks small cell lung cancer growth in vitro and in vivo. *Cancer Res*, Vol. 69, pp. 8645–8651.

Perry, M.C., Eaton, W.L., Propert, K.J. et al. (1987) Chemotherapy with or without radiation therapy in limited small-cell carcinoma of the lung. N Engl J Med, Vol. 16, No. 15, (Apr 1987), pp. 912-918

Quoix, E., Fraser, R., Wolkove, N. et al. (1990) Small cell lung cancer presenting as solitary pulmonary nodule. *Cancer*, Vol. 66, pp. 577-82

Rea, F., Callegaro, D. & Favaretto, A. (1998) Long term results of surgery and chemotherapy in small cell lung cancer. *Eur J Cardio-Thoracic Surg*, Vol. 14, pp. 398–402

Ried, T. et al. (1994) Mapping of multiple DNA gains and losses in primary small cell lung carcinomas by comparative genomic hybridization. *Cancer Res*, Vol. 54, pp. 1801–1806

Rostad, H., Naalsund, A., Jacobsen, R. et al. (2004) Small cell lung cancer in Norway. Should more patients have been offered surgical therapy? *Eur J Cardiothorac Surg*, Vol. 26, No. 4, (Oct 2004), pp. 782-786

Schreiber, D., Rineer, J., Weedon, J. et al. (2010) Survival outcomes with the use of surgery in limited-stage small cell lung cancer: should its role be re-evaluated? Cancer, Vol. 116, No. 5 (Mar 2010), pp. 1350-1357

Seute, T., Leffers, P., Velde, G.P.M., et al. (2008) Detection of brain metastases from small cell lung cancer - consequences of changing imaging techniques (CT versus MRI). *Cancer*, Vol. 112, pp. 1827-1834

Shepherd, F.A., Crowley, J., Van Houtte, P. et al. (2007) The International Association for the Study of Lung Cancer Lung Cancer Staging Project: Proposal regarding the clinical staging of small cell lung cancer in the forthcoming (seventh) edition of the Tumor, Node, Metastasis classification for lung cancer. *J Thorac Oncol*, Vol. 2, pp. 1067-1077

Shepherd, F.A., Ginsberg, R.J., Evans, W.K., et al. (1983) Reduction in local recurrence and improved survival in surgically treated patients with small cell lung cancer. *J Thorac Cardiovasc Surg*, Vol. 86, No. 4, pp. 498-506

Shepherd, F.A., Ginsberg, R., Patterson, G.A., et al. (1991) Is there ever a role for salvage operations in limited small-cell lung cancer? *J Thorac Cardiovasc Surg*, Vol. 101, pp. 196–200

Shepherd, F.A. (2010) Surgery for Limited Stage Small Cell Lung Cancer. *J Thoracic Onc*, Vol. 5, No. 2, pp. 147-149

Shields, T.W. (1982) Surgical therapy for carcinoma of the lung. *Clin Chest Med*, Vol. 3, No. 2, (May 1982), pp. 369-387

Stahel, R.A., Ginsberg, R., Havemann, K. et al. (1989) Staging and prognostic factors in small cell lung cancer: a consensus report.. *Lung Cancer*, Vol. 5, pp. 119-126

Stahel, R.A. (1991) Diagnosis, staging, and prognostic factors of small cell lung cancer. Curr Opin Oncol, Vol. 3, No. 2, pp. 306-311

Thomson, D., Hulse, P., Lorigan, P., et al. (2011) The role of positron emission tomography in management of small cell lung cancer. *Lung cancer* (Apr 2011) doi:10.1016/j.lungcan.2011.03.013

Travis, W.D., Brambilla, E., Müller-Hermelink, H.K. et al. World Health Organization classification of tumours: pathology and genetics: tumours of the lung, pleura, thymus and heart. Vol. 10.

Travis, W.T., Brambilla, E., Muller-Hermelink, K. & Harris, C.C. (2004) Tumours of the lung, pleura, thymus and heart. In: http: www.iarc.fr/en/publications/pdfs-online/pat-gen/bb10/bb10-cover.pdf

Tsuchiya, R.., Suzuki, K. & Ichinose, Y. (2005) Phase II trial of postoperative adjuvant cisplatin and etoposide in patients with completely resected stage I-IIIa small cell lung cancer: the Japan Clinical Oncology Lung Cancer Study Group Trial (JCOG9101). *Thorac Cardiovasc Surg*, Vol. 129, No. 5, (May 2005), pp. 977-983

Turrisi, A.T., Kim, K., Blum, R., Sause, W.T., et al. (1999) Twice-daily compared with once-daily thoracic radiotherapy in limited small-cell lung cancer treated concurrently with cisplatin and etoposide. *N Engl J Med*, Vol. 340, No. 4 (January 1999), pp. 265-271

Usuda, J., Ichinose, S., Ishizumi, T. et al. (2011) Klotho predicts good clinical outcome in patients with limited-disease small cell lung cancer who received surgery. *Lung Cancer*, (April 2011) doi:10.1016/j.lungcan.2011.03.004

Van Loon, J., De Ruysscher, D., Wanders, R., et al. (2010) Selective nodal irradiation on basis of 18FDG-PET scans in limited-disease small-cell lung cancer: a prospective study. Int J Radiat Oncol Biol Phys, Vol. 77, pp. 329-336

Van Meerbeeck, J.P., Fennell, D.A. & De Ruysscher, D.K. (2011) Small-cell lung cancer. *Lancet*, (May 2011) doi:10.1016/S0140-6736(11)60165-7

Varlotto, J.M., Recht, A., Flickinger, J.C., et al. (2011) Lobectomy leads to optimal survival in early-stage small cell lung cancer: a retrospective analysis. *J Thorac Cardiovasc Surg*, (June 2011) doi:10.1016/j.jtcvs.2010.11.062

Whang-Peng, J. et al. (1982) Specific chromosome defect associated with human small-cell lung cancer; deletion 3p(14–23). *Science*, Vol. 215, pp. 181–182

Zelen, M. (1973) Keynote address on biostatistics and data retrieval. *Cancer Chemother Rep*, Vol. 4, No. 31-42

Part 3

Immunity and Infection

14

Interleukin-17 and T Helper 17 Cells in Mucosal Immunity of the Lung

M.S. Paats, P.Th.W. van Hal, C.C. Baan, H.C. Hoogsteden,
M.M. van der Eerden and R.W. Hendriks
Erasmus Medical Center, Rotterdam
The Netherlands

1. Introduction

In all mammals, including humans, the immune system is responsible for the protection against potentially hazardous pathogens, such as bacteria, viruses, parasites and fungi. In this remarkably effective defense system leukocytes, which mediate both innate and adaptive immune responses, play a central role.

The innate immune system comprises granulocytes (neutrophils, eosinophils and basophils), natural killer (NK) cells, mast cells and macrophages. These cells are the first line of defense and provide the immediate response against pathogens. Neutrophils and macrophages can eliminate a pathogen directly by phagocytosis. Moreover, their pattern-recognition receptors, recognizing structurally conserved molecules derived from microbes such as bacterial lipopolysaccharides, unmethylated CpG, or viral double-stranded RNA, allow them to respond to a wide variety of microbial invaders, e.g. by producing cytokines that activate T lymphocytes of the adaptive immune system.

Acquired or adaptive immunity is characterized by a slower but highly specific immune response. Three major cell types are involved in adaptive immunity: antigen presenting cells (APCs), T lymphocytes and B lymphocytes. Dendritic cells (DCs) are the most potent APCs. They act as messengers between the innate and the adaptive immune system by taking up, processing and presenting antigens to T lymphocytes. In response to presented antigens, T lymphocytes may react in different ways: $CD4^+$ T helper cells produce various cytokines that direct the immune response, whereas $CD8^+$ cytotoxic T cells produce toxic granules that induce death of infected cells. B cells are able to respond to pathogens by terminal differentiation into plasma cells after which they produce large quantities of antibodies. Modulation of B cell function and antibody production by $CD4^+$ T cells is an important step in coordinating immune responses. Upon activation, B cells can migrate to germinal centers, which are specialized structures in secondary lymphoid organs, where they interact with T cells and DCs. Costimulatory signals from T cells then facilitate selection of B cells with high affinity for immunoglobulins and control class switching of the immunoglobulin (Ig) to IgG, IgA and IgE.

Following pathogen elimination, lymphocytes leave a lasting legacy of the antigens they have come across represented by memory cells. As a result, lymphocytes are able to mount a faster and stronger immune response in future encounters with the same antigen. Defective T cell function can increase susceptibility to infections, allergies and autoimmune diseases. T lymphocytes can however also be manipulated to either eradicate tumor or control graft rejection after organ transplantation. Therefore, in addition to basic biological interest, knowledge on T cell biology is important to the understanding of the etiology of a wide variety of diseases and may improve current therapies.

During activation in a particular cytokine milieu, naïve $CD4^+$ T cells can differentiate into one of the several subsets of T helper (Th) cells. Already in 1986, Mosmann and Coffman introduced the concept of distinct types of T helper cells, which was based on the distinct cytokines profiles that T cells produce when they are stimulated to differentiate (Mosmann and Coffman 1989). They described two types of Th lymphocytes, type 1 helper T cells (Th1 cells) and type 2 helper T cells (Th2 cells). Th1 cells produce large quantities of interferon (IFN)γ, induce delayed hypersensitivity reactions, activate macrophages, and are essential for the defense against intracellular pathogens. Th2 cells produce mainly interleukin (IL)-4 and are important in inducing IgE production, recruiting eosinophils to sites of inflammation, and helping to clear parasitic infections. Cytokines produced by cells of the innate immune system govern the differentiation of these T helper cells. IFNγ and IL-12 drive naive T cells into the Th1 pathway, whereas IL-4 initiates the differentiation of naive T cells into Th2 cells. At a molecular level, the differentiation of Th1 and Th2 cells requires specific transcription factors: T-bet for Th1 cells (Szabo et al. 2000) and GATA3 for Th2 cells (Zheng and Flavell 1997) (Figure 1). An additional T helper subset was recently identified which restrains excessive effector T cell responses and therefore accounts for the maintenance of immune homeostasis and prevention of immunopathology. These cells are called regulatory T (Treg) cells and are naturally present in the immune system as a functionally distinct $CD4^+$ T cell expressing the forkhead transcription factor FoxP3 and producing the cytokines IL-10 and transforming growth factor (TGF)-β. The differentiation of naïve T cells towards this lineage is driven by IL-2 and TGF-β (Weaver and Hatton 2009) (Figure 1). T follicular helper (Tfh) cells are yet another $CD4^+$ T cell population (Nurieva et al. 2008; Vogelzang et al. 2008). They are important for the formation of germinal centers. Once these germinal centers are formed, Tfh cells are needed to maintain and regulate B cell differentiation into plasma cells and memory B cells. The signals that specifically instruct the differentiation of human Tfh cells remain unclear, but IL-12 and IL-21 seem to be required. Tfh cells express Bcl6 as their master transcription factor and may produce IL-21 and IL-4 (Yusuf et al. 2010; Ma et al. 2009; Crotty 2011) (Figure 1).

Interestingly, in recent years T cells were shown to produce proinflammatory cytokines that could not be classified according to this Th1-Th2 scheme. IL-17 is the most prominent amongst these cytokines, and T cells that preferentially produce IL-17 but not IFNγ or IL-4 were named Th17 cells. The discovery of this new subset of helper T cells that selectively produces IL-17 has provided better and exciting insights into immunoregulation, host defense and the pathogenesis of autoimmune diseases. In particular, it now appears that Th17 cells do not only play a key role in chronic inflammatory lung disorders, but also mediate protective immunity against various pathogens at respiratory mucosal sites.

2. Interleukin 17 and T helper 17 cells

IL-17 (also denoted IL-17A) was cloned in 1993 and initially called CTLA-8 (Rouvier et al. 1993). In 1995, it was renamed as IL-17, its receptor was cloned and it was identified as a cytokine expressed by T cells, exerting effects on epithelial, endothelial, and fibroblast cells (Yao et al. 1995). IL-17 has diverse biological functions, but the best characterized functions

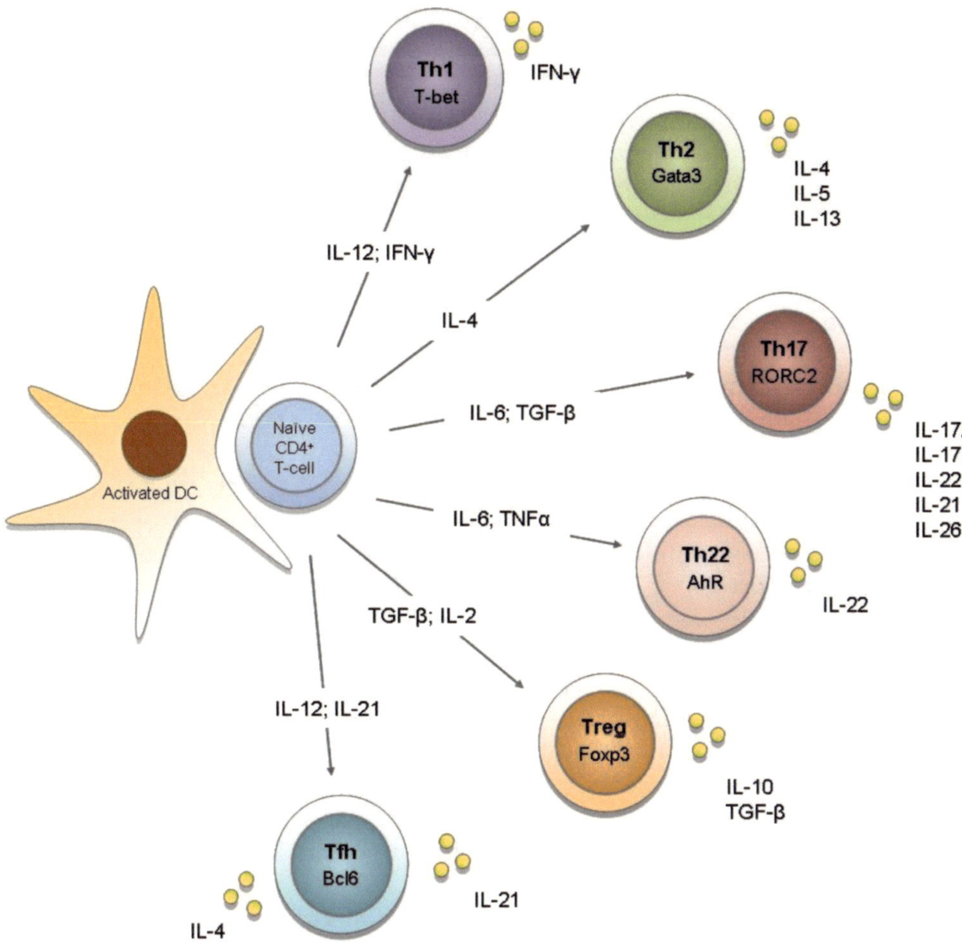

Fig. 1. Overview of human CD4+ effector T cell differentiation.
Upon activation in a particular cytokine milieu, naïve CD4+ T cells may differentiate into one of several lineages of T helper (Th) cells, including Th1, Th2, Th17, and Treg cells. These separate lineages are characterized by their distinct cytokine production pattern. The differentiation pathways are mainly based on the induction of transcription factors that serve as master regulators of specific lineages. However, cytokine production by Th cells seems to be more flexible than previously believed and recently new cells, such as Th22 and Tfh cells have been described. Whether these new subsets represent distinct lineages remains to be elucidated.

relate to its proinflammatory effects. Specifically, IL-17 recruits neutrophils via effects on granulopoiesis (Schwarzenberger et al. 1998; Fossiez et al. 1996) and CXC chemokine induction, including CXCL8/IL-8 (Laan et al. 1999). Furthermore, it acts on macrophages to promote their recruitment and survival and stimulates the production of proinflammatory cytokines and anti-microbial peptides, particularly β-defensins, from a variety of immune and non-immune cells (Kolls and Linden 2004; Weaver et al. 2007; Ouyang, Kolls, and

Zheng 2008; Crome, Wang, and Levings 2010). By now we know that the IL-17 family includes 6 family members: IL-17A, IL-17B, IL-17C, IL-17D, IL-17E and IL-17F. IL-17A and IL-17F are the most closely related isoforms, sharing 55% homology with each other. Because of their structural and functional similarities and the fact that they are both produced by Th17 cells, IL-17A and IL-17F have been most thoroughly studied and characterized. Although it was known for more than 15 years that IL-17 is a product of activated $CD4^+$ T cells, it was not until 2005 that the Th17 cell was described as a distinct $CD4^+$ T-cell subset, critically responsible for the production of IL-17 in the context of autoimmunity (Harrington et al. 2005).

2.1 Phenotype and differentiation of Th17 cells

IL-17A is the hallmark cytokine for Th17 cells. Nevertheless, these cells also produce other cytokines, such as IL-21, IL-22, tumor necrosis factor (TNF)-α, other members of the IL-17 family and, specifically in humans, IL-26 (Dong 2008). As with Th1 and Th2 cells, no single surface marker is specific for Th17 cells. However, human Th17 cells are thought to preferentially express CD161 on the cell surface (Cosmi et al. 2008). Additionally, the selective expression of chemokine receptors in subsets of human memory T cells has been useful in defining lineages with different effector functions and migratory capacity (Sallusto, Mackay, and Lanzavecchia 2000). It has been shown that human Th17 cells express the chemokine receptor CCR6 and its ligand CCL20 (Dong 2008; Wilson et al. 2007). Coexpression of CCR4 and CCR6 further defines human T cells that produce IL-17 but not IFNγ (Acosta-Rodriguez, Rivino et al. 2007). In contrast, expression of CCR6 and CXCR3 identifies a more heterogeneous effector T cell population that produces both IFNγ and IL-17 (Acosta-Rodriguez, Rivino et al. 2007). These patterns of chemokine receptors appear to be biologically significant, as memory Th17 cells specific for *Candida albicans* are mainly $CCR6^+CCR4^+$ positive, whereas those that recognize *Mycobacterium tuberculosis* antigens are present in the $CCR6^+CXCR3^+$ subgroup producing both IFNγ and IL-17 (Acosta-Rodriguez, Rivino et al. 2007; Annunziato et al. 2007).

The combination of cytokines that stimulate differentiation of Th17 cells has been subject of much debate. Initial studies on human T cell differentiation indicated that T cell activation in the presence of IL-1β, IL-6 and/or IL-23 was sufficient to induce Th17 cells, and that TGF-β inhibited this process (Acosta-Rodriguez, Napolitani et al. 2007; Chen et al. 2007; Crome, Wang, and Levings 2010; Wilson et al. 2007). In subsequent studies, however, TGF-β was reported to be important for the development of human IL-17 producing cells (Manel, Unutmaz, and Littman 2008; Volpe et al. 2008; Yang, Anderson et al. 2008). This discrepancy could be explained by more recent reports showing that the requirement for TGF-β in the differentiation process is indirect and relates to suppression of Th1 differentiation (Crome, Wang, and Levings 2010; Santarlasci et al. 2009). In the current view, the combination of IL-1β and IL-6 is essential for proper human Th17 cell differentiation whereas IL-23 is important for both expansion and survival of lineage-committed Th17 cells (Wilson et al. 2007). In addition to cytokine-driven Th17 lineage commitment, it has also been shown that prostaglandin E2 (PGE2), which is a mediator of tissue inflammation, directly promotes differentiation, expansion and proinflammatory function of human and mouse Th17 cells (Yao et al. 2009). In humans, PGE2 induces up-regulation of the IL-23 and IL-1 receptors (IL-23R and IL-1R, respectively) and by synergism with IL-1β, IL-6 and IL-23 (Boniface et al. 2009).

The observation that Th17 cells are a distinct lineage of cells with a unique cytokine and chemokine/chemokine receptor profile, led to the discovery of RORγt in mice (Ivanov et al. 2006). RORγt encodes the retinoid orphan nuclear receptor, and this transcription factor is required for the differentiation of Th17 cells. In the human system it has also been shown that forced over-expression of RORC2 (the human equivalent of RORγt) in human naïve T cells induces a Th17-like phenotype, by inducing IL-17A, IL-17F, IL-26 and CCR6 expression and down-regulating IFNγ secretion (Manel, Unutmaz, and Littman 2008; Crome et al. 2009) (Figure 1). Activation of RORγt also causes expression of the IL23R, indicating that IL-23 acts on T cells that are already committed to the Th17 lineage. Exposure of developing Th17 cells to IL-23 not only enhances the expression of IL-17 but also induces IL-22 and suppresses IL-10 and IFNγ (McGeachy et al. 2007). Yet, RORC2 alone can induce IL-17 production in only 20% of the T cell population (Chen and O'Shea 2008) indicating that it acts in cooperation with other transcription factors for full commitment of precursors to the Th17 lineage. In addition to RORC2, the most specific and master transcription factor, at least four other transcription factors are linked to the human Th17 cell fate. These include signal transducer and activator of transcription-3 (STAT3), interferon regulatory factor-4 (IRF4), runt box transcription factor-1 (Runx1), and the aryl hydrocarbon receptor (AhR) (Chen and O'Shea 2008). Together they form a sophisticated network with positive and negative feedback loops. In addition, Th17 cells are inhibited by IL-2 (produced by Treg cells), IFNγ (produced by Th1 cells), and IL-4 (produced by Th2 cells) but also by other negative regulators such as retinoic acid (Elias et al. 2008).

Although this scheme of T helper cell differentiation might seem complex (Figure 1), it is in fact an oversimplification. Recent studies on T helper cell differentiation have revealed more plasticity in cytokine production than predicted by conventional models of T helper cell lineage commitment. Activated memory T cells preserve plasticity to alter their cytokine program according to the stimuli they receive. A cytokine restricted to one T helper subset can therefore be secreted by another subset under changing stimulation conditions. This feature is also observed in human Th17 cells (Chen and O'Shea 2008). Acquisition of IFNγ-producing potential by Th17 cells, particularly the simultaneous production of IFNγ and IL-17, is common (Chen et al. 2007; Wilson et al. 2007) (see Figure 2). Additionally, Th17 cells can even stop producing IL-17 and become selective IFNγ producers resulting in a complete subset switch (O'Shea and Paul 2010). Although Th1 cells do not become IL-17 producers, under particular circumstances they can make IL-13 (Hayashi et al. 2007). Th17 cells produce IL-22, but cells that make IL-22 and not IL-17 ("Th22 cells") have recently been identified as well (Duhen et al. 2009; Trifari et al. 2009). Simultaneous production of IL-22 and IFNγ has also been described (O'Shea and Paul 2010). This plasticity even concerns master regulators: FoxP3 expression within Treg cells is heterogeneous and transient and former.

Treg cells have the capacity to produce proinflammatory cytokines such as IL-17 (Bluestone et al. 2009).

Moreover, also multiple master regulators can be expressed, such as Gata3 and FoxP3 in Tregs (Mantel et al. 2007), or a combination of RORC2 and FoxP3 (mixed Th17-Treg) (O'Shea and Paul 2010). Therefore, expression of master regulators should not be simplified as mutually exclusive but rather as a gradient of transcription factors (O'Shea and Paul 2010). It remains to be shown whether there are preferential directions for plasticity or whether effector T cells can change in any direction from every starting point (Bluestone et al. 2009). Plasticity could be an answer to the evolution of pathogens, allowing a proper response to new threats.

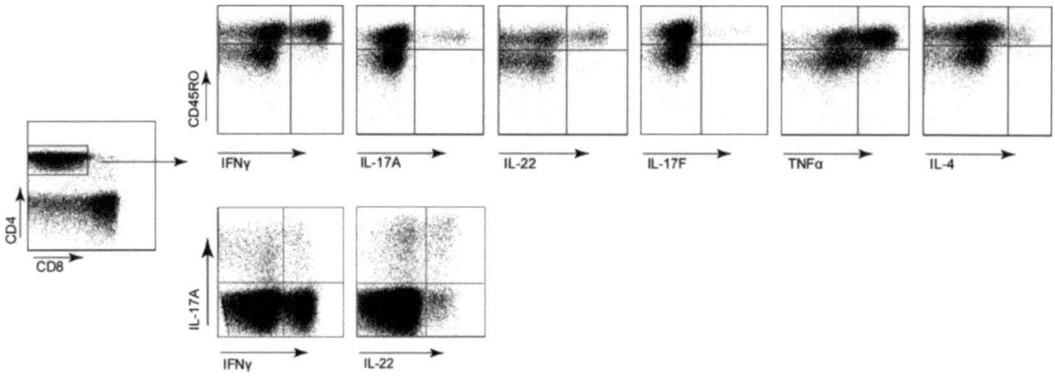

Fig. 2. Flow cytometric analysis of cytokine production by $CD4^+$ T helper cells.
With the use of a technique called flow cytometry, it is possible to depict the cytokine producing potential of individual cells. In this experiment peripheral blood mononuclear cell (PBMC) suspensions were stained with monoclonal antibodies specific for CD3, CD4, CD8, and the indicated cytokines. Live $CD4^+$ $CD3^+$ T cells were gated and analyzed for the presence of the indicated cytokines in combination with the CD45R0 marker for memory T cells. Results are shown as dot plots and illustrate that $CD4^+$ T helper cells are capable of producing all of the tested cytokines (top row, right upper quadrants). Moreover, $CD4^+$ T helper cells have the potential to be simultaneously positive for IL-17 and IFNγ, and IL-17A and IL-22 respectively (bottom row, right upper quadrants).

2.2 IL-17 producing cells other than Th17 cells

Th17 cells are not the exclusive producers of IL-17 nor is this production their only function. Other cell populations capable of producing IL-17 include both adaptive and innate immune cells.

Within the adaptive arm of the immune system, a subset of $CD8^+$ cytotoxic T cells is also capable of producing IL-17. Studies have shown that these cells develop under conditions that are similar to those required by Th17 cells, but different from those required by IFNγ producing $CD8^+$ T cells (Kondo et al. 2009). However, adaptive immune responses cannot explain the early IL-17-mediated immune responses that have crucial roles during stress responses and host defense. Early responses are induced within hours following tissue injury or exposure to pathogens (Ferretti et al. 2003; Happel et al. 2003; Zheng et al. 2008), which is not enough time to allow for Th17 differentiation, indicating that innate immune cells play a crucial role in these early responses. The key feature of this innate IL-17 response is the early neutrophil recruitment. This results in a more efficient resolution of infection, in the maintenance of mucosal barrier integrity, but also in the potential induction of autoimmunity (2). Recent studies have shown that γδ T cells are important innate-like IL-17-producing cells during infectious diseases and autoimmune inflammation (Aujla, Dubin, and Kolls 2007; Sutton et al. 2009; Ito et al. 2009). Additionally, innate(-like) IL-17-producing cells described in literature include $CD3^+$ invariant natural killer T (iNKT) cells, lymphoid tissue inducer (LTi)-like cells, natural killer (NK) cells and myeloid cells (Cella et al. 2009; Cua and Tato 2010; Michel et al. 2007).

The γδ T cell subset is an innate-like immune cell population that has an important role at the mucosal barrier. These cells do not express the classical αβ T cell receptor (TCR) but a γδ TCR instead. They bind to epitopes in much the same way as antibodies do and provide a rapidly available source of IL-17 (Sutton et al. 2009). Like γδ T cells, iNKT cells play a pivotal role in immunity as they provide a rapid response, with the capacity to critically amplify and regulate adaptive immune responses (Godfrey et al. 2004). Initially, they have been divided into subsets that produce either IL-4 or IFNγ, but recently a new IL-17-producing subset that develops in the thymus has been described. This subset seems already committed to making IL-17 (Michel et al. 2008). The LTi cell represents a primitive precursor of NK, NKT, and $CD4^+$ T cells. Specifically immature ($CD127^+$) NK cells are closely related to LTi cells (Eberl et al. 2004). LTi cells promote the formation of lymphoid organs and sustain primed $CD4^+$ T cell memory responses (Eberl et al. 2004). Thus, like IL-17 producing γδ T cells and NKT cells, LTi cells provide a rapidly available source of IL-17. Interestingly, it was recently recognized that innate lymphoid cells (ILCs) can be considered a family of non-T/non-B lymphocytes that includes not only NK and LTi cells, but also cells that produce IL-5, IL-13, IL-17 or IL-22. These ILC subsets are developmentally related and require cytokine signals through the common γ-chain of the IL-2 receptor. The distinct ILC subsets, which seem to have important roles in protective immunity analogous to helper T cell subsets, were recently reviewed by Spits and DiSanto (Spits and Di Santo 2011). Next to LTi and NK cells, other innate IL-17 producers have been postulated, including macrophages and neutrophils (reviewed by (Cua and Tato 2010; Song et al. 2008), however data is limited and further studies are needed to understand more of their role in mucosal tissue.

2.3 Interactions between Th17 and other cells of the immune system

Cells of the immune system modulate each other's function. Many cells may interact with Th17 cells including APCs, other T helper subsets, B cells and neutrophils (Figure 3). APCs play a central role in directing immune responses by secreting cytokines that polarize $CD4^+$ T cells into distinct lineages. Several studies support the hypothesis that changes in APC function probably precede inappropriate development and expansion of Th17 cells. For example, monocytes from inflamed joints of rheumatoid arthritis patients promote the development to Th17 cells but not Th1 or Th2 cells via a cell-contact-dependent mechanism (Evans et al. 2009). Furthermore, it was found that monocyte-derived DCs from patients with multiple sclerosis secrete elevated levels of IL-23 when compared to healthy controls (Vaknin-Dembinsky, Balashov, and Weiner 2006). Additionally, in psoriasis DCs secrete IL-1β, IL-23 and CCL20, promoting both the development of Th17 cells and their migration to the skin (Kryczek et al. 2008). However, the initial stimuli that polarize APCs to produce cytokines that promote Th17 cells are still unclear.

It has long been known that Th1 and Th2 cells antagonize each other's differentiation and function. Not surprisingly, IFNγ produced by Th1 cells and IL-4 produced by Th2 cells inhibit Th17 development (Bettelli, Oukka, and Kuchroo 2007). For Treg cells and Th17 cells there appears to be an even closer developmental relationship because the differentiation of both of these cell types require transforming growth factor (TGF)β (Veldhoen et al. 2006). Additionally, Th17 differentiation is inhibited by Treg cells, via the production of IL-2. Th17 cells can also modulate B cell function as has been shown by their ability to promote antibody production (IgM, IgG and IgA but not IgE) (Acosta-Rodriguez, Napolitani et al. 2007).

There is growing evidence that T cells are involved in orchestrating sustained mobilization of neutrophils. In the lungs for instance, in a subpopulation of COPD patients there is an accumulation of $CD4^+$ and $CD8^+$ T cells, which is associated with the presence of neutrophils

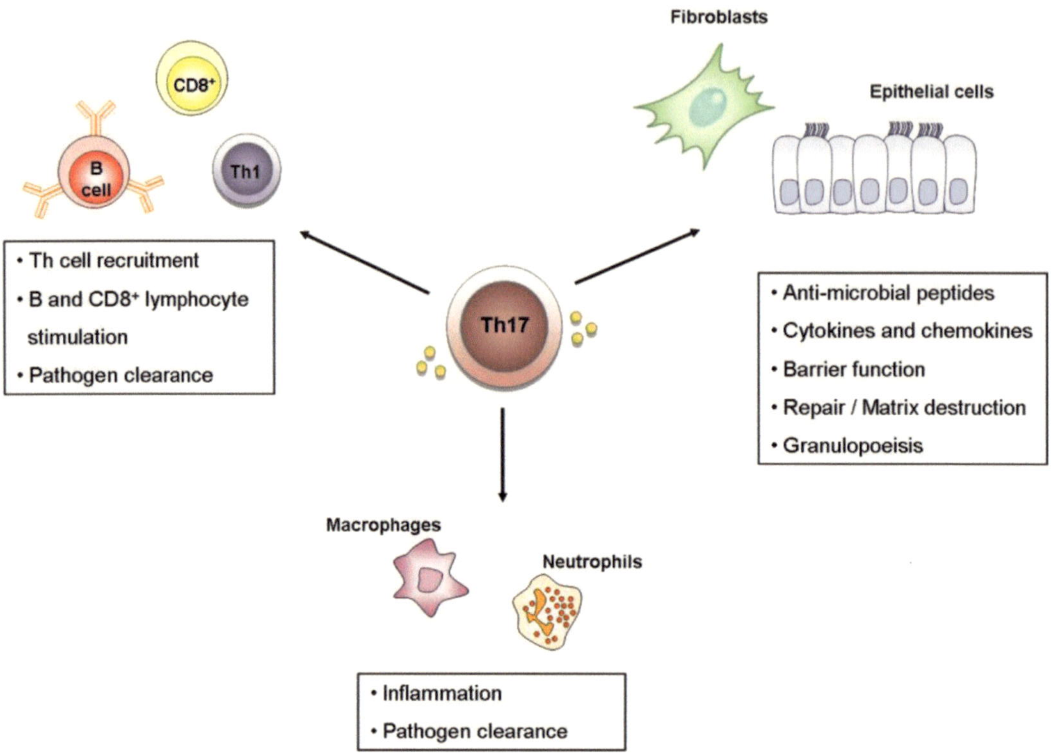

Fig. 3. Th17 cells act on other immune cells and on cells of non-hematopoietic origin. Cytokines produced by Th17 cells have the ability to act on other cells. This allows for a crosstalk between immune and non-immune cells to provide protection and promote inflammation.

(Turato et al. 2002). IL-17 seems to be an important mediator of linking activated T cells to accumulation of neutrophils, although solid data on T helper cells and neutrophils are lacking. In vitro work confirmed that IL-17 orchestrated neutrophilic influx by the production of CXCL8 (IL-8), CXCL1 (GRO-a), and granulocyte-macrophage colony stimulating factor (GM-CSF) in airway epithelial cells, smooth muscle cells, endothelial cells, and fibroblasts (Murphy et al. 2008). So, the importance of Th17 cells in neutrophilic inflammation lies in the ability of IL-17 to induce granulopoiesis, neutrophil chemotaxis, and the anti-apoptotic properties of G-CSF (Kolls and Linden 2004; Ouyang, Kolls, and Zheng 2008). Accordingly, administration of IL-17A to the lung induces robust neutrophil recruitment (Laan et al. 1999), although - by contrast - chronic IL-17A/F overexpression resulted in enhanced lymphocyte and macrophage but not neutrophil numbers (Park et al. 2005; Yang, Chang et al. 2008).

3. IL-17 in lung diseases

Although Th17 cells have only recently been recognized as a distinct lineage of CD4+ T cells, associations between IL-17 and human disease have been known for many years. Particularly disorders previously classified as typical Th1 disease, such as rheumatoid arthritis (Kotake et al. 1999), inflammatory bowel disease (Fujino et al. 2003), and psoriasis (Arican et al. 2005), are now considered to be primarily Th17-driven. For that reason (chronic) lung conditions previously believed to be Th1 cell disorders deserve special attention as Th17 cells might contribute to their pathogenesis. Moreover, immunity mediated by Th17 cells seems particularly important at epithelial and mucosal surfaces, as indicated by the distinct pattern of expression of Th17 subset-associated chemokine and cytokine receptors (Aujla et al. 2008; Ouyang, Kolls, and Zheng 2008).

Because Th17 cells and IL-17 play a role in regulating neutrophilic and macrophage inflammation in the lung, a potential role in many different lung diseases including asthma and chronic obstructive pulmonary disease (COPD), cystic fibrosis (CF), pulmonary infectious diseases, sarcoidosis and other interstitial lung diseases and rejection after lung transplantation, seems legitimate. Asthmatics were shown to have elevated levels of IL-17A mRNA and protein levels in induced sputum and these levels were positively correlated with disease severity (Bullens et al. 2006; Molet et al. 2001; Al-Ramli et al. 2009). In COPD, recent studies showed increased expression of Th17 cytokines in bronchial mucosa and sputum (Di Stefano et al. 2009; Doe et al. 2010). Airway neutrophilia is a major feature of CF exacerbations and it is shown that sputum IL-17 is upregulated and correlates with *Pseudomonas aeruginosa* colonization (Dubin and Kolls 2007). In infection models in mice, there is considerable evidence that IL-17 and/or IL-23 are important in host responses against *Klebsiella pneumoniae* (Tesmer et al. 2008). Furthermore, several studies have now linked IL-17 to fibrosis in the lung in mouse models of pulmonary fibrosis and idiopathic pulmonary fibrosis in humans (Braun et al. 2010; Kurasawa et al. 2000; Wilson et al. 2010). Similarly, Th17 cells and IL-17 may be important regulators of the airway fibrotic response driving the development of bronchiolitis obliterans syndrome (BOS) upon lung transplantation.

For functional analysis of IL-17 producing cells in relation to other immune cells or epithelial cells, it is important to consider their anatomical localization. Obviously, bronchoscopy-guided or surgically guided biopsies allow histopathologically examination in situ, but are not frequently performed because they are invasive techniques. Bronchoalveolar lavage (BAL) is again not commonly performed except in lung transplantation and interstitial lung disease. For this reason sputum and nasopharyngeal washes are often studied. Blood and serum might be ideal to study because they are easily accessible. However, it is not always clear to what extend these compartments reflect what is happening in the lung. The methodology to study IL-17$^+$ T cells in biopsies or in serum and BAL represents only indirect evidence of Th17 cells. Flow cytometry does provide direct evidence as it can combine several parameters (Figure 2). In this way, identification of distinct IL17$^+$ T cells and even separate subpopulations is relatively simple.

3.1 COPD and asthma

COPD and asthma represent two classes of chronic obstructive lung disorders that may share some similar immunological disease mechanisms. COPD is marked by a progressive and irreversible airway obstruction and emphysematic changes in the lung. In asthma the airway obstruction is reversible and there is a marked airway hyperresponsiveness and airway inflammation. Recent studies on the immunological mechanisms of COPD and asthma pathogenesis point towards a role for IL-17 and Th17 cells in both diseases.

3.1.1 COPD

In COPD, chronic inhalation of toxic particles and gases causes destruction of lung parenchyma, activates epithelial cells, increases mucus production and stimulates migration of many inflammatory cells (Hogg 2004; Hogg et al. 2004). This results in an abnormal inflammatory response in the small airways and alveoli. It is believed that both the innate and the adaptive immune system are involved in this inflammatory process (Barnes 2008; Hogg et al. 2004). Progression of the disease is associated with the presence of lymphoid follicles, a histological hallmark of an adaptive immune response and termed bronchus-associated lymphoid tissue (BALT) collections. The presence of neutrophils, BALT collections, autoantibodies in the lungs, and also autoreactive T cells in the periphery, indicate $CD4^+$ T cell involvement in the pathogenesis of COPD (Curtis, Freeman, and Hogg 2007; Feghali-Bostwick et al. 2008; Hogg et al. 2004; Vanaudenaerde et al. 2011). A potential role for adaptive immune responses in COPD has also been suggested in studies that show expansion of lung T and B cells with oligoclonality in patients with COPD and in murine emphysema models (Motz et al. 2010; Sullivan et al. 2005). To date, there are only few studies examining the expression of IL-17A and IL-17F in COPD. However, since neutrophilic inflammation (including elevated CXCL8 levels) is a common feature of COPD (Barnes 2000), and infiltrating $CD4^+$ T cells in COPD were previously considered to be Th1 cells, it is expected that Th17 cells play an important role in this disease.

Although direct evidence for the role of IL-17 and Th17 cells in COPD remains largely absent, the importance of IL-17 in stimulating chemokine production and the role of neutrophils and macrophages in promoting COPD pathogenesis have led to interest in a potential connection (Curtis, Freeman, and Hogg 2007). Another possible link derives from the ability of IL-17 to drive matrix metalloproteinases (MMP)9 production, a protein which is involved in the breakdown of extracellular matrix, as is observed in emphysema (Prause et al. 2004). It is also known that IL-17-mediated signalling induces target cells to produce various inflammatory mediators such as TNF-α, IL-6 and IL-1β. Interestingly, increased levels of IL-6 and TNFα are found in sputum and BAL fluid and have been associated with disease severity in patients with COPD (Hacievliyagil et al. 2006). TNFα promotes CXCL8 expression from airway epithelial cells. Elevated levels of serum TNFα have also been linked to exacerbations in COPD patients (Calikoglu et al. 2004). In addition TNFα production by mast cells is increased due to IL-17A, leading to neutrophil infiltration in the airways (Feldmann et al. 2001). Furthermore, IL-17 is capable of increasing mucin production from airway epithelial cells (Prause et al. 2004) and excessive mucus production is one of the characteristic of COPD. Recently it was shown that patients with stable COPD exhibited elevated numbers of IL-22- and IL-23-positive cells in the bronchial epithelium and IL-17-positive cells in the submucosa when compared to healthy controls (Di Stefano et al. 2009; Doe et al. 2010; Chang et al. 2011). Additionally, airway smooth muscle cells from COPD patients express IL-17RA and respond to IL-17 by inducing CXCL8 production (Rahman et al. 2005). In contrast to these findings, the levels of IL-17 in sputum from patients with COPD do not differ from control subjects (Barczyk, Pierzchala, and Sozanska 2003). In addition to human studies, mice exposed to cigarette smoke exhibit enhanced IL-17 production (Melgert et al. 2007; Harrison et al. 2008). Experiments on murine lung epithelial cells have also shown that overexpression of IL-17A induces a COPD-like lung inflammation (Park et al. 2005). Taken together, these findings indicate a role for Th17 cells in COPD, but it is still unclear whether and how these cells contribute to disease pathogenesis or progression. Moreover, to what extend Th1 and Th17-mediated immune responses affect airway obstruction, emphysematic changes, inflammation or COPD exacerbations are questions that need to be addressed.

3.1.2 Asthma

Asthma is usually characterized by concurrent airway inflammation, cytokine production, and airway hyperresponsiveness to relevant antigens and a specific trigger. The central role of the Th2 subset in the disease, inducing airway eosinophilia and bronchial hyperresponsiveness, is well accepted. Individually, the Th2 cytokines can explain many of the salient features of asthma, including IgE induction in B cells (IL-4), airway eosinophilia (IL-5) goblet cell hyperplasia (IL-4, IL-13) and bronchial hyperreactivity (IL-13 acting on bronchial smooth muscle cells) (Wills-Karp et al. 1998). However, some individuals with asthma display airway neutrophilia rather than eosinophilia (Anderson 2008). It appears that in those patients with asthma in which inflammation is nonatopic, non-IgE-dependent, and noneosinophilic, airway neutrophilia is correlated with asthma severity. This suggests a major role for neutrophils, at least in this subset of patients with asthma (Louis et al. 2000). Neutrophilic inflammation has also been described in sudden-onset fatal asthma and neutrophil numbers are highly elevated in status asthmaticus (Lamblin et al. 1998). These observations suggest a role for these cells in severe and fatal asthma (Cosmi et al. 2011). With the involvement of neutrophils, several studies tried to find an association between Th17 lymphocytes and asthma.

Asthmatics have elevated levels of IL-17A mRNA and protein in breath condensate, sputum, BAL, and airway biopsies (Bullens et al. 2006; Pene et al. 2008; Molet et al. 2001). Furthermore, increased IL-17A and IL-17F levels are positively correlated to disease severity, suggesting an important role for IL-17A and IL-17F in severe asthma (Al-Ramli et al. 2009). Indeed, elevated IL-17A levels also correlate to increased neutrophilic inflammation, a characteristic of severe and steroid-resistant asthma (Bullens et al. 2006). One could also hypothesize that IL-17 may have opposite pathophysiological roles in different disease stages, as would be supported by findings in an asthma mouse model, indicating that IL-17A is required for induction of disease but negatively regulates established asthma (Schnyder-Candrian et al. 2006). IL-17F may also play an important role in the development of asthma, as a polymorphism in IL-17F which results in a loss-of-function mutation, is inversely related to asthma risk (Hizawa et al. 2006). In these studies however, the cellular source of IL-17 remained unknown, but recent studies attributed the production of IL-17 primarily to $CD4^+$ T cells (Pene et al. 2008; Tesmer et al. 2008). A novel subset of Th2 memory cells that co-express the key Th2 and Th17 transcription factors, GATA3 and RORCT, respectively, and coproduce Th2 and Th17 cytokines was recently described (Wang et al. 2010). Interestingly, the number of $IL\text{-}17^+$ Th2 cells was significantly increased in peripheral blood of atopic asthma patients. Compared with classical Th17 or Th2 cells, these $IL\text{-}17^+$ Th2 cells had an increased capacity to induce influx of inflammatory leukocytes, and therefore are thought to represent key pathogenic cells promoting exacerbation of allergic asthma.

3.2 Pulmonary infections

There is considerable evidence that IL-17 and other Th17 cytokines are important in pulmonary host responses to infection by a variety of different bacteria, fungi and protozoa, and viruses. Also in infection, the major function of IL-17 appears to be to promote chemokine and pro-inflammatory cytokine production and consequent recruitment and activation of neutrophils and macrophages. Additionally, Th17 cytokines can control the infection by induction of anti-microbial peptides during the early immune responses at mucosal sites. Upon stimulation with various microbial agents, activated DCs secrete cytokines which determine the type of adaptive immunity that develops, i.e., whether the immune response is skewed toward Th1 or Th17 cells. Nevertheless, Th17 responses do not always seem to have a protective effect in mucosal infections. Current studies suggest that limited and correctly timed Th17 responses are protective, when appropriately balanced with concurrent Th1 immunity, but that uncontrolled Th17 cell activity could lead to a counterproductive level of organ inflammation (Tesmer et al. 2008).

Human studies on the role of IL-17 and Th17 cells in pulmonary infections are limited. The best human "model" demonstrating the role of IL-17 and Th17 cells in clearing pulmonary infections is Job's syndrome or the hyper-IgE syndrome. This syndrome is caused by loss-of-function mutations in STAT3, resulting in the inability of naïve T cells to differentiate into Th17 cells. These patients manifest chronic, recurrent and severe bacterial and fungal infections (Milner et al. 2008). Although other factors such as disturbed neutrophil chemotaxis are also involved in hyper-IgE syndrome (Hill et al. 1974), the Th17 cell deficiency is prominent. This therefore suggests an essential role for Th17 cells in the host immune system.

3.2.1 Bacteria

The host response to bacteria is largely triggered by Toll like receptor (TLR) ligands stimulating the production of inflammatory mediators, such as the pro-inflammatory cytokines IL-1β, IL-6 and TNFα, and the recruitment of phagocytic cells to the lung (Akira, Uematsu, and Takeuchi 2006). Several components of the innate immune system have been identified as key mediators of bacterial clearance such as neutrophils and macrophages. The role of Th17 cells in bacterial pneumonia is less clear. However, HIV patients with depleted $CD4^+$ T cells are more susceptible to bacterial infections in the lung (Wolff and O'Donnell 2003), indicating a role for T cells in bacterial pneumonia.

One of the best studied bacterial pathogens in pulmonary host defense is *Klebsiella pneumoniae*. *Klebsiella pneumoniae* is a virulent Gram-negative pathogen that can cause pneumonia. In mice infected with this organism, TLR4 activation in the lung leads to production of IL-23 by DCs, which then stimulates $CD4^+$, $CD8^+$ and even γδ T cells to release IL-17 (Happel et al. 2003). Interestingly, both IL17A and IL17F are induced in a dose-dependent fashion (Aujla et al. 2008; Happel et al. 2005). Accordingly, the protective effects of IL-17 in host defense against bacterial pathogens were shown in studies that compared the susceptibility of IL-17R-deficient and control mice to *K. pneumoniae* infection (Ye et al. 2001). After intranasal infection, IL-17R-deficient mice were more susceptible to lung infection with *K. pneumoniae* (Happel et al. 2005; Ye et al. 2001). The increased bacteraemia and mortality observed in these mice were associated with delayed neutrophil recruitment and reduced expression levels of CXCL1, CXCL2, and G-CSF in the lung 12–24 hrs after infection. Related experiments demonstrated the essential role of IL-23 in triggering IL-17 production during this infection. Also IL-23-deficient mice are highly susceptible to *K. pneumoniae* and do not upregulate IL-17 in response to infection, whereas IL-17 production readily occurs after infection in control mice (Happel et al. 2005). Furthermore, administration of recombinant IL-17 restores the early chemokine response, enhances local production of TNFα and IL-1β, and reduces the bacterial burden in IL-23-deficient mice after *K. pneumoniae* infection (Happel et al. 2005; Ye et al. 2001). Together, these findings demonstrate that IL-17 produced in an IL-23-dependent fashion is essential for early recruitment of neutrophils and other inflammatory cells to provide immunity to *K.*

pneumoniae infection. In these studies it was also shown that in addition to IL-17 also IL-22 is measurable during infection. In contrast to gene deletion of IL-17, which results in a substantial reduction of CXCL1 and G-CSF in response to bacterial challenge, antibody neutralization of IL-22 causes an even more profound defect in mucosal immunity that leads to rapid dissemination of bacteria from the lung to the spleen (Aujla et al. 2008). The loss of mucosal immunity was not associated with defects in G-CSF or CXCL1 but with loss of barrier function and anti-microbial protein expressed in lung epithelium. Thus while IL-17 production by Th17 cells is critically important in host defense against *K. pneumoniae* infection in the airway because of its role in neutrophil recruitment and activation, IL-22 acts by augmenting the barrier defense against pathogens by triggering the production of anti-microbial peptides and enhancing healing of the epithelium should it be breached (Aujla et al. 2008). Importantly, not only Th17 responses are necessary for optimal protective immunity to *K. pneumonia*. Also IL-12-driven Th1 responses, resulting in efficient IFNγ production, contribute to the optimal bacterial clearance in a mouse model of *K. pneumonia* (Happel et al. 2005).

Following these initial studies with *K. pneumoniae*, the importance of IL-23 and IL-17 in host defense has been further established for a growing list of pathogens. Similar to *K. pneumoniae*, in mice infected with *Mycoplasma pneumoniae*, infiltration of the lungs by neutrophils is dependent on IL-23–induced upregulation of IL-17 (Wu et al. 2007). Additionally, accumulating evidence suggests that another Gram-negative extracellular respiratory pathogen, *Bordetella pertussis* which causes the whooping cough, may bias the host response towards the production of Th17 cytokines by preferentially inhibiting IL-12 and inducing IL-23 (Fedele et al. 2008). The above-referenced studies clearly demonstrate a protective role for Th17 effector cytokines in host defense against primary challenges with specific extracellular Gram-negative pathogens. Th17 response may also play a role in controlling primary infection with intracellular pathogens such as *Mycobacterium tuberculosis*, although a much more limited one when compared with extracellular bacterial pathogens. It was shown that although Th17 cells are not critical to the primary response to *M. tuberculosis*, Th17 activation is clearly involved in response to vaccination against tuberculosis (Khader et al. 2007). In addition to this Th17-mediated vaccine-induced immunity to *M. tuberculosis*, Th17 cytokine responses have also been implicated in vaccine-induced immunity against *B. pertussis* (Higgins et al. 2006) and *Streptococcus pneumoniae* (Malley et al. 2006). This indicates that the host Th17 effector cytokines have evolved as protective immune mechanisms against extracellular bacteria but are dispensable for primary protection against most intracellular pathogens that require a Th1 pathway for protection, such as in tuberculosis infection.

Pseudomonas aeruginosa is another Gram-negative pathogen. Although not as virulent as *K. pneumoniae*, *P. aeruginosa* is a highly adaptable pathogen that causes both acute and chronic pulmonary infections. Chronic colonization and infection in the lung is associated with pre-existing airway disease such as CF. CF is a disease characterized by the excessive production of aberrantly hydrated mucus in the airways, resulting from mutations in the ion channel cystic fibrosis transmembrane conductance regulator (CFTR). This increased mucus production, blocks normal ciliary function and thereby enhances recurrent pulmonary infections. During pulmonary exacerbation, CF patients exhibit airway neutrophilia and elevated levels of IL-23 and both IL-17A and IL-17F in bronchoalveolar lavage fluid and sputum (McAllister et al. 2005). Recently it was shown that $CD4^+$ Th17 cells are prominently featured in the airway walls of CF patients but that NKT cells and γδ T cells are also sources of IL-17 in patients with CF (Tan et al. 2011). In the latter study, IL-17^{+} cells were correlated with CF and non-CF bronchiectasis, but not with the presence of *P. aeruginosa*. It has been shown that clearance of *P. aeruginosa* is dependent on Th17 responses (Dubin and Kolls 2007).

3.2.2 Fungi, viruses and other opportunistic pathogens

Several reports from mouse and human studies have shown that Th17 cells are important for clearing opportunistic infections such as *Cryptococcus neoformans, Pneumocystis jirovecii* and *Candida albicans*. E.g. patients with Job's syndrome are extremely susceptible to mucocutaneous fungal infections caused by Candida species. It has been suggested that Th17 cytokines, particularly IL-17, contribute to tissue pathology in invasive *Aspergillus* infection in the lung particularly in the setting of NADPH oxidase deficiency (Romani et al. 2008). In respiratory tract models of fungal infections using *P. jirovecci*, induction of IL-23 and IL-17 following pathogen challenge is protective, since IL-23KO mice or neutralization of the IL-23/IL-17 axis resulted in impaired clearance of the pathogen (Rudner et al. 2007).
Human viruses can induce IL-17 responses, as shown for herpes simplex virus (Maertzdorf, Osterhaus, and Verjans 2002) and respiratory syncytial virus (Hashimoto et al. 2005). Human rhinovirus infections are associated with exacerbations of asthma and COPD and IL-17 was shown to function synergistically with human rhinovirus to induce IL-8 from epithelial cells. This may contribute to the recruitment of neutrophils, immature DCs and memory T cells to the lung contributing to severe inflammatory profiles seen during viral exacerbations of airway disease (Wiehler and Proud 2007).
Taken together, there is accumulating evidence for the involvement of IL-17 in bacterial, fungal and viral infection in the respiratory system in the mouse, whereas in human the role of IL-17 or Th17 cells is largely unexplored.

3.3 Sarcoidosis, pulmonary fibrosis and other interstitial lung diseases

Interstitial lung diseases (ILD) refer to a very heterogeneous group of lung diseases affecting the lung parenchyma. The exact nature of the initiating event and the subsequent cascade of mechanistic proceedings are most likely different in every single ILD. Multiple factors are likely to be involved but it is now clear that the immune system plays a major part in the pathogenesis of ILD. A similarity in every ILD is the interaction of growth factors, cytokines, and other mediators with cells that reside in the lung which seem to form part of the cascade of events that have been identified in the pathogenesis.
Recent data point to a potential role of IL-17 and Th17 cells in a number of ILD. E.g. Wegener granulomatosis (Abdulahad et al. 2008), Langerhans histiocytosis (Coury et al. 2008), and hypersensitivity pneumonitis (Joshi et al. 2009; Simonian et al. 2009) have been reported to be linked to IL-17. Pulmonary IL-17 producing γδ T cells have also been detected in response to bleomycin-induced tissue damage, a model for induced pulmonary fibrosis (Braun et al. 2010). Conversely, a particular subset of γδ T cells secreting IL-17 has been shown to contribute to hyperinflammatory granulomatous disease and fatal lung tissue damage during pulmonary aspergillosis (Romani et al. 2008). Recently, also sarcoidosis was suggested as a Th1/Th17 multisystem disorder (Facco et al. 2011), based on the presence of IL-17 positive CD4^{+} T cells in sarcoid lung tissue and their ability to respond to the chemotactic stimulus CCL20. Moreover IL-17A was expressed by macrophages infiltrating

sarcoid tissue. Sarcoidosis is a systemic inflammatory disease characterized by non-caseating granulomas in various organs with pulmonary involvement in over 90% of patients (ATS 1999). These granulomas are compact, organized collections of macrophages and epithelioid cells, surrounded by and infiltrated with T lymphocytes, but the pathological processes that result in granulomatous inflammation are largely unknown. The accumulation in the lung of apparently oligoclonal IFNγ-producing T helper cells in sarcoidosis indicated an antigen-driven Th1 response (Rosen 2007; Zaba et al. 2010). Also because IL-17A has been implicated in the formation of a mycobacterial infection-induced granuloma in the lung (Curtis and Way 2009), we investigated Th17 cells by intracellular flow cytometry and immunohistochemistry in blood, BAL and bronchial mucosal biopsies from a cohort of newly diagnosed sarcoidosis patients and healthy controls. These studies provided evidence for the involvement of the Th17 lineage in sarcoidosis: IL-17A-expressing T cells were present in and around the granuloma and IL-22-expressing T cells were found in the subepithelial lamina propria in mucosal biopsies of sarcoidosis patients (Figure 4). This was accompanied by the presence of IL-17A$^+$, IL-17A$^+$IFNγ$^+$ and IL-17A$^+$IL-4$^+$ memory T helper cells in BAL and by a significant increase in the proportions of these cells in the circulation (ten Berge et al. 2011).

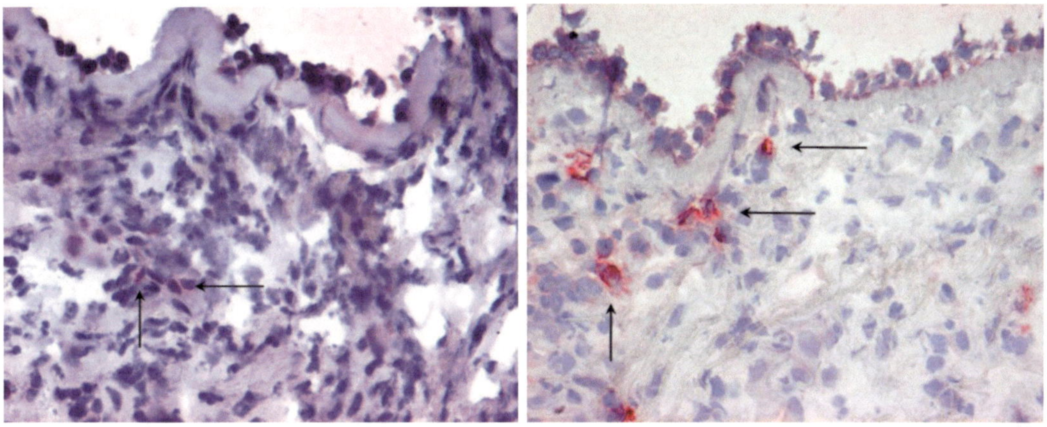

Fig. 4. IL-17A$^+$ and IL-22$^+$ cells in sarcoidosis lung biopsies containing granulomas. Hematoxylin nucleus staining and IL-17A (left) and IL-22 (right) staining of lung mucosal frozen sections from a granuloma-containing sarcoidosis biopsy (40 x magnifications). Arrows indicate IL-17A$^+$ cells as well as diffuse IL-17A staining in red (left) and IL-22$^+$ cells as well as diffuse IL-22 staining in the epithelium in red (right).

3.4 IL-17 in transplantation

Organ transplantation is currently a valid treatment option for selected patients with end-stage disease. Graft rejection is still the most severe complication following organ transplantation. In lung transplantation, episodes of acute rejection (AR) tend to lead to chronic rejection, which is the main cause of late graft loss and poor long-term survival (Lee, Christie, and Keshavjee 2010; Burton et al. 2007). The diagnosis of AR is based on clinical findings and/or histological confirmation in transbronchial biopsies (Vanaudenaerde et al. 2006). It has been shown that in addition to the frequency and severity of AR, also other risk factors such as ischemia-reperfusion injury (Lee, Christie, and Keshavjee 2010), gastro-oesophageal reflux (King et al. 2009), CMV pneumonitis and other infections (Valentine et al. 2009) are associated with an increased risk of chronic rejection. Chronic graft rejection, clinically known as BOS is defined as a progressive decline in lung function with other underlying conditions being absent (Estenne et al. 2002). More than 50% of the patients surviving five years after lung transplantation suffer from BOS (Christie et al. 2010).

Classically, graft rejection has been shown to be mediated by $CD4^+$ and $CD8^+$ T cells (Heeger 2003). Th1 cells were associated with graft rejection, whereas Th2 cells were considered to protect against rejection (Piccotti et al. 1997). Evidence is accumulating for an important role of IL-17 in allograft rejection, both in rodent models and humans. Prior to the first description of Th17 cells, IL-17 was implicated in the process of allograft rejection. Blocking IL-17 function in a rat cardiac allograft transplantation model increased graft survival significantly (Antonysamy et al. 1999). Around that same period, a number of reports highlighted the importance of IL-17 in the context of renal transplantation. Already in 1998 it was shown that IL-17 was detectable by immunofluorescent staining of acutely rejecting human renal transplant biopsies, but not in healthy kidneys or pre-transplant biopsies (Van Kooten et al. 1998). Moreover, elevated IL-17 mRNA and protein levels could be detected in renal biopsy specimens and urinary sediment from patients found to have subclinical rejection when compared with control samples without any evidence of rejections (Loong et al. 2002). Additionally, elevated IL-17 mRNA and protein levels were detectable as early as the second post-operative day in a rat renal allograft model and its appearance is followed by the local production of pro-inflammatory molecules known to be induced by IL-17 (Hsieh et al. 2001).

It is important to keep in mind that transplantation procedures themselves may have a direct effect on the cytokine profile within the graft. Following an organ harvest the ischemia-reperfusion injury results in the release of a number of inflammatory mediators. These mediators include some of the cytokines that are important in T cell differentiation such as TGFβ (Basile et al. 2001). A recent study demonstrated that factors released by human endothelial cells as a consequence of ischemia-reperfusion injury could enhance the production of both IL-17 and IFNγ by $CD4^+$ T cells (Rao, Tracey, and Pober 2007). These findings indicate that perioperative factors might result in increased Th17 activity within the graft.

3.4.1 IL-17 in lung transplantation

In lung transplantation, IL-17 has been implicated in ischemia reperfusion injury, acute rejection, infection and BOS (Bobadilla et al. 2008; Vanaudenaerde, De Vleeschauwer et al. 2008; Yoshida et al. 2006). At day 28 after lung transplantation, IL-17 mRNA levels were found to be elevated in the bronchoalveolar lavage (BAL) fluid from patients with acute rejection when compared with those without rejection. This difference disappeared at longer follow up (Vanaudenaerde et al. 2006). These increased IL-17 levels were associated with increased numbers of both BAL lymphocytes and neutrophils and correlated with the severity of rejection (Vanaudenaerde et al. 2006). However, such a correlation with severity of rejection could not be confirmed in another study even though this study did show increased numbers of IL-17 positive cells in endobronchial biopsies early after lung transplantation (Snell et al. 2007). These apparently conflicting results may be explained by differences in the time of sampling, suggesting that early events after transplantation may be critical for inducing IL-17 production or that patient selection is crucial (Shilling and

Wilkes 2011). Additionally, patient heterogeneity may also cause conflicting results, e.g. by including both unilateral and bilateral transplant patients or by not discriminating between primary lung diseases.

Protein levels of IL-6 and IL-1β and mRNA levels for TGF-β, IL-17, IL-23 and IL-8 in BAL fluid were increased in lung transplant recipients with BOS when compared to controls (Vanaudenaerde, Wuyts et al. 2008). CXCL8, a potent chemoattractant for neutrophils, has previously been associated with BOS, but it was unclear whether the presence of neutrophils was just a marker of general inflammation or a key mediator of obliterative bronchiolitis (McDyer 2007). Since IL-17 promotes neutrophil chemotaxis, the presence of neutrophils has been suggested to be secondary to a Th17-mediated alloimmune or autoimmune response (Shilling and Wilkes 2011). In a mouse model increased levels of IL-6 and IL-17 also correlated with tracheal obliteration, and blockade of IL-6 decreased both allograft fibrosis and IL-17 transcripts (Nakagiri et al. 2010). Increased neutrophilic inflammation of the airways with upregulation of IL-8 is common in the BAL of BOS patients. However, there are also many of these patients without considerable BAL neutrophilia despite the fact that they seem to be in an identical clinical condition with progressive decline in lung function, compatible with BOS. This may indicate the existence of different phenotypes within BOS with possible different treatment strategies. BAL neutrophilia might therefore be an important tool to select patients who might benefit from azithromycin treatment, since it has been demonstrated that azithromycin significantly reduces airway neutrophilia and CXCL8 in patients with BOS (Gottlieb et al. 2008).

Th17 cell responses may also trigger BOS by facilitating autoimmune responses, because autoantibodies against collagen type V have been described to be involved in lung allograft rejection (Burlingham et al. 2007). Immunohistochemical analysis indicated that collagen V becomes exposed in the lung matrix after ischemia-reperfusion injury in rat lung isografts and allografts (Yoshida et al. 2006), and that collagen V peptides are released in the BAL (Haque et al. 2002). Additionally, in humans it has been shown that pre-transplant patients who exhibit collagen V reactivity have an increased incidence of early graft dysfunction following lung transplantation (Bobadilla et al. 2008).

Recent observations in our own group indicate that not only in BOS but also in stable lung transplantation patients IL-17 and other Th17 cytokines might play a role. We found enhanced Th17 differentiation of peripheral blood mononuclear cells (PBMC) in a group of stable lung transplantation patients, compared with both healthy individuals and patients on the waiting list for a lung transplantation. The increase in the proportions of circulating Th17 cells was not linked to donor-specific haploreactivity. Interestingly, increased proportions of circulating IL-17A$^+$ CD4$^+$ T cells co-expressing IFNγ were found, indicating that specific Th17 subpopulations may have a functional role in stable lung transplantation patients (Paats *et al.*, unpublished data).

4. Therapeutic potential

Accumulating evidence suggests that IL-17 and other cytokines involved in the Th17 pathway play an important role in the pathogenesis of various lung diseases. Interference with the activity of Th17 cells or the inflammatory mediators that either induce them (IL-1β, IL-6, and IL-23), act in concert with IL-17 (TNFα and IL-1β), or work downstream of IL-17 could be an effective treatment modality. One of these novel treatment modalities is cell blockade by monoclonal antibodies. Most antibody therapies have not yet been tested in lung pathology, which is remarkable because of the lung's continuous exposure to external triggers and pathogens. The risks of monoclonal antibody therapies must also be kept in mind. Adverse effects including infections, cancer and autoimmune disease are all issues that need consideration before antibody treatment can be introduced (Hansel et al. 2010).

The most direct way to control the biologic effects of Th17 cells would be to target production of their effector cytokines. Monoclonal antibodies against IL-17 or the IL-17R and a soluble IL-17R have been developed for clinical application. Administration of LY2439821, an anti-IL-17 monoclonal antibody, has been described in RA and improved signs and symptoms of the disease, without significant adverse events (Genovese et al. 2010). Additionally, it is promising that clinical trials with the fully human antibody, AIN457, in RA, psoriasis and noninfectious uveitis, show that targeting IL-17A interrupts inflammation and reduces disease activity (Hueber et al. 2010). Inhibitors of other products of Th17 cells such as IL-21 and IL-22 have not reached the clinical setting (Ma et al. 2008; Young et al. 2007). Another option might be to down-regulate IL-1β, IL-6 and IL-23, the cytokines that induce Th17 differentiation. Targeting the IL-6R with a monoclonal antibody (e.g., tocilizumab, a humanized monoclonal antibody against the receptor) and neutralizing the IL-1R with an antagonist (e.g., anakinra, a recombinant human IL-1R antagonist) are two effective approaches to the treatment of rheumatoid arthritis and other autoimmune inflammatory diseases (Dinarello 2005; Yokota et al. 2005). A monoclonal antibody (ustekinumab) targeting the shared IL-12/IL-23 p40 subunit, blocks both Th1 and Th17 cells and was shown to be efficient in the treatment of psoriasis and Crohn's disease (Griffiths et al. 2010). IL-17 induces the production of IL-1β and TNFα. Antibodies, antagonists or receptor antagonists to IL-1 and TNFα are already in use for a range of autoimmune and chronic inflammatory conditions (Sutton et al. 2009). Unfortunately, recurrence of immunoinflammatory disease when treatment with TNFα inhibitors is discontinued is common. A combination of IL-17 and TNFα inhibitors, administered either simultaneously or sequentially, might be a good alternative to better control inflammation (Nadkarni, Mauri, and Ehrenstein 2007; Miossec, Korn, and Kuchroo 2009). Targeting intracellular signaling molecules or transcriptional factors involved in the activation of IL-17 production e. g. by small molecule inhibitors is an alternative approach for the development of new drugs. However, it is complicated by the fact that many of the signaling pathways are not unique to the IL-23-IL-17 axis and may also inhibit responses of other cell types involved in protective immunity (Mills 2008).

Non-selective blockade of the adaptive immune system by the use of steroids or cyclosporine seem ineffective in patients with severe asthma, COPD and CF (Barnes 2008; Vanaudenaerde et al. 2011). This is probably due to the reported steroid resistance of the Th17 cell–neutrophil axis (McKinley et al. 2008). Other medication capable of dampening the innate immune system might be an alternative way to interfere with the Th17 pathway. The best documented therapy for reducing IL-17-T cell-mediated neutrophilia is macrolide therapy, which is being used effectively in clinical practice in patients with CF, asthma, COPD and BOS (Jaffe and Bush 2001; Seemungal et al. 2008). In addition, in vitro studies have shown that vitamin D inhibits Th17 cells (Mora, Iwata, and von Andrian 2008; Colin et al. 2010), hence vitamin D therapy might have potential in controlling Th17-mediated lung diseases. Clinical trials that could prove the importance of vitamin D in chronic lung diseases are currently in progress. Furthermore, other medication capable of interfering with the innate immune system, such as vitamin A or statins, merits attention (Vanaudenaerde et al. 2011).

5. Conclusions

We still have much to learn about the phenotype, function and regulation of human Th17 cells. It is however clear that IL-17 and other Th17 associated cytokines play a central role in regulating diverse immune responses. With their potential to induce a pronounced neutrophilic inflammation, which is a common feature of many pulmonary inflammatory conditions, Th17 cells are subject of great research interest. Important to realize is that besides Th17 cells there are also other sources of IL-17, including $CD8^+$ T cells, γδ T cells, NK T cells, and LTi cells. Depending on the timing, the tissue, and the local microenvironment, IL-17 secreting cells appear to be able to play both beneficial and detrimental roles in lung immunity and disease. The exact balance of these roles during the processes of many autoimmune and infectious diseases is however not fully understood yet. Therefore, the challenge lies in uncovering strategies to maximize the protective effect of IL-17 producing cells while simultaneously preventing these cells from causing immune-mediated host damage. At present, therapies that modulate the Th17 cell pathway are being tested in the clinic with promising results.

6. Acknowledgement

We thank Bernt van den Blink, Alex Kleinjan and Ingrid Bergen (Erasmus MC Rotterdam) for their assistance and stimulating discussions.

7. References

Abdulahad, W. H., C. A. Stegeman, P. C. Limburg, and C. G. Kallenberg. 2008. Skewed distribution of Th17 lymphocytes in patients with Wegener's granulomatosis in remission. *Arthritis Rheum* 58 (7):2196-205.

Acosta-Rodriguez, E. V., G. Napolitani, A. Lanzavecchia, and F. Sallusto. 2007. Interleukins 1beta and 6 but not transforming growth factor-beta are essential for the differentiation of interleukin 17-producing human T helper cells. *Nat Immunol* 8 (9):942-9.

Acosta-Rodriguez, E. V., L. Rivino, J. Geginat, D. Jarrossay, M. Gattorno, A. Lanzavecchia, F. Sallusto, and G. Napolitani. 2007. Surface phenotype and antigenic specificity of human interleukin 17-producing T helper memory cells. *Nat Immunol* 8 (6):639-46.

Akira, S., S. Uematsu, and O. Takeuchi. 2006. Pathogen recognition and innate immunity. *Cell* 124 (4):783-801.

Al-Ramli, W., D. Prefontaine, F. Chouiali, J. G. Martin, R. Olivenstein, C. Lemiere, and Q. Hamid. 2009. T(H)17-associated cytokines (IL-17A and IL-17F) in severe asthma. *J Allergy Clin Immunol* 123 (5):1185-7.

Anderson, G. P. 2008. Endotyping asthma: new insights into key pathogenic mechanisms in a complex, heterogeneous disease. *Lancet* 372 (9643):1107-19.

Annunziato, F., L. Cosmi, V. Santarlasci, L. Maggi, F. Liotta, B. Mazzinghi, E. Parente, L. Fili, S. Ferri, F. Frosali, F. Giudici, P. Romagnani, P. Parronchi, F. Tonelli, E. Maggi, and S. Romagnani. 2007. Phenotypic and functional features of human Th17 cells. *J Exp Med* 204 (8):1849-61.

Antonysamy, M. A., W. C. Fanslow, F. Fu, W. Li, S. Qian, A. B. Troutt, and A. W. Thomson. 1999. Evidence for a role of IL-17 in alloimmunity: a novel IL-17 antagonist promotes heart graft survival. *Transplant Proc* 31 (1-2):93.

Arican, O., M. Aral, S. Sasmaz, and P. Ciragil. 2005. Serum levels of TNF-alpha, IFN-gamma, IL-6, IL-8, IL-12, IL-17, and IL-18 in patients with active psoriasis and correlation with disease severity. *Mediators Inflamm* 2005 (5):273-9.

ATS, ERS, WASOG. 1999. Statement on sarcoidosis. Joint Statement of the American Thoracic Society (ATS), the European Respiratory Society (ERS) and the World Association of Sarcoidosis and Other Granulomatous Disorders (WASOG) adopted by the ATS Board of Directors and by the ERS Executive Committee, February 1999. *Am J Respir Crit Care Med* 160 (2):736-55.

Aujla, S. J., Y. R. Chan, M. Zheng, M. Fei, D. J. Askew, D. A. Pociask, T. A. Reinhart, F. McAllister, J. Edeal, K. Gaus, S. Husain, J. L. Kreindler, P. J. Dubin, J. M. Pilewski, M. M. Myerburg, C. A. Mason, Y. Iwakura, and J. K. Kolls. 2008. IL-22 mediates mucosal host defense against Gram-negative bacterial pneumonia. *Nat Med* 14 (3):275-81.

Aujla, S. J., P. J. Dubin, and J. K. Kolls. 2007. Th17 cells and mucosal host defense. *Semin Immunol* 19 (6):377-82.

Barczyk, A., W. Pierzchala, and E. Sozanska. 2003. Interleukin-17 in sputum correlates with airway hyperresponsiveness to methacholine. *Respir Med* 97 (6):726-33.

Barnes, P. J. 2000. Chronic obstructive pulmonary disease. *N Engl J Med* 343 (4):269-80.

2008. Immunology of asthma and chronic obstructive pulmonary disease. *Nat Rev Immunol* 8 (3):183-92.

Basile, D. P., D. Donohoe, K. Roethe, and J. L. Osborn. 2001. Renal ischemic injury results in permanent damage to peritubular capillaries and influences long-term function. *Am J Physiol Renal Physiol* 281 (5):F887-99.

Bettelli, E., M. Oukka, and V. K. Kuchroo. 2007. T(H)-17 cells in the circle of immunity and autoimmunity. *Nat Immunol* 8 (4):345-50.

Bluestone, J. A., C. R. Mackay, J. J. O'Shea, and B. Stockinger. 2009. The functional plasticity of T cell subsets. *Nat Rev Immunol* 9 (11):811-6.

Bobadilla, J. L., R. B. Love, E. Jankowska-Gan, Q. Xu, L. D. Haynes, R. K. Braun, M. S. Hayney, A. Munoz del Rio, K. Meyer, D. S. Greenspan, J. Torrealba, K. M. Heidler, O. W. Cummings, T. Iwata, D. Brand, R. Presson, W. J. Burlingham, and D. S. Wilkes. 2008. Th-17, monokines, collagen type V, and primary graft dysfunction in lung transplantation. *Am J Respir Crit Care Med* 177 (6):660-8.

Boniface, K., K. S. Bak-Jensen, Y. Li, W. M. Blumenschein, M. J. McGeachy, T. K. McClanahan, B. S. McKenzie, R. A. Kastelein, D. J. Cua, and R. de Waal Malefyt. 2009. Prostaglandin E2 regulates Th17 cell differentiation and function through cyclic AMP and EP2/EP4 receptor signaling. *J Exp Med* 206 (3):535-48.

Braun, R. K., A. Martin, S. Shah, M. Iwashima, M. Medina, K. Byrne, P. Sethupathi, C. H. Wigfield, D. D. Brand, and R. B. Love. 2010. Inhibition of bleomycin-induced pulmonary fibrosis through pre-treatment with collagen type V. *J Heart Lung Transplant* 29 (8):873-80.

Bullens, D. M., E. Truyen, L. Coteur, E. Dilissen, P. W. Hellings, L. J. Dupont, and J. L. Ceuppens. 2006. IL-17 mRNA in sputum of asthmatic patients: linking T cell driven inflammation and granulocytic influx? *Respir Res* 7:135.

Burlingham, W. J., R. B. Love, E. Jankowska-Gan, L. D. Haynes, Q. Xu, J. L. Bobadilla, K. C. Meyer, M. S. Hayney, R. K. Braun, D. S. Greenspan, B. Gopalakrishnan, J. Cai, D. D. Brand, S. Yoshida, O. W. Cummings, and D. S. Wilkes. 2007. IL-17-dependent cellular immunity to collagen type V predisposes to obliterative bronchiolitis in human lung transplants. *J Clin Invest* 117 (11):3498-506.

Burton, C. M., J. Carlsen, J. Mortensen, C. B. Andersen, N. Milman, and M. Iversen. 2007. Long-term survival after lung transplantation depends on development and severity of bronchiolitis obliterans syndrome. *J Heart Lung Transplant* 26 (7):681-6.

Calikoglu, M., G. Sahin, A. Unlu, C. Ozturk, L. Tamer, B. Ercan, A. Kanik, and U. Atik. 2004. Leptin and TNF-alpha levels in patients with chronic obstructive pulmonary disease and their relationship to nutritional parameters. *Respiration* 71 (1):45-50.

Cella, M., A. Fuchs, W. Vermi, F. Facchetti, K. Otero, J. K. Lennerz, J. M. Doherty, J. C. Mills, and M. Colonna. 2009. A human natural killer cell subset provides an innate source of IL-22 for mucosal immunity. *Nature* 457 (7230):722-5.

Chang, Y., J. Nadigel, N. Boulais, J. Bourbeau, F. Maltais, D. H. Eidelman, and Q. Hamid. 2011. CD8 positive T cells express IL-17 in patients with chronic obstructive pulmonary disease. *Respir Res* 12:43.

Chen, Z., and J. J. O'Shea. 2008. Regulation of IL-17 production in human lymphocytes. *Cytokine* 41 (2):71-8.

Chen, Z., C. M. Tato, L. Muul, A. Laurence, and J. J. O'Shea. 2007. Distinct regulation of interleukin-17 in human T helper lymphocytes. *Arthritis Rheum* 56 (9):2936-46.

Christie, J. D., L. B. Edwards, A. Y. Kucheryavaya, P. Aurora, F. Dobbels, R. Kirk, A. O. Rahmel, J. Stehlik, and M. I. Hertz. 2010. The Registry of the International Society for Heart and Lung Transplantation: twenty-seventh official adult lung and heart-lung transplant report--2010. *J Heart Lung Transplant* 29 (10):1104-18.

Colin, E. M., P. S. Asmawidjaja, J. P. van Hamburg, A. M. Mus, M. van Driel, J. M. Hazes, J. P. van Leeuwen, and E. Lubberts. 2010. 1,25-dihydroxyvitamin D3 modulates Th17 polarization and interleukin-22 expression by memory T cells from patients with early rheumatoid arthritis. *Arthritis Rheum* 62 (1):132-42.

Cosmi, L., R. De Palma, V. Santarlasci, L. Maggi, M. Capone, F. Frosali, G. Rodolico, V. Querci, G. Abbate, R. Angeli, L. Berrino, M. Fambrini, M. Caproni, F. Tonelli, E. Lazzeri, P. Parronchi, F. Liotta, E. Maggi, S. Romagnani, and F. Annunziato. 2008. Human interleukin 17-producing cells originate from a CD161+CD4+ T cell precursor. *J Exp Med* 205 (8):1903-16.

Cosmi, L., F. Liotta, E. Maggi, S. Romagnani, and F. Annunziato. 2011. Th17 cells: new players in asthma pathogenesis. *Allergy* 66 (8):989-98.

Coury, F., N. Annels, A. Rivollier, S. Olsson, A. Santoro, C. Speziani, O. Azocar, M. Flacher, S. Djebali, J. Tebib, M. Brytting, R. M. Egeler, C. Rabourdin-Combe, J. I. Henter, M. Arico, and C. Delprat. 2008. Langerhans cell histiocytosis reveals a new IL-17A-dependent pathway of dendritic cell fusion. *Nat Med* 14 (1):81-7.

Crome, S. Q., A. Y. Wang, C. Y. Kang, and M. K. Levings. 2009. The role of retinoic acid-related orphan receptor variant 2 and IL-17 in the development and function of human CD4+ T cells. *Eur J Immunol* 39 (6):1480-93.

Crome, S. Q., A. Y. Wang, and M. K. Levings. 2010. Translational mini-review series on Th17 cells: function and regulation of human T helper 17 cells in health and disease. *Clin Exp Immunol* 159 (2):109-19.

Crotty, S. 2011. Follicular helper CD4 T cells (TFH). *Annu Rev Immunol* 29:621-63.

Cua, D. J., and C. M. Tato. 2010. Innate IL-17-producing cells: the sentinels of the immune system. *Nat Rev Immunol* 10 (7):479-89.

Curtis, J. L., C. M. Freeman, and J. C. Hogg. 2007. The immunopathogenesis of chronic obstructive pulmonary disease: insights from recent research. *Proc Am Thorac Soc* 4 (7):512-21.

Curtis, M. M., and S. S. Way. 2009. Interleukin-17 in host defence against bacterial, mycobacterial and fungal pathogens. *Immunology* 126 (2):177-85.

Di Stefano, A., G. Caramori, I. Gnemmi, M. Contoli, C. Vicari, A. Capelli, F. Magno, S. E. D'Anna, A. Zanini, P. Brun, P. Casolari, K. F. Chung, P. J. Barnes, A. Papi, I. Adcock, and B. Balbi. 2009. T helper type 17-related cytokine expression is increased in the bronchial mucosa of stable chronic obstructive pulmonary disease patients. *Clin Exp Immunol* 157 (2):316-24.

Dinarello, C. A. 2005. Blocking IL-1 in systemic inflammation. *J Exp Med* 201 (9):1355-9.

Doe, C., M. Bafadhel, S. Siddiqui, D. Desai, V. Mistry, P. Rugman, M. McCormick, J. Woods, R. May, M. A. Sleeman, I. K. Anderson, and C. E. Brightling. 2010. Expression of the T helper 17-associated cytokines IL-17A and IL-17F in asthma and COPD. *Chest* 138 (5):1140-7.

Dong, C. 2008. TH17 cells in development: an updated view of their molecular identity and genetic programming. *Nat Rev Immunol* 8 (5):337-48.

Dubin, P. J., and J. K. Kolls. 2007. IL-23 mediates inflammatory responses to mucoid Pseudomonas aeruginosa lung infection in mice. *Am J Physiol Lung Cell Mol Physiol* 292 (2):L519-28.

Duhen, T., R. Geiger, D. Jarrossay, A. Lanzavecchia, and F. Sallusto. 2009. Production of interleukin 22 but not interleukin 17 by a subset of human skin-homing memory T cells. *Nat Immunol* 10 (8):857-63.

Eberl, G., S. Marmon, M. J. Sunshine, P. D. Rennert, Y. Choi, and D. R. Littman. 2004. An essential function for the nuclear receptor RORgamma(t) in the generation of fetal lymphoid tissue inducer cells. *Nat Immunol* 5 (1):64-73.

Elias, K. M., A. Laurence, T. S. Davidson, G. Stephens, Y. Kanno, E. M. Shevach, and J. J. O'Shea. 2008. Retinoic acid inhibits Th17 polarization and enhances FoxP3 expression through a Stat-3/Stat-5 independent signaling pathway. *Blood* 111 (3):1013-20.

Estenne, M., J. R. Maurer, A. Boehler, J. J. Egan, A. Frost, M. Hertz, G. B. Mallory, G. I. Snell, and S. Yousem. 2002. Bronchiolitis obliterans syndrome 2001: an update of the diagnostic criteria. *J Heart Lung Transplant* 21 (3):297-310.

Evans, H. G., N. J. Gullick, S. Kelly, C. Pitzalis, G. M. Lord, B. W. Kirkham, and L. S. Taams. 2009. In vivo activated monocytes from the site of inflammation in humans specifically promote Th17 responses. *Proc Natl Acad Sci U S A* 106 (15):6232-7.

Facco, M., A. Cabrelle, A. Teramo, V. Olivieri, M. Gnoato, S. Teolato, E. Ave, C. Gattazzo, G. P. Fadini, F. Calabrese, G. Semenzato, and C. Agostini. 2011. Sarcoidosis is a Th1/Th17 multisystem disorder. *Thorax* 66 (2):144-50.

Fedele, G., M. Nasso, F. Spensieri, R. Palazzo, L. Frasca, M. Watanabe, and C. M. Ausiello. 2008. Lipopolysaccharides from Bordetella pertussis and Bordetella parapertussis differently modulate human dendritic cell functions resulting in divergent prevalence of Th17-polarized responses. *J Immunol* 181 (1):208-16.

Feghali-Bostwick, C. A., A. S. Gadgil, L. E. Otterbein, J. M. Pilewski, M. W. Stoner, E. Csizmadia, Y. Zhang, F. C. Sciurba, and S. R. Duncan. 2008. Autoantibodies in patients with chronic obstructive pulmonary disease. *Am J Respir Crit Care Med* 177 (2):156-63.

Feldmann, M., F. M. Brennan, B. M. Foxwell, and R. N. Maini. 2001. The role of TNF alpha and IL-1 in rheumatoid arthritis. *Curr Dir Autoimmun* 3:188-99.

Ferretti, S., O. Bonneau, G. R. Dubois, C. E. Jones, and A. Trifilieff. 2003. IL-17, produced by lymphocytes and neutrophils, is necessary for lipopolysaccharide-induced airway neutrophilia: IL-15 as a possible trigger. *J Immunol* 170 (4):2106-12.

Fossiez, F., O. Djossou, P. Chomarat, L. Flores-Romo, S. Ait-Yahia, C. Maat, J. J. Pin, P. Garrone, E. Garcia, S. Saeland, D. Blanchard, C. Gaillard, B. Das Mahapatra, E. Rouvier, P. Golstein, J. Banchereau, and S. Lebecque. 1996. T cell interleukin-17 induces stromal cells to produce proinflammatory and hematopoietic cytokines. *J Exp Med* 183 (6):2593-603.

Fujino, S., A. Andoh, S. Bamba, A. Ogawa, K. Hata, Y. Araki, T. Bamba, and Y. Fujiyama. 2003. Increased expression of interleukin 17 in inflammatory bowel disease. *Gut* 52 (1):65-70.

Genovese, M. C., F. Van den Bosch, S. A. Roberson, S. Bojin, I. M. Biagini, P. Ryan, and J. Sloan-Lancaster. 2010. LY2439821, a humanized anti-interleukin-17 monoclonal antibody, in the treatment of patients with rheumatoid arthritis: A phase I randomized, double-blind, placebo-controlled, proof-of-concept study. *Arthritis Rheum* 62 (4):929-39.

Godfrey, D. I., H. R. MacDonald, M. Kronenberg, M. J. Smyth, and L. Van Kaer. 2004. NKT cells: what's in a name? *Nat Rev Immunol* 4 (3):231-7.

Gottlieb, J., J. Szangolies, T. Koehnlein, H. Golpon, A. Simon, and T. Welte. 2008. Long-term azithromycin for bronchiolitis obliterans syndrome after lung transplantation. *Transplantation* 85 (1):36-41.

Griffiths, C. E., B. E. Strober, P. van de Kerkhof, V. Ho, R. Fidelus-Gort, N. Yeilding, C. Guzzo, Y. Xia, B. Zhou, S. Li, L. T. Dooley, N. H. Goldstein, A. Menter, and Accept Study Group. 2010. Comparison of ustekinumab and etanercept for moderate-to-severe psoriasis. *N Engl J Med* 362 (2):118-28.

Hacievliyagil, S. S., H. Gunen, L. C. Mutlu, A. B. Karabulut, and I. Temel. 2006. Association between cytokines in induced sputum and severity of chronic obstructive pulmonary disease. *Respir Med* 100 (5):846-54.

Hansel, T. T., H. Kropshofer, T. Singer, J. A. Mitchell, and A. J. George. 2010. The safety and side effects of monoclonal antibodies. *Nat Rev Drug Discov* 9 (4):325-38.

Happel, K. I., P. J. Dubin, M. Zheng, N. Ghilardi, C. Lockhart, L. J. Quinton, A. R. Odden, J. E. Shellito, G. J. Bagby, S. Nelson, and J. K. Kolls. 2005. Divergent roles of IL-23 and IL-12 in host defense against Klebsiella pneumoniae. *J Exp Med* 202 (6):761-9.

Happel, K. I., M. Zheng, E. Young, L. J. Quinton, E. Lockhart, A. J. Ramsay, J. E. Shellito, J. R. Schurr, G. J. Bagby, S. Nelson, and J. K. Kolls. 2003. Cutting edge: roles of Toll-like receptor 4 and IL-23 in IL-17 expression in response to Klebsiella pneumoniae infection. *J Immunol* 170 (9):4432-6.

Haque, M. A., T. Mizobuchi, K. Yasufuku, T. Fujisawa, R. R. Brutkiewicz, Y. Zheng, K. Woods, G. N. Smith, O. W. Cummings, K. M. Heidler, J. S. Blum, and D. S. Wilkes. 2002. Evidence for immune responses to a self-antigen in lung transplantation: role of type V collagen-specific T cells in the pathogenesis of lung allograft rejection. *J Immunol* 169 (3):1542-9.

Harrington, L. E., R. D. Hatton, P. R. Mangan, H. Turner, T. L. Murphy, K. M. Murphy, and C. T. Weaver. 2005. Interleukin 17-producing CD4+ effector T cells develop via a lineage distinct from the T helper type 1 and 2 lineages. *Nat Immunol* 6 (11):1123-32.

Harrison, O. J., J. Foley, B. J. Bolognese, E. Long, 3rd, P. L. Podolin, and P. T. Walsh. 2008. Airway infiltration of CD4+ CCR6+ Th17 type cells associated with chronic cigarette smoke induced airspace enlargement. *Immunol Lett* 121 (1):13-21.

Hashimoto, K., J. E. Durbin, W. Zhou, R. D. Collins, S. B. Ho, J. K. Kolls, P. J. Dubin, J. R. Sheller, K. Goleniewska, J. F. O'Neal, S. J. Olson, D. Mitchell, B. S. Graham, and R. S. Peebles, Jr. 2005. Respiratory syncytial virus infection in the absence of STAT 1 results in airway dysfunction, airway mucus, and augmented IL-17 levels. *J Allergy Clin Immunol* 116 (3):550-7.

Hayashi, N., T. Yoshimoto, K. Izuhara, K. Matsui, T. Tanaka, and K. Nakanishi. 2007. T helper 1 cells stimulated with ovalbumin and IL-18 induce airway hyperresponsiveness and lung fibrosis by IFN-gamma and IL-13 production. *Proc Natl Acad Sci U S A* 104 (37):14765-70.

Heeger, P. S. 2003. T-cell allorecognition and transplant rejection: a summary and update. *Am J Transplant* 3 (5):525-33.

Higgins, S. C., A. G. Jarnicki, E. C. Lavelle, and K. H. Mills. 2006. TLR4 mediates vaccine-induced protective cellular immunity to Bordetella pertussis: role of IL-17-producing T cells. *J Immunol* 177 (11):7980-9.

Hill, H. R., H. D. Ochs, P. G. Quie, R. A. Clark, H. F. Pabst, S. J. Klebanoff, and R. J. Wedgwood. 1974. Defect in neutrophil granulocyte chemotaxis in Job's syndrome of recurrent "cold" staphylococcal abscesses. *Lancet* 2 (7881):617-9.

Hizawa, N., M. Kawaguchi, S. K. Huang, and M. Nishimura. 2006. Role of interleukin-17F in chronic inflammatory and allergic lung disease. *Clin Exp Allergy* 36 (9):1109-14.

Hogg, J. C. 2004. Pathophysiology of airflow limitation in chronic obstructive pulmonary disease. *Lancet* 364 (9435):709-21.

Hogg, J. C., F. Chu, S. Utokaparch, R. Woods, W. M. Elliott, L. Buzatu, R. M. Cherniack, R. M. Rogers, F. C. Sciurba, H. O. Coxson, and P. D. Pare. 2004. The nature of small-airway obstruction in chronic obstructive pulmonary disease. *N Engl J Med* 350 (26):2645-53.

Hsieh, H. G., C. C. Loong, W. Y. Lui, A. Chen, and C. Y. Lin. 2001. IL-17 expression as a possible predictive parameter for subclinical renal allograft rejection. *Transpl Int* 14 (5):287-98.

Hueber, W., D. D. Patel, T. Dryja, A. M. Wright, I. Koroleva, G. Bruin, C. Antoni, Z. Draelos, M. H. Gold, Group Psoriasis Study, P. Durez, P. P. Tak, J. J. Gomez-Reino, Group Rheumatoid Arthritis Study, C. S. Foster, R. Y. Kim, C. M. Samson, N. S. Falk, D. S. Chu, D. Callanan, Q. D. Nguyen, Group Uveitis Study, K. Rose, A. Haider, and F. Di Padova. 2010. Effects of AIN457, a fully human antibody to interleukin-17A, on psoriasis, rheumatoid arthritis, and uveitis. *Sci Transl Med* 2 (52):52ra72.

Ito, Y., T. Usui, S. Kobayashi, M. Iguchi-Hashimoto, H. Ito, H. Yoshitomi, T. Nakamura, M. Shimizu, D. Kawabata, N. Yukawa, M. Hashimoto, N. Sakaguchi, S. Sakaguchi, H. Yoshifuji, T. Nojima, K. Ohmura, T. Fujii, and T. Mimori. 2009. Gamma/delta T cells are the predominant source of interleukin-17 in affected joints in collagen-induced arthritis, but not in rheumatoid arthritis. *Arthritis Rheum* 60 (8):2294-303.

Ivanov, II, B. S. McKenzie, L. Zhou, C. E. Tadokoro, A. Lepelley, J. J. Lafaille, D. J. Cua, and D. R. Littman. 2006. The orphan nuclear receptor RORgammat directs the differentiation program of proinflammatory IL-17+ T helper cells. *Cell* 126 (6):1121-33.

Jaffe, A., and A. Bush. 2001. Anti-inflammatory effects of macrolides in lung disease. *Pediatr Pulmonol* 31 (6):464-73.

Joshi, A. D., D. J. Fong, S. R. Oak, G. Trujillo, K. R. Flaherty, F. J. Martinez, and C. M. Hogaboam. 2009. Interleukin-17-mediated immunopathogenesis in experimental hypersensitivity pneumonitis. *Am J Respir Crit Care Med* 179 (8):705-16.

Khader, S. A., G. K. Bell, J. E. Pearl, J. J. Fountain, J. Rangel-Moreno, G. E. Cilley, F. Shen, S. M. Eaton, S. L. Gaffen, S. L. Swain, R. M. Locksley, L. Haynes, T. D. Randall, and A. M. Cooper. 2007. IL-23 and IL-17 in the establishment of protective pulmonary CD4+ T cell responses after vaccination and during Mycobacterium tuberculosis challenge. *Nat Immunol* 8 (4):369-77.

King, B. J., H. Iyer, A. A. Leidi, and M. R. Carby. 2009. Gastroesophageal reflux in bronchiolitis obliterans syndrome: a new perspective. *J Heart Lung Transplant* 28 (9):870-5.

Kolls, J. K., and A. Linden. 2004. Interleukin-17 family members and inflammation. *Immunity* 21 (4):467-76.

Kondo, T., H. Takata, F. Matsuki, and M. Takiguchi. 2009. Cutting edge: Phenotypic characterization and differentiation of human CD8+ T cells producing IL-17. *J Immunol* 182 (4):1794-8.

Kotake, S., N. Udagawa, N. Takahashi, K. Matsuzaki, K. Itoh, S. Ishiyama, S. Saito, K. Inoue, N. Kamatani, M. T. Gillespie, T. J. Martin, and T. Suda. 1999. IL-17 in synovial fluids from patients with rheumatoid arthritis is a potent stimulator of osteoclastogenesis. *J Clin Invest* 103 (9):1345-52.

Kryczek, I., A. T. Bruce, J. E. Gudjonsson, A. Johnston, A. Aphale, L. Vatan, W. Szeliga, Y. Wang, Y. Liu, T. H. Welling, J. T. Elder, and W. Zou. 2008. Induction of IL-17+ T cell trafficking and development by IFN-gamma: mechanism and pathological relevance in psoriasis. *J Immunol* 181 (7):4733-41.

Kurasawa, K., K. Hirose, H. Sano, H. Endo, H. Shinkai, Y. Nawata, K. Takabayashi, and I. Iwamoto. 2000. Increased interleukin-17 production in patients with systemic sclerosis. *Arthritis Rheum* 43 (11):2455-63.

Laan, M., Z. H. Cui, H. Hoshino, J. Lotvall, M. Sjostrand, D. C. Gruenert, B. E. Skoogh, and A. Linden. 1999. Neutrophil recruitment by human IL-17 via C-X-C chemokine release in the airways. *J Immunol* 162 (4):2347-52.

Lamblin, C., P. Gosset, I. Tillie-Leblond, F. Saulnier, C. H. Marquette, B. Wallaert, and A. B. Tonnel. 1998. Bronchial neutrophilia in patients with noninfectious status asthmaticus. *Am J Respir Crit Care Med* 157 (2):394-402.

Lee, J. C., J. D. Christie, and S. Keshavjee. 2010. Primary graft dysfunction: definition, risk factors, short- and long-term outcomes. *Semin Respir Crit Care Med* 31 (2):161-71.

Loong, C. C., H. G. Hsieh, W. Y. Lui, A. Chen, and C. Y. Lin. 2002. Evidence for the early involvement of interleukin 17 in human and experimental renal allograft rejection. *J Pathol* 197 (3):322-32.

Louis, R., L. C. Lau, A. O. Bron, A. C. Roldaan, M. Radermecker, and R. Djukanovic. 2000. The relationship between airways inflammation and asthma severity. *Am J Respir Crit Care Med* 161 (1):9-16.

Ma, C. S., S. Suryani, D. T. Avery, A. Chan, R. Nanan, B. Santner-Nanan, E. K. Deenick, and S. G. Tangye. 2009. Early commitment of naive human CD4(+) T cells to the T follicular helper (T(FH)) cell lineage is induced by IL-12. *Immunol Cell Biol* 87 (8):590-600.

Ma, H. L., S. Liang, J. Li, L. Napierata, T. Brown, S. Benoit, M. Senices, D. Gill, K. Dunussi-Joannopoulos, M. Collins, C. Nickerson-Nutter, L. A. Fouser, and D. A. Young. 2008. IL-22 is required for Th17 cell-mediated pathology in a mouse model of psoriasis-like skin inflammation. *J Clin Invest* 118 (2):597-607.

Maertzdorf, J., A. D. Osterhaus, and G. M. Verjans. 2002. IL-17 expression in human herpetic stromal keratitis: modulatory effects on chemokine production by corneal fibroblasts. *J Immunol* 169 (10):5897-903.

Malley, R., A. Srivastava, M. Lipsitch, C. M. Thompson, C. Watkins, A. Tzianabos, and P. W. Anderson. 2006. Antibody-independent, interleukin-17A-mediated, cross-serotype immunity to pneumococci in mice immunized intranasally with the cell wall polysaccharide. *Infect Immun* 74 (4):2187-95.

Manel, N., D. Unutmaz, and D. R. Littman. 2008. The differentiation of human T(H)-17 cells requires transforming growth factor-beta and induction of the nuclear receptor RORgammat. *Nat Immunol* 9 (6):641-9.

Mantel, P. Y., H. Kuipers, O. Boyman, C. Rhyner, N. Ouaked, B. Ruckert, C. Karagiannidis, B. N. Lambrecht, R. W. Hendriks, R. Crameri, C. A. Akdis, K. Blaser, and C. B. Schmidt-Weber. 2007. GATA3-driven Th2 responses inhibit TGF-beta1-induced FOXP3 expression and the formation of regulatory T cells. *PLoS Biol* 5 (12):e329.

McAllister, F., A. Henry, J. L. Kreindler, P. J. Dubin, L. Ulrich, C. Steele, J. D. Finder, J. M. Pilewski, B. M. Carreno, S. J. Goldman, J. Pirhonen, and J. K. Kolls. 2005. Role of IL-17A, IL-17F, and the IL-17 receptor in regulating growth-related oncogene-alpha and granulocyte colony-stimulating factor in bronchial epithelium: implications for airway inflammation in cystic fibrosis. *J Immunol* 175 (1):404-12.

McDyer, J. F. 2007. Human and murine obliterative bronchiolitis in transplant. *Proc Am Thorac Soc* 4 (1):37-43.

McGeachy, M. J., K. S. Bak-Jensen, Y. Chen, C. M. Tato, W. Blumenschein, T. McClanahan, and D. J. Cua. 2007. TGF-beta and IL-6 drive the production of IL-17 and IL-10 by T cells and restrain T(H)-17 cell-mediated pathology. *Nat Immunol* 8 (12):1390-7.

McKinley, L., J. F. Alcorn, A. Peterson, R. B. Dupont, S. Kapadia, A. Logar, A. Henry, C. G. Irvin, J. D. Piganelli, A. Ray, and J. K. Kolls. 2008. TH17 cells mediate steroid-resistant airway inflammation and airway hyperresponsiveness in mice. *J Immunol* 181 (6):4089-97.

Melgert, B. N., W. Timens, H. A. Kerstjens, M. Geerlings, M. A. Luinge, J. P. Schouten, D. S. Postma, and M. N. Hylkema. 2007. Effects of 4 months of smoking in mice with ovalbumin-induced airway inflammation. *Clin Exp Allergy* 37 (12):1798-808.

Michel, M. L., A. C. Keller, C. Paget, M. Fujio, F. Trottein, P. B. Savage, C. H. Wong, E. Schneider, M. Dy, and M. C. Leite-de-Moraes. 2007. Identification of an IL-17-producing NK1.1(neg) iNKT cell population involved in airway neutrophilia. *J Exp Med* 204 (5):995-1001.

Michel, M. L., D. Mendes-da-Cruz, A. C. Keller, M. Lochner, E. Schneider, M. Dy, G. Eberl, and M. C. Leite-de-Moraes. 2008. Critical role of ROR-gammat in a new thymic pathway leading to IL-17-producing invariant NKT cell differentiation. *Proc Natl Acad Sci U S A* 105 (50):19845-50.

Mills, K. H. 2008. Induction, function and regulation of IL-17-producing T cells. *Eur J Immunol* 38 (10):2636-49.

Milner, J. D., J. M. Brenchley, A. Laurence, A. F. Freeman, B. J. Hill, K. M. Elias, Y. Kanno, C. Spalding, H. Z. Elloumi, M. L. Paulson, J. Davis, A. Hsu, A. I. Asher, J. O'Shea, S. M. Holland, W. E. Paul, and D. C. Douek. 2008. Impaired T(H)17 cell differentiation in subjects with autosomal dominant hyper-IgE syndrome. *Nature* 452 (7188):773-6.

Miossec, P., T. Korn, and V. K. Kuchroo. 2009. Interleukin-17 and type 17 helper T cells. *N Engl J Med* 361 (9):888-98.

Molet, S., Q. Hamid, F. Davoine, E. Nutku, R. Taha, N. Page, R. Olivenstein, J. Elias, and J. Chakir. 2001. IL-17 is increased in asthmatic airways and induces human bronchial fibroblasts to produce cytokines. *J Allergy Clin Immunol* 108 (3):430-8.

Mora, J. R., M. Iwata, and U. H. von Andrian. 2008. Vitamin effects on the immune system: vitamins A and D take centre stage. *Nat Rev Immunol* 8 (9):685-98.

Mosmann, T. R., and R. L. Coffman. 1989. TH1 and TH2 cells: different patterns of lymphokine secretion lead to different functional properties. *Annu Rev Immunol* 7:145-73.

Motz, G. T., B. L. Eppert, S. C. Wesselkamper, J. L. Flury, and M. T. Borchers. 2010. Chronic cigarette smoke exposure generates pathogenic T cells capable of driving COPD-like disease in Rag2-/- mice. *Am J Respir Crit Care Med* 181 (11):1223-33.

Murphy, D. M., I. A. Forrest, P. A. Corris, G. E. Johnson, T. Small, D. Jones, A. J. Fisher, J. J. Egan, T. E. Cawston, C. Ward, and J. L. Lordan. 2008. Simvastatin attenuates release of neutrophilic and remodeling factors from primary bronchial epithelial cells derived from stable lung transplant recipients. *Am J Physiol Lung Cell Mol Physiol* 294 (3):L592-9.

Nadkarni, S., C. Mauri, and M. R. Ehrenstein. 2007. Anti-TNF-alpha therapy induces a distinct regulatory T cell population in patients with rheumatoid arthritis via TGF-beta. *J Exp Med* 204 (1):33-9.

Nakagiri, T., M. Inoue, E. Morii, M. Minami, N. Sawabata, T. Utsumi, Y. Kadota, K. Ideguchi, T. Tokunaga, and M. Okumura. 2010. Local IL-17 production and a decrease in peripheral blood regulatory T cells in an animal model of bronchiolitis obliterans. *Transplantation* 89 (11):1312-9.

Nurieva, R. I., Y. Chung, D. Hwang, X. O. Yang, H. S. Kang, L. Ma, Y. H. Wang, S. S. Watowich, A. M. Jetten, Q. Tian, and C. Dong. 2008. Generation of T follicular helper cells is mediated by interleukin-21 but independent of T helper 1, 2, or 17 cell lineages. *Immunity* 29 (1):138-49.

O'Shea, J. J., and W. E. Paul. 2010. Mechanisms underlying lineage commitment and plasticity of helper CD4+ T cells. *Science* 327 (5969):1098-102.

Ouyang, W., J. K. Kolls, and Y. Zheng. 2008. The biological functions of T helper 17 cell effector cytokines in inflammation. *Immunity* 28 (4):454-67.

Park, H., Z. Li, X. O. Yang, S. H. Chang, R. Nurieva, Y. H. Wang, Y. Wang, L. Hood, Z. Zhu, Q. Tian, and C. Dong. 2005. A distinct lineage of CD4 T cells regulates tissue inflammation by producing interleukin 17. *Nat Immunol* 6 (11):1133-41.

Pene, J., S. Chevalier, L. Preisser, E. Venereau, M. H. Guilleux, S. Ghannam, J. P. Moles, Y. Danger, E. Ravon, S. Lesaux, H. Yssel, and H. Gascan. 2008. Chronically inflamed human tissues are infiltrated by highly differentiated Th17 lymphocytes. *J Immunol* 180 (11):7423-30.

Piccotti, J. R., S. Y. Chan, A. M. VanBuskirk, E. J. Eichwald, and D. K. Bishop. 1997. Are Th2 helper T lymphocytes beneficial, deleterious, or irrelevant in promoting allograft survival? *Transplantation* 63 (5):619-24.

Prause, O., S. Bozinovski, G. P. Anderson, and A. Linden. 2004. Increased matrix metalloproteinase-9 concentration and activity after stimulation with interleukin-17 in mouse airways. *Thorax* 59 (4):313-7.

Rahman, M. S., J. Yang, L. Y. Shan, H. Unruh, X. Yang, A. J. Halayko, and A. S. Gounni. 2005. IL-17R activation of human airway smooth muscle cells induces CXCL-8 production via a transcriptional-dependent mechanism. *Clin Immunol* 115 (3):268-76.

Rao, D. A., K. J. Tracey, and J. S. Pober. 2007. IL-1alpha and IL-1beta are endogenous mediators linking cell injury to the adaptive alloimmune response. *J Immunol* 179 (10):6536-46.

Romani, L., F. Fallarino, A. De Luca, C. Montagnoli, C. D'Angelo, T. Zelante, C. Vacca, F. Bistoni, M. C. Fioretti, U. Grohmann, B. H. Segal, and P. Puccetti. 2008. Defective tryptophan catabolism underlies inflammation in mouse chronic granulomatous disease. *Nature* 451 (7175):211-5.

Rosen, Y. 2007. Pathology of sarcoidosis. *Semin Respir Crit Care Med* 28 (1):36-52.

Rouvier, E., M. F. Luciani, M. G. Mattei, F. Denizot, and P. Golstein. 1993. CTLA-8, cloned from an activated T cell, bearing AU-rich messenger RNA instability sequences, and homologous to a herpesvirus saimiri gene. *J Immunol* 150 (12):5445-56.

Rudner, X. L., K. I. Happel, E. A. Young, and J. E. Shellito. 2007. Interleukin-23 (IL-23)-IL-17 cytokine axis in murine Pneumocystis carinii infection. *Infect Immun* 75 (6):3055-61.

Sallusto, F., C. R. Mackay, and A. Lanzavecchia. 2000. The role of chemokine receptors in primary, effector, and memory immune responses. *Annu Rev Immunol* 18:593-620.

Santarlasci, V., L. Maggi, M. Capone, F. Frosali, V. Querci, R. De Palma, F. Liotta, L. Cosmi, E. Maggi, S. Romagnani, and F. Annunziato. 2009. TGF-beta indirectly favors the development of human Th17 cells by inhibiting Th1 cells. *Eur J Immunol* 39 (1):207-15.

Schnyder-Candrian, S., D. Togbe, I. Couillin, I. Mercier, F. Brombacher, V. Quesniaux, F. Fossiez, B. Ryffel, and B. Schnyder. 2006. Interleukin-17 is a negative regulator of established allergic asthma. *J Exp Med* 203 (12):2715-25.

Schwarzenberger, P., V. La Russa, A. Miller, P. Ye, W. Huang, A. Zieske, S. Nelson, G. J. Bagby, D. Stoltz, R. L. Mynatt, M. Spriggs, and J. K. Kolls. 1998. IL-17 stimulates granulopoiesis in mice: use of an alternate, novel gene therapy-derived method for in vivo evaluation of cytokines. *J Immunol* 161 (11):6383-9.

Seemungal, T. A., T. M. Wilkinson, J. R. Hurst, W. R. Perera, R. J. Sapsford, and J. A. Wedzicha. 2008. Long-term erythromycin therapy is associated with decreased chronic obstructive pulmonary disease exacerbations. *Am J Respir Crit Care Med* 178 (11):1139-47.

Shilling, R. A., and D. S. Wilkes. 2011. Role of Th17 cells and IL-17 in lung transplant rejection. *Semin Immunopathol.*

Simonian, P. L., C. L. Roark, F. Wehrmann, A. K. Lanham, F. Diaz del Valle, W. K. Born, R. L. O'Brien, and A. P. Fontenot. 2009. Th17-polarized immune response in a murine model of hypersensitivity pneumonitis and lung fibrosis. *J Immunol* 182 (1):657-65.

Snell, G. I., B. J. Levvey, L. Zheng, M. Bailey, B. Orsida, T. J. Williams, and T. C. Kotsimbos. 2007. Interleukin-17 and airway inflammation: a longitudinal airway biopsy study after lung transplantation. *J Heart Lung Transplant* 26 (7):669-74.

Song, C., L. Luo, Z. Lei, B. Li, Z. Liang, G. Liu, D. Li, G. Zhang, B. Huang, and Z. H. Feng. 2008. IL-17-producing alveolar macrophages mediate allergic lung inflammation related to asthma. *J Immunol* 181 (9):6117-24.

Spits, H., and J. P. Di Santo. 2011. The expanding family of innate lymphoid cells: regulators and effectors of immunity and tissue remodeling. *Nat Immunol* 12 (1):21-7.

Sullivan, A. K., P. L. Simonian, M. T. Falta, J. D. Mitchell, G. P. Cosgrove, K. K. Brown, B. L. Kotzin, N. F. Voelkel, and A. P. Fontenot. 2005. Oligoclonal CD4+ T cells in the lungs of patients with severe emphysema. *Am J Respir Crit Care Med* 172 (5):590-6.

Sutton, C. E., S. J. Lalor, C. M. Sweeney, C. F. Brereton, E. C. Lavelle, and K. H. Mills. 2009. Interleukin-1 and IL-23 induce innate IL-17 production from gammadelta T cells, amplifying Th17 responses and autoimmunity. *Immunity* 31 (2):331-41.

Szabo, S. J., S. T. Kim, G. L. Costa, X. Zhang, C. G. Fathman, and L. H. Glimcher. 2000. A novel transcription factor, T-bet, directs Th1 lineage commitment. *Cell* 100 (6):655-69.

Tan, H. L., N. Regamey, S. Brown, A. Bush, C. M. Lloyd, and J. C. Davies. 2011. The th17 pathway in cystic fibrosis lung disease. *Am J Respir Crit Care Med* 184 (2):252-8.

ten Berge, B., M.S. Paats, I. Bergen, B. van den Blink, H. C. Hoogsteden, B. N. Lambrecht, R. W. Hendriks, and A. KleinJan. 2011. Increased IL-17A expression in granulomas and in circulating memory T cells in sarcoidosis. *Rheumatology* in press.

Tesmer, L. A., S. K. Lundy, S. Sarkar, and D. A. Fox. 2008. Th17 cells in human disease. *Immunol Rev* 223:87-113.

Trifari, S., C. D. Kaplan, E. H. Tran, N. K. Crellin, and H. Spits. 2009. Identification of a human helper T cell population that has abundant production of interleukin 22 and is distinct from T(H)-17, T(H)1 and T(H)2 cells. *Nat Immunol* 10 (8):864-71.

Turato, G., R. Zuin, M. Miniati, S. Baraldo, F. Rea, B. Beghe, S. Monti, B. Formichi, P. Boschetto, S. Harari, A. Papi, P. Maestrelli, L. M. Fabbri, and M. Saetta. 2002. Airway inflammation in severe chronic obstructive pulmonary disease: relationship with lung function and radiologic emphysema. *Am J Respir Crit Care Med* 166 (1):105-10.

Vaknin-Dembinsky, A., K. Balashov, and H. L. Weiner. 2006. IL-23 is increased in dendritic cells in multiple sclerosis and down-regulation of IL-23 by antisense oligos increases dendritic cell IL-10 production. *J Immunol* 176 (12):7768-74.

Valentine, V. G., M. R. Gupta, J. E. Walker, Jr., L. Seoane, R. W. Bonvillain, G. A. Lombard, D. Weill, and G. S. Dhillon. 2009. Effect of etiology and timing of respiratory tract infections on development of bronchiolitis obliterans syndrome. *J Heart Lung Transplant* 28 (2):163-9.

Van Kooten, C., J. G. Boonstra, M. E. Paape, F. Fossiez, J. Banchereau, S. Lebecque, J. A. Bruijn, J. W. De Fijter, L. A. Van Es, and M. R. Daha. 1998. Interleukin-17 activates human renal epithelial cells in vitro and is expressed during renal allograft rejection. *J Am Soc Nephrol* 9 (8):1526-34.

Vanaudenaerde, B. M., S. I. De Vleeschauwer, R. Vos, I. Meyts, D. M. Bullens, V. Reynders, W. A. Wuyts, D. E. Van Raemdonck, L. J. Dupont, and G. M. Verleden. 2008. The role of the IL23/IL17 axis in bronchiolitis obliterans syndrome after lung transplantation. *Am J Transplant* 8 (9):1911-20.

Vanaudenaerde, B. M., L. J. Dupont, W. A. Wuyts, E. K. Verbeken, I. Meyts, D. M. Bullens, E. Dilissen, L. Luyts, D. E. Van Raemdonck, and G. M. Verleden. 2006. The role of interleukin-17 during acute rejection after lung transplantation. *Eur Respir J* 27 (4):779-87.

Vanaudenaerde, B. M., S. E. Verleden, R. Vos, S. I. Vleeschauwer, A. Willems-Widyastuti, R. Geenens, D. E. Raemdonck, L. J. Dupont, E. K. Verbeken, and I. Meyts. 2011. Innate and Adaptive Interleukin-17-producing Lymphocytes in Chronic Inflammatory Lung Disorders. *Am J Respir Crit Care Med* 183 (8):977-86.

Vanaudenaerde, B. M., W. A. Wuyts, N. Geudens, T. S. Nawrot, R. Vos, L. J. Dupont, D. E. Van Raemdonck, and G. M. Verleden. 2008. Broncho-alveolar lavage fluid recovery correlates with airway neutrophilia in lung transplant patients. *Respir Med* 102 (3):339-47.

Veldhoen, M., R. J. Hocking, C. J. Atkins, R. M. Locksley, and B. Stockinger. 2006. TGFbeta in the context of an inflammatory cytokine milieu supports de novo differentiation of IL-17-producing T cells. *Immunity* 24 (2):179-89.

Vogelzang, A., H. M. McGuire, D. Yu, J. Sprent, C. R. Mackay, and C. King. 2008. A fundamental role for interleukin-21 in the generation of T follicular helper cells. *Immunity* 29 (1):127-37.

Volpe, E., N. Servant, R. Zollinger, S. I. Bogiatzi, P. Hupe, E. Barillot, and V. Soumelis. 2008. A critical function for transforming growth factor-beta, interleukin 23 and proinflammatory cytokines in driving and modulating human T(H)-17 responses. *Nat Immunol* 9 (6):650-7.

Wang, Y. H., K. S. Voo, B. Liu, C. Y. Chen, B. Uygungil, W. Spoede, J. A. Bernstein, D. P. Huston, and Y. J. Liu. 2010. A novel subset of CD4(+) T(H)2 memory/effector cells that produce inflammatory IL-17 cytokine and promote the exacerbation of chronic allergic asthma. *J Exp Med* 207 (11):2479-91.

Weaver, C. T., and R. D. Hatton. 2009. Interplay between the TH17 and TReg cell lineages: a (co-)evolutionary perspective. *Nat Rev Immunol* 9 (12):883-9.

Weaver, C. T., R. D. Hatton, P. R. Mangan, and L. E. Harrington. 2007. IL-17 family cytokines and the expanding diversity of effector T cell lineages. *Annu Rev Immunol* 25:821-52.

Wiehler, S., and D. Proud. 2007. Interleukin-17A modulates human airway epithelial responses to human rhinovirus infection. *Am J Physiol Lung Cell Mol Physiol* 293 (2):L505-15.

Wills-Karp, M., J. Luyimbazi, X. Xu, B. Schofield, T. Y. Neben, C. L. Karp, and D. D. Donaldson. 1998. Interleukin-13: central mediator of allergic asthma. *Science* 282 (5397):2258-61.

Wilson, M. S., S. K. Madala, T. R. Ramalingam, B. R. Gochuico, I. O. Rosas, A. W. Cheever, and T. A. Wynn. 2010. Bleomycin and IL-1beta-mediated pulmonary fibrosis is IL-17A dependent. *J Exp Med* 207 (3):535-52.

Wilson, N. J., K. Boniface, J. R. Chan, B. S. McKenzie, W. M. Blumenschein, J. D. Mattson, B. Basham, K. Smith, T. Chen, F. Morel, J. C. Lecron, R. A. Kastelein, D. J. Cua, T. K.

McClanahan, E. P. Bowman, and R. de Waal Malefyt. 2007. Development, cytokine profile and function of human interleukin 17-producing helper T cells. *Nat Immunol* 8 (9):950-7.

Wolff, A. J., and A. E. O'Donnell. 2003. HIV-related pulmonary infections: a review of the recent literature. *Curr Opin Pulm Med* 9 (3):210-4.

Wu, Q., R. J. Martin, J. G. Rino, R. Breed, R. M. Torres, and H. W. Chu. 2007. IL-23-dependent IL-17 production is essential in neutrophil recruitment and activity in mouse lung defense against respiratory Mycoplasma pneumoniae infection. *Microbes Infect* 9 (1):78-86.

Yang, L., D. E. Anderson, C. Baecher-Allan, W. D. Hastings, E. Bettelli, M. Oukka, V. K. Kuchroo, and D. A. Hafler. 2008. IL-21 and TGF-beta are required for differentiation of human T(H)17 cells. *Nature* 454 (7202):350-2.

Yang, X. O., S. H. Chang, H. Park, R. Nurieva, B. Shah, L. Acero, Y. H. Wang, K. S. Schluns, R. R. Broaddus, Z. Zhu, and C. Dong. 2008. Regulation of inflammatory responses by IL-17F. *J Exp Med* 205 (5):1063-75.

Yao, C., D. Sakata, Y. Esaki, Y. Li, T. Matsuoka, K. Kuroiwa, Y. Sugimoto, and S. Narumiya. 2009. Prostaglandin E2-EP4 signaling promotes immune inflammation through Th1 cell differentiation and Th17 cell expansion. *Nat Med* 15 (6):633-40.

Yao, Z., W. C. Fanslow, M. F. Seldin, A. M. Rousseau, S. L. Painter, M. R. Comeau, J. I. Cohen, and M. K. Spriggs. 1995. Herpesvirus Saimiri encodes a new cytokine, IL-17, which binds to a novel cytokine receptor. *Immunity* 3 (6):811-21.

Ye, P., F. H. Rodriguez, S. Kanaly, K. L. Stocking, J. Schurr, P. Schwarzenberger, P. Oliver, W. Huang, P. Zhang, J. Zhang, J. E. Shellito, G. J. Bagby, S. Nelson, K. Charrier, J. J. Peschon, and J. K. Kolls. 2001. Requirement of interleukin 17 receptor signaling for lung CXC chemokine and granulocyte colony-stimulating factor expression, neutrophil recruitment, and host defense. *J Exp Med* 194 (4):519-27.

Yokota, S., T. Miyamae, T. Imagawa, N. Iwata, S. Katakura, M. Mori, P. Woo, N. Nishimoto, K. Yoshizaki, and T. Kishimoto. 2005. Therapeutic efficacy of humanized recombinant anti-interleukin-6 receptor antibody in children with systemic-onset juvenile idiopathic arthritis. *Arthritis Rheum* 52 (3):818-25.

Yoshida, S., A. Haque, T. Mizobuchi, T. Iwata, M. Chiyo, T. J. Webb, L. A. Baldridge, K. M. Heidler, O. W. Cummings, T. Fujisawa, J. S. Blum, D. D. Brand, and D. S. Wilkes. 2006. Anti-type V collagen lymphocytes that express IL-17 and IL-23 induce rejection pathology in fresh and well-healed lung transplants. *Am J Transplant* 6 (4):724-35.

Young, D. A., M. Hegen, H. L. Ma, M. J. Whitters, L. M. Albert, L. Lowe, M. Senices, P. W. Wu, B. Sibley, Y. Leathurby, T. P. Brown, C. Nickerson-Nutter, J. C. Keith, Jr., and M. Collins. 2007. Blockade of the interleukin-21/interleukin-21 receptor pathway ameliorates disease in animal models of rheumatoid arthritis. *Arthritis Rheum* 56 (4):1152-63.

Yusuf, I., R. Kageyama, L. Monticelli, R. J. Johnston, D. Ditoro, K. Hansen, B. Barnett, and S. Crotty. 2010. Germinal center T follicular helper cell IL-4 production is dependent on signaling lymphocytic activation molecule receptor (CD150). *J Immunol* 185 (1):190-202.

Zaba, L. C., G. P. Smith, M. Sanchez, and S. D. Prystowsky. 2010. Dendritic cells in the pathogenesis of sarcoidosis. *Am J Respir Cell Mol Biol* 42 (1):32-9.

Zheng, W., and R. A. Flavell. 1997. The transcription factor GATA-3 is necessary and sufficient for Th2 cytokine gene expression in CD4 T cells. *Cell* 89 (4):587-96.

Zheng, Y., P. A. Valdez, D. M. Danilenko, Y. Hu, S. M. Sa, Q. Gong, A. R. Abbas, Z. Modrusan, N. Ghilardi, F. J. de Sauvage, and W. Ouyang. 2008. Interleukin-22 mediates early host defense against attaching and effacing bacterial pathogens. *Nat Med* 14 (3):282-9.

15

Current Status of the Mollicute (Mycoplasma) Lung Disease: Pathogenesis, Diagnostics, Treatment and Prevention

Silvia Giono-Cerezo[1,*], Guadalupe Estrada-Gutiérrez[2], José Antonio Rivera-Tapia[3], Jorge Antonio Yáñez-Santos[3] and Francisco Javier Díaz-García[4]

[1]*Departamento de Microbiología, Escuela Nacional de Ciencias Biológicas, IPN*
[2]*Departamento de Infectología, Instituto Nacional de Perinatología, México, D.F.,*
[3]*Benemérita Universidad Autónoma de Puebla, Puebla, México*
[4]*Departamento de Salud Pública, Facultad de Medicina, UNAM*
México

1. Introduction

The microorganisms referred as mycoplasmas ("mushroom form") are eubacteria included within the Class Mollicutes (from latin *mollis* ="soft", *cutis*= "skin"), which comprises the smallest self-replicating bacteria, showing distinctive features such as: a) lack of a rigid cell wall envelope, b) sterol incorporation into their own plasma membrane, and c) Reduced cellular (0.3 - 0.8 μm diameter) and genome sizes (0.58-2.20 Mb). Some genera use the UGA stop codon to encode tryptophan [Bove, 1993; Razin et al., 1998].

The term "mycoplasmas" will be used herein when referring to any species within the Class *Mollicutes*. Due to their reduced genome sizes, the mycoplasmas exhibit restricted metabolic and physiological pathways for replication and survival [Razin et al., 1998]. This makes evident why these bacteria display strict dependence to their hosts for acquisition of aminoacids, nucleotides, lipids and sterols as biosynthetic precursors. [Baseman & Tully, 1997; Razin et al., 1998].

Recognized human pathogenic mycoplasma species mostly belongs to the *Mycoplasma* and *Ureaplasma* genera (Table 1). Acute or fulminant diseases are rarely caused by these bacteria, instead they produce subclinical or covert infections that become chronic and/or persistent [Baseman & Tully, 1997; Razin et al., 1998]. Cell surface colonization and in some cases subsequent invasion and intracellular residence have been well documented for several *Mycoplasma* species which infect humans [Andreev et al., 1995; Baseman et al., 1995; Díaz-García et al., 2006; Giron et al., 1996; Jensen et al., 1994; Lo et al., 1993; Taylor-Robinson et al., 1991].

The primary habitats of the mycoplasmas infecting humans are the mucosal surfaces of the respiratory and genitourinary tracts [Cassell et al., 1994a; Taylor-Robinson, 1996]. Moreover,

* Corresponding Author

the mycoplasmas display host- and tissue-specific tropism, reflecting their nutritional demands and parasitic lifestyle [Razin et al., 1998]. Thus, *M. pneumoniae* is found principally in the respiratory tract, whereas *M. genitalium, Ureaplasma spp., M. hominis, M. fermentans* and *M. penetrans* are primarily urogenital residents, but exceptionally they can be isolated from other unusual tissues and organs, especially in immunocompromised patients or in patients undergoing solid organ transplantation [Waites & Talkington, 2004; Waites et al., 2005; Waites, 2008].

Mycoplasmal respiratory infections in humans can be ascribed mainly to *M. pneumoniae* and, in fetuses or newborns, to *Ureaplasma* species. *M. pneumoniae* is a well-known pathogen in atypical and community-acquired pneumonia, whereas *U. urealyticum* and *U. parvum* have been associated with vertically-transmitted intrauterine and neonatal pneumonia [Taylor-Robinson, 1996; Waites et al., 2005].

Species	Primary colonization sites		Substrate utilization		
	Oropharyngeal tract	Urogenital tract	Glucose	Arginine	Urea
Mycoplasma fermentans	✓	✓	✓	✓	×
M. genitalium	✓	✓	✓	×	×
M. hominis	✓	✓	×	✓	×
M. penetrans	×	✓	✓	✓	×
M. pneumoniae	✓	×	✓	×	×
Ureaplasma parvum	✓	✓	×	×	✓
U. urealyticum	✓	✓	×	×	✓

✓ Present; × Absent
Modified from Taylor-Robinson, 1996.

Table 1. Mycoplasma species pathogenic for humans.

A worldwide rise in the frequency of *M. pneumoniae*-associated lower respiratory tract disease has been observed, from 6 - >30% in the 1990s, to 0 - 66.7% in 2010 [Reviewed by Loens et al., 2003, 2010]. Therefore the pathogenic role of *M. pneumoniae* in respiratory disease has been proved in persons of all ages, sometimes causing severe respiratory disease, and it may induce clinically significant manifestations in extrapulmonary sites by direct invasion and/or immunologic effects. Only in the USA, *M. pneumoniae* is responsible for more than 100,000 hospitalizations of adults each year [Waites & Talkington, 2004; Waites, 2008]. This close interplay between *M. pneumoniae* and the host's respiratory epithelium induces local damage and in turn elicits release of inflammatory mediators by the host. The magnitude of the later response appears to be related to the severity of disease [Waites, 2008].

Respiratory tract colonization with *Ureaplasma* spp., and rarely with *M. hominis,* in preterm infants has been associated with higher incidence of pneumonia, severe respiratory failure, bronchopulmonary dysplasia, and ultimately with death [Viscardi et al., 2002]. These bacteria can be transmitted from infected females to their fetus or newborn by three main different routes: a) Ascending intrauterine infection from vaginal colonization; b) Hematogenous spreading from placental infection, and c) Acquisition of the microorganism by the neonate during passage through an infected maternal birth canal. [Viscardi et al., 2002; Waites et al., 2005]. An inverse correlation between ureaplasmal vertical transmission rate and gestational age has been established, and this increases with duration of premature rupture of membranes. Improved molecular detection of colonizing *Ureaplasma* in respiratory tract specimens suggests a higher frequency of colonization in very low birth weight infants than that previously reported with culture-based studies (25–48% vs. 20%) [Viscardi & Hasday, 2009].

Infrequently, *M. fermentans* has been detected in adults who developed respiratory distress syndrome and/or from bronchoalveolar lavage in AIDS patients with pneumonia, highlighting the potential of this species to cause lower respiratory tract disease in susceptible hosts [Waites &Talkington, 2004].

2. Taxonomic characterization of Mollicutes

Modern mycoplasmal taxonomy relies on combined data from phenotypic traits and phylogeny based on the 16S rRNA gene sequences [Brown et al., 2007; International Committee on Systematics of Prokaryotes- Subcommittee on the taxonomy of Mollicutes (ICSP-STM), 2010]. Among the phenotypic characteristics, there are few useful metabolic markers including the ability to ferment glucose, the ability to hydrolyze urea and arginine, and dependence on cholesterol for growth and anaerobiosis. Despite the high rate of surface antigenic variation, serologic relatedness at the species level is still used in routine identification of mycoplasmas [Brown et al., 2007; ICSP-STM, 2010; Razin et al., 1998]. There are currently more than 200 species allocated into four orders, five families and eight genera within the class *Mollicutes* (Figure1), including the undefined *candidatus Phytoplasma* [Brown et al., 2007; ICSP-STM, 2010].

2.1 Phylogeny, genome content and molecular analysis

The Mollicutes 16S rRNA-based phylogenetic tree is monophyletic arising from a single branch of the *Clostridium ramosum* branch. The Mollicutes split into two major branches: the AAP branch, containing the *Acholeplasma*, *Anaeroplasma* and *Asteroleplasma* genera, and the *Candidatus Phytoplasma* phyla; the other is the SEM branch that includes the *Spiroplasma*, *Entomoplasma*, *Mesoplasma*, *Ureaplasma* and *Mycoplasma* genera [Johansson et al., 1998; Maniloff 1992; Razin et al., 1998). Interestingly, the genus *Mycoplasma* is polyphyletic, with species clustering within the Spiroplasma, Pneumoniae and Hominis phylogenetic groups [Behbahani et al., 1993; Johansson et al., 1998, Maniloff 1992]. Nevertheless, additional phylogenetic markers such as the elongation factor EF-Tu (*tuf*) gene, ribosomal protein genes, the 16S/23S rRNA intergenic sequences, etc, have been already used as complementary comparative data, thus there is no unique phylogenetic tree for *Mollicutes* [Razin et al., 1998].

The mycoplasmas may have evolved through regressive evolution from closely related Gram positive bacteria with low content of guanine plus cytosine (G+C), probably the Clostridia or *Erysipelothrix* [Bove, 1993; Brown et al., 2007; Razin et al., 1998]. The massive gene losses (i.e. genes involved in cell wall and aminoacid biosynthesis) had left mycoplasmas with a coding repertoire of 500 to 2000 genes [Sirand-Pugnet et al., 2007]. The G+C content in DNA of mycoplasmas varies from 23 to 40 mol%, while genome size range is 580–2200 Kbp, much smaller than those of most walled bacteria [Razin et al., 1998].

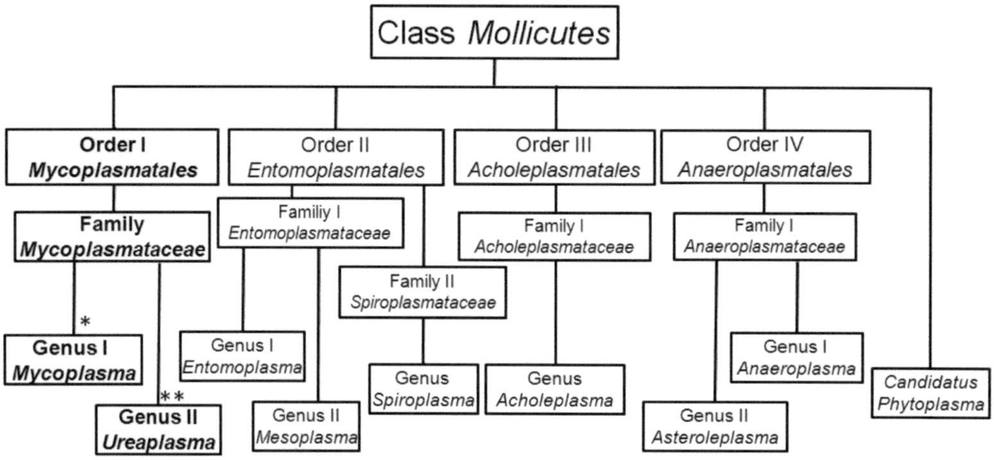

* Includes more than one hundred species. At present five species are recognized human pathogens.
** Includes seven species, two of them are pathogenic for humans.
Adapted from: Razin et al, 1998.

Fig. 1. Taxonomy of Class Mollicutes.

From a comparative analysis of the complete genome sequences from 17 mycoplasma species, Sirand-Pugnet et al., 2007, identified 729 clusters of orthologous groups of proteins (COGs) that represent 21 categories of diverse cellular functions. This analysis revealed that mycoplasmas shared a limited core genome (i.e. the essential translation machinery), while there is a wide diversity of COGs that are only found in one or a few species. Moreover, frequent chromosomal rearrangements occurring at specific loci involved in expression of surface proteins were also identified [Momynaliev & Govorun, 2001; Sirand-Pugnet et al., 2007].

3. Immune response

Host defense in respiratory mycoplasmosis is dependent on both innate and humoral immunity. In general terms, mycoplasmas reaching the lower respiratory tract may be opsonized by antibody and complement, and then activated macrophages begin phagocytosis and migration to the site of infection by chemotaxis. Finally, complement-mediated cytolysis may then play a role in limiting the growth of the mycoplasmas. However, immunity against mycoplasmal infection is typically short-lived, hence infection recurrence is common (Waites et al., 2007, 2008).

3.1 Innate and adaptive immune response

M. pneumoniae infection is able to activate the host innate immune system, so the inflammatory event elicited by accounts for the early signs and symptoms of the infection. After become opsonized, *M. pneumoniae* is susceptible to complement-mediated cytolysis, probably through both the alternative and classical pathways [Waites et al., 2007]. It has been suggested that innate immune recognition of *M. pneumoniae* has also a pivotal role for mucin expression in the airway, at both mRNA and protein levels, since blockage of the toll-like receptor (TLR)-2 signaling pathway results in marked reduction of mucin expression [Chu et al., 2005]. Moreover, *M. pneumoniae* is capable of interact with mast cells and surfactant protein (SP)-A, resulting in cytokine production and bacterial growth inhibition, respectively [Waites et al, 2007].

After primary encounter with *M. pneumoniae*, the immune system of an immunocompetent host responds by rapidly producing antibodies (mainly directed against the P1 adhesin and glycolipid antigens) that peak after 3 to 6 weeks, followed by a gradual decline over months to years [Waites & Talkington, 2004]. The onset of symptoms may coincide with demonstrable antibody titers due to prolonged incubation period. Acute infection can often be difficult observed by evidence of rising *M. pneumoniae*-specific IgM antibodies, especially in pediatric populations. [Waites, 2007, 2008]. IgA antibodies are produced early in the course of disease, rise quickly to peak levels, and decrease earlier than IgM or IgG [Waites & Talkington, 2004].

Adaptive immunity, characterized by both B and T lymphocyte responses, has a major impact on the progression of *M. pneumoniae* respiratory disease. Mycoplasmas activate the immune system by inducing non-specific proliferation of B- and T-lymphocyte populations (mitogenic stimulation), thereby inducing autoimmune responses with concurrent production of cytokines (Table 2). Immune responses that develop after infection often fail

Organism	Cells / Experimental system	Cytokine(s) released
M. pneumoniae	• Lung Alveolar type II pneumocytes	Interleukin (IL)-1β, tumour necrosis factor (TNF)-α, IL-8.
	• Nasal epithelial cells/peripheral blood macrophages	IL-2, IL-6, RANTES, intercellular adhesion molecule (ICAM)-1, transforming growth factor (TGF)-β1 and TNF-α
	• Peripheral blood mononuclear cells	IL-1β, IL-2/IL-2R, IL-6, Interferon (IF)-γ, and TNF-α.
	• Lung ephitelial carcinoma A549 cells	IL-1β, IL-8, and TNF-α.
	• *M. pneumoniae*-infected patients	IL-2/IL-2R, IL-4, IL-5, IL-6, IL-8, IL-12, IL-18, IF-γ, and TNF-α.
Ureaplasma spp.	• Neonatal fibroblasts	IL-6 and IL-8.
	• Peripheral blood/Cord blood monocytes	TNF-α, IL-8, IL-6, and IL-10.
	• THP-1-derived macrophages / Human lung fibroblasts	TNF-α, IL-6, ICAM-1, and vascular endothelial growth factor (VEGF).
	• THP-1 monocytes	IL-1α, TNF-α, and IL-8.

Data from Dakhama et al., 2003; Kazachkov et al., 2002; Li et al., 2000a; Manimtim et al., 2001; Peltier et al., 2008 ; Stancombe et al., 1993; Yang et al, 2004.

Table 2. Mycoplasma-induced cytokine secretion.

to eliminate the mycoplasma, indicating that adaptive immunity apparently has a limited effect on clearance of an established infection, thus leading to asymptomatic carriage for variable periods of time. Cytokine production and lymphocyte activation may either minimize disease through the enhancement of host defense mechanisms and subsequent elimination of the infecting organisms, or exacerbate disease through the development of immunologic hypersensitivity [Waites et al, 2007, 2008]. It has been suggested that there is no correlation between severity of pneumonia caused by *M. pneumoniae* and T-cell deficiencies, thus cell-mediated defense against respiratory mycoplasmosis appears to be rather limited [Cartner et al, 1998].

Molecular mimicry, survival within cells and phenotypic plasticity (antigenic variation) are the major mechanisms by which mycoplasmas evade the immune response [Chambaud et al, 1999; Razin et al., 1998; Rottem & Naot, 1998]. Furthermore, a transient impairment of T-lymphocyte function, or depletion of CD4+ T cells, can be induced by *M. pneumoniae* [Waites et al., 2007].

In the context of perinatal pneumonia, very low birth weight infants have relative deficiencies in mucosal barrier function and in both the innate and adaptive immune responses. These immature hosts may generate poor immune responses, including secretory IgA, serum complement components, defensins, fibronectin, and altered cytokine production. Impaired chemotaxis, phagocytosis, and microbial killing by neonatal immune cells highlight the vulnerability of preterm neonates to systemic infections, and partially explain the eventual systemic spread of bacteria [Waites et al., 2005].

3.2 Cell culture models

Mycoplasmas possess an impressive capability of maintaining a dynamic surface architecture that is antigenically and functionally versatile, contributing to their capability to adapt to a large range of habitats and cause diseases that are often chronic in nature [Rottem, 2003]. The probable role of mycoplasmas in chronic respiratory diseases has been studied *in vitro* using diverse cell culture models. Several of these models are focusing in the study of adherence, invasion and fusion as the strategies to induce damage to the host cells [Baseman et al., 1995; Razin, 1999; Rottem, 2003].

M. pneumoniae is the most extensively studied system with respect to adhesions and receptors [Rottem, 2003] because of its significance as pathogen for humans. Models in human lung cells analyzed by inmunofluorescence and confocal microscopy reveal that *M. pneumoniae* parasitize cells surface, enter the intracellular spaces and locate throughout the cytoplasmic and perinuclear regions within 2 hr postinfection [Baseman et al., 1995]. The microorganism can survive within the host cells for prolonged periods of time, well protected from the immune system and from de action of many antibiotics and may explain its pathogenic potential [Yavlovich et al., 2004]. Another *in vitro* studies show that this microorganism has a polar, tapered cell extension at one of the poles containing an electron-dense core in the cytoplasma. This structure, termed the tip organelle, functions both as an attachment organelle and as the leading end in gliding motility [Baseman et al., 1995; Razin, 1999; Rottem, 2003; Svenstrup et al., 2002]. Host-pathogen studies in an air-liquid culture of differentiated human airway epithelial cells revealed that the microorganism bounds initially to ciliated epithelial cells, but colonization become more evently distributed over the entire surface with time [Krunkosky et al., 2007]. We recently studied the adherence of *U. urealyticum* to a respiratory epithelial cell line, as a virulence factor for lung disease. We describe that *U. urealyticum* induce changes in cell morphology mediated probably by the loss of microvilli, and that the microorganism invades the cell forming vacuoles [Torres-Morquecho et al., 2010].

Since chronic lung disease is characterized by an early increased number of activated neutrophils and alveolar macrophages, with later architectural epithelial and endothelial cell damage [Li et al., 2002], all of these cells represent excellent targets for the study of mycoplasmal infections. As the key processes occurring in all respiratory diseases are the exacerbation of lung inflammation and injury, most of the *in vitro* models have been developed to study the inflammatory response mediated primarily by cytokines.

Different studies have demonstrated that the release of Interleukin (IL)-2, IL-6 RANTES, ICAM-1, TGF-β1 and TNF-α by human nasal epithelial cells and peripheral monocytes infected with *M. pneumoniae* could be implicated in the asthma exacerbation in children and may play a role in the pathogenesis of chronic asthma [Dakhama et al., 2003; Kazachkov et al., 2002; Krunkosky et al., 2007]. Additionally, it has been recently demonstrated that *M. pneumoniae* infection induces reactive oxygen species and DNA damage in human lung cells [Sun et al., 2008].

A number of studies show that *Ureaplasma urealyticum* induce the production of TNF-α, IL-8, IL-6 [Li et al., 2000a; Manimtim et al., 2001; Peltier et al., 2008], NF-κB and nitric oxide [Li et al., 2000b] by human macrophages and monocytes. Infection assays in macrophages performed in combination with LPS showed that *U. urealyticum* enhances the proinflammatory response to a second infection by blocking expression of counterregulatory cytokines (IL-6 and IL-10), predisposing the preterm infant to prolonged and dysregulated inflammation, lung injury, and impaired clearance of secondary infections [Manimtim et al., 2001]. Furthermore, *U. urealyticum* stimulates macrophages to produce vascular endothelial grow factor (VEGF) and intercellular adhesion molecule-1 (ICAM-1) *in vitro*, which are potentially associated with both early and later pathological changes in the lung during the development of chronic lung disease [Li et al., 2002a]. The same raise in proinflammatory cytokine release is observed when *U. urealyticum* interacts with neonatal pulmonary fibroblast [Stancombe et al., 1993], suggesting a role in the development of bronchopulmonary dysplasia. Finally, it has been demonstrated that *U. urealyticum* induces apoptosis in human lung epithelial cells and macrophages [Li et al., 2002b], involving in impairing lung structure observed in chronic lung disease.

4. Lung disease in humans

4.1 *Mycoplasma pneumoniae*

Respiratory infections due to *M. pneumoniae* can affect either the upper or the lower tract, or both simultaneously. This pathogen is responsible for up to 40% of cases of community-acquired pneumonia [Atkinson, et al., 2008]. Nearly 50% of the *M. pneumoniae*-infected patients show non-specific signs and symptoms, often similar to those produced by other respiratory pathogens such as *Chlamydophila pneumoniae, Streptococcus pneumoniae* and some viruses, and although these infections are usually mild or asymptomatic, they are not always self-limiting [Waites & Talkington, 2004; Waites et al., 2008].

Symptomatic disease emerges gradually within few days post-infection and persists for several weeks or months. Upper respiratory tract symptoms include sore throat, fever, cough, headache, coryza, myalgias, chills, earache and malaise. Clinical manifestations of lower respiratory tract infections generally include: non-productive cough which later turns productive with non-hemorrhagic sputum, dyspnoea, adenopathy, wheezing and, rarely, respiratory failure [Waites & Talkington, 2004; Waites et al., 2008].

4.1.1 Pathogenesis

Occurrence of airway disease initiates from the close interplay between the microorganism and the mucosal epithelium as a result of cytadherence, the main virulence factor of the bacterium, which is mediated through a polarized tip attachment organelle. This tip structure comprise the main protein adhesin, named P1, along with several other adhesins and accessory proteins (High Molecular Weight [HMW]-1, HMW-2, HMW-3, Protein [P]-90, P-40 and P-30) [Waites et al., 2008].

Unlike other bacterial lung pathogens (*S. pneumoniae, Pseudomonas aeruginosa* and *Haemophilus influenzae*) which bind specifically to glycolipids containing unsubstituted GalNAcβ1-4Gal residues, *M pneumoniae* attaches to host cells either through a sialic acid-free glycoprotein or sulfated glycolipids containing terminal Gal($3SO_4$)_1 residues. It is worthy to note that the apical microvillar border and cilia of the epithelium express the sialoglycoconjugate-type receptors, thus allowing the selective attachment of *M. pneumoniae* to the ciliated cells [Krivan et al., 1988, 1989; Roberts, D.D. et al, 1989; Olson & Gilbert, 1993; Rottem & Naot, 1998].

Cytadhered *M. pneumoniae* is able to cause damage through generation of reactive oxygen species (ROS), which act in concert with host's endogenous ROS to induce oxidative stress. Bacteria-derived superoxide anions act to inhibit catalase in host cells, thereby reducing the enzymatic breakdown of peroxides, rendering the host cell more susceptible to oxidative damage [Rottem & Naot, 1998; Waites et al., 2004]. Mycoplasmal species exert primarily deleterious effects on the host respiratory epithelium, such as ciliostasis and apoptosis, resulting in localized damage and an immune response which, although often robust, is poorly efficacious in terms of clearing the organism or preventing subsequent reinfections [Waites et al., 2004].

Recently, a *M. pneumoniae* protein homolog to the pertussis toxin S1 subunit was identified and it showed specific binding to surfactant protein A [Kannan et al., 2005] This protein also showed protein:ADPribosyltransferase activity, inducing vacuolation and ciliostasis in cultured host cells. This immunodominant protein has been named as community-acquired respiratory distress syndrome toxin (CARDS TX). Host-cell targets for CARDS TX remain unidentified at present, as does how the toxin's function might relate to its specific binding to surfactant protein A [Kannann & Baseman, 2006; Waites et al., 2004, 2008].

Cytopathic effects observed in *M. pneumoniae*-infected host cells include loss of ciliated epithelia, cell vacuolation, reduced oxygen consumption, reduced glucose utilization, diminished amino acid uptake and macromolecular synthesis, ultimately leading to exfoliation. Clinically, the above mentioned events in the lung tissues are noticeable by the persistent hacking cough [Waites et al., 2004, 2008].

Some clinical characteristics of *M. pneumoniae* infections are consistent with an intracellular location of the pathogen, mainly the establishment of latent or chronic infections, limited efficacy of some antimicrobials, necessity for prolonged treatment to eradicate infection in some instances and circumvention of the host immune response [Waites & Talkington, 2004]

4.1.2 Role in COPD and asthma

Chronic obstructive pulmonary disease (COPD) is an inflammatory disorder of the lungs that leads to blockage of the airways which eventually interferes with the exchange of oxygen and carbon dioxide, making breathing progressively more difficult. It is mainly associated with long-term smoking, but presence of persistent bacterial infections has been related to the etiology, pathogenesis and clinical course of COPD [Blasi, 2004; Sethi, 2000].

Well-known bacterial pathogens such as *Streptococcus pneumoniae, Haemophilus influenzae,* and *Moraxella catarrhalis* have been associated with acute exacerbations in COPD and asthma. [Guilbert & Denlinger, 2010; Sethi, 2000; Waites & Talkington, 2004]. Since late 1970's, several authors suggested a relationship between COPD and *M. pneumoniae* infection [Buscho *et al.*, 1978; Gump *et al.*, 1976; Smith *et al.*, 1980], but it was until late 1990's and early 2000's that several studies based on serology brought attention once more on this issue. [Lieberman et al., 2001, 2002; Mogulkoc *et al.*, 1999]. It is well known that mycoplasmas species pathogenic for humans have the ability to induce chronic disease states in which clearance of the bacteria is extremely difficult. [Rottem & Naot, 1998].

A growing body of evidence indicates that there is a link between *M pneumoniae* infection and COPD. In a Yemeni study, *M. pneumoniae* infection was demonstrated by culture and serologic methods in 20.4% (11/54) of COPD patients [Al-Moyed & Al-Shamahy, 2003]. In a group of 144 Dutch patients with CAP, 12.5 % were infected with *M. pneumoniae* and less than 40% of these *M. pneumoniae*-infected patients had COPD, even though specific serologic tests were mainly negative [Dorigo-Zetsma *et al.*, 2001]. In contrast. *M. pneumoniae* was the most frequent pathogen (22.7%, alone or in association with other microorganisms) among CAP patients that required hospitalization related to COPD, asthma and/or pulmonary fibrosis. [Caberlotto *et al.*, 2003].

A rather weak association between *M. pneumoniae* infection and acute asthma has been suggested on the basis of contradictory data about mycoplasma infection frequencies from several trials. Conversely, strong associations of this pathogen with chronic asthma have been established [Guilbert & Denlinger, 2010; Sutherland & Martin, 2007]. Evidence for this association includes the following: a) Higher prevalence of *M. pneumoniae* in asthmatics than in healthy subjects; b) Improved pulmonary function in mycoplasma-infected asthmatic patients after treatment with macrolide antibiotics; c) Demonstration of long-term airway dysfunction consistent with a persistent infection; and d) *M. pneumoniae*-induced production of inflammatory mediators (IgE, substance P and neurokinin 1, and IL-5) implicated in the pathogenesis of asthma [Waites & Talkington, 2004].

By means of murine models of chronic respiratory infection, it has been demonstrated *M. pneumoniae* can produce pneumonia, with consistent immunologic responses in term of specific IgM antibodies [Wubbel et al., 1998]. Other findings revealed post-infection time-dependent differential cytokine production, with increased expression of TNF-α, IL-1, IL-6, and IFN-γ in the acute phase, whereas IL-2 and IL-2 receptor gene expression was seen only during reinfection. [Pietsch et al., 1994].

Relationship between the timing of Mycoplasma infection, allergic sensitization, and subsequent pulmonary physiologic and immune response was assessed by Chu et al., 2003. Before ovalbumin sensitization, experimental *M. pneumoniae* infection resulted in reduced airway hyperresponsiveness (AHR), reduced lung inflammatory cell recruitment, and a predominantly Th1 response. In contrast, *M. pneumoniae* infection post-sensitization initially caused a transient reduction in AHR, followed by augmented AHR, and a Th2-dominant airway inflammatory process that potentiates organism survival in the lungs. Further characterization of the *M. pneumoniae* effects on ovoalbumin sensitized mice, long-term infection provoked collagen deposition in airway wall accompanied by augmented expression of TGF-β1 in the lungs [Chu et al., 2005].

4.2 *Mycoplasmas* in immunocompromised hosts

Association between immunodeficiency and mycoplasmal infections has been reported since the mid 1970s to the date. Mycoplasmas can disseminate from localized infections and cause invasive diseases, especially in hypogammaglobulinemic subjects. Significance of mycoplasma species other than *M. pneumoniae* or *Ureaplasma* spp. in respiratory diseases is a matter of controversy [Cassell et al., 1994a].

4.2.1 *Mycoplasma fermentans* associated to lung diseases

It has been well documented that *M. pneumoniae* produces respiratory disease in adults; it is also worthy of consideration as a cause of respiratory infections in persons of all age groups, though very few attempts have been made to determine whether it occurs in neonates and young infants [Waites et al., 2005]. However, due to their fastidious growth requirements and presumably less frequent occurrence than *Ureaplasma* spp. or *M. hominis*, much less is known about the epidemiology and disease associations of organisms such as *M. fermentans*, *M. genitalium*, and *M. penetrans* in humans. Waites and Talkington, 2005, recently reviewed the importance of *M. fermentans* in human diseases and provided more detail on the conditions described above as well as others [Waites et al., 2005].

The role of *M. fermentans* as a pathogen is unclear, it has been associated with the pathogenesis of rheumatoid arthritis [Williams et al., 1970]. However, the potential importance of *M. fermentans* in human diseases has recently been further demonstrated. Isolation of about 30 strains of *M. fermentans* from previously healthy non-AIDS patients who had a sudden onset of a severe and often fatal form of respiratory distress syndrome was recorded by R. Dular in Ottawa, Canada [unpublished, as cited by Hu et al., 1998]. Also they have reported the detection by PCR of *Mycoplasma fermentans* in the respiratory tract of children with pneumonia [Cassell et al., 1994b]. It has been demonstrated that a wild strain of *M. fermentans* isolated from the respiratory tract of an asthma patient was able to produce severe experimental respiratory disease in hamsters [Yáñez, 1997]. Román-Méndez et al., 2007, have showed that *Mycoplasma fermentans* persisted in the respiratory tract of hamsters during 120 days and all hamsters developed histological evidence of pulmonary inflammation. Lo et al., 1993, have reported the presence of infections due to *Mycoplasma fermentans* in patients with adult respiratory distress syndrome with or without systemic disease. *M. fermentans* can be detected in the upper and lower urogenital and respiratory tracts and bone marrow, and has been associated with a variety of systemic conditions in adults including inflammatory arthritis and pneumonia [Ainsworth et al., 2000a, 2001; Gilroy et al., 2001; Lo et al., 1989; Schaeverbeke et al.,1996; Taylor-Robinson, 1996; Tully, 1993; Waites & Talkington, 2005]

It has been recovered from the throats of 16% of children with community-acquired pneumonia, some of whom had no other etiologic agent identified, but the frequency of its occurrence in healthy children is not known. [Taylor-Robinson, 1996].

M. fermentans has also been detected in adults with an acute influenza-like illness who developed respiratory distress syndrome, and from bronchoalveolar lavage in AIDS patients with pneumonia, sometimes as the sole microbe, so it clearly has the potential to cause respiratory tract disease in susceptible hosts [Lo et al., 1993; Ainsworth et al., 2001]. This mycoplasma is also known to colonize mucosal surfaces in healthy persons, complicating efforts to understand its role in disease [Ainsworth et al., 2000b].

Mycoplasma fermentans, isolated decades ago from the urogenital tract, has been implicated in several disease conditions. Interest in this organism has recently increased because of its possible role in the pathogenesis of rheumatoid arthritis. Over the last decade, intensive studies have been carried out in order to understand the strategy employed by *M. fermentans* to interact with host cells and to avoid or subvert host protective measures [Rechnitzer et al., 2011].

Attention was focused on *M. fermentans* in the late 1980's because of reports that it may be important as a mediator or cofactor in the development of AIDS [Lo et al., 1989; Saillard et al., 1990]. The identification of mycoplasmal membrane components that participate in the adhesion of the parasite and the finding that some mycoplasmas can reside intracellularly [Rottem, 2003] open up new horizons in the study of the role of mycoplasma and host surface molecules in mycoplasma–host cell interactions [Rechnitzer et al., 2011].

Unlike *M. pneumoniae, M. fermentans* lacks a well-defined terminal attachment tip to mediate attachment and cell invasion. Since intracellular organisms are resistant to host defense mechanisms and to antibiotic treatment, this feature may account for the difficulty in eradicating mycoplasmas from cell cultures. A study by Yavlovich et al., 2001, demonstrated that *M. fermentans* binds plasminogen and converts it to plasmin, where upon mycoplasmal cell surface proteins are altered to promote its internalization. The role of plasminogen activation as a virulence factor and other aspects of *M. fermentans* pathogenesis, including the importance of membrane surface proteins that mediate cell fusion, cytadherence, and antigenic variation, are discussed by Rottem, 2003. The fusion of *M. fermentans* with eukaryotic host cells raises exciting questions on how microinjection of mycoplasmal components into eukaryotic cells affects host cells [Rottem, 2003].

The fusion process as well as the invasion of host cells by *M. fermentans* brings up an emerging theme in mycoplasma research, the subversion by *M. fermentans* of host cell functions mainly in signal-transduction pathways and cytoskeletal organization [As cited by Rechnitzer et al., 2011].

4.2.2 *Mycoplasma penetrans, Mycoplasma pirium* and Human Immunodeficiency Virus (HIV) disease

M. penetrans was first isolated from urine of homosexual men infected with (HIV), but not from healthy age-matched subjects. Subsequent studies suggested an association of this mycoplasma with Kaposi's sarcoma, but later findings did not confirm such association. This organism has been detected in HIV-negative persons, and despite its ability to invade epithelial cell, there is no conclusive evidence of any significant role in human disease [Yañez et al., 1999; Waites et al, 2005; Baseman & Tully, 1997].

Initial isolation of *M. pirum* from human peripheral blood lymphoid cells of HIV-positive patients, along with *M. penetrans* and *M. fermentans*, lead scientists to suggest a role as cofactor in acquire immunodeficiency syndrome (AIDS) progression. However, despite *M. pirum* was detected in rectal specimens of homosexual men and in urine of patients with AIDS, no conclusive evidence of its pathogenic role in human disease has been found. [Waites et al, 2005; Baseman & Tully, 1997]. Taking into account that *M. penetrans* and *M. pirum* have been associated with immune compromise, extragenital dissemination in infected patients, including respiratory disease, should be considered.

4.3 *Ureaplasma urealyticum and Ureaplasma parvum* in urogenital and respiratory tract infections

Although *U. urealyticum* and *U. parvum* are common commensals of the urogenital tract of humans, they are considered as important pathogens associated with infertility and nongonococcal urethritis in men, multiple obstetrical complications in women, and neonatal lung disease [Viscardi, 2010; Volgmann et al., 2005; Waites et al., 2005).

Genital ureaplasmas are natural residents of male urethra contaminating the semen during ejaculation. However, these microorganisms, particularly *U. urealyticum*, play and etiologic role in both genital infections and male infertility (Gdoura et al., 2008). Recent studies reveal that *U. urealyticum* strains are isolated more often in men with non-gonococcal urethritis than in healthy men (Deguchi et al., 2004; Maeda et al., 2004; Povlsen et al., 2002). Ureaplasmas are widespread among the male partners of infertile couples (Gdoura et al., 2007, 2008), and their presence is correlated with the alteration of some characteristics of semen, such as density, sperm motility, concentration, and probably morphology (Naessens et al., 1986; Reichart et al., 2000; Wang et al., 2006). The attachment to sperm and the induction of germ cell apoptosis have been proposed as mechanisms by which *U. urealyticum* affects sperm quality (Shang et al., 1999; Waites et al., 2005).

The infection of the female urinary tract with *U. urealyticum* is frequently overlooked. However, since a high isolation rate of this microorganism has been observed in urine and urethral samples from women with unexplained chronic urinary symptoms, treatment of the infection is now indicated (Baka et al., 2009; Potts et al., 2000).

Genital ureaplasmas can be found in vaginal flora in 40% of sexually inactive and 67% sexually active women (Viscardi, 2010). The infection is generally asymptomatic in nature, and is sexually transmitted between partners. Ureaplasmas can survive in the reproductive tract for many years, undetected, until the patient is specifically tested for the infection.

U. urealyticum is recovered from the lower genital tract of 70-80% of pregnant women (Carey et al., 1991; Volgmann, 2005), but vaginal carriage is not reliably predictive of preterm birth (Kafetzis et al., 2004; Povlsen et al., 2001). However, there is a consistent association when the infection is present in the amniotic fluid, chorioamnion or placenta (Eschenbach, 1993; Kundsin et al., 1996; Yoon et al., 2000, 2003). The secretion of phospholipases A and C has been suggested to be the means by which ureaplasmas may initiate preterm labor by liberating arachidonic acid and altering prostaglandin synthesis (De Silva & Quinn, 1986). In addition, recently we reported that the interaction between *U. urealyticum*, intrauterine leukocytes and fetal membranes results in the secretion of high amounts of IL-1b and prostaglandin E2, which could induce uterine contraction leading to preterm labor (Estrada et al., 2010). Isolation of *U. urealyticum* from chorioamnion has been consistently associated with histological chorioamnionitis and is inversely related to birth weight, even when adjusting for duration of labor, rupture of the fetal membranes, and the presence of other bacteria [Cassel et al., 1993; Waites et al., 2005].

There is accumulating epidemiologic and experimental evidence that intrauterine or postnatal infection with genital ureaplasmas is a significant risk factor for complications of extreme preterm birth such as bronchopulmonary dysplasia (BDP) and intraventricular hemorrhage [Kafetzis, et al., 2004; Viscardi, 2010]. *Ureaplasma* spp can be transmitted from an infected mother to the fetus or neonate by ascending intrauterine infection, hematogenous route involving umbilical vessels, or through passage of an infected maternal birth canal with resultant colonization of the skin, mucosal membranes or respiratory tract [Waites, 2005].

Among premature infants, respiratory tract colonization with genital ureaplasmas has been associated with pneumonia, chronic lung disease, infant wheezing, respiratory distress syndrome, acute respiratory insufficiency, and increased mortality [Cultrera et al., 2006;

Kafetzis et al., 2004]. For some infants, ureaplasmal infection triggers a vigorous response in the lungs involving the elevation of adhesion molecules, collagenases, proinflammatory cytokines and neutrophil activation and migration, which increase the risk of developing bronchopulmonary dysplasia characterized by delayed alveolarization, chronic inflammation, and fibrosis [Manimtim et al., 2001; Schelonka & Waites, 2007]. Additionally, free radical generation and oxidative injury induced by recruited neutrophils could contribute to lung damage [Buss et al., 2003]. Apoptosis of pneumocytes and pulmonary mesenchymal cells has been shown to occur as part of the pathogenesis of *U. urealyticum* [Li et al., 2002], while *U. parvum* lipoproteins activate NF-kB and induce TNF-α in macrophages, favoring the inflammatory response (Shimizu et al., 2008). Apparently, there is no trend in the prevalence of either species between infants with or without bronchopulmonary dysplasia [Katz et al., 2005].

5. Diagnostic procedures

Much of the mycoplasmal respiratory diseases, especially those caused by *M. pneumoniae,* are underdiagnosed because the laboratory diagnostic strategies are quite different than those for fast-growing bacteria. It is noteworthy that mycoplasmal etiology of respiratory diseases is considered only after failure of diagnosis of other common bacterial etiologies. In addition, there are few specialized or reference laboratories and skilled personnel [Cassell et al., 1994a; Waites et al., 2000].

5.1 Types of specimens, transport and collection

Detection or isolation of mycoplasmas in clinical specimens requires careful consideration of the type of specimen available and the organism (species) sought [Cassell et al., 1994a]. Specimens appropriate for laboratory diagnosis of respiratory mycoplasmal infections include: Bronchoalveolar lavage (BAL), sputum, pleural fluid, nasopharyngeal and throat swabs, endotracheal aspirates (ETA) and lung biopsies. Liquid specimens or tissues do not require special transport media if culture can be performed within 1 hour, otherwise specimens should be placed in transport media, such as SP-4 broth, 10B broth or 2SP broth. When swabbing is required, aluminum- or plastic-shafted calcium alginate or dacron swabs should be used, taking care to obtain as many cells as possible [Atkinson et al., 2008; Cassell et al., 1994a; Waites et al., 2002].

Other specimens such as blood, cerebrospinal fluid, pericardial fluid and synovial fluid must be considered when extrapulmonary disease is suspected, thus specimen collection should reflect the site of infection and/or the disease process. [Atkinson et al., 2008, Waites & Talkington, 2004].

5.2 Culture

Routine culture methods for isolation/detection of most mycoplasma species are time-consuming, thus emission of results may delay up to 5-6 weeks. Furthermore, there is no ideal formulation of culture media for all pathogenic species, mainly due to their different substrate and pH requirements [Waites et al., 2000]. Modified SP-4 media (broth and agar) [Lo et al., 1993], containing both glucose and arginine, can support the growth of all human pathogenic *Mycoplasma* species, including the fastidious *M. pneumoniae* and *M. genitalium.* A set of Shepard´s 10B broth and A8 agar can be used for cultivation of *Ureaplasma* species and *M. hominis.*

For cultivation, specimens in transport media should be thoroughly mixed, and then should be 10-fold serially diluted in broth (usually up to 10^{-6}) in order to overcome potential inhibitory substances, and to allow semiquantitative estimation of mycoplasmal load. Subcultures in agar media should be also performed. [Cassell et al., 1994a]. All inoculated media are incubated under microaerophilic atmosphere at 37°C.
Detection of *M. pneumoniae* in broth culture is based on its ability to ferment glucose, causing an acidic shift after 4 or more days, readily visualized by the presence of the phenol red pH indicator. Broths with any color change, and subsequent blind broth passages, should be subcultured to SP4 agar, incubated, and examined under the low-power objective of the light microscope in order to look for development of typical "fried egg"-like colonies of up to 100 µm in diameter (Figure 2). Examination of agar plates must be done on a daily basis during the first week, and thereafter every 3 to 4 days until completing 5 weeks or until growth is observed [Waites et al., 2000, 2004]. *M. genitalium*, *M. fermentans* and *M. penetrans* are also glucose-fermenting and formed colonies morphologically indistinguishable from those of *M. pneumoniae*, thus serologic-based definitive identification can be done by growth inhibition, metabolic inhibition, and mycoplamacidal tests [Cassel et al., 1993].

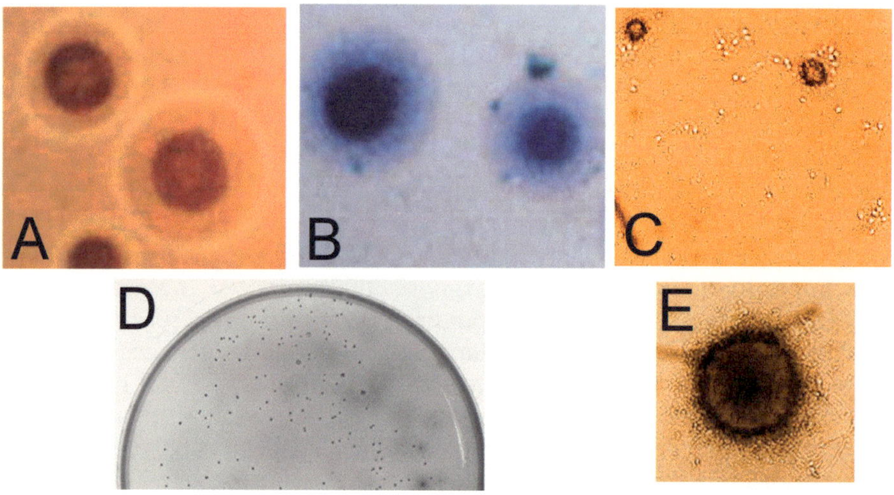

A) Typical "Fried-egg" appearance of *Mycoplasma* spp. colonies on SP-4 agar. B) Dienes-stained mycoplasma colonies. C) Tiny brown-colored ureaplasmal colonies on modified SP-4 agar. D) Macroscopic view of Dienes-stained mycoplasma colonies growth on SP-4 agar in 30 mm-diameter Petri dishes. E) Closer view of an ureaplasma colony.

Fig. 2. Morphology of mycoplasma colonies in culture.

Hidrolysis of urea by Ureaplasma and hidrolysis of arginine by *M. hominis* cause an alkaline shift, turning the colour of 10B broth from yellow to pink. Tiny brown or black irregular colonies of *Ureaplasma* species develop between 1 -5 days on A8 agar plates, due to urease production in the presence of manganese sulfate (Figure 2). Typical fried egg colonies are produced by *M. hominis* in this medium [Cassell et al., 1994a, Waites et al., 2000].

5.3 Immunodiagnosis by serological tests

As culture of *M. pneumoniae* is slow and insensitive, the laboratory diagnosis of *M. pneumoniae* infection has largely relied on serological testing. Seroconversion or rising specific antibody titers are observed among *M. pneumoniae*-infected patients. This immunologic response can be measured by several tests, including: metabolic inhibition assay, complement fixation or enzyme-linked immunoassays (EIA). Serum samples are easy to collect and handle, but it is required paired acute- and convalescent-phase specimens. Commercial assay formats include indirect immunofluorescence, particle agglutination assay, and EIA [Atkinson et al., 2008, Cassell et al., 1994a; Waites & Talkington, 2004].

Prior to the widespread availability of commercialized antibody assays, presence of cold agglutinins (IgM antibodies that are produced 1 to 2 weeks after initial infection in about half of *M. pneumoniae*-infected subjects) was used to confirm primary atypical pneumonia (Waites & Talkington, 2004). Although there have been recent improvements, the sensitivity and specificity of antibody detection is still suboptimal. Nevertheless, the complex and time-consuming nature of many of the serological assays that have been used in the past have limited acceptance of serology for routine diagnostic testing. [Cassell et al., 1994a; Waites et al., 2000].

At present, besides research laboratories, no serologic tests assays for mycoplasmas other than *M. pneumoniae* have been standardized for diagnostic purposes in routine clinical microbiology laboratories nor made commercially available elsewhere. [Cassell et al., 1994a, Waites et al., 2005].

5.4 PCR and other molecular tests

Nucleic acid amplification techniques (NAATs) are more sensitive, and considerably more rapid than culture, showing a fair to good correlation with serology. PCR testing for species-specific mycoplasmal infection are suitable for both upper and lower respiratory samples. Interestingly, sample processing prior amplification must be optimized depending of the type of specimen to overcome the presence of PCR inhibitors (i.e., nasopharyngeal samples have higher rate of PCR inhibition than throat swabs). Differential sample preparation from the same specimen has been done when testing separate single-species PCRs on BAL [De Barbeyrac et al., 1993]. A culture-enhanced PCR approach has also been suggested to overcome the effect of inhibitors in the amplification process [Abele-Horne et al., 1998].

In early 2000s, Loens et al.(2003) stated that the development and application of new nucleic acid amplification techniques (NAATs) in diagnostic mycoplasmology required proper validation and standardization, and performance of different NAATs must be compared with each other in order to define the most sensitive and specific tests. The NAATs have demonstrated their potential to produce rapid, sensitive and specific results, and are now considered the methods of choice for direct detection of *M. pneumoniae, M. genitalium,* and *M. fermentans* [Cassell et al., 1994a]. There is a great variation in methods used from study to study, including variability of target gene sequences (P1, 16S RNA, ATPase, *tuf*), assay format (single, multiplex) or technologies (Real-time PCR, NASBA) [Loens et al., 2003a, 2010]. Also, different specimens have been used, such as sputum, nasopharyngeal or pharyngeal swabs, brochoalveolar lavages or pleural fluid, and then it is difficult to compare these data. A comprehensive review about the use of NAATs for the detection of *M. pneumoniae* in clinical samples was done by Loens et al., 2003b, 2010, and by Ieven, 2010. Table 3, shows a selection of primers sets developed in the 1990s for testing diverse clinical samples.

Organism	Primer sets		Sequence (5′→3′)	Target	Amplicon size (bp)	Ref.
Mollicutes-specific	FW:	GPO-1	ACT CCT ACG GGA GGC AGC AGT A	rDNA 16S	715	Van Kuppeveld *et al.*, 1992
	RV:	MGSO	TGC ACC ATC TGT CAC TCT GTT AAC CTC			
M. fermentans	FW:	RW005	GGT TAT TCG ATT TCT AAA TCG CCT	IS-like element	206	Wang *et al.*, 1992
	RV:	RW004	GGA CTA TTG TCT AAA CAA TTT CCC			
	IP:	RW006	GCT GTG GCC ATT CTC TTC TAC GTT			
	FW:	Mf-1	GAA GCC TTT CTT CGC TGG AG	rDNA 16s	272	Van Kuppeveld *et al.*, 1992
	RV:	Mf-2	ACA AAA TCA TTT CCT ATT CTG TC			
	IP:	GPO-1	ACT CCT ACG GGA GGC AGC AGT A			
M. genitalium	FW:	MGS-1	GAG CCT TTC TAA CCG CTG C	MgPa adhesion gene	673	De Barbeyrac *et al.*, 1993
	RV:	MGS-2	GTG GGG TTG AAG GAT GAT TG			
	IP:	MGS-I	AAG CAA CGT AGT AGC GTG AGC			
	FW:	MGS-1	GAG CCT TTC TAA CCG CTG C	MgPa adhesion gene	371	De Barbeyrac *et al.*, 1993
	RV:	MGS-4	GTT GTT ATC ATA CCT TCT GAT			
	IP:	MGS-I	AAG CAA CGT AGT AGC GTG AGC			
M. hominis	FW:	MYCHOMP	ATA CAT GCA TGT CGA GCG AG	rDNA 16s	170	Grau *et al.*, 1994
	RV:	MYCHOMN	CAT CTT TTA GTG GCG CCT TAC			
	IP:	MYCHOMS	CGC ATG GAA CCG CAT GGT TCC GTT G			
	FW:	Mh-1	TGA AAG GCG CTG TAA GGC GC	rDNA 16s	281b	Van Kuppeveld *et al.*, 1992
	RV:	Mh-2	GTC TGC AAT CAT TTC CTA TTG CAA A			
	IP:	GPO-1	ACT CCT ACG GGA GGC AGC AGT A			
M. penetrans	FW:	MYCPENETP	CAT GCA AGT CGG ACG AAG CA	rDNA 16s	407	Grau *et al.*, 1994
	RV:	MYCPENETN	AGC ATT TCC TCT TCT TAC AA			
	IP:	MYCPENETS	CAT GAG AAA ATG TTT AAA GTC TGT TTG			
M. pneumoniae	FW:	MP5-1	GAA GCT TAT GGT ACA GGT TGG	Unknown gene	144	Bernet *et al.*, 1989
	RV:	MP5-2	ATT ACC ATC CTT GTT GTA AGG			
	IP:	MP5-4	CGT AAG CTA TCA GCT ACA TGG AGG			
	FW:	MP-P11	TGC CAT CAA CCC GCG CTT AAC	P1 adhesin gene	466	De Barbeyrac *et al.*, 1993
	RV:	MP-P12	CCT TTG CAA CTG CTC ATA GTA			
	IP:	MP-I	CAA ACC GGG CAG ATC ACC TTT			
Ureaplasma spp.	FW:	U5	CAA TCT GCT CGT GAA GTA TTA C	Urease genes	429	Blanchard *et al.*, 1993
	RV:	U4	ACG ACG TCC ATA AGC AAC T			
	IP:	U9	GAG ATA ATG ATT ATA TGT CAG GAT CA			
	FW:	Uu-1	TAA ATG TCG GCT CGA ACG AG	rDNA 16s	311	Van Kuppeveld *et al.*, 1992
	RV:	Uu-2	GCA GTA TCG CTA GAA AAG CAA C			
	IP:	UUSO	CAT CTA TTG CGA CGC TA			
U. parvum U. urealyticum	FW:	UMS-125	GTA TTT GCA ATC TTT ATA TGT TTT CG	MBA gene	402,403 (Up) 443 (Uu)	Kong *et al.*, 1999
	RV:	UMA-226-	CAG CTG ATG TAA GTG CAG CAT TAA ATT C			

bp, Base pairs; FW, Forward; RV, Reverse; IP, Internal probe.

Table 3. Selected primer sets used for detection of mycoplasmas in clinical specimens

6. Treatment and prevention

Due to absence of the cell wall envelope, mycoplasmas are insensitive to β-lactam antibiotics. However, antibiotics targeting protein synthesis or DNA modification molecules are highly effective against these bacteria. Macrolides, tetracyclines and fluoroquinolones eliminate mycoplasmas efficiently both *in vivo* and *in vitro* [Cassell et al., 1994a; Waites et al., 2000, 2008].

Mycoplasmal infections in the upper respiratory tract are usually self-limiting, so antibiotic treatment is not generally recommended, even though some clinicians recommend it to prevent the risk of recurrence of respiratory illness [Waites & Talkington, 2004]

The antimicrobial of choice for treating lower respiratory tract *M. pneumoniae* infections are the macrolides in both adults and children. Patients receiving macrolides of recent generation showed improved tolerance, require fewer doses and have shorter treatment duration than older compounds. However, empirical antimicrobial treatment for *M. pneumoniae*-infected ambulatory patients is more practical; hence if hospitalization is required and/or patient has underlying risk factor, antimicrobial susceptibility testing is recommended. Use of tetracycline and fluoroquinolones is restricted to treat adult patients and should not be used in children aged <8 years [Cassell et al., 1994a; Waites et al., 2000]. A potential problem in the antimicrobial management of *M. pneumoniae* infections is the emergence of macrolide resistance [Atkinson et al., 2008; Waites et al., 2008].

The recovery of *Ureaplasma spp* and/or *M. hominis* in pure or mixed cultures from clinical specimens of symptomatic patients, in absence of associated biota, should be considered sufficient to initiate antimicrobial therapy. These microorganisms are resistant to sulfonamides and trimethoprim, and often exhibit resistance to aminoglycosides and chloramphenicol. *Ureaplasma spp* is resistant to clindamycin and susceptible to erythromycin, whereas *M. hominis* shows the opposite susceptibility profile. While tetracyclines are the antibiotics of choice for treating ureaplasmal infections in adults, erythromycin therapy is recommended for neonates. In contrast, *M. hominis* infections other than central nervous system in children under 8 years of age can be treated with clindamycin [Cassell et al., 1994a; Waites et al., 2000, 2005].

Since strains from several mycoplasma species rapidly acquire resistance to antimicrobials, prevention of mycoplasmal infections via chemoprophylaxis is not recommended [Razin et al, 1998].

6.1 Mycoplasmal susceptibility testing

As antibiotic-resistant strains of mycoplasmas have appeared and become more common, antibiotic susceptibility testing for these microorganisms has become important. [Roberts, M.C., 1992]. However there are no official guidelines for performance, interpretation, or quality control of *in vitro* susceptibility tests for human mycoplasmas [Waites & Talkington, 2004].

The broth dilution method is the most widely used. Prior to test, pure cultures should be passage in appropriate broth and the color-changing units (CCU) or colony-forming units (CFU) quantitative method. For the assay, bacterial cultures should be adjusted to 1000 - 10000 CCU in 0.2 mL, followed by a 2-hour incubation at 37°C, to begin active growth. The broth microdilution assay involves the addition of 100-µL aliquots of adjusted cultures to wells 2 - 12, then 100 µL of broth containing the highest concentration of the antibiotics is added to wells 1 and 2, followed by 2-fold serial dilutions up to well 12 (concentration range 256-0.008 µg/mL). Positive and negative controls should be included. The initial minimal inhibitory concentration (MIC) is defined as the lowest dilution of antibiotic in which metabolism of the organism is inhibited, as evidenced by lack of color change in the media at the time the control organism well first shows color change. Presumptive MICs for ureaplasmas will be available at 16 to 24 h and those for *M. hominis* will be at 36 to 48 h but *M. pneumoniae* may require 5 days or more until evidence of grow in the control wells is evident [Cassell et al., 1994a; Waites et al., 2000].

There are commercial kits for mycoplasma susceptibility testing such as: Mycoplasma IST, Mycoplasma SIR, Mycofast "All In", and MYCOKIT ATB, although they are available only in Europe.

Reports of macrolide resistance in *M. pneumoniae* strains have been published since the past decade. These resistant strains were shown to possess gene mutations in the 23S rRNA. The impact of macrolide resistance on the clinical course of infections is still unclear, but PCR assays have been developed to detect some of these mutations in order to identify these resistant strains [Atkinson et al., 2008].

Tetracycline resistance among *Ureaplasma spp* and *M. hominis* isolates can be distinguished by broth- or agar-based methods since the resistant strains consistently have MICs of ≥ 8 µg/mL whereas susceptible strains have MICs of ≤ 2 µg/mL, with no overlapping between the two populations [Waites et al., 2000; Cassell et al., 1994a]. Tetracycline resistance among *M. hominis* and *Ureaplasma spp.* isolates has been associated with the presence of Tet M determinant which codes for production of a ribosome-binding protein that prevents tetracycline binding to ribosomes [Roberts, M.C., 2002].

6.2 Vaccines

The initial vaccine candidate for *M. pneumoniae* was formalin-inactivated bacteria, but their protective efficacy results were generally disappointing, since some immunized volunteers developed more severe illness after experimental challenge with live mycoplasmas. Development of live attenuated vaccines never made it to human use due to concern over residual virulence of the vaccine strain of *M. pneumoniae* [Waites et al., 2008]. Other vaccine candidates have included acellular protein and polysaccharide components and recombinant DNA. While the importance of the P1 adhesin in mediating *M. pneumoniae* cytadherence and initiation of disease cannot be denied, animal studies using P1 as a vaccine antigen have not demonstrated protective efficacy [Razin et al., 1998; Waites & Talkington, 2004].

As higher rates of surface antigenic variation among several human mycoplasmas have been described, whenever promising antigens are selected as vaccine candidates they are rapidly discarded. The three types of antigenic variation are: 1) Phase variation, a feature involving selective turning on/off of gene transcription; 2) Size variation as a result of variation in the number of tandem repeats near the 5′ end; and 3) Differential masking of surface antigens by the lipid moiety of lipoproteins [Chambaud et al., 1999; Momynaliev & Govorun, 2001].

The availability of the full genome sequences of several human mycoplasmas, will allow better understanding of the structure and functionality of these bacteria, including virulence factors and immunogenic molecules.

7. Concluding remarks

It is undeniable the ability of *Mycoplasma pneumoniae* and *Ureaplasma* spp. to cause pneumonia. Other mycoplasma species are potential respiratory pathogens, especially in conjunction with immune compromise. There is strong evidence that mycoplasmal respiratory infections elicit inflammatory responses that can result chronic lung injury both in adults and neonates. Improvement of laboratory methods for research and diagnostic purposes in mycoplasmology has allowed establishing associations with pulmonary diseases such as COPD, asthma, and BPD. However additional work must be done for prevention, treatment strategies and vaccine development.

8. Acknowledgements

This work was supported by grants from:
Research Fellow System of SNI-CONACYT (SGC, GEG, JART, FJDG); EDI-COFAA grant by SEP-IPN, ICYT-DF (SGC); PRIDE C grant by DGAPA-UNAM (FJDG).
Corresponding author: Dra. Silvia Giono-Cerezo. Laboratorio de Bacteriología Médica, Departamento de Microbiología, ENCB-IPN. Carpio y Plan de Ayala S/N, Col. Casco de Sto. Tomás, C.P. 11340, México D.F.México. Phone: +52(55)57296300 ext. 62374.
Email: sgiono@yahoo.com

9. References

Abele-Horn, M., Busch, U., Nitschko, H., Jacobs, E., Bax, R., Pfaff, F., Schaffer, B., & Heesemann, J. (1998). Molecular Approaches to Diagnosis of Pulmonary Diseases Due to *Mycoplasma pneumoniae*. *Journal of Clinical Microbiology,* Vol. 36, No. 2 (February 1998), pp. 548–551, ISSN 0095-1137

Ainsworth, J.G., Clarke, J., Goldin, R., & Taylor-Robinson, D. (2000a). Disseminated *Mycoplasma fermentans* in AIDS Patients: Several Case Reports. *International Journal of STD & AIDS,* Vol. 11, No. 11 (November 2000), pp. 751-755, ISSN 0956-4624

Ainsworth, J.G., Hourshid, S., Webster, A.D., Gilroy, C.B., & Taylor-Robinson, D. (2000b). Detection of *Mycoplasma fermentans* in Healthy Students and Patients with Congenital Immunodeficiency. *Journal of Infection,* Vol. 40, No. 2 (March 2000), pp. 138-140, ISSN 0163-4453

Ainsworth, J.G., Easterbrook, P.J., Clarke, J., Gilroy, C.B., & Taylor-Robinson, D. (2001). An Association of Disseminated *Mycoplasma fermentans* in HIV-1 Positive Patients with Non-Hodgkin's Lymphoma. *International Journal of STD & AIDS,* Vol. 12, No. 8 (August 2001), pp. 499-504, ISSN 0956-4624

Al-Moyed, K.A., & Al-Shamahy, H.A. (2003). *Mycoplasma pneumoniae* Infection in Yemen: Incidence, Presentation and Antibiotic Susceptibility. *Eastern Mediterranean Health Journal,* Vol. 9, No. 3 (May 2003), pp. 279-290, ISSN 1020-3397

Andreev, J., Borovsky, Z., Rosenshine, I., & Rottem, S. (1995). Invasion of HeLa Cells by *Mycoplasma penetrans* and the Induction of Tyrosine Phosphorylation of a 145 kDa Host Cell Protein. *FEMS Microbiology Letters,* Vol. 132, No. 3 (October 1995), pp. 189-194. ISSN 0378-1097

Atkinson, T.P., Balish, M.F., & Waites, K.B. (2008). Epidemiology, Clinical Manifestations, Pathogenesis and Laboratory Detection of *Mycoplasma pneumoniae* Infections. *FEMS Microbiology Reviews,* Vol. 32 No. 6 (November 2008), pp. 956–973, ISSN 0168-6445

Baka, S., Kouskouni, E., Antonopoulou, S., Sioutis, D., Papakonstantinou, M., Hassiakos, D., Logothetis, E., & Liapis, A. (2009). Prevalence of *Ureaplasma urealyticum* and *Mycoplasma hominis* in Women with Chronic Urinary Symptoms. *Urology,* Vol.74. No.1 (July 2009), pp. 62-66, ISSN: 0090-4295.

Baseman, J.B., Lange, M., Criscimagna, N.L., Giron, J.A., & Thomas, C.A. (1995). Interplay Between *Mycoplasmas* and Host Target Cells. *Microbial Pathogenesis, Vol. 19,* No. 2 (August 1995), pp. 105-116, ISSN 0882-4010

Baseman, J.B., & Tully, J.G. (1997). *Mycoplasmas*: Sophisticated Reemerging and Burdened by Their Notoriety. *Emerging Infectious Diseases,* Vol. 3, No. 1 (January-March 1997), pp. 21-32, ISSN 1080-6040

Bernet, C., Garret, M., de Barbeyrac, B., Bebear, C., & Bonnet, J. (1989). Detection of *Mycoplasma pneumoniae* by Using Polymerase Chain Reaction. *Journal of Clinical Microbiology,* Vol. 27, No. (1989), pp. 2492-2496, ISSN 0095-1137

Blasi, F. (2004). Atypical Pathogens and Respiratory Tract Infections. *European Respiratory Journal,* Vol. 24, No. 1 (July 2004), pp. 171–181, ISSN 0903-1936

Bové, J.M. (1993). Molecular features of *Mollicutes*. *Clinical Infectious Diseases,* Vol. 17, Supplement 1 (August 1993), pp. S10-S31, ISSN 1058-4838

Brown, D.R., Whitcomb, R.F., & Bradbury, J.M. (2007). Revised Minimal Standards for Description of New Species of the Class *Mollicutes* (Division Tenericutes). *International Journal of Systematic and Evolutionary Microbiology,* Vol. 57, No. 11 (November 2007), pp. 2703–2719. ISSN 1466-5026

Buscho, R.O., Saxtan, D., Shultz, P.S., Finch, E., & Mufson, M.A. (1978). Infections with Viruses and *Mycoplasma pneumoniae* During Exacerbations of Chronic Bronchitis. *Journal of Infectious Diseases,* Vol. 137, No. 4 (April 1978), pp. 377–383, ISSN 0022-1899

Buss, I.H., Senthilmohan, R., Darlow, B.A., Mogridge, N., Kettle, A.J., & Winterbourn, C.C. (2003). 3-Chlorotyrosine as a Marker of Protein Damage by Myeloperoxidase in Tracheal Aspirates from Preterm Infants: Association with Adverse Respiratory Outcome. *Pediatric Research,* Vol. 53, No. 3 (March 2003), pp. 455-462. ISSN: 0031-3998

Caberlotto, O.J., Cadario, M.E., Garay, J.E., Copacastro, C.A., Cabot, A., & Savy, V.L. (2003). Community-Acquired Pneumonia in Patients in 2 Hospital Populations. *Medicina (B Aires)* Vol. 63, No. 1 (January-February 2003), pp. 1-8, ISSN 0025-7680

Carey, J.C., Blackwelder, W.C., Nugent, R.P., Matteson, M.A., Rao, A.V., Eschenbach, D.A., Lee, M.L., Rettig, P.J., Regan, J.A., & Geromanos, K.L. (1991). Antepartum Cultures for *Ureaplasma urealyticum* are not Useful in Predicting Pregnancy Outcome. The Vaginal Infections and Prematurity Study Group. *American Journal of Obstetrics and Gynecology,* Vol. 164, No. 3 (March 1991), pp.728-733. ISSN: 0002-9378.

Cartner, S.C., Lindsey, J. R., Gibbs-Erwin, J., Cassell, G.H., & Simecka. J.W. (1998). Roles of Innate and Adaptive Immunity in Respiratory Mycoplasmosis. *Infection and Immunity,* Vol. 66, No. 8 (August1998), pp. 3485–3491, ISSN 0019-9567

Cassell, G.H.; Waites, K.B.; Watson, H.L.; Crouse, D.T. & Harasawa, R. (1993). *Ureaplasma urealyticum* Intrauterine Infection: Role in Prematurity and Disease in Newborns. *Clinical Microbiology Reviews,* Vol.6. No.1. (January-March 1993), pp.69-87, ISSN 0893-8512.

Cassell, G.H., Blanchard, A., Duffy, L., Crabb, D., & Waites, K.B. (1994a). *Mycoplasmas*, In: *Clinical and Pathogenic Microbiology*, B.J. Howard, J.F. Keiser, A.S. Weissfeld, T.F. Smith, & R.C. Tilton (Eds), pp. 491-502, Mosby, ISBN 978-0801664267, Boston, USA.

Cassell, G.H., Yáñez, A., Duffy, L. B., Moyer, J., Cedillo, L., Hammerschlag, M.R., Rank, R.G., & Glass, J.I. (1994b). Detection of *Mycoplasma fermentans* in the Respiratory Tract of Children with Pneumonia. 10th International Congress of the International Organization for Mycoplasmology (IOM), Bordeaux, France, July 1994. In *IOM Letters* Vol. 3, p. 456, ISSN 1023-1226

Chambaud, I., Wróblewski, H., & Blanchard, A. (1999). Interactions Between Mycoplasma Lipoproteins and the Host Immune System. *Trends in Microbiology,* Vol. 7, No. 12 (December 1999), pp. 493-499, ISSN 0966-842X

Chu, H.W., Honour, J.M., Rawlinson, C.A., et al. (2003). Effects of Respiratory *Mycoplasma pneumoniae* Infection On Allergen-Induced Bronchial Hyperresponsiveness and Lung Inflammation in Mice. *Infection and Immunity,* 2003; Vol. 71, No 3 (March 2003), pp. 1520-1526, ISSN 0019-9567

Chu H.W., Jeyaseelan S., Rino J.G., Voelker D.R., Wexler R.B., Campbell K., Harbeck R.J., & Martin, R.J. (2005a). TLR2 Signaling Is Critical for *Mycoplasma pneumoniae*-Induced Airway Mucin Expression. *Journal of Immunology,* Vol. 174, No. 9 (May 2005), pp. 5713–5719, ISSN 0022-1767

Chu, H. W., Rino, J. G., Wexler, R.B., Campbell, K., Harbeck, R. J., & Martin, R. J. (2005b) *Mycoplasma pneumoniae* Infection Increases Airway Collagen Deposition in a Murine Model of Allergic Airway Inflammation. *American Journal of Physiology, Lung Cellular and Molecular Physiology,* Vol. 289, No. 1 (July 2005), pp. L125-L133, ISSN 1040-0605

Cultrera, R., Seraceni, S., Germani, R., & Contini, C. (2006). Molecular Evidence of *Ureaplasma urealyticum* and *Ureaplasma parvum* Colonization in Preterm Infants During Respiratory Distress Syndrome. *BMC Infectious Diseases,* Vol.21. No. 6 (November 2006), pp. 166, ISSN 1471-2334

Dakhama, A., Kraft, M.,Martin, R.J., & Gelfand, E.W. (2003). Induction of Regulated Upon Activation, Normal T cells Expressed and Secreted (RANTES) and Transforming Growth Factor-Beta 1 in Airway Epithelial Cells by *Mycoplasma pneumoniae. American Journal of Respiratory Cellular and Molecular Biology,* Vol. 29, No. 3 (September 2003), pp. 344-351, ISSN 1044-1549

De Barbeyrac, B., Bernet-Poggi, C., Febrer, F., Renaudin, H., Dupon, M., & Bebear, C. (1993). Detection of *Mycoplasma pneumoniae* and *Mycoplasma genitalium* in Clinical Samples by Polymerase Chain Reaction. *Clinical Infectious Diseases,* Vol. 17, Suppl 1 (August 1993), S83-S89, ISSN 1058-4838

De Silva, N.S., & Quinn, P.A. (1986). Endogenous Activity of Phospholipases A and C in *Ureaplasma urealyticum. Journal of Clinical Microbiology.* Vol. 23, No. 2 (February 1986), pp. 354-359, ISSN 0095-1137

Deguchi, T., Yoshida, T., Miyazawa, T., Yasuda, M., Tamaki, M., Ishiko, H., & Maeda, S. (2004). Association of *Ureaplasma urealyticum* (Biovar 2) with Nongonococcal Urethritis. *Sexually Transmitted Diseases,* Vol.31. No.3 (March 2004), pp. 192-195. ISSN 0148-5717.

Díaz-García, F.J., Herrera-Mendoza, A.P., Giono-Cerezo, S., & Guerra-Infante, F. (2006). *Mycoplasma hominis* Attaches to and Locates Intracellularly On Human Spermatozoa. *Human Reproduction,* Vol. 21, No. 6 (June 2006), pp. 1591-1598, ISSN 0268-1161

Dorigo-Zetsma, J.W., Verkooyen, R.P., van Helden, H.P., van der Nat, H., & van den Bosch, J.M. (2001). Molecular Detection of *Mycoplasma pneumoniae* in Adults with Community-Acquired Pneumonia Requiring Hospitalization. *Journal of Clinical Microbiology,* Vol. 39, No. 3 (March 2001), pp. 1184-1186, ISSN: 0095-1137

Eschenbach, D.A. (1993). *Ureaplasma urealyticum* and Premature Birth. *Clinical Infectious Diseases.* Vol. 17 Suppl. 1 (August 1993), pp. S100-S106, ISSN 1058-4838

Estrada-Gutierrez, G., Gomez-Lopez, N., Zaga-Clavellina, V., Giono-Cerezo, S., Espejel-Nuñez A., Gonzalez-Jimenez, M.A., Espino y Sosa, S., Olson, D.M., & Vadillo-Ortega, F. (2010). Interaction Between Pathogenic Bacteria and Intrauterine

Leukocytes Triggers Alternative Molecular Signaling Cascades Leading to Labor in Women. *Infection and Immunity*,.Vol.78. No.11. pp.4792-4799. ISSN: 0019-9567.

Gdoura, R., Kchaou, W., Chaari, C., Znazen, A., Keskes, L., Rebai, T., & Hammami, A. (2007). *Ureaplasma urealyticum, Ureaplasma parvum, Mycoplasma hominis* and *Mycoplasma genitalium* Infections and Semen Quality of Infertile Men. *BMC Infectious Diseases*. Vol.7. pp.129. ISSN 1471-2334.

Gdoura, R., Kchaou, W., Ammar-Keskes, L., Chakroun, N., Sellemi, A., Znazen, A., Rebai, T., & Hammami, A. (2008). Assessment of *Chlamydia trachomatis, Ureaplasma urealyticum, Ureaplasma parvum, Mycoplasma hominis,* and *Mycoplasma genitalium* in Semen and First Void Urine Specimens of Asymptomatic Male Partners of Infertile Couples. *Journal of Andrology*. Vol.29. No.2. pp. 198-206. ISSN:0196-3635.

Gilroy, C. B., Keat, A., & Taylor-Robinson, D. (2001). The Prevalence of *Mycoplasma fermentans* in Patients with Inflammatory Arthritides. *Rheumatology (Oxford),* Vol. 40, No. 12 (December 2001), pp. 1355-1358, ISSN 1462-0324

Girón, J.A., Lange, M., & Baseman, J. B. (1996). Adherence, Fibronectin Binding, and Induction of Cytoskeleton Reorganization in Cultured Human Cells by *Mycoplasma penetrans. Infection and Immunity,* Vol. 64, No. 1 (January 1996), pp. 197-208, ISSN 0019-9567

Guilbert T.W., & Denlinger, L.C. (2010). Role of Infection in the Development and Exacerbation of Asthma. *Expert Reviews in Respiratory Medicine,* Vol. 4, No. 1 (February 2010), pp. 71–83, ISSN 1747-6348

Gump, D.W., Phillips, C.A., Forsyth, B.R., McIntosh, K., Lamborn, K.R., & Stouch, W.H. (1976). Role of Infection in Chronic Bronchitis. *American Review of Respiratory Disease,* Vol. 113, (April 1976), pp. 465–474, ISSN 0003-0805

Hu, W.S., Hayes, M.M., Wang, R.Y., Shih, J.W., & Lo, S-H. (1998) High-Frequency DNA Rearrangements in the Chromosomes of Clinically Isolated *Mycoplasma fermentans. Current Microbiology,* Vol. 37, No. 1 (July1998), pp. 1–5, ISSN 0343-8651

Ieven, M. (2007). Currently Used Nucleic Acid Amplification Tests for the Detection of Viruses and Atypicals in Acute Respiratory Infections. *Journal of Clinical Virology,* Vol. 40, No. 4 (December 2007), pp. 259-276, ISSN 1386-6532

International Committee on Systematics of Prokaryotes- Subcommittee on the taxonomy of Mollicutes (ICSP-STM). (2011). *International Journal of Systematic and Evolutionary Microbiology,* Vol. 61, No. 3 (March 2011), pp. 695–697, ISSN 1466-5026.

Jensen, J.S., Blom, J., & Lind, K. (1994). Intracellular Location of *Mycoplasma genitalium* in Cultured Vero Cells as Demonstrated by Electron Microscopy. *International Journal of Experimental Pathology, Vol. 75,* No. 2 (April 1994), pp. 91-98, ISSN ISSN 0959-9673

Johansson K. E., Heldtander, M. U. K., & Petterson, B. Characterization of Mycoplasmas by PCR and Sequence Analysis with Universal 16S rDNA Primers, p. 145-165. In: Miles R & Nicholas R, *Mycoplasma protocols*. Humana Press.1998. ISBN 0-89603-525-5, Totowa, NJ, USA.

Kafetzis, D.A.; Skevaki, C.L.; Skouteri, V.; Gavrili, S.; Peppa, K.; Kostalos, C.; Petrochilou, V. & Michalas, S. (2004). Maternal Genital Colonization with *Ureaplasma urealyticum* Promotes Preterm Delivery: Association of the Respiratory Colonization of Premature Infants with Chronic Lung Disease and Increased Mortality. *Clinical Infectious Diseases*. Vol.39. No.8. pp.1113-1122. ISSN: 1058-4838.

Kannan, T.R., & Baseman, J.B. (2006). ADP-Ribosylating and Vacuolating Cytotoxin of *Mycoplasma pneumoniae* Represents Unique Virulence Determinant Among Bacterial Pathogens. *Proceedings of the National Academy of Sciences of U.S.A.,* Vol. 103, No. 17 (April 2006), pp.6724-6729. ISSN 0027-8424

Kannan, T.R., Provenzano, D., Wright, J.R., & Baseman, J.B. (2005). Identification and Characterization of Human Surfactant Protein A Binding Protein of *Mycoplasma pneumoniae. Infection and Immunity,* Vol. 73, No. 5 (May 2005), pp. 2828-2834, ISSN 0019-9567

Katz, B.; Patel, P.; Duffy, L.; Schelonka, R.L.; Dimmitt, R.A. & Waites, K.B. (2005). Characterization of Ureaplasmas Isolated from Preterm Infants with and without Bronchopulmonary Dysplasia. *Journal of Clinical Microbiology.* Vol.43. No.9. pp.4852-4854. ISSN: 0095-1137.

Kazachkov, M.Y.; Hu, P.C.; Carson, J.L.; Murphy, P.C.; Henderson, F.W., & Noah, T.L. (2002). Release of Cytokines by Human Nasal Epithelial Cells and Peripheral Blood Mononuclear Cells Infected with *Mycoplasma pneumoniae. Experimental biology and medicine (Maywood),* Vol. 227, No. 5 (May 2002), pp. 330-335, ISSN: 1525-1373

Krivan, H. C., Roberts, D. D., & Ginsburg, V. (1988) Many Pulmonary Pathogenic Bacteria Bind Specifically to the Carbohydrate Sequence GalNAc Beta 1-4Gal Found in Some Glycolipids. *Proceedings of the National Academy of Sciences of U.S.A.,* Vol. 85, No. 16 (August 1988), pp. 6157-6161, ISSN 0027-8424

Krivan, H.C.; Olson, LD; Barile, MF, Ginsberg, V & Roberts, D (1989). Adhesion of *Mycoplasma pneumoniae* to Sulfated Glycolipids and Inhibition by Dextran Sulfate. *Journal of Biological Chemistry,* Vol. 264, No. pp. 9283-9288, ISSN 0021-9258

Krunkosky, T.M.; Jordan, J.L.; Chambers, E., & Krause, D.C. (2007). *Mycoplasma pneumoniae* Host-Pathogen Studies in an Air-Liquid Culture of Differentiated Human Airway Epithelial Cells. *Microbial Pathogenesis,* Vol. 42, No. 2-3 (February-March 2007), pp. 98-103, ISSN 0882-4010

Kundsin, R.B., Leviton, A., Allred, E.N., & Poulin, S.A. (1996). *Ureaplasma urealyticum* Infection of the Placenta in Pregnancies that Ended Prematurely. *Obstetrics and Gynecology,* Vol. 87, No. 1 (January 1996), pp.122-127, ISSN: 0029-7844.

Li, Y.H.; Brauner, A.; Jensen, J.S. & Tullus, K. (2002). Induction of Human Macrophage Vascular Endothelial Growth Factor and Intercellular Adhesion Molecule-1 by *Ureaplasma urealyticum* and Downregulation by Steroids. *Biol Neonate.* Vol.82. No.1. pp.22-28. ISSN: 0006-3126

Li, Y.H.; Brauner, A.; Jonsson, B.; van der Ploeg, I.; S√∂der, O.; Holst, M., & Jensen, J.S. (2000). Lagercrantz H, Tullus K. *Ureaplasma urealyticum*-Induced Production of Proinflammatory Cytokines by Macrophages. *Pediatric Research,* Vol. 48, No. 1 (July 2000) pp.114-119. ISSN: 0031-3998

Li, Y.H., Chen, M., Brauner, A., Zheng, C., Jensen, J.S., & Tullus, K. (2002). *Ureaplasma urealyticum* Induces Apoptosis in Human Lung Epithelial Cells and Macrophages. *Biology of the Neonate,* Vol. 82, No. 3, pp. 166-173. ISSN: 0006-3126.

Li, Y.H.; Yan, Z.Q.; Jensen, J.S.; Tullus, K., & Brauner, A. (2000). Activation of nuclear factor kappaB and induction of inducible nitric oxide synthase by *Ureaplasma urealyticum* in macrophages. *Infection and Immunity,* Vol. 68, No. 12 (December 2000), pp. 7087-7093, ISSN 0019-9567

Lieberman, D., Ben-Yaakov, M., Lazarovich, Z., Hoffman, S., Ohana, B., Friedman, M.G., Dvoskin, B., Leinonen, M., & Boldur, I. (2001). Infectious Etiologies in Acute Exacerbation of COPD. *Diagnostic Microbiology and Infectious Diseases,* Vol. 40, No. 3 (July 2001), pp. 95–102, ISSN 0732-8893

Lieberman, D., Ben-Yaakov, M., Shmarkov, O., Gelfer, Y., Varshavsky, R., Ohana, B., Lazarovich, Z., & Boldur, I. (2002). Serological Evidence of *Mycoplasma pneumoniae* Infection in Acute Exacerbation of COPD. *Diagnostic Microbiology and Infectious Diseases,* Vol. 44, No. 1 (September 2002), pp.1–6, ISSN 0732-8893

Lo, S.C., Wear, D.J., Green, S.L., Jones, P-G., & Legier, J.F. (1993). Adult Respiratory Distress Syndrome With or Without Systemic Disease Associated With Infections Due to *Mycoplasma fermentans. Clinical Infectious Diseases,* Vol. 17, Suppl. 1 (August 1993), pp. S259-S263, ISSN 1058-4838

Lo, S.C., Dawson, M.S., Wong, D.M., Newton 3rd, P.B., Sonoda, M.A., Engler, W.F., Wang, R.Y., Shih, J.W., Alter, H.J., & Wear, D.J. (1989) Identification of *Mycoplasma incognitus* Infection in Patients with AIDS: an Immunohistochemical, *in situ* Hybridization and Ultrastructural Study. *American Journal of Tropical Medicine, and Hygiene,* Vol. 41, No. 5 (November 1989), pp. 601-616, ISSN 0002-9637

Lo, S-C; Hayes, MM & Kotani, H (1993). Adhesion Onto and Invasion Into Mammalian Cells by *Mycoplasma penetrans* - A Newly Isolated Mycoplasma From Patients with AIDS. *Modern Pathology, Vol. 6,* No. 3 (May 1993), pp. 276-280, ISSN 0893-3952

Loens, K., Goossens, H., & Ieven. M. (2010). Acute Respiratory Infection Due to *Mycoplasma pneumoniae*: Current Status of Diagnostic Methods. *European Journal of Clinical Microbiology and Infectious Diseases,* Vol. 29, No. 9 (September 2010), pp. 1055–1069, ISSN 0934-9723

Loens, K., Ieven, M., Ursi, D., Beck, T., Overdijk, M., Sillekens, P., & Goossens, H. (2003a). Detection of *Mycoplasma pneumoniae* by Real-Time Nucleic Acid Sequence-Based Amplification. *Journal of Clinical Microbiology,* Vol. 41, No. 9 (September 2003), pp. 4448-4450, ISSN ISSN: 0095-1137

Loens, K., Ursi, D., Goossens, H., & Ieven, M. (2003b). Molecular Diagnosis of *Mycoplasma pneumoniae* Respiratory Tract Infections. *Journal of Clinical Microbiology,* 2003 Vol. 41, No. 11(November 2003), pp. 4915-4923; ISSN ISSN: 0095-1137

Macfarlane, J., Holmes, W., Gard, P., Macfarlane, R., Rose, D., Weston, V., Leinonen, M., Saikku, P., & Myint, S. (2001). Prospective study of the Incidence, Aetiology and Outcome of Adult Lower Respiratory Tract Illness in the Community. *Thorax,* Vol. 56, No. 2 (February 2001), pp. 109-114, ISSN 0040-6376

Maeda, S., Deguchi, T., Ishiko, H., Matsumoto, T., Naito, S., Kumon, H., Tsukamoto, T., Onodera, S., & Kamidono, S. (2004). Detection of *Mycoplasma genitalium, Mycoplasma hominis, Ureaplasma parvum* (Biovar 1) and *Ureaplasma urealyticum* (Biovar 2) in Patients with Non-gonococcal Urethritis Using Polymerase Chain Reaction-Microtiter Plate Hybridization. *International Journal of Urology,* Vol.11. No.9. pp.750-754. ISSN: 0919-8172.

Maniloff, J. (1992). Phylogeny of Mycoplasmas. In: *Mycoplasmas: Molecular biology and Pathogenesis,* J. Maniloff, R.N. McElhaney, L.R. Finch & J.B. Baseman (Eds.), pp. 549-559, American Society for Microbiology, ISBN1-55581-050-0, U.S.A.

Manimtim, W.M., Hasday, J.D., Hester, L., Fairchild, K.D., Lovchik, J.C., & Viscardi, R.M. (2001). *Ureaplasma urealyticum* Modulates Endotoxin-Induced Cytokine Release by

Human Monocytes Derived from Preterm and Term Newborns and Adults. *Infection and Immunity*, Vol. 69, No. 6 (June 2001), pp. 3906-3915, ISSN: 0019-9567.

Mogulkoc, N., Karakurt, S., Isalska, B., Bayindir, U., Celikel, T., Korten, V., & Colpan, N. 1999. Acute Purulent Exacerbation of Chronic Obstructive Pulmonary Disease and *Chlamydia pneumoniae* Infection. *American Journal of Respiratory Critical Care Medicine*, Vol. 160, No. 1 (July 1999), pp. 349–353, ISSN 1073-449X

Momynaliev, K.T., & Govorun, V.M. (2001). Mechanisms of genetic instability in Mollicutes (mycoplasmas). *Russian Journal of Genetics;* Vol. 37, No. 9 (2001), pp. 979–992, ISSN 1022-7954

Naessens, A.; Foulon, W.; Debrucker, P.; Devroey, P. & Lauwers, S. (1986). Recovery of Microorganisms in Semen and Relationship to Semen Evaluation. *Fertility and Sterility*. Vol.45. No.1. pp.101-105. ISSN: 0015-0282.

Olson, LD & Gilbert, AA (1993). Characteristics of *Mycoplasma hominis* adhesion. *Journal of Bacteriology*, Vol. 175, No. 10 (October 1993), pp. 3224-3227, ISSN 0021-9193

Peltier, M.R.; Tee, S.C., & Smulian, J.C. (2008). Effect of Progesterone on Proinflammatory Cytokine Production by Monocytes Stimulated with Pathogens Associated with Preterm Birth. *American Journal of Reproductive Immunology*, Vol. 60, No.4, pp. 346-353, ISSN 1046-7408

Pietsch, K., Ehlers, S., & Jacobs, E. (1994). Cytokine Gene Expression in the Lungs of BALB/c Mice During Primary and Secondary Intranasal Infection with *Mycoplasma pneumoniae. Microbiology*, Vol. 140, (August 1994), pp. 2043-2048, ISSN 1350-0872

Potts, J.M.; Ward, A.M. & Rackley, R.R. (2000). Association of Chronic Urinary Symptoms in Women and *Ureaplasma urealyticum*. *Urology*, Vol. 55, No. 4, pp. 486-489, ISSN 0090-4295

Povlsen, K.; BjÃ¸rnelius, E.; Lidbrink, P. & Lind, I. (2002). Relationship of *Ureaplasma urealyticum* Biovar 2 to Nongonococcal Urethritis. *European Journal of Clinical Microbiology and Infectious Diseases*,Vol. 21, No. 2, pp.97-101, ISSN: 0934-9723

Povlsen, K.; Thorsen, P. & Lind, I. (2001). Relationship of *Ureaplasma urealyticum* Biovars to the Presence or Absence of Bacterial Vaginosis in Pregnant Women and to the Time of Delivery. *European Journal of Clinical Microbiology and Infectious Diseases*, Vol. 20, No. 1, pp. 65-67, ISSN: 0934-9723.

Razin, S. (1999). Adherence of Pathogenic Mycoplasmas to Host Cells. *Bioscience Reports*, Vol. 19, No.5 (October 1999), pp.367-372, ISSN 0144-8463

Razin, S; Yoguev, D., & Naot, Y. (1998). Molecular Biology and Pathogenicity of Mycoplasmas. *Microbiology and Molecular Biology Reviews*, Vol. 62, No. 4 (December 1998), pp. 1094-1156, ISSN 1092-2172

Rechnitzer, H., Brzuszkiewicz, E., Strittmatter, A., Liesegang, H., Lysnyansky, I., Daniel, R., Gottschalk, G., & Rottem, S. (2011). Genomic Features and Insights Into the Biology of *Mycoplasma fermentans*. *Microbiology*, Vol. 157, pp. 760-773. ISSN: 1350-0872

Roberts, D.D., Olson, L.D., Barile, M.F., Ginsburg, V., & Krivan, H.C. (1989). Sialic Acid-Dependent Adhesion of *Mycoplasma pneumoniae* to Purified Glycoproteins. *Journal of Biological Chemistry*, Vol. 5, No. 264 (June 1989), pp. 9289-9293, ISSN 0021-9258

Roberts, M.C. (1992). Antibiotic Resistance. In: *Mycoplasmas: Molecular biology and Pathogenesis*, J. Maniloff, R.N. McElhaney, L.R. Finch & J.B. Baseman (Eds.), pp. 513-523, American Society for Microbiology, ISBN1-55581-050-0, U.S.A.

Román-Méndez, C., Santellán-Olea, M.R., Cedillo, L., & Rivera-Tapia, J.A.. (2007). Alteraciones histológicas a nivel pulmonar inducidas por *Mycoplasma fermentans. Revista Mexicana de Patología Clínica*, Vol. 54, No 1, pp. 40-46.

Rottem, S., & Naot, Y. (1998). Subversion and Exploitation of Host Cells by Mycoplasmas. *Trends in Microbiology,* Vol 6, No. 11 (November 1998), pp. 436-440, ISSN 0966-842X

Rottem, S. (2003). Interaction of Mycoplasmas with Host Cells. *Physiology Reviews*, Vol. 83, No.2 (Apr 2003), pp. 417-432, ISSN 0031-9333

Saillard, C., Carle, P., Bove, J.M., Bebear, C., Lo, S.C., Shih, J.W., Wang, R.Y., Rose, D.L., & Tully, J.G. (1990). Genetic and Serologic Relatedness Between *Mycoplasma fermentans* Strains and a Mycoplasma Recently Identified in Tissues of AIDS and Non-AIDS Patients. *Research in Virolology,* Vol. 141, No. 3 (May-June 1990), pp. 385-395, ISSN 0923-2516

Schaeverbeke, T., Gilroy, C.B., Bebear, C., Dehais, J., & Taylor-Robinson, D. (1996). *Mycoplasma fermentans,* but not *M penetrans,* detected by PCR assays in synovium from patients with rheumatoid arthritis and other rheumatic disorders. *Journal of Clinical Pathology,* Vol. 49, pp. 824-828, ISSN 0021-9746

Schelonka, R.L., & Waites, K.B. (2007). Ureaplasma Infection and Neonatal Lung Disease. *Seminars in Perinatology,* Vol. 31, No.1, pp. 2-9, ISSN: 0146-0005.

Sethi S. 2000. Bacterial Infection and the Pathogenesis of COPD. *Chest,* Vol. 117, No. 5, Suppl. 1 (May 2000), pp. 286-291, ISSN 0012-3692

Shang, X.J., Huang, Y.F., Xiong C.L., Xu, J.P., Yin, L. & Wan, C.C. (1999). *Ureaplasma urealyticum* Infection and Apoptosis of Spermatogenic Cells. *Asian J Androl.* Vol.1. No.3. pp.127-129. ISSN: 1008-682X.

Shimizu, T.; Kida, Y. & Kuwano, K. (2008). *Ureaplasma parvum* Lipoproteins, Including MB Antigen, Activate NF-{kappa}B through TLR1, TLR2 and TLR6. *Microbiology.* Vol.154. No.5. pp.1318-1325. ISSN: 1350-0872.

Sirand-Pugnet, P., Citti. C., Barré, A., & Blanchard, A. (2007), Evolution of Mollicutes: Down a Bumpy Road with Twists and Turns. *Research in Microbiology* 158 (2007) 754-766. ISSN 0923-2508

Smith, C. B., Kanner, R.E., Golden, C.A., Klauber, M.R., & Renzetti Jr., A.D. (1980). Effect of Viral Infections on Pulmonary Function in Patients with Chronic Obstructive Pulmonary Diseases. *Journal of Infectious Diseases,* Vol. 141, No. 3 (March 1980), pp. 271–280, ISSN 0022-1899

Stancombe, B.B.; Walsh, W.F.; Derdak, S.; Dixon, P., & Hensley, D. (1993). Induction of Human Neonatal Pulmonary Fibroblast Cytokines by Hyperoxia and *Ureaplasma urealyticum. Clinical Infectious Diseases,* Vol. 17, Suppl 1 (August 1993), pp. S154-S157, ISSN 1058-4838

Sun, G.; Xu, X.; Wang, Y.; Shen, X.; Chen, Z., & Yang, J. (2008). *Mycoplasma pneumoniae* Infection Induces Reactive Oxygen Species and DNA Damage in A549 Human Lung Carcinoma Cells. *Infection and Immunity,* Vol. 76, No. 10 (October 2008), pp. 4405-4413, ISSN 0019-9567

Svenstrup, H.F.; Nielsen, P.K.; Drasbek, M.; Birkelund, S. & Christiansen, G. (2002). Adhesion and Inhibition Assay of *Mycoplasma genitalium* and *M. pneumoniae* by Immunofluorescence Microscopy. *Journal of Medical Microbiology,* Vol. 51, No. 5 (May 2002), pp. 361-373, ISSN 0022-2615

Taylor-Robinson, D., Davies, H. A., Sarathchandra, P., & Furr, P. M. (1991). Intracellular Location of *Mycoplasmas* in Cultured Cells Demonstrated by Immunocytochemistry and Electron Microscopy. *International Journal of Experimental Pathology,* Vol. 72:, pp. 705-714. ISSN 0959-9673

Taylor-Robinson, D. (1996). Infections Due to Species of *Mycoplasma* and *Ureaplasma*: an Update. *Clinical Infectious Diseases, 23*: 671-684. ISSN 1058-4838

Torres-Morquecho, A., Rivera-Tapia, A., González-Velazquez, F., Torres, J., Chávez-Munguia, B., Cedillo-Ramírez, L., & Giono-Cerezo, S. (2010). Adherence and Damage to Epithelial Cells of Human Lung by *Ureaplasma urealyticum* strains biotype 1 and 2. *African Journal of Microbiology Research,* Vol. 4, No. 6 (March 2010), pp. 480-491, ISSN 1996-0808

Tully, J. G. 1993. Current Status of the Mollicute Flora of Humans. *Clinical Infectious Diseases,* Vol. 17, Suppl. 1(August 1993), pp. S2-S9, ISSN 1058-4838

Van Kuppeveld, F.J.M., Van Der Logt, J.T.M., Angulo, A.F., van Zoest ,M.J., Quint, W.G., Niesters, H.G., Galama, J.M., & Melchers, W.J. (1992). Genus- and Species-Specific Identification of Mycoplasmas by 16S rRNA Amplification. *Applied and Environmental Microbiology,* Vol. 58, No. 8 (August 1992), pp. 2606-2615, ISSN 0099-2240

Viscardi, R.M. (2010). *Ureaplasma* Species: Role in Diseases of Prematurity. *Clinics in Perinatology,* Vol.37. No.2 (June 2010). pp.393-409, ISSN 0095-5108.

Viscardi, R.M., Manimtim, W.M., Sun, C.-C.J., Duffy, L., & Cassell, G.H. (2002). Lung Pathology in Premature Infants with *Ureaplasma urealyticum* Infection. *Pediatric and Developmental Pathology,* Vol. 5, No. 2 (March-April 2002), pp. 141-150, ISSN 1093-5266

Volgmann, T.; Ohlinger, R. & Panzig, B. (2005). *Ureaplasma urealyticum*-Harmless Commensal or Underestimated Enemy of Human Reproduction? A review. *Archives of Gynecology and Obstetrics,* Vol. 273, No.3 (December 2005), pp. 133-139, ISSN: 0932-0067.

Waites, K.B., Bebear, C.M., Robertson, J.A., Talkington, D.F., & Kenny, G.E. Laboratory Diagnosis of Mycoplasmal Infections. Cumitech 34. (2000). *Coordinating ed. FS Nolte.* Washington: American Society for Microbiology.

Waites, K.B., & Talkington, D.F. (2004). *Mycoplasma pneumoniae* and Its Role as a Human Pathogen. *Clinical Microbiology Reviews,* Vol. 17, No. 4 (October 2004), pp. 697–728, ISSN 0893-8512

Waites, K.B., & Talkington, D.F. (2005). New Developments in Human Diseases Due to Mycoplasmas. In: *Mycoplasmas: pathogenesis, molecular biology, and emerging strategies for control,* A. Blanchard & G. Browning (ed.), p. 289-354, Horizon Scientific Press, ISBN 0849398614, Norwich, United Kingdom.

Waites, K.B., Katz, B., & Schelonka, R. (2005). Mycoplasmas and Ureaplasmas as Neonatal Pathogens. *Clinical Microbiology Reviews,* Vol. 18, No. 4 (October 2005), pp. 757–789, ISSN 0893-8512

Waites, K.B., Simecka, J.W., Talkington, D.F., & Atkinson, T.P. (2007). Pathogenesis of *Mycoplasma pneumoniae* Infections: Adaptive Immunity, Innate Immunity, Cell Biology, and Virulence Factors. In: *Community-Acquired Pneumonia,* N. Suttorp, T. Welte,& R. Marre (Eds.), pp. 183-198, Birkhäuser Verlag Basel, ISBN 3-7643-7562-0, Switzerland

Waites K. B., Balish M. F., & Atkinson T. P. New Insights Into the Pathogenesis and Detection of *Mycoplasma pneumoniae* Infections. *Future Microbiology*, Vol. 3, No. 6 (2008): pp. 635–648. ISSN 1746-0913

Wang, R.Y., Hu, W.S., Dawson, M.S., Shih, J.W., & Lo, S.C. (1992). Selective Detection of *Mycoplasma fermentans* by Polymerase Chain Reaction and By Using a Nucleotide Sequence Within the Insertion Sequence-Like Element. *Journal of Clinical Microbiology*, Vol. 30, No. 1 (January 1992), pp. 245-248, ISSN: 0095-1137

Wang, Y.; Liang, C.L.; Wu, J.Q.; Xu, C.; Qin, S.X. & Gao, E.S. (2006). Do *Ureaplasma urealyticum* Infections in the Genital Tract Affect Semen Quality? *Asian Journal of Andrology*, Vol. 8, No. 5, pp. 562-568, ISSN: 1008-682X.

Williams, M. H., Brostoff, J. & Roitt, I. M. (1970). Possible Role of *Mycoplasma fermentans* in Pathogenesis of Rheumatoid Arthritis. *Lancet, Vol.* 2, No. 7667 (August 8 1970), pp. 277–280, ISSN 0140-6736

Wubbel, L., Jafri, H. S., Olsen, K., et al *Mycoplasma pneumoniae* Pneumonia in a Mouse Model. *Journal of Infectious Diseases*, 1998;178,1526-1529, ISSN 0022-1899

Yang, J., Hooper, W.C., Phillips, D.J., & Talkington, D.F. (2004). Cytokines in *Mycoplasma pneumoniae* Infections. *Cytokine and Growth Factor Reviews*, Vol. 15, No. 2-3 (April-June 2004), pp. 157-168, ISSN1359-6101

Yáñez, A. 1997. Some aspects of the pathogenicity of *Mycoplasma fermentans* in the Respiratory Tract of Hamsters and Rabbit's Joints. Doctoral dissertation. National School of Biological Sciences, National Polytechnic Institute, Mexico.

Yáñez, A., Cedillo, L., Neyrolles, O., Alonso, E., Prévost, M.C., Rojas, J., Watson, H.L., Blanchard, A,, & Cassell, G.H. (1999). *Mycoplasma penetrans* Bacteremia and Primary Antiphospholipid Syndrome. *Emerging Infectious Diseases*, Vol. 5, No. 1 (January-February 1999), pp. 164-167, ISSN: 1080-6059

Yavlovich, A., A. A. Higazi, and S. Rottem. 2001. Plasminogen Binding and Activation by *Mycoplasma fermentans. Infection and Immunity*, Vol. 69, No. 4 (April 2001), pp. 1977-1982, ISSN 0019-9567

Yavlovich, A.; Tarshis, M., & Rottem, S. (2004). Internalization and Intracellular Survival of *Mycoplasma pneumoniae* by Non-Phagocytic Cells. *FEMS Microbiology Letters*, Vol. 233, No. 2 (April 2004), pp. 241-246, ISSN: 1574-6968

Yoon, B.H.; Romero, R.; Kim, M.; Kim, E.C.; Kim, T.; Park, J.S. & Jun, J.K. (2000). Clinical Implications of Detection of *Ureaplasma urealyticum* in the Amniotic Cavity with the Polymerase Chain Reaction. *American Journal of Obstetrics and Gynecology*, Vol.183, No.5 (November 2000), pp. 1130-1137, ISSN: 0002-9378.

Yoon, B.H.; Romero, R.; Lim, J.H.; Shim, S.S.; Hong, J.S.; Shim, J.Y. & Jun, J.K. (2003). The Clinical Significance of Detecting *Ureaplasma urealyticum* by the Polymerase Chain Reaction in the Amniotic Fluid of Patients with Preterm Labor. *American Journal of Obstetrics and Gynecology*. Vol. 189, Vol. 4 (October 2003), pp. 919-924, ISSN: 0002-9378.

Pulmonary Paracoccidioidomycosis: Clinical, Immunological and Histopathological Aspects

Luz E. Cano[1,2,*], Ángel González[1,2], Damaris Lopera[1], Tonny W. Naranjo[1,3] and Ángela Restrepo[1]
[1]*Corporación para Investigaciones Biológicas (CIB),*
[2]*Escuela de Microbiología, Universidad de Antioquia (UdeA),*
[3]*Escuela Ciencias de la Salud, Universidad Pontificia Bolivariana (UPB),*
Medellín,
Colombia

This chapter is dedicated to the memory of a great scientist, a man of vision, a true mentor, Professor Henrique Leonel Lenzi, Emeritus Professor, Laboratory of Pathology, Instituto Oswaldo Cruz (Fiocruz), Rio de Janeiro, Brazil

1. Introduction

The systemic endemic mycoses are a group of microbial pathologies affecting primarily the lower respiratory tract, often overlooked in the evaluation of community-acquired pneumonia. They form a heterogeneous group caused by dimorphic fungi that share similar characteristics. All of them have the respiratory tract as the portal of entry and from the lungs they may disseminate to the mucous membranes, the skin, and many other organs. Nonetheless, each fungal disease has specific characteristics concerning its clinical course, diagnosis, and management. Interestingly, specific geographical areas of the world have been associated with acquisition of these mycoses. The diagnosis may be difficult and delayed owing to the varied manifestations and the multitude of differential diagnoses (Bonifaz et al., 2011; Hsu et al., 2010).

The major endemic systemic mycoses include histoplasmosis, coccidioidomycosis, blastomycosis, paracoccidioidomycosis (PCM), and penicilliosis. All of them can cause disease in both immunocompetent and immunocompromised hosts, in particular, AIDS and organ transplantation patients, and more recently recipients of biological therapies, such as TNF inhibitors or antagonists. These mycoses have similar clinical and radiologic presentations but require different treatments. Furthermore, when they have spread to the lymph nodes or skin, they may mimic other pathologies such as leishmaniasis, lymphoma, and syphilis, among others (Bonifaz et al., 2011).

* Corresponding Author

In addition, some of them have been reported outside of the endemic areas (Europe, Japan, USA), all cases occurring in immigrants, tourists, or workers returning from endemic countries (Buitrago et al., 2011; Poisson et al., 2007).
For these reasons, it is essential that physicians around the world be informed of the clinical characteristics of these fungal diseases in order to include them in their differential diagnosis of patients coming from or visiting the recognized endemic areas.

2. Defining paracoccidioidomycosis (PCM)

Paracoccidioidomycosis (PCM) is an endemic systemic mycosis caused by the thermally dimorphic fungus, *Paracoccidioides brasiliensis*. The infection is acquired after inhalation of the infectious particles (conidia) produced by the fungus's mycelia form present in its as yet unknown natural habitat (Restrepo & Tobón, 2009; Restrepo et al., 2011). This fungal pathogen has two morphotypes, a mold at temperatures under 28°C that frequently reveals chlamydoconidia and more rarely conidia (size <5 µm): the latter can transform into yeast cells under the influence of body temperature. In tissues and cultures at 35°C–37°C, this fungus grows as a yeast resembling a pilot's wheel due to its multiple buds (Figure 1). Yeast cells are round to oval but quite variable in size (4–40 µm).

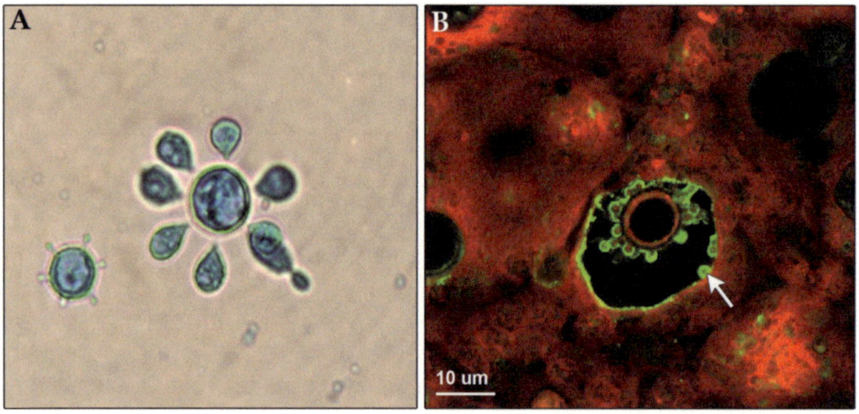

Fig. 1. *P. brasiliensis* budding yeast cells. (A) Pilot's wheel-like appearance of yeasts observed in a lactophenol cotton blue preparation from a colony grown at 36ºC. (B) Multiple budding yeast cells observed in lung tissue with small spheric buds (arrow), attached to or released (arrow) from a large mother cell. Confocal indirect immunofluuorescence for fibronectin-covered *P.brasiliensis* yeast cells.

P.brasiliensis is only known in its asexual (anamorph) stage, but through molecular techniques it has been classified in the phylum Ascomycota, order Onygenales, family Onygenacea, close to *Histoplasma capsulatum*, *Blastomyces dermatitidis*, and *Emmonsia parva* phylogenetic tree, all of which have a teleomorphic, sexual stage in the genus *Ajellomyces* (Bialek et al., 2000b; Brummer et al., 1993).
More recently, the presence and expression of the mating type locus in several isolates of this fungus have been reported (Torres et al., 2010). Other studies have revealed that there are at least three distinct phylogenetic species, or clades, which are recognized within the genus (PS2, PS3, and S1) (Matute et al., 2006). In addition and based on high polygenetic

diversity and exclusive morphogenetic characteristics, a different species, designated as *P.lutzi*, has been proposed (Teixeira et al., 2009).

2.1 General concepts on ecology

Geography sets PCM apart from other endemic mycoses of the Americas, such as histoplasmosis and coccidioidomycosis, as it is strictly confined to Latin America from Mexico at 23° North to Argentina at 34° South (Colombo et al., 2011; Nucci et al., 2009; Restrepo et al., 2011). The endemic areas are thus contained within the Tropics of Cancer and Capricorn (Bonifaz, 2010). PCM, however, is much more frequently reported in South- than in Central-American countries respecting Chile, Surinam, the Guyana, Nicaragua and Belize and with rare exceptions (one case each in Trinidad, Grenada and Guadeloupe), also the Caribbean Islands (Lacaz et al., 2002; Restrepo et al., 2011). Brazil accounts for over 80% of all reported cases with Venezuela, Colombia, Ecuador, Bolivia and Argentina informing lesser proportion of cases (Colombo et al., 2011; Restrepo et al., 2011).

Additionally, this mycosis is not distributed homogeneously within a particular endemic territory but is concentrated in tropical and subtropical regions with abundant forests and waterways, high annual rainfall indices (1400–2999 mm), and mild temperatures (17°C–24°C) predominating throughout the year (Borelli, 1972; Calle et al., 2001; Restrepo et al., 2001). Soil texture and moisture availability are also important (Conti-Díaz, 2007; Restrepo et al., 2001), as found in Brazil by spatial and ecologic correlate analyses (Simões et al., 2004). Studies on this aspect discovered a cluster of juvenile patients with the acute or subacute form who were potentially connected to the 1982–83 El Niño Southern Oscillation (ENSO) climatic anomalies (Barrozo et al., 2010).

P. brasiliensis's microniche has not been pinpointed precisely because the few isolations from natural sources have been sporadic, with soil being the substrate most frequently mentioned (Franco et al., 2000). Presently, there are indications that the habitat is to be found near waterways or in humid areas also propitious to agricultural crops such as coffee, tobacco and sugar cane (Calle et al., 2001; Restrepo et al., 2001). One hypothesis postulated that fish and aquatic birds would be required around the microniche to allow survival and dispersion of the fungus in nature (Conti-Díaz, 2007). Of ecological importance is the regular isolation of the fungus from armadillos (*Dassypus novemcinctus, Cabassous centralis*) captured in the endemic areas, some of which revealed internal lesions (Bagaggli et al., 2003). Dogs and other domesticated and feral animals have also been implicated (Ricci et al., 2004; Richini-Pereira et al., 2008). Nonetheless, *P. brasiliensis*'s microniche remains unknown despite many attempts to isolate it from suspected sites such as the permanent areas of residence of patients, in and around armadillos' burrows and their foraging areas (Restrepo et al., 2001).

Another circumstance that has hindered tracing the habitat has been the lack of information on outbreaks, which could have facilitated detection of the common source of infection (Lacaz et al., 2002; Restrepo et al., 2001). An increased number of childhood cases in areas where this disorder had previously been considered rare was noted by Coimbra et al. (1994) and Gonçalves et al. (1998), who suggested that colonization, gradual felling of the original native forests or changes in agricultural practices had probably exposed children to aerosolized fungal propagules, leading to increased disease rates. By the same token, in their study of 1,000 patients, Bellissimo-Rodrigues et al. (2011) pinpointed an area with the highest number of juvenile PCM cases, all of whom had resided close to coffee plantations, thereby raising the possibility of aerosol infection through agriculture-related work. None of the above reports, however, mentioned attempts at isolating the fungus from the environment.

Another important blocking factor in the search for the fungus's habitat is its capacity to enter prolonged quiescent stages, which has been demonstrated by the approximately 90 imported cases reported from nonendemic countries, as exemplified by the patients recently diagnosed in Europe (Buitrago et al., 2011; Mayayo et al., 2007; Poisson et al., 2007). All patients corresponded to emigrants living in Japan, the USA, Canada or several of the European countries where they had lived for a mean of 14 years after abandoning their native PCM-endemic homelands (Lacaz et al., 2002; Nucci et al., 2009; Shankar et al., 2011). These data clearly reveal *P. brasiliensis*'s ability to enter prolonged latency, to revive without notice and cause clinically manifested disease. This latency period prompted Borelli to create the term *reservarea* to indicate the site where the primary infection is thought to have occurred and distinguishing it from the site, the *endemic* area, where the infection was diagnosed (Borelli 1972).

2.2 General concepts on epidemiology

2.2.1 Distribution by age

The disease is relatively uncommon in children and adolescents with approximately 2% of all patients less than 10 years of age and 8% less than 20 years old. (Bellissimo-Rodrigues et al., 2011; Paniago et al., 2003; Shankar et al., 2011). Clinically manifested PCM occurs, consequently, more often (>80%) in adult patients 30–60 years old with the fourth decade of life presenting the largest number of cases (Colombo et al., 2011; Nucci et al., 2009; Paniago et al., 2003). The predominance of adult patients is reflected in higher mortality rates for those within this age group (Bittencourt et al., 2005; Coutinho et al., 2002; Prado et al., 2009; Santo, 2008). Although co-existence of the mycosis with HIV infection is relatively uncommon, 4%-5% according to data in the two largest series of cases published in Brazil (Belissimo-Rodrigues et al., 2011; Morejon et al., 2009), this dual infection has introduced a significant change in age distribution as these patients are younger (mean, 34 years of age) than the PCM non-AIDS cases (mean, 45 years of age).

2.2.2 Distribution by gender

Gender differences are also important markers of this fungal disorder, with adult males exhibiting overt disease much more often than females (Bellisimo-Rodrigues et al., 2011; Lacaz et al., 2002; Restrepo et al., 2011). Data taken from different series encompassing 5,500 patients revealed that 5,045 were males and 455 females for a male-to-female ratio of 11.1 to 1 (Shankar et al., 2011). In the largest Brazilian series totaling 1,000 patients, the male-to-female ratio was lower: 6 to 1. It should be noted that important variations have become apparent when comparing the series with the lowest ratio of 5.3 to 1 reported in Brazil by Blotta et al. (1999) and the highest 70.6 to 1 reported by Shankar et al. (2011) for Colombia. These findings indicate that present knowledge is insufficient to explain the male-to-female differences according to country of residence and indicate that inter-country variability needs further study.

The difference in the incidence of overt PCM between adult men and women has also been explained on hormonal grounds. In 27 women with the mycosis, 70% had menopausal signs and in 11% hysterectomy had been performed (Severo et al., 1998). Interestingly, in a series of 95 children with PCM collected from various Brazilian reports, there were 51 boys and 44 girls for a 1.16 to 1 ratio (Shankar et al., 2011). Such results contrast sharply with the 11.1 to 1 ratio recorded for overt PCM in adults. Since in children hormonal expression has not yet been fully developed, the finding of an almost equal gender distribution in prepubertal patients strengthens the protective role of hormones in this fungal disorder.

Additionally, in the experimental mouse model of PCM infection, differences in male and female animals have been noted. The fungus secretes a 17 beta estradiol-binding protein that attaches to the female hormone, regulating protein expression and hindering the mycelia to yeast transition so that in females fungal development is halted and the infection is controlled. On the other hand, in males conidia transform promptly into yeast cells and these multiply actively, resulting in progressive infection (Shankar et al., 2011). Additionally and as will be explained below, females exhibit a more active cellular immune response capable of halting the progress of the infection.

2.2.3 Distribution by occupation

Approximately 60% of the patients with active PCM work or have worked in agriculture-related jobs, notably in tobacco, coffee and sugarcane fields (Calle et al., 2001; Colombo et al., 2011; Nucci et al., 2009; Paniago et al., 2003). Other occupations mentioned in large series are masonry, bricklaying and mining, as well as lumberjacking in indigenous forests. These occupations are, ultimately, associated with inhalation of dust (Conti-Diaz & Calegari, 1979; Lacaz et al., 2002; Paniago et al., 2003; Restrepo et al., 2011). Even though residence in rural areas is a common trait among PCM patients, migration to urban settlements would be accompanied by a change in jobs so that when the diagnosis is established in these secondary localities, the medical history may record a different, non-PCM-related occupation. Additionally, recent land exploitation methods rely on insecticide application and soil burning, as done in sugarcane plantations, which should kill the fungus if present in the soil (Nucci et al., 2009; Restrepo et al., 2011). As a consequence, human exposure would no longer be as common; however, further observations are required to fully understand this point.

2.2.4 Incidence and prevalence

Despite the measures being implemented in Brazil, PCM is not yet a reportable disease, with the exception of the States of Mato Grosso do Sul, Minas Gerais and São Paulo (Bellissimo-Rodrigues et al., 2011). Consequently, prevalence and incidence rates are not fully dependable. Coutinho et al. (2002) reported an annual incidence rate of 1–3 per 100,000 inhabitants, and, based on 3,181 deaths known to have occurred as a result of PCM, a mean annual mortality rate of 1.45 per million inhabitants was estimated with a nonhomogenous spatial distribution among Brazil's regions and states. The authors concluded that PCM was important because it was the eighth cause of death from predominantly chronic or recurrent types of infections and parasitic diseases. It also had the highest mortality rate among the systemic mycoses but had low visibility. The great majority of deaths occurred in males (84.75%) and in the older age groups.

Bittencourt et al. (2005) analyzed 551 deaths of the mycosis in Parana State, Brazil, with an average annual mortality rate of 3.48 per million inhabitants, accounting not only for the fifth cause of death among the predominantly chronic infectious diseases, but also the highest mortality rate among the systemic mycoses. Santo (2008) reviewed 1,950 PCM death certificates finding that the largest number of deaths had occurred in men in the older age groups and among rural workers. The largest series of cases ever published (Bellissimo-Rodrigues et al., 2011) analyzed 1,000 Brazilian PCM patients and indicated that in the 1980–1999 period, the incidence rates for the Riberão Preto district in São Paulo State were equivalent to a mean of 2.70 cases per 100,000 inhabitants. Colombian estimates show a much lower incidence rate, with the highest being 0.24 per 100,000 inhabitants. Since these were annual mean mortality rates calculated on the basis of 7,482 deaths reported to be caused by PCM, the figures varied from 1.45 to 3.48 per one million inhabitants (Bellissimo-Rodrigues et al., 2011).

The importance of this mycosis can be inferred by the high burden of deaths occurring among the working population in individuals aged 30–60 years, mostly men engaged in agriculture (Bellissimo-Rodrigues et al., 2011).

2.3 Clinical presentations

PCM presents a gamut of clinical manifestations grouped according to the organs involved and the duration of the disease (Franco et al., 1987; Restrepo et al., 2008). Depending on the age and immune status of the host and on the size of the inhaled fungal inoculum, infection could be asymptomatic or may give rise to several different forms of disease. In immunocompetent individuals, they usually overcome fungal invasion; nonetheless, the fungus could remain quiescent, and a latent infection may be established. Four different clinical presentations are recognized, as follows.

2.3.1 Subclinical infection

After inhalation of the fungal particles, individuals may develop minor pulmonary symptoms that cannot be differentiated from those produced by other agents of pneumonia. The clinical manifestations often resolve spontaneously without medical intervention; however, the fungus could persist in a latent form and may later give rise to disease through endogenous reactivation, an event that may coincide with an alteration of the host's immune response (Benard et al., 2005). In some cases, the initial infection may leave a residual lung lesion. The latter situation presents the so-called regressive form of PCM. The latency process is known to exist and is frequently prolonged (mean, 14 years), as revealed by the cases reported outside the endemic areas (Buitrago et al., 2011; Walker et al., 2008; Shankar et al., 2011).

2.3.2 Acute/subacute or juvenile-type disease

This form of the mycosis is the result of the progression of a unresolved initial infection. The *acute/subacute progressive form* is seen mainly in undernourished children and adults less than 30 years of age and is the form observed in immunosuppressed individuals, such as those with HIV infection. The *juvenile form* is characterized by predominant involvement of the reticuloendothelial system. The mean duration of symptoms at consultation is 60 days and the most frequently involved organs are lymph nodes, skin, liver and spleen; less frequently bone marrow, stomach, small bowel, bones and joints are also invaded (Benard et al., 1994; Londero et al., 1996; Mendes, 1994; Morejon et al., 2009; Pereira et al., 2004).

2.3.3 Chronic or adult-type disease

This is the most frequently reported form of PCM, it has a prolonged course (months to years) and is diagnosed mainly in patients ranging from 30 to 50 years of age. This clinical form is characterized by significant lung damage as well as extrapulmonary manifestations. The respiratory symptoms become apparent only after several years with productive cough seen in 50% of the patients. Physical examination reveals few abnormalities even if extensive radiographic alterations are noted. The scarcity of respiratory symptoms explains why patients seek medical consultation based mainly on extrapulmonary manifestations, such as the presence of mucosal and skin lesions (Gomes et al., 2008; Marchiori et al., 2011; Mendes, 1994; Tuder et al., 1985). Besides the lungs, the most frequently compromised organs are the oral mucosa (involving oropharynx and larynx), skin and adrenal glands. Less frequently, the nasal and anal mucosa, genital organs and central nervous system may also be attacked. Mucosal lesions may be single or multiple, are progressive and destructive, giving rise to bleeding and pain, and are accompanied by dysphonia, dysphagia and sialorrhea.

2.3.4 Residual form

This form manifests the sequelae of prior disease at a moment when fungal growth has been arrested and the patient has overexpressed his immune responses to the point of developing fibrosis. This is exemplified by the *chronic form* of the mycosis where the lungs support the most prominent fibrotic changes, a complication recorded in approximately 60% of the patients (Funari et al., 1999; Naranjo et al., 1990; Tobón et al., 1995, 2003; Tuder et al., 1985). The chronic progressive adult form often precedes the establishment of the *residual form*. In most cases, when the patient is finally diagnosed, this sequela is already present, reflecting the corresponding structural and functional alterations (Benard et al., 2005; Bethlem et al., 1999; Lacaz et al., 2002; Restrepo et al., 2008). It is noteworthy that residual lesions do not respond to antifungal treatment. Pulmonary fibrosis is an incapacitating disorder that may lead to core pulmonale and, finally, to death (Tobón et al., 2003; Tuder et al., 1985).
In the differential diagnosis of PCM, various diseases including tuberculosis, histoplasmosis, leishmaniasis, malignancies, lymphomatous disorders and certain abdominal syndromes should be considered (Campos et al., 2008; Nogueira et al., 2006; Ramos & Saraiva, 2008). It is important to note that PCM may coexist with tuberculosis in approximately 10% of the cases (Gomes et al., 2008; Quagliato et al., 2007).

2.4 Establishing the diagnosis

Diagnosis of PCM is based on the identification and isolation of the fungus. The microscopic visualization in representative clinical samples (including respiratory specimens or biopsies) of multiple budding yeast cells with a pilot's wheel-like appearance by direct KOH preparations or special stains, establishes the diagnosis (Lacaz et al., 2002; Nucci et al., 2009; Restrepo et al., 2009, 2011). Isolation of the fungus in culture is considered the gold standard and is successful in 60–85% of the cases. Additionally, serologic and immune-based tests [including agar gel immunodiffusion, complement fixation, enzyme-linked immunosorbent assays (ELISA) and antigen detection] are also frequently employed. These laboratory tests have great value and can also be employed in follow-up studies (Gómez et al., 1997, 1998; Lacaz et al., 2002; Nucci et al., 2009; Restrepo et al., 2009, 2011). In addition, in the last decade, molecular tests to diagnose PCM have been implemented; these tests require further research (Buitrago et al., 2011; Gomes et al., 2000; Bialek et al., 2000a; Koishi et al., 2010).

2.5 Therapeutic options

Treatment of PCM should be implemented according to the disease form; in addition, adequate nutrition, control of associated diseases, and measures to stop smoking must be implemented. Treatment of this mycosis includes sulfonamides, amphotericin B and azoles (Quagliato et al., 2007). Thus, in the case of minor and moderate forms of PCM, the combination of trimethoprim-sulfamethoxazole can be used (Shikanai-Yasuda et al., 2008). In cases of severe illness, treatment must be implemented using amphotericin B and continued with an oral antifungal, preferably itraconazole (Quagliato et al., 2007). Among the azoles, the latter is the drug of choice as it is effective in 98% of cases, irrespective of the clinical form, and has a low relapse rate (3%) (Naranjo et al., 1990; Shikanai-Yasuda et al., 2002). Nonetheless, it may not be possible to eradicate the etiologic agent completely, and the risk of endogenous reactivation may persist. Treatment of PCM is prolonged, usually taking 6 months to 1 or maximum 2 years, but in general it should continue until clinical manifestations are resolved, except for those due to residual fibrotic sequelae (Hahn et al., 2000; Shikanai-Yasuda et al., 2002).

3. Pathogenesis of experimental PCM in mice

Animal models are excellent tools to study the pathogenesis of the different infectious diseases. In order to understand the pathogenesis of PCM, different animal models of this mycosis have been established, using different hosts such as mice (Calich et al., 1985; Cano et al., 2000; Defaveri et al., 1982; McEwen et al., 1987; Moscardi & Franco, 1980), hamsters (Essayag et al., 2002; Iabuki & Montenegro, 1979; Peraçoli et al., 1982), guinea pigs (Fava-Netto et al., 1961) and rats (Iovannitti et al., 1999). All of these are powerful tools to explore the molecular and cellular aspects of PCM pathogenesis. The ability to control multiple variables in the establishment of the experimental models allows simulation of the human disease states and monitoring their course quantitatively. Therefore, animal models are a useful alternative to study the kinetics of the mechanisms involved in the pathogenesis of PCM.

3.1 Establishment of a pulmonary PCM model induced by *Pb*-conidia

Problems determining the initial stages of the host–*P. brasiliensis* interaction in humans when the fungal habitat is unknown indicate that an animal model of pulmonary PCM that would mimic, as closely as possible, human disease is needed. Such a model was established by the intranasal administration of *Pb*-conidia to male BALB/c mice to be studied sequentially during the course of infection (McEwen et al., 1987; Restrepo et al., 1992). In this model, we have determined certain immune, histological and radiological aspects of pulmonary lesions by histopathology (early and chronic periods) (González et al., 2008a, b, c; Lopera et al., 2010, 2011) as well as by high-resolution computed tomography-HRCT (chronic periods) (Lopera et al., 2010). The local immune response has been measured by determining different cytokines in supernatants of pulmonary homogenates (González et al., 2003, 2005b, 2008d; Naranjo et al., 2010).

3.2 Early immunological and histopathological findings in the model

It has been hypothesized that once *P. brasiliensis* conidia reach the lung, they interact initially with the extracellular matrix (ECM) proteins (expressed predominantly in lung tissue), lung epithelial cells (which also express these ECM proteins on their own surface), alveolar macrophages (Mϕs) and pulmonary dendritic cells. In addition, it has been reported that the different fungal morphotypes of *P. brasiliensis* (conidia, yeast cells and mycelia) exhibit on their surface adhesin-type molecules that allow both binding to several ECM proteins –

mainly fibronectin, fibrinogen and laminin - and adherence to epithelial cells (Caro et al., 2008; González et al., 2005a, 2008a, b; Hernández et al., 2010). Activation of pulmonary cells, mainly Mϕs, took place after fungal interaction, thus initiating the inflammatory process through production of pro-inflammatory cytokines and chemokines, which in turn induced the expression of adhesion molecules on the leukocytes' surface (González et al., 2003, 2005b).

3.2.1 Early pulmonary inflammatory process

During the first 4 days post-infection, an acute inflammatory process, composed mainly of polymorphonuclear neutrophils (PMNs) and Mϕs, was observed in the lungs (Cock et al., 2000; González et al., 2003, 2005b; Restrepo et al., 1992). At the histopathological level, this inflammatory event concurred with a bronchopneumonic process in which PMNs and Mϕs accumulated and fused with each other to constitute extensive, ill-defined masses, located inside the alveolar and the surrounding peribronchiolar spaces, resulting in involvement of approximately 40% of the lung's area (Cock et al., 2000; González et al., 2005b; Restrepo et al., 1992). It should be noted that during the first 3 days post-challenge, eosinophils and lymphocytes were also observed at the perivascular level (González et al., 2005b). After the 4th day post-challenge, the cellular infiltrate was replaced by mononuclear cells, mainly Mϕs. The results of additional studies conducted in bronchoalveolar lavage fluids (BALs) coincided with the *in situ* description, with predominance of PMNs and Mϕs during the period indicated (González et al., 2003). Interestingly, at the end of the 2nd week post-infection, the inflammatory process decreased, indicating transient control of fungal invasion (González et al., 2005b).

Similarly, high levels of pro-inflammatory cytokines [interleukin (IL)-1β, IL-6, tumor necrosis factor-alpha (TNF-α) and chemokine, macrophage inflammatory protein (MIP)-2)] were recorded, especially in the pulmonary compartments and during the first 4 days post-challenge, (González et al., 2003). The production of these molecules by both inflammatory and endothelial cells accounted for the recruitment of certain inflammatory cells indirectly through induction of adhesion molecule expression, which in turn mediated migration of the inflammatory cells into the injured tissue (Tracey & Cerami, 1994). In accordance with the above results, a significant decrease in the mouse pulmonary fungal burden occurred after the first 2 days post-challenge (Cock et al., 2000; González et al, 2005b).

3.2.2 Expression of adhesion molecules and extracellular matrix proteins in the lungs

Adhesion molecules expressed on the cell's surface of both leukocytes and endothelial cells are important mediators in the recruitment of leukocytes to sites of inflammation including the lungs (Albeda et al., 1994; Pilewski & Albelda, 1993). Expression of these adhesion molecules is induced by the production of pro-inflammatory cytokines such as TNF-α and IL-1 (Osborn et al., 1989; Masinovsky et al., 1990), which have been reported as important inflammatory components in a variety of lung diseases including those caused by fungi (Hamacher & Schaberg, 1994; Izzo et al., 1998; Yokomura et al., 2001; Yu & Limper, 1997). In our PCM mouse model, we have observed that lungs of mice infected intranasally with *P.brasiliensis* conidia show a higher expression of adhesion molecules during the first 4 days post-challenge. Thus, the intercellular adhesion molecule-1 (ICAM-1) was overexpressed mainly on bronchiolar epithelium, vascular endothelium, pneumocytes and Mϕs; the vascular cell adhesion molecule-1 (VCAM-1) was also overexpressed but only in the vascular endothelial cells, while CD18 and Mac-1, two molecules belonging to the β_2 integrin family, were strongly expressed on PMNs and Mϕs (González et al., 2005b).

In lungs of mice infected with *P. brasiliensis* conidia, an initial deposition of fibrin-like material was detected after 2 days post-infection. In addition, an increased deposition and rearrangement of the following ECM proteins - laminin, fibronectin, fibrinogen, collagen and proteoglycans - were observed not only at the beginning of infection, but also during the late periods of fungal infection (González et al., 2008c). Interestingly, this increased deposition of ECM proteins in the lungs of infected mice was accompanied by a marked afflux of pro-inflammatory cells (González et al., 2008c).

In addition, *P. brasiliensis* is known to express adhesin-like molecules on its surface that recognize and bind to ECM proteins (Barbosa et al., 2006; González et al., 2005a). More recently, in elegant experiments using antisense technology, the role of a *P. brasiliensis*-adhesin molecule was confirmed when a 32-kDa protein, a putative adhesion member of the haloacid dehalogenase (HAD) superfamily of hydrolases, conferred both adherence capacity to pulmonary human epithelial cells and virulence in a mouse model of infection (Hernández et al., 2010)

The observations described above may suggest that ECM proteins modulate the pathogenesis of PCM by means of two mechanisms: 1) participation in the migration of pro-inflammatory cells into the lungs and 2) serving as a binding protein for *P. brasiliensis* expressing on its surface adhesin-like molecules (receptors). These interactions may serve the fungus both for attachment to host tissue (evading the physical barriers) and dissemination to other organs, contributing in this manner to the establishment of the disease process.

3.2.3 Expression by pulmonary phagocytes of microbicidal molecules

During any infectious process, phagocytic cells are the main effector cells, which upon their activation (e.g., by cytokines), produce microbicidal substances [i.e., degradative enzymes, defensins, lysozymes, reactive oxygen intermediates (ROS) and reactive nitrogen intermediates (RNI)] capable of inhibiting and destroying several pathogens (Nathan & Shiloh, 2000; Newman et al., 2000).

Taking into account that both PMN and Mϕs are the principal components of the pulmonary inflammatory infiltrate of mice infected with *P. brasiliensis* conidia, the expression of microbicidal molecules produced by these phagocytic cells in the PCM model was determined. *In vivo* studies failed to detect nitric oxide (NO) production or inducible nitric oxide synthase (iNOS, the enzyme responsible for NO production) during the early days post-challenge in the lungs of mice infected with *P. brasiliensis*. Interestingly, as will be described below, a higher expression of iNOS was observed in the late periods of infection (González et al., 2008d). In additional studies, we observed an increase of *in situ* lysozyme expression (PMN and Mϕs) in the lungs of mice infected with *P. brasiliensis* conidia during the first 4 days post-challenge. This expression was accompanied by a decrease in the number of fungal propagules (González et al., 2008), observations suggesting that lysozymes may exert an antifungal effect against *P. brasiliensis*.

Altogether, the above observations led us to propose a description of the initial mechanism triggered by the infection with *P. brasiliensis* conidia:

1. Once the conidia reach the lungs, they adhere to both ECM proteins and epithelial cells through the interaction with adhesins present on their own surface; in addition, the

fungal cells may interact with alveolar Mϕs or dendritic cells present on the alveolar space.

2. Once the adhesion process or the cellular interaction takes place, induction of the production of pro-inflammatory cytokines takes place, which in turn stimulates the expression of adhesion molecules with such expression modulating the migration of circulating inflammatory cells into the lung tissue. This event triggers a strong inflammatory process, enhancing cytokine and chemokine production as well as increasing the deposition and rearrangement of ECM proteins.
3. *P. brasiliensis* conidia will experience a transitional process to yeast cells if no inhibitory mechanism intervenes in such process.
4. Once the phagocytes are activated, they will express, or produce, microbicidal molecules capable of destroying the fungus.
5. If the fungus is able to overcome the fungicidal mechanisms exerted by the host's defenses, dissemination to other organs will occur, perhaps using their adhesins to bind to ECM proteins or by producing degradative enzymes able to cleave such ECM proteins. Finally, the disease process will become established.

3.3 Chronic immune responses in the model

The intranasal inoculation of *P. brasiliensis* conidia into BALB/c male mice resulted in a progressive disease characterized by an increase of CFUs in the lungs, with maximal values at the 12th and 16th week's post-infection (Franco et al., 1998). In addition, extrapulmonary dissemination to the spleen (week 4) and liver (week 12) will take place, as indicated by the isolation in culture of the fungus from these organs (McEwen et al., 1987).

Then, during the infectious process corresponding to the chronic stages, different immunological mechanisms such as inflammatory responses, cytokine production, metalloproteinase expression, nitric oxide participation, granuloma formation and, finally, the chronic pulmonary sequelae characterized by fibrosis enter into play, as described below.

3.3.1 Production of cytokines

Additionally, several studies on the cytokines implicated in the chronic stages of experimental PCM have demonstrated, through ELISA assays and the Multiplex system, that from the 4th to the 8th week post-challenge, infected mice exhibited a significant increase in IL-1β, TNF-α, IL-12p40, RANTES, MIG, PDGF-b, IL-13 and TGF-β. Even though these cytokines have been implicated in the formation and maintenance of granuloma, some of them (IL-1β, TNF-α, IL-13 and TGF-β) are also directly involved in fibrosis generation (Franco et al., 1998; Lopera et al., 2011; Naranjo et al., 2011; Wynn, 2007).

Other authors, using both male and female mice in a PCM experimental model, have shown different immune responses that are gender-dependent with high production of Th1 cytokines and T-beta expression by the paracoccin-stimulated cultures of spleen cells from infected female mice; in contrast, cells from infected males produced higher levels of the Th2 cytokines and expressed GATA-3 (Pinzan et al., 2010). These results were confirmed using mice that had been submitted to gonadectomy followed by inverse hormonal reconstitution, where spleen cells derived from castrated males reconstituted with estradiol had produced higher levels of IFN-γ and lower levels of IL-10 than normal males in response to paracoccin stimulus. In contrast, spleen cells from castrated female mice that had been treated with testosterone produced more IL-10 and less IFN-γ than cells from normal females (Pinzan et al., 2010). In conclusion, these results reveal that the sexual hormones had a profound effect on the biology of immune cells, with estradiol favoring protective responses against *P.brasiliensis* infection.

3.3.2 iNOS expression and nitric oxide (NO) production in the lungs

In this PCM pulmonary model, the role of the NO system was determined during the chronic immune response by means of lung biopsies from infected mice. We developed an immunohistochemical stain for iNOS (NOS2) and observed that this enzyme was expressed mainly *in vivo* by the epithelioid histiocytes, with its maximal expression occurring 12 weeks after infection (González et al., 2008d). The expression of iNOS correlated significantly (r=0.77891) with the number of granulomas present in the pulmonary parenchyma (González et al., 2008d), suggesting that at this stage iNOS induction may depend on factors or mechanisms related to the environment in the granuloma (Goldman et al., 1996).

In addition, the *in vivo* administration of aminoguanidine (a highly specific inhibitor of iNOS) to *P. brasiliensis*-infected and noninfected mice induced in the former a significant reduction of their survival in comparison with negative control mice. These results suggest that during the chronic stages (12–17 weeks post-infection), the NO system played an important protective role against fungal infection (González et al., 2008d). This effect has also been observed in a model of latent tuberculosis (Flynn et al., 1998). However, Nascimento et al. (2002) proposed a dual role for nitric oxide in another experimental PCM model, where NOS2-derived NO would be essential for resistance to the fungus, but its overproduction would be associated with susceptibility.

Using NOS2-deficient mice, Livonesi et al. (2009) demonstrated that this enzyme is to be considered as a resistance factor during experimental PCM because it controls fungal proliferation, cytokine production, development of a high inflammatory response and consequently formation of necrosis. Other authors demonstrated that NO has an important role in granuloma modulation, by controlling osteopontin and MMP production, as well as by inducing loose granuloma formation and fungal dissemination, resulting, at later phases, in progression of experimental PCM (Nishikaku et al., 2009). However, iNOS-derived NO seems not to be the sole factor responsible for the immunosuppression observed during the infections caused by *P. brasiliensis*.

3.3.3 Granulomatous inflammation in the lungs during experimental PCM

The granuloma is the histologic hallmark of a variety of infectious and noninfectious processes, including PCM, all of which elicit chronic granulomatous inflammation. The word "granuloma" is derived from the Latin word *granulum*, which means a small particle of grain and, traditionally, is microscopically described as a compact, rounded aggregate of Mϕs usually surrounded by a rim of lymphocytes that results in a response to chronic antigenic stimulation. Aggregation of Mϕs is the minimum requirement of a granuloma, regardless of whether the lesion also contains necrosis, lymphocytes, plasma cells, or multinucleated giant cells (Mukhopadhyay & Gal, 2010). The granuloma functions both as a niche in which some microorganisms can grow or persist and as an immunologic microenvironment in which cells interact to control and prevent dissemination of the eliciting pathogen (Flynn et al., 2011).

Pulmonary granulomatous inflammation in experimental PCM is a dynamic process that goes from dispersal parenchymal inflammation, to well-defined nodules, from periarterial sheath inflammation to pseudotumoral masses (Figure 2) (Lopera et al., 2011). The lung's area occupied by the inflammatory reaction increases gradually from 8 to 12 weeks after *P.brasiliensis* infection, involving up to 40% of the lung's area. In the following subsections, we will describe the structure and cellular composition of granuloma during the experimental infection; review the formation and maintenance of the granuloma reported in the literature and compare the main features of human and experimental pulmonary histopathology during the course of *P. brasiliensis* infection.

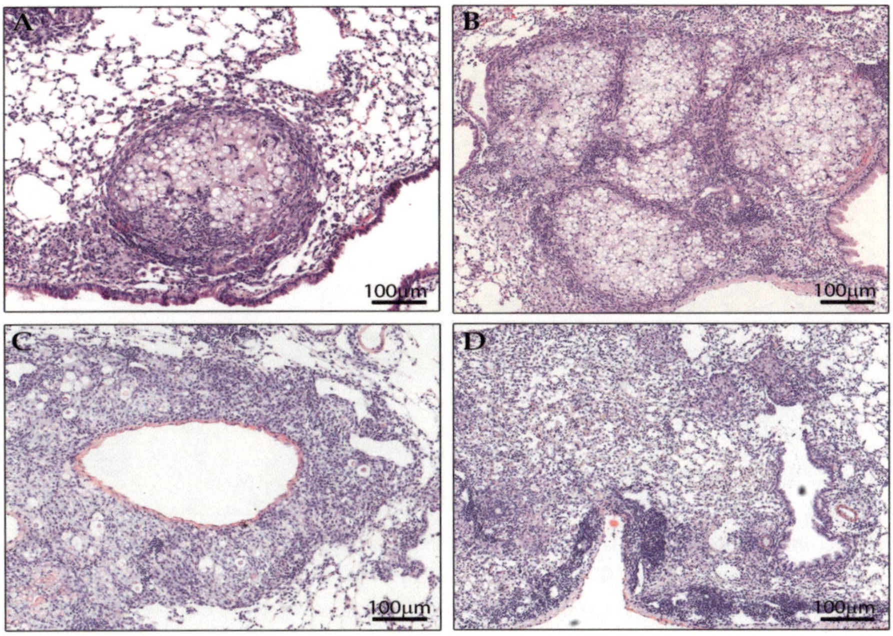

Fig. 2. Pulmonary lesions observed in BALB/c mice infected with *P. brasiliensis* conidia. (A) Well-defined nodules. (B) Confluent granulomas. (C) Periarterial sheath inflammation. (D) Dispersed parenchymal inflammation. H&E stained slides, 10X.

Structure and cellularity of pulmonary lesions: The well-defined granuloma or the nodular pattern corresponds to multiple sphere-like or oval parenchymal granulomas adjacent to terminal bronchioles, about 400 μm in diameter, sometimes isolated but becoming confluent as infection progresses. This is the predominant pattern throughout the infectious process in the lungs of BALB/c mice infected with *P. brasiliensis* conidia. In humans and experimental PCM, the general structure of granuloma consists in two distinct zones: one noncollagenic central zone composed of *P. brasiliensis* yeasts and Mϕs, and one peripheral zone composed by lymphocytes and fibroblastoid-like cells (Kerr et al., 1988). However, the cellularity and pattern of lesions change as infection progresses. A summary of the main structural and cellular changes in the granulomas sequentially observed in the experimental model of PCM is presented below (Lopera et al., 2011).

During the early stages of granuloma development, 4 weeks post-infection in our experimental model, granulomas were composed of a central core or zone of Mϕs and fungi with a frequent and intense infiltration by PMNs, sometimes presenting an apoptotic aspect. Some Mϕs formed multinucleated giant cells. The central zones of the granulomas were surrounded by a fibroblast-like layer expressing concentric layers of reticular fibers with a lesser amount of interstitial collagen. The peripheral zone consisted of a noncontinuous halo of small lymphocytes, at times forming pseudofollicular lymphocyte aggregates. At this time, an intense and diffuse parenchymal inflammation, disposed near or around the granulomas, accompanied the pulmonary response to *P. brasiliensis*.

During the most chronic stages of the infection (8, 12 and 16 weeks), Mϕs acquired a xanthomatous aspect, cholesterol crystals appeared in the central zone of the granuloma and a large number of mature plasma cells located at the periphery and mixed with the fibroblastic-like cells were observed. Besides well-defined granulomas, the peak of inflammation (8–12 weeks p.i.) was characterized by periarterial inflammation accompanied by lymphatic dilatation and edema. The cellular infiltrate defined the periarterial inflammatory sheaths with dispersed fungi (Figure 3) and more mature plasmocytes and eosinophils in comparison with the granuloma.

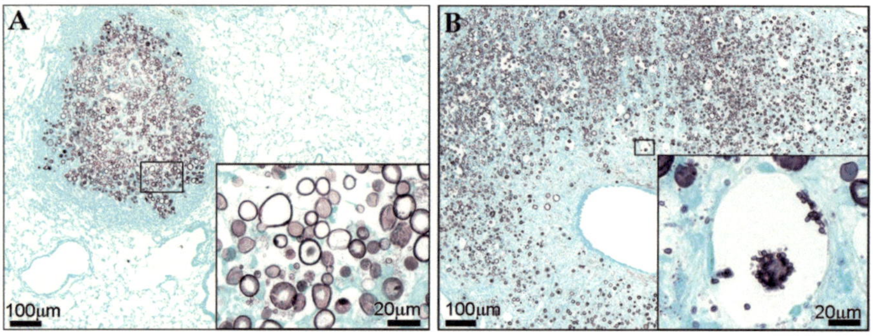

Fig. 3. Fungal aspects as seen in the lesions of a mouse with experimental pulmonary PCM. (A) Nodule full of fungi in the central area (10X), that present multiple-budding yeast cells with varying sizes (insert 100X). (B) Numerous fungi spread all over the periarterial space (10X), several of them presenting a special perifungal space (insert 100X). Grocott's stained slides.

Multiple granulomas fused and formed pseudotumoral masses or "paracoccidioidomas" five to six times larger than nodules (2,000 ± 194 μm in length) were observed in the final period of evaluation (16 weeks p.i.) in this experimental model.

Formation and maintenance of P. brasiliensis-induced granuloma: The mechanisms that drive the migration of cells that will form and maintain the granuloma around *P. brasiliensis* have begun to be explored. However, important differences in the experimental models as concerns the infective propagules (conidia, yeast cells) and the fungal isolates used, as well as the route of inoculation and the experimental host's genetic background, makes conclusions difficult. **Table 1** presents the main results of research that has analyzed the cells and mediators involved in *P. brasiliensis*-induced granulomatous inflammatory response centered on pulmonary findings.

The major biological significance of granuloma is the limitation of the infection to a local area . However, diffuse and loose granulomatous inflammation does not limit infection and is associated with incapacity to control the disease, as shown by the large number of fungal cells and the diminished survival time of infected animals (Livonesi et al., 2008, 2009).

An inflammatory response is necessary for disease control but it is also responsible for the typical immunopathology caused by diseases such as PCM that include tissue necrosis and cavitations in the center of granulomas.

Experimental model	Main results	Reference
Male BALB/c mice infected *i.n.* with 26×10^6 viable or heat-killed *P.brasiliensis* yeasts; or inoculated with 6.5×10^6 nonviable fragmented yeast cells	Granuloma formation required viable yeast cells or conidia. Heat-killed *Pb* yeasts or yeast fragments did not induce granuloma formation.	(Bedoya et al., 1986; Cock et al., 2000)
Rats infected *i.p.* with *P.brasiliensis* yeasts	Although most lesions developed in peritoneal cavity, granulomas also appeared in lung. Pulmonary granulomas were less collagenic than those observed in omentum, diaphragm and liver.	(Kerr, et al., 1988)
Male C57Bl/6 mice and IFN-γ and TNF receptor p55-deficient mice infected *i.v.* with 1×10^6 *P.brasiliensis* yeast cells	IFN-γ and TNF receptor p55-deficient mice were not able to build organized granulomas, presented greater number of fungi and high rates of mortality.	(Souto et al., 2000)
Male C57BL/6 and ICAM-1KO mice infected *i.t.* with 1×10^6 *Pb* 18 yeast cells	ICAM-1 was required for the early formation of granulomas. In the absence of ICAM-1, granuloma development delayed 60 days vs. 30 days in control mice.	(Moreira et al., 2006)
In vitro granuloma model induced by gp43-coated beads	*In vitro* granuloma formation required B1-cells and Mϕs interaction. Mϕs alone were not able to migrate to the beads and form granulomas. Soluble gp43 antigen-enhanced granuloma-like structure formation.	(Vigna et al., 2006)
BALB/c and BALB/Xid mice infected *i.t.* with 1×10^6 *Pb*18 yeast cells	Mice deficient in B1-cells (BALB/Xid mice) exhibited smaller pulmonary granulomas with less fungi and longer survival. Therefore, B1-cells participated in the exacerbation of granulomatous lesions and increased host susceptibility to infection.	(Popi et al., 2008)
C57BL/6 IL-12p40$^{-/-}$ and WT mice infected *i.v.* with 1×10^6 *Pb*18 yeast.	In the absence of the IL-12p40 subunit, involved in both IL-12 and IL-23 formation, mice developed high number of pulmonary granulomas without defined delimitations associated with high number of yeast cells.	(Livonesi et al., 2008)
C57BL/6 iNOS$^{-/-}$ and WT mice infected *i.v.* with 1×10^6 *Pb*18 yeast	iNOS$^{-/-}$ mice showed granulomas with high inflammatory response, central necrotic areas, diffuse distribution of cells, incipient reticulin fiber pattern and high number of yeast cells.	(Livonesi et al., 2009)
BALB/c male mice infected *i.n.* with 4×10^6 *P.brasiliensis* conidia	Extracellular matrix proteins overexpressed and suffered rearrangement process during the course of infection. These ECM proteins localized surrounding the granuloma.	(Gonzalez et al., 2008c)

Abbreviations: *i.n.*: intranasally, *i.p.*: intraperitoneally, *i.t.*: intratracheally *i.v.*: intravenously, *Pb: P. brasiliensis,* WT: wild-type

Table 1. Contribution of cell subsets and molecules in pulmonary granuloma formation following infection with *P. brasiliensis.*

3.3.4 Fibrosis as sequelae of PCM disease

Pulmonary fibrosis is detected in several disorders with known or unknown etiologies (Datta et al., 2011). In this sense, this progressive and prominent complication is also observed in approximately 60% of patients suffering from the chronic form of PCM (Restrepo et al., 2008). Given that the *P. brasiliensis* microniche remains uncharacterized and taking into consideration the prolonged latency observed in PCM, the characteristics of the primary infection have not been defined, and great difficulties have arisen when sequentially evaluating the development of fibrosis attributed to this infection in humans. However, results from the experimental pulmonary PCM model have given convincing evidence as to the progress of this disease (González et al., 2008b).

In contrast with idiopathic pulmonary fibrosis (IPF) for which current research indicates that inflammation is of lesser importance with fibrosis appearing primarily as a disorder of fibroblast proliferation and activation in response to an as yet unknown trigger (Meltzer & Noble, 2008), the development of fibrosis in PCM is a progressive event, resulting from a persistent antigenic stimulus leading to chronic inflammation and establishment of fibrosis mainly located in the perihilar region, the main bronchi and their branches, and the large pulmonary vessels (Restrepo et al., 2011). The functional limitation caused by the development of fibrosis may advance toward cor pulmonale, progressive lung incapacity and finally death (Restrepo et al., 2008; Tobón et al., 2003; Tuder et al., 1985).

The fibrosis process begins with acute injury caused by the interaction of *P. brasiliensis* conidia with ECM proteins and lung epithelial cells; this interaction is followed by chronic granulomatous inflammation with fibroblast proliferation and activation, an increase in ECM proteins predominantly composed of fibronectin, fibrinogen, collagen type I and III, as observed in the surroundings of the granulomas.

These EM proteins contribute to the establishment of fibronodular lesions that continue to advance even after appropriate antifungal therapy with itraconazole, a medication that effectively controls the active stage of this mycosis but does not hinder lung fibrosis (González et al., 2008a, c; Naranjo et al., 2010; Tobón et al., 2003).

Even though patients with chronic PCM show well-established pulmonary lesions at diagnosis, all of them are not in the same stage of infection development, explaining why, although not sequentially, several studies have been able to describe certain histological patterns present during the development of fibrosis in humans. Tuder et al. (1985) described the lungs of 12 patients with chronic PCM in histopathological terms and concluded that chronic pulmonary PCM is a disease that affects both lungs equally and that fibrosis is mainly related to the progressive course of the granulomatous reaction to cicatrization and, to a lesser degree, is probably due to direct induction by the fungi. This study described extensive areas of dense fibrosis close to the hilar region and involved structures such as the bronchi and lymph nodes with fibrosis extending as fibrous septa of variable thickness throughout the lung parenchyma (Tuder et al., 1985).

With the development of HRCT, several studies have been published demonstrating the correlation between histopathological and radiological findings, thus providing a more precise characterization of the pattern and magnitude of the lung abnormalities, as well as better follow-up of patients with chronic pulmonary PCM. In regards to fibrotic findings on chest tomography, this process has been described as thickening of interlobular and alveolar septa, primarily those interconnecting the granulomas (Marchiori et al., 2011). This has been correlated histopathologically with prominent collagen deposition, especially near the hilar regions, comprising lymph nodes, bronchi and the main pulmonary artery branches; additionally, pulmonary architectural alterations were also observed (Funari et al., 1999; Marchiori et al., 2011; Souza et al., 2006).

Notwithstanding, in some patients, fibrosis development has been recorded in the absence of a clearly established granulomatous reaction, thus allowing speculation that the fungus itself might induce an active and higher collagen deposition (Marchiori et al., 2011; Tuder et al., 1985).

In reference to PCM animal models, several have been developed with the purpose of understanding the complete course of the disease; despite differences on the inoculum used (infective forms and concentration), fungal isolates, route of inoculation and host genetic background, the results have made it possible to define certain common phases during the granulomatous inflammation process (Burger et al., 1996; Calich et al., 1985; Da Silva et al., 2009; Xidieh et al., 1999). However, only the murine model of chronic pulmonary PCM in male BALB/c mice induced by the intranasal inoculation of naturally infective conidia has provided a reproducible model to observe in detail not only the characteristics of the inflammatory response induced by *P. brasiliensis* conidia, but also the important components of the PCM residual form (Cock et al., 2000; González et al., 2008a; Restrepo et al., 1992).

In the murine model described above, it was determined that at 4 weeks post-infection, when the granuloma are well shaped, thin fibers of collagen and reticulin became evident, suggesting the beginning of a fibrotic process, which progressed simultaneously with the presence of leukocyte infiltrates surrounding the granuloma (Lopera et al., 2010). After the 8th week post-infection, thick fibers of collagen and reticulin became evident as an indicator of established fibrosis; fibers of both proteins gradually increasing up to 12 weeks post-infection indicated the collagenesis process reaching its highest intensity, with particular involvement of the periarterial space and the surrounding area of the granuloma (Figure 4), whether or not it was confluent. Observations made in the 16th week post-infection revealed a well-established pulmonary fibrosis process (González et al., 2008b, c; Lopera et al., 2010; Naranjo et al., 2010).

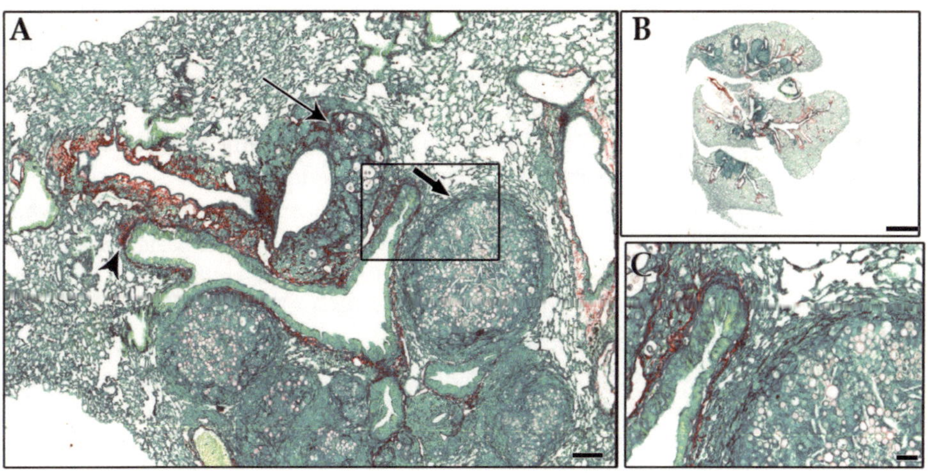

Fig. 4. Characteristics of lung fibrosis in *P. brasiliensis* infected mice. (A) Increased collagen (red fibers) noticed in the periarterial inflammatory reaction (thin arrow), in the periphery of granulomas (thick arrow) and in the bronchial wall (arrow's head). (B) Panoramic view of the entire lung. (C) Detail of collagen fibers deposition in the periphery of a granuloma and around a bronchus. Picrosirius and fast green (PIFG) stained lung sections. (Scale bars: A = 100μm, B = 2mm and C = 30μm).

One of the pathogenic mechanisms involved in the progressive accumulation of collagen and later development of fibrosis could be the disproportion between synthesis and degradation of ECM components such as reticulin and collagen, primarily due to an imbalance among the mediators of matrix degradation, metalloproteinases (MMPs) and their inhibitors (Garcia-de-Alba et al., 2010; Pardo & Selman, 2006). The presence of MMPs, specifically collagenase MMP-1 and gelatinase-A MMP-2, and the tissue inhibitors of MMPs (TIMP-1) was evaluated using immune stain in the murine model of pulmonary PCM. The results indicated that 4 weeks after *P. brasiliensis* intranasal inoculation, 85% of infected mice expressed MMP-1 as MMP-2 and 71% of them expressed TIMP-1, both with moderate intensity; at 16 weeks post-infection, almost all them showed equally positive immune stains to the TIMP-1 and MMPs evaluated, with the difference that close to 37% of them exhibited high stain intensity (Bárcenas et al., 2004). The immune stain was observed on epithelial alveolar cells and alveolar Mϕs located in peribronchial tissue, although by immune staining, it was not possible to observe an imbalance between MMPs and TIMP-1. This study suggested that as more collagen becomes deposited, more activity of MMPs and their inhibitors will be present.

Although much remains to be done, the results offered by animal models have contributed greatly to understanding the genesis of the fibrotic process in PCM.

3.3.5 Experimental attempts to control fibrosis

Although currently several antifungal drugs are available for the treatment of PCM, as mentioned above in the diagnosis and treatment sections, the majority of them require prolonged therapies oscillating between 1 and 2 years (Borges-Walmsley et al., 2002). Additionally and even though these antifungal drugs can arrest the progression of the infection by restricting fungal proliferation, the principal sequelae of PCM, pulmonary fibrosis, persists, and it has been observed in both humans and murine models (Naranjo et al., 2010; Tobón et al., 2003). The fibrosis process generates progressive lung incapacity and it is probably a source of *P. brasiliensis* in future relapses of the disease (Borges-Walmsley et al., 2002). For these reasons, the need to search for new drugs or for the implementation of combined therapies has been indicated (Pappas, 2004), including experiments aiming to prevent or at least reduce the appearance of this serious sequela.

According to the recommendations given by the American Thoracic Society, the basic therapy for the treatment of patients suffering from pulmonary fibrosis includes certain immunosuppressive drugs based on the theory that the development of fibrosis is attributable to persistent inflammatory stimulus. However, the effect of using this kind of medication in humans with the chronic form of PCM remains unknown.

Recently, we evaluated the effect of two combined therapies (itraconazole + prednisolone) and (itraconazole + pentoxifylline) on the development of fibrosis using our murine model of pulmonary PCM, which reproduces the human infection from its inception until reaching the chronic form (Naranjo et al., 2011). In this study, the azolic derivative (itraconazole) was used because it is the antifungal treatment of choice for PCM (Restrepo et al., 2011; Shikanai-Yasuda et al., 2006). In reference to the combined itraconazole + prednisolone therapy, the authors reported that although a significant reduction in both granulomatous inflammation and development of fibrosis was observed when this combined therapy was used, once it was ended, the fibrotic process reappeared and progressed over the levels observed when treatment with itraconazole alone was given. On the contrary, the use of itraconazole combined with pentoxifylline, a methylxanthine compound with recognized immune modulatory properties (Inoue et al., 2004; Tong et al., 2004) and antifibrotic effects when acting on fibroblast cells (Fang et al., 2003; Romanelli et al., 1997; Valente et al., 2003), generated good results.

The combined itraconazole + pentoxifylline therapy promptly reduced the granulomatous inflammation and caused a significant and rapid decrease of both thin reticulin and collagen fibers. The most important result was that thick fiber deposition of these proteins, which are considered fibrosis indicators, was reduced to normal levels, as seen in the uninfected mice, and remained low even after the end of the treatment. Considering fungal loads, it was demonstrated that the addition of pentoxifylline to itraconazole treatment did not produce additional deleterious effects on itraconazole antifungal activity; on the contrary, a tendency towards a faster reduction of fungal burdens was observed when the combined therapy was used (Naranjo et al., 2011). These beneficial effects were noted even when such combined therapy was started belatedly at 8 weeks post-infection, a time at which the fibrosis process was already established in the murine model.

The fact that in mice the combined itraconazole + pentoxifylline therapy promptly reduced the development of pulmonary fibrosis to levels lower than those seen with antifungal therapy alone, and that this effect was maintained even after treatment termination, presents a promising advance in the development and establishment of adjunctive immunotherapies for the treatment not only of pulmonary chronic PCM but also of several disorders or chronic infections that lead to the development of fibrosis.

These findings could imply not only a reduction of treatment costs but, more importantly, improvement in the chronic pulmonary PCM patients' quality of life.

4. Pulmonary histopathology in patients with PCM: The counterpart of the experimental infection

Reports on the pathologic features of pulmonary lesions in patients with the chronic adult form of PCM are scarce in the literature. The classical report was published by Tuder et al. (1985), who described five main pathologic aspects in the lungs of 12 patients with PCM as follows:

1. Pneumonic reaction characterized by acute alveolitis with histiocytes, few PMNs, lymphocytes and plasma cells;
2. Early granulomatous formation described as circumscribed epithelioid granulomas with reticulin fibers but with no dense collagen layer surrounding them;
3. Mature and healed granuloma with collagen in their periphery;
4. Mixed pattern (early and mature granuloma in the same pulmonary area);
5. Pulmonary fibrosis.

In addition, the pulmonary lesions could be either diffuse or circumscribed (Machado, 1965).

Most recently, a study that included 23 patients with lung samples obtained by surgical biopsy or at necropsy showed similar pathological features that included alveolar wall and interlobular septal thickening, as determined by the accumulation of inflammatory cells or, less frequently, by fibrosis; filling of the alveolar spaces with inflammatory exudate; granulomas with or without fibrosis; and other evidence of fibrosis, such as architectural distortion and honeycombing. Cavitation secondary to necrosis was also a common finding (Marchiori et al., 2011).

As mentioned before, the PCM experimental animal models revealed a chronic, progressive infection that closely resembled human lesions but that did not reproduce certain histopathological aspects such as cavitated nodules, emphysema and the honeycombing pattern.

5. Radiological aspects of PCM in humans and experimental mice

Conventional HRCT has been applied as a noninvasive tool to evaluate and quantify pulmonary damage occurring in our experimental model of PCM (Lopera et al., 2010). This work has revealed that noninvasive conventional medical x-ray tomography is adequate to follow the sequential lung lesions in experimental PCM in mice. This procedure allowed detection of the main pathological patterns, the differential topographic distribution of the pulmonary lesions in both lungs, and their intensity.

The intensity of the inflammatory reaction, evaluated by histomorphometry, increased until the 12th week of infection, with a subsequent decrease due to the tendency to form predominantly compact and more isolated pseudotumoral masses. This histopathological behavior was also detected by HRCT, as expressed by lung density measures (Hounsfield units, HU) that showed a significant correlation, mainly in the upper or hilar lung region (Figure 5).

When the mice were followed up sequentially, HRCT showed that 80% of them had peribronchial consolidations that persisted throughout the evaluation periods. Pulmonary consolidations were associated with a significant increase in upper lung density as compared with controls, −263±29 vs. −426±8 HU at week 4 (*p<0.001*), −191±25 vs. −403±17 HU at week 8 (*p<0.001*), and −269±43 vs. −445±12 at week 12 (*p<0.001*). At week 16, upper consolidations tended to decrease as well as the corresponding density, −356±33 vs. −466±9 (*p<0.01*).

Histopathological analysis revealed that consolidation, as assessed by HRCT, was equivalent histologically to a confluent granulomatous reaction, while nodules corresponded to individual compact granulomas. During the same period of infection, confluent granulomas formed pseudotumoral masses that obstructed large bronchi. Discrete focal fibrosis was visible gradually around granulomas, but this finding was only evident with histopathology.

Comparing the above results with radiological findings in patients is difficult because the size of lungs, the resolution of the topographer and the protocols used.

In humans, assessment of disease progression and treatment outcome normally includes chest x-rays and then CT studies. At the time of diagnosis and in patients with active disease, chest x-ray revealed interstitial and alveolar-interstitial infiltrates, often bilateral and symmetrical, occasionally confluent, located preferentially in the central and basal areas of the lung (pattern in butterfly wings) (do Valle et al., 1992; Trad et al., 2006). A study of radiological monitoring carried out in 173 patients with chronic PCM reported presence of reticular interstitial infiltrates in 89.3% of the cases and nodular in 54.5%, bilateral alveolar in 45.4%, and mixed (in butterfly wings) in 44.7%. Emphysema was reported in 34.1%, septal lines by 25.7%, pleural thickening by 7.5%. Nine cases (6.8%) presented cavitations and three cases (2.2%) giant nodules or masses (Trad et al., 2006).

CT proved superior to conventional radiographs in demonstrating early interstitial reticular and nodular infiltrates and showed abnormal findings in the majority of patients with chronic pulmonary PCM (more than 93%).

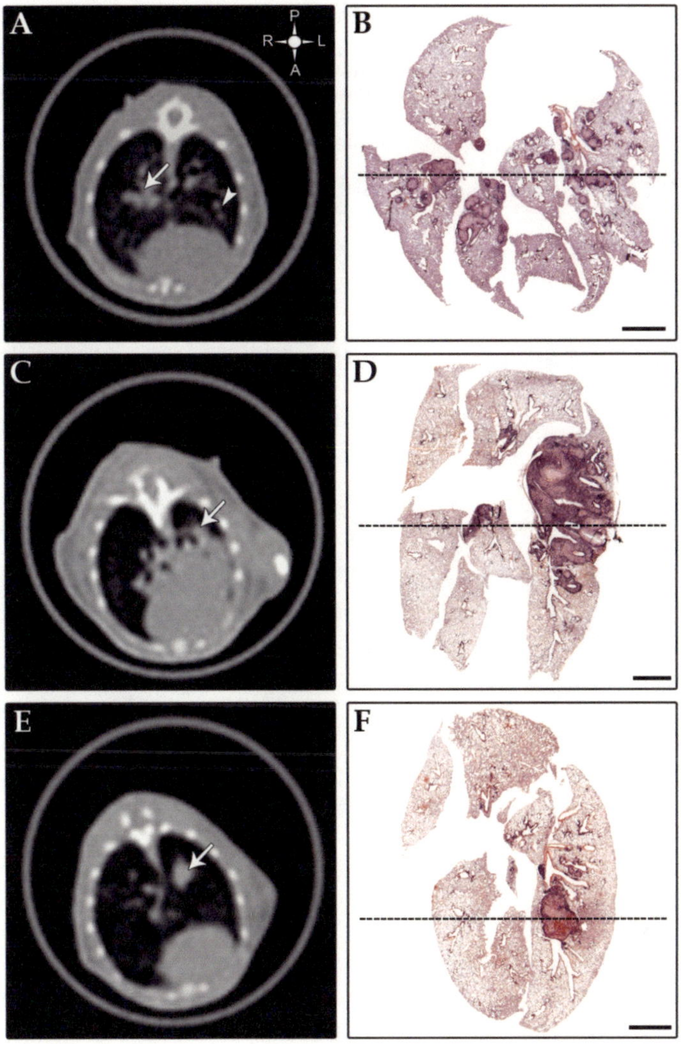

Fig. 5. Patterns of the main lung lesion as detected by conventional medical HRCT and histopathological methods in the experimental mouse PCM model. A, C, E correspond to HRCT images and B, D, F show the corresponding histopathological lesions taken in a coronal plane. The upper right symbol in (A) indicates posterior or dorsal (P), anterior or ventral (A), left (L) and right (R) regions. Dotted lines in B, D and F show an approximated position of the tomographic section. (A) Large nodular lesion represented by a peri-bronquial consolidation (arrow) is located at right hilar region and other left small nodules are indicated by arrowhead. (B) Several nodules with varied sizes. (C) Confluent lesion expressed by left central peri-bronchial consolidation (arrow) extended from the hilum to large area of the parenchyma. (D) Consolidated areas of perivascular and justabronchial granulomatous lesions. (E) Pseudotumoral lesion defining a left central pulmonary mass (arrow). (F) Left central pseudotumoral mass obstructing the bronchus. Scale bar for HRCT images = 1 cm. Scale bar for histopathological images = 2 mm. Adapted from PLoS Negl Trop Dis 4(6): e726. doi:10.1371/journal.pntd.0000726.g005.

The most frequent HRCT findings in patients with pulmonary PCM were ground-glass attenuation areas; small centrilobular, cavitated and large nodules; parenchymal bands; airspace consolidations; interlobular septal thickening; architectural distortion; traction bronchiectasis; paracicatricial emphysema and fibrosis. Most of those HRCT findings concentrated in the periphery and posterior regions involving all lung zones, with slight increased intensity in the middle zones (Funari et al., 1999; Marchiori et al., 2008, 2009; Muniz et al., 2002; Souza et al., 2006). The radiologic patterns described above in patients with pulmonary PCM were dependent on the stage of the disease and on the exclusion or inclusion of patients who had received previous treatment were excluded.

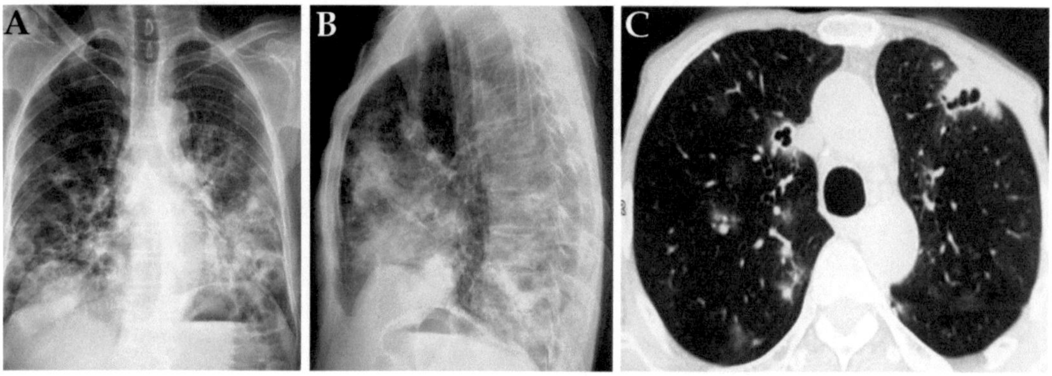

Fig. 6. Radiological findings in a patient with chronic pulmonary PMC at diagnosis.
(A, B) Postero-anterior chest and lateral radiographs showing bilateral reticulonodular and ground-glass opacities with cavitations. (C) HRCT shows consolidations, ground glass attenuations and cavitated masses.

6. Final remarks

Infection by *P. brasiliensis* is, no doubt, acquired only in the endemic areas of Central and South America, especially in Brazil. However, as the fungus exhibits the capacity to remain dormant in the tissues of the infected human host for extended periods and is, likewise, able to regain its vitality giving rise to overt disease, one may encounter the mycosis in individuals living in non-autochthonous areas, distant from those where the primary infection was acquired.

This is why it is imperative to keep informed physicians and other health-related professionals on this endemic mycosis and be prepared to include it among the differential diagnoses of disorders compatible with PCM. A detailed interrogation on the patient's former places of residence or visit should be obtained in order to focus the diagnosis. On the same token, *P. brasiliensis* should be taken into considerations whenever clinical samples and biopsies are being analyzed. It is only through knowledge that the specific diagnosis will be made in these difficult to diagnose non-autochthonous cases.

One of the main aims of this chapter was educational, namely, informing pneumologists and related professionals of the existence of this "tropical" disorder. It should be remembered that *P. brasiliensis* travels along with its host to any part of the world and that this host, now ill, may well be your own patient.

7. References

Albeda, S.M., Smith, C.W. & Ward, P.A. (1994). Adhesion molecules and inflammatory injury. *FASEB J*, Vol.8: 504–512, ISSN 0892-6638.

Bagaggli, E., Franco, M., Bosco, S. de M., Hebeler-Barbosa, F., Trinca, L.A. & Montenegro, M.R. (2003). High frequency of *Paracoccidioides brasiliensis* infection in armadillos (*Dasypus novemcinctus*): an ecological study. *Med Mycol*,Vol. 41, No. 3, pp. 217-223, ISSN 1369-3786.

Barbosa, M. S., Bao, S. N., Andreotti, P. F., de Faria, F. P., Felipe, M. S., dos Santos-Feitosa, L., Mendes-Giannini, M. J. & Soares, C. M. (2006). Glyceraldehyde-3-phosphate dehydrogenase of *Paracoccidioides brasiliensis* is a cell surface protein involved in fungal adhesion to extracellular matrix proteins and interaction with cells. *Infect Immun*, Vol. 74, No. 1, pp. 382–389, ISSN0019-9567.

Bárcenas, C., Cano, L. E., Cock A. M., Martínez, A. R. & Restrepo, A. (2004). Expresión de metaloproteinas y sus inhibidores de tejido en un modelo murino de fibrosis pulmonar. *Med-UNAB*, Vol. 7, No.19, pp. 9-14, ISSN 0123-7047.

Barrozo, L.V., Benard, G., Silva, M.E., Bagagli, E., Marques, S.A. & Mendes, R.P. (2010). First description of a cluster of acute/subacute paracoccidioidomycosis cases and its association with a climatic anomaly. *PLoS Negl Trop Dis*.Vol. 4: e643. ISSN 1935-2735.

Bedoya, V., McEwen, J.G., Tabares, A.M., Jaramillo, F.U. & Restrepo, A. (1986). Pathogenesis of paracoccidioidomycosis: a histopathological study of the experimental murine infection. *Mycopathologia*, Vol. 94, No.3, pp. 133-144, ISSN 0301-486X.

Bellissimo-Rodrigues, F., Machado, A. & Martinez, R. (2011). Paracoccidioidomycosis: epidemiological features of a 1,000 cases series from a hyperendemic area on the Southeast of Brazil. *Am J Trop Med Hyg*, Vol. 85, No.3, pp.546-50. ISSN 0002-9637.

Benard, G., Orii, N. M., Marques, H. H., Mendonça, M., Aquino, M. Z., Campeas, A. E., del Negro, G. B., Durandy, A. & Duarte, A. J. (1994). Severe acute paracoccidioidomycosis in children. *Pediatr Infect Dis J*, Vol. 13, No. 6, pp. 510-515, ISSN 0891-3668.

Benard, G., Kavakama, J., Mendes-Giannini, M. J., Kono, A., Duarte, A. J. & Shikanai-Yasuda, M. A. (2005). Contribution to the natural history of paracoccidioidomycosis: identification of the primary pulmonary infection in the severe acute form of the disease--a case report. *Clin Infect Dis*, Vol. 40, No. 1, pp. e1-4. ISSN1537-6591.

Bethlem, E. P., Capone, D., Maranhao, B., Carvalho, C. R. & Wanke, B (1999). Paracoccidioidomycosis. *Curr Opin Pulm Med*, Vol.5, No. 5, pp. 319-325, ISSN 1070-5287.

Bialek, R., Ibricevic, A., Aepinus, C., Najvar, L. K., Fothergill, A. W., Knobloch, J. & Graybill, J. R. (2000a). Detection of *Paracoccidioides brasiliensis* in tissue samples by a nested PCR assay. *J Clin Microbiol*, Vol. 38, No. 8, pp. 2940-2942, ISSN0095-1137.

Bialek, R., Ibrecevic, A., Fothergill, A. & Begerow, D. (2000b). Small subunit ribosomal DNA sequences shows *Paracoccidioides brasiliensis* closely related to *Blastomyces dermatitidis*. *J Clin Microbiol*, Vol.38, No. 9, pp. 3190-3193, ISSN0095-1137.

Bittencourt, J.I., de Oliveira R.M. & Coutinho Z.F. (2005). Paracoccidioidomycosis mortality in the State of Parana, Brazil, 1980/1998. *Cad Saude Publica*, Vol. 21, No. 6, pp. 1856 - 1864, ISSN 0102-311X.

Blotta, M. H., Mamoni, R. L., Oliveira, S. J., Nouer, S. A., Papaiordanou, P. M., Goveia,A. & Camargo, Z.P. (1999). Endemic regions of paracoccidioidomycosis in Brazil: a clinical and epidemiologic study of 584 cases in the southeast region. *Am J Trop Med Hyg,* Vol. 61, No. 3, pp. 390-394, ISSN0002-9637.

Bonifaz, A. (2010). Chapter 219: Paracoccidioidomicosis, *in* Bonifaz, A. (ed.), *Micología Médica Básica,* 3rd Ed. McGrow Hill, Mexico, pp. 259-270.

Bonifaz, A., Vázquez-González, D. & Perusquía-Ortiz, A.M. (2011). Endemic systemic mycoses: coccidioidomycosis, histoplasmosis, paracoccidioidomycosis and blastomycosis. *J Dtsch Dermatol Ges.* Vol. 9, No. 9, pp.705-14. ISSN 1610-0387.

Borelli, D. (1972). Some ecological aspects of paracoccidioidomycosis. *Proceedings Panamerican Symposium on Paracoccidioidomycosis,* Washington: Pan American Health Organization, Washington, D:C., PAHO Scientific Publication N° 254, pp. 59-64.

Borges-Walmsley, M. I., Chen, D., Shu, X. & Walmsley, A. R. (2002). The pathobiology of *Paracoccidioides brasiliensis.Trends Microbiol,* Vol. 10, No.2, pp. 80-87, ISSN 0966-842X.

Brummer, E., Restrepo, A., Stevens, D.A., Azzi, R., Gómez, A.G., Hoyos, G., McEwen, J.G., Cano, L.E. & de Bedout, C. (1984). Murine model of paracoccidioidomycosis production of fatal acute pulmonary or chronic pulmonary and disseminated disease. Immunological and pathological observations. *J Exp Pathol,* Vol.1, No. 3, pp. 241–255, ISSN0730-8485.

Brummer, E., Castañeda, E. & Restrepo, A. (1993). Paracoccidioidomycosis: an update. *Clin Microbiol Rev,* Vol. 6, No. 2, pp. 89-117, ISSN 0893-8512.

Buitrago, M.J., Bernal-Martinez, L., Castelli, M.V., Rodríguez-Tudela, J.L. & Cuenca-Estrella, M. (2011). Histoplasmosis and paracoccidioidomycosis in a non-endemic area: a review of cases and diagnosis. *J Travel Med,* Vol.18, No. 1, pp. 26-33, ISSN 1708-8305.

Burger, E., Miyaji, M., Sano, A., Calich, V. L., Nishimura, K. & Lenzi, H. L. (1996). Histopathology of paracoccidioidomycotic infection in athymic and euthymic mice: a sequential study. *Am J Trop Med Hyg,* Vol. 55, No.2, pp. 235-242, ISSN 0002-9637.

Calich, V. L., Singer-Vermes, L. M., Siqueira, A. M. & Burger, E. (1985). Susceptibility and resistance of inbred mice to *Paracoccidioides brasiliensis. Br J Exp Pathol,* Vol. 66, No.5, pp. 585-594, ISSN 0007-1021.

Calle, D., Rosero, S., Orozco, L.C., Camargo, D., Castañeda, E. & Restrepo, A. (2001). Paracoccidioidomycosis in Colombia: an ecological study. *Epidemiology Infection,* Vol. 126, No. 2, pp. 309-315, ISSN 0950-2688.

Calvi, S. A., Soares, A. M., Peraçoli, M. T.,Franco, M., Ruiz, R. L. Jr., Marcondes-Machado, J., Fecchio, D., Mattos, M. C. & Mendes, R. P. (2003). Study of bronchoalveolar lavage fluid in paracoccidioidomycosis: cytopathology and alveolar macrophage function in response to gamma interferon; comparison with blood monocytes. *Microbes Infect,* Vol. 5, No. 15, pp. 1373-1379, ISSN 1286-4579.

Campos, M. V., Penna, G. O., Castro, C. N., Morales, M. A., Ferreira, M. S. & Santos, J. B. (2008). Paracoccidioidomycosis at Brasilia's university hospital. *Rev Soc Bras Med Trop,*Vol. 41, No. 2, pp. 169-172, ISSN 0037-8682.

Cano, L.E., Singer-Vermes, L.M., Costa, T.A., Mengel, J.O., Xidieh, C.F., Arruda, C., André, D.C., Vaz, C.A., Burger, E. & Calich, V.L. (2000). Depletion of CD8 (+) T cells *in vivo* impairs host defense of mice resistant and susceptible to pulmonary paracoccidioidomycosis. *Infect Immun,* Vol.68, No. 1, pp. 352-359, ISSN 0019-9567.

Carlos, T. M. & Harlan, J. M. (1990). Membrane proteins involved in phagocyte adherence to endothelium. *Immunol Rev,*Vol. 114, No. 1, pp. 5–27, ISSN 0105-2896.

Caro, E., González, A., Muñoz, C., Urán, M. E., Restrepo, A., Hamilton, A. J. & Cano, L.E. (2008). Recognition of laminin by *Paracoccidioides brasiliensis* conidia: a possible mechanism of adherence to human type II alveolar cells. *Med Mycol,* Vol. 46, No. 8, pp. 795-804, ISSN 1369-3786.

Cock, A. M., Cano, L. E., Vélez, D., Aristizábal, B. H., Trujillo, J. & Restrepo, A. (2000). Fibrotic sequelae in pulmonary paracoccidioidomycosis: histopathological aspects in BALB/c mice infected with viable and non-viable *Paracoccidioides brasiliensis* propagules. *Rev Inst Med Trop Sao Paulo,* Vol. 42, No. 2, pp. 59-66, ISSN 0036-4665.

Coimbra, Jr. C.E., Wanke, B., Santos, R.V., do Valle, A.C., Costa, R.L. & Zancope-Oliveira, R.M. (1994). Paracoccidioidin and histoplasmin sensitivity in Tupi-Monde Amerindian populations from Brazilian Amazonia. *Ann Trop Med Parasitol,* Vol. 88, No. 2, pp. 197-207, ISSN 0003-4983.

Colombo, A. L., Tobón, A., Restrepo, A., Queiroz-Telles, F. & Nucci, M. (2011). Epidemiology of endemic systemic fungal infections in Latin America. *Med Mycol,* Vol. 49, No. 8, pp.785-98. ISSN1460-2709.

Conti-Díaz, I.A. & Calegari L.F. (1979). Paracoccidioidomycosis in Uruguay: its status and current problems. *Bol Oficina Sanit. Panam,* Vol. 86, No. 3, pp. 219–229, ISSN0030-0632.

Conti-Díaz, I. (2007). Point of view on the unknown ecological niche of *Paracoccidioides brasiliensis*. Our hypothesis of 1989: Present status and perspectives. *Rev. Inst. Med. Trop. S. Paulo,* Vol. 49, No. 2, pp. 131-134, ISSN0036-4665.

Coutinho, Z.F., Silva, D., Lazera, M., Petri, V., Oliveira, R.M., Sabroza, P. C. & Wanke, B. (2002). Paracoccidioidomycosis mortality in Brazil (1980-1995). *Cad Saude Publica,* Vol. 18, No. 5, pp. 1441-1454, ISSN 0102-311X.

Da Silva, F. C., Svidzinski, T. I., Patussi, E. V., Cardoso, C. P., De Oliveira Dalalio, M. M. & Hernandes, L. (2009). Morphologic organization of pulmonary granulomas in mice infected with *Paracoccidioides brasiliensis*. *Am J Trop Med Hyg,* Vol. 80, No.5, pp. 798-804, ISSN 1476-1645.

Da Silva, M. B., Marques, A. F., Nosanchuk, J. D., Casadevall, A.,Travassos, L. R. & Taborda, C. P. (2006). Melanin in the dimorphic fungal pathogen *Paracoccidioides brasiliensis*: effects on phagocytosis, intracellular resistance and drug susceptibility. *Microbes Infect,* Vol. 8, No. 1, pp. 197–205, ISSN1286-4579.

Datta, A., Scotton, C. J. & Chambers, R. C. (2011). Novel therapeutic approaches for pulmonary fibrosis. *Br J Pharmacol,* Vol. 163, No.1, pp. 141-72, ISSN 1476-5381.

Defaveri, J., Rexkallah-Iwasso, M.T. & Franco, M.F. (1982). Experimental pulmonary paracoccidioidomycosis in mice: morphology and correlation of lesions with humoral and cellular immune response. *Mycophatologia,* Vol. 77, No. 1, pp. 3–11, ISSN 0301-486X.

Essayag, S.M., Landaeta, M.E., Hartung, C., Magaldi, S., Spencer, L., Suárez, R., García, F. & Pérez, E. (2002). Histopathologic and histochemical characterization of calcified structures in hamsters inoculated with *Paracoccidioides brasiliensis*. *Mycoses,* Vol.45, No.(9-10), pp. 351-357, ISSN0933-7407.

Fang, C. C., Lai, M. N., Chien, C. T., Hung, K. Y., Tsai, C. C., Tsai, T. J. & Hsieh, B. S. (2003). Effects of pentoxifylline on peritoneal fibroblasts and silica-induced peritoneal fibrosis. *Perit Dial Int,* Vol. 23, No.3, pp. 228-36, ISSN 0896-8608.

Fava-Netto, C., De Brito, T. & Lacaz, C.S. (1961). Experimental South American blastomycosis of the guinea pig. *Pathol Microbiol,* Vol. 24, No. 2, pp. 192–206, ISSN0031-2959.

Flynn, J.L., Scanga, C.A., Tanaka, K.E. & Chan, J. (1998). Effects of aminoguanidine on latent murine tuberculosis. *J Immunol,* Vol. 160, No.4 pp. 1796–1803, ISSN 0022-1767.

Flynn, J.L., Chan, J. & Lin, P.L. (2011). Macrophages and control of granulomatous inflammation in tuberculosis. *Mucosal Immunol,* Vol.4, No.3, pp. 271-278, ISSN 1935-3456.

Fornazim, M. C., Balthazar, A., Quagliato, R., Mamoni, R. L., Garcia, C. & Blotta, M. H. S. L. (2003). Evaluation of bronchoalveolar cells in pulmonary paracoccidioidomycosis. *Eur Respir J,* Vol. 22, No. 6, pp. 895–899, ISSN 0903-1936.

Franco, L., Najvar, L., Gómez, B. L., Restrepo, S., Graybill, J. R. & Restrepo, A. (1998). Experimental pulmonary fibrosis induced by *Paracoccidioides brasiliensis* conidia: measurement of local host responses. *Am J Trop Med Hyg,* Vol. 58, No.4, pp. 424-30, ISSN 0002-9637.

Franco, M., Montenegro, M. R., Mendes, R. P., Marques, S. A., Dillon, N. L. & Mota, N. G. (1987). Paracoccidioidomycosis: a recently proposed classification of its clinical forms. *Rev Soc Bras Med Trop,* Vol. 20, No. 2, pp.129-132, ISSN 0037-8682.

Franco, M., Bagagli, E., Scapolio, S. & da Silva Lacaz, C. (2000). A critical analysis of isolation of *Paracoccidioides brasiliensis* from soil. *Med Mycol,* Vol. 38, No. 3, pp. 185-191, ISSN 1369-3786.

Funari, M., Kavakama, J., Shikanai-Yasuda, M. A., Castro, L. G., Bernard, G., Rocha, M. S., Cerri, G. G. & Muller, N. L. (1999). Chronic pulmonary paracoccidioidomycosis (South American blastomycosis): high-resolution CT findings in 41 patients. *AJR Am J Roentgenol,* Vol. 173, No.1, pp. 59-64, ISSN 0361-803X.

Garcia-de-Alba, C., Becerril, C., Ruiz, V., Gonzalez, Y., Reyes, S., Garcia-Alvarez, J., Selman, M. & Pardo, A. (2010). Expression of matrix metalloproteases by fibrocytes: possible role in migration and homing. *Am J Respir Crit Care Med,*Vol. 182, No.9, pp. 1144-52, ISSN 1535-4970.

Gaur, N. K., Klotz, S. A. & Henderson, R. L. (1999). Overexpression of the *Candida albicans* ALA1 gene in *Saccharomyces cerevisiae* results in aggregation following attachment of yeast cells to extracellular matrix proteins, adherence properties similar to those of *Candida albicans. Infect Immun,* Vol. 67, No. 11, pp. 6040–6047, ISSN 0019-9567.

Goldman, D., Cho, Y., Zhao, M.L., Casadevall, A. & Lee, S.C. (1996). Expression of inducible nitric oxide synthase in rat pulmonary *Cryptococcus neoformans* granulomas. *Am J Pathol,* Vol. 148, No. 4, pp. 1275–1282, ISSN 0002-9440.

Gomes, E., Wingeter, M. A., & Svidzinski, T. I. (2008) Clinical-radiological dissociation in lung manifestations of paracoccidioidomycosis. *Rev Soc Bras Med Trop,* Vol. 41, No. 5, pp. 454-458, ISSN 1678-9849.

Gomes, G. M., Cisalpino, P. S., Taborda, C. P. & de Camargo, Z. P. (2000). PCR for diagnosis of paracoccidioidomycosis. *J Clin Microbiol,* Vol. 38, No. 9, pp. 3478-3480, ISSN 0095-1137.

Gómez, B. L., Figueroa, J. I., Hamilton, A. J., Diez, S., Rojas, M., Tobón, A. M., Hay, R. J. & Restrepo, A. (1998). Antigenemia in patients with paracoccidioidomycosis: detection of the 87-kilodalton determinant during and after antifungal therapy. *J Clin Microbiol*, Vol. 36, No. 11, pp. 3309-3316, ISSN0095-1137.

Gómez, B.L., Figueroa, J.I., Hamilton, A.J., Ortiz, B., Robledo, M.A., Hay, R.J. & Restrepo, A. (1997). Use of monoclonal antibodies in diagnosis of paracoccidioidomycosis: new strategies for the detection of circulating antigens. *J ClinMicrobiol*, Vol. 35, No. 12, pp. 3278-3283, ISSN 0095-1137.

Gonçalves, A. J., Londero, A. T., Terra, G. M., Rozenbaum, R., Abreu, T. F. & Nogueira, S. A. (1998). Paracoccidioidomycosis in children in the state of Rio de Janeiro (Brazil). Geographic distribution and the study of a "reservarea". *Rev Inst Med Trop São Paulo*, Vol. 40, No. 1, pp. 11-13, ISSN 0036-4665.

González, A., Sahaza, J. H., Ortiz, B. L., Restrepo, A. & Cano, L. E. (2003). Production of pro-inflammatory cytokines during the early stages of experimental *Paracoccidioides brasiliensis* infection. *Med Mycol*, Vol. 41, No. 5, pp. 391-399, ISSN1369-3786.

González, A., Gómez, B. L., Díez, S., Hernández, O., Restrepo, A., Hamilton, A. J. & Cano, L. E. (2005a). Purification and partial characterization of a *Paracoccidioides brasiliensis* protein with capacity to bind to extracellular matrix proteins. *Infect Immun*, Vol. 73, No. 5, pp. 2486-2495, ISSN 0019-9567.

González, A., Lenzi, H. L., Motta, E. M., Caputo, L., Sahaza, J. H., Cock, A. M., Ruiz, A. C., Restrepo, A. & Cano, L. E. (2005b).Expression of adhesion molecules in lungs of mice infected with *Paracoccidioides brasiliensis* conidia. *Microbes Infect*, Vol. 7, No. 4, pp. 666-673, ISSN 1286-4579.

González, A., Caro, E., Muñoz, C., Restrepo, A., Hamilton, A. J. & Cano, L .E. (2008a). *Paracoccidioides brasiliensis* conidia recognize fibronectin and fibrinogen which subsequently participate in adherence to human type II alveolar cells: involvement of a specific adhesin. *Microb Pathog*, Vol. 44, No. 5, pp. 389-401, ISSN 0882-4010.

González, A., Gómez, B. L., Muñoz, C., Aristizábal, B. H., Restrepo, A., Hamilton, A. J. & Cano, L. E. (2008b). Involvement of extracellular matrix proteins in the course of experimental paracoccidioidomycosis. *FEMS Immunol Med Microbiol*, Vol. 53, No. 1, pp. 114-125, ISSN 0928-8244.

González, A., Lenzi, H. L., Motta, E. M., Caputo, L., Restrepo, A., & Cano, L. E. (2008c). Expression and arrangement of extracellular matrix proteins in the lungs of mice infected with *Paracoccidioides brasiliensis* conidia. *Int J Exp Pathol*, Vol. 89, No. 2, pp. 106-116, ISSN 1365-2613.

González, A., Restrepo, A. & Cano, L. E. (2008d). Pulmonary immune responses induced in BALB/c mice by *Paracoccidioides brasiliensis* conidia. *Mycopathologia*, Vol. 165, No. 4-5, pp. 313-330, ISSN 0301-486X.

Hahn, R. C., & Hamdan, J. S. (2000). Effects of amphotericin B and three azole derivatives on the lipids of yeast cells of *Paracoccidioides brasiliensis*. *Antimicrob Agents Chemother*, Vol. 44, No. 7, pp. 1997-2000, ISSN 0066-4804.

Hamacher, J. & Schaberg, T. (1994). Adhesion molecules in lung diseases. *Lung*, Vol. 172, No. 4, pp. 189–213, ISSN 0341-2040.

Hernández, O., Almeida, A. J., González, A., García, A. M., Tamayo, D., Cano, L. E., Restrepo, A. & McEwen, J. G. (2010). A 32-kilodalton hydrolase plays an important role in *Paracoccidioides brasiliensis* adherence to host cells and influences pathogenicity. *Infect Immun,* Vol. 78, No. 12, pp. 5280-5286, ISSN 1098-5522.

Hsu, L.Y., Ng, E.S. & Koh, L.P. (2010). Common and emerging fungal pulmonary infections. *Infect Dis Clin North Am,* Vol. 24, No. 3, pp. 557-577, ISSN 1557-9824.

Iabuki, K. & Montenegro, M.R. (1979). Experimental paracoccidioidomycosis in the Syrian hamster: morphology, ultrastructure and correlation of lesions with presence of specific antigens and serum levels of antibodies. *Mycopathologia,* Vol. 67, No. 3, pp. 131–141, ISSN0301-486X.

Inoue, K., Takano, H., Yanagisawa, R. & Sakurai, M. (2004). Anti-inflammatory Effect of Pentoxifylline. *Chest,* Vol. 126, No.1, pp. 321, ISSN 0012-3692.

Iovannitti, C.A., Finquelievich, J.L., Negroni, R. & Elías-Costa, M.R. (1999). Histopathological evolution of experimental paracoccidioidomycosis in Wistar rats. *Zentralbl Bakteriol,* Vol.289, No. 2, pp. 211-216, ISSN0934-8840.

Izzo, A. A., Lovchik, J. A. & Lipscomb, M. F. (1998). T and B cell independence of endothelial cell adhesion molecule expression in pulmonary granulomatous inflammation. *Am J Respir Cell MolBiol,* Vol. 19, No. 4, pp. 588–597, ISSN 1044-1549.

Kerr, I.B., de Oliveira, P.C. & Lenzi, H.L. (1988). Connective matrix organization in chronic granulomas of experimental paracoccidioidomycosis. *Mycopathologia,* Vol. 103, No.1, pp. 11-20, ISSN 0301-486X.

Koishi, A. C., Vituri, D. F., DionízioFilho, P. S., Sasaki, A. A., Felipe, M. S. & Venancio, E. J. (2010). A semi-nested PCR assay for molecular detection of *Paracoccidioides brasiliensis* in tissue samples. *Rev Soc Bras Med Trop,* Vol. 43, No. 6, pp. 728-730, ISSN 1678-9849.

Lacaz, C. S., Porto, E., Martins, J.E.C., Heins-Vaccari, E.M. & Melo, N.T. (2002). Paracoccidioidomicose, *in* Lacaz C, Porto E, Martins JEC., Heins-Vaccari, E.M., Melo, N.T. (eds.), *Tratado de Micología Médica Lacaz.* 9th ed. Servier. São Paulo, Brazil, pp. 639-729.

Livonesi, M.C., Souto, J.T., Campanelli, A.P., Maffei, C.M., Martinez, R., Rossi, M.A. & Da Silva, J.S. (2008). Deficiency of IL-12p40 subunit determines severe paracoccidioidomycosis in mice. *Med Mycol,* Vol. 46, No.7, pp. 637-646, ISSN 1369-3786.

Livonesi, M.C., Rossi, M.A., de Souto, J.T., Campanelli, A.P., de Sousa, R.L., Maffei, C.M., Ferreira, B.R., Martinez, R. & da Silva, J.S. (2009). Inducible nitric oxide synthase-deficient mice show exacerbated inflammatory process and high production of both Th1 and Th2 cytokines during paracoccidioidomycosis. *Microbes Infect,* Vol. 11, No.1, pp. 123-132, ISSN 1286-4579.

Londero, A. T. (1986). Paracoccidioidomicose: Patogenia, formas clinicas, manifestacões pulmonares e diagnostico. *J Pneumol (Brazil),* Vol. 12, No. 1, pp. 41–57, ISSN0102-3586.

Londero, A. T., Rios-Gonçalves, A. J., Terra, G. M. & Nogueira, S. A. (1996). Paracoccidioidomycosis in Brazilian children. A critical review (1911–1994). *Arq Bras Med,* Vol. 70, No. 4, pp. 197–203, ISSN.0365-0723 .

Lopera, D., Naranjo, T., Hidalgo, J. M., de Oliveira Pascarelli, B. M., Patiño, J. H., Lenzi, H. L., Restrepo, A. & Cano, L. E. (2010). Pulmonary abnormalities in mice with paracoccidioidomycosis: a sequential study comparing high resolution computed tomography and pathologic findings. *PLoS Negl Trop Dis,* Vol. 4, No.6, pp. e726, ISSN 1935-2735.

Lopera, D., Naranjo, T. W., Cruz, O. G., Restrepo, A., Cano, L. E. & Lenzi, H. L. (2011). Structural and topographic dynamics of pulmonary histopatology and local cytokine profiles in mice infected with *Paracoccidioides brasiliensis* conidia. *PLoS Neglected Tropical Diseases,* Vol.5, No.7, pp. e1232, ISSN 1935-2735.

Machado, J.M.J. & Teixeira G.A. (1965). Das sequelas da blastomicose Sul-Americana. *Hospital,* Vol. 68, No. X, pp.141–147.

Marchiori, E., Escuissato, D.L., Souza, A.S.Jr., Barillo, J.L., Warszawiak, D. & de Souza, A.S. (2008). Computed tomography findings in patients with tracheal paracoccidioidomycosis. *J Comput Assist Tomogr,* Vol. 32, No.5, pp. 788-791, ISSN 1532-3145.

Marchiori, E., Valiante, P.M., Mano, C. M., Zanetti, G., Escuissato, D. L., Souza, A. S. Jr., & Capone, D. (2011). Paracoccidioidomycosis: High-resolution computed tomography-pathologic correlation. *Eur J Radiol,* Vol. 77, No. 1, pp. 80-84, ISSN 1872-7727.

Masinovsky, B., Urdal, D. & Gallatin, W. M. (1990). IL-4 acts synergistically with IL-1 beta to promote lymphocyte adhesión to microvascular endothelium by induction of vascular cell adhesion molecule-1. *J Immunol,* Vol. 145, No. 9, pp. 2886–2895, ISSN0022-1767.

Matute, D. R., Sepulveda,V. E., Quesada, L. M., Goldman, G. H., Taylor, J. W., Restrepo, A. & McEwen, J. G. (2006). Microsatellite analysis of three phylogenetic species of *Paracoccidioides brasiliensis. J Clin Microbiol,* Vol.44, No. 6, pp. 2153-2157, ISSN.

Mayayo, E., Lopez-Aracil, V., Fernandez-Torres, B., Mayayo, R. & Dominguez, M. (2007). Report of an imported cutaneous disseminated case of paracoccidioidomycosis. *Rev Iberoam Micol,* Vol.24, No.1, pp. 44-46, ISSN 1130-1406.

McEwen, J.G., Bedoya, V., Patiño, M.M., Salazar, M.E. & Restrepo, A. (1987). Experimental murine paracoccidioidomycosis induced by the inhalation of conidia. *J Med Vet Mycol,* Vol. 25, No. 3, pp. 165–175, ISSN0268-1218.

McMahon, J. P., Wheat, J., Sobel, M. E., Pasula, R., Downing, J. F. & Martin, W. J. (1995). Murine laminin binds to *Histoplasma capsulatum.* A possible mechanism of dissemination. *J Clin Invest,* Vol. 96, No. 2, pp. 1010-1017, ISSN0021-9738.

Meltzer, E. B. & Noble, P. W. (2008). Idiopathic pulmonary fibrosis. *Orphanet J Rare Dis,* Vol. 3, No. 1, pp. 8, ISSN 1750-1172.

Mendes, R. P. (1994). The gamut of clinical manifestations, *in* Franco, M., Lacaz, C., Restrepo, A., & del Negro, G (eds). *Paracoccidioidomycosis,* CRC Press, Boca Raton, FL, pp. 233–258.

Moreira, A. P., Campanelli, A. P., Cavassani, K. A., Souto, J. T., Ferreira, B. R., Martinez, R., Rossi, M. A. & Silva, J. S. (2006). Intercellular adhesion molecule-1 is required for the early formation of granulomas and participates in the resistance of mice to the infection with the fungus *Paracoccidioides brasiliensis. Am J Pathol,* Vol. 169, No. 4, pp. 1270-1281, ISSN0002-9440.

Morejon, K.M., Machado, A.A. & Martinez, R. (2009). Paracoccidioidomycosis in patients infected with and not infected with human immunodeficiency virus: a case-control study. *Am J Trop Med Hyg,* Vol. 80, No. 3, pp. 359-366, ISSN1476-1645.

Moscardi, M.& Franco, M.F. (1980). Experimental paracoccidioidomycosis in mice. I. Immunopathological aspects of intraperitoneal infection. *Rev Inst Med Trop Sao Paulo,* Vol.22, No.6, pp. 286-293, ISSN 0036-4665

Mukhopadhyay, S. & Gal, A.A. (2010). Granulomatous lung disease: an approach to the differential diagnosis. *Arch Pathol Lab Med,* Vol.134, No.5, pp. 667-690, ISSN 1543-2165.

Muniz, M.A., E, M., Magnago, M., Moreira, L.B. & de Almeida Junior, J. (2002). Paracoccidioidomicose pulmonar - aspectos na tomografia computadorizada de alta resolução. *Radiol Bras,* Vol. 35, No.3, pp. 147-154, ISSN 0100-3984

Naranjo, M. S., Trujillo, M., Múnera, M. I., Restrepo, P., Gómez, I., & Restrepo, A. (1990). Treatment of paracoccidioidomycosis with itraconazole. *J Med Vet Mycol,* Vol. 28, No. 1, pp. 67-76, ISSN 0268-1218.

Naranjo, T. W., Lopera, D. E., Diaz-Granados, L. R., Duque, J. J., Restrepo, A. & Cano, L. E. (2010). Histopathologic and immunologic effects of the itraconazole treatment in a murine model of chronic pulmonary paracoccidioidomycosis. *Microbes Infect,* Vol. 12, No.14-15, pp. 1153-62, ISSN 1769-714X.

Naranjo, T. W., Lopera, D. E., Diaz-Granados, L. R., Duque, J. J., Restrepo, A. & Cano, L. E. (2011). Combined itraconazole-pentoxifylline treatment promptly reduces lung fibrosis induced by chronic pulmonary paracoccidioidomycosis in mice. *Pulm Pharmacol Ther,* Vol. 24, No.1, pp. 81-91, ISSN 1522-9629.

Nascimento, F.R.F., Calich, V.L.G., Rodrigues, D. & Russo, M. (2002). Dual role of nitric oxide in paracoccidioidomycosis: essential for resistance but overproduction associated with susceptibility. *J Immunol,* Vol. 168, No.9 , pp. 4593–4600, ISSN 0022-1767.

Nathan, C., & Shiloh, M. U. (2000). Reactive oxygen and nitrogen intermediates in the relationship between mammalian host and microbial pathogens. *Proc Natl Acad Sci USA,* Vol.97, No. 16, pp. 8841-8848, ISSN 0027-8424.

Newman, S. L., Goote, L., Gabay, J. E. & Selsted, M. E. (2000).Identification of constituents of human neutrophil azurophil granules that mediated fungistasis against *Histoplasma capsulatum. Infect Immun,* Vol. 68, No. 10, pp. 5668–5672, ISSN0019-9567.

Niño-Vega, G. A., Calcagno, A. M., San-Blas, G., San-Blas, F., Gooday, G. W. & Gow, N. A. (2000). RFLP analysis reveals marked geographical isolation between strains of *Paracoccidioides brasiliensis. Med Mycol,* Vol. 38, No. 6, pp. 437-441, ISSN1369-3786.

Nishikaku, A. S., Sanchez-Molina, R. F., Ribeiro, L. C., Scavone, R., Albe, B. P., Silva-Cunha, C. & Burger, E. (2009). Nitric oxide participation in granulomatous response induced by *Paracoccidioides brasiliensis* infection in mice. *Med Microbiol Immunol,* Vol. 198, No. 2, pp.123–135, ISSN 1432-1831.

Nogueira, M. G., Andrade, G. M., & Tonelli, E. (2006). Clinical evolution of paracoccidioidomycosis in 38 children and teenagers. *Mycopathologia,* Vol. 161, No. 2, pp. 73-81, ISSN 0301-486X.

Nucci, M., Colombo, A.L. & Queiroz-Telles, F. (2009). Paracoccidioidomycosis. *Curr Fungal Infect Rep.,* Vol. 3, No. 1, pp. 15-20, ISSN 1936-3761.

Osborn, L., Hession, C., Tizard, R., Vasallo, C., Luhowsky, S., Chi-Rosso, G. & Lobb, R. (1989).Direct expression of vascular cell adhesion molecule-1, a cytokine-induced endotelial protein that binds to lymphocytes. *Cell,* Vol. 59, No. 6, pp. 1203–1211, ISSN0092-8674.

Pappas, P. G. (2004). Immunotherapy for invasive fungal infections: from bench to bedside. *Drug Resist Updat,* Vol. 7, No.1, pp. 3-10, ISSN 1368-7646.

Pardo, A. & Selman, M. (2006). Matrix metalloproteases in aberrant fibrotic tissue remodeling. *Proc Am Thorac Soc,* Vol. 3, No.4, pp. 383-388, ISSN 1546-3222.

Peraçoli, M.T.S., Mota, N.G.S. & Montenegro, M.R. (1982). Experimental paracoccidioidomycosis in the Syrian hamster. Morphology and correlation of lesions with humoral and cell mediated immunity. *Mycopathologia,* Vol. 79, No. 1, pp. 7-17, ISSN0301-486X.

Pereira, R. M., Bucaretchi, F., Barison-Ede, M., Hessel, G. & Tresoldi, A. T. (2004). Paracoccidioidomycosis in children: clinical presentation, follow-up and outcome. *Rev Inst Med Trop São Paulo,* Vol. 46, No. 3, pp. 127-131, ISSN 0036-4665.

Pilewski, J. M. & Albelda, S. M. (1993). Adhesion molecules in the lung. An overview. *Am Rev Respir Dis,* Vol. 148, No. 6, pp. S31-37, ISSN0003-0805.

Pinzan, C.F., Ruas, L.P., Casabona-Fortunato, A.S., Carvalho, F.C. & Roque-Barreira, M. C. (2010). Immunological basis for the gender differences in murine *Paracoccidioides brasiliensis* infection. PLoS ONE, Vol. 5, No. 5, pe10757. ISSN 1932-6203.

Poisson, D., Heitzmann, A., Mille, C., Muckensturm, B., Dromer, F., Dupont, B. & Hocqueloux, L. (2007). *Paracoccidioides brasiliensis* in a brain abscess: First French case. *J Mycol Med,* Vol. 17, pp. 114-118, ISSN1156-5233.

Popi, A.F., Godoy, L.C., Xander, P., Lopes, J.D. & Mariano, M. (2008). B-1 cells facilitate *Paracoccidioides brasiliensis* infection in mice via IL-10 secretion. *Microbes Infect,* Vol.10, No.7, pp. 817-824, ISSN 1286-4579.

Prado, M., da Silva, M. B., Laurenti, R., Travassos, L. R. & Taborda, C. P. (2009). Mortality due to systemic mycoses as a primary cause of death or in association with AIDS in Brazil: a review from 1996 to 2006. *Mem Inst Oswaldo Cruz,* Vol.104, No. 3, pp. 513-521, ISSN 1678-8060.

QuagliatoJr, R., Grangeia, A. T., de Massucio, R. A., De Capitani, E. M., RezendeSde, M. & Balthazar, A. B. (2007). Association between paracoccidioidomycosis and tuberculosis: reality and misdiagnosis. *J Bras Pneumol,* Vol.33, No. 3, pp. 295-300, ISSN 1806-3756.

Ramos, E. S, & Saraiva, L. E. (2008). Paracoccidioidomycosis. *Dermatol Clin,* Vol. 26, No. 2, pp. 257-269, ISSN 0733-8635.

Restrepo, A., McEwen, J.G. & Castañeda, E. (2001). The habitat of *Paracoccidioides brasiliensis*: how far from solving the riddle? *Med Mycol,* Vol. 39, No. 3, pp. 233-241, ISSN 1369-3786.

Restrepo, A., Benard, G., de Castro, C. C., Agudelo, C. A. & Tobón, A. M. (2008). Pulmonary paracoccidioidomycosis. *Semin Respir Crit Care Med,* Vol. 29, No.2, pp. 182-97, ISSN 1069-3424.

Restrepo, A., & Tobón, A.M. (2009). *Paracoccidioides brasiliensis, in* Mandell, G. L., Bennett, J. E., & Dolin, R., (eds), *Mandell, Douglas and Bennett's Principles and Practice of Infectious Diseases, 7th ed.* Elsevier, Philadelphia, pp. 3357-3363.

Restrepo, A., González, A. & Agudelo, C.A. (2011). Chapter 21: Paracoccidioidomycosis, *in*W. Dismukes, C. Kauffman, P. Pappas, J. Sobel (eds): *Essentials of Medical Mycology,* 2nd Ed.: Springer, N.Y, N.Y., pp 367-385.

Restrepo, S., Tobón, A., Trujillo, J. & Restrepo, A. (1992). Development of pulmonary fibrosis in mice during infection with *Paracoccidioides brasiliensis* conidia. *J Med Vet Mycol,* Vol.30, No. 3, pp. 173–184, ISSN0268-1218.

Ricci, G., Mota, F. T., Wakamatsu, A., Serafim, R. C., Borra, R. C. & Franco, M. (2004). Canine paracoccidioidomycosis. *Med Mycol,* Vol.42, No. 4, pp. 379-383, ISSN1369-3786.

Richini-Pereira, V.B., Bosco, S.M.G., Griese, J., Theodoro, R.C., Macoris, S.A.G., Silva, R.J., Barrozo, L., Tavares, P.M.S. & Zancopé-Oliveira, R.M. (2008). Molecular detection of *Paracoccidioides brasiliensis* in road-killed wild animals. *Med Mycol,* Vol.46, No. 1, pp. 35-40, ISSN1369-3786.

Rodrigues, M. L., Dos Reis, G., Puccia, R., Travassos, L. R. & Alviano, C. S. (2003). Cleavage of human fibronectin and other basement membrane-associated proteins by a *Cryptococcus neoformans* serine proteinase. *Microb Pathog,* Vol. 34, No. 2, pp. 65–71, ISSN0882-4010.

Romanelli, R. G., Caligiuri, A., Carloni, V., De Franco, R., Montalto, P., Ceni, E., Casini, A., Gentilini, P. & Pinzani, M. (1997). Effect of pentoxifylline on the degradation of procollagen type I produced by human hepatic stellate cells in response to transforming growth factor-beta 1. *Br J Pharmacol,* Vol. 122, No.6, pp. 1047-54, ISSN 0007-1188.

San-Blas, G., Niño-Vega, G. & Iturriaga, T. (2002). *Paracoccidioides brasiliensis* and paracoccidioidomycosis: Molecular approaches to morphogenesis, diagnosis, epidemiology, taxonomy and genetics. *Med Mycol,* Vol.40, No. 3, pp. 225-242, ISSN1369-3786.

Santo, A.H. (2008). Paracoccidioidomycosis-related mortality trend, state of São Paulo, Brazil: a study using multiple causes of death. *Rev Panam Salud Publica,* Vol.23, No.5, pp. 313-324, ISSN 1020-4989.

Severo, L. C., Roesch, E. W., Oliveira, E. A., Rocha, M. M. & Londero, A. T. (1998). Paracoccidioidomycosis in women. *Rev. Iberoam. Micol.,* Vol. 15, No. 2, pp. 88–89, ISSN1130-1406.

Shankar, J., Restrepo, A., Clemons, K.V. & Stevens, D.A. (2011). Paracoccidioidomycosis: hormones and the resistance of women. *Clinical Microbiology Reviews,* Vol. 24, No. 2, pp. 296-313, ISSN1098-6618.

Shikanai-Yasuda, M. A., Benard, G., Higaki, Y., Del Negro, G. M., Hoo, S., Vaccari, E. H., Gryschek, R. C., Segurado, A. A., Barone, A. A. & Andrade, D. R. (2002). Randomized trial with itraconazole, ketoconazole and sulfadiazine in paracoccidioidomycosis. *Med Mycol,* Vol. 40, No. 4, pp. 411-417, ISSN1369-3786.

Shikanai-Yasuda, M., Queiroz-Telles, F., Poncio, R., Lopes, A. & Moretti, M. (2006). Guideliness in paracoccidioidomycosis. *Rev. Soc. Bras. Med. Trop,* Vol. 39, No.3, pp. 297-310, ISSN 0037-8682.

Shikanai-Yasuda, M. A., Conceição, Y. M., Kono, A., Rivitti, E., Campos, A. F. & Campos, S. V. (2008). Neoplasia and paracoccidioidomycosis. *Mycopathologia,* Vol. 165, No. 4-5, pp. 303-312, ISSN 0301-486X.

Simões, L.B., Marques, S.A. & Bagagli, E. (2004). Distribution of paracoccidioidomycosis: determination of ecologic correlates through spatial analyses. *Med Mycol,* Vol. 42, No. 6, pp. 517-523, ISSN1369-3786.

Soares, A.M., Rezkallah-Iwasso, M.T., Oliveira, S.L., Peraçoli, M.T., Montenegro, M.R. & Musatti, C.C. (2000). Experimental paracoccidioidomycosis in high and low antibody responder mice of Selection IV-A. *Med Mycol.* Vol. 38, No.4, pp. 309-315, ISSN1369-3786.

Souto, J.T., Figueiredo, F., Furlanetto, A., Pfeffer, K., Rossi, M.A. & Silva, J.S. (2000). Interferon-gamma and tumor necrosis factor-alpha determine resistance to *Paracoccidioides brasiliensis* infection in mice. *Am J Pathol,* Vol.156, No.5, pp. 1811-1820, ISSN 0002-9440.

Souza, A.S., Jr., Gasparetto, E.L., Davaus, T., Escuissato, D.L. & Marchiori, E. (2006). High-resolution CT findings of 77 patients with untreated pulmonary paracoccidioidomycosis. *AJR Am J Roentgenol,* Vol. 187, No.5, pp. 1248-1252, ISSN 1546-3141.

Teixeira, M. M., Theodoro, R. C., de Carvalho, M. J., Fernandes, L., Paes, H. C., Hahn, R. C., Mendoza, L., Bagagli, E., San-Blas, G. & Felipe, M. S. (2009). Phylogenetic analysis reveals a high level of speciation in the *Paracoccidioides* genus. *Mol Phylogenet Evol,* Vol. 52, No. 2, pp. 273-283, ISSN1095-9513.

Tobón, A. M., Gómez, I., Franco, L. & Restrepo, A. (1995). Seguimiento post-terapia en pacientes con paracoccidioidomicosis tratados con itraconazol. *Rev Colomb Neumol,* Vol. 7, No. X, pp. 74–78, ISSN0121-5426.

Tobón, A. M., Agudelo, C. A., Osorio, M. L., Alvarez, D. L., Arango, M., Cano, L. E. & Restrepo, A. (2003). Residual pulmonary abnormalities in adult patients with chronic paracoccidioidomycosis: prolonged follow-up after itraconazole therapy. *Clin Infect Dis,* Vol. 37, No. 7, pp. 898-904, ISSN1537-6591.

Tong, Z., Chen, B., Dai, H., Bauer, P. C., Guzman, J. & Costabel, U. (2004). Extrinsic allergic alveolitis: inhibitory effects of pentoxifylline on cytokine production by alveolar macrophages. *Ann Allergy Asthma Immunol,* Vol. 92, No.2, pp. 234-239, ISSN 1081-1206.

Torrado, E., Castañeda, E., de la Hoz, F. & Restrepo A. (2000). Paracoccidioidomicosis: definición de las áreas endémicas de Colombia. *Biomédica,* Vol.20, No. 4, pp. 327-334, ISSN.0120-4157.

Torres, I., García, A. M., Hernández, O., González, A., McEwen, J. G., Restrepo, A. & Arango, M. (2010). Presence and expression of the mating type locus in *Paracoccidioides brasiliensis* isolates. *Fung Genet Biol.* Vol. 47, No. 4, pp. 373-380, ISSN1096-0937.

Tracey, K. J. & Cerami, A. (1994). Tumor necrosis factor: a pleiotropic cytokine and therapeutic target. *Ann Rev Med,* Vol. 45, No. 1, pp. 491–503, ISSN0066-4219.

Trad, H.S., Trad, C.S., Junior, J.E. & Muglia, V.F. (2006). Revisão radiológica de 173 casos consecutivos de paracoccidioidomicose. *Radiol Bras,* Vol.39, No.3, pp. 175-179, ISSN 0100-3984.

Tuder, R. M., el Ibrahim, R., Godoy, C. E. & De Brito, T. (1985). Pathology of the human pulmonary paracoccidioidomycosis. *Mycopathologia,* Vol. 92, No. 3, pp. 179-188, ISSN0301-486X.

Valente, E. G., Vernet, D., Ferrini, M. G., Qian, A., Rajfer, J. & Gonzalez-Cadavid, N. F. (2003). L-arginine and phosphodiesterase (PDE) inhibitors counteract fibrosis in the Peyronie's fibrotic plaque and related fibroblast cultures. *Nitric Oxide,* Vol. 9, No.4, pp. 229-44, ISSN 1089-8603.

Vigna, A.F., Almeida, S.R., Xander, P., Freymuller, E., Mariano, M. & Lopes, J.D. (2006). Granuloma formation *in vitro* requires B-1 cells and is modulated by *Paracoccidioides brasiliensis* gp43 antigen. *Microbes Infect,* Vol.8, No.3, pp. 589-597, ISSN 1286-4579.

Walker, S. L., Pembroke, A. C., Lucas, S. B. & Vega-Lopez, F. (2008). Paracoccidioidomycosis presenting in the UK. *Br J Dermatol,* Vol. 158, No. 3, pp. 624-626, ISSN0007-0963.

Wasylnka, J. A. & Moore, M. M. (2000). Adhesion of *Aspergillus* species to extracellular matrix proteins: evidence for involvement of negatively charged carbohydrates on the conidial surface. *Infect Immun,* Vol. 68, No. 6, pp. 3377–3384, ISSN0019-9567.

Wynn, T. A. (2007). Common and unique mechanisms regulate fibrosis in various fibroproliferative diseases. *J Clin Invest,* Vol. 117, No.3, pp. 524-529, ISSN 0021-9738.

Xidieh, C. F., Lenzi, H. L., Calich, V. L. & Burger, E. (1999). Influence of the genetic background on the pattern of lesions developed by resistant and susceptible mice infected with *Paracoccidioides brasiliensis. Med Microbiol Immunol,* Vol. 188, No.1, pp. 41-9, ISSN 0300-8584.

Yokomura, I., Iwasaki, Y., Nagata, K., Nakanishi, M., Natsuhara, A., Harada, H., Kubota, Y., Ueda, M., Inaba, T. & Nakagawa, M. (2001). Role of intercellular adhesion molecule 1 in acute lung injury induced by candidemia. *Exp Lung Res,* Vol. 27, No. 5, pp. 417–431, ISSN0190-2148.

Yu, M. L. & Limper, A. H. (1997). *Pneumocystis carinii* induces ICAM-1 expression in lung epithelial cells through a TNF-alpha-mediated mechanism. *Am J Physiol,* Vol. 273, No. 6, pp. L1103–1111, ISSN0002-9513.

17

Nocardia Infection in Lung Transplantation

Pilar Morales[1], Ana Gil-Brusola[2] and María Santos[2]
[1]*LungTrasplant Unit,* [2]*Microbiology Department,*
Hospital Universitario La Fe, Valencia
Spain

1. Introduction

Organ transplant recipients (OTR) in general and, in particular, lung transplant recipients (LTx) - due to their underlying disease, extensive surgery, and the continual and profound immunosuppression to which they are subjected - become perfect targets for the development of infections. These are more frequent and severe than in the non-transplanted population, and may be caused by either common or less frequent opportunistic pathogens such as the *Nocardia* species.

Nocardia are ubiquitous bacteria found mainly in soil, organic matter and water (Lerner, 1996). Based on the available literature and on our own experience, we know that they can cause infections in both immunocompetent (40%) and immunocompromised patients (B.L. Beaman & L. Beaman, 1994), with a low frequency in transplantations in general , which is somewhat higher in LTx. Onset of disease is generally insidious and it is difficult to diagnose and treat. It produces mainly respiratory symptoms, but complications can occur, spreading to other organs and causing high mortality. In this chapter, we intend to review various epidemiological, clinical, diagnostic, therapeutic and prophylactic aspects of *Nocardia* infections in adult LTx.

2. Epidemiology and pathogenesis

2.1 General aspects

The genus *Nocardia* includes aerobic, gram-positive, weakly acid-fast bacteria of the order Actinomycetales. Other microorganisms that belong to this order are *Corynebacterium*, *Rhodococcus, Gordonia, Tsukamurella, Actinomadura* and *Mycobacterium*, particularly rapidly growing nontuberculous mycobacteria (Sorrell et al., 2005), which can also cause infections in humans. More than 50 species of *Nocardia* have been defined either phenotypically or by molecular methods (Brown-Elliott et al., 2006). Originally, only 10-12 species were known to cause disease in humans, the most frequently described being *N. asteroides, N. nova, N. farcinica, N. transvalesis, N. brasiliensis, N. pseudobrasiliensis, N. otitidiscaviarum* and *N. brevicatena complex*, with variations according to different environments and authors. Nowadays, taxonomy of this genus has undergone considerable changes due to modern molecular techniques, such as identification by 16S ribosomal RNA gene sequencing. New species have been described, such as *N. cryacigeorgica* (Schlaberg et al., 2008), *N. veterana* (Pottumarthy et al., 2003), *N. abscessus* (Yassin et al., 2000), *N. paucivorans* (Eisenblatter et al.,

2002) and *N. kruczakiae* (Conville et al., 2004), which should be taken into account in case of isolation in LTx samples.

Immune response to *Nocardia* is T-cell mediated (Deem, 1983). Therefore, the reduced cellular immune response of solid OTR is one of the major factors predisposing a patient to infection; in fact, 60% of cases occurs in immunocompromised patients.

2.2 Frequency

Estimated frequency of *Nocardia* infection among solid OTR globally ranges from 0.1 to 3.5 (Peleg et al., 2007a). In the past, these cases were more frequent in kidney, heart and liver transplantations, and less in LTx (Husain et al., 2002), but recently infections in the latter have been described as the most frequent (3.5%, Peleg et al., 2007a; 1.8%, Santos et al., 2011; 1.9%, Ponyagariyagorn et al., 2008). This increased risk of *Nocardia* infection in LTx may be due to several factors: a) the graft may have anatomical deficiencies, including lung denervation, reduced cough reflex and poor mucociliary clearance (Kramer et al., 1993; Husain et al., 2002); b) the organ has been continuously exposed to the atmosphere, with constant stimulation of the lung by environmental antigens and an increased risk of rejection; and, therefore, c) a need for more intense immunosuppression than in other solid OTR. Moreover, high average levels of calcineurin inhibitors 30 days prior to infection have been independently associated with subsequent infection by *Nocardia* (Hewagama et al., 2011).

The most frequently reported species of *Nocardia* in LTx, with variations in percentage in different studies, are *N. nova*, *N. farcinica*, *N. asteroides* and *N. brasiliensis*.

2.3 Risk factors

There are two multivariate studies (Peleg et al., 2007a; Martinez-Tomás et al., 2007) which investigate the influence of several variables as risk factors for *Nocardia* infection in solid OTR. Among them, three have been described as independent: a) the doses of immunosuppressive therapy, as already mentioned; b) chronic use of corticosteroids; and c) cytomegalovirus disease in the previous 6 months (Paya, 1999).

The relationship between opportunistic infections, including nocardiosis, and alemtuzumab, a monoclonal antibody that targets the antigen D52 and is used to prevent graft rejection (Basu et al., 2005; Peleg et al., 2007 b) by causing profound lymphopaenia, has been also reported. Moreover, the use of rituximab (Kundranda et al., 2007), another immunomodulator that targets the CD20 protein found on B cells and used in solid OTR to prevent or treat antibody-mediated rejection, has also been described.

Finally, hypogammaglobulinaemia, combined with immunosuppression, may favour the development of *Nocardia* infections (Corales et al., 2000), as has been observed in heart transplantation.
Renal failure, prolonged respiratory support and early graft rejection may also be risk factors but have not yet been demonstrated in multivariate analysis.

2.4 Transmission

The main route for *Nocardia* infection is inhalation of aerosolised microorganisms. From the respiratory tract, bacteria can then move to other organs, the most commonly and seriously affected being the central nervous system (CNS). Involvement of skin and subcutaneous tissue, bones and joints, retina and, less frequently, other organs or structures (heart, kidney, peritoneum, endocardium, testicles, etc.) is also possible. Primary cutaneous infection can occur by direct inoculation in both immunocompetent and immunocompromised patients (Brown-Elliot et al., 2006). There is no evidence for human-to-human transmission and disease presents mainly as isolated cases, although an outbreak related to contamination by dust pollution (Sahathevan et al., 1991) in a liver transplantation unit and some spread by contamination of hands in a cardiovascular surgery unit (Wenger et al., 1998) have been documented based on molecular data.

3. Symptoms and radiology

Time of onset of infection after transplantation is variable, but tends to be late. It rarely occurs in the first month and may range from 1 to 28 years (Santos et al., 2011). The greatest risk is within the first year (Peleg et al., 2007a, Clark, 2009), but later cases have also been described (Peraira et al., 2003, Oszoyoglu et al., 2007). Pulmonary presentation is the most common, with subacute and insidious pneumonia. Less frequent is the cutaneous form, following a minor injury or by direct inoculation (Ambrosioni et al., 2010). Symptoms are usually non-specific and include fever, fatigue, dyspnoea, cough and pleuritic pain (Patel & Payá, 1997; Minero et al., 2009). Common radiographic abnormalities include irregular nodular lesions which may cavitate, diffuse interstitial infiltrates and lung consolidation with parapneumonic pleural effusion (Balikian et al., 1978; Morales et al., 2011) (Figure 1). Both lungs are usually affected, without significant anatomical or zonal distribution (Oszoyoglu et al., 2007). In the case of single-lung transplantation, *Nocardia* can infect both the native and the transplanted organ (Husain et al., 2002).

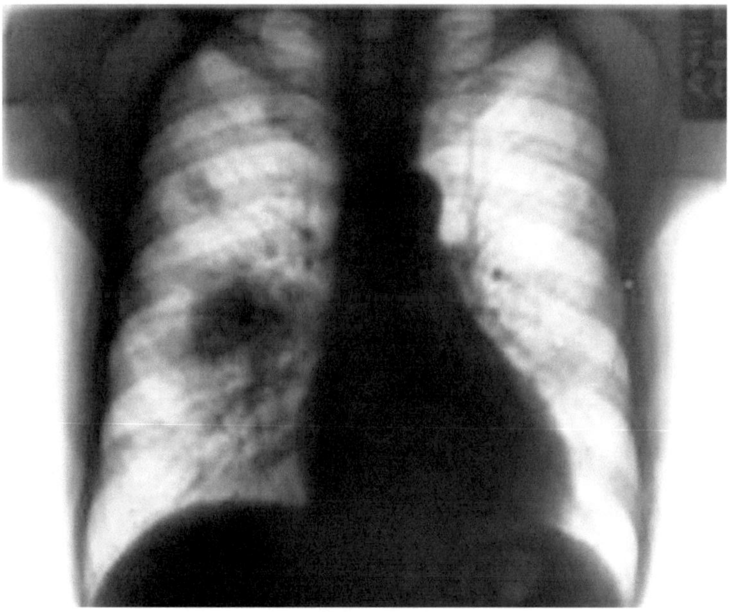

Fig. 1. Radiographic changes associated with Nocardia infection.

Haematogenous spread has been reported in up to 50% of cases (Clark, 2009), so it is important to exclude *Nocardia* clinically and/or radiologically in other organs, especially in the CNS (Singh & Husain, 2000). Moreover, and especially when the patient has a central venous catheter, blood should be cultured to rule out *Nocardia*. Cerebral involvement may be asymptomatic, therefore requiring neuroimaging with magnetic resonance or high resolution computed tomography (Ambrosini et al., 2010), or symptomatic, with headache, vomiting, altered level of consciousness, focal signs and seizures. Multiple radiographic cerebral lesions are observed in 40% (Singh & Husain, 2000). Meningitis is uncommon. Other forms of presentation of dissemination are cutaneous, ocular, intestinal, testicular and bone and joint disorders. Primary as well as disseminated cutaneous forms may present as subcutaneous nodules, cellulitis, abscess, mycetoma and sporotrichoid skin changes (Merigou et al., 1998). In this location, *N. brasiliensis* is the most common. The presence of the cutaneous form in organ transplant recipients should be followed by the exclusion of other forms of presentation of nocardiosis.

We must take into account the possible and frequent co-infections that occur with common and opportunistic bacteria, viruses, especially CMV, and fungi, mainly *Aspergillus* (Cabada et al., 2010) that make the patient's clinical and therapeutic management difficult (Santos et al., 2011). Differential diagnosis of pulmonary infection and brain nodule must include *Nocardia, Aspergillus* spp., *Cryptococcus neoformans, Mycobacteria, Rhodococcus equi*, post-transplant lymphoproliferative disease and primary lung cancer with metastasis.

4. Microbiological diagnosis

Definitive diagnosis of nocardiosis requires microscopic observation, isolation or nucleic acid detection of *Nocardia* in one or more samples from a suspected site. Specimen collection can be spontaneous, such as in the case of sputum (which is useful in up to 53% of cases), superficial such as in the case of a skin smear, or may require deeper samples such as bronchoaspirate, bronchoalveolar lavage or tissue biopsies. Smear staining with Gram stain, Ziehl-Neelsen (ZN) and modified ZN is the most useful and fastest diagnostic method. It can provide a diagnosis within the first few hours, showing abundant gram-positive or partially acid-fast branched bacilli (Figure 2), which are very characteristic of *Nocardia*, with moderate or abundant leukocytes resulting from the inflammatory response.

Differential diagnosis with *Rhodococcus, Gordonia* and rapidly growing mycobacteria must be considered, as discussed above. This information provides a reliable presumptive diagnosis and may guide empiric antibiotic therapy. Although *Nocardia* may grow in non-selective culture media, samples that can be contaminated with normal flora, such as those from the respiratory tract, should also be cultured in selective media such as Thayer-Martin agar with antibiotics (Shawar et al., 1990). Typical colonies appear chalky white (Figure 3) with aerial hyphae. Its growth is aerobic and may take from 2 to 5 days, sometimes even a week.

Species identification may by phenotypic, at least for the most common *Nocardia*, but genotypic methods such as polymerase chain reaction (PCR), restriction endonuclease analysis and sequencing of a portion of the 16S rRNA gene provide a safer and more accurate diagnosis. These techniques, however, are carried out by a limited number of laboratories (Brown-Elliot et al., 2006).

Identification of the species can be useful to guide treatment, since some have intrinsic resistance to several antibiotics, or to predict prognosis, since some species, such as *N.*

farcinica, are more virulent. In cases in which disseminated nocardiosis is suspected, *Nocardia* can also be isolated from a blood culture, although this is rare.

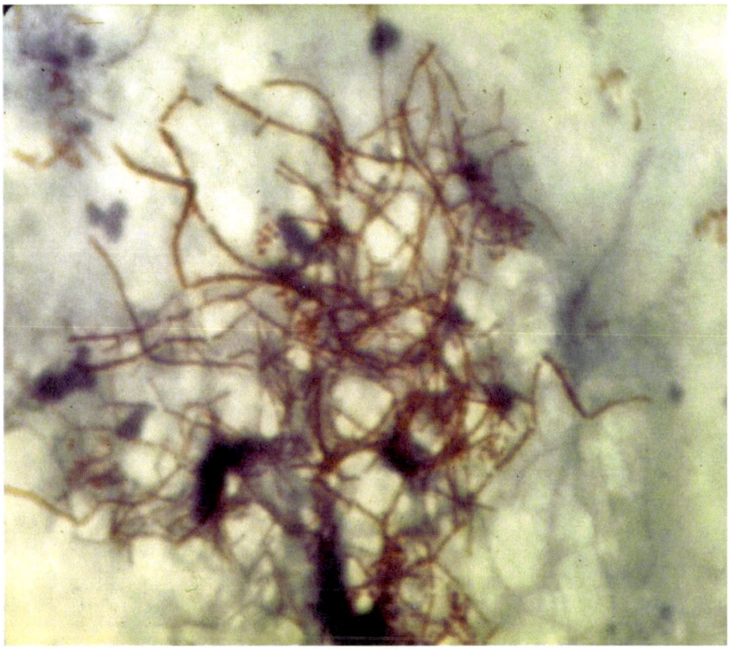

Fig. 2. Nocardia ZN stain.

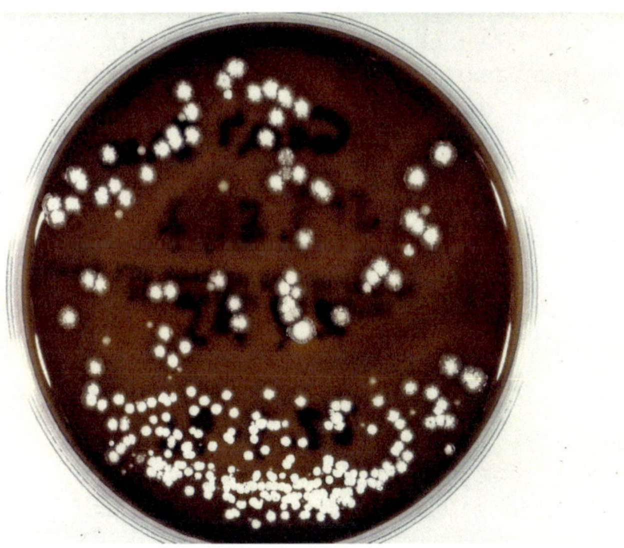

Fig. 3. Colonies of Nocardia.

Antimicrobial susceptibility testing of the *Nocardia* isolate is strongly recommended by the Clinical Laboratory Standard Institute (CLSI), which published the first approved methods in 2003 (Wayne, 2003). Primary susceptibility testing must include amikacin, amoxicillin/clavulanic acid, ceftriaxone, ciprofloxacin, clarithromycin, imipenem, linezolid, minocycline, trimethoprim-sulfamethoxazole (TMP/SMX) and tobramycin. Secondary recommendations include cefepime, cefotaxime, doxycycline, gentamicin and moxifloxacin. Some species of *Nocardia* have more predictable susceptibility patterns or, in other words, there are patterns of known resistance, such as *N. otitidiscaviarum* to imipenem, or the multi-resistance of *N. farcinica*, so it is sometimes necessary to perform *in vitro* synergy studies. The susceptibility patterns of the most common *Nocardia* can be seen in table 1.

	N. asteroides	***N. nova***	***N. farcinica***	***N. brasiliensis***
TMP/SMX	S (91-100)	S (89-100)	S (89-100)	S (100)
AMC	R (0-70)	R (3-50)	S (40-100)	S (65-100)
CEF	S (75-100)	S (70-100)	S (70-100)	V (50-100)
IMP	S (70-100)	S (100)	S (100)	V (0-100)
AMK	S (85-100)	S (100)	S (100)	S (100)
LZD	S (100)	S (100)	S (100)	S (100)
MIN	V (25-100)	V (29-100)	V (12-96)	S (0-100)
CIP	R(0-98)	R (0)	S (50-100)	R (0-30)
MXF	(50)	-	(88)	-

Table 1. Expected and reported antimicrobial susceptibility of selected *Nocardia* species (% of isolates susceptible in various series). Composite data from references (Clark, 2009; Hewagama et al., 2011; Brown-Elliott et al., 2001). TMP/SMX, trimethoprim-sulfamethoxazole; AMC, amoxicillin/clavulanic acid; CEF, ceftriaxone; IMP, imipenem; AMK, amikacin; LZD, linezolid; MIN, minocycline; CIP, ciprofloxacin; MXF, moxifloxacin; S, sensitive; R, resistant; V, variable.

5. Treatment and evolution

5.1 General aspects

Treatment of *Nocardia* infections in LTx is based primarily on antibiotics. In some cases, such as brain or cutaneous abscesses that do not respond to initial antibacterial therapy, surgical drainage is also required and, whenever possible, especially in more severe cases, a reduction of immunosuppressive therapy should be applied. The best treatment has not yet been determined. In the past, the antimicrobial of choice was TMP/SMX, but since the development of new antibiotics, *in vitro* synergy studies, the insidious nature of the disease and its high mortality, the recommendation is a combination of two or three drugs (Clark, 2009).

There are few studies correlating susceptibility data with clinical outcome (Sorrell et al., 2005), so the best combination is uncertain. Nevertheless, it is often chosen on the basis of: a) the species of *Nocardia* isolated; b) its sensitivity to antibiotics and possible interactions with the complex medication of transplanted patients; c) the location, extent and severity of the infection; and d) the experts' opinion and documented experience in the literature.

5.2 Empiric therapy

According to clinical experience, TMP/SMX remains the antimicrobial agent of choice for many *Nocardia* infections (Hewagama et al., 2011), supported by the *in vitro* synergy of its two components, the fact that it reaches high levels in lung, brain, skin and bone (Smego et al., 1983) and that it can be used as intravenous or oral maintenance therapy (Table 2). The main side effects include rash, nausea, vomiting, erythema multiforme, bone marrow suppression, hyperkalaemia and crystalluria, which may limit its use. Some species - *N. farcinica*, *N. otitidiscaviarum* and *N. nova* - may be resistant to sulphonamides, so it is important to determine the species and its *in vitro* susceptibility. These resistances and possible allergies to sulphonamides promoted the search for alternative antibiotics. Amikacin is universally active against most *Nocardia* species, except for *N. transvaliensis* and *N. brasiliensis*. The main limitations for its use are optical and renal toxicity. The combination of imipenem and amikacin is accepted as initial therapy in patients with severe nocardiosis (Minero et al., 2009) while the antibiogram is pending. This antibiotic combination is additive and synergic *in vitro* (Kanemitsu et al., 2003), maintains synergy when associated with sulphonamides (Gombert et al., 1986) and is effective in humans, so this triple combination has also been recommended as first-line treatment in patients with severe disease including dissemination to the CNS, where it is always better to use at least two drugs with good intracranial diffusion and, when severe, a triple combination (Ambrosioni et al., 2010). During the administration of amikacin and imipenem, doses should be adjusted according to renal function and auditory function should be monitored. In addition, in LTx, co-administration of cyclosporine or tacrolimus with amikacin may enhance the nephrotoxicity of aminoglycosides.

INFECTION	PRIMARY THERAPY	ALTERNATIVE THERAPY
Primary cutaneous	TMP/SMX*	TMP/SMX+ Fluoroquinolone
Pulmonary stable	TMP/SMX iv or po	Imipenem+amikacin or minocycline or linezolid
Pulmonary critical	Imipenem+amikacin or TMP/SMX	Linezolid
Cerebral	Imipenem+amikacin or TMP/SMX	Linezolid or ceftriaxone or cefotaxime or minocycline
Disseminated	Imipenem+amikacin or TMP/SMX	Ceftriaxone, cefotaxime, linezolid or minocycline

Table 2. Antibiotics suggested for Nocardia infections in organ recipients (Clark, 2009, Ambrosioni et al., 2010, modified). TMP/SMX, trimethoprim-sulfamethoxazole.

As regards the carbapenems, imipenem and meropenem have a similar spectrum of activity and effectiveness and, although the latter is somewhat less effective against *N. asteroides complex* (NAC) and more effective against *N. brasiliensis* and *N. otitidiscaviarum*, it is preferred in cases with CNS involvement, since imipenem has been associated with seizures. Ertapenem has slightly less activity against several species of *Nocardia* and doripenem, with a similar spectrum of antibiotic activity to meropenem (Lai et al., 2009) but without CNS penetration, has not been tested.

Other beta-lactam antibiotics such as the third-generation cephalosporins ceftriaxone or cefotaxime, due to their good CNS penetration, may be combined with other antimicrobials for treatment of intracranial infections with good results, depending on the species of *Nocardia*, since some may be intrinsically resistant (Garlando et al., 1992; Durmaz et al., 2001).

5.3 Other alternatives

The literature includes experiences of varying degrees of success with other antibiotic treatments, including minocycline and tigecycline, macrolides, ampicillin, piperacillin/ tazobactam, fluoroquinolones (ciprofloxacin, moxifloxacin and gatifloxacin), but experiences are limited and there is not enough scientific basis to include them in general recommendations. With moxifloxacin, which is active against *N. farcinica* (Hanse et al., 2008), good results have been obtained in some cases; however, in others there has been recurrence in the CNS, despite its activity and having achieved high levels of drug in the abscess material (Dahan et al., 2006).

In recent years, the oxazolidinone linezolid has been gathering attention due to its excellent activity against all species of *Nocardia*, including *N. farcinica* (Brown-Elliot et al., 2001). It has been used successfully, even in monotherapy, in six patients with disseminated nocardiosis (Moylett et al., 2003) and also in combination with other antimicrobials (Lewis et al., 2003; Rivero et al., 2008). It has extensive intravenous and oral bioavailability, crosses the blood-brain barrier, does not require renal or liver dose adjustments and has few interactions with immunosuppressive agents (Jodlowski et al., 2007), which makes it a very reasonable alternative as first- or second-line treatment of *Nocardia* infections in LTx (especially in cases of kidney involvement). Limitations on long-term use are conditioned by its high cost and possible toxicity, since, in addition to its minor adverse effects such as rash, nausea and vomiting, it may also induce, less frequently, thrombocytopaenia, aplastic anaemia, peripheral neuropathy, lactic acidosis and serotonin syndrome (Beekmann et al., 2008).

5.4 Duration of treatment

The optimal duration of treatment has not been standardised, but should be several months due to the difficulty of eradicating *Nocardia* and frequency of relapse (Sorrell et al., 2005). Most patients begin to improve in 1-2 weeks, but more severe cases must follow an additional 3 to 4 weeks of intravenous therapy before switching to oral treatment. Cerebral nocardiosis requires at least 9-12 months of treatment, whereas soft tissue and lung presentations require 6-12 months, depending on the clinical course and response to treatment (Clark, 2009). If the infection is associated with a central venous catheter, this must be removed and followed by administration of antibiotic treatment for several months.

5.5 Consolidation therapy

When the patient improves and intravenous treatment can be withdrawn, oral alternatives may include amoxicillin-clavulanate, TMP/SMX, linezolid, clarithromycin, ciprofloxacin and moxifloxacin as consolidation therapy. There are no trials comparing the effects of these antibiotics. Some studies recommend a dual oral combination after severe infections, such as those involving the CNS (Sullivan & Chapman, 2010).

After discontinuation of treatment, the patient should be monitored for a minimum of one year to detect possible relapses. In some hospitals, prophylaxis is maintained for as long as the patient remains immunosuppressed (King et al., 1993; Poonyagariyagorn et al., 2008).

5.6 Evolution

Despite combined treatment, the prognosis is variable and depends heavily on: the extent of infection, the underlying conditions of the organ recipients and co-infections that precede or coincide with *Nocardia* infection (Peleg et al., 2007b). Overall mortality is around 40% (Husain et al., 2002). In CNS infections it is 30-55% (Mamelak et al., 1994) and in the lung about 14-18% (Poonyagariyagorn et al., 2008; Morales et al., 2011). The prognosis is better in isolated skin lesions, in which some studies report up to 90% healing.

Delayed diagnosis and discontinuation of treatment has also been associated with poor prognosis. There is little information on the crude mortality rate, because in many cases the patient died due to multiple causes and it is difficult to determine the impact of *Nocardia* infection on the final outcome.

6. Prevention/Prophylaxis

Given the low incidence of *Nocardia* infection in LTx and that its onset tends to be late, primary chemoprophylaxis is not indicated. However, in patients with solid organ transplant in general, TMP/SMX is administered daily for at least six months post-transplant and then on alternate days indefinitely to prevent infection by *Pneumocystis jiroveci* (Hewayama et al., 2011). Some works suggest that this prophylaxis reduces infection by *Nocardia* and this benefit extends to other microorganisms. Nevertheless, there is an increasing number of reports of TMP/SMX susceptible *Nocardia* isolations in transplant recipients taking this antibiotic as prophylaxis (Roberts et al., 2000; Husain et al., 2002; Poonyagariyagorn et al., 2008; Khan et al., 2008; Minero et al., 2009). This fact raises doubts concerning the prophylactic role of TMP/SMX to prevent nocardiosis. The lack of efficacy may be due to different protocols in SOT recipients. Relapse has also been documented in LTx (Poonyagariyagorn, 2008; Roberts et al., 2000) after one cycle of antibiotic treatment, possibly due to short-term duration or interruption, but the data are controversial with regard to recommending secondary prophylaxis. Long-term prophylaxis to prevent these relapses is only suggested in a few hospitals.

Moreover, considering that *Nocardia* is a ubiquitous microorganism, it is important to teach LTx to alter their lifestyle and adopt a careful and alert attitude in order to reduce their high epidemiological risk of exposure, especially in the community. Recently, Avery and Michaels have published an excellent guide to strategies for avoiding infection following solid organ transplantation (Avery & Michaels, 2009).

7. Peri-Transplant considerations

7.1 Pre-Transplant

The future LTx may have had an infection that has already been treated or that is still active during the pre-transplant evaluation period. In fact, this happens with some frequency in patients with cystic fibrosis (CF). Neither situation, according to most experts and to our own experience, is an absolute contraindication for transplantation. Nevertheless, the patient must be monitored closely, being aware of possible relapses, complications or dissemination of infection, and ensuring full compliance with treatment.

7.2 Post-Transplant

Considerations are similar when nocardiosis occurs after transplantation, as we have previously discussed in the text, paying special attention to possible relapses.

7.3 Donor

Even though there is no documented case of *Nocardia* infection in the organ donor, nocardiosis would hypothetically be a relative contraindication for transplantation. In any case, treatment would be obligatory.

8. Final considerations

The practice of organ transplantation in general and lung transplantation in particular is a growing technique in the clinical setting and transplant recipients inevitably need immunosuppressive treatment. Therefore, the appearance of opportunistic infections, specifically nocardiosis, is expected. Given the nonspecific clinical and radiological signs, diagnosis of these infections is based on high clinical suspicion, proper sample collection and rapid microbiological diagnostic methods to confirm it and properly orient the antibiotic treatment as early as possible. The future challenge seems to be the application of molecular methods directly on the sample (Couble et al., 2005) and perhaps fewer but more effective and less toxic antibiotics, less aggressive immunosuppressive therapy and, overall, to try to avoid infection with a healthy lifestyle.

9. References

Avery, RK., Michaels, MG., & AST Infectious Diseases Community of Practice. 2009. Strategies for safe-living following solid organ transplantation. *Am J Transplant,* Vol 9, No 4 Suppl, (December 2009), pp. S252-S257.

Ambrosioni, J., Lew, D., Garbino, J. 2010. Nocardiosis: updated clinical review and experience at a tertiary center. *Infection,* Vol 38, No 2, (April 2010), pp. 89-97.

Balikian, JP., Herman, PG., & Kopit, S. 1978. Pulmonary nocardiosis. *Radiology,* Vol 126, No 3, (Mars 1978), pp. 569-573.

Basu, A., Ramkumar, M., Tan, HP., Marcos, A., Fung, JJ., Starzl, TE., Shapiro, TE., Khan A, & McCauley J. 2005. Reversal of acute cellar rejection after renal transplantation with Campath-1H. *Transplant Proc,* Vol 37, No 2, (Mars 2005), pp. 923-926.

Beaman, BL., & Beaman, L. 1994. Nocardia species: host-parasite relationships. *Clin Microbiol Rev,* Vol 7, No 2, (April 1994), pp. 213-264.

Beekmann, SE., Gilbert, DN., & Polgreen, PM. 2008. Toxicity of extended courses of linezolid: results of an Infectious Diseases Society of America Emerging Infections Network survey. *Diagn Microbiol Infect Dis,* Vol 62, No 4, (December 2008), pp. 407-410.

Brown-Elliott, BA., Ward, SC., Crist, CJ., Mann, LB., Wilson, RW., & Wallace, RJ, Jr. 2001. In vitro activities of linezolid against multiple Nocardia species. *Antimicrob Agents Chemother,* Vol 45, No 4, (April 2001), pp. 1295-1297.

Brown-Elliott, BA., Brown, JM., Conville, PS., & Wallace, RJ Jr. 2006. Clinical and laboratory features of the *Nocardia* spp. based on current molecular taxonomy. *Clin Microbiol Rev,* Vol 19, No 2, (April 2006), pp. 259-282.

Cabada, MM., Nishi, SP., Lea, AS., Schnadig, V., Lombrad, GA., Lick, SD., & Valentine, VG. 2010. Concomitant pulmonary infection with *Nocardia transvalensis* and *Aspergillus ustus* in lung transplantation. *J Heart Lung Transplant,* Vol 29, No 8,(August 2010), pp. 900-903.

Clark, NM., and the AST infectious diseases community of practice. 2009. *Nocardia* in solid organ transplant recipients. *Am J Transp,* Vol 9, No 4 Suppl, (December 2009), pp. S70-S77.

Conville, PS., Brown, JM., Steigertwalt, AG., Lee, JW., Anderson ,VL., Fishbain, JT., Holland, SM., & Witebsky, FG. 2004. *Nocardia kruczakiae* sp. nov., a pathogen in immunocompromised patients and a member of the *"N. nova complex"*. *J Clin Microbiol,* Vol 42, No 11, (November 2004), pp. 5139-5145.

Corales, R., Chua, J., Mawhorter, S., Young, JB., Starling, R., Tomford, JW., McCarthy, P., Braun, WE., Smedira, N., Hobbs, R., Haas, G., Pelegrin, D., Majercik, M., Hoercher, K., Cook, D., & Avery, RK. 2002. Significant post-transplant hypogammaglobulinemia in six heart transplant recipients: An emerging clinical phenomenon? *Transpl Infect Dis,* Vol 2, No 3, (September 2002), pp. 133-139.

Couble, A., Rodriguez-Nava, V., de Montclos, MP., Boiron, P., & Laurent F. 2005. Direct detection of *Nocardia* spp. In clinical samples by a rapid molecular method. *J Clin Microbiol,* Vol 43, No 4, (April 2005), pp. 1921-1924.

Dahan, K., El Kabbaj, D., Venditto, M., Pastural, M., & Delahousse, M. 2006. Intracraneal Nocardia recurrence during fluorinated quinolones therapy. *Transpl Infect Dis,* Vol 8, No 3, (September 2006), pp. 161-165.

Deem, RL., Doughty, FA., & Beaman, BL. 1983. Immunologically specific direct T lymphocyte-mediated killing of *Nocardia asteroides*. *J Immunol,* Vol, 130, No 5, (May 1983), pp. 2401-2406.

Durmaz, R., Atasoy, MA., Durmaz, G., Adapinar, B., Arslantas, A., Aydinli, A., & Tel E. 2001. Multiple nocardial abscesses of cerebrum, cerebellum and spinal cord, causing quadriplegia. *Clin Neurol Neurosurg,* Vol 103, No 1, (April 2001), pp. 59-62.

Eisenblätter, M., Disko, U., Stoltenburg-Didinger, G., Scherübl, H., Schaal, KP., Roth, A., Ignatius, R., Keitz, M., Hahn, H., & Wagner, J. 2002. Isolation of Nocardia paucivorans from the cerebrospinal fluid of a patient with relapse of cerebral nocardiosis. *J Clin Microbiol,* Vol 40, No 9, (September 2002), pp. 3532-3534.

Garlando, F., Bodmer, T., Lee, C., Zimmerli, W., & Pirovino, M. 1992. Successful treatment of disseminated nocardiosis complicated by cerebral abscess with ceftriaxone and amikacin. Case Report. *Clin Infect Dis,* Vol 15, No 6, (December 1992), pp. 1039-1040.

Gombert, ME., Aulicino, TM., duBouchet, L., Silverman, GE., & Sheinbaum, WM. 1986. Therapy of experimental cerebral nocardiosis with imipenem, amikacin, trimethoprim sulfamethoxazole and minocycline antimicrob agents chemother. *Antimicrob Agents _Chemother,* Vol 30, No 2, (August 1986), pp. 270-273.

Hansen, G., Swanzy, S., Gupta, R., Cookson, B., & Limaye, AP. 2008. *In vitro* activity of fluoroquinolones against clinical isolates of *Nocardia* identified by partial 165 rRNAsequencing. *Eur J Clin Microbiol Infect Dis,* Vol 27, No 2, (February, 2008), pp. 115-120.

Hewagama, S., Langan, K., Nishi, SP., Valentine, VG., & Peleg AY. Chapter 17. Elsevier Inc.. ISHLT Monographseries. Diagnosis and management of infectious diseases in cardiothoracic transplantation and mechanical circulatory support. ed. Mooney ML, Hannan MM, Husain S, Kirklin JK. 2011, vol 5. pp 175-186. ISSN 1930-2134. Philadelphia.

Husain, S., McCurry, K., Dauber, J., Singh, N., & Kusne, S. 2002. *Nocardia* infection in lung transplant recipients. *J Heart Lung Transplant,* Vol 21, No 3, (Mars 2002), pp. 354-359.

Jodlowski, TZ., Melnychuk, I., & Conry, J. 2007. Linezolid for the treatment of *Nocardia* spp. infections. *Ann Pharmacother,* Vol 41, No 10, (October 2007), pp. 1694-1699.

Kanemitsu, K., Kunishima, H., Saga, T., Harigae, H., Ishikawa, S., Takemura, H., & Kaku, M. 2003. Efficacy of amikacin combinations for nocardiosis. *Tohoku J Exp Med,* Vol 201, No 3, (November, 2003), pp. 157-163.

Khan, BA., Duncam, M., Reynolds, J., & Wilkes, DS. 2008. *Nocardia* infection in lung transplant recipients. *Clin Transplant,* Vol 22, No 5, (September-October 2008), pp. 562-566.

King, CT., Chapman, SW., & Butkus, DE. 1993. Recurrent nocardiosis in a renal transplant recipient. *South Med J,* Vol 86, No 2, (February 1993), pp. 225-228.

Kramer, MR., Marshall, SE., Starnes, VA., Gamberg, P., Amitai, Z., & Theodore, J. 1993. Infectious complications in heart lung transplantation. Analysis of 200 episodes. *Arch Intern Med,* Vol 153, No 17, (September 1993), pp. 2010-2016.

Kundranda, MN., Spiro, TP., Muslimani, A., Gopalkrishna, KV., Melaragno, MJ., & Daw, HA. 2007. Cerebral nocardiosis in a patient with NHL treated with rituximab. *Am J Hematol,* Vol 82, No 11, (November, 2007), pp. 1033-1034.

Lai, CC., Tan, CK., Lin, SH., Liao, CH., Chou, CH., Hsu, HL., Huang, YT., & Hsueh, PR. 2009. Comparative in vitro activities of nemonxacin, doripenem, tigecycline, and 16 antimicrobials against *Nocardia brasiliensis, Nocardia asteroides* and unusual *Nocardia* species. *J Antimicrobial Chemother,* Vol 64, No 1, (July 2009), pp. 73-78.

Lerner, PI. 1996. Nocardiosis. *Clin Infect Dis,* Vol 22, No 6, (June 1996), pp. 891-903.

Lewis, KE., Ebden, P., Wooster, SL., Rees, J., & Harrison, GA. 2003. Multisystem infection with *Nocardia farcinica*-therapy with linezolid and minocycline. *J Infect,* Vol 46, No 3, (April 2003), pp. 199-202.

Mamelak, AN., Obana, WG., Flaherty, JF., & Rosenblum ML. 1994. Nocardial brain absceess: treatment strategies and factors influencing outcome. *Neurosurgery,* Vol 35, No 4, (October 1994), pp. 622-631.

Martinez-Tomás, R., Menéndez-Villanueva, R., Reyes-Calzada, S., Santos-Durantez, M., Vallés-Tarazona, JM., Modesto-Alapont, M., & Gobernado-Serrano, M. 2007. Pulmonary Nocardiosis: risk factors and outcomes. *Respirology,* Vol 12, No 3, (May 2007), pp. 394-400.

Merigou, D., Beylot-Barry, M., Ly, S., Doutre, MS., Texier-Maugein, J., Billes, P., & Beylot, C. 1998. Primary cutaneous *Nocardia asteroides* infection after heart transplantation. *Dermatology,* Vol 196, No,2, pp. 246-247.

Minero, MV., Marín, M., Cerenado, E., Rabadán, PM., Bouza, E., & Muñoz, P. 2009. Nocardiosis at the turn of the century. *Medicine (Baltimore)*, Vol 88, No 4, (July 2009), pp. 250-261.

Morales, P., Gil-Brusola, A., & Santos, M. 2011. *Nocardia* infection in lung transplant recipients: Twenty years review. *Am J Crit Care Med,* Vol 183, No 1, (May 2011), A4648.

Moylett, EH., Pacheco, SE., Brown-Elliott, BA., Perry, TR., Buescher, ES., Birmingham, MC., Schentag, JJ., Gimbel, JF., Apodaca, A., Schwartz, MA., Rakita, RM., & Wallace, RJ Jr. 2003. Clinical experience with linezolid for the treatment of *Nocardia* infection. *Clin Infect Dis,*Vol 36, No 3 (February 2003), pp. 313-318.

Oszoyoglu, AA., Kirsch, J., & Mohammed, TL. 2007. Pulmonary nocardiosis after lung transplantation: CT findings in 7 patients and review of literature. *J Thorac Imaging,* Vol 22, No 2, (May 2007), pp. 143-148.

Patel, R., & Payá, CV. 1997. Infections in solid-organ transplant recipients. *Clin Microbiol Rev,* Vol 10, No1, (January 1997), pp. 86-124.

Paya CV. 1999. Indirect effects of CMV in the solid organ transplant patient. *Transpl Infect Dis,* Vol 1, (suppl 1), pp. 8-12.

Peleg, AY., Husain, S., Qureshi, ZA., Silveira, FP., Sarumi, M., Shutt, KA., Kwak, EJ., & Paterson, DL. 2007. Risk factors, clinical characteristics, and outcome of *Nocardia* infection in organ transplant recipients: a matched case-control study. *Clin Infect Dis,* Vol 44, No 10, (May 2007), pp. 1307-1314.

Peleg, AY., Husain, S., Kwak, EJ., Silveira, FP., Ndirangu, M., Tran, J., Shutt, KA., Shapiro, R., Thai, N., Abu-Elmagd, K., McCurry, KR., Marcos, A., & Paterson, DL. 2007. Opportunistic infections in 547 organ transplant recipients receiving alemtuzumab, a humanized monoclonal CD-52 antibody. *Clin Infect Dis,* Vol 44, No 2, (January 2007), pp. 204-212.

Peraira, JR., Segovia, J., Fuentes, R., Jiménez-Mazuecos, J., Arroyo, R., Fuertes, B., Mendaza, P., & Pulpon, LA. 2003. Pulmonary nocardiosis in heart transplant recipients: treatment and outcome. *Transplant Proc,* Vol 35, No 5, (August 2003), pp. 2006-2008.

Poonyagariyagorn, HK., Gershman, A., Avery, R., Minai, O., Blazey, H., Asamoto, K., Alster, J., Murthy, S., Mehta, A., Petterson, G., Mason, DP., & Budev M. 2008. Challenges in the diagnosis and management of *Nocardia* infections in lung transplant recipients. *Transpl Infect Dis,* Vol 10, No 6, (December 2008), pp. 403-408.

Pottumarthy, S., Limaye, AP., Prentice, JL., Houze, YB., Swanzy, SR., & Cookson, BT. 2003. *Nocardia veterana,* a new emerging pathogen. *J Clin Microbiol,* Vol 41, No 4, (April 2003), pp. 1705-1709.

Roberts, SA., Franklin, JC., Mijch, A., & Spelman, D. 2000. Nocardia infection in heart-lung transplant at Alfred Hospital, Melbourne, Australia, 1989-1998. *Clin Infect Dis,* Vol 31, No 4, (October, 2000), pp. 968-972.

Rivero, A., García-Lázaro, M., Pérez-Camacho, I., Natera, C., del Carmen Almodovar, M., Camacho, A., & Torre-Cisneros J. 2008. Successful long-term treatment for dissemitad infection with multiresistant *Nocardia farcinica. Infection,* Vol 36, No 4, (August 2008), pp. 389-391.

Sahathevan, M., Harvey, FA., Forbes, G., O'Grady, J., Gimson, A., Bragman, S., Jensen, R., Philpott-Howard, J., Williams, R., & Casewell, MW. 1991. Epidemiology, bacteriology and control of an outbreak of *Nocardia asteroides* infection on a liver unit. *J Hosp Infect,* Vol 18, Suppl A, (June 1991), pp. 473-80.

Santos, M., Gil-Brusola, A., & Morales, P. 2011. Infection by *Nocardia* in solid organ transplantation: thirty years of experience. *Transplant Proc,* (in press).

Schlaberg, R., Huard, RC., & Della-Latta, P. 2008. *Nocardia cyriacigeorgica,* an emerging pathogen in the United States. *J Clin Microbiol,* Vol 46, No 1, (January 2008), pp. 265-273.

Shawar, RM., Moore, DG., & LaRocco, MT. 1990. Cultivation of *Nocardia* spp on chemically defined media for selective recovery of isolates from clinical specimens. *J Clin Microbiol,* Vol 28, No 3, (Mars 1990), pp. 508-512.

Singh, N., Husain, S. 2000. Infections of the central nervous system in transplant recipients. *Transpl Infect Dis,* Vol 2, No 3, (September 2000), pp. 101-11.

Smego, RA Jr., Moeller, MB., & Gallis, HA. 1983. Trimetoprim-sulfamethoxazole therapy for *Nocardia* infections. *Arch Intern Med,* Vol 143, No 4, (April, 1983), pp. 711-718.

Sorrell, TC., Mitchell, DH., & Iredell, JR. In: Mandel GL, Bennett JE, Dolin R, eds. Principles and Practice of Infectious Diseases. 6th Ed. Philadelphia, PA: Churchill Livingstone 2005, pp. 2916-2914.

Sullivan, DC., & Chapman, SW. 2010. Bacteria that masquerade as fungi: actinomycosis/ nocardia. *Proc Am Thorac Soc,* Vol 7, No 3, (May 2010), pp. 216-221.

Wayne, PA. 2003. Susceptibility testing of mycobacteria, nocardiae and other aerobic actinomycetes. M24-A. Clinical and Laboratory Standards Institute (CLSI/NCCLS).

Wenger, PN., Brown, JM., McNeil, MM., & Jarvis, WR. 1998. *Nocardia farcinica* sternotomy site infections in patients following open heart surgery. *J Infect Dis,* Vol, 178, No 5, (November, 1998), pp. 1539-1543.

Yassin, AF., Rainey, FA., Mendrock, U., Brzezinka, H., & Schaal, KP. 2000. *Nocardia abscessus* sp. nov. *Int J Syst Evol Microbiol,* Vol 50, No 4, (July, 2000), pp. 1487-1493.

18

In Vivo Models of Lung Disease

Tracey L. Bonfield
Inflammatory Mediator and Cystic Fibrosis Lung Disease Modeling CORE Center
Department of Pediatric Pulmonology
Case Western Reserve University
Cleveland, Ohio
USA

1. Introduction

Development of new therapeutics for lung diseases requires good modeling systems in which to test hypotheses. Often, how lung diseases are modeled *in vivo*, are not at all initiated by the same events that cause the disease in humans. The models for interstitial pulmonary fibrosis or chronic obstructive lung disease for example, require the use of toxic reagents and models for asthma do not use the same antigenic stimuli. What this means is what is used to initiate disease *in vivo* using animal models is not necessarily totally responsible for the same disease in humans. Even in situations of generating genetic models focusing on identified genes associated with specific disease entities modeled *in vivo*, the disease in the animal model is still not the same as the disease in humans even if the gene is most certainly involved. The focus of this chapter is to describe a variety of the animal models that have been developed to study specific lung disease entities including understanding the strength and the weaknesses of the *in vivo* modeling systems. The main goal of animal modeling is to provide an *in vivo*_complex scenario which allows for the pursuit of defining the underlying mechanisms of diseases or importantly to provide a format for studying new interventional therapeutics. The focus of the chapter will start with basic anatomy, physiological differences and immunological responses which either enhance the selection of the model or are used to study specific components of the disease process.

Anatomy and Lung Models: For an *in vivo* model to provide the appropriate conditions, modeling the anatomy and the physiology of the lung model must first be considered. Whether dealing with small rodents such as mice, rats, and ferrets or larger animal such as pigs, sheep or monkeys, a detailed understanding of the model's anatomy and physiology must be considered for the correlation to human diseases (1,2). The issues to consider include the anatomical patterns of the alveolar spaces, the bronchial tree, milieu differences including the changes in the surfactant proteins, phospholipids, and physiological differences including the respiratory rate and airway clearance mechanisms (3,4). Some of the issues of correlating with human disease have to do with how the lung structure is different with the human lung and how this relates to differences in lung structure and function. This also relates to size, oxygenation and gaseous exchange. Another important issue is how the lung structure relates to the physiology and whether the mechanisms for homeostasis maintenance the same? This complicates things further since in most instances a direct cross-over between animal models and human disease is not complete. The relevant comparative anatomy of the lung would include all of the variables outlined in Figure 1.

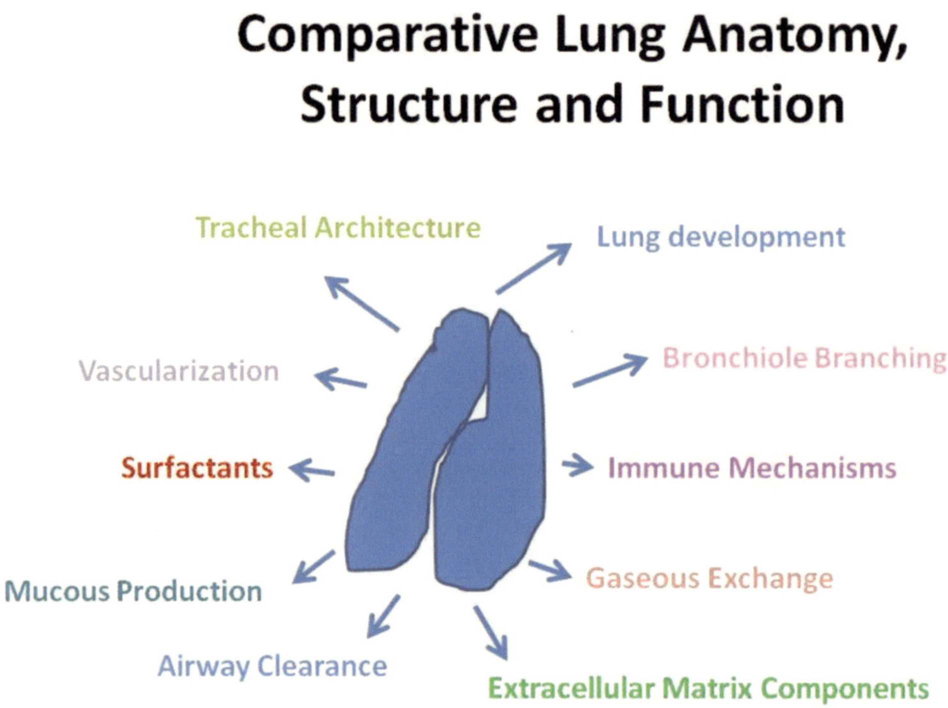

Fig. 1. Contributions to *In vivo* Lung Models. Here we show the lung and the variables associated with model selection regardless of the lung disease to be studied.

Function and Lung Model: The selection of an *in vivo* model must take into consideration not just the similarities and differences between the model and the human disease but also the question being asked in the disease application. The more common comparisons are listed in Table 1, when evaluating murine and rat models. Certainly, some animal models provide good *in vivo* correlates to the clinical situation; other are not so realistic. Choosing the model has to do with the question being answered and the reasoning behind selecting the model. For examples, cats and horses have been shown to develop spontaneous airway hyper-responsiveness, which would be consistent with human asthma (5,6). However, given the size of the animals, the inability to generate congenic species makes these models economically unrealistic. The opposite perspective is the ability to use mice for diseases such as asthma and cystic fibrosis (CF). Although the specific disease can be mimicked, the spectrum of the pathophysiology is different. For example, the mouse model for CF does not develop spontaneous lung disease (4,7). The model does provide an invaluable tool to study infection induced inflammation and in some case cell specific contribution of disease (8). In the murine asthma model, a variety of antigens can be used to induce disease, but it has been shown that many of the pathways associated with disease in humans are not played out in the murine model of the disease (9,10). It is a balance between the clinical or mechanistic question and the goal of the study for the selection of the appropriate model. Animal models afford the opportunity for investigators to experimentally manipulate a number of controlled variables such as strain of animal, and environment to investigate the molecular interactions involved in the pathogenesis of many lung diseases. The selection is based upon the basic pathophysiology, anatomy and the ability to induce the disease in a time sensitive fashion for comparative and economic consistency.

Mechanism of Study	Mouse	Rat
Lung Remodeling and Repair	Offers the ability to study specific genes associated with repair and remodeling. Depends on species susceptibility to either the Th_1 or Th_2 process.	Enhanced susceptibility to develop Th_2 driven cellular immune responses. Larger airways, easier to measure breathing dynamics.
Inflammation	Mechanisms involve similar but often different proteins. Careful experimental design for a focused approach on the similarities but remembering the differences.	Functionally similar but several components and events which are different. Understanding the similarities and differences are important in the context of disease.
Response to Infection	Similar processes and players with proteins being both the same and different. This all depends on protein homology or even presence.	Similar processes with players of proteins being often times similar. The issue is the availability of reagents for studying the mechanisms of interests.
Response to Injury	Injury response is relative to the total surface area at the air-liquid interface. Mouse models use chemicals, which are not the initiators in human disease.	Injury associated with chemicals of mechanical contributions can be used due to the size difference from the murine counterparts. Chemicals used are always associated with real human disease.

Table 1. In Vivo Models and Studies of Lung Disease Pathophysiology

Acute Lung Injury: Acute lung injury (ALI) and acute respiratory distress syndrome (ARDS) results from severe injury to the lung parenchyma (11). Animal modeling experiments of ALI and ARDS have been very useful in providing some directions into the mechanisms related to disease pathogenesis and providing opportunities to explore new and innovative therapeutic targets. As with most lung disease modeling systems, the design of the model and its manipulation is predominately dictated by the hypothesis and the focal point of pathology. The pathology associated with ALI and ARDS includes inflammatory cell recruitment, exudation with edema in the small airways potentially resulting in alveolar collapse (12). The recruitment of inflammatory cells, the changes in tonicity at the tissue interface are all pathologies which contribute to the injurious process. This occurs through enhancing the production of inflammatory proteins, proteases and reactive oxygen radicals at the tissue interface. This gets to the mechanisms associated with the development of ALI and ARDS including the processes involving the injury and down-stream response to the injury which also contributes to tissue damage (13,14). There are three different models that are used for inducing different aspects of ALI and ARDS. These include the surfactant washout (LAV) model, oleic acid intravenous injection (OAI) model and the lipopolysaccharide (LPS) model (15). The LAV model utilizes a series of broncholaveolar lavages which requires larger animals like rats and ferrets. In the surfactant washout models, the focus is removing the protective anti-inflammatory molecules such as surfactant protein A (SP-A) potentially altering the air-liquid interface surface tension, resulting in changes in oxygenation efficiency. The change in surface milieu signals the production of pro-inflammatory cytokines with results in recruitment of inflammatory cells which ultimately ctonritbutes to interstitial tissue damage (15). The OAI model uses an infusion of oleic acid into the central vein or the right atrium (16,17), necessitating the requirement of larger animals. There is considerable diversity in terms of the dosing and the timing of the administration of OAI, making the model highly variable and not well accepted. The precise mechanisms by which the oleic acid induces lung edema, and the mechanisms associated with the recruitment of inflammatory cells and injury are not completely understood. The response of the animal to the oleic acid, results in a series of inflammatory events that create ALI/ARDS which has been theroretically associated with anhanced pro-inflammatory cytokine production.

The production of the pro-inflammatory cytokines in the LPS model is the common process involved with ALI development, as discussed in reference to the OAI and LAV models. The LPS model uses the product of gram negative bacteria (LPS) to induce cytokines and the down-stream events which result in inefficiency in the ability to resolve infection (15,18). In a sense it is a process that confuses the immune system so that it is unable to perform efficiently. The LPS is usually extracted from *Escherichia coli*, but could be from other gram negatives such as *Pseudomonas aeruginosa*, a common pathogen associated with community acquired pneumonia and ventilator associated pneumonia (19,20). The development of stable lung injury is dependent on dosage, time, route of administration and size of the model selected. In the murine models of the ALI/ARDS the LPS is administered intra-tracheally. The process of infection induced ALI and/or ARDS may include sepsis in the animal model but also in human disease. In fact, about 50% of sepsis cases ultimately account for ALI and ARDS ventilator support (21). The development of sepsis, results from a sustained and uncontrolled inflammatory response to the infectious insult contributing to dysfunction of at least one organ system. The sequences of events which lead to sepsis are unknown as well as the events that result in pulmonary failure (22,23). In the models of sepsis induced ALI/ARDS, LPS is administered intra-tracheally or induced by surgically clipping the gastrointestinal tract (11,15).

In Vivo Models, Clinical Relevance and Limitations. Histologically, human ALI/ARDS can be sub-divided into an exudative and fibroproliferative phase (24). The exudative phase is characterized by the accumulation of inflammatory proteins containing neutrophils (25), followed by the accumulation of macrophages initiating the fibroproliferative phase of the disease (26,27). In some patients the process and side-effects of the acute inflammatory response completely resolves whereas others progress with chronic inflammation, fibrosis and neovascularization (28). Each of the different models used to develop ALI/ARDS have both valid and controversial contributions to studying these diseases *in vivo*. How these models compare and provide insight into ALI/ARDS is outlined in Figure 2. In the surfactant washout model, it is a useful tool in studying the importance of surfactant maintenance in airway-interface surface tension and pathophysiology of ALI. The issue is that most clinical conditions do not result in clinically significant surfactant abnormalities in the adult population (29). In the OAI model, the ability to induce the pathophysiology of ALI/ARDS is dependent on using injectable oleic acid, which is obviously not similar to the *in vivo* clinical development of the disease. However, it is still a useful model for studying the pathology of ARDS especially with a focus on membrane injury (16,17). Since infection has been closely associated with the development of ALI/ARDS, the LPS model seems to be the most translatable. However the other two models probably represent up-stream events in the exposure, specificity and sensitivity of the development of infection based ALI/ARDS (30-32). As with most *in vivo* animal models it does not appear that the model is consistent with all of the components of the human disease. The LPS model does not appear to develop the fibroproliferative phase of ALI/ARDS; which limits the use of these models for studying the secondary issues associated with ALI/ARDS chronic inflammation and fibrosis (15,30).

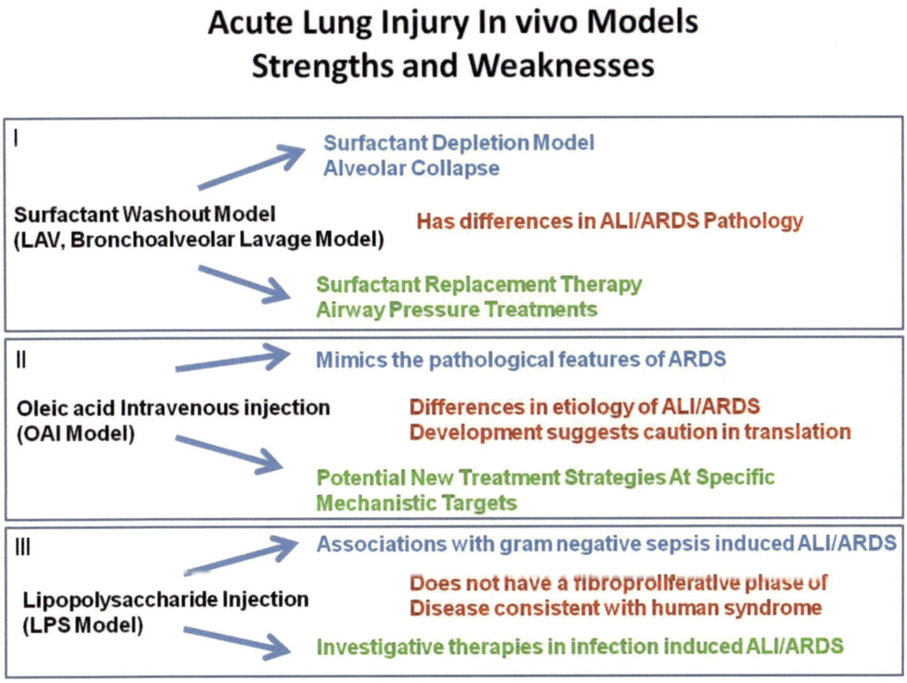

Fig. 2. In Vivo Models of Acute Lung Injury. Three principal models exist for studying ALI/ARDS. In each case the model has important contribution to the pathophysiology shown in blue, and potential therapies shown in green. The important caveats and limitations are shown in red.

Chronic Obstructive Pulmonary Disease (COPD) and Emphysema: COPD is the fifth leading cause of death worldwide and is associated with pollution and smoking history (33). COPD is a very complex disease with four described traits: emphysema, small airway remodeling, chronic bronchitis and pulmonary hypertension (34). The underlying pathophysiology of COPD is dependent on the structure and function of the lung along with the immunological processes that occur post-insult. Although patients present with variations and combinations of these pathologies, all patients progress into severe pulmonary failure. The kinetics of disease progression is dependent on the patient, patient compliance to therapeutic intervention and the ability to respond to current therapeutics. In this case the animal model of choice should require a close attention to lung anatomy and physiology since these play very important roles in the overall development of COPD and emphysema (35), especially as it relates to the overall development of new therapeutics. Besides the basics of understanding the similarities and differences between lung anatomy of the animal model and that of the human disease some consideration must also be given to the overall lung mechanics.

The *in vivo* model most commonly used to study COPD includes cigarette smoke (36). The issue lies with the ability to deliver a homogenous dosing of cigarette smoke over a defined time range, and that these models do not completely recapitulate the human disease. Further, since there are genomic differences which increase susceptibility to COPD, the translatable ability is always in the background. Additionally, the pulmonary pathology produced in the context of the cigarette model produces subtle pathologies which may also introduce subjective interpretation in quantifying the histopathology (37). Better computerized-microscopic programs need to be developed that can better quantify and minimize subjective interpretation of the studies (26,38).

Non-specific inflammation is another indicator of COPD, with a predominance of neutrophils and the inflammation approach to studying COPD focuses on apoptosis and elastase (39,40). The apoptosis model focuses on the failure of the COPD lung to repair itself post-injury focusing on dysregulated normal lung tissue turnover. The mechanism associated with apoptosis induced COPD has been linked to the production of vascular endothelial growth factor (VEGF) and/or the VEGF receptor (40). It is not clear whether this VEGF/VEGF receptor dysfunction is by itself critical for inducing endothelial cell apoptosis and the processes that result in decreased vascularization in the lung or whether it is in the context of a variety of other factors which ultimately contribute to COPD.

The elastase model uses a product of the inflammatory response to initiate and perpetuate the inflammatory response seen in COPD. The original hypothesis for the importance of elastase came patients α_1-anti-trypsin deficiency (41,42). Individuals with this disease develop emphysema and COPD. These patients are treated with exogenous α_1-anti-trypsin, the endogenous inhibitor of elastase. In COPD/emphysema, the recruitment of inflammatory cells and the disproportionate production of proteases without the appropriate anti-protease counter-part ultimately results in extracellular matrix degradation, inflammatory cell recruitment, matrix metalloprotease activity, cellular activation which all contribute to the lung damage similar to the mechanisms in α_1-anti-trypsin deficiency (43,44). The disadvantage of the elastase model, is that the function of elastase and cigarette smoke in COPD emphysema are potentially mediated through very different pathophysiological mechanisms which again brings up the issue of clinical translation. It is efficient to have a very specific inducer of emphysema for investigating specific mechanisms and therapeutic development. However, results obtained from specific products need to be taken into consideration as compared to the complex *in vivo* environment post complex insult (45,46). Some investigators have used LPS to induce airway and parenchymal changes, although the pathophysiology is more reminiscent of ALI/ARDS than COPD (33,47). Table 2 lists the pros and cons of each of the COPD models.

Model	**Pathology**	**Positives of Model**	**Negatives of Model**
Cigarette Induced COPD	Dilated alveolar ducts, abnormal parenchyma and increased numbers of goblet cells. Pulmonary function tests show decrease in effectiveness.	The most similar to the human disease in terms of inducing agent that produces emphysema.	It is not debilitating in animals. Lesions do not progress beyond a certain point to mimic the human disease.
Apoptosis Induced COPD	Induction of air space enlargement. Matrix breakdown.	Induces enlarged airspaces in short period of time.	Pathophysiological mechanisms are not permanent.
Elastase Induced COPD	Increased numbers of neutrophils, elevated elastase.	Rapid and easy onset, easy to measure functional changes and possibly relevant to the repair and remodeling issues in COPD.	Mechanism of disease induction is secondary to the initiators of clinical COPD.
Starvation-Induced COPD	Decreased lung volume, changes in lung structure and function.	Limited variability and short term impact on disease development.	Compassionate care of animals. The pathology may be due to decreased repair mechanisms.
LPS Induced COPD	Produces enlarged airways in chronic scenarios. Matrix metalloproteinase production	Short-term model with parenchymal changes.	Inflammatory differential is not the same as pollutant induced insult which may reflect different mechanisms of pathophysiology.

Table 2. Models of COPD

Bronchopulmonary Dysplasia: Bronchopulmonary dysplasia (BPD) remains the leading cause of respiratory morbidity and mortality in severely pre-term infants (48,49). The treatment of prematurity itself induces BPD, which complicates matters including ventilator induced surfactant deficiency and inflammation (44,50). Intrinsic BPD is characterized by immaturity, decreased growth, and immature vascularization (51). The main model for BPD is hyperoxic exposure in animal models such as rats and mice (49). Hyperoxia inhibits the normal budding and branching of the bronchi (52) leading to arrest in lung development resembling pre-term infant BPD (53). In these studies, it appears that both the airways and capillary vessels are affected requiring ventilation which can also contribute to inflammation and dysplasia (48,49,51). To understand the mechanisms and outcomes in BPD, animal models must contain elements of the normal fetal lung and the mechanisms associated with development and function. For the pulmonary mechanics studies, the *in vivo* models consist of larger animal models including lamb, rabbits and guinea pigs (49). The change in lung mechanics and the accumulation of fluid, changes the airway surface tension contributing to robust inflammatory cytokine production contributing further to the histopathology. Using these models, studies have provided avenues for understanding the role of surfactant therapy, decreased tidal volumes, improved control of oxygenation on BPD development and translation clinically (49,54).

Alveolar Proteinosis: The lung faces physical and environmental challenges, due to changing in lung volumes as well as exposure to foreign pathogens. The pulmonary surfactant system is integral in protecting the lung from these challenges via two different and distinct groups of surfactant proteins (55). Surfactant protein (SP)-B and SP-C are small molecular weight hydrophobic surfactant proteins that regulate air liquid interface surface tension. SP-A and SP-D are the larger hydrophilic surfactant proteins which aide in surface tension but which also have microbicidal function. Additionally, there are other non-surfactant proteins called defensins which also aid in inflammation and host defense (56). Pulmonary alveolar proteinosis (PAP) is a process by which there is a surfactant accumulation in the lungs potentially due to the inability to catabolize surfactant (57). There are three forms of the disease: genetic, exposure induced and idiopathic (58). The genetic disease specifically impacts children, and is associated with mutations in some of the surfactant protein genes (59-61). Exposure induced PAP is found in scenarios of particulate inhalation including silica and titanium (62-65). The idiopathic form is associated with circulating auto-antibodies against the macrophage growth and differentiation factor granulocyte-macrophage colony stimulating factor (GM-CSF) (66,67). Clinical studies have correlated the presence of the neutralizing antibody to PAP (66,68,69). Clinical trials of GM-CSF, plasmapheresis and whole lung lavage have shown limited successes with some sustainable relief, but none of the treatments are curative (70). In terms of animal models, most have been done with mice since the defects are most often associated with the absence of surfactant or GM-CSF proteins and murine GM-CSF knockout development of alveolar proteinosis (71-73). The surfactant protein knockouts develop diseases very reminiscent of pediatric interstitial proteinosis (50). The GM-CSF knockout mouse has many pathophysiological outcomes which are reminiscent of the human PAP adult disease (74). The nice part of these models is that they do not have to be induced, so there is relatively little variability between animal to animal. There have been some attempts to develop an autoimmune model of idiopathic PAP using monkeys and mice (75,76). These efforts have provided important insight into the potential mechanisms of development in early and late stages of PAP due to autoimmunity against GM-CSF.

Agent utilized	Pathology	Advantages	Disadvantages
Bleomycin	Induced lung damage and repair.	Ease of administration.	Requires specific dosing regimen. Toxic to investigators.
Silica	Chronic inflammatory response and repair mechanisms associated with fibrosis.	Sustained inflammation since silica is not resolved by macrophages.	Not a natural inducer of fibrosis. The mechanisms may not be translatable.
FITC	Inflammatory response and repair mechanisms. Natural hapten induced inflammatory mechanisms.	Visualize areas of repair and fibrosis.	Some characteristics of the lung disease are absent. There is significant variability depending on the FITC batch.
Irradiation	Induces direct cell death via DNA damage with a subsequent influx of inflammatory cells. The radiation may also directly induce the fibrotic processes.	Ease of study, no chemical requirement. Mimics human process in terms of initiation and progress.	Long time for the fibrosis to develop, limited to modeling radiation induced pneumonitis.
Viral Induced Transgenes	Viruses used to up-regulate mediators of fibrosis.	Specific *in vivo* molecules associated with IPF formation such as TNF or TGFB.	Deal with potential mechanisms but is not realistic to defining disease process.

Table 2. In vivo Models for Interstitial Pulmonary Fibrosis

Interstitial Pulmonary Fibrosis. Fibrosis is an important cause of morbidity and mortality in a variety of lung diseases, but it has a very prominent role in idiopathic pulmonary fibrosis (IPF)–(77). IPF presents with a homogenous phenotype with both definable physiologic and radiographic presentation but without identifiable etiology (78) although, the literature suggests that alveolar type II cell injury is an important early feature in the pathogenesis of pulmonary fibrosis (79). The source of injury is unknown. Different approaches to modeling pulmonary fibrosis have been used by investigating exposure to bleomycin, silica, fluorescein isothiocyannate (FITC) and irradiation (77). At the genetic level, some models of IPF have included over-expression of 'hypothesized" genes in the pathogenesis of IPF or utilization of transgenics for cell specific contribution to IPF. Bleomycin is the most frequently used agent in modeling IPF (80,81). The advantage of bleomycin is the ease with which it can be administered and the consistency of the IPF pathophysiology. Bleomycin is a chemotherapeutic agent which induces lung damage through direct DNA strand breakage and the generation of free radicals. The response to the injury is healing and fibrosis. Silica aerosolized into the lung induces pulmonary fibrosis through inducing chronic inflammation and frustrated phagocytosis by macrophages (77,82). Post-ingestion, the macrophages constitutively produce pro-fibrotic cytokines (83). The greatest advantage of the silica based system is that the silica particles are not easily cleared from the lungs creating a persistent stimulus and a non-reversible fibrotic process. Regardless of the model fibrosis is dependent on the strain of animals, suggesting immune dependent contribution to the overall susceptibility of IPF development. FITC is another chemical used to induce pulmonary fibrosis (77,84). Fluorescein, delivered directly into the airway acts as a hapten attaching to lung proteins providing a depot for continuous lung exposure to antigen. The advantage of the FITC model is the ability to actually image the processes as they occur in the lung.

Asthma: Asthma is a very complex and heterogeneous disease affecting 300 million people worldwide especially in Westernized countries (85). Why developing countries seem to be somewhat protective has been the foundation for the hygiene hypothesis (86). Asthma is a complex trait caused by multiple environmental factors with the main characteristics being airway inflammation and airway hyper-reactivity (AHR) (87). The pathogenesis of asthma is associated with many environmental factors, many cell types and several molecular and cellular pathways. Some specific presentations of asthma are outlined in Figure 3 (88,89). The majority of the induced asthmas are due to exposure to an irritant such as air pollution, allergen or viral exposure. Even aspirin and drug induced asthma can be associated with changes in the pulmonary milieu upon dosing. Interestingly, some asthma phenotypes are not associated with identifiable exposures, such as exercise induced and metabolic syndrome associated asthma.

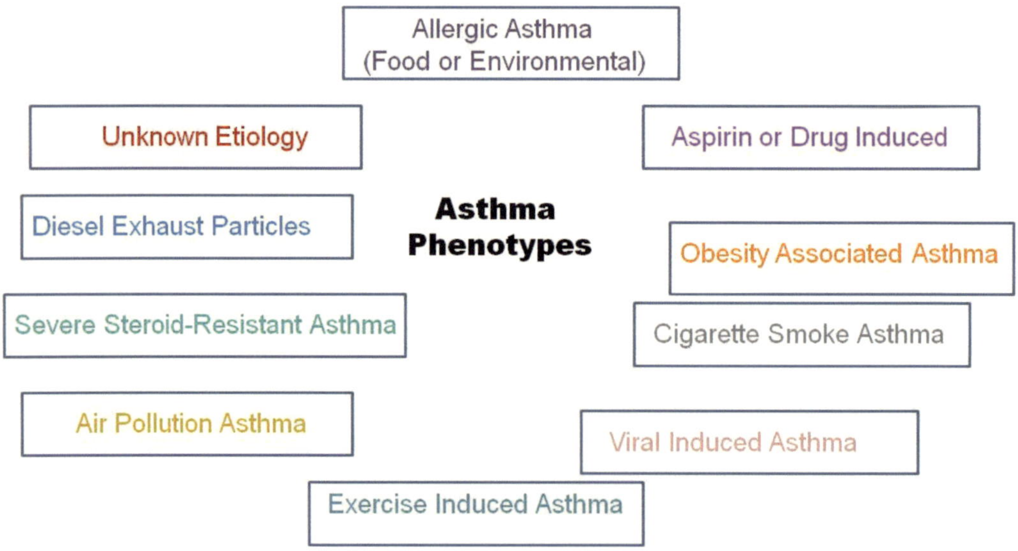

Fig. 3. Asthma Phenotypes. Asthma is a heterogeneous disease with multiple factors associated with the development and response to therapy. Given these issues, designing experiments and translating into clinical significance become a challenge.

These different pathways and phenotypes probably suggest mechanisms that are co-existent but also synergistic depending on the patient, environment, compliance and documentation.

Animal models of asthma have helped to clarify some of the underlying pathophysiological mechanisms contributing to the development of asthma (5,9,10). Much of the focus of these models is on T cell driven allergic responses contributing to understanding of the heterogeneity of asthma (90). The murine model of asthma using Balb/C mice has defined the important role of allergen-specific Th_2 cells in recruiting eosinophils into the airway, their activation and the release of histamine associated with atopic airway reactive disease. The major caveat in the murine asthma studies is that the allergen sensitization process does not completely recapitulate the allergic response in humans complicating the ability to utilize these models for therapeutic development (91). This has been quite frustrating in asthma therapy development, even though certain biomarkers have been identified in the *in vivo* models they have ultimately not translated into efficient therapeutic care for patients with asthma (10). The inability to translate the observations from the animal models to patient care were very disappointing and increased the lack of the appreciation of the animal models toward mechanisms and pathogenesis of asthma. The fortunate component of the murine asthma model is the ability to sensitize the animals to a variety of foreign proteins and to use transgenic animals for studying mechanisms and response to different exposures. In most scenarios, the challenge results in a Th_2 polarization and enhanced allergen-specific IgE production (92). Pathologically the lungs have eosinophilia, mucus secretion and goblet cell hyperplasia, airway hyper-responsiveness and remodeling with fibrosis (5,88). These asthmatic phenomena have suggested that cytokines and cells other than T-cells, such as IFNγ, IL-17 and/or neutrophils, may also play a significant role in the lung pathology (93,94). Further, Th_2 targeted therapies have not been as effective as hoped in many clinical trials of asthma, suggesting alternative pathways to the lung inflammation and remodeling. These have resulted in several distinct alternatives to the traditional allergen challenge model. Table 3 outlines the different animal models currently available to study various aspects of the pathophysiology associated with asthma.

Lung Cancer: Several *in vivo* models exist which provide the opportunity to study cancer (95). The complications in these models are their inability to completely correlate with histologic patterns of the malignancies, natural strain susceptibility and time frames for cancer induction in humans. One important difference between the animal models and the human disease is that these animals have higher basal metabolic rates changing metastatic potential (33). Failure to develop specific tumor types is probably due to the variability of the transgene expression early in lung development. The most common compound utilized for the development of tumors in animal models is urethane (96). Mouse models have been used to study the roll of mutant oncogenes in the genesis of lung adenocarcinomas (97-99). These models have also proven useful for studying potential therapeutics. The development of a tyrosine kinase inhibitor which blocks epidermal growth factor receptor (EGFR) was found to benefit some patients after testing in mouse models. The deletion of other genes associated with human small-cell lung cancers could also be mimicked in a murine lung model aiding in therapeutic development of inhibitors (33,95).

Malignant mesothelioma is a cancer associated with environmental exposure to asbestos (95). The disease has a poor prognosis, with little to offer patients in terms of therapy. Mouse models of pleural mesothelioma have been produced by exposing mice to asbestos

Model	Advantage	Disadvantage	Pathology Association	Translation into the Clinic
Allergen Challenge	Similar to atopic induced asthmatic disease. Can be defined by the route, dosage and duration of the sensitization and challenge regime.	The model does not recapitulate all of the components of the allergic disease.	Airway hyper-reactivity, systemic IgE, mucous production, goblet cell hyperplasia.	Variability in species, sensitization/challenge regimes, and duration of studies. Has introduced some clinical failures.
Viral Respiratory Infection	Independent of Th_2 mechanism, Induced using sendai virus (parainfluenza) or respiratory syncitial virus (RSV).	Maybe considered a contributor to the human disease but may precede the start of asthma symptoms in humans.	Airway hyper-reactivity, alternatively activated macrophages and natural killer cells.	Evidence for viruses has been found in patients with severe asthma and in children with asthma with pre-exposure to RSV.
Air Pollution	Ozone is a common inducer. This appears to be concentration, route and dosage dependent.	Difficult to obtain consistency due to inhalation variability.	Severe airway hyper-reactivity associated with neutrophils. Also requires the presence of IL-17.	May lead to some understanding of the down-stream event in severe chronic asthma.
Intrinsic AHR	Requires strain specific manipulation and is associated with specific proteases.	Is strain specific and appears to associate with the asthma susceptibility gene.	Appears to regulate the control of airway hyper-reactivity through smooth muscle cell activation and bronchospasm.	The association of the proteases to human asthma.

Table 3. In Vivo Models for the Versatility of the Asthma Phenotypes

fibers. A wide range of natural and synthetic fibers, chemicals and metals have also been shown to induce pleural and peritoneal mesotheliomas (100,101). Recently the technology of xenographic transplantation of human malignant mesotheliomas into rats or mice has been used to study new chemotherapeutic agents including immunotherapy, gene therapy and multimodality therapy (95). Asbestos-induced malignant mesotheliomas produced in rodents resemble the human disease with respect to latency and growth of the tumor cells. Even with these similarities, mice are not perfect models for humans.

Cystic Fibrosis: Cystic fibrosis (CF) is the result of defects in the gene encoding the cystic fibrosis transmembrane regulator (CFTR) and is the most common genetic disease among Caucasians (102).. Even though new therapeutics including correctors and activators like VX-770 has shown great promise in new phases of CF therapy, the cure has been elusive (103). The development of the *in vivo* models has focused on four major points of pathophysiology: anatomy, physiology, airway clearance and intrinsic and/or induced inflammation. The mouse model been the main model in CF research for several years, however, the model does not develop spontaneous lung disease requiring the introduction of bacteria to initiate the pathophysiological events associated with CF infection and inflammation (104). There are several different models of CFTR deficiency ranging from the complete absence of CFTR (null) to the partial expression and/or function (4). There have also been murine models developed in which the lung mutation remains but the gastrointestinal phenotype is corrected or it is cell specific (105). The reason for these later series of animals is that the murine CFTR null mutant consistently has gastrointestinal blockage once the mice have been weaned, increasing mortality and expense of the animals. To prevent obstruction, the animals are put on a laxative. Investigators have a choice whether to use laxative treated animals or gut corrected animals. In either case, it is likely that gastrointestinal obstruction is important in the overall immunity and host response to infection in CF. Therefore, observations in the gut corrected mouse may ultimately have to be verified in the null mouse depending on the focus of the studies. Even with the differences in the gastrointestinal constitution, the severity of the different murine models is defined by CFTR protein function related to the mRNA expressed, protein synthesis or folding of the complete CFTR protein (4). In addition to the gastrointestinal obstruction, most of the models display inflammation (106), failure to thrive (107), decreased survival (108,109) and hyper-responsiveness to stimulation (110). To improve the ability to look at CF globally, larger models of CFTR deficiency have been developed to better investigate the airway pathogenesis and progression of lung disease. Further, unique models have been developed using transgenic technology to induce CFTR deficiency in specific cell types, allowing for the sequential investigation of all of the contributing cellular abnormalities and how they contribute to the CF pathophysiology (105,107,111).

The pig has become an exciting new direction for CF model development. The pig lungs and human lungs have similar comparative anatomy (112,113) and have been used to study a variety of aspects of lung pathophysiology including surfactant homeostasis, airway hyper-responsiveness and lung injury (114). The first studies have shown that there were no differences in the newborn pig birth weight or appearance (4). Deficient CFTR in the pigs did not appear to alter normal birth weight, appearance and/or lung anatomy or function. The absence of CFTR however, did result in defective nasal transepithelial cell potential and all piglets developed severe gastrointestinal obstruction. Further, with piglet aging there appears to changes in lung physiology and function resembling that of infant with CF. However, the development of lung disease is still being investigated as to whether it is an intrinsic phenomena due to the absence of CFTR, or the result of environmental exposure (112). The pig is a great model for studies in CF lung pathophysiology, however husbandry and cost and reproductive cycle play a major part in being able to conduct several studies with reasonable numbers of animals.

The ferret has been shown to also be a good animal model for studying CFTR lung biology (7,115). The ferret lung shows CFTR expression in the airway epithelium and submucosal glands, identical to that in humans (4,7). Like the pig model, the majority of the CFTR deficient ferrets also developed gastrointestinal obstruction with "failure to thrive" (115,116).

To study CF, the availability of three established *in vivo* model systems provides ample ability to study various components of CF pathophysiology. Besides CFTR deficient mice, pigs and ferrets, other models have also been developed or observed (117) including the sheep (118) and monkey models (119). These have been less studied for a variety of reasons. Although these models have provided invaluable insight into the development of new CF therapeutics, new model systems should be considered to get even closer to the overall mechanisms associated with CF.

Summary: Human lung disease is a major cause of morbidity and mortality in the world. The pulmonary dysfunction may be primary or secondary to a variety of events. The pathophysiological mechanisms associated with the disease processes are different depending upon whether the insult is external as in the case of infection or injury or internal as in the case of genetic anomalies associated with important pulmonary or secretion functions. Studying lung disease requires models that attempt to recapitulate the human phenomena. There are no perfect models, and the selection for studies must be based upon the criteria of study and the ability of the model to meet the needs of the study. In this chapter we have highlighted a variety of pulmonary diseases and syndromes with a focus on the models used to study the various pathophysiological mechanisms associated with that specific disease entity. In the end, model development and usage will continue as a conduit with which to test mechanisms and to explore the development of new and innovative therapeutics.

2. References

[1] Hoymann, H. G. 2006. New developments in lung function measurements in rodents. *Exp. Toxicol. Pathol.* 57 Suppl 2: 5-11.

[2] Sadikot, R. T., J. W. Christman, and T. S. Blackwell. 2004. Molecular targets for modulating lung inflammation and injury. *Curr. Drug Targets.* 5: 581-588.

[3] Fisher, J. H., V. Sheftelyevich, Y. S. Ho, S. Fligiel, F. X. McCormack, T. R. Korfhagen, J. A. Whitsett, and M. Ikegami. 2000. Pulmonary-specific expression of SP-D corrects pulmonary lipid accumulation in SP-D gene-targeted mice. *Am. J. Physiol Lung Cell Mol. Physiol* 278: L365-L373.

[4] Fisher, J. T., Y. Zhang, and J. F. Engelhardt. 2011. Comparative biology of cystic fibrosis animal models. *Methods Mol. Biol.* 742: 311-334.

[5] Braun, A., and T. Tschernig. 2006. Animal models of asthma: innovative methods of lung research and new pharmacological targets. *Exp. Toxicol. Pathol.* 57 Suppl 2: 3-4.

[6] Herszberg, B., D. Ramos-Barbon, M. Tamaoka, J. G. Martin, and J. P. Lavoie. 2006. Heaves, an asthma-like equine disease, involves airway smooth muscle remodeling. *J. Allergy Clin. Immunol.* 118: 382-388.

[7] Li, Z., and J. F. Engelhardt. 2003. Progress toward generating a ferret model of cystic fibrosis by somatic cell nuclear transfer. *Reprod. Biol. Endocrinol.* 1: 83.

[8] Mueller, C., S. A. Braag, A. Keeler, C. Hodges, M. Drumm, and T. R. Flotte. 2011. Lack of cystic fibrosis transmembrane conductance regulator in CD3+ lymphocytes leads to aberrant cytokine secretion and hyperinflammatory adaptive immune responses. *Am. J. Respir. Cell Mol. Biol.* 44: 922-929.

[9] Braun, A., T. Tschernig, and D. A. Groneberg. 2008. Editorial: Experimental models of asthma. *J. Occup. Med. Toxicol.* 3 Suppl 1: S1.

[10] Kumar, R. K., and P. S. Foster. 2002. Modeling allergic asthma in mice: pitfalls and opportunities. *Am. J. Respir. Cell Mol. Biol.* 27: 267-272.

[11] Jugg, B. J., A. J. Smith, S. J. Rudall, and P. Rice. 2011. The injured lung: clinical issues and experimental models. *Philos. Trans. R. Soc. Lond B Biol. Sci.* 366: 306-309.

[12] Matthay, M. A. 2008. Treatment of acute lung injury: clinical and experimental studies. *Proc. Am. Thorac. Soc.* 5: 297-299.

[13] Rubenfeld, G. D., E. Caldwell, E. Peabody, J. Weaver, D. P. Martin, M. Neff, E. J. Stern, and L. D. Hudson. 2005. Incidence and outcomes of acute lung injury. *N. Engl. J. Med.* 353: 1685-1693.

[14] Matthay, M. A. 1999. Conference summary: acute lung injury. *Chest* 116: 119S-126S.

[15] Wang, H. M., M. Bodenstein, and K. Markstaller. 2008. Overview of the pathology of three widely used animal models of acute lung injury. *Eur. Surg. Res.* 40: 305-316.

[16] Wang, H. M., M. Bodenstein, B. Duenges, S. Ganatti, S. Boehme, Y. Ning, B. Roehrig, and K. Markstaller. 2010. Ventilator-associated lung injury superposed to oleic acid infusion or surfactant depletion: histopathological characteristics of two porcine models of acute lung injury. *Eur. Surg. Res.* 45: 121-133.

[17] Davidson, K. G., A. D. Bersten, H. A. Barr, K. D. Dowling, T. E. Nicholas, and I. R. Doyle. 2000. Lung function, permeability, and surfactant composition in oleic acid-induced acute lung injury in rats. *Am. J. Physiol Lung Cell Mol. Physiol* 279: L1091-L1102.

[18] Liu, D. D., Y. H. Hsu, and H. I. Chen. 2007. Endotoxin-induced acute lung injury is enhanced in rats with spontaneous hypertension. *Clin. Exp. Pharmacol. Physiol* 34: 61-69.

[19] Cash, H. A., D. E. Woods, B. McCullough, W. G. Johanson, Jr., and J. A. Bass. 1979. A rat model of chronic respiratory infection with Pseudomonas aeruginosa. *Am. Rev. Respir Dis.* 119: 453-459.

[20] Carrillo-Marquez, M. A., K. G. Hulten, W. Hammerman, L. Lamberth, E. O. Mason, and S. L. Kaplan. 2011. Staphylococcus aureus pneumonia in children in the era of community-acquired methicillin-resistance at Texas Children's Hospital. *Pediatr. Infect. Dis. J.* 30: 545-550.

[21] Lever, A., and I. Mackenzie. 2007. Sepsis: definition, epidemiology, and diagnosis. *BMJ* 335: 879-883.

[22] Fisher, C. J., and S. B. Yan. 2000. Protein C levels as a prognostic indicator of outcome in sepsis and related diseases. *Crit. Care Med.* 28: S49-S56.

[23] Lyn-Kew, K., and T. J. Standiford. 2008. Immunosuppression in sepsis. *Curr. Pharm. Des* 14: 1870-1881.

[24] Morrison, R. J., and A. Bidani. 2002. Acute respiratory distress syndrome epidemiology and pathophysiology. *Chest Surg. Clin. N. Am.* 12: 301-323.

[25] Chollet-Martin, S., C. Gatecel, N. Kermarrec, M. Gougerot-Pocidalo, and D. M. Payen. 1996. Alveolar neutrophil functions and cytokine levels in patients with the adult respiratory distress syndrome during nitric oxide inhalation. *Am. J. Respir. Crit. Care Med.* 153: 985-990.
[26] Desai, S. R. 2002. Acute respiratory distress syndrome: imaging of the injured lung. *Clin. Radiol.* 57: 8-17.
[27] Matute-Bello, G., W. C. Liles, F. Radella, K. P. Steinberg, J. T. Ruzinski, L. D. Hudson, and T. R. Martin. 2000. Modulation of neutrophil apoptosis by granulocyte colony-stimulating factor and granulocyte/macrophage colony-stimulating factor during the course of acute respiratory distress syndrome. *Crit. Care Med.* 28: 1-7.
[28] Mosser, D. M., and J. P. Edwards. 2008. Exploring the full spectrum of macrophage activation. *Nat. Rev. Immunol.* 8: 958-969.
[29] Anzueto, A., R. Baughman, K. Guntupalli, J. Weg, H. Wiedemann, A. Raventos, F. Lemaire, W. Long, D. Zaccardelli, and E. Pattishall. 1996. Aerosolized surfactant in adults with sepsis-induced acute respiratory distress syndrome. *N. Engl. J. Med.* 334: 1417-1421.
[30] Cockcroft, D. W. 2001. Defining the lung's response to endotoxin. *Am. J. Respir. Crit. Care Med.* 163: 1520-1523.
[31] Andersson, U., and K. J. Tracey. 2003. HMGB1 in sepsis. *Scand. J. Infect. Dis.* 35: 577-584.
[32] O'Grady, N. P., H. L. Preas, J. Pugin, C. Fuiza, M. M. Tropea, D. Reda, S. M. Banks, and A. F. Suffredini. 2001. Local inflammatory responses following bronchial endotoxin instillation in humans. *Am. J. Respir. Crit. Care Med.* 163: 1591-1598.
[33] Green, F. H., V. Vallyathan, and F. F. Hahn. 2007. Comparative pathology of environmental lung disease: an overview. *Toxicol. Pathol.* 35: 136-147.
[34] Hansel, N. N., L. Gao, N. M. Rafaels, R. A. Mathias, E. R. Neptune, C. Tankersley, A. V. Grant, J. Connett, T. H. Beaty, R. A. Wise, and K. C. Barnes. 2009. Leptin receptor polymorphisms and lung function decline in COPD. *Eur. Respir. J.* 34: 103-110.
[35] Winkler, A. R., K. H. Nocka, T. H. Sulahian, L. Kobzik, and C. M. Williams. 2008. In vitro modeling of human alveolar macrophage smoke exposure: enhanced inflammation and impaired function. *Exp. Lung Res.* 34: 599-629.
[36] Martin, J. G., and M. Tamaoka. 2006. Rat models of asthma and chronic obstructive lung disease. *Pulm. Pharmacol. Ther.* 19: 377-385.
[37] Tuder, R. M., T. Yoshida, I. Fijalkowka, S. Biswal, and I. Petrache. 2006. Role of lung maintenance program in the heterogeneity of lung destruction in emphysema. *Proc. Am. Thorac. Soc.* 3: 673-679.
[38] McCullough, B., X. Ying, T. Monticello, and M. Bonnefoi. 2004. Digital microscopy imaging and new approaches in toxicologic pathology. *Toxicol. Pathol.* 32 Suppl 2: 49-58.
[39] Taraseviciene-Stewart, L., I. S. Douglas, P. S. Nana-Sinkam, J. D. Lee, R. M. Tuder, M. R. Nicolls, and N. F. Voelkel. 2006. Is alveolar destruction and emphysema in chronic obstructive pulmonary disease an immune disease? *Proc. Am. Thorac. Soc.* 3: 687-690.
[40] Marwick, J. A., C. S. Stevenson, J. Giddings, W. MacNee, K. Butler, I. Rahman, and P. A. Kirkham. 2006. Cigarette smoke disrupts VEGF165-VEGFR-2 receptor signaling complex in rat lungs and patients with COPD: morphological impact of VEGFR-2 inhibition. *Am. J. Physiol Lung Cell Mol. Physiol* 290: L897-L908.

[41] Petrache, I., I. Fijalkowska, T. R. Medler, J. Skirball, P. Cruz, L. Zhen, H. I. Petrache, T. R. Flotte, and R. M. Tuder. 2006. alpha-1 antitrypsin inhibits caspase-3 activity, preventing lung endothelial cell apoptosis. *Am. J. Pathol.* 169: 1155-1166.

[42] Karaaslan, C., H. Hirakawa, R. Yasumatsu, L. Y. Chang, R. A. Pierce, J. D. Crapo, and S. Cataltepe. 2011. Elastase Inhibitory Activity of Airway alpha1-Antitrypsin Is Protected by Treatment With a Catalytic Antioxidant in a Baboon Model of Severe Bronchopulmonary Dysplasia. *Pediatr. Res.* 70: 363-367.

[43] Stolk, J., B. Veldhuisen, L. Annovazzi, C. Zanone, E. M. Versteeg, T. H. van Kuppevelt, W. Nieuwenhuizen, P. Iadarola, J. H. Berden, and M. Luisetti. 2006. Correction: Short-term variability of biomarkers of proteinase activity in patients with emphysema associated with type Z alpha-1-antitrypsin deficiency. *Respir. Res.* 7: 20.

[44] Podowski, M., C. L. Calvi, C. Cheadle, R. M. Tuder, S. Biswals, and E. R. Neptune. 2009. Complex integration of matrix, oxidative stress, and apoptosis in genetic emphysema. *Am. J. Pathol.* 175: 84-96.

[45] Rohrer, J., B. R. Wuertz, and F. Ondrey. 2010. Cigarette smoke condensate induces nuclear factor kappa-b activity and proangiogenic growth factors in aerodigestive cells. *Laryngoscope* 120: 1609-1613.

[46] Rose, J. E., F. M. Behm, T. Murugesan, and F. J. McClernon. 2010. Silver acetate interactions with nicotine and non-nicotine smoke components. *Exp. Clin. Psychopharmacol.* 18: 462-469.

[47] Barnes, P. J. 2004. Alveolar Macrohages as Orchestrators of COPD., 1 ed. 59-70.

[48] Cerny, L., J. S. Torday, and V. K. Rehan. 2008. Prevention and treatment of bronchopulmonary dysplasia: contemporary status and future outlook. *Lung* 186: 75-89.

[49] Bourbon, J. R., O. Boucherat, J. Boczkowski, B. Crestani, and C. Delacourt. 2009. Bronchopulmonary dysplasia and emphysema: in search of common therapeutic targets. *Trends Mol. Med.* 15: 169-179.

[50] Kishore, U., A. L. Bernal, M. F. Kamran, S. Saxena, M. Singh, P. U. Sarma, T. Madan, and T. Chakraborty. 2005. Surfactant proteins SP-A and SP-D in human health and disease. *Arch. Immunol. Ther. Exp. (Warsz.)* 53: 399-417.

[51] Abman, S. H. 2008. The dysmorphic pulmonary circulation in bronchopulmonary dysplasia: a growing story. *Am. J. Respir. Crit Care Med.* 178: 114-115.

[52] Baleeiro, C. E. O., S. E. Wilcoxen, S. B. Morris, T. J. Standiford, and R. Paine. 2003. Sublethal hyperoxia impairs pulmonary innate immunity. *J. Immunol.* 171: 955-963.

[53] Paine, R., III, S. E. Wilcoxen, S. B. Morris, C. Sartori, C. E. Baleeiro, M. A. Matthay, and P. J. Christensen. 2003. Transgenic overexpression of granulocyte macrophage-colony stimulating factor in the lung prevents hyperoxic lung injury. *Am. J. Pathol.* 163: 2397-2406.

[54] Soll, R. F., and F. Blanco. 2003. Natural surfactant extract versus synthetic surfactant for neonatal respiratory distress syndrome. *The Cochrane Library* 1: 1-35.

[55] Clark, H. W., K. B. M. Reid, and R. B. Sim. 2000. Collectins and innate immunity in the lung. *Microbes and Infection* 2: 273-278.

[56] Krasnodembskaya, A., Y. Song, X. Fang, N. Gupta, V. Serikov, J. W. Lee, and M. A. Matthay. 2010. Antibacterial effect of human mesenchymal stem cells is mediated in part from secretion of the antimicrobial peptide LL-37. *Stem Cells* 28: 2229-2238.

[57] DeMello, D. E., and Z. Lin. 2001. Pulmonary alveolar proteinosis: a review. *Pediatr. Pathol. Mol. Med.* 20: 413-432.

[58] Presneill, J. J., K. Nakata, Y. Inoue, and J. F. Seymour. 2004. Pulmonary alveolar proteinosis. *Clin. Chest Med.* 25: 593-613, viii.

[59] Mahut, B., C. Delacourt, P. Scheinmann, J. de Blic, T. M. Mani, J. C. Fournet, and G. Bellon. 1996. Pulmonary alveolar proteinosis: experience with eight pediatric cases and a review. *Pediatrics* 97: 117-122.

[60] Nogee, L. M., D. E. de Mello, L. P. Dehner, and H. R. Colten. 1993. Brief report: deficiency of pulmonary surfactant protein B in congenital alveolar proteinosis. *N. Engl. J. Med.* 328: 406-410.

[61] Nogee, L. M. 2004. Alterations in SP-B and SP-C expression in neonatal lung disease. *Annu. Rev. Physiol* 66: 601-623.

[62] Carnovale, R., J. Zornoza, A. M. Goldman, and M. Luna. 1977. Pulmonary alveolar proteinosis: its association with hematologic malignancy and lymphoma. *Radiology* 122: 303-306.

[63] Cordonnier, C., J. Fleury-Feith, E. Escudier, K. Atassi, and J. F. Bernaudin. 1994. Secondary alveolar proteinosis is a reversible cause of respiratory failure in leukemic patients. *Am. J. Respir. Crit Care Med.* 149: 788-794.

[64] Keller, C. A., A. Frost, P. T. Cagle, and J. L. Abraham. 1995. Pulmonary alveolar proteinosis in a painter with elevated pulmonary concentrations of titanium. *Chest* 108: 277-280.

[65] McCunney, R. J., and R. Godefroi. 1989. Pulmonary alveolar proteinosis and cement dust: a case report. *J. Occup. Med.* 31: 233-237.

[66] Kitamura, T., N. Tanaka, J. Watanabe, K. Uchida, S. Kanegasaki, Y. Yamada, and K. Nakata. 1999. Idiopathic pulmonary alveolar proteinosis as an autoimmune disease with neutralizing antibody against granulocyte/macrophage colony-stimulating factor. *J. Exp. Med.* 190: 875-880.

[67] Bonfield, T. L., D. Russell, S. Burgess, A. Malur, M. S. Kavuru, and M. J. Thomassen. 2002. Autoantibodies against granulocyte macrophage colony-stimulating factor are diagnostic for pulmonary alveolar proteinosis. *Am. J. Respir. Cell Mol. Biol.* 27: 481-486.

[68] Seymour, J. F., I. R. Doyle, K. Nakata, J. J. Presneill, O. D. Schoch, E. Hamano, K. Uchida, R. Fisher, and A. R. Dunn. 2003. Relationship of anti-GM-CSF antibody concentration, surfactant protein A and B levels, and serum LDH to pulmonary parameters and response to GM-CSF therapy in patients with idiopathic alveolar proteinosis. *Thorax* 58: 252-257.

[69] Bonfield, T. L., M. S. Kavuru, and M. J. Thomassen. 2002. Anti-GM-CSF titer predicts response to GM-CSF therapy in pulmonary alveolar proteinosis. *Clin. Immunol.* 105: 342-350.

[70] Kavuru, M. S., T. L. Bonfield, and M. J. Thomassen. 2003. Plasmapheresis, GM-CSF, and alveolar proteinosis. *Am. J. Respir. Crit. Care Med.* 167: 1036.

[71] Trapnell, B. C., and J. A. Whitsett. 2002. GM-CSF regulates pulmonary surfactant homeostasis and alveolar macrophage-mediated innate host defense. *Annu. Rev. Physiol.* 64: 775-802.

[72] Trapnell, B. C., J. A. Whitsett, and K. Nakata. 2003. Pulmonary alveolar proteinosis. *N. Engl. J. Med.* 349: 2527-2539.

[73] Shibata, Y., Y. P. Berclaz, Z. C. Chroneos, M. Yoshida, J. A. Whitsett, and B. C. Trapnell. 2001. GM-CSF regulates alveolar macrophage differentiation and innate immunity in the lung through PU.1. *Immunity* 15: 557-567.

[74] Reed, J. A., M. Ikegami, L. Robb, C. G. Begley, G. Ross, and J. A. Whitsett. 2000. Distinct changes in pulmonary surfactant homeostasis in common beta-chain- and GM-CSF-deficient mice. *Am. J. Physiol Lung Cell Mol. Physiol* 278: L1164-L1171.

[75] Sakagami, T., D. Beck, K. Uchida, T. Suzuki, B. C. Carey, K. Nakata, G. Keller, R. E. Wood, S. E. Wert, M. Ikegami, J. A. Whitsett, M. Luisetti, S. Davies, J. P. Krischer, A. Brody, F. Ryckman, and B. C. Trapnell. 2010. Patient-derived granulocyte/macrophage colony-stimulating factor autoantibodies reproduce pulmonary alveolar proteinosis in nonhuman primates. *Am. J. Respir. Crit Care Med.* 182: 49-61.

[76] Uchida, K., K. Nakata, B. C. Trapnell, T. Terakawa, E. Hamano, Y. Inoue, A. Mikami, I. Matsushita, J. F. Seymour, M. Oh-eda, I. Ishige, Y. Eishi, T. Kitamura, Y. Yamada, K. Hanaoka, and N. Keicho. 2004. High affinity autoantibodies specifically eliminate granulocyte-macrophage colony stimulating factor activity in the lung of patients with idopathic pulmonary alveolar proteinosis. *Blood* 103: 1089-1098.

[77] Degryse, A. L., and W. E. Lawson. 2011. Progress toward improving animal models for idiopathic pulmonary fibrosis. *Am. J. Med. Sci.* 341: 444-449.

[78] Cook, D. N., D. M. Brass, and D. A. Schwartz. 2002. A matrix for new ideas in pulmonary fibrosis. *Am. J. Respir. Cell Mol. Biol.* 27: 122-124.

[79] Lawson, W. E., J. E. Loyd, and A. L. Degryse. 2011. Genetics in pulmonary fibrosis--familial cases provide clues to the pathogenesis of idiopathic pulmonary fibrosis. *Am. J. Med. Sci.* 341: 439-443.

[80] Hattori, N., J. L. Degen, T. H. Sisson, H. Liu, B. B. Moore, R. G. Pandrangi, R. H. Simon, and A. F. Drew. 2000. Bleomycin-induced pulmonary fibrosis in fibrinogen-null mice. *J. Clin. Invest.* 106: 1341-1350.

[81] Swaisgood, C. M., E. L. French, C. Noga, R. H. Simon, and V. A. Ploplis. 2000. The development of bleomycin-induced pulmonary fibrosis in mice deficient for components of the fibrinolytic system. *Am. J. Pathol.* 157: 177-187.

[82] Barbarin, V., Z. Xing, M. Delos, D. Lison, and F. Huaux. 2005. Pulmonary overexpression of IL-10 augments lung fibrosis and Th2 responses induced by silica particles. *Am. J. Physiol Lung Cell Mol. Physiol* 288: L841-L848.

[83] Kang, J. L., K. Lee, and V. Castranova. 2000. Nitric oxide up-regulates DNA-binding activity of nuclear factor-κB in macrophages stimulated with silica and inflammatory stimulants. *Mol. Cell. Biol.* 215: 1-9.

[84] Cochand, L., P. Isler, F. Songeon, and L. P. Nicod. 1999. Human lung dendritic cells have an immature phenotype with efficient mannose receptors. *Am J Respir Cell Mol. Biol.* 21: 547-554.

[85] Belvisi, M. G., D. J. Hele, and M. A. Birrell. 2004. New advances and potential therapies for the treatment of asthma. *BioDrugs.* 18: 211-223.

[86] Elias, J. A., C. G. Lee, T. Zheng, B. Ma, R. J. Homer, and Z. Zhu. 2003. New insights into the pathogenesis of asthma. *J Clin. Invest* 111: 291-297.

[87] Brutsche, M. H., L. Joos, I. E. A. Carlen Brutsche, R. Bissinger, M. Tamm, A. Custovic, and A. Woodcock. 2002. Array-based diagnostic gene-expression score for atopy and asthma. *J. Allergy Clin. Immunol.* 109: 271-273.

[88] Ballow, M. 2006. Biologic immune modifiers: Trials and tribulations--are we there yet? *J. Allergy Clin. Immunol.* 118: 1209-1215.
[89] Boyton, R. J., and D. M. Altmann. 2004. Asthma: new developments in cytokine regulation. *Clin. Exp. Immunol.* 136: 13-14.
[90] Shapiro, S. D. 2006. Animal models of asthma: Pro: Allergic avoidance of animal (model[s]) is not an option. *Am. J. Respir. Crit Care Med.* 174: 1171-1173.
[91] Finotto, S., M. F. Neurath, J. N. Glickman, S. Qin, H. A. Lehr, F. H. Green, K. Ackerman, K. Haley, P. R. Galle, S. J. Szabo, J. M. Drazen, G. T. De Sanctis, and L. H. Glimcher. 2002. Development of spontaneous airway changes consistent with human asthma in mice lacking T-bet. *Science* 295: 336-338.
[92] Shaver, J. R., J. G. Zangrilli, S. Cho, R. A. Cirelli, M. Pollice, A. T. Hastie, J. E. Fish, and S. P. Peters. 1997. Kinetics of the development and recovery of the lung from IgE-mediated inflammation. *Am. J. Respir. Crit. Care Med.* 155: 442-448.
[93] Elias, J. A., R. J. Homer, Q. Hamid, and C. G. Lee. 2005. Chitinases and chitinase-like proteins in TH2 inflammation and asthma. *J. Allergy Clin. Immunol.* 116: 497-500.
[94] D'Ambrosio, D., P. Panina-Bordignon, and F. Sinigaglia. 2003. Chemokine receptors in inflammation: an overview. *J Immunol. Methods* 273: 3-13.
[95] Hoenerhoff, M. J., H. H. Hong, T. V. Ton, S. A. Lahousse, and R. C. Sills. 2009. A review of the molecular mechanisms of chemically induced neoplasia in rat and mouse models in National Toxicology Program bioassays and their relevance to human cancer. *Toxicol. Pathol.* 37: 835-848.
[96] Taguchi, A., K. Politi, S. J. Pitteri, W. W. Lockwood, V. M. Faca, K. Kelly-Spratt, C. H. Wong, Q. Zhang, A. Chin, K. S. Park, G. Goodman, A. F. Gazdar, J. Sage, D. M. Dinulescu, R. Kucherlapati, R. A. Depinho, C. J. Kemp, H. E. Varmus, and S. M. Hanash. 2011. Lung cancer signatures in plasma based on proteome profiling of mouse tumor models. *Cancer Cell* 20: 289-299.
[97] Naltner, A., S. Wert, J. A. Whitsett, and C. Yan. 2000. Temporal/spatial expression of nuclear receptor coactivators in the mouse lung. *Am. J. Physiol Lung Cell Mol. Physiol* 279: L1066-L1074.
[98] Heissig, B., S. Rafii, H. Akiyama, Y. Ohki, Y. Sato, T. Rafael, Z. Zhu, D. J. Hicklin, K. Okumura, H. Ogawa, Z. Werb, and K. Hattori. 2005. Low-dose irradiation promotes tissue revascularization through VEGF release from mast cells and MMP-9-mediated progenitor cell mobilization. *J. Exp. Med.* 202: 739-750.
[99] Rozakis-Adcock, M., R. Fernley, J. Wade, T. Pawson, and D. Bowtell. 1993. The SH2 and SH3 domains of mammalian Grb2 couple the EGF receptor to the Ras activator mSos1. *Nature* 363: 83-85.
[100] Kane, A. B. 2006. Animal models of malignant mesothelioma. *Inhal. Toxicol.* 18: 1001-1004.
[101] Altomare, D. A., C. A. Vaslet, K. L. Skele, R. A. De, K. Devarajan, S. C. Jhanwar, A. I. McClatchey, A. B. Kane, and J. R. Testa. 2005. A mouse model recapitulating molecular features of human mesothelioma. *Cancer Res.* 65: 8090-8095.
[102] Konstan, M. W., D. R. VanDevanter, L. Rasouliyan, D. J. Pasta, A. Yegin, W. J. Morgan, and J. S. Wagener. 2010. Trends in the use of routine therapies in cystic fibrosis: 1995-2005. *Pediatr. Pulmonol.* 45: 1167-1172.
[103] Shah, S. 2011. VX-770, a CFTR potentiator, may have a potential clinical benefit in a subgroup of people with cystic fibrosis. *Thorax.*

[104] Chroneos, Z. C., S. E. Wert, J. L. Livingston, D. J. Hassett, and J. A. Whitsett. 2000. Role of cystic fibrosis transmembrane conductance regulator in pulmonary clearance of Pseudomonas aeruginosa in vivo. *J. Immunol.* 165: 3941-3950.

[105] Hodges, C. A., C. U. Cotton, M. R. Palmert, and M. L. Drumm. 2008. Generation of a conditional null allele for Cftr in mice. *Genesis.* 46: 546-552.

[106] Bruscia, E. M., P. X. Zhang, E. Ferreira, C. Caputo, J. W. Emerson, D. Tuck, D. S. Krause, and M. E. Egan. 2009. Macrophages directly contribute to the exaggerated inflammatory response in cystic fibrosis transmembrane conductance regulator-/- mice. *Am. J. Respir. Cell Mol. Biol.* 40: 295-304.

[107] Hodges, C. A., B. R. Grady, K. Mishra, C. U. Cotton, and M. L. Drumm. 2011. Cystic Fibrosis growth retardation is not correlated with loss of Cftr in the intestinal epithelium. *Am. J. Physiol Gastrointest. Liver Physiol.*

[108] van Heeckeren, A. M., M. D. Schluchter, W. Xue, and P. B. Davis. 2006. Response to acute lung infection with mucoid Pseudomonas aeruginosa in cystic fibrosis mice. *Am. J. Respir. Crit Care Med.* 173: 288-296.

[109] van Heeckeren, A. M., J. Tscheikuna, R. W. Walenga, M. W. Konstan, P. B. Davis, B. Erokwu, M. A. Haxhiu, and T. W. Ferkol. 2000. Effect of Pseudomonas infection on weight loss, lung mechanics, and cytokines in mice. *Am. J. Respir. Crit Care Med.* 161: 271-279.

[110] van Heeckeren, A. M., and M. D. Schluchter. 2002. Murine models of chronic Pseudomonas aeruginosa lung infection. *Lab Anim* 36: 291-312.

[111] Hodges, C. A., M. R. Palmert, and M. L. Drumm. 2008. Infertility in females with cystic fibrosis is multifactorial: evidence from mouse models. *Endocrinology* 149: 2790-2797.

[112] Wine, J. J. 2010. The development of lung disease in cystic fibrosis pigs. *Sci. Transl. Med.* 2: 29ps20.

[113] Rogers, C. S., D. A. Stoltz, D. K. Meyerholz, L. S. Ostedgaard, T. Rokhlina, P. J. Taft, M. P. Rogan, A. A. Pezzulo, P. H. Karp, O. A. Itani, A. C. Kabel, C. L. Wohlford-Lenane, G. J. Davis, R. A. Hanfland, T. L. Smith, M. Samuel, D. Wax, C. N. Murphy, A. Rieke, K. Whitworth, A. Uc, T. D. Starner, K. A. Brogden, J. Shilyansky, P. B. McCray, Jr., J. Zabner, R. S. Prather, and M. J. Welsh. 2008. Disruption of the CFTR gene produces a model of cystic fibrosis in newborn pigs. *Science* 321: 1837-1841.

[114] Meyerholz, D. K., D. A. Stoltz, E. Namati, S. Ramachandran, A. A. Pezzulo, A. R. Smith, M. V. Rector, M. J. Suter, S. Kao, G. McLennan, G. J. Tearney, J. Zabner, P. B. McCray, Jr., and M. J. Welsh. 2010. Loss of cystic fibrosis transmembrane conductance regulator function produces abnormalities in tracheal development in neonatal pigs and young children. *Am. J. Respir. Crit Care Med.* 182: 1251-1261.

[115] Sun, X., H. Sui, J. T. Fisher, Z. Yan, X. Liu, H. J. Cho, N. S. Joo, Y. Zhang, W. Zhou, Y. Yi, J. M. Kinyon, D. C. Lei-Butters, M. A. Griffin, P. Naumann, M. Luo, J. Ascher, K. Wang, T. Frana, J. J. Wine, D. K. Meyerholz, and J. F. Engelhardt. 2010. Disease phenotype of a ferret CFTR-knockout model of cystic fibrosis. *J. Clin. Invest* 120: 3149-3160.

[116] Rogers, C. S., W. M. Abraham, K. A. Brogden, J. F. Engelhardt, J. T. Fisher, P. B. McCray, Jr., G. McLennan, D. K. Meyerholz, E. Namati, L. S. Ostedgaard, R. S. Prather, J. R. Sabater, D. A. Stoltz, J. Zabner, and M. J. Welsh. 2008. The porcine

lung as a potential model for cystic fibrosis. *Am. J. Physiol Lung Cell Mol. Physiol* 295: L240-L263.

[117] Spadafora, D., E. C. Hawkins, K. E. Murphy, L. A. Clark, and S. T. Ballard. 2010. Naturally occurring mutations in the canine CFTR gene. *Physiol Genomics* 42: 480-485.

[118] Williams, S. H., V. Sahota, T. Palmai-Pallag, S. J. Tebbutt, J. Walker, and A. Harris. 2003. Evaluation of gene targeting by homologous recombination in ovine somatic cells. *Mol. Reprod. Dev.* 66: 115-125.

[119] Wine, J. J., D. Glavac, G. Hurlock, C. Robinson, M. Lee, U. Potocnik, M. Ravnik-Glavac, and M. Dean. 1998. Genomic DNA sequence of Rhesus (M. mulatta) cystic fibrosis (CFTR) gene. *Mamm. Genome* 9: 301-305.

19

Inhibition of Adhesion and Invasion of *Pseudomonas aeruginosa* to Lung Epithelial Cells: A Model of Cystic Fibrosis Infection

Ayman M. Noreddin, Ghada Sawy,
Walid Elkhatib, Ehab Noreddin and Atef Shibl
Hampton University,
Hampton, VA,
USA

1. Introduction

Cystic Fibrosis is a lethal autosomal recessive lung disorder resulting from a mutation in the transmembrane conductance regulator (CFTR) protein. The CFTR is a chloride channel encoded by a single gene on chromosome 7. More than 1200 mutations have been identified that result in defective or absent CFTR protein [1]. The most common mutation is ΔF508 (deletion of phenylalanine 508). This deletion leads to a non-functional, misfolded protein that is subsequently degraded [2]. While multiple organ systems are affected, CF is most often characterized by thickened mucus secretions and an inability to clear the lungs [1, 3-4]. In recent decades, improvements in life expectancy were achieved by new methods of antibiotic delivery as well as addition of new treatments to thin lung fluids. An example is the use of DNase to clear the buildup of extracellular DNA that occurs in the CF lung. This also relieves some of the exaggerated inflammatory response that is a characteristic of the CF lung [5].

Over their life time, CF patients experience multiple infections by various pneumonia-causing bacteria [6]. With more patients surviving to adulthood, chronic infections with *Pseudomonas aeruginosa* are coming to the forefront as a leading cause of death [7]. Problems presented by infected CF lung are multi-dimensional; the electrolyte balance and pH of the fluids are abnormal. The mucus is thick and of an alternative composition compared to normal lung and may contribute to colonization with *Pseudomonas aeruginosa* [2, 3, 5]. As such, research is multi-pronged and includes gene therapy to correct the defective protein, amelioration of inflammatory response and thinning of alveolar surface fluids [8, 9]. Significantly, Pseudomonas bacteria colonize the CF lung far easier than normal lung. Normal lung tissue has several naturally occurring defenses that work in concert with commonly prescribed antibiotics for recovery from lung infections [4, 10]. The CF patient appears to lack these natural defenses [1, 7].

Pseudomonas aeruginosa biofilms are difficult to treat due to multi-drug resistance. Many aspects of biofilms from physical structure to genetics and protein expression are under heavy investigation to elucidate the mechanisms by which biofilms develop antibiotic resistance. Within the biofilm matrix, bacteria are well protected from hostile environmental elements and host defenses. Cells in different areas of the biofilm take on various patterns of gene expression, as such; biofilms are described as a community or as functioning similar to a multi-cellular organism [3]. Biofilms develop slowly, destroy surrounding tissue and evade even healthy immune systems. Standard dose antibiotic therapy can reduce biofilm as well as planktonic cells shed from the biofilm, but rarely eradicate the entire biofilm. This allows a cycle of subsequent regrowth and new shedding of planktonic cells which possess altered antibiotic resistance [11]. Some theories describe the heavy matrix, flow channels and oxygen gradients within the biofilm structure as contributing to problems with penetration of antibiotics into the biofilm. Others describe a counteraction of host defenses or alterations in gene and protein expression not only within the biofilm, but also in the CF host [11-13]. In this proposal we will discuss a novel experimental approach to study the pharmacodynamics of antibiotics used to treat *Pseudomonas aeruginosa* biofilms in CF lung versus normal lung.

Pseudomonas aeruginosa is an important human pathogen that can cause a wide range of infectious diseases that are associated with high morbidity and mortality rates [14]. Exposed tissue surfaces lined with epithelia are the most common targets of that pathogen *e.g.* epithelial surface of the eye and airways.

Adhesion of *Pseudomonas aeruginosa* to the airway cellular receptors is the initial event to establish respiratory colonization and infection [12, 15-16]. Interestingly, the affinity of *Pseudomonas aeruginosa* to bind to the inflamed or injured epithelial cells (CF or mechanically ventilated patients) is significantly higher than that to bind normal cell surfaces; thus preventing bacterial adherence may minimize lung pathology for high-risk patients [16].

The exploit of natural compounds, especially carbohydrates, to prevent infection has been considered in lung infectivity studies; since bacteria associated with pneumonia is known to bind the carbohydrate receptors on the pulmonary epithelium [12]. Dextran, a polymer of α (11,16) linked D- glucose (branched at the 3 position), is a widely available polysaccharide that has been used in the *in vitro* and *in vivo* infection models to block the adherence of *Pseudomonas aeruginosa*, *Hemophilus influenza* and *Staphylococcus aureus* [12, 15]. Berries of *Vaccinium* family (include cranberry) and their extracts that contain a saccharide effective in preventing the attachment of *Escherichia coli* to the uroepithelial receptors are well-known examples as well [12].

Recent studies suggested that many pathogenic organisms have the ability to invade and reside in the host cells during the early stage of infection. The discovery of antibiotic-resistant intracellular *Heamophilus influenzae* in the lung of individuals with Chronic Obstructive Pulmonary Disease (COPD) implicates intracellular bacteria as an important reservoir for the persistent infection [17]. *Pseudomonas aeruginosa* can also survive for up to 24 hours inside the lung epithelium without inducing cytotoxicity and is known to develop resistance to the treatments afterwards [17]. Accordingly, it is equally substantial to combat bacterial adhesion and invasion as a preventive step of the infection as well as the development of bacterial resistance.

It has been reported that some inexpensive natural extracts (e.g. Berries of *Vaccinium* family and dextran) have shown promising anti-adhesion properties with some micro-organisms (e.g. *Escherichia coli*) in the urinary tract infections, therefore, they might worth testing as topical therapeutics for prevention of *Pseudomonas aeruginosa* adhesion and invasion to lung epithelial cells [18-19].

In this study, the efficacy of some natural extracts with potential anti-adhesion properties and their combinations with ciprofloxacin was evaluated as blocking agents for the adhesion and the invasion of *Pseudomonas aeruginosa* PAO1 to A549 lung epithelial cells.

2. Building CF infection model

Ciprofloxacin and gentamicin sulfate were purchased from Sigma/Aldrich (St. Louis, MO, USA) and their stock solutions were prepared in 0.1N HCl (32 mg/ml) and water (32 mg/ml), respectively, and stored at -80°C. Before use; the antibiotic dilutions were made in F12-K cell culture medium (Cellgro, Mediatech, Inc, Manassas, VA, USA). Other Cell culture reagents were also obtained from Cellgro, Mediatech Inc. (Manassas, VA, USA). Dextran of molecular weight (MW) 40,000 was provided by Dr. John Brekke (University of Minnesota Duluth, MN, USA). Bacterial culture reagents were obtained from Difco Laboratories (Detroit, MI, USA).

The commercially available *Vaccinium macrocarpon* (cranberries) and *Glycine max* (soybean) were blended and extracted with distilled water (1:1 and 1:3.5, respectively) at room temperature.

Both crude mixtures were left to decant overnight at 4°C. Their supernatants were then subjected to two steps centrifugation at 4750 rpm for 20 min followed by 12,000 rpm for 10 min. The resultant supernatants were membrane filtered (0.22 µm, Millipore Corp. Billerica, MA). The sterile extracts were then stored at -80°C in 1ml aliquots till they were used in the adhesion or invasion assays.

The concentrations of the solid contents of such extracts were determined by evaporating the water content at 40°C and weighing the solid residues until constant weights were achieved.

Pseudomonas aeruginosa strain PAO1 was purchased from American Type Culture Collection (ATCC, Rockville, MD). *P. aeruginosa* PAO1 was grown until achieving the exponential growth phase over 16 hours at 37°C in Cation Adjusted Muller Hinton Broth (CAMHB) (Sigma-Aldrich, St. Louis. MO) from which 0.5 McFarland (1.5×10^8 CFU/ml) was prepared in F12-K tissue culture medium to initiate adhesion or invasion assays.

A549 lung epithelial cell line was obtained from American Type Culture Collection (ATCC, Rockville, MD). The cells were passed in 75 cm^2 flasks (BD Falcon, San Jose, CA), and then 1.5×10^5 cells were counted using the Hemocytometer and seeded into 12 well tissue culture plates (Becton Dickinson, NJ, USA). The cells were incubated in F12-K medium supplemented with 10% (vol/vol) Fetal Bovine Serum (FBS) at 37°C in the presence of 5% CO_2 to achieve confluence over 48 hours.

Minimum Inhibitory Concentration (MIC) and Minimum Cytotoxic Concentration (MCC) were two factors controlled the choice of the extract or ciprofloxacin concentrations selected in the adhesion and invasion assays. In order to prevent adhesion or invasion, the bacterial cells need to be alive but incapable of clinging to or intruding into the lung epithelial cells; therefore, sub-MIC had to be determined prior to the assays. On the other hand, the lung cells integrity was kept intact via using sub-MCC of the different tested agents. MICs were determined according to the Clinical and Laboratory Standards Institute (CLSI, M7-A7 and M100-S16, Criteria for *Pseudomonas aeruginosa*). Cytotoxicity of the tested agents against the A549 lung epithelial cell line was determined using crystal violet nuclei staining method as described by Gillies, *et al.* (1986) [10] with minor modifications. Briefly, confluent monolayer of A549 lung epithelial cell was incubated for 2 hrs with 200 µl of two-fold serial dilutions of different tested agents prepared in F12-K Medium, and then the cells were washed twice with phosphate-buffered saline (PBS). After rinsing, the cells were fixed with 1% (vol/vol) gluteraldehyde (Sigma/Aldrich, St. Louis, MO) and stained with 0.1% crystal violet (Fisher Scientific, Pittsburgh, PA) for 15 min. The dye was removed through multiples sterile water rinsing and the absorbed crystal violet was then dissolved with 0.5% (vol/vol) Triton X-100 (Sigma/Aldrich, St. Louis, MO).

Absorbance was measured at λ590 nm using Synergy™2 Microplate Reader (BioTech Instruments, Inc. Vermont, USA). Absorbance data were analyzed using Excel spread sheet and sub-MCCs were determined for different agents.

For SEM analysis, A549 lung epithelial cells were challenged with PAO1 cells for 1 hour, washed 3 times with F12-K medium and subsequently fixed with 5% (vol/vol) gluteraldehyde over 24 hours. The cells were then flushed with sterile deionized water to remove salts and dried before scanning with JSM-6490LV SEM (Peabody, Massachusetts) equipped with a tungsten filament, an accelerating voltages of 15-20 kV and a chamber pressure of 60-70 Pa according to the method described by Carterson *et al* with minor modifications [11]. All infectivity studies were carried out in a sterile class II biological safety cabinet (Sterilgard III Advance, Baker Company, Sanford, Maine, USA) according to the method described Plotkowski, *et al* [12] with some modifications. Initially, the confluent monolayer of A549 lung epithelial cells was incubated with 500μl fresh F12-K cell culture medium (control wells), 500μl of the natural extract or combination solutions (natural extract and ciprofloxacin) in F12-K medium at 37°C for 15 min followed by mixing with 500μl of 0.5 McFarland (1.5×10^8 CFU/ml) suspension of *P. aeruginosa* PAO1 prepared in F12-K medium for one minute to achieve homogenous bacterial distribution in Multiwell™ 12-well tissue culture plate (Becton Dickinson, NJ, USA). Ciprofloxacin (0.0625 μg/ml), dextran (50.0 mg/ml), and the aqueous extracts of soybean (42.8 mg/ml), and cranberry (25.4 mg/ml) as well as the combinations of the three later agents with ciprofloxacin were applied as potential anti-adhesion agents in the aforementioned assay. The mixture was incubated at 37°C for 1 hour to establish bacterial adhesion. Each plate had a control well and all experiments were carried out in triplicates.

At the end of the incubation time, cells were gently washed thrice with FBS free F12-K medium to eliminate the non-adhered bacterial cells of *P. aeruginosa* PAO1 and then lysis of the mammalian cells was carried out with 1ml of 1% (vol/vol) tween-20 (Astoria-Pacific, Clackamas, Oregon, USA) at 37°C for 30 min.

After lysis, ten-fold serial dilutions for the *P. aeruginosa* PAO1 suspension in each well followed by plating onto Cation Adjusted Muller Hinton II (CAMHII) agar were carried out. All CAMHII agar plates were incubated at 37°C for 18 hours for determining CFU/ml through viable cell counting for different treatments as well as for the untreated control. Percentage adhesion for each treatment relative to the untreated control was calculated and the averages of triplicate experiments were expressed graphically ± standard deviations (S.D). Data analysis was carried out using Graphpad prism 5 (GraphPad Software Inc. La Jolla, CA) that utilized One Way Analysis of Variance (ANOVA) followed by Dunnett Multiple Comparison test to determine the significant treatment differences as compared to the untreated control.

Parallel experiments were carried out as described under adhesion assay except for an extra step performed to assess *P. aeruginosa* PAO1 invasion into A549 lung epithelial cells. After 15 min incubation with 500 μL of the drug or the combination solutions in F12-K medium at 37°C, bacterial suspension (500 μL of 0.5 McFarland) was added and mixed with the aforementioned solutions for 1min in Multiwell™ 12-well tissue culture plates. The plates were incubated at 37°C for 2 hours to allow for invasion. Gentamicin exclusion method as described by Fleiszig *et al* [13] was then used to kill the adherent bacterial cells. This step involved washing of the adherent cells with FBS free F12-K medium followed by incubation of the infected cells with fresh F12-K medium containing 300µg/ml gentamicin for 1 hour at 37°C. After incubation, the dead bacteria were washed thrice with FBS free F12-K medium and the lung epithelial cells A549 were lysed with 1% (vol/vol) Tween-20 solution to determine the count of internalized *P. aeruginosa* PAO1 cells. The resultant cell suspensions were tenfold serially diluted, plated onto CAMHII agar plates, and incubated as previously described under adhesion assay.

Percentage invasion for each treatment relative to the control was calculated and the averages of triplicate experiments were expressed graphically ± standard deviations (S.D). Data analyses were carried out using Graphpad Prism 5 (GraphPad Software Inc. La Jolla, CA) that utilized the one way ANOVA followed by Dunnett Multiple Comparison adjustment to determine the significance of treatment differences on the invasion of *P. aeruginosa* PAO1 as compared to the control.

Adhesion of *P. aeruginosa* PAO1 to lung epithelial cells A549 was visualized using Scanning Electron Microscopy (SEM). Imaging revealed that *P. aeruginosa* PAO1 could adhere to the lung epithelial cells without disrupting the lung cells morphology (Figure 1).

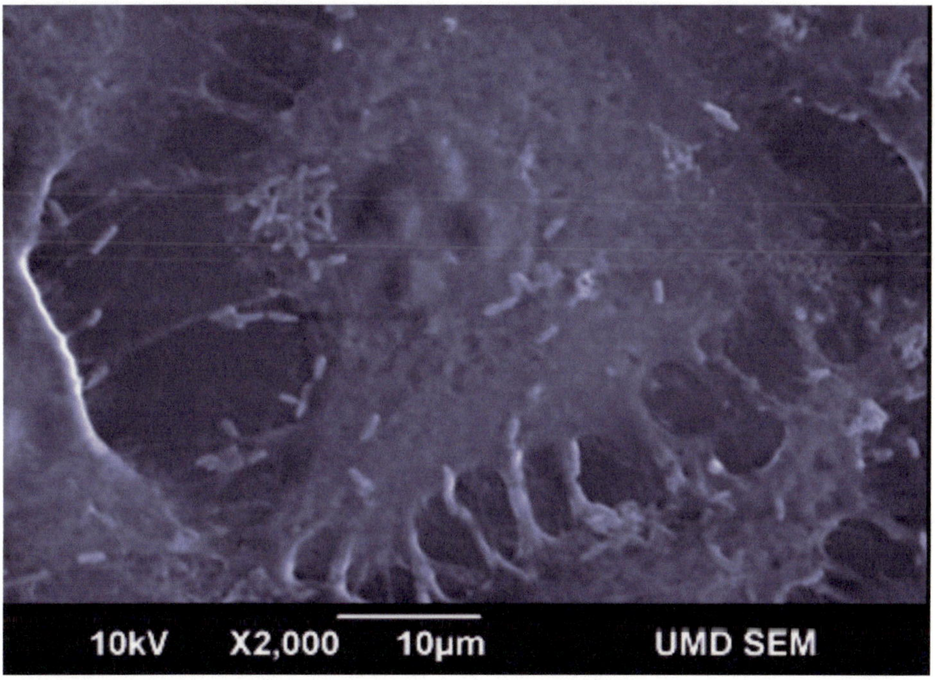

Fig. 1. Scanning Electron Micrograph illustrating the adherence of *Pseudomonas aeruginosa* PAO1 to A549 lung epithelial cells.

The soluble solid ingredients for the applied extracts were determined as described under Materials and Methods and their concentrations were 50.9 mg/ml and 85.7 mg/ml for the aqueous extracts of cranberry, and soybean respectively. Dextran was applied at a concentration level of 50.0 mg/ml.

MIC of ciprofloxacin and natural extracts against *P. aeruginosa* PAO1 and MCC of the same agents on A549 lung epithelial cells were determined according to CLSI criteria and the method described by Gillies *et al.* [10], respectively. The results showed that all the tested natural extracts had relatively high concentrations of MICs against *P. aeruginosa* PAO1 and of MCC on A549 lung epithelial cells (Table 1). These results may indicate that these agents are relatively non-toxic to the A549 lung epithelial cells as well as they cannot inhibit the growth of *P. aeruginosa* PAO1 at the tested concentrations.

Treatment	MIC[a] (μg/ml)	MCC[b] (μg/ml)
Ciprofloxacin	0.125	> 64
Dextran	>10000	>10000
Cranberry Extract	>5090	>5090
Soybean Extract	>8570	>8570

[a]Minimum Inhibitory Concentration
[b]Minimum Cytotoxic Concentration

Table 1. MIC and MCC (μg/ml) values for ciprofloxacin and different natural extracts against *P. aeruginosa* PAO1 and A549 lung epithelial cells, respectively.

Based on the data shown in table (1), sub-MIC and sub-MCC concentrations of both ciprofloxacin and the natural extracts were selected in the adhesion and invasion assays to evaluate their effects, as single agents or in combination with ciprofloxacin, on *P. aeruginosa* PAO1 adhesion and invasion without interfering with the viability of the bacterial or mammalian cells. Accordingly, ciprofloxacin (0.0625 μg/ml), dextran (50.0 mg/ml), cranberry extract (25.5 mg/ml), and soybean extract (42.8 mg/ml) were selected at their subMIC/subMCC for testing the effects of the single treatments on *P. aeruginosa* PAO1 adhesion and invasion to the lung epithelial cells. In combination treatments, the effect of ciprofloxacin (0.0625 μg/ml) on the adhesion and invasion of *P. aeruginosa* PAO1 was assessed with halves of the aforementioned concentrations of the tested single agents.

2.1 Effect of natural extracts and their combinations with ciprofloxacin on the adhesion of *P. aeruginosa* PAO1 to A549 lung epithelial cells

Adhesion of the *P. aeruginosa* PAO1 to the lung epithelial cells was assessed through viable cell counting of the bound bacteria to the cell surface from each independent triplicate experiment and the untreated controls. Adhesion of *P. aeruginosa* PAO1 to A549 lung epithelial cells in the presence of different natural extracts, as single agents and in combination with ciprofloxacin, was expressed as the percentage of adhered bacterial cells to the epithelial cell surface and normalized to that of the untreated controls. In that regard, ciprofloxacin (0.0625 μg/ml), dextran (50.0 mg/ml), cranberry extract (25.5 mg/ml), soybean extract (42.8 mg/ml) could reduce *P. aeruginosa* PAO1 adhesion by 26.3%, 16.4%, 54.5%, and 45%, respectively compared to the untreated control. On the other hand, ciprofloxacin combination with dextran (25.0 mg/ml), cranberry extract (12.7 mg/ml), soybean extract (21.4 mg/ml) could reduce *P. aeruginosa* PAO1 adhesion by 87.5%, 100%, and 72%, respectively as compared to that of the control (Figure 2). Interestingly, combination of ciprofloxacin (0.0625 μg/ml) with cranberry extract (12.7 mg/ml) could completely inhibit the adhesion (0.0%) of *P. aeruginosa* PAO1 to A549 lung epithelial cells. Although dextran was relatively the least effective single anti-adhesion treatment (83.6%±12.1%), it achieved a significant higher effect upon combination with ciprofloxacin (12.5%±4.2%).

Soybean extract was an effective anti-adhesion agent (55.0%±6.4%) compared to ciprofloxacin (73.7%±2.08%) and their combination could synergistically (28.03%±0.65%) and significantly (P<0.0001) reduce the ability of *P. aeruginosa* PAO1 to adhere to the A549 lung epithelial cells (Figure 2).

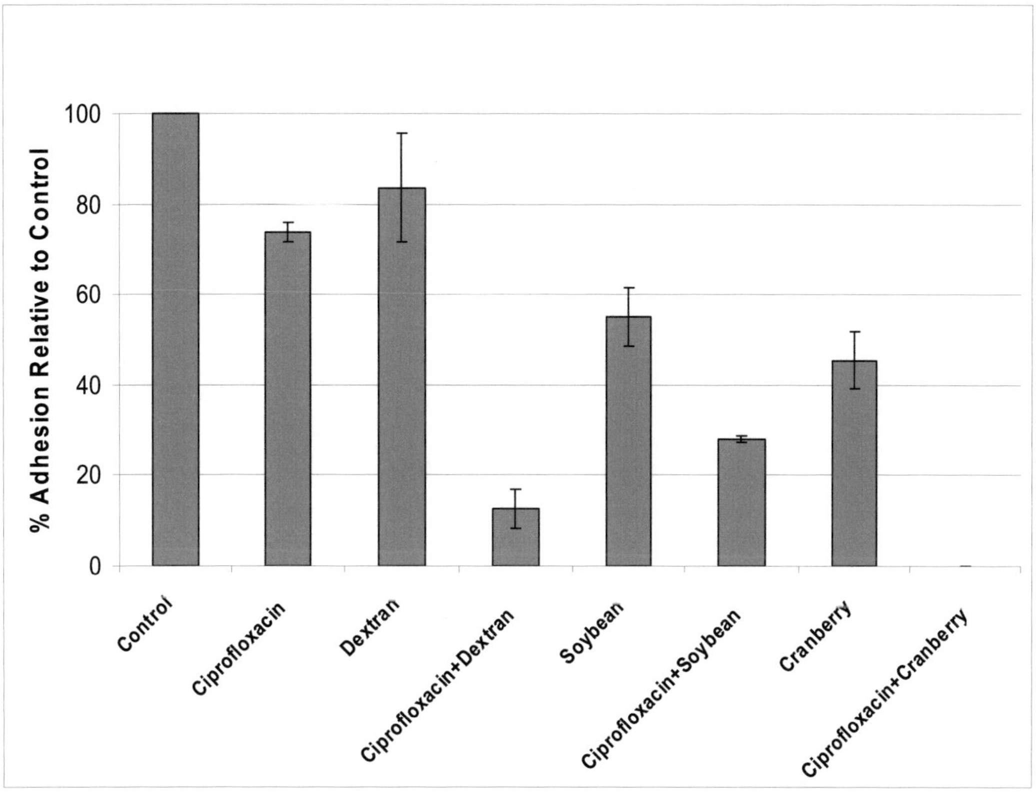

Fig. 2. The effect of different natural extracts alone and in combination with ciprofloxacin on the adhesion of *P. aeruginosa* PAO1 to A549 lung epithelial cells as compared to the untreated control.

2.2 Effect of natural extracts and their combinations with ciprofloxacin on the invasion of *P. aeruginosa* PAO1 to A549 lung epithelial cells

The ability of the adhered bacterial cells to internalize into the lung epithelial cells in the presence of different natural extracts, as single agents or in combination with ciprofloxacin, was assessed through calculation of percentage invasion of *P. aeruginosa* PAO1 from three independent experiments relative to the untreated controls. The results of gentamicin exclusion assay are believed to reflect the count of bacteria that has invaded cells [4, 13] with different treatments. Expectedly, both single cranberry and combination with ciprofloxacin were able to completely abrogate the invasion of *P. aeruginosa* PAO1 to the lung cells (0.0%). Although 45.5%±6.7% of the initial bacterial inoculum was able to bind to the epithelial cells after treatment in the presence of cranberry extract, none of this adhered population was able to penetrate the lung epithelial cells. Following the synergistic effect of cranberry extract, the combination of ciprofloxacin with both of soybean (17.6%±7.12%) and dextran

(11.8%±2.1%) achieved comparable and significant ($P<0.0001$) anti-invasion effects compared to the control. Similar to the results for the adhesion assay, dextran and soybean were more effective in combination with ciprofloxacin in preventing invasion rather than the single agents (75.5%±2.1%) and (17.6%±11.8%) as shown in figure (3).

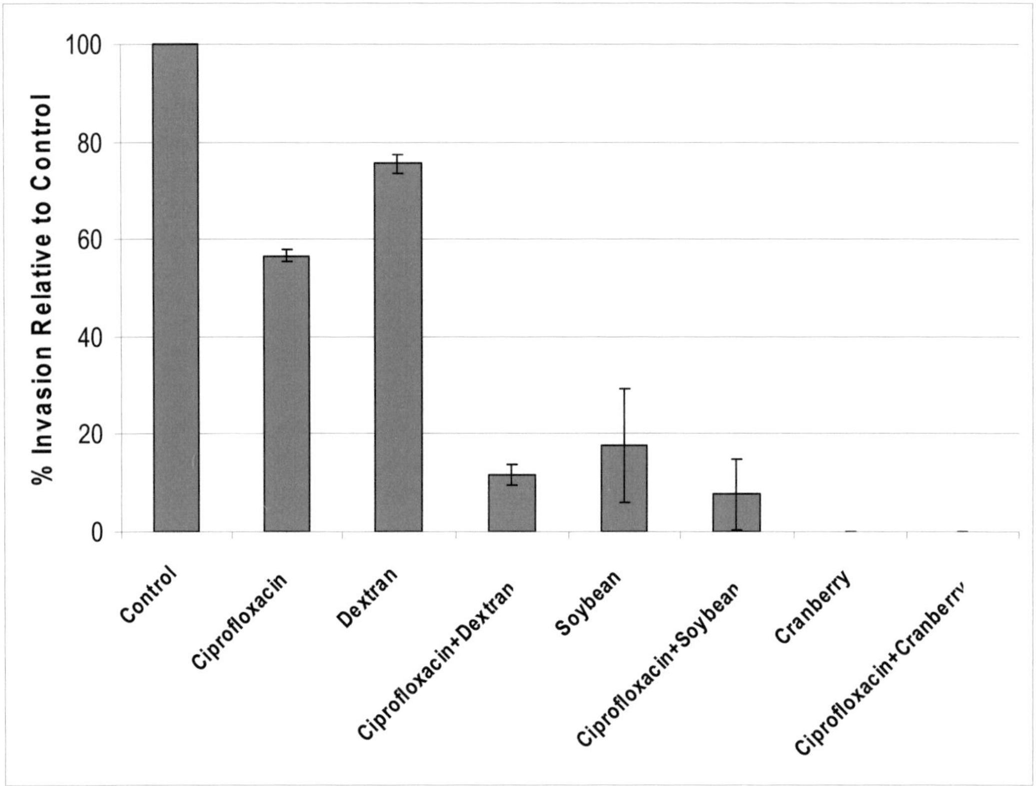

Fig. 3. The effect of different natural extracts alone and in combination with ciprofloxacin on the invasion of *P. aeruginosa* PAO1 to A549 lung epithelial cells as compared to the untreated control.

3. Discussion

Pseudomonas aeruginosa is a major cause for mortality seen in CF patients [6]. Adhesion and subsequent invasion of that organism to the lung epithelial cells are considered as the initial and substantial steps in the lung infection [5, 14-16]. Once the colonization of the organism is established, it is rarely eradicated. Several strategies have been developed to prevent *P. aeruginosa* infection in CF patients through different antibiotics and immunizations, but were not successful [8, 17-19]; therefore, development of other prophylactic measures as anti-adhesion and anti-invasion approaches is required. Ciprofloxacin, a fluoroquinolone, is considered as an antibiotic of choice for the treatment of the lung infections with *Pseudomonas aeruginosa* [7]. The current study aimed at introducing a new strategy to prevent *Pseudomonas aeruginosa* adhesion and invasion to the lung epithelial cells using different combinations of ciprofloxacin and aqueous extracts from widely available natural products such as cranberry, and soybean. Dextran, which has been tested before in many occasions and found to be an effective anti-adhesion agent [2, 8, 11], was tested on that epithelial cell infection model as well to assess its anti-adhesion and anti-invasion activities compared to the other natural products, alone and in combination with ciprofloxacin.

The virulence factors of different *Pseudomonas aeruginosa* strains were attributed either to their direct host cell cytotoxicity or ability to adhere, invade, and survive within the epithelial cells. *P. aeruginosa* PAO1 virulence is categorized under the second types of isolates and invasion of that strain was suggested to contribute to biofilm formation and establishment of chronic lung infections [7]. Interestingly, the binding of *Pseudomonas aeruginosa* to the uninjured epithelial surfaces was found to be minimal. However, the binding ability of the organism increases dramatically in presence of epithelial surface inflammation or injury (such as in CF patients) [6, 20]. Scanning electron microscopy imaging revealed establishment of *P. aeruginosa* PAO1 binding to lung epithelial cells as the first step of *Pseudomonas aeruginosa* infection. Such binding did not affect the cells integrity or morphology (Figure1). Similarly, Fleiszig *et al.* [13] noted that integrity of the infected cells remains unaffected since the strain *P. aeruginosa* PAO1 does not use cytotoxicity as a virulence mechanism against the lung epithelial cells.

In order to exclude the inhibitory effect of ciprofloxacin and the applied natural extracts on *P. aeruginosa* PAO1 and A549 lung epithelial cells, the MICs of ciprofloxacin and the natural extracts against *P. aeruginosa* PAO1 and the MCCs of the same agents were determined to aid selection of the concentrations of different agents that will be tested on the adhesion and invasion models.

Unsurprisingly, the MICs and MCCs values could not be reached within the tested concentration levels for the different natural extracts, which were relatively high compared to ciprofloxacin, indicating that they are relatively non-toxic to the A549 lung epithelial cells as well as to *P. aeruginosa* PAO1. It has been reported that extracts of the natural sources are considered as endless reservoirs of safe and relatively inexpensive bioactive agents [9].

Dextran is a widely available polysaccharide that has been used in clinical settings as plasma expander [2]. It was previously tested as a carbohydrate treatment that blocks the epithelial glycoconjugates and impedes the bacterial legends from binding to pulmonary epithelial cell receptors [2]. Aerosolized dextran has been examined in a mouse infection model to prevent pneumonia caused by *Pseudomonas aeruginosa* and it could significantly reduce the development of pneumonia in the treated group relative to the untreated control animals, being an immuno-stimulant and a sputum rheology enhancer [2].

The combination treatment of dextran with ciprofloxacin disabled the internalization abilities of 85% of the bacterial population that adhered in the control experiments. Application of dextran resulted in an average of 14% reduction in both adhesion and invasion of *P. aeruginosa* PAO1 to the lung epithelia. This reduction is slightly less than that was found by Bryan *et al.* [2] who reported 35% reduction on *P. aeruginosa* PAO1 adhesion to nasal polyp primary culture cells when pretreated with dextran. Factors such as difference in the cell culture type or the experimental conditions may provide an explanation for the disparity in the activities. The same authors proposed that the likely mechanism through which dextran blocks bacterial adhesion was through the non-specific interaction with the epithelial cells; since pre-incubation of *P. aeruginosa* PAO1 with dextran before performing the infection abolished its anti-adhesion properties [2]. Consequently, the inhibitory action of dextran might not only involve *P. aeruginosa* PAO1 adhesion, but also other potential pathogens especially those targeting respiratory epithelia.

To our knowledge, there were no previous studies that reported the utilization of soybean extract as a potential anti-adhesion or anti-invasion treatment. The present study, however, proposes that the aqueous extract of soybean (*Glycine max*) is an additional promising treatment against adhesion and invasion of *P. aeruginosa* PAO1 to the lung epithelial cells. Compared to the control treatment, 28% and 17% of the applied bacterial inoculum were able to adhere and invade the lung epithelial cells, respectively, upon application of soybean extract combination with ciprofloxacin. These results suggest that on average half of the bacterial population that were able to adhere after treatment with soybean extract were not capable to invade the lung epithelial cells

Aqueous extract of cranberry (*Vaccinium macrocarpon*) was by far the most effective anti-adhesion and anti-invasion treatment when used in combination with ciprofloxacin. Cranberry belongs to *Vaccinum* family that has a wide spectrum of *in vitro* antimicrobial activity [21]. Many reports have demonstrated that proanthocyanidines and saccharides of cranberry were able to inhibit adhesion and invasion of some pathogenic microbes *in vitro*, and that cranberry juice clinically prevents urinary tract infection in women by inhibiting *Escherichia coli* adhesion to uroepithelial glycolipid receptors [3, 9]. The activity of the cranberry extract extended to provide protection against resistant strains of *Escherichia coli* by a mechanism that is unlikely to increase the selective pressure associated with antibiotics resistance [3]. Therefore, combining cranberry extract with ciprofloxacin sub-MIC may block the initial steps of infection, adhesion and invasion, as well as minimizing the development of bacterial resistance.

The results of this study may indicate that cranberry extract could turn the adhered bacteria unable to invade the lung epithelial cells since 45% of *P. aeruginosa* PAO1 population that were able to adhere to the lung cells under treatment with cranberry were, simultaneously, incapable of invading those cells and further molecular studies are required to elucidate this interesting point.

In published randomized clinical trial, cranberry juice was found to only affect harmful bacteria leaving normal bacterial flora unaffected; an observation that could suggest the therapeutic benefits of cranberry without having major unexpected side effects [21]. Cranberry juice, capsules and powder were also found to reduce urinary tract infection recurrences as well as the salival counts of the bacteria causing dental carries [21-24].

The significance of proposing the anti-adhesion treatments emanates from the fact that the earlier the establishment of airway infection is prevented the better the expected therapeutic outcome; since the persistence of intracellular bacteria causes sloughing of epithelial cells containing these bacteria and may contribute to spreading of the infection, establishment of the biofilm, rendering the bacterial eradication by the antibiotics difficult and favoring the bacterial endurance in the host airway [7].

In light of these *in vitro* anti-adhesion and anti-invasion effects of the promising natural extracts, further *in vivo* studies are required to explore their putative applications as an alternative strategy to combat the respiratory infections and the potential reduction of the antibiotic resistance rates.

4. Abbreviations

CF: Cystic Fibrosis
COPD: Chronic Obstructive Pulmonary Disease
CAMHB: Cation Adjusted Muller Hinton Broth

MIC: Minimum Inhibitory Concentration
MCC: Minimum Cytotoxic Concentration
CLSI: Clinical and Laboratory Standards Institute
SEM: Scanning Electron Microscopy
ANOVA: Analysis of Variance

5. References

[1] Gambardella S, Biancolella M, D'Apice MR et al. Gene expression profile in CFTR mutated bronchial cell lines.*Clin Exp Med* 2006; 6:157-165.

[2] Soferman R. Immunopathophysiologic mechanisms of cystic fibrosis lung disease. *IMAJ* 2006; 8:44-48.

[3] Singh AP, Chauhan SC, Andrianifahanana M, et al. MUC4 expression is regulated by cystic fibrosis transmembrane conductance regulator in pancreatic adenocarcinoma cells via transcriptional and post-translational mechanisms. *Oncogene* 2007; 26:30-41.

[4] Moskwa P, Lorentzen D, Excoffon KJ, et al. A novel host defense system of airway is defective in cystic fibrosis.*Am J Respir Crit Care Med* 2007; 175:174-183.

[5] Blau H. Cystic fibrosis lung disease: interplay of a microbial microcosm and extremes of inflammation *IMAJ* 2006; 8:58-59.

[6] Bilton D, Henig N, Morrissey B and Golfried Ml. Addition of inhaled tobramycin to ciprofloxacin for acute exacerbations of Pseudomonas aeruginosa infection in adult bronchiectasis. *Chest* 2006; 130:1503-1510.

[7] Smyth A. Update on treatment of pulmonary exacerbations in cystic fibrosis *Curr Opin Pulm Med* 2006; 12:440-444.

[8] McLachlan G, Baker A, Tennant P, et al. Optimizing aerosol gene delivery and expression in the ovine lung .*Molecular Therapy* 2007; 15:348-354.

[9] Fischer AC, Smith CL, Cebotaru L, Zhang X, et al. et al. Expression of a truncated cystic fibrosis transmembrane conductance regulator with an AAV5-pseudotyped vector in primates. *Molecular Therapy, 15(4):756-63.*

[10] Delgado MA, Poschet JF, Deretic Vl. Nonclassical pathway of Pseudomonas aeruginosa DNA-induced interleukin-8 secretion in cystic fibrosis airway epithelial cells.*Infection and Immunity* 2006; 74(5):2975-2984.

[11] Bavington C, and Page C. Stopping bacterial adhesion: a novel approach to treating infections. Respiration 2005;72: 335-344.

[12] Bryan R, Feldman M, Jawetz SC et al. The effects of aerosolized dextran in a mouse model of *Pseudomonas aeruginosa* pulmonary infection. J Infect Dis 1999;179: 1449-1458.

[13] Howell AB, Vorsa N, Der Marderosian A, Foo LY. Inhibition of the adherence of P-fimbriated *Escherichia coli* to uroepithelial-cell surfaces by proanthocyanidin extracts from cranberries. N Engl J Med 1998;339:1085-1086.

[14] Angus AA, Lee AA, Augustin DK et al. *Pseudomonas aeruginosa* induces membrane blebs in epithelial cells, which are utilized as a niche for intracellular replication and motility. Infect Immun 2008;76:1992-2001.

[15] Imundo L, Barasch J, Prince A, Al-Awqati Q. Cystic fibrosis epithelial cells have a receptor for pathogenic bacteria on their apical surface. Proc Natl Acad Sci U.S.A 1995;92:3019-3023.

[16] Swanson B, Savel R, Szoka F, Sawa T,Wiener-Kronish J. Development of a high throughput *Pseudomonas aeruginosa* epithelial cell adhesion assay. J Microbiol Methods 2003;52:361-366.
[17] Garcia-Medina R, Dunne WM, Singh PK, Brody SL. *Pseudomonas aeruginosa* acquires biofilm-like properties within airway epithelial cells. Infect Immun 2005;73:8298-8305.
[18] Barghouthi S, Guerdoud LM, Speert DP. Inhibition by dextran of *Pseudomonas aeruginosa* adherence to epithelial cells. Am J Respir Crit Care Med 1996;154:1788-1793.
[19] Howell AB, and Foxman B. Cranberry juice and adhesion of antibiotic-resistant uropathogens. JAMA 2002;287:3082-3083.
[20] Gillies RJ, Didier N, Denton M. Determination of cell number in monolayer cultures. Anal Biochem 1986;159:109-113.
[21] Carterson AJ, Honer Bentrup K, Ott CM et al. A549 lung epithelial cells grown as three-dimensional aggregates: alternative tissue culture model for *Pseudomonas aeruginosa* pathogenesis. Infect Immun 2005;73:1129-1140.
[22] Plotkowski MC, Saliba AM, Pereira SH, Cervante MP, Bajolet-Laudinat O. *Pseudomonas aeruginosa* selective adherence to and entry into human endothelial cells. Infect Immun 1994;62:5456-5463.
[23] Fleiszig SM, Zaidi TS, Preston MJ, Grout M, Evans DJ et al. Relationship between cytotoxicity and corneal epithelial cell invasion by clinical isolates of *Pseudomonas aeruginosa*. Infect Immun 1996;64:2288-2294.
[24] Beachey EH. Bacterial adherence: adhesin-receptor interactions mediating the attachment of bacteria to mucosal surface. J Infect Dis 1981;143:325-345.
[25] Kallenius G, Mollby R, Svenson SB, Winberg J. Microbial adhesion and the urinary tract. Lancet 1981;318(8251):866.
[26] Boren T, Falk P, Roth KA, Larson G, Normark S. Attachment of *Helicobacter pylori* to human gastric epithelium mediated by blood group antigens. Science 1993;262:1892-1895.
[27] Speert DP. Prevention of severe lower respiratory infections in patients with cystic fibrosis. Semin Respir Infect 1989;4:266-271.
[28] Pennington JE, Reynolds HY, Wood RE, Robinson RA, Levine AS. Use of a *Pseudomonas Aeruginosa* vaccine in pateints with acute leukemia and cystic fibrosis. Am J Med 1975;58:629-636.
[29] Wood RE, Pennington JE, Reynolds HY. Intranasal administration of a *Pseudomonas* lipopolysaccharide vaccine in cystic fibrosis patients. Pediatr Infect Dis 1983;2:367-369.
[30] Bentzmann S, Roger P, Puchelle E. *Pseudomonas aeruginosa* adherence to remodelling respiratory epithelium. Eur Respir J 1996;9:2145-2150.
[31] Kontiokari T, Salo J, Eerola E, Uhari M. Cranberry juice and bacterial colonization in children: a placebo-controlled randomized trial. Clin Nutr 2005;24:1065-1072.
[32] Weiss EI, Kozlovsky A, Steinberg D, Lev-Dor R, Bar Ness GR. et al. A high molecular mass cranberry constituent reduces mutans streptococci level in saliva and inhibits *in vitro* adhesion to hydroxyapatite. FEMS Microbiol Lett 2004;232:89-92.
[33] Avorn J, Monane M, Gurwitz JH, Glynn RJ, Choodnovskiy I. et al. Reduction of bacteriuria and pyuria after ingestion of cranberry juice. JAMA 1994;271:751-754.
[34] Stothers L. A randomized trial to evaluate effectiveness and cost effectiveness of naturopathic cranberry products as prophylaxis against urinary tract infection in women. Can J Urol 2002;9:1558-1562.

Part 4

Paediatrics

20

Bronchitis in Children

Christian Peiser
*Department for Pediatric Pneumology and Immunology,
Charité, Medical University Berlin,
Germany*

1. Introduction

For a paediatrician, children with bronchitis are part of the daily work. Infections of the respiratory system are the most common reason for children presenting at the doctor´s practice. Almost all infants and younger school children become sick several times a year with a bronchitis. In most cases with the beginning of day nursery or nursery school there is an abrupt accumulation and many parents have the feeling that their child is permanently ill. That bronchitis occurs much more frequently in winter than in summer, as everyone knows from personal experience. The cold air outside and the dry heated air indoors, increases the vulnerability of the mucosa for pathogens. Whether the clinical course of a bronchitis is uncomplicated or associated with a bronchial obstruction, is partly caused by the genetic predisposition of the child. Depending on family history of bronchial asthma and allergies, the risk may be increased many times over. The health damage due to exposure to tobacco smoke is a major point which should not be underestimated.

The following pages describe in the form of a brief overview symptoms and signs of bronchitis in children. The different types and stages of bronchitis are shown. The most common viruses that cause bronchitis are described, in particular the respiratory syncytial virus. One chapter deals with bronchopulmonary dysplasia, an important risk factor for bronchitis in children. Furthermore, some important differential diagnoses are presented, which can become manifest with the typical symptoms of a bronchitis. The laboratory diagnosis with the aim of differentiating between viral and bacterial bronchitis is discussed. Finally, therapeutic options are mentioned.

2. Signs and symptoms of bronchitis in children

2.1 Cough

The main symptom of bronchitis is a cough. At the beginning of the disease it tends to be dry and unproductive. With increasing production of secretion the mucus becomes less viscous, which makes coughing more effective. Some children have such severe coughing attacks that vomiting can be induced. An adequate supply of volume and inhalation therapy with 0.9% NaCl can help to make the mucus more fluid, enabling it to be brought up more easily by coughing. There are medications, usually in the form of so-called cough syrups, which will also assist mucolytic activity. After regression of an acute bronchitis, an unpleasant dry cough can still remain for several days or weeks. This is caused by a transient hyperreactivity of the bronchial system due to the infection-induced inflammation.

2.2 Tachypnoea and dyspnoea

If secreted mucus, an oedema of the bronchial mucosa or a spasm of the bronchial musculature induce bronchial obstruction, tachypnoea and dyspnoea may belong to the acute disorders. Typical clinical signs for dyspnoea are movement of the nostrils, inter- or subcostal retractions, use of accessory respiratory muscles, an upright upper body position, and in the auscultation wheezing and sometimes also rales. In this situation inhalation therapy with bronchodilatatory agents and the systemic administration of steroids may be helpful. Because the expiration is more difficult that the inspiration, an emphysema may be formed due to air trapping. Children with respiratory distress may become anxious and excited, which makes the situation worse. The excitement and anxiety of the parents may also be transferred to the child. In the case of severe respiratory distress, the oxygen saturation in the blood may decrease critically, making oxygen substitution necessary. Measurement of vital parameters and blood gas analyses are standard procedures. The suctioning of secretions and mucus, or the application of respiratory supportive procedures, such as CPAP or intubation and ventilation, should be made immediately possible.

2.3 Pain

Pain in the context of bronchitis can be caused by an inflammatory involvement of the trachea or pleura. In the case of retrosternal pain during coughing, a tracheitis is most probable. Respiratory-dependent, especially in deep inspiration increasing pain, which is localized more laterally in one or both sides of the chest, makes a pleuritis more probable. Especially the dry chafing of inflamed visceral pleura and parietal pleura against each other is very painful. If the child develops shallow breathing to avoid the pain, an insufficient ventilation of the lung may result with the increased risk of a secondary bacterial infection. For this reason, an appropriate analgesia is strongly recommended.

2.4 Fever

Fever is a general clinical sign, which may occur in any infection, including one of the respiratory system. The increase of body temperature is a non-specific symptom and can range from low-grade fever up to hyperpyrexia with acute physical stress for the child. In the case of an infection of the upper respiratory tract, additionally clinical signs (in addition to the cough, tachydyspnea, pain and fever) are sniffing (rhinitis), a sore throat (pharyngitis) and earache (otitis media). Furthermore, swollen and aching cervical lymph nodes are a common local response to the inflammation process.

3. Different types of bronchitis in children

3.1 Acute, complicated, chronic, recurrent

The average duration of an acute bronchitis is about 1 week with the range from ½ week up to 2 weeks. Afterwards a nervous cough may remain for several days or a few weeks. The acute bronchitis has a very high rate of complete recovery; the prognosis is very good. An exception is an acute bronchitis caused by adenovirus; in this case complications in the clinical course or a chronification of the bronchitis are described.

If the symptoms and signs of an acute bronchitis persist for 4 – 6 weeks, we call it complicated bronchitis. If an acute bronchitis is followed by another one, they can be taken for a complicated bronchitis by mistake. Approximately 20% of acute bronchitis has a complicated course. One possible complication is the secondary bacterial superinfection of a primary viral infection. In this case the child needs to be treated with antibiotics. Another possible complication is the transition from bronchitis into bronchopneumonia. In many cases this is detectable by pulmonary auscultation, but to confirm the diagnosis, a chest X-ray is necessary. A primary bacterial bronchitis usually presents clinically as a complicated bronchitis.

Signs and symptoms of a bronchitis persisting for more than 3 months are called chronic bronchitis.

If children repeat lots of acute bronchitis over months, it is called recurrent bronchitis. Mainly children in day nursery or nursery school are affected quite often, because the risk of infection is particularly high there. In the cold seasons bronchitis occurs more frequently compared to the warm seasons.

3.2 Non-obstructive or obstructive

Bronchitis can be associated more or less with bronchial obstruction. The risk of an obstruction depends on the lumen of the inflamed bronchus; the smaller the lumen, the more likely is a clinically relevant obstruction. For this reason, the terms "obstructive bronchitis" and "bronchiolitis" were sometimes used as synonyms. Bronchial obstruction can be caused by the following pathophysiological alterations:

1. The smooth muscles of the bronchus get contracted, which can lead to an acute shortness of breath.
2. The mucosa of the respiratory epithelium is swollen due to the inflammation, which narrows the bronchial lumen.
3. The increased production of mucus clogs the lumen as well. Furthermore, due to the inflammation in the respiratory epithelium, the function of the cilia is reduced, and mucus cannot be transported adequately.

Auscultation of the lung shows wheezing. A so-called silent lung is typical for a severe bronchial obstruction with air trapping and emphysema. In this case the resting expiratory position is shifted to the inspiration, what may create a circulus vitiosus.

3.3 Non-allergic or allergic

Bronchitis is an inflammatory disease of the bronchial mucosa. In most cases the inflammation is caused by an infection. Also allergens may cause an acute or chronic bronchitis, they act mostly as a trigger. The presence of one or more allergies increases the statistical risk for the development of bronchial asthma. Relevant inhalation allergens are dust mites, animal dander, mould fungus and pollen.

As their zoological name "Dermatophagoides" indicates, dust mites feed on epithelia from the skin, of which one person loses about 1.5 grams per day. They are, depending on the type, 0.1 - 0.5 mm in size and they live in normal house dust. They are found in carpets, curtains, upholstered furniture, mattresses, duvets and pillows, stuffed animals etc. The allergen comes from the faeces of the mites. In order to avoid exposure, the following protections should be carried out: the use of an encasing such as a mattress cover, monthly washing of duvets and pillows, occasional freezing of soft toys at -20 °C, followed by rinsing, no long carpets, regular vacuuming and avoidance of dust turbulence.

With regard to animal dander, those species which are most relevant and which human beings have close contact with are especially dogs, cats, guinea pigs, hamsters, horses and birds. The allergen concentration varies within a species, depending on the breed. For this reason it could happen that someone tolerates contact with one cat very well, whereas contact with another cat induces an acute bronchial obstruction. In the case of a clinically relevant allergy against an animal, the contact should be avoided.

The spores of mould fungus can also cause an allergic reaction, like bronchial hyperreactivity or bronchial obstruction. If at home the walls are infested with mould fungus, the house has to be renovated.

Among the pollen, early flowering plants (birch, alder, hazel, willow) and grasses are most relevant. The occurrence of pollen-induced disorders, namely rhinoconjunctivitis and bronchial asthma, are strongly season-dependent and time-limited. On the basis of cross-reactions, for example between birch pollen and apple, in the case of an allergy against birch pollen, an allergic reaction against apple in the form of an oral allergy syndrome may occur. In the case of pollen, allergen avoidance is almost impossible. In order to reduce the intensity of pollen-induced allergy symptoms, desensitization is recommended.

3.4 Special forms: Bronchitis fibroplastica, bronchioloitis obliterans

A special form of bronchitis in childhood is the bronchitis fibroplastica. Older synonyms are fibrinous bronchitis, pseudomembranous bronchitis or Hoffmann's bronchitis. It is characterized by obstruction of the bronchi, usually a lobe or segment, consisting of mucin, which forms large endobronchial casts of rubber-like consistency. Pre-existing pathological conditions, such as bronchial asthma or cystic fibrosis, which are attended by hypersecretion of viscous mucus, may act as triggers. Childhood tuberculosis or primary immunodeficiency seem to be associated with a higher incidence of bronchitis fibroplastica as well. However, exact epidemiological data are still missing. Main symptoms are a cough and dyspnoea, and sometimes pleuritic pain and fever occur. In pulmonary auscultation over the affected area of the lung the breath is quiet or absent; sometimes wheezing or rales can be heard. X-rays of the chest typically show an atelectatic area next to an emphysematic one. The therapy consists in the prompt removal of the sticky casts consisting of mucin via rigid bronchoscopy. If they are not removable, administration of N-acetylcysteine or DNase may be helpful. If a child without known pre-existing diseases falls ill with bronchitis fibroplastica, additional diagnostic investigations should be carried out: sweat tests, tuberculin tests, allergy tests.

Another special form of bronchitis in children is the bronchiolitis obliterans. An inflammation of the small airways induces a pathologic tissue remodelling with granulations, which obstruct the lumen of the bronchioles. This process may be triggered by infections, inhalation of toxic agents, autoimmune diseases or a chronic rejection after lung transplantation. In the group of long-term survivors after lung transplantation, bronchioltis obliterans is the most frequent cause of death. The clinical signs and symptoms are quite unspecific: a cough and reduced general condition. In pulmonary auscultation the breath is quiet and rales can be heard. The X-ray of the chest eventually shows some infiltration or it looks normal. The disease may begin rapidly or slowly and the clinical course may be progressive or stable. Therapeutic options are a high-dose glucocorticoid administration, and in the case of lung transplantation, an increase in the dosage of the immunosuppressive medication.

4. Different stages of bronchitis in children

4.1 Bronchial hyperreactivity

Bronchial hyperreactivity is a chronic inflammation of the bronchial mucosa with recurrent bronchial obstruction, which may be triggered by infections, allergens or nonspecific stimuli, such as cold air, physical or even emotional stress. The inflammatory activity causes a swelling of the bronchial mucosa with a reduction of the bronchial lumen consecutively. The smaller the lumens are physiologically, such as in infants, the more relevant is its reduction regarding clinical symptoms. Furthermore, inflammation of the bronchial mucosa increases the vulnerability to viruses or bacteria.

To make the diagnosis "bronchial hyperreactivity", an accurate and detailed medical history is the most important step. Additionally, measurement of the lung function may confirm the diagnosis, in particular in the case of a reduced flow in the smaller airways; after administration of a beta-sympathomimetic via inhalation the bronchial obstruction should be reversible, at least partly. The lung function test can be carried out with children who are old enough to participate actively. Furthermore, measurement of the NO-exhalation may be useful to monitor the amount of bronchial inflammation. In some cases it may be helpful to carry out a bronchial provocation test via inhalation of methacholine, histamine or carbachol. Of course, all emergency tools have to be available.

4.2 Bronchitis

Bronchitis is a clinically apparent inflammation of the bronchi, triggered by a bronchial hyprerreactivity, by viruses or bacteria or by allergens. The symptoms (cough, tachypnoea and dyspnoea, pain, fever), the different courses (acute, complicated, chronic, recurrent) and different forms (non-obstructive, obstructive) have been described.

4.3 Bronchiolitis

Bronchiolitis is an inflammation of the smallest bronchi and bronchioles. Due to the small lumens of these airways, swelling of bronchial mucosa may induce severe obstruction quite rapidly, in most cases associated with pulmonary hyperinflation. This can lead to the phenomenon of the so-called silent obstruction, that means barely wheezing, humming or whistling, but fine bubble rales at the end of inspiration. Bronchiolitis is a typical disease of infancy, the age peak is between 4 and 6 months.

4.4 Bronchopneumonia

Bronchopneumonia is a possible course of a complicated bronchitis. Whereas a primary pneumonia normally is localized to one segment or lobe of the lung, in the case of a bronchopneumonia there is a disseminated inflammation from the bronchi down to the alveoli.

4.5 Bronchial asthma

Bronchial asthma is a disease with chronic inflammation of the respiratory system with bronchial hyperreactivity and variable airway obstructions. In many children and adolescents we find a positive family history for asthma and/or allergies. The restriction of the air flow, mainly during the expiration, is caused by spastic contraction of the smooth muscle in the bronchial wall, oedematous swelling of the bronchial mucosa and hypersecretion of viscous mucus. In addition to these pathological mechanisms, a tissue remodelling may take place after bronchial asthma over several years, which makes the airways less elastic. In most cases patients have an allergic bronchial asthma; case of non-allergic asthma and mixed forms are possible as well.

Criteria for the diagnosis of bronchial asthma in children and adolescents are a relative forced ventilation capacity (FEV1/VK) < 75% of age- and gender-related norm and a 15 % increase with prolonged expiratory time, or after inhalation of a short-acting beta-sympathomimetic. A further criterion is a decrease in respiratory resistance (R) > 50% of baseline after inhalation of a short-acting beta-sympathomimetic. If the lung function measurement shows a normal result, but the clinical history is typically for bronchial asthma, then a circadian variability of the measured peak expiratory flow (PEF) > 20% confirms the diagnosis. If the doctor is still in doubt with the diagnosis, a provocation test (for example physical stress or inhalation of metacholine) may be helpful to make the right diagnosis.

The therapy of bronchial asthma is successful if clinical signs and symptoms of the disease are under control, so that the affected children or adolescents feel free from disorders if they are able to partake in sport without any restriction, if there are no side effects of the medications and if no long-term injury will occur. Taken together, if the children or adolescents just have a normal life with this chronic disease. Parts of the therapy are prevention (for example not smoking, either actively or passively, avoidance of allergens, if possible), general procedures (for example participation on training courses of instruction, doing sports, doing physiotherapy), pharmacotherapy and rehabilitation, if it is required. The prescription of drugs should be carried out in accordance with an algorithm, which has various steps depending on the severity of the bronchial asthma and gives the opportunity to step up or step down. Standard drugs in pharmacotherapy of bronchial asthma are low-dose inhaled glucocorticoids and orally administered leukotriene antagonists (additionally or alternatively) for long-term therapy, as well as inhaled short-acting beta-sympathomimetics for acute therapy. Because of this treatment, severe asthma attacks have become very rare incidents.

5. Common viruses causing bronchitis in children

Acute bronchitis is almost (in approximately 90%) induced by viruses. The most common ones are respiratory syncytial, parainfluenza-, influenza-, adeno-, rhino-, metapneumo- and human bocavirus. Acute bronchitis, which is induced by bacteria primary, is rare (approximately 10%). In 15% of viral bronchitis a secondary bacterial infection will happen.

5.1 Respiratory syncytial virus (RSV)

It is a member of the family of paramyxoviridae, has a single-stranded RNA and is enveloped. We distinguish two serological groups A and B from each other. The pathogenicity of the virus depends crucially on two glycoproteins on the viral surface: glycoprotein G enables the docking with the host cell, such as pneumocytes, glycoprotein F is responsible for the endocytosis into the cell. The fact that the affected cell undergoes a fusion with neighbouring cells and form syncytia has given the virus its name. Further details of incubation time, infection and clinical signs and symptoms are in the section "Characteristics of RSV infection."

5.2 Parainfluenzavirus

It belongs to the family of paramyxoviridae, has a single-stranded RNA and an envelope. It is (in contrast to the influenza viruses) genetically stable. There are 4 different types. The transmission of the virus proceeds via droplet or smear infection. The incubation period is 3 - 6 days. At the age of 2 years, almost all children have been sick at least once with a parainfluenza infection. In infancy and early childhood parainfluenza virus causes an acute laryngotracheobronchitis with typical croup symptoms.

5.3 Influenzavirus

It is assigned to the family of orthomyxoviridae. It is divided into the 3 types A, B and C, of which A and B are most relevant for infections of humans. The genome of influenza viruses type A and B consists of eight single-stranded RNA segments. This creates a high genetic variability of antigenic drift and antigenic shift, in the case of a dual infection. The eight RNA segments contain the genetic information for 11 proteins, of which one is the neuraminidase. Transmission paths of the virus are aerosols and saliva, as well as contact with contaminated surfaces. The incubation period is 1 - 4 days. Typically we see a high incidence of influenza during the winter months. The epidemic often has its origin in the nursery, kindergarten or school. Because of the high contagiosity, pandemics with high lethality may occur, recently caused by the H1N1 subtype, the so-called "swine flu". In contrast to the common cold, the clinical course of the influenza infection is characterized by significantly reduced general condition, high fever and a much higher complication rate. Children with a disease of the respiratory tract, a heart failure or a deficiency of the immune system have an especially high risk for severe complications. The diagnosis of influenza can be made with a rapid test (usually an Elisa) or by RT-PCR, which is more sensitive and specific, from a nasal or throat swab or corresponding rinse water.

In the case of a severe or complicated clinical course, treatment with an antiviral compound is indicated. In childhood, the neuraminidase inhibitors oseltamivir (oral administration, approved from the first year of life) and zanamivir (inhalation, approved from the fifth year of life) are used. Safety studies were carried out in order to extend the approval of oseltamivir on the first year of life. The vaccination against influenza provides the best protection. Because of the high genetic variability of the virus, the vaccination has to be repeated each year with a current antigen mixture. In addition to the self-protection, the collective protection is of great importance.

5.4 Adenovirus

It is a member of the family of adenoviridae. It is a double-stranded DNA virus with a strong environmental resistance. More than 50 serotypes with various clinical manifestations have been identified so far. The transmission proceeds via droplet or smear infection. The incubation time is between 2 and 10 days. Most adenovirus-induced diseases occur in the age between 6 months and 5 years, usually in the form of a common cold. However, it can lead to complicated clinical courses with severe obstruction, pneumonia or persistent bronchial hyperreactivity for months.

5.5 Rhinovirus

It belongs to the family of picornaviridae, the RNA is single stranded. We know about 100 subtypes; the genetic variability is large. Rhinovirus is transmitted primarily via aerosol. The incubation period is 2 - 5 days. In the first years of life, the incidence of infection with the virus is around 1 - 2 times per year. Whereas in adults rhinovirus infections usually cause a common cold, in infants and small children obstructive bronchitis appear quite often.

5.6 Metapneumovirus

It is a member of the paramyxoviridae, a RNA virus and enveloped. We know 2 subtypes A and B, each with two sub-groups A1 and A2, as well as B1 and B2. Droplet and smear infections are the transmission paths. Incubation time is 4 – 6 days. During the first year of life about one quarter of infants become infected with the metapneumovirus; by the time children start school, almost everyone has had an infection with this ubiquitous virus. Most prevalent symptoms are rhinitis and bronchitis.

5.7 Human bocavirus

The human bocavirus was discovered only in 2005. It belongs to the Parvoviridae family and has a single-stranded DNA. The transmission of the virus proceeds via droplet or smear infection. Accurate epidemiological data are yet to be collected. Clinically, acute respiratory symptoms are most relevant.

6. Characteristics of RSV infection in children

6.1 Risk factors

An RSV infection, which occurs in infancy, may have a severe clinical course. Not only in infancy, but until the age of 5 years, RSV infection may cause disorders of clinical relevance. The majority of children undergo one or more RSV infections during the first 2 years of life, usually without a severe or complicated course. Risk factors for a severe or complicated clinical course are small, narrow airways (this is the reason why infants suffer worse than older children). Boys are affected slightly more often than girls. Another risk factor, which should not be underestimated, is the exposure to tobacco smoke. Furthermore, the family history to allergies has an adverse influence. Pre-term birth or chronic diseases of the lung increase the risk for a complicated course of a RSV infection considerably. We see a seasonal accumulation with endemic-like clusters of RSV infections during the cold autumn and winter months. The transmission occurs by droplet and smear infection. The incubation time is at 3 - 6 days.

6.2 Severity of the clinical course

If the RS virus affects the respiratory epithelium of the smallest bronchi and bronchioles with desquamation of the epithelial cells and oedema of the mucosa, the main symptom is bronchial obstruction. Distal to an obstructed airway, atelectatic areas may be formed, next to emphysematic areas. If this causes a mismatch between ventilation and perfusion, the main symptom is tachydyspnoea with partial or even global respiratory insufficiency. In this case, the infant needs to get hospitalized for oxygen substitution and, if necessary, with respiratory support or even mechanical ventilation. An additional reason for hospitalization is the risk, especially in very young infants, of apnoea and death due to apnoea.

6.3 Diagnosis

The diagnosis can be carried out using a rapid test, which is based on the immunofluorescence method. The inflammation parameters in the blood are only slightly increased. The X-ray of the chest often shows diffuse infiltrations of the lung and a partial reduction of the transmission due to emphysema.

6.4 Limitation of therapeutic options

The therapeutic options are very limited. Because the replication of the RS virus takes place inside the epithelial cells of the lung, bronchodilatatory agents show no positive effect. Treatment with steroids has no effect as well, what is confirmed by meta-analysis. An antiviral therapy with the nucleoside analogue ribavirin is not recommended for the following reasons: firstly, there seems to be no relevant effect; secondly, it is teratogenic and has to be administered via aerosol, which could lead to an exposure of pregnant women who are in contact to the child. There is only one agent with a small, but significant benefit in the case of an RSV bronchitis or bronchiolitis; it is the leukotriene receptor antagonist montelukast. Additionally, supportive therapy, such as inhalation with 0.9% NaCl or decongestant nose drops may be helpful.

6.5 Indications for palivizumab

Palivizumab is a monoclonal antibody against the RS virus. It can be used for passive immunization. It binds to the glycoprotein F, the fusion protein, and thereby prevents the virus entering the cell. During the months with high incidence of RSV infections, palivizumab has to be injected every 4 weeks. Palivizumab is indicated for significant prematurity, bronchopulmonary dysplasia and hemodynamic relevant congenital heart failures. The prophylactic immunization with palivizumab reduces severity and duration of the disease significantly; the hospitalization frequency is halved.

6.6 Recent research on an active immunization

Previous research on an active vaccine, already carried out in the 1960s, was not successful. Currently there are new research activities in this area. A life vaccine against RSV and PIV3 (parainfluenza virus type 3) is in phase 1 / 2 study.

7. Bronchopulmonary dysplasia as a risk factor for bronchitis in children

7.1 Definition and pathophysiology

Today bronchopulmonary dysplasia (BPD) is more relevant than ever. Because of the major advances in neonatology with high survival rates of extremely immature preterm infants, there is an increase of diseases and complications, which are typically associated with prematurity, like BPD. If very preterm infants are born, their lungs are not completely developed, neither structurally nor functionally, especially with respect to the synthesis of surfactant. Because of the respiration prior to maturity, the lung tissue undergoes a fibrotic remodelling process of the alveoli. Prenatal and postnatal factors, such as inflammation, infection, hyperoxia and mechanical ventilation, have an additional adverse effect.

Because the morphological alterations are not visible and the radiological ones do not correlate well with the clinical severity, the BPD is defined by the duration of oxygen supplementation for longer than 28 days. Depending on the amount of oxygen supplementation and the requirement of breathing support, we distinguish mild, moderate and severe BPD.

7.2 Prophylaxis and therapy

The following prophylactic procedures may reduce the severity of BPD: the prenatal anti-inflammatory treatment via administration of beta-dexamethasone to the mother, the so-called "lung maturation", is standard. The application of surfactant as soon as possible is very important. A patent ductus arteriosus with hemodynamic relevance should be treated early, if possible pharmacologically, if necessary via ligature. A protective effect of vitamin A has been demonstrated, although the effect is only minor.

Therapeutic procedures are avoidance of hyperoxia, moderate infusion or even forced diuresis. high-caloric nutrition, gentle ventilation mode, physiotherapy, and in very rare cases, the postnatal application of corticosteroids.

7.3 Prognosis

The BPD also affects the future life of the children: they suffer more frequently with bronchial hyperreactivity and asthma, they have an increased risk for the incidence of respiratory infections, and in the first year of life they are more often hospitalized for acute respiratory problems. Even if they have no symptoms, the measurement of lung function will show worse values.

8. Differential diagnoses of bronchitis in children

8.1 Croup

In distinction from the original diphtheritic croup (which has become very rare thanks to the vaccination), the common croup is a subglottic laryngitis with an inflammatory oedema of the mucosa in the context of a viral infection of the respiratory system. The main prevalence is at the age between 6 months and 6 years. Typically in the late evening or during the night in the cold winter, the affected infants and children get an acute attack with a barking cough, hoarseness, inspiratory stridor and dyspnoea. We divide the croup into 4 different degrees of severity, from just cough and hoarseness without dyspnoea to dramatic dyspnoea with the feeling of combustion.

What are the urgent measures in the case of a croup attack? The first step is to reassure the anxious and excited child. It should be kept in an upright position, in order to allow the use of the thoracal muscles for breathing. The child should be brought into the fresh and cold air, which may reduce the swelling of the respiratory mucosa. If available, a glucocorticoid suppository can be administered by the parents. Prophylactically, a moistening of the air indoors is recommended. In many cases of a moderate croup episode, these easy measures may stabilize the situation, that the parents are able to manage it at home without any professional help. However, in severe cases or in any cases of doubt, the ambulance should be called immediately. The emergency doctor can initiate an inhalation with adrenaline, an oxygen supplementation and an intravenous application of a glucocorticoid. If necessary, the child can be hospitalized and monitored via pulse oximetry. In very rare cases, the sedation of a child (for example with chloral hydrate) is unavoidable. In extreme severe and complicated clinical courses, the treatment of the child at an intensive care unit is recommended.

In the extremely rare case of a diphtheritic croup, the treatment with diphtheria antitoxin has to start immediately. Also extremely rare (thanks to the haemophilus vaccination), a bacterial epiglottitis occurs. But because of its rarity, the risk of misinterpretation as a normal croup is quite high. In contrast to the croup, the epiglottitis usually is associated with high fever, a very poor general condition, a septic clinical course, an increased salivation and dysphagia. An epiglottis is always a peracute emergency. Inspection of the pharynx using a spatula is strictly contraindicated, because the slightest mechanical provocation can induce a complete occlusion of the epiglottis without any possibility for an intubation. Then only cricothyrotomy or tracheostomy can be carried out, to save the life of the child.

8.2 Aspiration

Aspiration of gastric juice or of a foreign body causes coughing. Common foreign bodies are small pieces of an apple or a carrot, half or whole peanuts and all sorts of small parts made of plastic or metal, quite often from the toys, the child has played with. We distinguish between the acute and the chronic foreign body aspiration.

In the case of an acute aspiration the child has an abrupt coughing attack and dyspnoea. Because the beginning of the right main bronchus from the trachea is angulated to a lesser extent compared with the left one, it is preferentially affected. Over the affected side the breath is quiet and wheezing can be heard. Radiologically, a mediastinal shift to the healthy side can be seen.

In contrast to an acute aspiration, which is associated with an abrupt coughing attack and dyspnoea, in the case of a chronic aspiration the clinical symptoms are milder and less severe. In most cases the foreign body is smaller compared to those of an acute aspiration, so that it can slide into a segmental bronchus, settle there and maintain an inflammatory response, which occurs as a chronic cough. This is the reason why chronic aspirations quite often get misinterpreted as a chronic bronchitis of infectious or allergic origin.

For treatment the bronchoscopical removal of the foreign body is necessary, almost always in the form of a rigid bronchoscopy.

8.3 Tuberculosis

In the case of a chronic cough it is important to take the possibility of a pulmonary tuberculosis as a differential diagnosis into account, especially in children who come from high-incidence countries, or if they have had or still have close contact with people coming from such areas. The mycobacterium tuberculosis is transmitted via the aerosols, which comes from coughing people with an open pulmonary tuberculosis. Children are generally less contagious, even if they have an open pulmonary tuberculosis, because there are only a few bacteria in the sputum. This phenomenon is called paucibacillary tuberculosis.

At the slightest suspicion of a tuberculosis infection, an appropriate diagnostic investigation has to be made: next to an accurate medical history and physical examination, immunological tests have to be carried out. These are an intracutanously applied tuberculin test and an IGRA (interferon-gamma release assay) from the blood. The combination of both tests results in an optimal specifity. Additionally, an X-ray from the chest at two levels belongs to the standard diagnostic. The microscopical and microbiological analysis is made from induced sputum or from gastric juice, because children younger than 10 years usually are not able to give sputum spontaneously.

If, in the case of an exposure to tuberculosis, all diagnostic investigations have a negative result, a chemoprophylaxis with isoniazid for 3 months is recommended. If the immunological tests are positive, but the clinical course, the X-ray and the analysis of induced sputum or gastric juice show normal results, then a preventive chemotherapy with either isoniazid as monotherapy for 9 months or alternatively with isoniazid and rifampicin as dual therapy for 4 months should be carried out. If a child has signs or symptoms of a tuberculosis, if pulmonary or extra-pulmonary, a combination therapy with at least 3 tuberculostatic drugs has to be initiated, for example with isoniazid, rifampicin and pyrazinamide. In most cases, after 2 months of treatment the medication can be reduced to an isoniazid/rifampicin - dual therapy. The total duration of the treatment depends on the clinical course and the severity of complication and is at least 6 months. Of course the choice of the tuberculostatic drugs has to be adjusted to possible resistances.

8.4 Cystic fibrosis (CF)

If infants have recurrent obstructive bronchitis with a chronic cough and problems to dissolve the mucus, one differential diagnosis, which has to be taken into account, is CF. Even though it is a rare disease, it is still one of the most common hereditary diseases. The mode of inheritance is autosomal recessive and caused by a mutation in the CFTR (cystic fibrosis transmembrane conductance regulator) - gene, which encodes a chloride ion channel. More than 1500 mutations have been known. The mutation deltaF508 describes the deletion of 3 base pairs, what causes the lack of phenylalanine at position 508 of the protein chain, and is with 70% by far the most frequent one. Depending on the amount of the CFTR defect, there are milder and more severe clinical courses of the disease. Due to the dysfunction of the chloride ion channel, the epithelial fluid film becomes hyperosmolar and the produced mucus gets dyscrinic.

The clinical course is characterized by this problem. Shortly after birth, due to the viscous intestinal secretion, a meconium ileus can be the first complication of a CF. The same problem may occur in later life as distal intestinal obstruction syndrome (DIOS). The most important focus in the progress of the CF is the respiratory system. The viscous sputum cannot be mobilized and brought out adequately, what gives bacteria a good medium for colonization, unfortunately quite often with mucoid pseudomonas aeruginosa and other multi-resistant bacteria. Also pulmonary mycoses (for example an aspergillosis) may occur. These permanent inflammatory processes lead to an irreversible tissue remodelling of the respiratory tract. At the end, atelectatic areaes and emphysematic bullae, insufficient for ventilation or diffusion, replace the normal tissue. Haemoptysis and pneumothoraces are dreaded complications. About 90% of all patients with CF develop an exocrine pancreatic insufficiency with the consequence of an inadequate intestinal absorption of proteins, fats and fat-soluble vitamins, which leads to dystrophy of the affected patients. With further progress of the disease, an endocrine pancreatic insufficiency may occur, which is why about 15% of all patients with CF develop an insulin-dependent diabetes mellitus.

Therapeutical tools are the removal of bronchial secretions by autogenic drainage, physiotherapy, inhalations, mucolysis and ample fluid intake, the antibacterial treatment by intravenous antibiotics, the stimulation of the digestion by dietary fibre enriched food and physical activity, the improvement of the intestinal absorption by replacement of enzymes (porcine pancreas powder) and substitution of vitamins, and the counteraction of dystrophy by high-caloric nutrition.

In the most patients with CF, the life limiting factor is the global respiratory insufficiency. Often, lung transplantation is the only life-prolonging option. Because of the enormous medical progress, especially in the development of new antibiotics, the life expectancy of people with CF increases steadily and rapidly. CF as a disease which occurs exclusively in childhood is part of medical history.

8.5 Primary ciliary dyskinesis

A primary ciliary dyskinesis often causes recurrent bronchitis. It is a genetically determined (usually autosomal recessive) disorder of the respiratory ciliated epithelium and other ciliated cells, resulting in a reduction in mucociliary clearance. Typical clinical symptoms are chronic rhinitis and sinusitis with much secretion, chronic bronchitis with a productive cough and recurrent pneumonia. Additional possible abnormalities are the formation of a hydrocephalus (due to the lack of ciliary motility of the ependymal cells), infertility in male (due to the lack of motility of the sperms) and in female patients (due to the lack of motility of the cilia of the fallopian tube) or a situs inversus (due to the absence of a directed cilia beat during the embryogenesis). A situs inversus occurs in 50% of the patients who are affected by the primary ciliary dyskinesis and it is called Kartagener's syndrome. In the diagnostic investigation of the primary ciliary dyskinesis the measurement of exhaled NO and the analysis of the ciliary function using a light microscope are purposeful tools. For confirmation of the diagnosis, an analysis via an electron microscope is needed. Therapeutic options are physiotherapy, inhalation and antibiotic treatment in the case of bacterial infections.

8.6 Vocal cord dysfunction

The vocal cord dysfunction (VCD) is a functional disorder with an acute spasm of the vocal cords. In most cases school children are affected. A VCD attack can range from a mild dyspnoea to the feeling of suffocation. Fortunately, such episodes are not life threatening, because despite the vocal cord spasm a small air gap still remains. Possible triggers for a VCD attack are coughing, physical exertion, inhalation of cigarette smoke or reflux of gastric juice, postnasal drip syndrome and general stress.

8.7 Gastroesophageal reflux

In the case of a recurrent or chronic cough, of course at first everybody thinks of a disease of the respiratory system. However, a gastroesophageal reflux may also cause such symptoms. Especially in the first months of life, chyme and gastric juice can flow back into the oesophagus and induce an inflammation of the mucosa there. Clinical symptoms may be heartburn, regurgitation, vomiting, feeding problems and finally dystrophia. Further symptoms may be a cough, hoarseness, bronchial obstruction, episodes with apnoea and cyanosis, as well as pneumonia due to aspiration. In order to avoid the gastroesophageal reflux in infants, the nutrition can be thickened and the feeding portions can be reduced by increasing the feeding frequency. In addition, the upper body should be slightly elevated. Potential drugs are antacids or proton pump blockers.

9. Inflammation parameters in the case of bronchitis in children

9.1 C-reactive protein (CRP)

CRP is an annular pentamer with sub-units composed of 206 amino acids each. It is synthesized in the liver and then secreted into the blood. Its concentration in the blood increases within 6 to 48 h in the case of any systemic inflammation. That can be an infectious disease, an immune reaction of non-infectious etiology or large tissue damage. Thus, CRP is an unspecific marker for inflammation and its increase starts with delay. Depending on the laboratory, a plasma concentration up to 0.1 - 1 mg/dl is in the normal range. Concentrations between 1 - 10 mg/dl are typical for mild to moderate concentrations, > 10 mg/dl for severe inflammation. Because of the reasonably long half-life of approximately 24 h, CRP is ideal for the follow-up monitoring of an inflammatory process which can help to evaluate the effectiveness of a treatment.

9.2 Interleukin-6 (IL-6)

IL-6 is a proinflammatory cytokine consisting of 184 amino acids. It is released primarily by monocytes, but also by T-lymphocytes, as well as endothelial and epithelial cells. Infections, non-infectious immunological reactions, tissue hypoxia and trauma induce the release of IL-6 within 6 h. Thus, IL-6 is an unspecific marker for various forms of inflammation as well, but its increase starts much faster. Depending on the laboratory, a plasma concentration up to 10 - 50 ng/l is in the normal range. The half-life in the blood is just a few minutes. Because of this very short half-life, the kinetics shows a narrow peak with the risk of false negative results in the case of measurements outside this peak.

9.3 Complete blood count (CBC)

The CBC may also be helpful in the diagnosis of an inflammation. High increases in the amount of the leucocytes occur in bacterial infections, but also in other inflammatory processes. Like CRP and IL-6, CBC is a non-specific marker of general inflammation. The increase of the leucocytes needs several hours and starts a little bit earlier than the increase of the CRP level. The standard value of the amount of leucocytes depends on the age of life: for adults 4 - 10 / nl, for school children 5 - 15 / nl, for small children 6 - 17,5 / nl and for newborns even 9 - 30 / nl are physiological. The differential blood count shows a reactive shift to the immature leucocytes, because their reinforced presence in the peripheral blood induces an enhanced release of still premature leucocytes from the bone marrow.

9.4 Erythrocyte sedimentation rate (ESR)

The ESR is a very non-specific marker for any kind of inflammation. The pathophysiological mechanisms, which lead to a higher ESR, are as follows: in the case of an inflammatory condition, erythrocytes form aggregates, which have a lower flow resistance compared to the sum of each separate erythrocyte. Furthermore, higher concentrations of acute phase proteins (like CRP), of fibrinogen or of immunoglobulins in the plasma, increase the ESR. It takes several weeks, after an inflammation has taken place, until an increased ESR gets normalized again. Standard value for boys or male adolescents is a sedimentation of 15 mm during 1 h, for girls or female adolescents 20 mm during 1 h.

9.5 Procalcitonin (PCT)

PCT is a protein which is constructed from 116 amino acids. It is produced mainly in the parafollicular C cells of the thyroid gland and in various neuroendocrine cells. Under physiological conditions, it acts as a prohormone of calcitonin. It is known that the release of PCT increases in the case of an infection, which is caused by bacterials, fungi or parasites. In this special condition, PCT is secreted predominantly in cells other the thyroid gland, including leukocytes, adipocytes, myocytes and hepatocytes. Stimuli for the synthesis of PCT in these cells are bacterial endotoxins (lipopolysaccharides = LPS) and cytokines (Interleukin - 1 beta, tumour necrosis factor - alpha). The pathophysiological significance of PCT increase has not yet been clarified. Anyway, there is no effect on the thyroid gland.

The PCT level in the blood increases within 3 h after stimulation by endotoxins or cytokines. The maximum of the PCT level is reached after 8 – 24 h and will be stable for another 24 h. Then the PCT amount will decrease again with a quite long half-life of 20 – 24 h. In healthy individuals, the physiological PCT level is < 0.5 µg/l. Values from 0.5 to 2.0 µg/l are associated with a mild respective moderate systemic infection, values from 2.0 to 10.0 µg/l with a severe systemic infection and values > 10.0 µg/l are in the majority of cases a sign of a sepsis. The amount of PCT correlates with the severity of the infectious disease and the mortality rate. In other very severe diseases, such as multiple trauma, large-scale burning, cardiogenic shock or multiple organ failure, the PCT level increases as well.

PCT remains nearly unaffected in the case of a localized, a viral, an autoimmunological or an allergic inflammation. For this reason it is an excellent marker for the rapid differentiation between viral and bacterial systemic (= antibiotic-requiring) infections.

Furthermore, PCT is well suited for the monitoring of the course of a systemic bacterial infection.

A big advantage of PCT, compared to CRP, CBC and ESR, is its much faster increase, which allows a very early detection of a systemic bacterial infection. Moreover, its predictive value for prediction of sepsis with 0.93 is much better than that of CRP, which is only 0.68. Furthermore, the interference by a therapy with steroids is much lower. One advantage compared to IL-6 is the better biological stability with a much longer half-life, what reduces the risk of false negative results. Additionally, in contrast to IL-6, autoimmunological inflammations do not interfere with PCT.

The measurement of the PCT level in patients with a febrile infection may be helpful to decide whether or not a patient needs an antibiotic treatment. In a clinical study it has been shown that by using a simple algorithm, the knowledge of the PCT level could reduce the administration of antibiotics from 80% previously to 44%.

On the one hand one wants to avoid the "treatment" of a viral infection with antibiotics, on the other hand one wants to assure the start of a required antibiotic therapy in time. Especially newborns and young infants may undergo fulminant clinical courses in the form of severe sepsis, for which reason this age group is very critical, and it is not acceptable to delay the start of an antibiotic treatment. Generally, it seems to be useful to give the measurement of PCT a higher priority than is currently given.

10. Therapeutic concepts for bronchitis in children - pro and contra

In general, a bronchitis may be treated symptomatically, because in most cases it is caused by an viral infection, and there exists no specific treatment. But the importance of the so-called household remedies should not be underestimated: an adequate fluid intake and inhalation of 0.9% NaCl may help to keep the bronchial mucosa moist and to liquefy the mucus. Sage drops may reduce the tussive irritation. The inhalation of essential oils, which are suitable for children, may also help to reduce discomfort, but it should be noted that there is a small risk of sensitization. In addition, there are a number of drugs (some are available in the pharmacy without prescription, some have to be prescribed), which have a reasonably proficient efficacy.

10.1 Sympathomimetic

For the treatment of an acute bronchial obstruction beta 2 - agonists are used, which have a selective effect on the respiratory system, in order to minimize beta 1 – receptor - mediated adverse effects on the heart. The binding of the drug to its receptor activates the adenylyl cyclase whereby ATP is converted to cAMP. That leads to a relaxation of the smooth musculature via a reduction in calcium ion concentration in the cells, and it leads to an inhibition of the release of mediators from mast cells. Generally, short-acting beta 2 - agonists, such as salbutamol, are used. In most cases salbutamol is applied in the form of inhalation, the common dosage is about ½ drop per kg body weight in about 2 ml 0.9% NaCl, administered with an ultrasonic nebulizer. Alternatively, especially en route, 1 – 2 puffs of a spray via a spacer can be used. The frequency of inhalation depends on the severity of bronchial obstruction. 3 - 6 applications in 24 hours are an average frequency during an acute obstructive bronchitis, but it can be increased, if necessary. The oral administration of salbutamol is possible, but because of a lower efficacy and an increase of adverse effects due to a higher intake into the blood this is not recommended as a first choice. Common adverse effects are restlessness, heart palpitations and shakiness. These symptoms are induced by an increased sympathetic activity and can be reduced by reduction of the single dosage or the frequency of administration. In pregnant female adolescents, salbutamol can induces tocolysis via the beta 2 - receptor.

10.2 Anticholinergic

Anticholinergics inhibit acetylcholine due to competition on the muscarinic acetylcholine receptors and antagonize its bronchoconstrictive effect. They were applicated via inhalation. In comparison to the sympathomimetics, their effect is weaker and occurs with a delay. Ipratropium bromide is used most frequently, usually in addition to a beta 2 - agonist, if the sympathomimetic effect is not sufficient. Possible side effects include dry mouth, a bitter taste, tachycardia and arterial hypertension.

10.3 Methylxanthine

The exact mechanism of action of methylxanthines, such as theophylline, is not fully known. Several different mokecularbiological pathways seem to be involved: methylxanthines inhibit the phosphodiesterase, increase intracellular cAMP and antagonize effects on the adenosine receptors. Due to these mechanisms, methylxanthines have bronchodilatatory and anti-inflammatory effects and they stimulate the respiratory centre in the brain stem. They are rarely used, mainly as reserve medication for severe asthma - attacks. Theophylline is then usually given as a continuous infusion. The side effects can be serious: tachycardia, extrasystoles, arterial hypertension, restlessness, insomnia, gastrointestinal disorders or increased diuresis.

10.4 Glucocorticoid

Glucocorticoids induce the secretion of lipocortin, a glycoprotein which inhibits the phospholipase A2 and thereby reduces the release of arachidonic acid. Due to this mechanism, the cyclooxygenase pathway produces less prostaglandins and the lipoxygenase pathway less leukotrienes. Several cytokines, particularly interleukin-1, interleukin-2 and tumour necrosis factor - alpha, are produced in a reduced amount as well. In the peripheral blood the number of monocytes is decreased and also their bactericidal and chemotactic effects, as well as their migration are reduced. All these changes have a non-specific anti-inflammatory effect. Depending on the half-life, glucocorticoids are divided into short-acting (for example cortisone and cortisol), medium-acting (for example prednisone, prednisolone and methyl prednisolone) and long-acting (for example dexamethasone) substances. The systematic administration of glucocorticoids over a short time period may be necessary in the case of an acute severe bronchial obstruction. In infants and young children the application can be carried out in the form of a suppository, which can be done at home by the parents. If a child with an acute severe bronchial obstruction is brought into the emergency room, the intravenous application is part of the standard therapy. The long-term treatment with a glucocoticoid should be done topically, that is via inhalation. Commonly used corticosteroids for an inhalation therapy are budesonide, beclomethasone and fluticasone. The dosages are here in the microgram range; that means, they are by a factor of 100 - 1000 lower than the systemically given dosages. Thereby any side effects are reduced to a minimum. Parents who are afraid of the possible adverse effects of corticoids from long-term treatment should have an informative consultation. If they have the relevant knowledge, then their worries should be placated. If there are local side effects , for example the development of an oral thrush these can arise after inhalation if the mouth is not rinsed with water.

10.5 Leukotriene antagonist

Leukotrienes, products of the arachidonic acid metabolism, are synthesized in mast cells, macrophages, eosinophils and basophils. They have a very strong bronchoconstrictive effect (1000-fold more potent than histamine), induce an oedema of the bronchial mucus via increasing the capillary permeability and increase the production of mucus. Additionally, leukotrienes have a chemotactic influence on inflammatory cells, especially the eosinophils, which sensitizes the nerve fibres occurring in the respiratory tract, resulting in a bronchial hyperreactivity. The most common leukotriene antagonist is montelukast. Because its structure is similar to the leukotriene D4, it acts as a selective competitor at the receptor without the effects mentioned above. Montelukast is used as a long-term anti-inflammatory therapy, often in combination with a topical corticosteroid. Montelukast is administered orally in the evening. The adverse effects that may occur include headache and abdominal pain.

10.6 Mucolytic

Mucolytic respective secretolytic drugs are expectorants. In contrast to secretomotoric drugs, which increase the activity of the ciliated epithelium, expectorants should cause a liquefaction of the bronchial mucus to make it easier to cough it up. Among the mucolytics are acetylcysteine, bromhexin and ambroxol. Acetylcysteine cleaves the disulfide bonds of the mucopolysaccharides. Furthermore, it has an anti-inflammatory effect due to catching free radicals with its reactive SH group. Bromhexin activates enzymes, which cleave the molecules of the mucus and stimulate the glandular cells to increase the mucus production, reduce the viscosity. Ambroxol is a metabolite of bromhexin. In addition to the effects of bromhexin, it stimulates the synthesis of surfacant. Some herbal substances, such as ivy, also belong to mucolytic drugs. Generally, the therapeutic significance of all these so-called cough syrups should not be overestimated. It is much more important that the children drink enough and make inhalations.

10.7 Antitussive

Antitussives reduce the cough by acting on the brain stem. Opiates, like codeine, dihydrocodeine, hydrocodone or noscapine, are the most common drugs against tussive irritation. There are newer substances, such as pentoxiverin, which have the advantage of lacking a sedative effect or an addiction potential. Pentoxiverin is an agonist at the sigma receptor and also acts antagonistically at the muscarinic M1 receptor. Potential side effects are nausea, vomiting and diarrhoea. It is contraindicated in children younger than 2 years because a depressant effect on the respiration cannot be excluded, and in pregnant women because there are no sufficient safety data. However, in childhood antitussives, these should be prescribed only in rare cases with a non-productive cough. Otherwise, if a productive cough is inhibited, the mucus remains in the airways, increasing the risk of secondary bacterial infections with bronchopneumonia.

10.8 Antibiotic

In the case of a bacterial infection treatment with antibiotics is recommended. The choice of the appropriate antibiotic depends on the age of the child, because in different age groups there are different spectra of bacteria. After receiving the antibiogram, the antibiotic therapy can be specified in accordance to sensitivities and resistances of the bacterium. Between community-acquired and nosocomial infections, bacterial spectra differ as well. Sometimes it is not possible to distinguish between a viral and a bacterial infection, since the clinical course and the blood parameters can be quite similar. In this situation it may be that a child will be treated with an antibiotic, although it is just a viral infection with high fever.

10.9 Oxygen supplementation

In the case of severe bronchial obstruction with spasms of the bronchial musculature, with oedema of the bronchial mucosa and production of viscous secretions, ventilation in the airways and diffusion in the alveoli may be disturbed. This can cause a partial (hypoxia, normocapnia) or global (hypoxia, hypercapnia) respiratory insufficiency. If the transcutanously measured oxygen saturation in the blood is too low, the supplementation of oxygen is necessary. Usually the oxygen is supplied via nasal prongs. If small children do not tolerate nasal prongs, a mask can be placed in front of the face, especially during sleep.

In the treatment of premature infants with a respiratory distress syndrome, we have different procedures, because there the toxic effect of oxygen on the immature organs has to be taken into account. Complications caused by oxygen can be BPD, the retinopathy of prematurity and an apoptosis-mediated neurodegeneration. The monitoring of the premature infants should contain a capnometric analysis next to the measurement of the oxygen saturation.

10.10 Physiotherapy

Physiotherapy is required in the case of chronic diseases of the respiratory system (for example cystic fibrosis or primary ciliary dyskinesis), but also in the case of acute pneumological problems (for example the formation of an atelectasis as a complication of pneumonia). The aims of physiotherapy are to attain effective ventilation of all lung sections and an effective drainage of secretion.

10.11 Nasal drops

0.9% NaCl - nose drops are used to moisten and clean the nasal mucosa. Decongestant nose drops (dependent on age 0.25%, 0.5% or 1% xylometazoline) should be given, if the eustachian tube is swollen in response to an infection of the upper airways, in order to guarantee the ventilation of the middle ear. These nose drops should not be given for longer than 7 days, otherwise they could lead to an irreversible damage of the mucosa. A stuffy nose is not a good reason for the application of decongestant nose drops. Depending on the age of the child, a nose spray may be used instead of nose drops.

11. References

Brodzinski H, Ruddy RM. (2009). Review of new and newly discovered respiratory tract viruses in children. *Pediatr Emerg Care,* 25 (5), 51-63, ISSN 0749-5161

Bundesärztekammer (BÄK), Kassenärztliche Bundesvereinigung (KBV), Arbeitsgemeinschaft der Wissenschaftlichen Medizinischen Fachgesellschaften (AWMF). (2011). *Nationale VersorgungsLeitlinie Asthma – Kurzfassung, 2. Auflage. Version 1.3,* available from: http://www.versorgungsleitlinien.de/themen/asthma

Deutsche Gesellschaft für Pädiatrische Infektiologie (DGPI) e. V. (2009). *DGPI Handbuch, Infektionen bei Kindern und Jugendlichen,* Thieme-Verlag, ISBN 978-3-13-144715-9, Stuttgart

Deis JN, Creech CB, Estrada CM, Abramo TJ. (2010). Procalcitonin as a marker of severe bacterial infection in children in the emergency department. *Pediatr Emerg Care,* 26 (1), 51-63, ISSN 0749-5161

Global Initiative for Asthma (GINA). (2010). *Global Strategy for Asthma Management and Prevention,* available from: http://www.ginasthma.org

Mitchell I. (2009). Treatment of RSV bronchiolitis: drugs, antibiotics. *Pediatr Respir Rev,* 10 Suppl 1, 14-15, ISSN 1526-0542

Ramanuja S, Kelkar PS. (2010). The approach to pediatric cough. *Ann Allergy Asthma Immunol,* 105 (1), 3-8

Rieger C, von der Hardt H, Sennhauser FH, Wahn U, Zach M (Eds.). (2004). *Pädiatrische Pneumologie,* Springer-Verlag, ISBN 3-540-43627-8, Berlin

Wainwright C. (2009). Acute viral bronchiolitis in children – a very common condition with few therapeutic options. *Pediatr Respir Rev,* 11, 39-45, ISSN 1526-0542

Bronchopulmonary Dysplasia

Shou-Yien Wu[1,2], Sachin Gupta[1],
Chung-Ming Chen[3,4] and Tsu-Fuh Yeh[3,4,5,*]
[1]*Division of Neonatology, Dept. of Ped. John Stroger Hospital of Cook County*
[2]*Rosalind Franklin University of Medicine and Science, Chicago, Illinois*
[3]*Dept. of Pediatrics*
[4]*Maternal Child Health Research Center, Taipei Medical University, Taipei*
[5]*Dept. of Ped. China Medical University, Taichung*
[1,2,3]*USA*
[4,5]*Taiwan*

1. Introduction

Bronchopulmonary dysplasia (BPD) continues to be the most common and most important complication in preterm infants with RDS. The incidence varies from 20 to 60 % in preterm infants whose weight are < 1500 gram. The presence of BPD is often associated with significant mortality and short term and long term morbidity, including growth failure and neurodevelopment delay.

The exact mechanism and pathogenesis of BPD is not completely understood. However, epidemiology study suggests a changing prevalence and clinical features in recent years. The traditional descriptions of BPD (so call classic or old BPD) are essentially related to lung injuries following mechanical ventilation while the recent description of BPD (new BPD) is probably related more to prematurity of the lungs. The relation between these two types of BPD is not clear. Recent studies indicated that inflammation may play an important role for both the classic and new BPD. Once lung injuries have established, managements are essentially supportive, therefore every effort should be focus on prevention. Proper respiratory care is the most essential in preventing lung injury. Other medications, either to improve the pulmonary function or to reduce the lung inflammation, have been tried with various successes. There is no magic bullet to cure the disease.

2. Definition

The original definition of bronchopulmonary dysplasia by Northway was base on radiological and pathological characteristics in prematurely born infants with respiratory distress syndrome (RDS) who were treated with mechanical ventilation and oxygen supplementation. Subsequently, the definition of BPD was changed to respiratory sequelae in infants requiring oxygen supplementation more than 28 days after birth since BPD may occur in tiny premature infants who have not previously had RDS. This definition was not

* Corresponding Author

without debate, because it includes a wide range of infants, i.e. from those ultimately appear to have no residual problems to those with severe BPD. A more practical definition was used: respiratory sequelae in infants who reach term age but are oxygen or mechanical ventilation dependent. The introduction of antenatal steroid prophylaxis, postnatal surfactant treatment caused revolutionary care of premature infants. Nowadays, more extreme low birth weight infants with birth weight < 1000gm and gestation age 23-28 weeks survived, they experienced a mild initial respiratory course, but required a low concentration of oxygen for a long time. In 2001, the United States National Institute of Child Health and Human Development (NICHD) conducted a workshop. A new definition, which categorizes the severity of BPD, was proposed.

2.1 Classic bronchopulmonary dysplasia (Classic BPD)

As described above, the classic BPD was defined as a chronic lung disease occurs in premature infants who had respiratory distress after birth, require oxygen supplementation or mechanical ventilator support at 28 postnatal days or 36 weeks postmenstrual age (PMA). Four stages I, II, III and IV are classified base on radiological findings and associated pathologic changes. Stage I and II describe acute and subacute course of respiratory distress syndrome. Stage III and IV often represent changes associated with chronic lung disease.

Stage I (2-3 days) is a period of acute RDS. The radiologic picture is similar to RDS.

Stage II (4-10 days) is a period of regeneration. The chest radiograph shows complete opacity of the lung obscuring the heart and lung borders.

Stage III (10-20 days) is a period of transition to chronic disease. The early radiographic changes are replaced by areas of coarse, irregular shaped densities and areas of cyst lesions. Areas of density are caused by interstitial edema or atelectasis due to obstruction of small bronchioles with luminal debris. The cysts represent foci of emphysema.

Stage IV (beyond 1 month) is a period of chronic disease. Chest radiograph shows large cysts and marked fibrosis and edema with areas of consolidation and areas of overinflation.

This definition becomes less relevant in current practice, since the improvement care of RDS, and survival of very tiny babies, classic BPD is uncommonly seen now, instead a new form of BPD (new BPD) is much increased.

2.2 New bronchopulmonary dysplasia (New BPD)

BPD is now defined clinically as a chronic lung disease occurring in premature infants who need for supplemental O2 for at least 28 days after birth, and its severity is graded according to the oxygen concentration and positive pressure of respiratory support at near term. For gestation age 32 weeks or more, the time of determination varies between 28 days to 56 days before discharge. For gestation age less than 32 week, the time of determination is 36 weeks postmenstrual age 36 weeks. A physiologic test such as pulse oximetry saturation is recommended to confirm the requirement of oxygen supplementation at the time of assessment (Table 1). Again, this definition is made clinically and the incidence of BPD can be various from hospital to hospital.

3. Epidemiology

The incidence of BPD varies among different institutions. This is due to differences in neonatal risk factors among different populations, patient care management and the discrepancies in the definition of BPD. Incidence figures must be interpreted with caution.

Gestation age	< 32 weeks	> 32 weeks
Time point of assessment	36 wk PMA or discharge to home, whichever comes first	28 d to 56 d postnatal age or discharge to home, whichever comes first
	Treatment with oxygen > 21% for at least 28 d plus	
Mild BPD	Breathing room air at 36 wk PMA or discharge, whichever comes first	Breathing room air by 56 d postnatal age or discharge, whichever comes first
Moderate BPD	Need for <30% oxygen at 36 PMA or discharge, whichever comes first	Need for < 30% oxygen at 56 d postnatal age or discharge, whichever comes first
Severe BPD	Need for $\geq$ 30% oxygen and/or positive pressure (PPV or NCPAP) at 36 wk PMA or discharge, whichever comes first	Need for $\geq$ 30% oxygen and/or positive pressure (PPV or NCPAP) at 56 d postnatal age or discharge, whichever comes first

Adapt from Jobe A. Bancalarie E. Bronchopulmonary Dysplasia. Am J Respir Crit Care Med 2001; 163: 1723-1729.

Table 1. Definition of New Bronchopulmonary Dysplasia: Diagnostic Criteria

For example, better prenatal and postnatal care increase survival of the very tiny infants, more infants who previously would have died now survive and remain oxygen/ventilator dependent at 28 days of age, the overall rate of BPD may increase, but the severity is much less. The denominator may also be different, some reports used all live births of premature infants as denominator; while others used only survived infants.

Parker et al reported the incidence of BPD increased from 10.6% in 1976 through 1980, to 21.7% (981 through 1985), and to 32.9% (1986 through 1990) in very low birth weight neonates (1500 g or less) admitted to a regional newborn care center in USA, while there was concurrent decline of neonatal death during the same periods (26.4%, 18.3%, and 15.9%, respectively). The diagnosis of BPD was given if neonates were treated supplemental oxygen for at least 28 days as a surrogate for oxygen treatment on postnatal day 28.

In 2007, a report from NICHD Neonatal Research Network database of USA shows the survival rate and the incidence of BPD (defined by supplemental O2 at 36 weeks PMA) in infants with birth weight of 501-1500g almost unchanged between1997and 2002. The survival increases slightly (from 84 to 85%) and the incidence of BPD decreases by 1% (from 23 to 22%). Tiny infants have highest rate and severity of BPD: 6% in 1250-1500g; 14%in 1001-1240g; 33% in750-1000g and 46% in 501 to 750g.

Since the release of a consensus statement by the American Academy of Pediatrics and the Canadian Pediatric Society in 2002, the use of postnatal corticosteroid has decreased. There was concern that the decreased use of postnatal steroid might increase the risk of BPD. A recent report from America which includes 77520 premature infants born at $\leq$32 weeks gestation in California, the overall rate of BPD increased over the decade: 20% in 1997-1999, 24% in 2000-2003 and 25.4% in 2004-2006. The rate of severe BPD also increased significantly: 3.6% 1997-1999, 5.1% in 2000-2003, and 9.5% in 2004-2006.

4. Pathology of bronchopumonary dysplasia

The characteristic changes of classic BPD are airway injury and inflammation, airway epithelial cell metaplasia, and parenchymal fibrosis. In contrast, the characteristic morphology of "new" BPD is disruption of lung development (Figure 1).

4.1 Classic bronchopumonary dysplasia

Four stages are classified according to the severity and anatomic component involved.

Stage I alveolar and interstitial edema with hyaline membranes, atelectasis, and necrosis of bronchial mucosa are present.

Stage II atelectasis becomes more evident, alternating with areas of emphysema. There is widespread necrosis and repair of bronchial mucosa. Cellular debris fills the airways.

Stage III extensive bronchial and bronchiolar metaplasia and hyperplasia evolve. Areas of emphysema are surrounded by areas of atelectasis, accompanied by massive interstitial edema with thickening of the basement membranes.

Stage IV massive fibrosis of the lung with destruction of alveoli and airways are present. In addition, there is hypertrophy of bronchial smooth muscle and metaplasia of airway mucosa. Finally, there is actual loss of pulmonary arterioles and capillaries and medial muscular hypertrophy of remaining vessels.

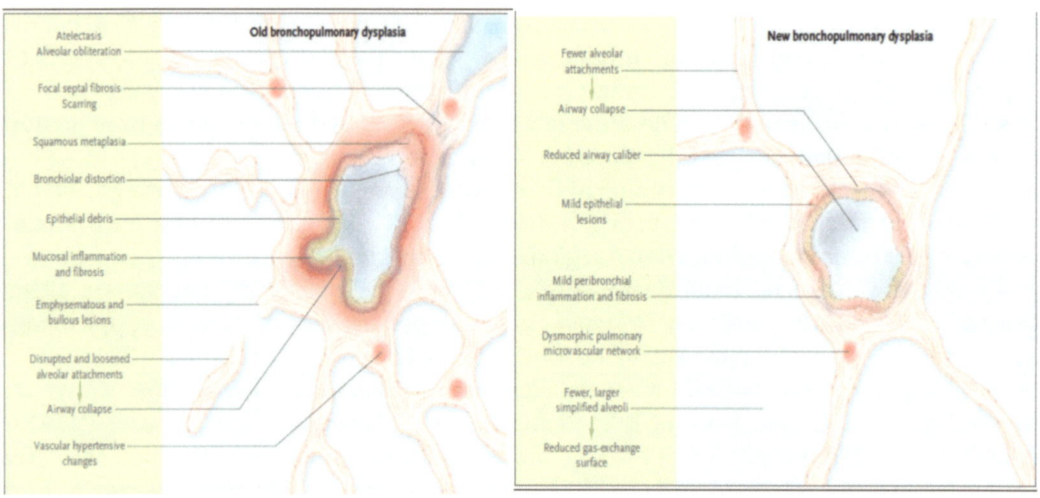

Fig. 1. Airway and Parenchymal Damage in Old and New BPD. „Old" and „new" BPD are two different morphologic outcomes of variable combinations of factors capable of injuring lungs of differing maturity. In old BPD, intense inflammation and disruption of normal pulmonary structures lead to a nonhomogeneous airway and parenchymal disease. In contrast, the main feature of new BDP is diffusely reduced alveolar development, which is associated with a clinically significant loss of surface area for gas excange, with airway injury, inflammation, and fibrosis that are usually milder than in old BPD.
(From Baraldi E., Filippone M. Chronic Lung Disease after Premature Birth. N Engl J M. 2007, 357(8);1951)

4.2 New bronchopulmonary dysplasia

Hislop et al. reported that mechanical ventilation of low birth weight infants leads to fewer alveoli. Husain et al. reported that extremely premature infants (gestation age ranged 24 to 32 weeks) dying of BPD had partial to complete arrest in acinar development whether infants received surfactant treatment or not. The alveolar structures are larger, simplified, and fewer in numbers. The amount of alveolar septal fibrosis is substantially less and tends to be more diffuse in surfactant-treated infants than in infants who did not have surfactant treatment. Coalson studied the autopsy lung specimens from infants who had received both prenatal steroids and surfactant treatment and have found the following findings: enlarged air spaces with minimal alveolization, dysmorphic capillary configuration and variable alveolar wall cellularity and fibrosis. Airway and vascular lesions, when present, tend to be present in infants, who over time develop more severe disease.

5. Pathogenesis

The pathogenesis of BPD is multifactorial. The original concepts of risk factors include: (1) prematurity; (2) respiratory distress; (3) mechanical ventilation; (4) oxygen supplementation. These factors still play an important role in the development of new BPD. However, infection and inflammation, pulmonary edema as result of and patent ductus arteriosus (PDA) or fluid overloading, nutritional deficiencies and genetic factors may also contribute to lung injury. Classic BPD is heavily influenced by injury inflammation and fibrosis; while new primarily is an arrest of development, disorder or delayed modeling and remodeling. (Figure 2)

5.1 Prematurity

Bronchopulmonary dysplasia occurs most commonly in premature infants. Extreme low birth weight infants have a deficiency of surfactant and immature lung parenchyma, compliant chest wall , inadequate respiratory drive and immature antioxidant enzyme system. Most of these infants need supplemental oxygen and assisted ventilation after birth to achieve adequate gas exchange. The functional and structural immaturity increases the risk of lung injury and disruption of normal alveolar development from antenatal and postnatal insults.

Infants born at 23-28 weeks gestation are just beginning to alveolarize the distal saccule of the lung in parallel with the development of the alveolar capillary bed. Alveolar development can be delayed with hypoxia, hyperoxia, inflammations, glucocorticoids, and poor nutrition.

Patent ductus arteriosus (PDA) is present in most ELBW infants. PDA shunt increases pulmonary blood flow, and may result in pulmonary edema. Lung compliance is reduced and lung resistance is increased, creating a need for more vigorous and protracted ventilator support.

5.2 Oxygen toxicity

Inspiration of high oxygen concentration is a major factor in the pathogenesis of BPD, though the precise concentration and duration of oxygen that is toxic to the immature lung has not been established. Any concentration in excess of room air might increase the risk of lung damage when administered over a period of time. Early pulmonary change caused by oxygen toxicity consists of atelectasis, edema, alveolar hemorrhage, inflammation, fibrin deposition, and thickening of alveolar membrane. Continuous high oxygen exposure causes influx of polymorphonuclear leukocytes containing proteolytic enzymes which causes inflammatory reaction and cytotoxic damage.

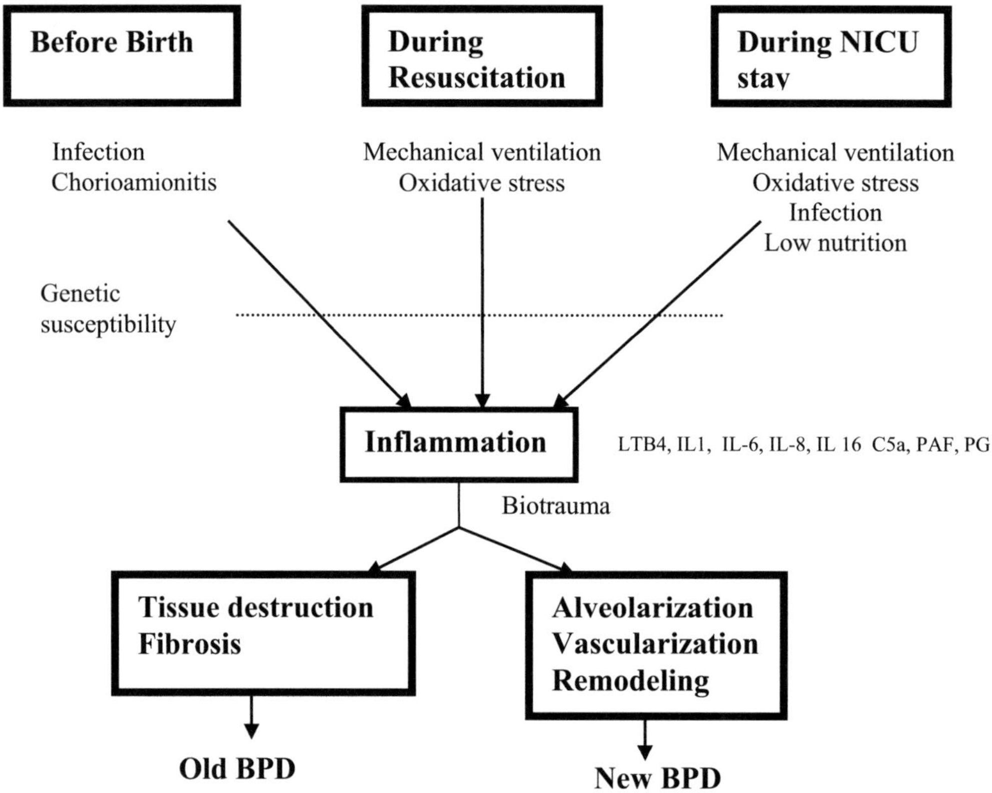

Fig. 2. Pathogenesis of Bronchopulmonary Dysplasia

The fetal lung is exposed to relatively low oxygen tension around 20 to 30 mmHg. Immediately after birth, the arterial oxygen tension climbs to 100 mmHg. The sudden increase of oxygen tension cause substantial oxidative stress. The principle mechanism involves the univalent reduction of molecular oxygen and formation of free oxygen radicals such as superoxide free radical (O_2^-), hydrogen peroxide (H_2O_2), hydroxyl free radical (OH) and singlet oxygen ($^1O_2$). These oxygen free radicals are highly reactive molecules that can cause oxidative damage to lung tissue and trigger the inflammatory reaction. Premature infants have inadequate antioxidant defense system because their antioxidant enzymes such as superoxide dismutase (SOD), catalase (CAT), glutathione peroxidase (GP) are not mature and nutrients deficiencies (vitamin E, vitamin C, beta-carotene, uric acid) are common, thus they are vulnerable to develop lung injury from oxygen toxicity.

5.3 Mechanical ventilation-barotrauma and volutrauma

Barotrauma is the lung injury caused by the pressure used to inflate the lung. The inspiratory pressures needed to inflate the surfactant-deficiency premature lungs often fivefold greater than the physiologic pressure of the normal lung. The alveoli are not homogenous inflated; some units remain collapsed and require higher pressure to reopen, whereas others become over distended. The resistance of collapsed alveoli to inflate leads to over distension of distal bronchioles during peak inflation and damage of bronchiolar epithelium. These over distension of airways and irregular aeration of alveoli lead to inflammation and release of cytokine.

Barotrauma produces alveolar shear stress, disruption of alveolarization, pulmonary air leak, and release of damaging cytokine and other biologically substances. High ventilator pressure has long been considered as a major cause of BPD, but tissue damage is now more attributed to over-distension of the lung from high tidal volume ventilation (volutrauma). In an animal experiment, Dreyfuss et al. demonstrated the most severe lung injury was seen with high tidal volume with high or low pressure. There were no abnormalities with low volume at high pressure. In clinical settings, however, high pressure usually delivers high volume, which in turn stretches alveolar wall and capillaries.

5.4 Inflammation

Inflammation plays the central role in the development of BPD. Inflammatory reaction may be triggered by factors including infection before or after birth, oxygen free radicals, barotraumas or volutrauma from mechanical ventilation, and pulmonary edema. Neutrophils and macrophages are recruited in the airway and pulmonary tissues. The activated neutrophils adhere to the endothelium of the pulmonary vascular system and thus initiate a sequence of pathogenetic events. Infants who subsequently develop BPD are found to have high concentration of proinflammatory and chemotactic factors in the tracheobronchial aspirate such as leukotrine B_4, interleuleukin-1β, interleukin-8, soluble ICAM-1, anaphylatoxin C5a, platelet aggregation factor and prostaglandin. Pulmonary inflammation affects normal alveolization and angiogenesis, these may further lead to remodeling of developing lung resulting in BPD. Leukotrienes may remain elevated in BPD infants even at 6 months of age and cause bronchoconstrictoin, vasoconstriction, edema, neutrophils chemotaxis and mucus production.

5.5 Prenatal and postnatal infection

5.5.1 Chorioamnionitis

Premature infants who were exposed to maternal chorioamnionitis and required mechanical ventilation after birth have higher incidence of BPD. Proinflammatory mediators IL-1, IL-6 and IL-8 were detected in the early tracheal aspirates from these infants, suggesting lung inflammation occurred before birth. Ureaplasma urealyticum is the most common organism associated with chorioamnionitis. Several studies have suggested an association between Ureaplasma urealyticum tracheal colonization and the development of severe respiratory failure and BPD in very low birth weight infants, but results have not been consistent.

5.5.2 Postnatal infection

Very low birth weight infants with early onset systemic infection or local pneumonia usually present with respiratory signs including cyanosis and apnea which required oxygen therapy or ventilator support. Intubated infants are prone to develop nosocomial infection with deteriorating gas exchange, and are at great risk for development of BPD. The presence of a systemic infection in premature infants was noted to increase the risk of late ductal reopening and failure to respond to medical treatment with indomethacin. Infants with infection and those with PDA had higher levels of 6-ketoprostaglandin F1-α than did control subjects. Levels of tumor necrosis factor-α were also elevated in infants with infection and in those with late PDA. The risk of BPD is enhanced if there is active PDA present at the time of infection.

5.6 Pulmonary edema, patent ductus arteriosus and fluid overloading

Increases pulmonary blood flow from left-to-right shunt blood flow crossing patent ductus arteriosus may result increasing interstitial fluid and pulmonary edema. Pulmonary compliance is reduced and resistance is increased, creating a need for prolonged ventilator support with higher oxygen concentration and ventilation pressure. Clinical evidence suggests that infants with RDS who receive great fluid intake or who do not show a diuretic phase during the first few days of life have a high incidence of BPD. This may be because high fluid intake increases the incidence of PDA. Elevated concentration of myeloperoxidase was noted in the tracheal fluid of infants with PDA, suggesting the increased pulmonary blood flow may result in damage of the pulmonary endothelium and adhesion and migration of polymorphonuclear cells into the lung tissue.

5.7 Nutrition, Vitamin A

Premature infants are undernutrition for days and weeks after birth due to critically ill state, intolerance of enteral feeding and fluid restriction. Sick infants have high caloric demand for growth, increased work of breathing and metabolism. Inadequate nutrition may amplify the lung injury of mechanical ventilation, oxygen toxicity and hinder the repair and recovery course. Vitamin C scavenges free oxygen radicals, as well as it interacts with vitamine E. Vitamin A is important in regulating early lung development and alveolar formation. Vitamin A deficiency may promote chronic lung disease by impairing lung healing, increasing the loss of cilia and squamous-cell metaplasia, increasing susceptibility to infection, and decreasing the number of alveoli.

5.8 Genetics

Studies in VLBW twins demonstrated that BPD status in one twin was a highly significant predictor of BPD in the other twin, irrespective of birth order, Apgar scores and other factors. Monozygotic twins had more BPD and a long duration of hospitalization. Lung development is regulated by a variety of genes that balance between pro- and anti-inflammation, oxygen toxicity, cell injury and death, tissue repair, and infection. Specific genes that are known to be involved in these biologic pathways have been evaluated for their potential contribution to BPD. Approximately half of the initial genetic-association studies have not been replicated.

6. Clinical course

Most infants who develop BPD usually have various degree of respiratory insufficiency resulting from RDS, pneumonia or poor respiratory effort after birth. Oxygen therapy or mechanical support is needed to maintain adequate gas exchange. Their pulmonary condition may show improvement in the first few days but deteriorate later. The pulmonary resistance increases gradually and blood gas shows carbon dioxide retention. Infants require more concentrated oxygen and more ventilator support. The deterioration may be triggered by (1)systemic or local infection; (2) the presence of pulmonary edema associated with PDA, fluid overload or congestive heart failure; (3) severe airway obstruction caused by bronchospasm or tracheobronchomalasia. BPD is often anticipated when mechanical ventilation and oxygen supplementation extend beyond10 to 14 days.

Some infants who have mild or moderate BPD show a slow but steady improvement and wean from support after 28 days old. On the other hand, some deteriorate and ultimately require months of oxygen supply and ventilator support. Respiratory acidosis with high PCO2 greater than 55 mmHg associated with compensated metabolic alkalosis is common. Hypoxemia and hypercarbia result from ventilation-perfusion mismatch and alveolar hypoventilation.

The oxygen requirement decrease gradually as the disease process improves, but it can increase during feeding, physical activity or episode of infection. Intubated infants are easily agitated either because of discomfort or airway obstruction; they are also prone to get nosocomial infection. Growth failure with poor weight gain is common due to insufficient enteral intake and increase work of breathing. Some infants with severe BPD develop pulmonary hypertension, right ventricular hypertrophy and eventually die of right-side heart failure (cor pulmonale).

Radiologic manifestation of mild BPD usually appears normal or mild haziness lung field. Moderate to severe BPD may show hyperinflation, lobar or segmental atelectasis, gas trapping with pulmonary interstitial emphysema (PIE) and increased lung streaking. Fibrosis band and enlarged cyst usually occurs in severe BPD.

Supplemental oxygen and /or ventilator dependent
Recurrent respiratory infection
Lung atelectasis
Gastrointestinal reflux
Aspiration pneumonia
Apnea
Hypertension
Wheezing and bronchospasm
Signs of inappropriate ADH
Signs of pulmonary hypertension and cor-pulmonale
Poor postnatal growth
Increase incidence of sudden infant death
Increase fetal hemoglobin
Neurodevelopmental delay

Table 2. Clinical features associated with BPD

7. Prevention of bronchopulmonary dysplasia

As stated above, the pathogensis of BPD has been linked to immature lung tissue, barotraumas and volutrauma resulting from mechanical ventilation, oxygen injury, and proinflammatory factors. Reduction of the incidence and severity of BPD may be possible through reduction of the causes of BPD. Among many strategies studied in the past, antenatal corticosteroids treatment, postnatal surfactant therapy, and gentle ventilation have been proved to be the most effective methods to target the development of BPD and decrease its severity.

7.1 Pharmacologic agents

7.1.1 Antenatal corticosteroid

Antenatal corticosteroid (ANC) was noted to be the most successful agent in reducing respiratory syndrome and increasing survival in premature infants by Liggins and Howie in 1972. It was not widely used until 1994 when the Consensus Development Conference Statement of National Institute of Health was published. Now women are at risk of preterm birth between 24 and 34 weeks'gestation are routinely given a course of corticosteroid before delivery. A single course of antenatal corticosteroids treatment is associated with an overall reduction of neonatal death, RDS, intraventricular hemorrhage, necrotizing enteritis, respiratory support, intensive care admissions and systemic infections in the first 48hoursof life. Long term follow up study demonstrates improvement of neurodevelopmental outcomes. Steroids accelerate structural maturation and surfactant synthesis of the lung, thus decrease the severity of RDS and BPD. The overall incidence of BPD in the population is not decreased due to increased survival of tiny babies.

Antenatal corticosteroid is most effective if given more than 24 hours after and up to 7 days after administration of the second dose of antenatal corticosteroids. Treatment for less than 24 hours is still associated with better outcome, ANC should be given unless immediately delivery is anticipated or there is evidence corticosteroid will have an adverse effect on the mother. Caution should be exercised when giving corticosteroid therapy to women with systemic infection including tuberculosis and infection.

Betamethasone is the steroid of choice, when available, to be given in a course of two doses of 12mg administered intramuscularly 24 hours apart. An alternative regimen would be four doses of 6mg dexamethasone intramuscularly every 12 hours. Betamethasone is associated with a greater reduction in the risk of death than dexamethasone; it also decreases risk of periventricular leukomalacia which was not found with dexamethasone treatment. Weekly repeat course of ANC reduce the occurrence and severity of RDS, but the short benefits are upset with a reduction in weight and head circumference. Weekly repeat course of ANC are not recommended. Prenatal steroid may decrease airway septation and aveolarization in animal, it is not clear if prenatal steroid itself or the associated increased survival of tiny infant would contribute to the recently high incidence of new BPD.

7.1.2 Postnatal surfactant therapy

The surfactant deficiency lung of premature infants is highly susceptible to lung injury and significant inflammatory reaction. The function of surfactant is to recruit alveoli and prevent atelectasis. Surfactant replacement reduces initial inspired oxygen and ventilation requirements as well as the incidence of respiratory distress syndrome, death, pneumothorax, pulmonary interstitial emphysema and the combined outcome of death or BPD. Combined use of prenatal steroid and postnatal surfactant therapy has proved to have an additive effect in improving lung function. As results of these treatments, the severe classic BPD is rarely seen today.

7.1.3 Methylxanthines

Apnea of prematurity occurs in at least 85 percent of infants who are less than 34 weeks gestation. Widely used treatments include application of continuous positive airway pressure and the prescription of methylxanthines. In fact, methylxanthines - caffeine, theophylline and aminophylline are one of the most common drugs used in premature infants. They inhibit

sleepiness-inducing adenosine and improve respiratory drive, reduce the frequency of apnea and the need for mechanical ventilation. Methylxanthines also inhibit TNF-α and leukotriene synthesis, thereby reducing inflammation and innate immunity.
Toxicity with theophylline is more common than with caffeine. Side effects are usually associated with plasma level over 20ug/ml. Serum levels less than 10ug/ml is not beneficial as an aid to wean the ventilator. Because of the narrow range of therapeutic levels of theophylline, caffeine is the drug of choice in the treatment of apnea of prematurity. Davis at el demonstrated an improvement in minute ventilation, an increase in tidal volume, a decrease in lung resistance and improved lung compliance 1 hour following 10 mg/kg of caffeine. In a randomized study by Schmidt et al, infant who received caffeine were less likely to use oxygen at 36 weeks postmenstrual age, and more likely to have ventilator discontinued earlier.

7.1.4 Postnatal corticosteroid

Because inflammation plays a central role in the pathogeneses of BPD, systemic corticosteroids especial dexamethasone have long been used for prevention and treatment of BPD. Lung inflammation is down-regulated by dexamethasone therapy. Dexamethasone is a potent, long acting steroid with almost exclusive glucocorticoid effect. Compared to hydrocortisone, dexamethasone is 25-50 times more potent. The half-life is 36-54 hours. Dexamethasone has been extensively studied in neonatal medicine and has shown to improve pulmonary function, facilitate extubation and decrease the incidence of BPD. However; many associated adverse side effects prevent the routine use of dexamethasone. The short term side effects include hyperglycemia, hypertension, hypertrophic cardiomyopathy, growth failure, GI bleeding and perforation. The risk of GI perforation increases with concomitant indomethacin treatment. There is also a concern of the chronic suppression of the hypothalamic-pituitary-adrenal axis, and long term neurodevelopmental delay.
Striking evidence from multiple studies of the adverse effects of dexamethasone and its long-term neurological effects on preterm infants prompted the American Academy of Pediatrics and the Canadian Pediatric Society to strongly discourage the use of corticosteroids to prevent or treat BPD in 2002. Since the release of this consensus statement, the use of corticosteroids has decreased significant, the incidence and severity of BPD increased significantly during this decade. To each gestation age, the time-related increase in BPD is inversely related to the decrease of dexamethasone use. The decline in use of dexamethasone associated with a concomitant increase in the use hydrocortisone. However, the use of hydrocortisone did not have any impact on the rate and severity of BPD.

7.2 Gentle ventilation

Mechanical ventilation both causes and treats BPD. When used, lowest ventilator setting to obtain adequate ventilation must be applied to minimize the barotrauma-volutrama and oxygen toxicity.

7.2.1 Tidal volume, inspiratory pressure and target range of oxygen saturation

In premature infants with lung disease, functional residual volume is reduced and some parts of alveoli are collapsed. The ideal tidal volume would be that open these collapsed area without over-distend the other areas. In general, initial PIP is set 16-20 cmH_2O in order to achieve a tidal volume of 4-6 ml/Kg in ELBW with respiratory failure. Peak inspiratory

pressure >20 mmHg is rarely needed. Peak end expiratory pressure is usually set at 4 cmH_2O, and short inspiratory time 0.3-0.4 seconds are used.
Oxygen saturation monitored by pulse oximetry offers the most reliable estimate of arterial oxygenation and easy to use. The ranges of oxygen saturation should be targeted between 91 to 95%. Oxygen therapy is very toxic for preterm babies, and maintaining even slightly high oxygen saturation contributes to retinopathy of prematurity and increases the duration of oxygen treatment. The STOP-ROP (Supplemental Therapeutic Oxygen for prethreshold Retinopathy of Prematurity) research group showed that newborn babies who had received oxygen supplementation to maintain saturation at 96-99% presented more pneumonia and a greater incidence of chronic lung disease than did those whose saturation was maintained at 89-94%. The results of the Surfactant, Positive Pressure, and Oxygenation Randomized Trial (SUPPORT) demonstrated that lower target range of oxygenation at 85to 89% did not significantly decrease the combined risk of death or BPD, but it resulted in an increase in mortality.

7.2.2 Permissive hypercarbia

Higher levels of PCO2 45-65 mmHg with pH above 7.20 now are accepted, thus allowing gentle ventilation to minimize lung injury. Early studies suggest that BPD occur more often among newborn infants with PaCO2 below 40mmHg. A randomized, controlled study of NICH Neonatal network demonstrated that mechanical ventilated extremely low birth weight infants who were assigned to minimal ventilation (PCO2 target >52 mm Hg) required less ventilator support at 36 weeks compared with infants with routine ventilation (PCO_2 target <48 mm Hg) (1% vs. 16% respectively, $p<0.01$). Unfortunately, after enrollment of 220 patients, the trial was halted because of unanticipated non-respiratory adverse events related to dexamethasone therapy. The relative risk for death or BPD at 36 weeks in both groups is no difference.

7.2.3 Nasal continuous positive pressure (nCPAP)

Nasal continuous positive pressure supports the breathing through a number of mechanisms: (1). splinting the airway thereby preventing airway obstruction, (2). dilating the airways and reducing resistance to airflow and so diminishing work of breathing, (3) aiding lung expansion and so reducing ventilation perfusion mismatch and improving oxygenation. Nasal CPAP used after extubation can prevent the instability associated with possible respiratory failure and reintubation.
Nasal CPAP, rather than intubation and ventilation, might be started shortly after birth for infants born at 25 to 28weeks' gestation. In the randomized, controlled Continuous Positive Airway Pressure or Intubtion at Birth (COIN) trial, there were fewer days of ventilation in the CPAP group, and a few CPAP infants received oxygen therapy at 28 days, but not at 36 PMA weeks. The early CPAP group did not significantly reduce the rate of death or BPD. Pneumothorax occurs in 6% of the CPAP infants and 3 % in the intubated group. Report from SUPPORT study, infants born 24-28 weeks of gestation, were randomly assigned to intubation and surfactant treatment, or to CPAP treatment initiated in the delivery room. There is no significant difference of death or BPD at 36 weeks. Infants who received CPAP treatment, as compared with infants who received intubation and surfactant treatment, less frequently required intubation or postnatal corticosteroids for BPD, and required fewer days of mechanical ventilation.

The value of early CPAP as a replacement of intubation and ventilation apparently to be established. Surfactant treatment is most effective if given shortly after birth. Tiny infants with respiratory distress receive nCPAP alone after bith may miss the benefit of prophylactic surfactant therapy. In our practice, we intubate these infants soon after birth, give a dose of surfactant treatment, then extubated and change to CPAP support if infants can tolerate, to avoid mechanical ventilation.

8. Management of BPD

Despite of the recent advances of neonatal medicine, little progress has been made in treatment of BPD. Cornerstones of treatment are pulmonary support to maintain optimal oxygen saturation and prevent complications and nutritional support to promote growth. Most patients with mild to moderate BPD gradually improve as healing occurs and lung growth continues. Infants with severe BPD especial who are ventilator dependent are more likely to have acute episodes of pulmonary decompensation secondary due to nosocomial infection, severe airway constriction, pulmonary air leak, increased pulmonary edema and the development of tracheobronchmalacia or cor pulmonale. Physical examination, radiographic survey, laboratory tests and echocardiogram are important in differential diagnosis and guide for specific treatment.

Respiratory support

Infants with established BPD who are ventilator dependent, gentle ventilation are preferred to avoid further lung injury. Oxygen saturation should be kept within 90-95%. Inappropriate low oxygen tension may induce pulmonary vasoconstriction and /or bronchospasm with resultant increase frequency of apnea and hypoxia. Higher PCO2 (55 to 65 mmHg) is accepted if pH is in normal range. Weaning these from mechanical ventilation is difficult and must be accomplished gradually. Caffeine or theophylline are usually used during the weaning phase to stimulate respiratory drive. Nasal CPAP may be applied to infants after extubation.
Infants with BPD who are not on oxygen therapy may experience oxygen desaturation with feeding or physical activity, additional oxygen supply might be need.

Phamacologic agents

Most medications used for treatment of BPD are targeted on one of the following pathophysiologic mechanisms of BPD: (1) bronchopulmonary constriction and airway hyperreactivity, (2) pulmonary edema, (3) airway inflammation, and (4) chronic lung injury and repair.

Bronchodilators

Infants with BPD have increased airway resistance due to peribronchial smooth muscle hypertrophy and airway hyperactivity. Acute bronchospasm in response to hypoxia event could lead to sudden deteriorating pulmonary status. Bronchodilators have been shown to reduce airway resistance, improve lung compliance and increase tidal volume in infants with BPD during acute episodes of bronchospasm. However, their effects are usually short-lived, and many drugs have significant cardiovascular side effects. Inhaled β-2 agonists such as albuterol or levalbuterol have shown to reverse acute episodes of bronchoconstriction and cause few cardiovascular side effects. An initial trial dose can be administered through a meter-dose inhaler with a spacer device or as a nebulized solution. If patients show improvement of gas exchange, the β-2 agonists can be given up to 48hours duration.

Chronic use of β-2 agonists is not recommended since there is no long term benefit in treatment or prevention of BPD in preterm infants. Ipratropium bromide is another anticholinergic preparation that dilates airway.

Methylxanthines are competitive nonselective phosphodiesterase inhibitors, prevent breakdown of cyclic AMP and cyclic GMP. This leads to raise intracellular c-AMP and c-GMP. They also inhibit TNF-α and leukotriene synthesis, thereby reducing inflammation and innate immunity. Methylxanthines are nonselective adenosine receptor antagonists. Adenosine can cause broncho-constriction and potentiate immunologically induced mediator release from lung mast cells. Inhibition of this action will cause bronchodilatation. Theobromine, a metabolic product of caffeine and theophylline, causes vasodilatation and increases urine volume. But methylxanthines are weak bronchodilators with mild diuretic effect, and are infrequently used in the treatment for acute bronchospasm.

Corticosteroid

As discussed above, systemic corticosteroids improve lung function and reduce the need of mechanical ventilation, but because the concern of long term adverse neurological outcome, now this treatment is reserved for infants with severe BPD who cannot be weaned from ventilator support. Dexamethsone with lower dose and shorter duration are usually used to facilitate extubation. A recent pilot study by Yeh et al , has shown that intratracheal instillation of budesonide by using surfactant as vehicle can effectively deliver budesonide to the lung and suppress the lung inflammation and improves pulmonary outcome without significant short term and long term side effects. More studies are needed before it can be recommended.

Nutrition and fluid supply

Adequate nutrition is difficult to achieve in infants with BPD because of high caloric demand, poor tolerance of enteral feeding and restriction of fluid intake. Impaired growth is common in these infants. Malnutrion can delay somatic growth and the development of new alveoli, making successful weaning from ventilator less likely. Infants with poor nutrition are also susceptible to infection. Also, there are special nutrients and vitamins that are frequently deficient in these infants and their lack may increase the risk of lung injury.

Many infants with BPD experience increased energy needs. The reasons for this are not entirely clear; increased work of breathing, catecholamine release due to stress, increased energy requirements for feeding, and the effects of medications probably all play a role. It is not unusual for infants with BPD to require 130 or even 160 Kcal/kg/day to support adequate growth. It may be difficult to provide adequate calories for these infants. They may have ongoing fluid restrictions due to concerns about pulmonary edema. They may experience fatigue with feeding or delayed gastric emptying. Increasing the caloric density of formula or breast milk with a balanced proportion of carbohydrate and fat may be helpful. A high carbohydrate load increases production of CO_2 which may be a concern in infants with respiratory compromise. Excess carbohydrate may also lead to osmotic diarrhea. Excess dietary fat may delay gastric emptying and exacerbate gastroesopageal reflux.

Diuretics

Infants with chronic lung disease tend to retain interstitial fluid which results in increased respiratory distress, increase in oxygen requirement, increase in ventilator settings, hypoxemia and hypercarbia. Diuretics mobilize fluid, improve lung compliance and decrease resistance.

Furosemide

Furosemide is the most commonly used diuretic. It is a potent and rapid acting loop diuretic. It can be used orally and intravenously. The main benefit of the intravenous route is a quick response.
Mechanism of Action: At the ascending loop of Henle, furosemide inhibits active reabsorption of chloride resulting in lower sodium and water reabsorption. It also acts against antidiuretic hormones, and increases urine aldosterone excretion. Furosemide decreases left ventricular filling pressure by increasing venous capacitance. Furosemide helps in chronic lung disease by both diuretic and vasculature effects.
Adverse effects: Main adverse effects of chronic furosemide therapy are hypercalciuria, nephrocalcinosis and hypochloremia. Electrolytes should be monitored carefully. Ototoxicity is related to plasma concentration and is usually reversible after cessation of therapy. Other side effects include: osteopenia, cholelithiasis, displacement of bilirubin and hyperparathyroidism.
According to Cochrane review in preterm infants < 3 weeks of age with BPD, intravenous furosemide administration has either inconsistent effects or no detectable effect. In infants less than 3 weeks of age with BPD, a single intravenous dose of 1 mg/kg of furosemide transiently improves pulmonary mechanics. Chronic enteral or intravenous furosemide administration improves both oxygenation and pulmonary mechanics. The Cochrane review concluded that there is little evidence to support any benefit of fu- rosemide administration with respect to ven- tilatory support, length of hospital stay, survival or long-term outcome. Accordingly, routine or sustained uses of systemic loop diuretics in infants with BPD cannot be recommended.
Inhaled furosemide has been shown to transiently improve pulmonary function. No long-term outcomes have been studied. More trials are needed before this delivery method can be recommended for routine use.

Thiazide Diuretics

Thiazides work by inhibiting sodium reabsorption in the distal tubule. In contrast to furosemide, thiazides decrease calcium excretion.

Potassium Sparing Diuretic

Spironolactone is a competitive antagonist of aldosterone. It is a weak diuretic and is usually given in combination with thiazides. There are very few randomized control trials. By Cochrane reviewer's opinion, in infants less than 3 weeks of age with BPD, chronic administration of thiazide and spironolactone improves lung compliance at four weeks of treatment and reduces need for furosemide. Only one study showed long-term benefits such as decreased rates of death and artificial ventilation.

Diuretics				
Drug	Site of Action	Route	Onset	Dose
Furosemide	Loop diuretic	IV PO	15-30 min 30-60 min	1 mg/kg/dose 1-3 mg/kg/dose
Hydrochlorothiazide	Distal tubule	PO	1-2 hrs	2-4 mg/kg/day
Spironolactone	Aldosterone antagonist	PO	3-5 days	1.5-3 mg/kg/day

Table 3.

Inhaled Nitric Oxide (INO)

INO decreases pulmonary vascular resistance and improves oxygenation. It is pro- posed that INO will improve oxygenation, improve ventilation and will decrease respiratory support. Side effects include methemoglobinemia and direct pulmonary injury if excessive INO is used

Studies on INO were done with different doses, started at different ages, different durations of treatment, and in infants whose characteristics were different among the studies. INO was approved by FDA to term and near-term infants. AAP Committee on Fetus and Newborn recommended that centers that provide INO therapy should provide comprehensive long-term medical and neurodevelopment follow-up and should establish prospective data collection for treatment time, course, toxic effects, treatment failure, use of alternative therapies, and outcomes.

A systematic review which included 11 studies failed to show a significant benefit of INO on BPD. Cochrane database for systematic review by Keith J Barrington in 2006 concluded: INO as rescue therapy for the very ill ventilated preterm infant does not appear to be effective, and may increase the risk of severe IVH. Later use of INO to prevent BPD also does not appear to be effective. Early routine use of INO in mildly sick preterm infants may decrease serious brain injury, and may improve survival without BPD. Further studies are needed.

Antioxidants

Free radical and oxidant stress cause dam- age to DNA, cell membrane, protein and lipids. Free radicals are produced by many mechanisms such as mitochondrial electron transport chain, prostaglandin metabolism, ischemia-reperfusion, hypoxia, neutrophil and macrophage activations, and endothelial cell hypoxanthine-xanthine oxidation. There is a balance between free radical production and clearing by the antioxidant system. The antioxidant defense system includes enzymatic components such as Co-Zn superoxide dismutase (SOD) glutathione peroxidase, and a non-enzymatic components such as glutathione, selenium, zinc, vitamin E and vitamin C. Preterm infants have an immature antioxidant defense system, and are highly exposed to oxidant stress, therefore prone to get tissue damage. Many antioxidant agents have been tried to treat or prevent BPD in new-born. These include:

Vitamin E: Tocopherol is a fat-soluble, anti- oxidant and it decreases reactive oxygen species The American Academy of Pediatrics Committee on Nutrition has recommended daily supplementation of 5-25 IU of vitamin E in preterm infants. Supplementing very low birth weight infants with vitamin E as an anti- oxidant agent has been proposed for pre- venting or limiting retinopathy of prematurity, intracranial hemorrhage, and chronic lung disease. In clinical trials, vitamin E supplementation did not affect the incidence of BPD. Vitamin E supplementation significantly increased the risk for necrotizing enterocolitis and sepsis.

Superoxide dismutase: Intra-tracheal ad- ministration of CuZn SOD in preterm infants did not reduce BPD. It decreased the need for asthma medications, emergency department visits and hospitalizations during the one year follow-up.Rosenfeld et al showed that radiologic evidence, clinical signs of BPD and days of CPAP were less in patients treated with SOD, and no side effects were observed. Cochrane database concluded that there is insufficient evidence that super- oxide dismutase is efficient in preventing chronic lung disease of prematurity, but it is well-tolerated, and has no serious adverse effects.

N acetyl cysteine (NAC): NAC is a precursor of cysteine, which is essential in Glutathione synthesis. Glutathione is a non- enzymatic antioxidant. NAC treatment in preterm infants did not prevent BPD or death, and did not improve lung function at discharge from the hospital .

Allopurinol: Allopurinol is inhibitor of xanthine oxidase, an enzyme which generates superoxide radicals. It did not decrease BPD in preterm infants of 24-32 weeks' gestation.

Metaltonin: Metaltonin is a hormone that is found in all biological organisms, and is a potent free radical scavenger. Melatonin treatment reduced the proinflammatory cytokines (IL-6, IL-8 and tumor necrosis factor (TNF)-alpha), and improved the clinical out- come in mechanically ventilated newborns with respiratory distress.

Vitamin A: Vitamin A is very important for the health of epithelial tissues. It reduces ciliary loss, and is associated with increased alveoli. In animals studies, vitamin A deficiency has been associated with necrotizing tracheobronchiolitis and squamous metaplasia the changes akin to BPD. Very low birth weight infants are known to have low vitamin levels.

There have been several studies looking at vitamin A in the prevention of BPD. The largest study by Tyson et al showed significant decrease (from 62% to 55%) in combined outcome of death or chronic lung disease.

Meta-analysis also revealed similar results.

A follow-up study did not show any untoward outcome at 18 to 22 months of age. Many units routinely use vitamin A for prevention of BPD. Five thousand IU of Vitamin A has to be given by tri-weekly intramuscular injections for four weeks. In one study it was given by oral route but was not effective in preventing BPD. Intravenous emulsion preparation needs to be studied by randomized control trials.

Cimetidine: In animal studies, lung injury as result of induction of cytochrome P450 by oxygen exposure may result in the release of free radical oxidants and arachidonic acid metabolites, that can be reduced by cimetidine. In study by Cotton et al of infants weighing less than 1250 grams who were mechanically ventilated and required oxygen, Cimetidine had no significant effect on the severity of respira tory insufficiency at 10 day postnatal age, and did not affect the tracheal aspirate levels of inflammatory markers or arachidonic acid metabolites.

Azithromycin: A macrolid antibiotic, azithromycin, acts act as a free radical scavenger, inhibits cytokines, and inhibits neutrophil chemotaxis. In a study by Bal- lard HO et al on extremely premature infants requiring mechanical ventilation, azithromycin did not affect mortality, incidence of BPD and days on ventilator.

Alpha-1 protease inhibitor (A1PI): Matrix Metalloproteinase is a member of a family of extracellular enzymes that are essential in proteolysis activity against extra cellular matrix proteins such as collagen, elastic lamina and fibronectin. These enzymes are produced by variety of cells such as fibro- blasts, osteoblasts, macrophages, monocytes and neutrophils. These enzymes are essential in growth, tissue remodeling, angiogenesis and wound healing. If the balance between activation and inhibition of this enzymes is disturbed, many pathological conditions can occur such as bronchopulmonary dysplasia. In a study by Stiskal JA et al, the incidence of CLD in survivors was lower in infants treated with intravenous A1PI as compared with a placebo group, but the difference was not statistically significant. The incidence of pulmonary hemorrhage was lower in the treated group.

Thyroxine, did not reduce the incidence of BPD. Estradiol and progesterone hormonal replacements were studied in 83 infants, but did not show decrease in incidence of BPD.

9. Conclusion

BPD is disease of multi-etiology. A large number of extremely preterm infants who survive are developing BPD, but the severity of the lung damage is considerably less than that observed in the classic form of BPD. Because most of these infants have only mild initial respiratory distress and, therefore, do not receive aggressive ventilation, other factors must be involved in the pathogenesis of this new, milder type of BPD. Clinical and epidemiological data strongly suggest that infections, either prenatal or postnatal, and the presence of PDA are major factors in the development of BPD. For this reason, efforts to prevent BPD in extremely low-birth weight infants should include an aggressive approach in the prevention and effective treatment of infections and PDA. BPD has long term adverse pulmonary and neurodevelopment outcome. Steroids usage for treatment of BPD also has been shown to have adverse neurodevelopment. Available data are sometime conflicting and inconclusive; clinicians must use their own clinical judgment to balance the adverse effects of BP D with the potential adverse effects of steroids for each individual patient.. Very low birth weight infants who remain on mechanical ventilation after 1 to 2 weeks of age are at very high risk of developing BPD . When considering corticosteroid therapy for such an infant, clinicians might conclude that the risks of a short course of glucocorticoid therapy is warranted . This individualized decision should be made in conjunction with the infant's parents. Other treatment and management are largely been supportive and most of them have no long term benefits. A recent pilot study from Yeh et al indicated that intratracheal instillation of budesonide using surfactant as vehicle can effectively deliver budesonide into the lungs and can significantly suppress lung inflammation, improve pulmonary outcome and without immediate and long term adverse effect.. More studies are needed to prove this. Until that time, proper respiratory care and avoidance of NICU infection are the most important steps leading to lower incidence of BPD.

10. Acknowledgements

Supports in Part from National Health Research Institute (NHRI-EX-100-9818PI) Taiwan

11. References

Aaltonen R., Vahlberg T., Lehtonen L., Alanen A. Ureaplasma urealyticum: no independent role in the pathogenesis of bronchopulmonary dysplasia. *Acta Obstet Gynecol Scand* 2006;85(11):1354–1359.

Abele-Horn M., Genzel-Boroviczeny O., Uhlig T., Zimmermann A., Peters J., Scholz M. Ureaplasma urealyticum colonization and bronchopulmonary dysplasia: a comparative prospective multicentre study. *Eur J Pediatr* 1998;157(12):1004–1011.

ACOG Committee opinion committee on obstetric practice antenatal corticosteroid therapy for Fetal Maturation. October 1998 Number 210.

American Academy of Pediatrics, Committee on Fetus and Newborn. Postnatal corticosteroids totreat or prevent chronic lung disease in preterm infants. *Pediatrics* 2002;109(2):330 –338

Baraldi E, Filippone M, Chronic lung disease after premature birth. *N Engl J Med* 2007; 357:1946-55

Baud O, Foix-L'Helias L, Kaminski M et al, Audibert F, Jarreau PH, Papiernik E, Huon C, Lepercq J, Dehan M, Lacaze-Masmonteil T. Antenatal glucocorticoid treatment and cystic periventricular leukomalacia in very premature infants. *N Engl J Med* 1999; 341(16):1190-6.

Bhandari V, Gruen J R. The Genomics of Bronchopulmonary Dysplasia. *NeoReviews* Aug 2007; 8: e336 - e344.

Capers CC, Ward ES, Murphy JEetal. Use of theophylline in neonate as an aid to ventilator weaning. *Ther Drug Monit* 1992; 14 (6):471-4.

Carlo WA, Stark AR, Wright LL, et al. Minimal ventilation to prevent bronchopulmonary dysplasia in extremely-low-birth-weight infants. *J Pediatr* 2002 Sep;141(3):370-4.

Clark RH, Gerstmann DR, Jobe AH, et al. Lung injury in neonates: causes, strategies for prevention and long-term consequences. *J Pediatr* 2001;139:478-86

Coalson JJ : Pathology of Bronchopulmonary Dysplasia. *Semin Perinatol* 30:179-184

Coalson JJ, Winter V, deLemos RA. Decreased alveolarization in baboon survivors with bronchopulmonary dysplasia. *Am J Respir Crit Care Med* 1995;152:640–646

Davis JM, Bhutani VK, Stefano JL, Fox WW et al. Changes in pulmonary mechanics following caffeine administration in infants with bronchopulmonary dysplasia. *Pediatr Pumlonol* 1989;6 (1) 49-52.

Denjean A, Paris-Llado J, Zupan V, et al: Inhaled salbutamol and beclomethasone for preventing broncho-pulmonary dysplasia: a randomized double-blind study. *Eur J Pediatr* 157:926-931, 1998

Engle WA, and the Committee on Fetus and Newborn the American Academy of Pediatrics. Surfactant-Replacement Therapy for Respiratory Distress in the Preterm and Term Neonate. *Pediatr* 2008;121(2):419-432

Fanaroff AA, Stoll BJ, Wright LL, Carlo WA, Ehrenkranz RA, Stark AR, et al. Trends in neonatal morbidity and mortality for very low birth weight infants. *Am J Obstet Gynecol* 2007;196:147.e1-8.

Garland JS, Buck RK, Allred EN, Leviton A. Hypocarbia before surfactant therapy appears to increase bronchopulmonary dysplasia risk in infants with respiratory distress syndrome. *Arch Pediatr Adolesc Med* 1995;149:617-22.

Gonzalez A, Sosenko IRS, Chandar J, et al. Influence of infection on patent ductus arteriosus and chronic lung disease in premature infants weighting 1000 grams or less. *J Pediatr* 1996;128:470–478

Gronec P, Reuss D, Gotze-Speer B. Speer C.P.The effects of dexamethasone on chemotactic activity and inflammatory mediators intracheobroncheal aspirates of preterm infants at risk for chronic lung disease. *J Pedistr* 1993; 122:938-944

Groneck P, Speer CP. Inflammatory mediators and BPD. *Arch Dis Child Fetal Neonatal Ed* 1995; 73:F1-3

Hansen T., Corbet A. Chronic lung disease- Bronchopulmonary dysplasia. In Taeusch, Ballard and Avery (ed) Schaffer & Avery's Diseases of The Newborn. 6th ed. Saunders, 1991, p519

Hislop AA, Wigglesworth JS, Desai R, Aber V. The effects of preterm delivery and mechanical ventilation on human lung growth. *Early Hum Dev* 1987;15:147- 64

Hussain NA, Siddiqui NH, Stocker JR. Pathology of arrested acinar development in postsurfactant bronchopulmonary dysplasia. *Hum Pathol* 1998;29:710–717.

Jobe A, Ikegami M. Mechanisms initiating lung injury in the preterm. *Early Hum Dev* 1998;53:81–94

Jobe A. Bancalarie E. Bronchopulmonary dysplasia. *Am J Respir Crit Care Med* 2001; 163: 1723-1729.

Khilfeh M, Agrawal V, Yeh TF. Pharmacological treatment and prevention of chronic lung disease in preterm infants,*www.neonatologytoday.net/newsletters/nt-apr10.pdf*

Kraybill EN, Runyan DK, Bose CL, Khan JH. Risk factors for chronic lung disease in infants with birth weight of 751 to 1000 grams. *J Pediatr.* 1989;115:115-20.

Kuo HT, Lin HC, Tsai CH, Chouc IC, Yeh TF. A follow-up study of preterm infants given budesonide using surfactant as a vehicle to prevent chronic lung disease in preterm infants. J Pediatr. 2010 Apr;156(4):537-41. Epub 2010 Feb 6.

Lee B.H., Stoll BJ, McDonald SA, Higgins RD, Adverse Neonatal Outcomes Associated With Antenatal Dexamethasone Versus Antenatal Betamethasone . *Pediatrics* 2006;117;1503-1510

Liggins GC, Howie RN. A controlled trial of antepartum glucocorticoid treatment for prevention of the respiratory distress syndrome in premature infants. *Pediatrics* 1972;50:515-525

NIH Consensus Statement Effect of Corticosteroids for Fetal Maturation on Perinatal Outcomes 1994 Feb 28-Mar 2;12(2):1-24

Northway WH Jr, Rosan RC, Porter DY. Pulmonary disease following respirator therapy of hyaline membrane disease: Bronchopulmonary dysplasia. *N Engl J Med* 1967;276:357

Parker RA, Lindstrom DP, Cotton RB. Evidence from twin study implies possible genetic susceptibility to bronchopulmonary dysplasia. *Semin Perinatol* 1996;20 :206 –209

Parker RA, Lindstrom DP, Cotton RB. Improved survival accounts for aost, but not all, of the increase in bronchopulmonary dysplasia. *Pediatrics* 1992;90:663-668

RCOG Green-top Guideline No. 7. October, 2010 Antenatal Corticosteroids to Reduce Neonatal Morbidity and Mortality.

Rhen T,Cidlowski J. Antiinflammatory action of glucocorticoids-new mechanisms for old drugs. *N Engl J Med* 2005;353:1711-23

Schelonka R.L., Katz B., Waites K.B., Benjamin D.K. Critical appraisal of the role of Ureaplasma in the development of bronchopulmonary dysplasia with metaanalytic techniques. *Pediatr Infect Dis J* 2005;24(12):1033–1039

Schmidt B, Roberts RS, Davis P et al. Caffeine therapy for apnea of prematurity. *N Engl J Med* 2006; 354

Schmit B, Roberts RS, Davis Pet al. Long-Term effects of Caffeine therapy for apnea of prematurity. *N Engl j Med* 2007 357 (19) 1893-902

Shinwell E, Lerner-Geva, Lusky A, Reichman B. Less postnatal steroids, more bronchopulmonary dysplasia: a population-based study in very low birthweight infants. *Arch Dis Child Fetal Neonatal Ed.* 2007;92(1):F30-F33

Speer CP. Inflammation and bronchopulmonary dysplasia: a continuous story. *Semin Fetal Neonat Med* 2006; 11(5):354-362

Speer CP. New insights into the pathogenesis of pulmonary inflammation in preterm infants. *Biol Neonate* 2001;79:205–209

Stark AR, Carlo WA, Tyson JE, et al. Adverse effects of early dexamethasone in extremely-low-birth-weight infants: National Institute of Child Health and Human Development Neonatal Research Network. *N Engl J Med* 2001;344:95–101

SUPPORT Study Group of the Eunice Kennedy Shriver NICHD Neonatal Research Network. Early CPAP versus surfactant in extremely preterm infants. *N Engl J Med* 2010;362:1970-9.

SUPPORT Study Group of the Eunice Kennedy Shriver NICHD Neonatal Research Network. Target ranges of oxygen saturation in extremely preterm infants. *N Engl J Med* 2010;362:1959-69.

Tyson JE, Wright LL, Oh W, et al. Vitamin A supplementation for extremely-low-birth-weight infants. National Institute of Child Health and Human Development Neonatal Research Network. *N Engl J Med* 1999; 340:1962.

Van Marter LJ, Dammann O, Allred EN, et al. Chorioamnionitis, mechanical ventilation and postnatal sepsis as modulators of chronic lung disease in preterm infants. *J Pediatr* 2002;140:171–176

Van Marter LJ, et al. Hydration during the first days of life and the risk of bronchopulmonary dysplasia inlow birth weight infants. *J Pediatr* 1990;116:942

van Waarde W.M., Brus F., Okken A., Kimpen J.L. Ureaplasma urealyticum colonization, prematurity and bronchopulmonary dysplasia. *Eur Respir J* 1997;10(4):886–890

Varsila E, Hallman M, Venge P, et al. Closure of patent dutus arteriosus dereases pulmonary myeloperoxidase in premature infants with respiratory distress syndrome. and the risk of bronchopulmonary dysplasia in low birth premature infants with respiratory distress syndrome. *Biol Noonate* 1995:67:167-171 (20): 2112-21.

Watterberg K, Scott SM. Evidence of Early Adrenal Insufficiency in Babies Who Develop Bronchopulmonary Dysplasia. *Pediatrics* 1995; 95: 120-125

Watterberg KL, Demers LM, Scott SM, Murphy S. Chorioamnionitis and early lung inflammation in infants in whom bronchopulmonary dysplasia develops. *Pediatrics* 1996; 97: 210-215.

Watterberg KL, Gerdes JS, Gifford KL, Lin HM. Prophylaxis against early adrenal insufficiency to prevent chronic lung disease in premature infants. *Pediatrics* 1999;104 :1258 –1263.

Wu SY, Joseph T, Medha Kamat , Suma Pyaty Tsu-Fuh Yeh TF. Postnatal corticosteroid to prevent or treat chronic lung disease in preterm infants. *www.neonatologytoday.net/newsletters/nt-nov09.pdf*

Yeh TF, J. Lin YJ, HuangC C, Chen,Y J, Lin CH, Hong C. Lin HC, Hsieh WS, Lien YJ. Early Dexamethasone Therapy in Preterm Infants: A Follow-up Study. *Pediatrics* May 1998; 101: e7

Yeh TF, Lin YJ, Hsieh WS, Lin HC, Lin CH, Chen JY, Kao HA, Chien CH. Early postnatal dexamethasone therapy for the prevention of chronic lung disease in preterm Infants with respiratory distress syndrome: A multi-centers clinical trial. *Pediatrics* 1997; 100: e3

Yeh TF, Lin YJ, Lin HC, et al. Outcomes at school age after postnatal dexamethasone therapy for lung disease of prematurity. *N Engl J Med* 2004;350: 1304-13

Yeh TF, Torre JA, Rastogi A, Anyebuno MA, Pildes RS Early postnatal dexamethasone therapy in premature infants with severe respiratory distress syndrome: a double-blind, controlled study. *J Pediatr* 1990; 117:273-282

Yoder B, Harrison M, Clark R. Time-Related changes in steriod use and bronchopulmonary dysplasia in preterm infants. *Pediatrics* 2009;124: 673-679

Yeh TF, Lin H C, Chang C H., Wu T S, Su B H, Tsai C L, Pyati S, Tsai C H. Early Intratracheal Instillation of Budesonide Using Surfactant as a Vehicle to Prevent Chronic Lung Disease in Preterm Infants: A Pilot Study. Pediatrics 121 (5) e1-e9, May, 2008.

22

Bronchopulmonary Dysplasia: The Role of Oxidative Stress

Jean-Claude Lavoie and Ibrahim Mohamed
Université de Montréal
Canada

1. Introduction

One of the critical and chronic complications of preterm birth is bronchopulmonary dysplasia (BPD). The incidence of BPD is high, ranging from 40% to 70% of infants born before 28 completed weeks' gestation (Stoll et al., 2010). The disease is characterized by impaired alveolar and vascular maturation, with long-term consequences on a number of systems including neurodevelopment. Risk factors for BPD include gestational age at birth, sex, inflammation and/or infection, oxygen supplementation, mechanical ventilation, and parenteral nutrition. Although the etiology of BPD is not well understood, risk factors are all associated with oxidative stress. A modulation of the redox environment is believed to play a major role in the pathogenesis of BPD.

This chapter will start by describing BPD, and then focus on the molecules involved in oxidative stress, the aim being that a better understanding favours more effective clinical intervention. Each of the risk factors in turn will be discussed according to the implied redox modifications occurring during BPD development.

2. Description of BPD

2.1 Historical perspective

Prior to the era of mechanical ventilation, few infants of very low birth weight (less than 1500 g) survived, and neonatal mortality for extremely low birth weight infants (less than 1000 g) exceeded 90% (Behrman et al., 1971). Most survivors required little or no oxygen supplementation initially but later deteriorated to requirements of up to 40% in order to prevent cyanosis. On radiography, findings included microcystic changes as well as varying degrees of hyperinflation and flattening of the diaphragm. Some infants recovered spontaneously over weeks to months but others died, with postmortem examination revealing hyperaeration and reduced alveolar septa. Wilson and Mikity in 1960 were the first to describe this chronic pulmonary syndrome, in a case report of five very small preterm survivors (Wilson & Mikity, 1960). At that time, assisted ventilation was not used in preterm infants. An additional 29 babies with Wilson–Mikity syndrome (WMS) were identified at the same medical institution in 1969 (Hodgman et al., 1969), and many other cases worldwide.

After the introduction of mechanical ventilation to manage respiratory distress syndrome in the mid-1960s, reports began to appear of radiographic and pathological abnormalities that seemed to result from exposure to high concentrations of oxygen and mechanical ventilation. In 1967, Northway et al. coined the term "bronchopulmonary dysplasia" to describe findings of pulmonary complications following respiratory therapy for hyaline membrane disease (Northway et al., 1967). Northway et al. believed the critical factor to be exposure to an inspired oxygen concentration > 80% for longer than 150 hours.

The 1990s saw major changes in both obstetric and neonatal care for preterm labour, with surfactant administration and assisted ventilation. The outcome of most preterm infants improved in the first half of the decade, particularly for infants with very low birth weight, who benefitted from decreased mortality and morbidity (Horbar et al., 2002). Following these changes, classical BPD, which occurred as a result of injury to the immature lung, became less common. Chronic lung disease in preterm infants became increasingly attributable to the response of the immature lung to early air breathing rather than to damage from barotrauma or oxygen toxicity. In 1999, Jobe described the "new" BPD as occurring in immature infants who did not have extensive lung disease soon after birth (Jobe, 1999). Jobe attributed the "new" BPD to pulmonary anomalies resulting from an inhibition of alveolar and vascular development (Jobe, 1999).

2.2 Clinical definitions

With the change in clinical presentation over time, a variety of definitions of BPD have been used in the literature.

i. **Original criteria for BPD**: A U.S. National Institutes of Health (NIH) workshop held in 1979 proposed to define BPD as a "continued oxygen dependency during the first 28 days plus compatible clinical and radiographic changes" (Natl Inst Health Consens Dev Conf Summ, 1979).
ii. **Traditional definition**: Instead of the original definition, Shennan et al. (1988) suggested a more accurate predictor of BPD to be, "the requirement for additional oxygen at a corrected postnatal gestational age of 36 weeks in infants born with a birth weight of less than 1,500 g". This definition appears to also predict pulmonary outcome among infants with the "new" BPD (Davis et al., 2002).
iii. **Severity definition**: Participants at a joint U.S. National Institute of Child Health & Human Development (NICHD)-National Heart, Lung, and Blood Institute (NHLBI) workshop defined mild, moderate and severe BPD according to both 28 days' and 36 weeks' criteria (Jobe & Bancalari, 2001). Mild BPD was defined as the need for supplemental oxygen at 28 days after birth but not at 36 weeks' postmenstrual age (PMA); moderate BPD, the need for supplemental oxygen at 28 days and at a fraction of inspired oxygen (FiO_2) < 0.30 at 36 weeks' PMA; and severe BPD, the need for supplemental oxygen at 28 days and, at 36 weeks' PMA, the need for mechanical ventilation and/or FiO_2 > 0.30. In a validation study, the NICHD-NHLBI workshop definitions accurately predicted pulmonary outcomes including percent of patients needing treatment with pulmonary medications and rehospitalization for pulmonary causes (Ehrenkranz et al., 2005).
iv. **Physiological definition**: An inherent limitation of all previous definitions is that the need for oxygen is determined by individual physicians rather than on the basis of a physiologic assessment. The assumption that the criteria on which the decision to administer oxygen is uniform and applied similarly across institutions is erroneous because there is no consensus in the literature, neonatologists have widely divergent

practices regarding oxygen-saturation targets. Indeed, published literature cites acceptable saturation ranges from 84% to 98% (Garg et al., 1988; Moyer-Mileur et al., 1996; Sekar & Duke, 1991; Walsh, 2003; Zanardo et al., 1995). Accordingly, the physiological definition determined BPD at 36 weeks of correct age as follows: 1) In all infants treated with mechanical ventilation, continuous positive airway pressure, or supplemental oxygen at $FiO_2 > 0.30$, without additional testing; 2) If the $FiO_2 < 0.30$, infants are to be gradually weaned to room air, in a timed stepwise fashion; those who cannot maintain an $SaO_2 \geq 88\%$ are diagnosed with BPD, unless they pass a timed, continuously monitored oxygen reduction test. An oxygen saturation 80% to 87% for 5 minutes, or < 80% for 1 minute, indicates BPD. If all SaO_2 measurements over 15 minutes ≥ 96%, or if instead, all SaO_2 measurements in a 60-minute period > 88%, the infant is deemed not to have BPD (Walsh et al., 2003).

To evaluate the impact of the physiological definition on BPD rates, 1598 consecutively born preterm infants (birth weight 501–1249 g) in hospital at 36 weeks' PMA were prospectively assessed and assigned an outcome using both the clinical and physiological definitions of BPD. The NICHD neonatal network centers demonstrated that many babies who, according to the nursing staff, required oxygen were able to maintain an $SaO_2 > 90\%$ on room air. Though 560 (35%) had clinical BPD (oxygen use at 36 weeks), only 398 (25%) had physiological BPD (as defined above) (Walsh et al., 2004).

2.3 Structural lung changes

As described by Northway et al. (1967), the histological features of classical BPD included prominent interstitial fibrosis, alveolar overdistention alternating with regions of atelectasis, and airway abnormalities such as squamous metaplasia and excessive muscularization. On the other hand, the "new" BPD shows histological features consistent with developmental arrest and impaired alveolar development (Husain et al., 1998): alveoli are fewer in number and larger in diameter than normal; the fibrosis, squamous metaplasia and excessive airway muscularization seen in classical BPD are conspicuously absent; airway and microvascular growth are affected. A short comparative study by Bhatt et al. (2001) found decreased levels of vascular endothelial growth factor (VEGF) and angiogenic receptors Flt-1 and Tie-2 in infants who died from BPD vs. from other causes. The authors concluded that the lungs from infants with BPD showed abnormal development of alveolar microvessels (abnormal placement in the alveolar septa) and that the capillaries were frequently dilated, changes attributable to low VEGF and associated receptors (Bhatt et al., 2000, 2001). Controls were five children born at term who died at a mean of 3.4 ± 1.3 days, whereas the five BPD subjects were born at 27 ± 2 weeks' gestation, received $FiO_2 > 0.5$ during 37 ± 33 days, and died at 65 ± 34 days.

2.4 Epidemiology

BPD remains the most prevalent and one of the most serious long-term sequelae of preterm birth (Fanaroff et al., 2007). There is considerable variation in reported rates, however, depending upon the centre. Among 4213 infants born in 2003 at 24–31 weeks' gestation in 10 different European regions, the rate of BPD (oxygen requirement at 36 weeks' PMA) was anywhere from 10.5% to 21.5% (Zeitlin et al., 2008).

A 2010 NICHD Neonatal Research Network report on neonatal outcomes of extremely preterm infants assessed 9575 infants born at extremely low gestational ages (22–28 weeks) and very low birth weights (401–1500 g) at network centers between January 1, 2003 and December 31, 2007. Including babies with mild BPD (oxygen therapy for 28 days but use of room air at 36 weeks), the incidence of BPD as determined by the severity-based definition was 68%; traditional definition, 42%; physiologic definition, 40% (Stoll et al., 2010).

2.5 Demographic factors

Factors linked to BPD include: 1) low gestational age at birth (Kraybill et al., 1989; Darlow & Horwood, 1992; Antonucci et al., 2004; Ambalavanan & Novak, 2003), 2) low birth weight (Darlow & Horwood, 1992; Hakulinenet al., 1988; Avery et al., 1987; Ambalavanan et al., 2008), 3) growth restriction (small for gestational age) (Durrmeyer X et al., 2011; Lal Mk et al., 2003; Zeitlin J et al., 2010), 4) male sex (Kraybill et al., 1989; Darlow & Horwood, 1992; Ambalavanan & Novak, 2003; Avery et al., 1987), and 5) white race (Avery et al., 1987; Palta et al., 1991). In a recent cohort, BPD affected 85% of infants born at 22 weeks' gestation vs. 23% of those born at 28 weeks' (Stoll et al., 2010). Furthermore, of the infants affected by BPD in a large American study which included over 9.5 million very low birth weight infants between 1993 and 2006, 59.3% were male while 40.7% were female (male : female ratio = 1.46 : 1) (Stroustrup & Trasande, 2010).

2.6 Impact of perinatal lung injury later in life

Preterm infants with BPD commonly develop impaired health, neurodevelopment, and quality of life later on in childhood. Often noted are: 1) increased risk of postneonatal mortality (Van Marter, 2009), 2) higher rates of rehospitalization (Jeng et al., 2008), 3) long-term pulmonary impairments (Broström et al., 2010) such as asthma (Baraldi et al., 2009) and emphysema (Wong et al., 2008), 4) failure to thrive (Theile et al., 2011), and 5) cognitive impairment (Anderson & Doyle, 2006), cerebral palsy (Koo KY et al 2010; Majnemer et al., 2000), and global neurodevelopmental deficits (Short EJ et al, 2003).

3. The preterm lung: Set-up for injury

Human lung development proceeds in five regulated stages: embryonic (3–7 weeks' gestation), pseudoglandular (7–17 weeks'), canalicular (17–27 weeks'), saccular (28–36 weeks') and alveolar and microvascular maturation (36 weeks' gestation to at least 2 years after birth). The lungs of preterm infants born at 24–28 weeks' gestation are in the late canalicular or early saccular stages and therefore cannot support efficient gas exchange. Branching and expansion of air spaces to form saccules and thinning of mesenchyme occur later in gestation, as do the formation of alveoli and the synthesis of surfactant by type II alveolar cells which only commence in late gestation. Any injury to the lung at the early stages of development can potentially alter the developmental process, leading to long-term pulmonary sequelae (Chakraborty et al., 2010).

Whereas fetal development is predicated on a hypoxic environment, at birth the oxidative load is sharply increased. At the same time, oxygen demands increase abruptly. The baby born at term easily adapts to this transition in most cases but for the preterm infant, the intra- to extra-uterine transition is not without risks. Among the reasons why the preterm infant is more likely to experience oxidative injury than more mature newborns and older children are the following: 1) intracellular defences against oxidative stress are still poorly developed; 2) the preterm infant is often, for various reasons, exposed to high concentrations of supplemental oxygen; and 3) the fetus and premature infant are also susceptible to inflammation and infection that may lead to increased oxidative stress (Saugstad, 2010).

It may therefore be instructive to look at some of the molecules implicated in oxidative stress, while drawing parallels with the corresponding processes in BPD. This added insight will contribute to delimiting specific sources of oxidant molecules that may contribute to the development of BPD, a topic we will explore later in the chapter in relation to BPD risk factors.

4. Oxidative stress

In utero, the arterial pressure of oxygen (PaO_2) is close to 30 mm Hg. After birth, with the baby breathing in ambient air, the PaO_2 rises to 75 mm Hg. This greater oxygen load increases the concentration of dissolved oxygen available for oxidative phosphorylation in the mitochondria, organelles that release 1-3% of oxygen in the form of reactive oxygen species (ROS).

Inspired oxygen (O_2) is a diatomic molecule with two free electrons (•O-O•). This molecule has the highest half-cell reduction potential (E_{hc}) *in vivo* (E_{hc} for the $½O_2/H_2O$ couple = 0.816 V). Consequently, dissolved O_2 readily accepts an electron (•) from donors such as polyunsaturated fatty acids or ascorbic acid, generating the free radical superoxide anion (•O-O•• or $O_2{}^{\bullet -}$). This transformation of O_2 into $O_2{}^{\bullet -}$ is spontaneous, generating the oxidized form of vitamin C (dehydroascorbate, DHA) and/or the by-products of fatty acid oxidation (lipid peroxides, aldehydes such as malondialdehyde or 4-hydroxy-2-nonenal (HNE), or isoprostanes). The reaction may also be catalyzed by nicotinamide adenine dinucleotide phosphate (NADPH) oxidase. Thus, the inspiration of diatomic oxygen leads to an increase in the cellular concentration of free radicals ($O_2{}^{\bullet -}$) as well as free O_2, which will contribute to metabolic regulation by hydroxylation of several biologically active molecules. For instance, O_2 is essential for the degradation of hypoxia-inducible factor-1α (HIF-1α); HIF-1α activates transcription of the gene encoding VEGF, an important growth factor for angiogenesis. This process is impaired in BPD (Husain et al., 1998; Bhatt et al., 2000, 2001). Figure 1 shows a number of oxidative-reduction (redox) reactions of interest.

4.1 Superoxide anion

The dismutation of the superoxide anion ($O_2{}^{\bullet -}$) into O_2 and H_2O_2 (2 •O-O•• + $2H^+$ → •O-O• + H••O-O••H) may be either spontaneous or catalyzed by a superoxide dismutase (SOD). In preterm infants, the pulmonary activity of SOD is suspected to be immature. As reported by Lee Frank in several animal species (mice, hamster, rat, guinea pig), the pulmonary activity of SOD, catalase, and glutathione peroxidase are only 10-15% of that in term babies, in preterm newborns < 32 weeks of human-equivalent gestation (Frank & Sosenko, 1987a, 1987b; Frank, 1991). As a result, the levels of $O_2{}^{\bullet -}$ may be higher in preterm than term neonates. Furthermore, the oxidant property of $O_2{}^{\bullet -}$ is not related to the attraction of an electron from a common antioxidant such as ascorbate, but to the donation of an electron to a free transition metal such as ferric iron (Fe^{3+}) in a Haber-Weiss reaction ($O_2{}^{\bullet -} + Fe^{3+} \rightarrow O_2 + Fe^{2+}$). The resulting ferrous ion (Fe^{2+}) from this reaction reacts rapidly with hydrogen peroxide (H_2O_2) in a Fenton reaction to generate Fe^{3+}, OH^- and •OH. This hydroxyl radical (•OH) is among the most reactive of molecules, leading to the oxidation of proteins, lipids and DNAs. Therefore, high oxygen supplementation coupled with low SOD activity add to oxidative stress, and this may be evidenced by an increase in the by-products of lipid peroxidation (lipid peroxides, malondialdehyde, HNE, alkanes such as ethane and pentane, and isoprostanes) and/or of protein oxidation (carbonyl compounds, o-dityrosine). Newborn infants receiving O_2 supplementation have demonstrably elevated levels of markers of oxidative stress such as exhaled ethane and pentane (Nycyk et al., 1998; Pitkanen et al., 1990), serum HNE (Ogihara et al., 1999), F_{2a}-isoprostanes in tracheal aspirate (Cotton et al., 1996) or in plasma (Ahola et al., 2004), protein-carbonyl in bronchoalveolar fluid (Gladstone & Levine et al., 1994) or o-dityrosine in urine (Kelly & Lubec, 1995; Lubec et al., 1997). It has been suggested that some of these markers may be higher in the first few days of life in preterm infants who will develop BPD as compared to those who will not (Gladstone & Levine et al., 1994; Hodgman et al., 1969). Hence, reducing the $O_2{\bullet^-}$ levels in preterm neonates has been a seductive approach to BPD prevention. Indeed, a randomized study of human recombinant SOD administered intratracheally in the first 24 hours to preterm infants at high risk (birth weight 600-1200g) has been associated with a lower incidence of respiratory illnesses such as wheezing, asthma and pulmonary infections (Davis et al., 1993; Davis et al., 2003).

4.2 Hydrogen peroxide

As noted in Figure 1, H_2O_2 is generated following high oxygen supplementation. Chemically, H_2O_2 is a relatively stable molecule that can diffuse passively through cell membranes. Its oxidation reactions occur in two ways, one by accepting an electron from ferrous iron (Fe^{2+}) to generate the free radical hydroxyl (•OH), the other by oxidizing sulfhydryl or thiol groups (R-SH) on protein. By its high affinity for thiol, H_2O_2 is considered an important player in the regulation of several metabolic pathways (Winterbourn & Hampton, 2008). Of interest to BPD, H_2O_2 can activate nuclear factor kappa B (NF-kB) (Flohé et al., 1997; Haddad, 2002; Haddad & Land, 2000; Takada et al., 2003), upregulating the transcription of genes encoding pro-inflammatory cytokines (Randell et al., 1990). H_2O_2 also contributes to the stability of HIF-1α (Bonello et al., 2007; Chen Y Shi, 2008; Haddad, 2002; López-Lázaro, 2006; Simon, 2006), a transcription factor involved in angiogenesis. It is therefore important that the intracellular level of H_2O_2 be tightly regulated.

The intracellular concentration of H_2O_2 depends on the balance between production from the dismutation of superoxide anions catalyzed by manganese superoxide dismutase (MnSOD) (Buettner et al., 2006), and detoxification by catalase and/or glutathione peroxidase. Catalase has a high catalytic activity but relative low affinity for H_2O_2 (K_m of 1.1 M) (Jones & Suggett, 1968), whereas glutathione peroxidase has a K_m close to 1 μM (Flohéa & Branda, 1969). With the exception of erythrocytes (Gaetani et al., 1996), catalase is present in peroxisomes and mitochondria. Glutathione peroxidase, however, is present in the cytosol, where it is an efficient regulator of the intracellular level of H_2O_2. Reduction of H_2O_2 by glutathione peroxidase implies a conversion of glutathione (GSH) to its disulfide form (GSSG). The cell exerts tight control over the intracellular concentrations of GSH and GSSG in order to maintain the appropriate redox environment for the various cellular processes to occur efficiently. Indeed, the redox potential is a component of the Gibbs free energy equation that predicts the feasibility of a chemical reaction. Several biochemical pathways are dependent on the intracellular redox potential, including NF-κB activation and HIF-1α levels as discussed earlier (Bonello et al., 2007; Chen & Shi, 2008; Haddad et al., 2000; Haddad & Land, 2000; Land & Wilson, 2005; López-Lázaro, 2006; Roy et al., 2008). In the presence of a large peroxide load or sustained generation of peroxides, the formation of GSSG can exceed the capacity of glutathione reductase to recycle it into GSH, and the redox potential will change to a more oxidized state.

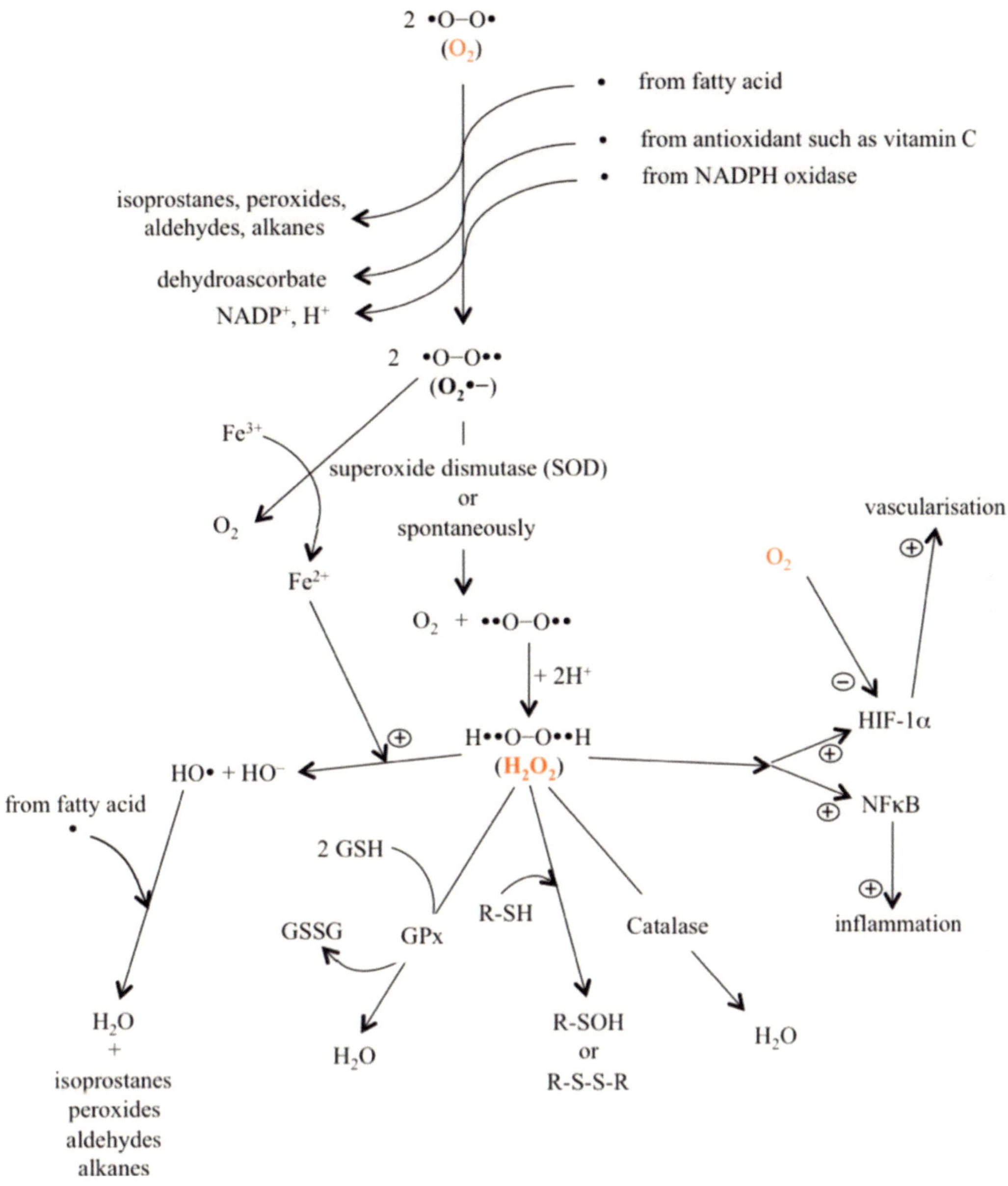

Fig. 1. Relationship between oxidant molecules and endogenous antioxidant defences.

Oxygen (O_2) supplementation as well as hydrogen peroxide (H_2O_2) from parenteral nutrition can lead to modulation of: 1) transcription factors such as hypoxia-inducible factor-1α (HIF-1 α) and nuclear factor kappa B (NF-κB), important players in the pathogenesis of BPD; 2) levels of oxidative stress markers (isoprostanes, peroxides, lipid aldehydes, alkanes); 3) activity of thiol-sensitive proteins (R-SH); and 4) redox potential of glutathione (GSH), as influenced by glutathione peroxidase (GPx) and the intracellular concentrations of reduced (GSH) and oxidized (GSSG) glutathione.

4.3 Redox potential of glutathione

The redox potential is dependent of the concentration of GSH and GSSG according to the Nernst equation: $\Delta E = \Delta E° \cdot (RT/nF) \cdot \log([GSH]^2/[GSSG])$ (Schafer & Buettner, 2001). In cells extracted from the endotracheal aspirate of intubated newborns, the level of glutathione increases with gestational age and female sex, being lower in preterm and male infants (Lavoie & Chessex, 1997). The sex is a significant risk factor for BPD, as BPD affects more boys than girls (Ambalavanan et al., 2008; Ambalavanan & Novak, 2003; Darlow & Horwood, 1992; Kraybill et al., 1989; Stroustrup & Trasande, 2010). The low glutathione concentration measured in preterm newborns (Lavoie & Chessex, 1997) is associated with an oxidized redox potential. Low blood level of glutathione were also reported in preterm neonates with chronic lung disease (White et al., 1994). Recently, Chessex et al. (2010) demonstrated a correlation between BPD severity in preterm infants (26 ± 1 weeks' gestation) and blood redox potential measured one week after birth: the more oxidized the redox potential, more severe the disease.

As previously reported (Schafer & Buettner, 2001), the redox potential acts as a switch for a number of metabolic pathways, inducing cellular proliferation, differentiation or death (apoptosis) (Figure 2). During organ development, cells must pass through the various cell cycle stages in order to allow for continued remodelling. This process is essential to proper lung development (Bruce et al., 1999; Luyet et al., 2000). Consequently, the redox potential must also cycle continuously (Figure 3). The proliferation phase is accompanied by a higher metabolic rate leading to increased generation of ROS. These ROS in turn favour a shift of the redox potential toward a more oxidized status, inducing the differentiation phase. Alternatively, the oxidized status may 1) induce apoptosis, which favours tissue remodelling, and 2) activate redox-sensitive factors inducing the transcription of genes that encode enzymes involved in glutathione synthesis and GSSG recycling (glutathione reductase). This last event will shift the redox potential toward a more reduced state, beginning a new cell cycle.

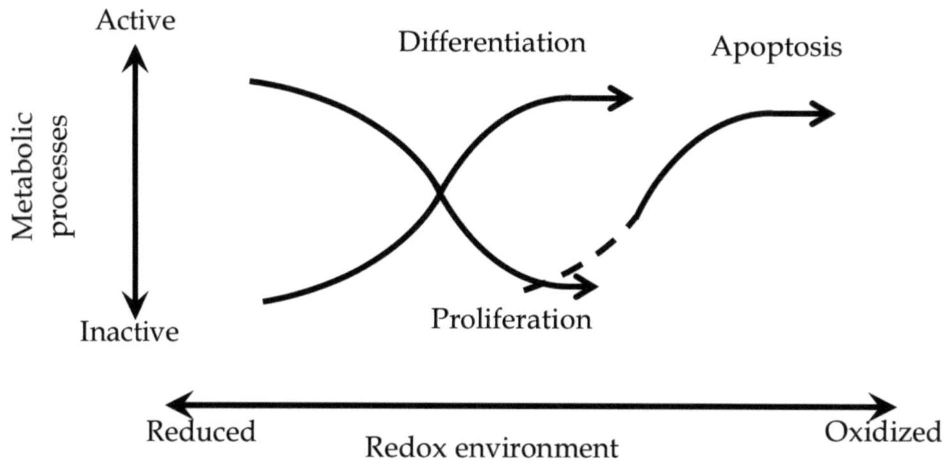

Fig. 2. The redox environment influences metabolic processes.
By modulation from a more reduced to a more oxidized state, the redox environment allows activation and inactivation of various metabolic processes controlling the cell cycle. A reduced state favours cellular proliferation whereas an oxidized state favours differentiation. A more oxidized state will also induce cell death by apoptosis.
(Adapted from Schafer FQ et al., 2001)

The link between redox potential and BPD can be explained by an exacerbated apoptosis rate caused by an abnormally elevated redox potential (Luyet et al., 2000). Lung samples from premature baboons with BPD (Das et al., 2004) showed a large number of apoptotic events. In newborn guinea pigs given parenteral nutrition for 4 days, the alveolar count was 20% lower when the nutritive solution was infused without light protection, peroxide concentration being higher in light-exposed solutions (Section 5.2 below) (Lavoie et al., 2004, 2005, 2008). On histology, 30% of alveolar cells were in an apoptotic state (Lavoie et al., 2004). During normal alveolar development, however, about 10% of cells die by apoptosis (Luyet et al., 2000), in order to thin the septa between alveoli for more efficient gas exchange (Bruce et al., 1999; Luyet et al., 2000).

Various factors may contribute to a shift in redox potential to a more oxidized state (Figure 3, dashed line). An induced or sustained oxidized status favours the apoptosis process, leading to a loss of tissue such as observed in BPD (Das et al., 2004; Lavoie et al., 2004, 2005, 2008). In preterm infants, these factors are oxygen supplementation, parenteral nutrition (containing peroxides), and inflammation.

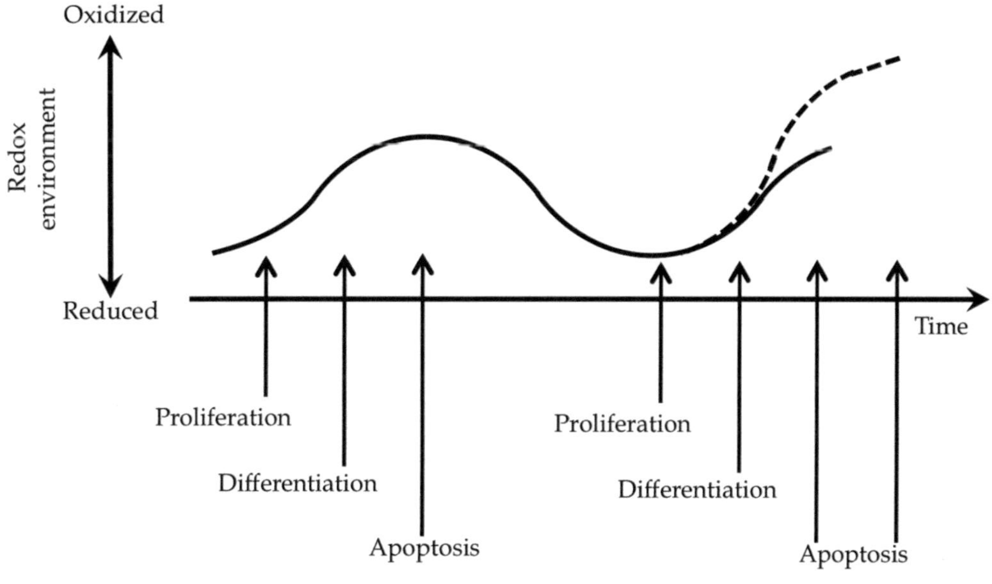

Fig. 3. The redox environment as a function of time.

A normal oscillation of the redox environment occurs over time, between a more reduced and a more oxidized state. As the environmental redox potential changes, pulmonary development is supported by cell proliferation, differentiation, and controlled apoptotic events. An excessively oxidized redox environment, such as that caused by oxidative stress, will favour an apoptotic phase, leading to loss of cells and impaired development.

5. Sources of oxidant molecules in BPD

Oxygen supplementation and parenteral nutrition are exogenous sources of oxidant molecules affecting the preterm neonate. Inflammation, however, is an endogenous source of oxidants and its role is complex. Indeed, inflammation can either be a source or consequence of oxidative stress. In this section, we will analyze each of these sources for their potential role in BPD.

5.1 Oxygen supplementation

Oxygen supplementation increases ROS generation in the lungs. For this reason, and because of the potential effect of oxidative stress on the development of BPD, it has been hypothesized that high O_2 concentration in inspired air is linked to the development of BPD in preterm neonates (Northway et al., 1967). This hypothesis is supported by animal studies. In rats, exposure to 95% O_2 during the first week of life resulted in a 13% reduction in pulmonary alveolar surface area at 40 days (Randell et al., 1990). However, the impact of oxygen has recently been questioned. Although major clinical advances such as the use of surfactant and continuous positive airway pressure (CPAP) have led to a reduction in oxygen supplementation, their impact on lessening the incidence of BPD has been only about 3% per year between 1993 and 2006, for a global reduction of 30% in 13 years (Stroustrup & Trasande, 2010). This relatively weak contribution was confirmed by studies in newborn preterm baboons, where a reduction in the fraction of inspired oxygen (FiO_2) from 80-100% to 21-50% had no significant impact on the levels of fibrosis and alveolar hypoplasia (Coalson et al., 1995, 1999). Similarly, a 2010 study of 1316 human infants born at less than 28 weeks' gestation reported a non-significant effect of ventilation strategy leading to a lower oxygen saturation (85-89% versus 91-95%) on the incidence of BPD (SUPPORT Study Group, 2010). Furthermore, The use of high-dose antioxidants scavenging free radicals (vitamins C and E) did not have any protective effect against alveolar hypoplasia (Berger et al., 1998). Free radicals were therefore not the major player in BPD.
If higher O_2 in inspired air could lead to a greater cellular concentration of H_2O_2 that is not quenched by vitamins C or E, the apparently weak effect of oxygen supplementation on BPD development must be explainable by another source of oxidant molecules masking the impact of O_2. It is noteworthy that the major risk factor for BPD is gestational age; the lower the age, the greater the incidence of BPD. Coincidentally, the more premature the infant, the greater is his dependence on parenteral nutrition. A 2011 study showed that preterm infants developing BPD received more parenteral than enteral nutrition (Wemhöner et al., 2011). In the various studies on BPD, including those in baboons, the gestation ages of the subjects were such that the infants likely required parenteral nutritive support, a major source of ROS and particularly of H_2O_2 (Laborie et al., 1998; Lavoie et al., 1997). In itself, parenteral nutrition may be sufficient to induce the development of BPD. In fact, however, it is highly probable that both parenteral nutrition and oxygen supplementation induce oxidative stress, by both increasing the intracellular concentration of H_2O_2 and modifying the redox potential of glutathione (Chessex et al., 2010).

5.2 Parenteral nutrition

Parenteral nutrition consists of the intravenous administration of a solution containing amino acids, dextrose, electrolytes, vitamins and lipids. Parenteral nutrition is essential for the nutritional support of the preterm infant, bypassing a gastrointestinal system whose immaturity severely limits the natural feeding process. Although parenteral nutrition is sufficient to support growth in the child, the instability of the nutrients in solution favours the generation of undesirable molecules. The admixture of redox-sensitive elements such as amino acids (tryptophan, tyrosine and others), polyunsaturated fatty acids, and vitamin C, in the presence of a strong oxidizing molecule such as dissolved oxygen, will induce oxidation of the nutrients and the formation of their consequent derivatives. For instance, peroxidation of omega-6 polyunsaturated fatty acids will yield lipid hydroperoxides and HNE (Massarenti et al., 2004; Silvers et al., 2001), while vitamin C and dissolved oxygen will produce H_2O_2 (Laborie et al., 1998; Lavoie et al., 1997). As vitamin C is the most powerful antioxidant found in parenteral nutrition, the main source of peroxides in parenteral nutrition would appear to be the multivitamin preparation (Laborie et al., 1998; Lavoie et al., 1997). Furthermore, this solution contains riboflavin, a photosensitive molecule. In the presence of light, photoexcited riboflavin catalyzes a peroxide-producing reaction (Laborie et al., 1998). The simple act of adequately shielding parenteral nutrition solutions from ambient light halved the concentration of peroxides in the infused solution (Chessex et al., 2001; Laborie et al., 1998, 1999, 2000; Lavoie et al., 1997, 2007) as well as in the urine of preterm infants (Bassiouny et al., 2009; Chessex et al., 2001). Adequate photoprotection of parenteral nutrition has also been reported to reduce the incidence of chronic lung disease (Bassiouny et al., 2009) or BPD (Chessex et al., 2007) in premature infants.

As administered in neonatal units, without adequate photoprotection, parenteral nutritive solutions are contaminated with several molecules having the potential to perturb the redox status of the lung, i.e. lipid hydroperoxides (Silvers et al., 2001), HNE (personal communication of Lavoie JC, 2011), ascorbylperoxide (Lavoie et al., 2004; Maghdessian et al., 2010), and H_2O_2 (Laborie et al., 1998; Lavoie et al., 1997; Silvers et al., 2001). All these molecules are detoxified by the glutathione system. Since glutathione levels are low in preterm infants (Lavoie & Chessex, 1997), these molecules can conceivably overwhelm the glutathione system, allowing the redox potential to shift toward an oxidized state. Infusion of parenteral nutrition without light protection for 4 days in newborn guinea pigs was associated with: 1) a loss of glutathione (Lavoie et al., 2000), 2) a more oxidized glutathione redox potential (Lavoie et al., 2008), and 3) a lower alveolar count (Lavoie et al., 2004, 2005, 2008), as compared to animals infused with a fully photoprotected solution. A recent study demonstrated that the blood glutathione redox potential measured in 7-day-old preterm infants (26 ± 1 weeks' gestation) was correlated with the severity of BPD; a more oxidized status was measured in the most severe cases (Chessex et al., 2010). Therefore, current knowledge suggests that each oxidant molecule affecting the glutathione system, whether from oxygen supplementation or from parenteral nutrition, may contribute to the development of BPD.

5.3 Inflammation

The third major risk factor for BPD is inflammation, a significant source of ROS (Federico et al., 2007; Pereda et al., 2006). Several pro-inflammatory cytokines have been detected in aspirated fluids from infants with BPD, the concentration increasing as a function of assisted ventilation duration and level of oxygen supplementation (Bose et al., 2008). As previously demonstrated, exposure to high amounts of O_2 favours the production of H_2O_2, a known activator of transcription factor NF-κB (Flohé et al., 1997; Haddad, 2002; Haddad & Land, 2000; Takada et al., 2003), which in turn upregulates the expression of several pro-inflammatory cytokine genes (Federico et al., 2007; Pereda et al., 2006). The oxygen-cytokine connection was further supported by research showing that oxygen supplementation induced an inflammatory response in preterm infants (Lavoie et al., 2010). The association between BPD and inflammation may therefore be explained by an initial oxidative stress followed by a local increase in H_2O_2 concentration. However, other researchers have argued that an inflammatory process independent of the variation in inspired oxygen concentration could also induce BPD, for example chorioamnionitis (Gien & Kinsella, 2011). Paananen R et al (2009) reported that elevated plasma concentrations of IL-6, a pro-inflammatory cytokine, and IL-10, an anti-inflammatory cytokine, on the first day of life were indicative of greater BPD risk, independently of previous exposure to chorioamnionitis (39% of the 128 preterm neonates in the cohort had had chorioamnionitis; incidence of BPD in cohort, 25%). The lack of correlation between an initial inflammatory process and BPD development was confirmed in 2010 in a study investigating the association between chorioamnionitis and BPD (Prendergast, et al., 2010). From the 71 preterm infants developing BPD, 41 had been exposed to chorioamnionitis and/or funisitis. Their results, however, showed a significant correlation between the severity of BPD and gestational age or birth weight. Thus, endogenous infection does not seem to be connected to the development of BPD while cytokines are, underlining a possible implication of oxidative stress early in life.

6. Strategies for prevention/treatment

Under the hypothesis that glutathione, by its very involvement in the cellular redox environment, could be a key player in BPD development, one strategy to prevent BPD development or reduce its severity would be to preserve or increase the intracellular concentration of glutathione. It is noteworthy that the low levels of glutathione observed in preterm infants (Lavoie & Chessex, 1997) are not due to a defective enzymatic process. Indeed, GSH synthesis is very active, even in newborns of 26 weeks' gestation (Lavoie & Chessex, 1998). The defect comes rather from the immaturity of the cellular transport system of cysteine (Lavoie et al., 2002), an amino acid whose low intracellular availability limits the synthesis of glutathione (Deneke & Fanburg, 1989). This fact may explain the failure of intravenous administration of N-acetylcysteine to prevent the development of BPD in extremely low birth weight newborns (Ahola et al., 2003).

If it is difficult to increase the intracellular concentration of glutathione, one must at least prevent its consumption by reducing oxidative stress. This can be partly achieved by monitoring blood oxygen saturation levels to prevent excessive oxygen supplementation. Prevention of inflammation will help as well. However, limiting peroxide contamination in parenteral nutrition is essential. Though photoprotection of the solution may be difficult to institute in the clinical setting, the process must be initiated in the pharmacy department at the time of compounding and continued until bedside. New nutritive strategies leading to improvements in the nutritive quality of parenteral products, reducing the oxidation of nutrients and preventing the generation of oxidant molecules, will have a positive impact on the incidence of BPD.

7. Conclusions/perspectives

Presently, no therapy exists for BPD (Gien & Kinsella, 2011) and its prevention is difficult. The etiology is multifactorial. This chapter focused on the part played by oxidative stress, in particular the glutathione redox potential. While a number of oxidant sources can contribute to the shift in redox potential toward a more oxidized state, several BPD-related factors were found to have an impact, among them oxygen supplementation, parenteral nutrition, and inflammation. Modification of even one of these factors may decrease the incidence of BPD, but the best practice remains to administer a combination of new measures, as suggested by Geary C et al. (2008), including early use of surfactant and nasal continuous positive airway pressure for ventilatory support, as well as lowered oxygen saturation targets and better nutritive support. It is remarkable that all associations between biochemical markers and BPD have been observed with parameters measured in the first days of life (Ahola et al., 2004; Geary et al., 2008; Gladstone & Levine, 1994; Lavoie et al., 2008; Ogihara et al., 1999; Pitkanen et al., 1990; Welty, 2001). The first week of life, in both infants and animal models, seems be a critical window during which all efforts to reduce oxidative stress must be pursued.

8. Acknowledgements

The authors are grateful to Danielle Buch, medical writer/editor at the Applied Clinical Research Unit of the Sainte-Justine Research Centre, for editing of this chapter.

9. References

Ahola T, Lapatto R, Raivio KO, Selander B, Stigson L, Jonsson B, Jonsbo F, Esberg G, Stôvring S, Kjartansson S, Stiris T, Lossius K, Virkola K, Fellman V. 2003. N-acetylcysteine does not prevent bronchopulmonary dysplasia in immature infants: a randomized controlled trial. J Pediatr 143:713-719.

Ahola T, Fellman V, Kjellemer I, Raivio KO, Lapatto R. 2004. Plasma 8-Isoprostane Is Increased in Preterm Infants Who Develop Bronchopulmonary Dysplasia or Periventricular Leukomalacia. Pediatr Res 56: 88–93.

Ambalavanan N, Novak ZE. 2003. Peptide Growth Factors in Tracheal Aspirates of Mechanically Ventilated Preterm Neonates. Pediatr Res 53: 240–244.

Ambalavanan N, Van Meurs KP, Perritt R, Carlo WA, Ehrenkranz RA, Stevenson DK, Lemons JA, Poole WK, Higgins RD; NICHD Neonatal Research Network, Bethesda, MD. 2008. Predictors of death or bronchopulmonary dysplasia in preterm infants with respiratory failure. J Perinatol 28:420-426.

Anderson PJ, Doyle LW. 2006. Neurodevelopmental outcome of bronchopulmonary dysplasia. Semin Perinatol 30:227-232.

Antonucci R, Contu P, Porcella A, Atzeni C, Chiappe S. 2004. Intrauterine smoke exposure: a new risk factor for bronchopulmonary dysplasia? J Perinat Med 32:272-277.

Avery ME, Tooley WH, Keller JB, Hurd SS, Bryan MH, Cotton RB, Epstein MF, Fitzhardinge PM, Hansen CB, Hansen TN, et al. 1987. Is chronic lung disease in low birth weight infants preventable? A survey of eight centers. Pediatrics 79:26-30.

Baraldi E, Carraro S, Filippone M. 2009. Bronchopulmonary dysplasia: definitions and long-term respiratory outcome. Early Hum Dev 85:S1-S3.

Bassiouny MR, Almarsafawy H, bdel-Hady H, Nasef N, Hammad TA, Aly H. 2009. A randomized controlled trial on parenteral nutrition, oxidative stress, and chronic lung diseases in preterm infants. J Pediatr Gastroenterol Nutr 48:363-369.

Behrman RE, Babson GS, Lessel R. 1971. Fetal and neonatal mortality in white middle class infants. Mortality risks by gestational age and weight. Am J Dis Child 121:486-489.

Berger TM, Frei B, Rifai N, Avery ME, Suh J, Yoder BA, et al. 1998. Early high dose antioxidant vitamins do not prevent bronchopulmonary dysplasia in premature baboons exposed to prolonged hyperoxia: a pilot study. Pediatr Res 43:719-726.

Bhatt AJ, Pryhuber GS, Huyck H, Watkins RH, Metlay LA, Maniscalco WM. 2001. Disrupted Pulmonary Vasculature and Decreased Vascular Endothelial Growth Factor, Flt-1, and TIE-2 in Human Infants Dying with Bronchopulmonary Dysplasia. Am J respir Crit Care Med 164:1971-1980.

Bhatt AJ, Amin SB, Chess PR, Watkins RH, Maniscalco WM. 2000. Expression of Vascular Endothelial Growth Factor and Flk-1 in Developing and Glucocorticoid-Treated Mouse Lung. Pediatr Res 47 :606-613.

Bonello S, Zähringer C, BelAiba RS, Djordjevic T, Hess J, Michiels C, KietzmannT , Görlach A. 2007. Reactive Oxygen Species Activate the HIF-1α Promoter Via a Functional NFκB Site. Arterioscler Thromb Vasc Biol 27:755-761.

Bose CL, Dammann CEL, Laughon MM. 2008. Bronchopulmonary dysplasia and inflammatory biomarkers in the premature neonate. Arch Dis Child Fetal Neonatal Ed 93:F455-F461.

Broström EB, Thunqvist P, Adenfelt G, Borling E, Katz-Salamon M. 2010. Obstructive lung disease in children with mild to severe BPD. Respir Med 104:362-370.

Bruce MC, Honaker CE and Cross RJ. 1999. Lung fibroblasts undergo apoptosis following alveolarization. Am J Respir Cell Mol Biol 20:228-236.

Buettner GR, Ng CF, Wang M, Rodgers VG, Schafer FQ. 2006. A new paradigm: manganese superoxide dismutase influences the production of H2O2 in cells and thereby their biological state. Free Radic Biol Med 41:1338-1350.

Chakraborty M, McGreal EP, Kotecha S. 2010. Acute lung injury in preterm newborn infants: mechanisms and management. Paediatr Respir Rev 11:162-170.

Chen H, Shi H. 2008. A reducing environment stabilizes HIF-2α in SH-SY5Y cells under hypoxic conditions. FEBS Lett 582:3899–3902.

Chessex P, Laborie S, Lavoie JC, Rouleau T. 2001. Photoprotection of solutions of parenteral nutrition decreases the infused load as well as the urinary excretion of peroxides in premature infants. Semin Perinatol 25:55-59.

Chessex P, Harrison A, Khashu M, Lavoie JC. 2007. In preterm neonates, is the risk of developing bronchopulmonary dysplasia influenced by the failure to protect total parenteral nutrition from exposure to ambient light? J Pediatr 151:213-214.

Chessex P, Watson C, Kaczala G, Rouleau T, Lavoie ME, Friel J, Lavoie JC. 2010. Determinants of oxidant stress in extremely low birth weight premature infants. Free Radic Biol Med 49:1380-6.

Coalson JJ, Winter V, DeLemos RA. 1995. Decreased alveolarization in baboon survivors with bronchopulmonary dysplasia. Am J Respir Crit Care Med 152:640-646.

Coalson JJ, Winter VT, Siler-Khodr T, Yoder BA. 1999. Neonatal chronic lung disease in extremely immature baboons. Am J Respir Crit Care Med 160:1333-1346.

Cotton RB, Morrow JD, Hazinski TA, Roberts LJ, Law AB, Steele S. 1996. F2-isoprostanes (F2-I) in tracheobronchial aspirate fluid (TBAF) indicate association between increased Fi02 and lipid peroxidation in the lungs of premature infants. *Pediatr Res* 39: 329A.

Darlow BA, Horwood LJ. 1992. Chronic lung disease in very low birthweight infants: a prospective population-based study. J Paediatr Child Health 28:301-305.

Das KC, Ravi D, Holland W. 2004. Increased apoptosis and expression of p21 and p53 in premature infant baboon model of bronchopulmonary dysplasia. Antioxid Redox Signal 6:109-116.

Davis JM, Rosenfeld WN, Sanders RJ, et al. 1993. Prophylactic effects of recombinant human superoxide dismutase in neonatal lung injury. J Appl Physiol 74:2234–2241.

Davis PG, Thorpe K, Roberts R, Schmidt B, Doyle LW, Kirpalani H, Trial of Indomethacin Prophylaxis in Preterms (TIPP) Investigators. 2002. Evaluating "old" definitions for the "new" bronchopulmonary dysplasia. J Pediatr 140:555-560.

Davis JM, Parad RB, Michele T, et al. 2003. Pulmonary outcome at one year corrected age in premature infants treated at birth with recombinant CuZn superoxide dismutase. Pediatrics 111:469–476.

Deneke SM, Fanburg BL. 1989. Regulation of cellular glutathione. Am J Physiol 257:L163-L173.

Durrmeyer X, Kayem G, Sinico M, Dassieu G, Danan C, Decobert F. 2011. Perinatal Risk Factors for Bronchopulmonary Dysplasia in Extremely Low Gestational Age Infants: A Pregnancy Disorder-Based Approach. J Pediatr Oct 31. [Epub ahead of print]

Egreteau L, Pauchard JY, Semama DS, Matis J, Liska A, Romeo B, Cneude F, Hamon I, Truffert P. 2001. Chronic oxygen dependency in infants born at less than 32 weeks' gestation: incidence and risk factors. Pediatrics 108:E26.

Ehrenkranz RA, Walsh MC, Vohr BR, Jobe AH, Wright LL, Fanaroff AA, Wrage LA, Poole K. 2005. Validation of the National Institutes of Health Consensus Definition of Bronchopulmonary Dysplasia. Pediatrics 116:1353–1360.

Fanaroff AA, Stoll BJ, Wright LL, et al; NICHD Neonatal Research Network. 2007. Trends in neonatal morbidity and mortality for very low birthweight infants. Am J Obstet Gynecol 196: 147.e1-8.

Federico A, Morgillo F, Tuccillo C, Ciardiello F, Loguercio C. 2007. Chronic inflammation and oxidative stress in human carcinogenesis. Int J Cancer 121:2381–2386.

Flohéa L, Branda I. 1969. Kinetics of glutathione peroxidase. Biochim Biophys Acta (BBA) – Enzymology 191:541-549.

Flohé L, Brigelius-Flohé R, Saliou C, Traber MG, Packer L. 1997. Redox regulation of NF-kappa B activation. Free Radic Biol Med 22:1115-1126.

Frank L, Sosenko IR. 1987a. Prenatal development of lung antioxidant enzymes in four species. J Pediatr 110:106-110.

Frank L, Sosenko IR. 1987b. Development of lung antioxidant enzyme system in late gestation: possible implications for the prematurely born infant. J Pediatr 110:9-14.

Frank L. 1991. Developmental aspects of experimental pulmonary oxygen toxicity. Free Radic Biol Med 11:463-494.

Gaetani GF, Ferraris AM, Rolfo M, Mangerini R, Arena S, Kirkman HN. 1996. Predominant role of catalase in the disposal of hydrogen peroxide within human érythrocytes. Blood 87:1595-1599.

Garg M, Kurzner SI, Bautista DB, Keens TG. 1988. Clinically unsuspected hypoxia during sleep and feeding in infants with bronchopulmonary dysplasia. Pediatrics 81:635-642.

Geary C, Caskey M, Fonseca R, Malloy M. 2008. Decreased incidence of bronchopulmonary dysplasia after early management changes, including surfactant and nasal continuous positive airway pressure treatment at delivery, lowered oxygen saturation goals, and early amino acid administration: a historical cohort study. Pediatrics 121:89-96.

Gien J, Kinsella JP. 2011. Pathogenesis and treatment of bronchopulmonary dysplasia. Current Opinion in Pediatrics 23:305–313.

Gladstone IM, Levine RL. 1994. Oxidation of proteins in neonatal lungs. Pediatrics 93:764-768.

Haddad JJ. 2002. Oxygen-sensing mechanisms and the regulation of redox-responsive transcription factors in development and pathophysiology. Respir Res 3:26.

Haddad JJE, Land SC. 2000. O2-evoked regulation of HIF-1a and NF-kB in périnatal lung epithelium requires glutathione biosynthesis. Am J Physiol Lung Cell Mol Physiol 278:L492-L503.

Haddad JJE, Olver RE, Land SC. 2000. Antioxidant/Pro-oxidant Equilibrium Regulates HIF-1α and NF-κB Redox Sensitivity. Evidence For Inhibition By Glutathione Oxidation In Alveolar Epithelial Cells J Biol Chem 275:21130-21139.

Hakulinen A, Heinonen K, Jokela V, Kiekara O. 1988. Occurrence, predictive factors and associated morbidity of bronchopulmonary dysplasia in a preterm birth cohort. J Perinat Med 16:437-446.

Hodgman JE, Mikity VG, Tatter D, Cleland RS. 1969. Chronic respiratory distress in the premature infant. Wilson-Mikity syndrome. Pediatrics 44:179-195.

Horbar JD, Badger GJ, Carpenter JH, Fanaroff AA, Kilpatrick S, LaCorte M, Phibbs R, Soll RF; Members of the Vermont Oxford Network. 2002. Trends in mortality and morbidity for very low birth weight infants, 1991-1999. Pediatrics 110:143-151.

Husain AN, Siddiqui NH, Stocker JT. 1998. Pathology of arrested acinar development in postsurfactant bronchopulmonary dysplasia. Hum Pathol 29:710-717.

Jeng SF, Hsu CH, Tsao PN, Chou HC, Lee WT, Kao HA, Hung HY, Chang JH, Chiu NC, Hsieh WS. 2008. Bronchopulmonary dysplasia predicts adverse developmental and clinical outcomes in very-low-birthweight infants. Dev Med Child Neurol 50:51-57.

Jobe AH. 1999. The New BPD: An Arrest of Lung Development. Pediatr Res 46:641-643.

Jobe AH, Bancalari E. 2001. Bronchopulmonary Dysplasia. Am J Respir Crit Care Med 163:1723–1729.

Jones P, Suggett A. 1968. The Catalase-Hydrogen Peroxide System. Kinetics Of Catalatic Action At High Substrate Concentrations. Biochem J 110 :617-620.

Kelly FJ, Lubec G. 1995. Hyperoxic injury of immature guinea pig lung is mediated via hydroxyl radicals. *Pediatr Res* 38: 786-791.

Kraybill EN, Runyan DK, Bose CL, Khan JH. 1989. Risk factors for chronic lung disease in infants with birth weights of 751 to 1000 grams. J Pediatr 115:115-120.

Koo KY, Kim JE, Lee SM, Namgung R, Park MS, Park KI, Lee C. 2010. Effect of severe neonatal morbidities on long term outcome in extremely low birth weight infants. Korean J Pediatr 53:694-700.

Laborie S, Lavoie JC, Chessex P. 1998. Paradoxical role of ascorbic acid and riboflavin in solutions of total parenteral nutrition: implication in photoinduced peroxide generation. Pediatr Res 43:601-606.

Laborie S, Lavoie JC, Pineault M, Chessex P. 1999. Protecting solutions of parenteral nutrition from peroxidation. JPEN J Parenter Enteral Nutr 23:104-108.

Laborie S, Lavoie JC, Pineault M, Chessex P. 2000. Contribution of multivitamins, air, and light in the generation of peroxides in adult and neonatal parenteral nutrition solutions. Ann Pharmacother 34:440-445.

Lal MK, Manktelow BN, Draper ES and Field DJ. 2003. Chronic lung disease of prematurity and intrauterine growth retardation: a population-based study. Pediatrics 111:483–487.

Land SC, Wilson SM. 2005. Redox Regulation of Lung Development and Perinatal Lung Epithelial Function. Antioxidants & Redox Signaling 7:92-107.

Lavoie JC, Belanger S, Spalinger M, Chessex P. 1997. Admixture of a multivitamin preparation to parenteral nutrition: the major contributor to in vitro generation of peroxides. Pediatrics 99:E6.

Lavoie JC, Chessex P. 1997. Gender and maturation affect glutathione status in human neonatal tissues. Free Radic Biol Med 23:648-657.

Lavoie JC, Chessex P. 1998. Development of glutathione synthesis and gamma-glutamyltranspeptidase activities in tissues from newborn infants. Free Radic Biol Med 24:994-1001.

Lavoie JC, Laborie S, Rouleau T, Spalinger M, Chessex P. 2000. Peroxide-like oxidant response in lungs of newborn guinea pigs following the parenteral infusion of a multivitamin preparation. Biochem Pharmacol 60 :1297-1303.

Lavoie JC, Rouleau T, Truttmann AC, Chessex P. 2002. Postnatal gender-dependent maturation of cellular cysteine uptake. Free Radic Res 36:811-817.

Lavoie JC, Chessex P, Rouleau T, Migneault D, Comte B. 2004. Light-induced byproducts of vitamin C in multivitamin solutions. Clin Chem 50:135-140.

Lavoie JC, Rouleau T, Chessex P. 2004. Interaction between ascorbate and light-exposed riboflavin induces lung remodelling. J Pharm Exp Ther 311: 634-639.

Lavoie JC, Rouleau T, Chessex P. 2005. Effect of coadministration of parenteral multivitamins with the lipid emulsion on lung remodeling in an animal model of TPN. Pediatr Pulmonol 40:53-56.

Lavoie JC, Rouleau T, Tsopmo A, Friel J, Chessex P. 2007. Influence of lung oxidant and antioxidant status on alveolarization: role of light-exposed TPN. Free Radic Biol Med 45:572-577.

Lavoie JC, Rouleau T, Tsopmo A, Friel J, Chessex P. 2008. Influence of lung oxidant and antioxidant status on alveolarization: role of light-exposed total parenteral nutrition. Free Radic Biol Med 45:572-577.

Lavoie P, Lavoie JC, Watson C, Rouleau T, Chang BA, Chessex P. 2010. Inflammatory response in preterm infants is induced early in life by oxygen and modulated by TPN. Pediatr Res 68:248-51.

López-Lázaro M. 2006. HIF-1: hypoxia-inducible factor or dysoxia-inducible factor? FASEB J 20:828–832.

Lubec G, Widness JA, Hayde M, Menzel D, Pollack A. 1997. Hydroxyl radical generation in oxygen treated infants. Pediatrics 100: 200-204.

Luyet C, Burri PH and Schittny JC. 2000. Pre- and postnatal lung development, maturation, and plasticity. Suppression of cell proliferation and programmed cell death by dexamethasone during postnatal lung development. Am. J Physiol Lung Cell Mol Physiol 282:L477-L483.

Maghdessian R, Cote F, Rouleau T, Ouadda AB, Levy E, Lavoie JC. 2010. Ascorbylperoxide contaminating parenteral nutrition perturbs the lipid metabolism in newborn guinea pig. J Pharmacol Exp Ther 334:278-284.

Majnemer A, Riley P, Shevell M, Birnbaum R, Greenstone H, Coates AL. 2000. Severe bronchopulmonary dysplasia increases risk for later neurological and motor sequelae in preterm survivors. Dev Med Child Neurol. 42:53-60.

Massarenti P, Biasi F, de FA, Pauletto D, Rocca G, Silli B, et al. 2004. 4-Hydroxynonenal is markedly higher in patients on a standard long-term home parenteral nutrition. Free Radic Res 38:73-80.

Moyer-Mileur LJ, Nielson DW, Pfeffer KD, Witte MK, Chapman DL. 1996. Eliminating sleep-associated hypoxemia improves growth in infants with bronchopulmonary dysplasia. Pediatrics 98:779-783.

Natl Inst Health Consens Dev Conf Summ. 1979. Antenatal diagnosis. Sponsored by the National Institute of Child Health and Human Development 2:11-15.

Northway WH Jr, Rosan RC, Porter DY. 1967. Pulmonary disease following respirator therapy of hyaline-membrane disease. Bronchopulmonary dysplasia. N Engl J Med 276:357-368.

Nycyk JA, Drury JA, Cooke RWI. 1998. Breath pentane as a marker for lipid peroxidation and adverse outcome in preterm infants. Arch Dis Child Fetal Neonatal Ed 79: F67–F69.

Ogihara T, Hirano K, Morinobu T, Kim HS, Hiroi M, Ogihara H, Tamai H. 1999. Raised concentration of aldehyde lipid peroxidation products in premature infants with chronic lung disease. Arch Dis Child Fetal Neonatal Ed 80: F21–F25.

Paananen R, Husa AK, Vuolteenaho R, et al. 2009. Blood cytokines during the perinatal period in very preterm infants: relationship of inflammatory response and bronchopulmonary dysplasia. J Pediatr 154:39–43.

Palta M, Gabbert D, Weinstein MR, Peters ME. 1991. Multivariate assessment of traditional risk factors for chronic lung disease in very low birth weight neonates. The Newborn Lung Project. J Pediatr. 119:285-292.

Pereda J, Sabater L, Aparisi L, Escobar J, Sandoval J, Viña J, López-Rodas G, Sastre J. 2006. Interaction between cytokines and oxidative stress in acute pancreatitis. Curr Med Chem 13:2775-2787.

Pitkanen OM, Hallman M, Andersson SM. 1990. Correlation of free oxygen radical-induced lipid peroxidation with outcome in very low birthweight infants. J Pediatr 116: 760-764.

Prendergast M, May C, Broughton S, Pollina E, Milner AD, Rafferty GF, Greenough A. 2010. Chorioamnionitis, lung function and bronchopulmonary dysplasia in prematurely born infants. Arch Dis Child Fetal Neonatal Ed 96:F270-F274.

Randell SH, Mercer RR, Young SL. 1990. Neonatal hyperoxia alters the pulmonary alveolar and capillary structure of 40-day-old rats. Am J Pathol 136:1259-1266.

Roy S, Khanna S, Sen CK. 2008. Redox regulation of the VEGF signaling path and tissue vascularization: Hydrogen peroxide, the common link between physical exercise and cutaneous wound Healing. Free Radic Biol Med 44:180-192.

Saugstad OD. 2010. Oxygen and oxidative stress in bronchopulmonary dysplasia. J Perinat Med 38:571-577.

Schafer FQ, Buettner GR. 2001. Redox environment of the cell as viewed through the redox state of the glutathione disulfide/glutathionne couple. *Free Radic Biol Med* 30:1191–1212

Sekar KC, Duke JC. 1991. Sleep apnea and hypoxemia in recently weaned premature infants with and without bronchopulmonary dysplasia. Pediatr Pulmonol 10:112-116.

Shennan AT, Dunn MS, Ohlsson A, Lennox K, Hoskins EM. 1988. Abnormal pulmonary outcomes in premature infants: prediction from oxygen requirement in the neonatal period. Pediatrics 82:527-523.

Short EJ, Klein NK, Lewis BA, Fulton S, Eisengart S, Kercsmar C, Baley J, Singer LT. 2003. Cognitive and academic consequences of bronchopulmonary dysplasia and very low birth weight: 8-year-old outcomes. Pediatrics 112:e359.

Silvers KM, Darlow BA, Winterbourn CC. 2001. Lipid peroxide and hydrogen peroxide formation in parenteral nutrition solutions containing multivitamins. JPEN J Parenter Enteral Nutr 25, 14-17.

Simon MC. 2006. Mitochondrial reactive oxygen species are required for hypoxic HIF alphastabilization. Adv Exp Med Biol 588:165-170.

Stoll BJ, Hansen NI, Bell EF, Shankaran S, Laptook AR, Walsh MC, hale EC, Newman NS, Schibler K, Carlo WA, Kennedy KA, Poindexter BB, Finer NN, Ehrenkranz RA, Duara S, Sanchez PJ, O'Shea M, Goldberg RN, Van Meurs KP, Faix RG, Phelps DL, Freantz ID, Watterberg KL, Saha S, Das A, Higgins RD, Eunice Kennedy Shriver National Institute of Child Health and Human Development Neonatal Research Network. 2010. Neonatal Outcomes of Extremely Preterm Infants From the NICHD NeonatalResearch Network. Pediatrics 126;443-456.

Stroustrup A, Trasande L. 2010. Epidemiological Characteristics and Resource Use in Neonates With Bronchopulmonary Dysplasia: 1993 -2006. Pediatrics 126:e291–e297.

SUPPORT Study Group of the Eunice Kennedy Shriver NICHD Neonatal Research Network, Finer NN, Carlo WA, Walsh MC, Rich W, Gantz MG, et al. 2010. Early CPAP versus surfactant in extremely preterm infants. N Engl J Med 362:1970-1979.

Takada Y, Mukhopadhyay A, Kundu GC, Mahabeleshwar GH, Singh S, Aggarwal BB. 2003. Hydrogen peroxide activates NF-kappa B through tyrosine phosphorylation of I kappa B alpha and serine phosphorylation of p65: evidence for the involvement of I kappa B alpha kinase and Syk protein-tyrosine kinase. J Biol Chem 278:24233-24241.

Theile AR, Radmacher PG, Anschutz TW, Davis DW, Adamkin DH. 2011. Nutritional strategies and growth in extremely low birth weight infants with bronchopulmonary dysplasia over the past 10 years. J Perinatol May 26 [Epub ahead of print].

Van Marter LJ. 2009. Epidemiology of bronchopulmonary dysplasia. Semin Fetal Neonatal Med. 14:358-366.

Walsh MC, Wilson-Costello D, Zadell A, Newman N, Fanaroff A. 2003. Safety, Reliability, and Validity of a Physiologic Definition of Bronchopulmonary Dysplasia. J Perinatology 23, 451–456.

Walsh MC, Yao Q, Gettner P, Hale E, Collins M, Hensman A, Everette R, Peters N, Miller N, Muran G, Auten K, Newman N, Rowan G, Grisby C, Arnell K, Miller L, Ball B,

McDavid G; National Institute of Child Health and Human Development Neonatal Research Network, 2004. Impact of a Physiologic Definition on Bronchopulmonary Dysplasia Rates. Pediatrics 114:1305–1311.

Welty SE. 2001. Is There a Role for Antioxidant Therapy in Bronchopulmonary Dysplasia? J. Nutr 131: 947S–950S.

Wemhöner A, Ortner D, Tschirch E, Strasak A, Rüdiger M. 2011. Nutrition of preterm infants in relation to bronchopulmonary dysplasia. BMC Pulmonary Medicine 11:7.

White CW, Stabler SP, Allen RH, Moreland S, Rosenberg AA. 1994. Plasma cysteine concentrations in infants with respiratory distress. J Pediatr 125:769-777.

Wilson MG, Mikity VG. 1960. A new form of respiratory disease in premature infants. AMA J Dis Child 99:489-499.

Winterbourn CC, Hampton MB. 2008. Thiol chemistry and specificity in redox signaling. Free Radic Biol Med 45:549-561.

Wong PM, Lees AN, Louw J, Lee FY, French N, Gain K, Murray CP, Wilson A, Chambers DC. 2008. Emphysema in young adult survivors of moderate-to-severe bronchopulmonary dysplasia. Eur Respir J 32:321-328.

Zanardo V, Trevisanuto D, Dani C, Bottos M, Guglielmi A, Cantarutti F. 1995. Oxygen saturation in premature neonates with bronchopulmonary dysplasia in a hammock. Biol Neonate 67:54-58.

Zeitlin J, Draper ES, Kollée L, Milligan D, Boerch K, Agostino R, Gortner L, Van Reempts P, Chabernaud JL, Gadzinowski J, Bréart G, Papiernik E; MOSAIC research group. 2008. Differences in rates and short-term outcome of live births before 32 weeks of gestation in Europe in 2003: results from the MOSAIC cohort. Pediatrics 121:e936-e944.

23

Partial Liquid Ventilation in the Extremely Preterm Infant: Potential Benefits and Harms

Mark William Davies
Grantley Stable Neonatal Unit, Royal Brisbane & Women's Hospital
Department of Paediatrics and Child Health, University of Queensland
Australia

1. Introduction

Preterm infants, especially the extremely preterm, require a large amount of support *ex utero*. They are often critically ill with greatly reduced chances of survival. Many die because of their overall immaturity with multiple organ systems that cannot adjust to extrauterine life, especially the lungs. Many die from their primary lung disease. The respiratory support they get from positive pressure ventilation almost always causes significant secondary lung injury.

Over the previous decades partial liquid ventilation has been put forward as an adjunct form of respiratory support for especially immature lungs and severe lung disease: not only to provide a superior form of respiratory support but to deliver that support with reduced lung injury. Recent studies have renewed the hope that partial liquid ventilation has great potential to change the course of neonatal lung disease and respiratory morbidity. (Blassnig, 2009)

Unfortunately, the extremely preterm infant is also at great risk of particular forms of brain injury (e.g., intraventricular haemorrhage, periventricular leucomalacia and other white matter injury). Disturbance of cerebral blood flow has been demonstrated to considerably increase the risk of these forms of brain injury.

One of the concerns with using partial liquid ventilation in the extremely preterm infant is its affect on cerebral blood flow which could lead to brain injury, especially at the start of partial liquid ventilation during the initial dosing of perfluorocarbon into the lungs. Any benefits of partial liquid ventilation might be outweighed by an increased risk of brain injury and the subsequent devastating consequences.

Before using partial liquid ventilation in human preterm infants it should be known to be safe with regard to its effects on cerebral blood flow during perfluorocarbon dosing. The effect of perfluorocarbon dosing at the start of partial liquid ventilation on cerebral blood flow can be mitigated to minimise or eliminate these adverse effects.

2. The consequences of lung disease in the extremely preterm neonate

2.1 Mortality

The extremely preterm infant, born at less than 26 weeks gestational age, is at great risk of dying. The risk increases with decreasing gestational age. The majority of these infants die because of general immaturity (including extremely immature lungs) or lung disease.

Data are available from Australia and New Zealand. All babies that are admitted to a newborn nursery who were born at less than 32 completed weeks gestation, or weighed <1,500 grams at birth, or received assisted ventilation (mechanical ventilation), or received major surgery are registered with the Australian and New Zealand Neonatal Network (ANZNN). The ANZNN reports annually on all registered babies. (ANZNN, 2009) The latest report of the ANZNN (ANZNN, 2009) is for births in 2006; of 339,271 live births there were 7,592 registered babies (2.2% of live births). There were 412 registered babies born at <26 weeks gestational age (5.4% of registered babies). Two thirds (276/412) survived to be discharged home - a mortality of 33%.

The EPICure study (Wood, 2000) is a large population based study designed to reveal outcomes for extremely preterm infants. They enrolled all babies born at less than 26 weeks gestational age, from March 1995 to December 1995, who were admitted to a neonatal intensive care unit in the United Kingdom of Great Britain and Northern Ireland and the Republic of Ireland. These infants are deemed to be extremely immature and at the limits of viability. About sixty percent (60%) of these infants died before discharge from hospital and about 70% of those deaths had a respiratory cause. (Costeloe, 2000) In an Australian study from around the same period (1992-1996) at the Royal Women's Hospital in Melbourne, about 28% of live born infants of 23 to 27 weeks gestational age died. Of those infants admitted to the intensive care nursery 60% of deaths had a respiratory cause. (Doyle, 1999)

Recent data are available from the Royal Brisbane and Women's Hospital in Brisbane, Australia. From 2003-2007 inclusive there were 163 infants admitted of less than 26 weeks gestational age: 58 (36%) died. Sixty-two percent (62%) of those deaths were either due to 'extreme prematurity' or a direct respiratory cause. (Cartwright, 2003; Cartwright, 2004; Cartwright, 2005; Cartwright, 2006; Cartwright, 2007)

2.2 Respiratory morbidity

Lung immaturity and/or lung disease not only carries a high mortality in extremely preterm babies, but it also causes significant morbidity. This includes the requirement for respiratory support, air leak and neonatal chronic lung disease. Mechanical ventilation often causes significant secondary lung injury due to barotrauma and volutrauma. This makes the acute lung disease much worse and, along with extreme prematurity, is a major factor in the subsequent progression to chronic lung disease. Neonatal chronic lung disease consists of distortion of the lung architecture, disturbed lung growth and chronic inflammation of the small airways and the lung parenchyma. Most patients with neonatal chronic lung disease are born extremely preterm. Infants with chronic lung disease have significant morbidity which manifests as a requirement for prolonged respiratory support and oxygen therapy, as well as an increased hospital stay. Chronic lung disease is also a major cause of late mortality.

Many extremely preterm infants need mechanical ventilation. About ninety percent (90%) of ANZNN registered babies in 2006 required some form of assisted ventilation. (ANZNN, 2009) The mean length of time of assisted ventilation was 11 days. Most babies required respiratory support for either hyaline membrane disease or non-specific respiratory distress. Intubation and positive pressure mechanical ventilation was required by ninety-seven percent (97%) of babies born <26 weeks gestation. The most extreme form of acute lung injury in ventilated neonates is air leak (pneumothorax, pulmonary interstitial emphysema, pneumomediastinum); it occurred in eight percent (8%) of infants <26 weeks gestational age.

The ANZNN defines chronic lung disease as any registered baby born less than 32 weeks gestational age who needs assisted ventilation for their initial lung disease and continues to require some form of respiratory support or oxygen therapy at 36 weeks corrected gestational age. Of babies born less than 26 weeks gestational age, who survived to 36 weeks corrected gestational age, 55% had chronic lung disease. Four percent (4%) of surviving registered babies born less than 32 weeks gestational age required prolonged oxygen therapy and went home on oxygen treatment. (ANZNN, 2009)

Local data from the Royal Brisbane and Women's Hospital (Cartwright, 2003; Cartwright, 2004; Cartwright, 2005; Cartwright, 2006; Cartwright, 2007) from 2003 to 2007 inclusive for 163 infants admitted of less than 26 weeks gestational age showed that:

- 99% were intubated and ventilated;
- the mean length of time of ventilation was 36 days (2001-2007 data only);
- 27% had an air leak;
- 74% had chronic lung disease; and
- 16% went home on oxygen treatment.

Three quarters (74%) of the EPICure cohort (Hennessy, 2008) had moderate to severe chronic lung disease; 36% went home on oxygen treatment. By two years of age almost two thirds of the cohort required hospital admission at least once for a respiratory illness. At six years many of the cohort had continuing respiratory symptoms, abnormal respiratory findings on physical examination and/or abnormal respiratory function tests.

2.3 Non-respiratory morbidity

Non-respiratory morbidity is very common in extremely preterm infants. This includes a number of different organ systems. The major morbidities include patent ductus arteriosus, necrotising enterocolitis, retinopathy of prematurity, intraventricular haemorrhage and periventricular leucomalacia.

Extremely preterm infants that survive also require a prolonged hospital stay (even when this is not because of respiratory disease). The long-term sequelae of extreme prematurity can include adverse neurodevelopmental outcomes such as developmental delay, cognitive and learning impairment, cerebral palsy, blindness and deafness.

Local data from the Royal Brisbane and Women's Hospital from 2003 to 2007 inclusive (Cartwright, 2003; Cartwright, 2004; Cartwright, 2005; Cartwright, 2006; Cartwright, 2007) shows that of the 163 infants admitted of less than 26 weeks gestational age:

- 61% had a patent ductus arteriosus;
- 46% had an intraventricular haemorrhage and/or periventricular leucomalacia;
- 16% had a severe intraventricular haemorrhage;
- 57% had retinopathy of prematurity (20% had severe retinopathy of prematurity); and
- the average length of stay in hospital was 127 days.

2.4 Mechanical ventilation

The management of lung disease in extreme preterm infants is predicate on the principle that respiratory support be provided until there is sufficient resolution of the lung disease and respiratory support is no longer required. Mechanical ventilation is a means of providing such support for babies with severe lung disease or extreme prematurity. Ventilation is provided to support gas exchange, i.e., oxygenation and carbon dioxide clearance.

The types of mechanical ventilation include-

1. Conventional mechanical ventilation - pressure controlled, time-cycled ventilation, including:
   - intermittent positive pressure ventilation;
   - synchronised intermittent positive pressure ventilation;
   - volume-targeted ventilation.
2. High frequency ventilation.
3. Volume-controlled ventilation - rarely used in neonates.

As can be seen from the above data the more usual forms of mechanical ventilation often don't work (babies still die from their extremely immature lungs and lung disease) and often damage the lungs causing significant respiratory morbidity (lung injury and subsequent chronic lung disease).

There is still a need for alternative forms of respiratory support that can provide ventilation and adequate gas exchange without damaging the lungs or put the infant at increased risk of brain injury.

3. The risk of brain injury in the extremely preterm infant

The developing brain is especially prone to injury and extremely preterm infants are at significant risk; this can result in long-term disability. (Vohr, 1996) The most common forms of brain injury arising in preterm infants are intraventricular haemorrhage, periventricular leukomalacia and other forms of white matter injury. Disturbance of cerebral blood flow have been demonstrated to substantially increase the risk of brain injury.

The germinal matrix lies in the subependymal region at the floor of the lateral ventricle and this is the site of intraventricular haemorrhage. It is especially prone to both under perfusion and over perfusion. The vascular structure of this region predisposes to damage from ischaemia and later reperfusion and/or over perfusion with subsequent venous haemorrhage. (Takashima, 2009) With severe grades of intraventricular haemorrhage there is additional haemorrhage in the periventricular white matter; both focal injury and more diffuse white matter injury. The white matter is especially susceptible because of the vulnerability of the glia (especially premyelinating oligodendrocytes) which is gestational age dependant. Also the periventricular area has a blood supply which is immature and watershed. The white matter is also particularly prone to hypoperfusion. (Takashima, 2009; Volpe, 2009a; Volpe, 2009b)

Given the vulnerability of the brain of the extremely preterm infant to both under and over perfusion it is not surprising that fluctuations of cerebral blood flow cause the most overt types of brain injury. (Ballabh, 2010; Perlman, 2009) Factors that lead to low cerebral blood flow also increase the risk of intraventricular haemorrhage and similarly those factors that lead to increased cerebral blood flow also increaese the risk of intraventricular haemorrhage. (Bassan, 2006) Periventricular leucomalacia can be easily produced in animal models of cerebral ischaemia. (Yoshioka, 1994; Ohyua, 1999)

Increased cerebral blood flow velocity increases the incidence of intraventricular haemorrhage and extension of existing intraventricular haemorrhage. (Van Bel, 1987) Low cerebral blood flow states increase the risk of intraventricular haemorrhage. (Kluckow 2000; du Plessis, 2008) The strongest link exists with the development of intraventricular haemorrhage and more variability in cerebral blood flow. (Vohr, 1996; Van Bel, 1987; Mullaart; 1994, Kissack, 2004; Perlman, 1983; Takashima 1995) In the beagle pup model

rapid changes in cerebral perfusion easily produce subependymal haemorrhages indistinguishable from those seen in human preterm infants. (Ment, 1982) Keeping cerebral blood flow fluctuations to a minimum must be a prime aim when caring for extremely preterm infants to prevent intraventricular haemorrhage. (du Plessis, 2008; Wells, 1995)
There are many factors that are known to alter cerebral blood flow in newborn infants (see Table 1). Because the preterm infant is more likely to have all the conditions listed in the left hand column of Table 1 it is not unreasonable to presume that fluctuations in cerebral blood flow are common particularly in the first few days of life. The preterm infant may also experience wide variations in cerebral blood flow because they do not have the normal autoregulation of cerebral blood flow. Thus periods of pressure-passive cerebral circulation are likely; the fluctuations in blood pressure that are common (Coughtrey, 1997) expose them to the extremes of cerebral blood flow and put them at risk of intraventricular haemorrhage. (du Plessis, 2008)

Factor	Effect
Cerebral perfusion pressure - arterial BP - venous pressure	**increased** perfusion pressure **increases** CBF … and vice versa - **increased** arterial pressure **increases** CBF … and vice versa - **decreased** venous pressure **increases** CBF … and vice versa
$PaCO_2$	**increased** $PaCO_2$ **increases** CBF … and vice versa
PaO_2	**increased** PaO_2 **increases** CBF … and vice versa
Patent ductus arteriosus	PDA with Left-to-Right shunt **decreases** diastolic flow which **decreases** CBF
Hypoglycaemia	**decreased** blood glucose **increases** CBF
Haemoglobin/blood viscosity	**increased** viscosity **decreases** CBF … and vice versa
Posthypoxic-ischaemic injury	vaso-dilatation **increases** CBF
Brain metabolism/activity	**increased** activity **increases** CBF … and vice versa
Autonomic nervous system	**increased** parasympathetic drive **increases** CBF … and vice versa **decreased** sympathetic drive **increases** CBF … and vice versa
Temperature	mild-moderate hyperthermia **increases** CBF hypothermia **decreases** CBF

Table 1. Factors known to alter cerebral blood flow. (Perlman, 2009; Pryds, 1996; Ito, 2005; Vavilala, 2002; Greisen, 2005; Volpe, 1982; Leahy, 1980; Rahilly, 1980) (CBF - cerebral blood flow; BP - blood pressure; CVP - central venous pressure; $PaCO_2$ - arterial carbon dioxide; PaO_2 - arterial oxygen; PDA - patent ductus arteriosus)

Many of the mechanisms listed in Table 1 put the extremely preterm infant at serious risk of significant cerebral blood flow alterations and intraventricular haemorrhage. Many respiratory problems or treatments are known to alter cerebral blood flow and/or increase the risk of intraventricular haemorrhage. These include:

- intratracheal surfactant instillation (has been shown to increase or decrease cerebral blood flow velocity on Doppler ultrasound (Schipper, 1997; Saliba, 1994; Kaiser, 2004);

- asynchronous breathing mechanical ventilation (increases the variability of cerebral blood flow (Rennie, 1987);
- endotracheal tube suction (has been shown to increase or decrease cerebral blood flow on near infrared spectroscopy (Limperopoulos, 2008;, Perlman, 1983; Kohlhauser, 2000);
- endotracheal tube retaping increases cerebral blood flow on near infrared spectroscopy (Limperopoulos, 2008);
- pneumothorax increases cerebral blood flow velocity on Doppler ultrasound, and increases the incidence of intraventricular haemorrhage. (Hill, 1982; Mehrabani, 1991)

The alterations in cerebral blood flow during the administration surfactant are of particular concern because surfactant administration is comparable to the intratracheal administration of perfluorocarbon when starting partial liquid ventilation. Any perfluorocarbon administration effects on cerebral blood flow may increase the risk of brain injury in the extremely preterm infant.

4. Liquid ventilation

Extremely preterm infants with immature lungs and severe lung disease could benefit greatly from alternative forms of respiratory support. New techniques are required because conventional forms of mechanical ventilation often don't work (babies still die from their extremely immature lungs and lung disease) and often damage the lungs causing significant respiratory morbidity (lung injury and subsequent chronic lung disease).
Liquid ventilation has been touted as an alternative form of respiratory support for numerous and varied types of lung disease. Extremely preterm infants with immature lungs and severe lung disease could benefit greatly from the technique of partial liquid ventilation. Recent studies have renewed the promise that partial liquid ventilation has significant potential to alter the course of neonatal lung disease and respiratory morbidity. (Blassnig, 2009)

4.1 History

Artificial respiration using liquid ventilation in mammals was initially tried in mice in the 1960s with solutions of saline in a hyperbaric environment. (Kylstra, 1962) Later experiments in the 1960s showed the successful use of fluorocarbons at atmospheric pressure for liquid ventilation in mice and cats. (Clark, 1966) At first experiments with perfluorocarbons were performed with immersion in perfluorocarbon liquid with spontaneously breathing animals or with gravity-assist bulk tidal flow of perfluorocarbon liquid. These techniques were not successful at removing sufficient carbon dioxide. (Kylstra, 1966; Schoenfish, 1973; Shaffer, 1978) Over the ensuing decades the use of time-cycled, pressure-limited mechanical ventilators allowed the development of the method of total liquid ventilation. (Shaffer, 1975) Total liquid ventilation can maintain adequate gas exchange in animals. (Wolfson, 1990) It has also been shown to improve lung function and gas exchange in experimental animal models of respiratory distress. (Shaffer, 1976; Shaffer, 1984; Shaffer, 1983; Wolfson, 1992) In 1991 Fuhrman *et al.* (Fuhrman, 1991) introduced the method of perfluorocarbon associated gas exchange using functional residual capacity volumes of perfluorocarbon with conventional gas ventilation. This technique is now best known as partial liquid ventilation and it is this technique which is most promising for practical clinical application.

4.2 Partial liquid ventilation

The technique of partial liquid ventilation entails pouring perfluorocarbon liquid into the endotracheal tube whilst ventilating the lung with gas ventilation (either conventional or high-frequency) continues. Customarily the starting volume of perfluorocarbon instilled into the lungs equals the estimated functional residual capacity and the perfluorocarbon is usually given slowly over 10 to 20 minutes. Repeated doses of perfluorocarbon are then given at intervals to keep a fluid level in the endotracheal tube at a positive end expiratory pressure (PEEP) of zero. Repeat doses are necessary because the functional residual capacity will increase as the liquid recruits collapsed alveoli, and to replace losses due to evaporation. Stopping partial liquid ventilation is achieved by ceasing further instillation of perfluorocarbon to allow it to evaporate into the expired gases. The technique is the same when used with high-frequency ventilation.

Perfluorocarbon liquids are a group of chemicals that are formed from the fluorination of organic compounds such as alkanes. They are odourless and colourless, and are chemically and biologically inert. Perfluorocarbons are almost insoluble in lipid and insoluble in water. They are more dense than water and soft tissue. Perfluorocarbon liquids can dissolve more than 20 times the oxygen, and three times the carbon dioxide, than water. They have a low surface tension and low viscosity, and most evaporate faster than water. (Shaffer, 1992; Degraeuwe, 1995)

The physical characteristics of perfluorocarbon liquids (see Table 2) determine the effects of partial liquid ventilation (Figure 1). During normal breathing and gas ventilation the inert gas nitrogen carries oxygen and carbon dioxide. During liquid ventilation perfluorocarbon replaces nitrogen as the carrier of oxygen and carbon dioxide. Perfluorocarbon liquids have a high oxygen carrying capacity and high solubility for carbon dioxide. (Shaffer, 1992; Meaney, 1997) The perfluorocarbon liquid is oxygenated and carbon dioxide removed by means of bulk tidal flow of gas provided by the gas ventilator. This occurs for either conventional or high frequency ventilation. The movement of perfluorocarbon in small peripheral airways is facilitated by its low viscosity.

The surface tension of perfluorocarbon liquids is low, (Shaffer, 1992) at around 15 to 18 millinewton per metre (mN/m). When the perfluorocarbon liquids goes into the lung the air/liquid alveolar interface (which in surfactant deficiency has a high surface tension of up to 50 mN/m (von Bismarck, 2007)) is abolished and surface tension decreases. This increases compliance and therefore alveolar recruitment improves. This allows the use of lower ventilator pressures and smaller tidal volumes; with reduction of barotrauma and volu-trauma respectively. Perfluorocarbons do not disturb natural surfactant production (Cleary, 1997) and they do not wash surfactant out of the lungs. (Rüfer, 1970; Modell, 1970)

Compared to water and soft tissue perfluorocarbon liquids have a high density (Shaffer, 1992) and will therefore mechanically recruit collapsed alveoli. This happens preferentially in the dependant portions of the lung therefore decreasing intra-pulmonary shunting by improving ventilation/perfusion matching. (Kelly, 1997)

Partial liquid ventilation has been known to have some anti-inflammatory effects. These were thought to be due mainly to the less injurious nature of liquid ventilation. However, it is now clear that perfluorocarbons have some direct anti-inflammatory action on cells (such as alveolar macrophages). Also this direct anti-inflammatory effect goes further than the perfluorocarbons acting as a simple barrier. (Heard, 2000) There is direct inhibition of the inflammatory response of alveolar macrophages in contact with perfluorocarbon liquids. (Smith, 1995; Thomassen, 1997) A recent study has shown that the disruption of lung development in newborn rats, caused by hyperoxia, can be prevented by a single daily dose of perfluorocarbon liquid into the lungs. (Blassnig, 2009)

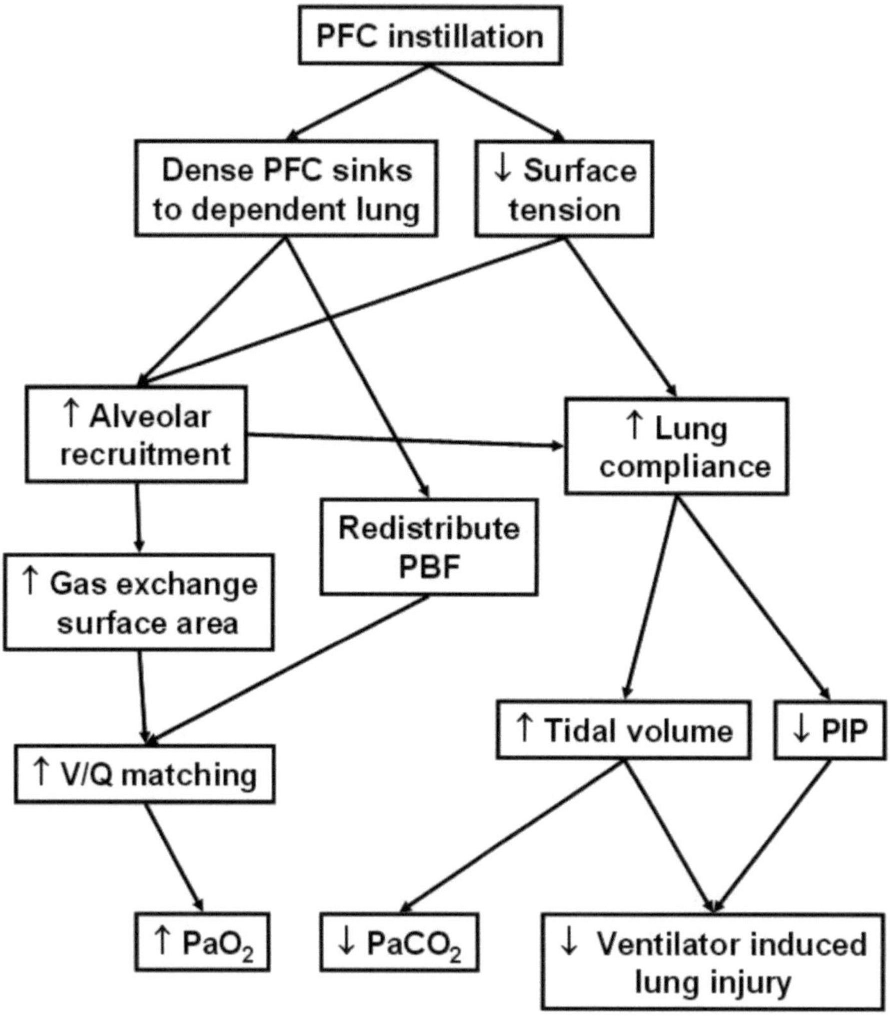

Fig. 1. The mechanical effects of partial liquid ventilation on respiratory function. (Davies, 2011) ($PaCO_2$ – arterial carbon dioxide; PaO_2 – arterial oxygen; PBF – pulmonary blood flow; PFC – perfluorocarbon; PIP – peak inspiratory pressure; Q – perfusion; V –ventilation)

4.3 Animal studies

Partial liquid ventilation has been touted as an alternative form of respiratory support for many types of lung disease because it improves gas exchange and lung function in the diseased and injured lung. Many animal studies using various models of lung injury and surfactant lack have shown improvement in oxygenation, carbon dioxide clearance and lung compliance. (Foust, 1996; Tutuncu, 1993; Smith, 1997a; Leach, 1993; Leach, 1995; Curtis, 1994a; Curtis, 1994b) Partial liquid ventilation is more effective in improving gas exchange and lung function than surfactant alone. (Leach, 1995) There is significantly less damage on

lung histology to lungs after partial liquid ventilation. (Foust, 1996; Smith, 1997a) Lower peak inspiratory pressures can be used to achieve adequate tidal volumes. (Degraeuwe, 1996) Partial liquid ventilation decreases intra-pulmonary shunting. (Zobel, 1996) Partial liquid ventilation increases oxygenation when combined with nitric oxide when treating pulmonary hypertension. (Zobel, 1996)
Most of the above studies have shown benefits of partial liquid ventilation over a few hours. Two studies have shown that it is feasible to use partial liquid ventilation for longer periods. Neonatal piglets with normal lungs have been ventilated for 24 hours with stable ventilation and blood gases with no haemodynamic deterioration. (Salman, 1995) Newborn piglets with surfactant deficiency demonstrated improved oxygenation and lung histology with up to 20 hours of partial liquid ventilation. (Smith, 1997a)

	Saline	**FC-77**	**Perflubron**
Density (g/mL)*	1.0	1.78	1.93
Kinematic viscosity (centistokes)*	1.0	0.8	1.10
Vapour pressure (mmHg)†	47	85	11
Surface tension (mN/m)*	72	15	18
Oxygen solubility (mL/100 mL)*	3.0	50	53
Carbon dioxide solubility (mL/100 mL) †	57	198	210

Table 2. Physical properties of two perfluorocarbon liquids compared with saline. (* 25°C; †37°C)

Partial liquid ventilation has also been used with high frequency ventilation. Animal studies investigating the effects of partial liquid ventilation with high frequency ventilation have shown the combined technique provides good gas exchange. (Smith, 1997a; Baden, 1997, Mrozek, 1998; Smith, 1997b; Sukumar, 1998) Smith *et al.* (Smith, 1997b) comparing various methods of high frequency partial liquid ventilation, showed that those forms of high frequency ventilation which allow volume recruiting manoeuvres, such as the addition of intermittent conventional breaths, gave superior gas exchange. It seems that, with the use of strategies aimed at maximal alveolar recruitment, high frequency partial liquid ventilation may not confer any additional benefit over high frequency ventilation alone. Davies *et al.* (Davies, 1999) demonstrated that if maximal recruitment is obtained with high frequency ventilation prior to starting high frequency partial liquid ventilation that the addition of partial liquid ventilation did not further improve oxygenation.

4.4 Human studies

4.4.1 Adult

A Cochrane systematic review (Davies, 2004a) of partial liquid ventilation in adults with acute lung injury and acute respiratory distress syndrome found one randomised, controlled trial. (Hirschl, 2002) Another randomised, controlled trial has since been published. (Kacmarek, 2006) There were no differences, in either study, in any clinically relevant outcomes in patients ventilated with partial liquid ventilation compared with conventional ventilation.

4.4.2 Paediatric

The Cochrane systematic review (Davies, 2004b), updated in 2009, of partial liquid ventilation in children with acute lung injury and acute respiratory distress syndrome found only one randomised, controlled trial as yet unpublished. (Fuhrman, 1998) This trial abstract report showed results from a clinical trial that was stopped early on paediatric acute respiratory distress syndrome (ARDS). The protocol underwent a number of changes during the trial which resulted in three different sets of inclusion criteria. The final set, with liberalised inclusion criteria, had an unexpected decrease in mortality in the control group so the trial was stopped to allow full data analysis to determine the safety of partial liquid ventilation in this group of patients. There were 182 patients enrolled (less than 20% of the target numbers) with an overall mortality of 24/91 (26%) in the partial liquid ventilation group and 18/91 (20%) in the conventional mechanical ventilation group. The authors concluded that partial liquid ventilation with perflubron was safe, however the trial was not powered to detect real differences in mortality and ventilator free days.

4.4.3 Neonatal

There have been several published reports of uncontrolled studies on the use of partial liquid ventilation in human neonates. (Meaney, 1997; Greenspan, 1989; Hirschl, 1995; Pranikoff, 1996; Garver, 1996; Leach, 1996; Bruch, 1997)

Pranikoff *et al.* (Pranikoff, 1996) reported the use of partial liquid ventilation in four infants with congenital diaphragmatic hernia, all of whom were on extra-corporeal life support at the time. There was improved oxygenation and total lung compliance with haemodynamic stability and no acute adverse effects.

Leach *et al.* (Leach, 1996) reported the use of partial liquid ventilation in 13 preterm infants from 24–33 weeks gestational age who had severe respiratory distress syndrome and failing conventional therapy. Ten infants had from 24 to 72 hours of partial liquid ventilation with improvement in oxygenation and lung compliance. Six of the 10 survived to 36 weeks corrected age. The partial liquid ventilation reportedly well tolerated without significant haemodynamic disturbance.

Two randomised controlled trials have been started in newborn infants but both were stopped before reaching their targeted numbers. Both remain unpublished. Hirschl wrote in a review on liquid ventilation of a randomised, controlled trial comparing conventional mechanical ventilation with partial liquid ventilation in preterm infants with severe lung disease. (Hirschl, 2004) Twenty-four patients were recruited to the study: 8 of 13 (62%) in the partial liquid ventilation group survived and all in the conventional ventilation group survived. Hirschl wrote that "This study was placed on hold concomitant with discontinuation of the paediatric trial and has not been resumed." (Hirschl, 2004) In another review Field wrote of a randomised, controlled trial where partial liquid ventilation was used in mature infants with respiratory failure; he wrote that "Twenty-four subjects were randomized before recruitment was unexpectedly and inexplicably suspended. The results have never been published." (Field, 2002)

5. Perfluorocarbon liquid instillation and the effect on cerebral blood flow

As discussed above one of the concerns with the use of partial liquid ventilation in extremely preterm infants is its possible effect on cerebral blood flow and the potential to cause brain injury, especially during the initial dosing of perfluorocarbon into the lungs at the start of partial liquid ventilation. It may well be that any of the benefits of partial liquid ventilation are outweighed by an increase in the risk of brain injury.

Davies et al (Davies, 2010a; Davies, 2010b) studied the effects of perfluorocarbon dosing, when initiating partial liquid ventilation, on haemodynamics and cortical cerebral blood flow in preterm lambs. They showed that compared with preterm lambs continuing to be ventilated with conventional gas mechanical ventilation, lambs that received a dose of tracheal perfluorocarbon liquid at the start of partial liquid ventilation had an increase in their cortical cerebral blood flow. This could not be reasonably explained by any related changes in haemodynamics or oxygenation. The lambs that had 30 mL/kg of tracheal perfluorocarbon had a minimal increase in arterial carbon dioxide over the 30 minute observation period, although arterial carbon dioxide was not measured continuously and the difference was not statistically significant. Overall, three different loading doses of perfluorocarbon liquid were studied: 20, 30 and 40 mL/kg. (Davies, 2010a; Davies, 2010b) There were no significant haemodynamic changes during perfluorocarbon dosing in any of the three different doses in preterm lambs; and whilst the cortical cerebral blood flow was increased in all three groups there was no difference between groups.

Davies (Davies, 2011) reported further studies in a rabbit model designed to investigate the effects of different dosing strategies on cerebral blood flow. These studies confirmed that when the dose of perfluorocarbon was given into the trachea at the start of partial liquid ventilation cerebral blood flow increased. The cerebral blood flow increased regardless of the volume of the dose of perfluorocarbon; either 10 or 20 mL/kg. Furthermore, if the arterial carbon dioxide was closely monitored and the ventilation adjusted to maintain target arterial carbon dioxide, or volume-controlled ventilation was used, then there was no increase in cerebral blood flow. There was no significant advantage in varying the duration of administration of the dose of perfluorocarbon within the range from 10 to 20 minutes, although it is probably best to avoid giving the dose over 5 minutes or less. There was no benefit in giving the dose of perfluorocarbon through a secondary lumen at the distal tip of the endotracheal tube. With differences in cerebral blood flow there were also differences in some of the variables that may explain these differences. There were no statistically significant differences seen in arterial carbon dioxide. Although, on the two occasions where the differences in arterial carbon dioxide were almost statistically significant there were significant differences in either carotid flow or cortical cerebral blood flow or both. On one of those occasions the differences in pH were statistically significant and the changes in arterial carbon dioxide mirrored changes in pH, as would be usual. There were associations between increasing cerebral blood flow (or its variability) and factors measured that might explain those increases. In those situations where cerebral blood flow were increased there were also consistent increases in blood pressure and arterial carbon dioxide, and decreases in arterial oxygen. The increases in arterial carbon dioxide were associated with decreases in tidal volumes delivered during perfluorocarbon dosing. The most compelling reason that it was simply decreased tidal volumes that caused increased arterial carbon dioxide was that during those dosing strategies where the tidal volumes did not decrease (when using volume-controlled ventilation or closely targeting arterial carbon dioxide by adjusting peak inspiratory pressure) the arterial carbon dioxide did not increase.

Burkhardt et al (Burkhardt, 2002) report the only other study that investigated the effects of perfluorocarbon dosing on surrogate measures of cerebral blood flow: cerebral concentration of total and oxygenated haemoglobin using near infrared spectroscopy. The cerebral concentration of oxygenated haemoglobin decreased initially (at 1 minute) when 30 mL/kg was given extremely rapidly (over about 40 seconds), with return to baseline by 3 min and an increase after 5 min. There was no decrease with 30 mL/kg given slowly (over about 16 minutes) nor when 10 mL/kg was administered. The cerebral concentration of oxygenated haemoglobin and the total cerebral haemoglobin concentration increased when 30 mL/kg of perfluorocarbon was given but not with 10 mL/kg. Similarly in both 30 mL/kg groups the arterial carbon dioxide increased and arterial oxygen decreased but not in the 10 mL/kg group. There was no control group, therefore conclusions cannot be drawn about the effect of perfluorocarbon dosing compared with gas ventilation alone. The study design makes direct comparisons between the two volumes of perfluorocarbon given difficult because the doses were also given over different durations. Interpretation is also difficult as they did not measure cerebral blood flow directly, did not record and report real-time haemodynamic variables during the perfluorocarbon liquid dosing, and only reported changes in cerebral oxygenation at discrete time points. Burkhardt et al (Burkhardt, 2002) concluded that giving perfluorocarbon extremely rapidly (20-30 times faster than the fastest dosing studied by Davies (Davies, 2011)) is not recommended because of the decrease in cerebral blood flow (as determined by total cerebral haemoglobin concentration) during perfluorocarbon dosing.

From the results of the above studies we can surmise that perfluorocarbon should best be administered whilst either monitoring arterial carbon dioxide continuously during perfluorocarbon dosing and keeping it under tight control or using volume-controlled ventilation. This will prevent any decrease in arterial blood pressure or oxygenation, or any increase in arterial carbon dioxide. This in turn will prevent any disturbance of cerebral blood flow. The lowest possible dose-volume of perfluorocarbon should be used (e.g., 10 mL/kg or smaller, larger volumes may be acceptable but shouldn't be given too fast), and the dose should not be given over 5 minutes or less.

Given the availability of a suitable product, randomised controlled trials of partial liquid ventilation in neonates are both feasible and desirable. Now the design of such trials can incorporate some of the data from the studies summarised above and ensure that the dosing procedure is as safe as it can be for use in extremely preterm infants.

6. Conclusions

As is demonstrated by the above studies partial liquid ventilation has great potential to disturb cerebral blood flow and increase the risk of brain injury. If partial liquid ventilation is to be used in extremely preterm infants it should be safe. The best protection for the extremely preterm brain is to start partial liquid ventilation safely without disturbing cerebral blood flow. Given the potential for harm associated with perfluorocarbon dosing in the most susceptible of preterm infants it is encouraging to know that there are ways of giving perfluorocarbon that can mitigate any increase in cerebral blood flow.

7. References

ANZNN (Australian and New Zealand Neonatal Network) 2009. Report of the Australian and New Zealand Neonatal Network 2006. Sydney, ANZNN.

Baden HP, Mellema JD, Bratton, SL, O'Rourke PP, Jackson JC. High-frequency oscillatory ventilation with partial liquid ventilation in a model of acute respiratory failure. Crit Care Med 1997; 25:299-302.

Ballabh P. Intraventricular hemorrhage in premature infants: mechanism of disease. Pediatr Res 2010; 67:1-8.

Bassan H, Feldman HA, Limperopoulos C, Benson CB, Ringer SA, Veracruz E, Soul JS, Volpe JJ, du Plessis AJ. Periventricular hemorrhagic infarction: risk factors and neonatal outcome. Pediatr Neurol 2006; 35:85-92.

Blassnig N, Dietl S, Tschirch E, Burkhardt W, Wemhöner A, Rüdiger M. Intratracheal application of PFC diminishes the hyperoxia-mediated impairment of postnatal lung development. Acta Paediatrica 2009; 98 (Suppl. 460):7.

Bruch LA, Flint A, Hirschl RB. Pulmonary pathology of patients treated with partial liquid ventilation. Mod Pathol 1997; 10:463-468.

Burkhardt W, Proquitté H, Krause S, Wauer RR, Rüdiger M. Cerebral oxygenation is affected by filling mode and perfluorochemical volume in partial liquid ventilation of healthy piglets. Biol Neonate 2002; 82:250-256.

Cartwright DW. Grantley Stable Neonatal Unit Royal Brisbane & Women's Hospital Annual Report 2005. Brisbane, GSNU.

Cartwright DW. Grantley Stable Neonatal Unit Royal Brisbane & Women's Hospital Annual Report 2006. Brisbane, GSNU.

Cartwright DW. Grantley Stable Neonatal Unit Royal Brisbane & Women's Hospital Annual Report 2007. Brisbane, GSNU.

Cartwright DW. Grantley Stable Neonatal Unit, Royal Brisbane and Women's Hospital Neonatology Report of Activities 2003. Brisbane, GSNU.

Cartwright DW. Grantley Stable Neonatal Unit, Royal Brisbane and Women's Hospital Neonatology Report of Activities 2004. Brisbane, GSNU.

Clark LC, Gollan F. Survival of mammals breathing organic liquids equilibrated with oxygen at atmospheric pressure. Science 1966; 152:1755-1756.

Cleary GM, Antunes MJ, Wu D et al. Disaturated phosphatidylcholine and surfactant protein B levels in healthy and meconium injured lungs after partial liquid ventilation. Pediatric Academic Societies' Annual Meeting, Abstracts-On-Disk®, 1997, 1479.

Costeloe K, Hennessy E, Gibson AT, Marlow N, Wilkinson AR. The EPICure study: outcomes to discharge from hospital for infants born at the threshold of viability. Pediatrics 2000;106:659-671.

Coughtrey H, Rennie JM, Evans DH. Variability in cerebral blood flow velocity: observations over one minute in preterm babies. Early Hum Dev 1997; 47:63-70.

Curtis SE, Peek JT. Effects of progressive intratracheal administration of perflubron during conventional gas ventilation in anesthetized dogs with oleic acid lung injury. Adv Exp Med Biol 1994b; 345:51-58.

Curtis SE, Tilden SJ, Bradley WE, Cain SM. Effect of continuous rotation on the efficacy of partial liquid (perflubron) breathing in canine acute lung injury. Adv Exp Med Biol 1994a; 361:449-456.

Davies MW, Dunster KR, Wilson K, Colditz PB. Perfluorocarbon dosing when starting partial liquid ventilation: haemodynamics and cerebral blood flow in preterm lambs. Neonatology 2010a; 97:144-153.

Davies MW, Dunster KR, Wilson K, Colditz PB. The effect of the dose volume of perfluorocarbon when starting partial liquid ventilation. J Paediatr Child Health 2010b;46(12):714–722.

Davies MW, Fraser JF. Partial liquid ventilation for preventing death and morbidity in adults with acute lung injury and acute respiratory distress syndrome. Cochrane Database Syst Rev 2004a, Issue 4. Art. No.: CD003707. DOI: 10.1002/14651858.CD003707.pub2.

Davies MW, Sargent PH. Partial liquid ventilation for the prevention of mortality and morbidity in paediatric acute lung injury and acute respiratory distress syndrome. Cochrane Database Syst Rev 2004b, Issue 4. Art. No.: CD003845. DOI: 10.1002/14651858.CD003845.pub2.

Davies MW, Stewart MJ, Souriel M, Chavasse R, Butt W. Oxygenation is not improved by partial liquid high frequency ventilation using a high lung volume strategy. An experimental study. Crit Care Resusc 1999;1(4):339–343.

Davies MW. Partial liquid ventilation and cerebral blood flow: the effects of the administration of a dose of perfluorocarbon liquid, when starting partial liquid ventilation, on cerebral blood flow (PhD Thesis). St Lucia, Qld: University of Queensland; 2011.

Degraeuwe PL, Vos GD, Blanco CE. Perfluorochemical liquid ventilation: From the animal laboratory to the intensive care unit. Int J Artif Organs 1995; 18:674–683.

Doyle LW, Gultom E, Chuang SL, James M, Davis P, Bowman E. Changing mortality and causes of death in infants 23-27 weeks' gestational age. J Paediatr Child Health 1999; 35(3):255–259.

du Plessis AJ. Cerebrovascular injury in premature infants: current understanding and challenges for future prevention. Clin Perinatol 2008; 35:609–641.

Field D. Alternative strategies for the management of respiratory failure in the newborn – clinical realities. Semin Neonatol 2002; 7:429–436.

Foust R, III, Tran NN, Cox C, Miller TF Jr, Greenspan JS, Wolfson MR, Shaffer TH. Liquid assisted ventilation: An alternative ventilatory strategy for acute meconium aspiration injury. Pediatr Pulmonol 1996; 21:316–322.

Fuhrman B, Blumer J, Toro-Figueroa L, Hernan L, Cox P, Curtis S, et al. Multicenter, randomized, controlled trial (RCT) of LiquiVent® partial liquid ventilation in paediatric ARDS. Proceedings of the Eleventh Annual Pediatric Critical Care Colloquium. Chicago, USA, 1998:A17.

Fuhrman BP, Paczan PR, DeFrancisis M. Perfluorocarbon associated gas exchange. Crit Care Med 1991; 19:712–722.

Garver KA, Kazerooni EA, Hirschl RB, DiPietro MA. Neonates with congenital diaphragmatic hernia: Radiographic findings during partial liquid ventilation. Radiology 1996; 200:219–223.

Greenspan JS, Wolfson MR, Rubenstein SD, Shaffer TH. Liquid ventilation of preterm baby. Lancet 1989; 2:1095.

Greisen G. Autoregulation of cerebral blood flow in newborn babies. Early Hum Dev 2005; 81:423–428.

Heard SO, Puyana JC. The anti-inflammatory effects of perfluorocarbons: let's get physical. Crit Care Med 2000. 28:1241–1242.

Hennessy EM, Bracewell MA, Wood N, Wolke D, Costeloe K, Gibson A, Marlow N, for the EPICure Study Group. Respiratory health in pre-school and school age children following extremely preterm birth. Arch Dis Child 2008; 93:1037–1043.

Hill A, Perlman JM, Volpe JJ. Relationship of pneumothorax to occurrence of intraventricular hemorrhage in the premature newborn. Pediatrics 1982; 69;144–149.

Hirschl R. Current experience with liquid ventilation. Paediatr Respir Rev 2004; 5(Suppl A):S339–S345.

Hirschl RB, Croce M, Gore D, Wiedemann H, Davis K, Zwischenberger J, Bartlett RH. Prospective, randomized, controlled pilot study of partial liquid ventilation in adult respiratory distress syndrome. Am J Resp Crit Care Med 2002;165:781–787.

Hirschl RB, Pranikoff T, Gauger P, Schreiner RJ, Dechert R, Bartlett RH. Liquid ventilation in adults, children, and full-term neonates. Lancet 1995; 346:1201–1202.

Ito H, Kanno I, Fukuda H. Human cerebral circulation: positron emission tomography studies. Ann Nucl Med 2005; 19:65–74.

Kacmarek RM, Wiedemann HP, Lavin PT, Wedel MK, Tütüncü AS, Slutsky AS. Partial liquid ventilation in adult patients with acute respiratory distress syndrome. Am J Respir Crit Care Med 2006; 173:882–889.

Kaiser JR, Gauss CH, Williams DK. Surfactant administration acutely affects cerebral and systemic hemodynamics and gas exchange in very-low-birthweight infants. J Pediatr 2004; 144:809–814.

Kelly KP. Partial liquid ventilation - turning back a PAGE on evolution (editorial). Br J Anaesth 1997; 78:1–2.

Kissack CM, Garr R, Wardle SP, Weindling AM. Postnatal changes in cerebral oxygen extraction in the preterm infant are associated with intraventricular hemorrhage and hemorrhagic parenchymal infarction but not periventricular leukomalacia. Pediatr Res 2004; 56:111–116.

Kluckow M, Evans N. Low superior vena cava flow and intraventricular haemorrhage in preterm infants. Arch Dis Child Fetal Neonatal Ed 2000; 82(3):F188–194.

Kohlhauser C, Bernert G, Hermon M, Popow C, Seidl R, Pollak A. Effects of endotracheal suctioning in high-frequency oscillatory and conventionally ventilated low birth weight neonates on cerebral hemodynamics observed by near infrared spectroscopy (NIRS). Pediatr Pulmonol 2000; 29:270–275.

Kylstra JA, Paganelli CV, Lanphier EH. Pulmonary gas exchange in dogs ventilated with hyperbarically oxygenated liquid. J Appl Physiol 1966; 21:177–184.

Kylstra JA, Tissing MO, Van der Maen A. Of mice as fish. ASAIO Transactions 1962; 8: 378–383.

Leach CL, Fuhrman BP, Morin FC, III, Rath MG. Perfluorocarbon associated gas exchange (partial liquid ventilation) in respiratory distress syndrome: A prospective, randomized, controlled study. Crit Care Med 1993; 21:1270–1278.

Leach CL, Greenspan JS, Rubenstein SD, Shaffer TH, Wolfson MR, Jackson JC, DeLemos R, Fuhrman BP. Partial liquid ventilation with perflubron in premature infants with severe respiratory distress syndrome. The LiquiVent Study Group. N Engl J Med 1996; 335:761–767.

Leach CL, Holm B, Morin FC III, Fuhrman BP, Papo MC, Steinhorn D, Hernan LJ. Partial liquid ventilation in premature lambs with respiratory distress syndrome: Efficacy and compatibility with exogenous surfactant. J Pediatr 1995; 126:412–420.

Leahy FAN, Cates D, MacCallum M, Rigatto H. Effect of CO2 and 100% O2 on cerebral blood flow in preterm infants. J Appl Physiol Respirat Environ Exercise Physiol 1980; 48:468–472.

Limperopoulos C, Gauvreau KK, O'Leary H, Moore M, Bassan H, Eichenwald EC, Soul JS, Ringer SA, Di Salvo DN, du Plessis AJ. Cerebral hemodynamic changes during intensive care of preterm infants. Pediatrics 2008; 122;e1006–e1013.

Meaney JF, Kazerooni EA, Garver KA, Hirschl RB. Acute respiratory distress syndrome: CT findings during partial liquid ventilation. Radiology 1997; 202:570–573.

Mehrabani D, Gowen CW, Kopelman AE. Association of pneumothorax and hypotension with intraventricular haemorrhage. Arch Dis Child 1991; 66:48–51.

Ment LR, Stewar WB, Duncan CC, Lambrecht R. Beagle puppy model of intraventricular hemorrhage. J Neurosurg 1982; 57:219–223.

Modell JH, Gollan F, Giammona ST, Parker D. Effects of fluorocarbon liquid on surface tension of pulmonary surfactant. Chest 1970; 57:263–265.

Mrozek JD, Bing DR, Meyers PA, Connett JE, Mammel MC. High frequency oscillation versus conventional ventilation following surfactant administration and partial liquid ventilation. Pediatr Pulmonol 1998; 26:21–29.

Mullaart RA, Hopman JCW, Rotteveel JJ, Daniëls O, Stoelinga GBA, De Haan AFJ. Cerebral blood flow fluctuation in neonatal respiratory distress and periventricular haemorrhage. Early Hum Dev 1994; 37:179–185.

Ohyua J, Marumob G, Ozawaa H, Takashimaa S, Nakajimac K, Kohsakac S, Hamaib Y, Machidab Y, Kobayashib K, Ryob E, Babad K, Kozumab S, Okaib T, Taketanib Y. Early axonal and glial pathology in fetal sheep brains with leukomalacia induced by repeated umbilical cord occlusion. Brain Dev 1999; 21:248–252.

Perlman JM, McMenamin JB, Volpe JJ. Fluctuating cerebral blood-flow velocity in respiratory-distress syndrome: relation to the development of intraventricular hemorrhage. N EngI J Med 1983; 309:204–209.

Perlman JM, Volpe JJ. Suctioning in the preterm infant: effects on cerebral blood flow velocity, intracranial pressure, and arterial blood pressure. Pediatrics 1983; 72;329–334.

Perlman JM. The relationship between systemic hemodynamic perturbations and periventricular-intraventricular hemorrhage—a historical perspective. Semin Pediatr Neurol 2009; 16:191–199.

Pranikoff T, Gauger PG, Hirschl RB. Partial liquid ventilation in newborn patients with congenital diaphragmatic hernia. J Ped Surg 1996; 31:613–618.

Pryds O, Edwards AD. Cerebral blood flow in the newborn infant. Arch Dis Child Fetal Neonatal Ed 1996; 74:F63–F69.

Rahilly PM. Effects of 2% carbon dioxide, 0.5% carbon dioxide, and 100% oxygen on cranial blood flow of the human neonate. Pediatrics 1980; 66;685–689.

Rennie JM, South M, Morley CJ. Cerebral blood flow velocity variability in infants receiving assisted ventilation. Arch Dis Child 1987; 62:1247–1251.

Rüfer R. Surfactant and alveolar surface forces after breathing of a fluorinated liquid. Fed Proc 1970; 29: 1813–1815.

Saliba E, Nashashibi M, Vaillant M-C, Nasr C, Laugier J. Instillation rate effects of Exosurf on cerebral and cardiovascular haemodynamics in preterm neonates. Arch Dis Child Fetal Neonatal Ed 1994; 71:F174–F178.

Salman NH, Fuhrman BP, Steinhorn DM, Papo MC, Hernan LJ, Leach CL, Fischer JE. Prolonged studies of perfluorocarbon associated gas exchange and of the resumption of conventional mechanical ventilation. Crit Care Med 1995; 23:919–924.

Schipper JA, Mohammad GI, van Straaten HLM, Koppe JG. The impact of surfactant replacement therapy on cerebral and systemic circulation and lung function. Eur J Pediatr 1997; 156:224–227.

Schoenfish WH, Kylstra JA. Maximum expiratory flow and estimated CO2 elimination in liquid ventilated dog's lungs. J Appl Physiol 1973; 35:117–121.

Shaffer TH, Douglas PR, Lowe CA, Bhutani VK. The effects of liquid ventilation on cardiopulmonary function in preterm lambs. Pediatr Res 1983; 17:303–306.

Shaffer TH, Ferguson JD, Koen PA, Moskowitz GD, Delioria-Papadopoulos GD. Pulmonary lavage in preterm lambs. Pediatr Res 1978; 12:695–698.

Shaffer TH, Lowe CA, Bhutani VK, Douglas PR. Liquid ventilation: Effects on pulmonary function in distressed meconium-stained lambs. Pediatr Res 1984; 18:47–52.

Shaffer TH, Moskowitz GD. An electromechanical demand regulated liquid breathing system. IEEE Trans Biomed Eng 1975; 22:412–417.

Shaffer TH, Rubenstein D, Moskowitz GD, Delioria-Papadopoulos M. Gaseous exchange and acid-base balance in premature lambs during liquid ventilation since birth. Pediatr Res 1976; 10:227–231.

Shaffer TH, Wolfson MR, Clark LC Jr. Liquid ventilation. Pediatr Pulmonol 1992; 14:102–109.

Smith KM, Bing DR, Meyers PA, Connett JE, Boros SJ, Mammel MC. Partial liquid ventilation: A comparison using conventional and high-frequency techniques in an animal model of acute respiratory failure. Crit Care Med 1997b; 25:1179–1186.

Smith KM, Mrozek JD, Simonton SC, Bing DR, Meyers PA, Connett JE, Mammel MC. Prolonged partial liquid ventilation using conventional and high-frequency ventilatory techniques: Gas exchange and lung pathology in an animal model of respiratory distress syndrome. Crit Care Med 1997a; 25:1888–1897.

Smith TM, Steinhorn DM, Thusu K, Fuhrman BP, Dandona P. A liquid perfluorochemical decreases the in vitro production of reactive oxygen species by alveolar macrophages. Crit Care Med 1995; 23:1533–1539.

Sukumar M, Bommaraju M, Fisher JE, Morin FC 3rd, Papo MC, Fuhrman BP, Hernan LJ, Leach CL. High-frequency partial liquid ventilation in respiratory distress syndrome: Hemodynamics and gas exchange. J Appl Physiol 1998; 84:327–334.

Takashima S, Iida K, Deguchi K. Periventricular leukomalacia, glial development and myelination. Early Hum Dev 1995; 43: 177–184.

Takashima S, Itoh M, Oka A. A history of our understanding of cerebral vascular development and pathogenesis of perinatal brain damage over the past 30 years. Semin Pediatr Neurol 2009; 16:226–236.

Thomassen MJ, Buhrow LT, Wiedemann HP. Perflubron decreases inflammatory cytokine production by human alveolar macrophages. Crit Care Med 1997; 25:2045–2047.

Tutuncu AS, Faithfull NS, Lachmann, B. Comparison of ventilatory support with intratracheal perfluorocarbon administration and conventional mechanical ventilation in animals with acute respiratory failure. Am Rev Resp Dis 1993; 148:785–792.

Van Bel F, Van de Bor M, Stijnen T, Baan J, Ruys JH. Aetiological role of cerebral blood-flow alterations development and extension of peri-intraventricular haemorrhage. Dev Med Child Neurol 1987; 29(5):601–614.

Vavilala MS, Lee LA, Lam AM. Cerebral blood flow and vascular physiology. Anesthesiol Clin North Am 2002; 20:247–264.

Vohr B, Ment LR. Intraventricular hemorrhage in the preterm infant. Early Hum Dev 1996; 44:1-16.

Volpe JJ, Perlman JM, Hill A, McMenamin JB. Cerebral blood flow velocity in the human newborn: the value of its determination. Pediatrics 1982; 70;147–152.

Volpe JJ. Brain injury in premature infants: a complex amalgam of destructive and developmental disturbances. Lancet Neurol 2009a; 8:110–124.

Volpe JJ. The encephalopathy of prematurity—brain injury and impaired brain development inextricably intertwined. Semin Pediatr Neurol 2009b;16:167–178.

von Bismarck P, Klemm K, Wistadt CF, Winoto-Morbach S, Uhlig U, Schutze S, Uhlig S, Lachmann B, Krause MF. Surfactant "fortification" by topical inhibition of nuclear factor-kappaB activity in a newborn piglet lavage model. Crit Care Med 2007; 35(10):2309–2318.

Wells JT, Ment LR. Prevention of intraventricular hemorrhage in preterm neonates. Early Hum Dev 1995; 42:209–233.

Wolfson MR, Greenspan JS, Deoras KS, Rubenstein SD, Shaffer TH. Comparison of gas and liquid ventilation: Clinical, physiological, and histological correlates. J Appl Physiol 1992; 72:1024–1031.

Wolfson MR, Shaffer TH. Liquid ventilation during early development: Theory, physiologic processes and application. J Dev Physiol 1990;13: 1–12.

Wood NS, Marlow N, Costeloe K, Gibson AT, Wilkinson AR. Neurologic and developmental disability after extremely preterm birth. EPICure Study Group. N Engl J Med 2000; 343:378–384.

Yoshioka H, Goma H, Nioka S, Ochi M, Miyake H, Zaman A, Masumura M, Sawada T, Chance B. Bilateral carotid artery occlusion causes periventricular leukomalacia in neonatal dogs. Developmental Brain Research 1994; 78:273–278.

Zobel G, Urlesberger B, Dacar D, Rödl S, Reiterer F, Friehs I. Partial liquid ventilation combined with inhaled nitric oxide in acute respiratory failure with pulmonary hypertension in piglets. Pediatr Res 1997; 41:172–177.

Part 5

Pulmonary Oedema: Cardiogenic and Non-Cardiogenic

24

Non-Cardiogenic Pulmonary Edema

J. Gonzales and A. Verin
Georgia Health Sciences University, Augusta, Georgia
United States

1. Introduction

Pulmonary edema (PE) remains one of the more common reasons for admission to the hospital. Pulmonary edema is either cardiac or non-cardiac. The cardiac causes of pulmonary edema occur because the cardiac pump function has failed and there is increased capillary hydrostatic pressure secondary to elevated pulmonary venous pressure. Cardiogenic pulmonary edema is the accumulation of fluid with a low-protein content in the lung interstitium and alveoli and occurs when the pulmonary venous and left atrial venous return exceeds left ventricular output. Most often this is due to left heart failure, cardiac valve disease, volume overload, kidney failure or cardiac tamponade. Non cardiogenic pulmonary edema (NCPE) is a condition that is associated with high morbidity and mortality. Pulmonary edema fluid accumulates in the lungs through damaged capillary endothelial cells and this leads to impaired gas exchange (oxygen and carbon dioxide) with hypoxia and respiratory failure. The best example of non-cardiogenic pulmonary edema is acute respiratory distress syndrome (ARDS) (Sartori et al, 2010). ARDS is a serious condition of hypoxia, bilateral lung infiltrates on chest roentgenogram with subsequent respiratory failure. The hallmark of ALI (acute lung injury)/ARDS on the cellular level is pulmonary capillary endothelial cell permeability and fluid leakage into the pulmonary parenchyma, followed by neutrophils, cytokines and an acute inflammatory response. It is associated with a high morbidity and 30-50% mortality. ARDS has multiple causes with the most common being sepsis or pneumonia, less common causes of ARDS with ensuing pulmonary edema are trauma or pancreatitis (Ware & Mathay, 2005). Other causes of NCPE in hospitalized patients are intravenous fluid with volume overload, neurogenic pulmonary edema, reperfusion pulmonary edema, re-expansion pulmonary edema, opiate overdose, salicylate toxicity. Less common, forms of NCPE are high altitude pulmonary edema (HAPE), immersion pulmonary edema and negative pressure pulmonary edema (NPPE).

2. Increased permeability pulmonary edema

NCPE causes direct injury to the lungs in several forms. Under normal conditions fluid outflow that occurs from the lung capillaries through tiny gaps in the vascular endothelial cell (EC) junction is removed from the interstitial space and returned to the circulation by the lymphatic system. Physiologically, the main forces regulating fluid balance in the lungs are the microvascular pressure of the capillaries. Fluid leaves the capillaries and enters the pulmonary interstitium in proportion to the net capillary hydrostatic pressure minus the net osmotic pressure across the vessel wall. The formula for filtration across the pulmonary capillary semi-permeable membrane is

$$Q=K\text{-}[CPmv\text{-}Ppmv)\text{-}(\pi mv\text{-}\pi pmv)]$$

which is different from the systemic capillary fluid exchange. Q=net transvascular flow of fluid, K=membrane permeability, Pmv=hydrostatic pressure in the microvessels, Ppmv=hydrostatic pressure in the peri-microvascular interstitium, πmv=plasma protein osmotic pressure in the circulation, πpmv=protein osmotic pressure in the peri-microvascular interstitium. This equation only reflects the known hydrostatic pressures without including the lymph hydrostatic pressure which has been studied but is unknown in relation to the Starling forces equation (Sartori et al, 2010). It is known that one of the main functions of the lymphatic system is to return plasma proteins from the interstitial tissue space to the bloodstream. Analyses of blood plasma and lymph have shown that all of the proteins that are found in the plasma are also found in the lymph although in lower concentrations (Ono et al, 2005). In normal circumstances, low pulmonary capillary hydrostatic pressure provides a "safety" factor against pulmonary edema across the lung tissue.

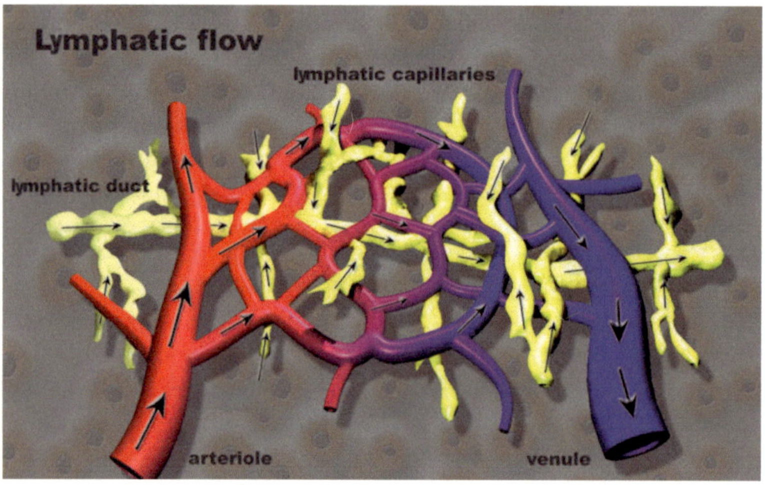

Fig. 1. Representation of the pulmonary arterial and venous capillary barrier and lymphatic flow.

Although hydrostatic pressures in the pulmonary arterial and venous system are known, the hydrostatic pressures of the interrelated pulmonary lymphatic system is unknown and largely unstudied. The illustration generously permitted by Dr. Davide Brunelli of Med-ars.it.

In some forms of NCPE such as ARDS disturbances of pulmonary capillary fluid balance and pulmonary permeability occur as a direct result of endotoxins and inflammation that cause disruption in the capillary EC barrier with barrier disruption and subsequent pulmonary venous congestion. As the volume excess initially enters the interstitium it is taken up by the lymphatic system to be returned to the vascular system. In normal circumstances the interstitial space can increase its volume by as much as 40% without resulting in pulmonary edema (Sartori et al, 2010). In pulmonary injury due to toxins or inflammation the fluid volume increase overwhelms the lymphatic drainage system and the hydrostatic forces become altered resulting in further injury to the pulmonary capillary endothelium. The result is persistent fluid accumulation that overwhelms the lymphatic drainage and tissue edema results. The final step occurs as the fluid volume overwhelms the hydrostatic forces and the excess fluid flows into the alveoli. The edema that is caused by the increasing fluid and vascular permeability is a hallmark of inflammation and tissue injury (Zimmerman & McIntyre, 2004). The edema formation can have severe consequences because the fluid and protein components in the edematous tissues and alveoli increase the diffusion barrier for oxygen and carbon dioxide with subsequent disruption of gas exchange thus precipitating hypoxia and respiratory failure. The rate of volume expansion is also a factor in pulmonary edema.

Other forms of NCPE such as HAPE, immersion pulmonary edema and NPPE may occur due to greatly altered thoracic pressures and are thought to have a largely hydrostatic non-inflammatory component (Fremont et al, 2007). The accelerated pulmonary edema that occurs with HAPE, immersion PE or NPPE is thought to be due to significant fluid shifts that come secondary to changes in intrathoracic pressure, and in the case of HAPE or immersion PE, possibly due to diminished atmospheric or oxygen inhalation pressures. Physiologically negative intrathoracic pressure is generated in the chest when a patient inspires against an obstructed airway. The rapid pressure change in the pulmonary venous circulation alters the transpulmonary fluid gradient. The increase in capillary hydrostatic pressure most likely causes capillary gap formation as well as transcellular fluid shifts. The fluid gradient is thus going from a high gradient to a low gradient. Although considered a second mechanism of the EC barrier disruption it is part of the capillary hydrostatic pressure. While it is unlikely that the rapidly resolved post obstructive PE and HAPE are of a different nature, it is more likely that all of the non-cardiogenic PE have the same hydrostatic mechanisms initially (Sartori et al, 2010 & Gantor et al, 2006). The NCPE in ARDS is ultimately a result of capillary permeability secondary to cellular damage, inflammatory cascades, and over inflation by mechanical ventilation resulting in endothelial permeability. The permeability from HAPE and scuba diving is not initiated by inflammation but rather stress failure occurring due to the increased pressures that occur at the capillary level in healthy subjects (Slade et al, 2001). The pulmonary capillary endothelial cell barrier is a semi-permeable membrane and is known to be an active biological interface between the blood and the surrounding tissue. The EC is a single layer of continuous endothelium lining the pulmonary capillaries and forms a single layer between blood and the pulmonary interstitium. The pulmonary capillaries have extremely thin walls to allow rapid exchange of respiratory gases across them (Costello et al, 1992).The endothelium modulates tone, growth, homeostasis and inflammation in the lungs and throughout the circulatory system (Ware & Matthay, 2005 & Umapathy et al, 2010). In NCPE due to diseases such as ARDS, the ensuing endotoxins and inflammatory markers induce capillary endothelial disarray and gap formations. This is followed by neutrophil chemotaxis, diapedesis and protein rich edema fluid leakage into the interstitial spaces. Inflammatory cascades are triggered and also enter into the interstitial milieu. As the capillary pressure increases there is damage of the capillary EC causing larger molecules such as proteins from the vascular space to flow into the interstitial space (Slade et al, 2001). NCPE in an ill patient with ARDS is a high protein pulmonary edema. The fluid/plasma ratio may be used to differentiate the etiology of pulmonary edema in NCPE and CPE. It is a measurement of the alveolar fluid, obtained by broncho- alveolar lavage (BAL), to the serum plasma during acute pulmonary edema and has been shown in studies to be sensitive enough to differentiate a low protein fluid that results from CPE or NCPE in a patient without illness compared to a high protein ratio NCPE such as occurs with illness such as endotoxin induced ARDS (Fremont et al, 2001; Ware et al, 2010). The protein concentration in the pulmonary interstitium of ARDS exceeds 60% of the plasma value whereas the protein concentration in HAPE, reperfusion PE, neurogenic PE and other non ARDS causes is less than 45% (Fein et al, 1079 & Staub et al, 1967). The result is capillary injury with gap formation and high permeability of the EC barrier with an increase of protein rich edema fluid into the interstitial space. The resulting pulmonary interstitial protein remains elevated compared to circulating blood plasma. At this point there is no longer a "quick" resolution possible.

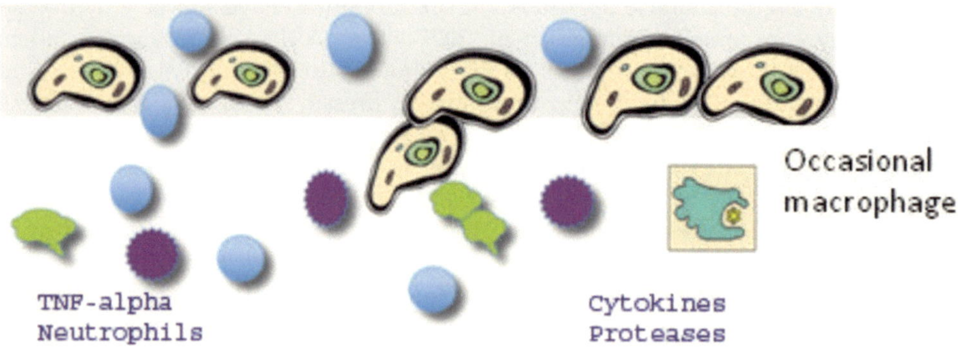

Fig. 2. Schematic representation of the endothelial barrier in inflammatory pulmonary edema.

NCPE causes direct injury to the lungs. The endothelial barrier is normally single layer of continuous endothelium lining the pulmonary capillaries. In ALI/ARDS the endotoxins recruited by the macrophages and neutrophils induce capillary endothelial disarray and gap formations. This is followed by neutrophil chemotaxis, diapedesis, proteases, cytokines and protein rich fluid into the interstitial spaces.

3. Neutrophils and molecular mechanisms in the endothelial and epithelial cell barrier in ALI/ARDS

Neutrophils play an important role in the development of pulmonary edema associated with ALI/ARDS. It is well known that neutrophils are prevalent in ARDS pulmonary edema and are central to the pathogenesis (Bdeir et al, 2010). Initially pulmonary macrophages are activated and recruit circulating neutrophils to the pulmonary microvascular system and the injured capillaries. The interaction of the neutrophils and the endothelium is initiated by adhesion receptors and by soluble or membrane bound chemoattractants. Intercellular adhesion molecules-1 (ICAM-1) and other proteins are known to be present but the specific role of these molecules and proteins is unclear (Downey et al, 1999). Once the neutrophils become activated and move subsequently into the pulmonary parenchymal interstitium, they sequester and initiate an important component of the inflammatory response in endotoxin induced ALI/ARDS. This activation and migration of neutrophils is a characteristic event in the progression of ALI and ARDS. Animal studies have shown that endothelial injury appears within minutes to hours after ALI initiation with resulting intercellular gaps of the EC. The EC gaps allow for permeability of fluid, neutrophils and cytokines into the pulmonary parenchymal space (Grommes & Soehnlein, 2011).

The neutrophils that infiltrate the lungs and migrate into the airways express pro-inflammatory cytokines such as TNF-α, IL-1β, IL-6 and contribute to both the endothelial and epithelial integrity disruption of the barriers (Bdeir et al, 2010; Grommes & Soehnlein, 2011; Abraham, 2003). It has also been well documented that the percentage of neutrophils correlates directly with the alveolar-arterial PO2 difference in ALI/ARDS pulmonary edema (Weiland et al, 1986). Neutrophil sequestration is aided by chemotactic factors and by the adhesion molecules on both the neutrophils and capillary endothelial cells (Hasko et al, 2006; Steinberg, 1994; Geerts et al, 2001). The activated neutrophils expressing IL-1β produce other pro-inflammatory cytokines after endotoxin administration. In fact, the removal of neutrophils after endotoxin administration almost entirely prevents an increase of IL-1β expression and attenuates endotoxin induced TNF-α. Neutrophils are the major source of IL-1β in murine models of the lung in ALI (Abraham, 2003). Another feature of the neutrophils that accumulate in the lung of murine models is increased activation of the transcriptional regulatory factor NF-κB. NF-κB is a protein complex that controls transcription of DNA and is involved in cellular responses to stimuli such as pulmonary edema due to ALI/ARDS. It is key in regulating the endotoxin induced immune response in neutrophils and produces increased amounts of pro-inflammatory cytokines whose transcription is dependent on NF-κB (Blackwell et al, 1996). Neutrophils also become an increasing liability in the edematous pulmonary interstitium as they release free radicals.

The alveolar-capillary barrier is a very thin membrane allowing oxygen CO_2 exchange for normal respiration. The major consequence of pulmonary edema is impaired gas exchange that interrupts the normal fluid exchange balance. The alveoli epithelium removes fluid by molecular mechanisms of sodium transport, however, the capillary endothelial barrier function has only incompletely defined pathways affecting the concurrent barrier disruption. Permeability of the EC in the capillaries with concurrent alveolar-capillary membrane damage and with leakage of fluid, neutrophils, proteases, cytokines and free radicals that all contribute to the ensuing pulmonary edema is a prominent feature of permeability edema and ALI/ARDS (Holter et al, 1986). The alveolar liquid clearance from the alveolus into the interstitium is based on active sodium transport largely through the highly regulated apical amiloride sensitive epithelial sodium channel complex (ENaC) with concomitant passive water transport and the Na^+, K^+ ATPase exchange (Ella et al, 2003; Folkesson & Matthay, 2006). The Na^+, K^+ ATPase exchange transports the alveolar liquid into the interstitium and ultimately into the lymphatic and blood vessels (Hamacher et al, 2010; Lucas et al, 2009). However, these transport processes are often impaired in ALI or ARDS.

It is likely that the induction of increased permeability of the pulmonary capillary bed is directly linked to reversible physical modifications of the pulmonary capillary endothelium (Kaner et al, 2000). The capillary endothelial regulation of endothelial permeability involves various pathways such as those involving reactive oxygen species (ROS), Rho GTPases, and tyrosine phosphorylation of junctional proteins all converge to regulate junctional permeability. They either affect the stability of junctional proteins or modulate their interactions (Lucas et al, 2009). The regulation of permeability at the junctions is mediated by active communication between the proteins of the adherens junctions and the actin cytoskeleton. Actin mediated endothelial cell contraction is the result of myosin light chain (MLC) phosphorylation by MLC kinase (MLCK) in Ca^{2+}/calmodulin- dependent manner. RhoA also potentiates MLC phosphorylation by inhibiting MLC phosphatase activity through its downstream effector Rho kinase (ROCK). As the actin/myosin driven contraction generates a contractile force it pulls VE-cadherin inward. This contraction will force VE-cadherin to dissociate from its adjacent partner causing endothelial gaps - the basic pathology in permeability pulmonary edema (Lucas et al, 2009).

4. Serum Biomarkers in permeability edema and ARDS

A complex progression of events is recognized in the development of permeability edema and ARDS but the exact nature of events is still an area of active study. A large variety of inflammatory mediators have been found to be elevated in ARDS including lung specific proteins, endotoxin binding proteins, tumor necrosis factor alpha (TNF-α), interleukins (ILs), chemokines and markers of endothelium activation such as adhesion molecules and von Willebrand factor antigen (VWF) (Tzouvelekis et al, 2005). A comprehensive review is beyond the scope of this article but some of the most widely known are discussed. There is an increased expression of the vascular endothelial growth factor VEGF gene in pulmonary edema. Although VEGF is widely expressed in the body, the highest level of expression in normal tissues is in the lung. Normally increased expression and angiogenesis is associated with lung tumors and has been studied as a target for therapy in lung cancer however VEGF also is known to stimulate actin stress fiber formation and new focal adhesions in endothelial cells suggesting a regulatory role in endothelial morphology (Kaner et al, 2000). A study by Kaner et al demonstrated that excess expression of VEGF within the murine lung was associated with increased permeability of pulmonary edema (Kaner et al, 2000). In addition to endotoxin effects on endothelial permeability there is strong evidence that cytokines such as tumor necrosis factor (TNF-α), interleukin (IL)-1β, IL-6, and IL-8 are associated with pulmonary edema. Shutte measured cytokine levels in patients with ARDS, severe pneumonia and cardiogenic pulmonary edema for comparison and found consistently higher levels of IL-8, IL-6 and TNF-α in the bronchoalveolar lavage fluid (BALF) and the serum of patients with ARDS and pneumonia compared to cardiogenic pulmonary edema (Schutte et al, 1996). Cytokines have various effects on activating endothelium inducing endothelial expression of adhesion molecules and leukocyte chemotaxis leading to a local inflammatory response in the lung. The cytokine, TNF-α induces macrophages and T_H1 cells and activates ECs and macrophages (Braun et al, 2005). Studies have been conflicting as far as elevation of TNF-α in patients with ARDS pulmonary edema, for example, Bauer demonstrated that TNF-α concentrations were significantly higher in patients with ARDS than those of pneumonia or of the control subjects (Bauer et al, 2000). Others, such as Hyers have found variability in the elevation of TNF-α, however, there is speculation that TNF-α is an acute phase cytokine and the timing of studies is important for its evaluation (Hyers, 1991). Although Bauer found that the TNF-α levels were significantly elevated it was also speculated that the elevation was more related to the severity of the lung disease and could not be extrapolated as a possible diagnostic marker for ARDS (Bauer et al, 2000). TNF-α is a known acute phase reactant and is also a cytokine involved in systemic inflammation. It is able to induce apoptotic cell death, inflammation, and inhibit tumorgenesis and viral replication. TNF-α is produced mainly by macrophages but can also be produced by other cells including endothelial cells (Schutte et al, 1996). Large amounts of TNF-α are released in response to LPS endotoxin, bacterial products and IL-1. TNF- α works with IL-1 and IL-6 to produce actions on various organ systems (Schutte et al, 1996; Braun et al, 2005; Bauer et al, 2000). TNF-α also induces EC activation and barrier dysfunction both of which occur in the pathogenesis of pulmonary edema and ALI/ARDS. It can promote edema by TNF receptor dependent chemokine production and adhesion molecule expression and leads to neutrophil chemotaxis (Braun et al, 2005; Ward, 1996). It also causes a decrease in transendothelial electrical resistance across human pulmonary artery EC (HPAEC) (Petrache et al 2003). The pulmonary capillary EC have a balanced system between contracting and tethering forces that normally act to protect the EC barrier from paracellular gaps. The balancing forces depend on cytoskeletal components such as actin based microfilaments, intermediate filaments and microtubules. TNF-α causes contraction via the actin filaments and this results in the formation of gaps and EC permeability (Braun 2005). In pulmonary edema associated with ARDS, TNF-α can mediate acute inflammation and edema formation. It can also have a beneficial effect by increasing alveolar fluid clearance via an amiloride sensitive, cAMP independent mechanism to enhance alveolar fluid clearance. This is accomplished by binding to its receptors or activating Na+ channels in the epithelium (Fukuda et al, 2001).

Other networks of cytokines regulate lung inflammation in lung injury and edema. Complement, C5a and or the membrane attack complex, C5b-9 can directly activate EC to up-regulate adhesion molecules (P-selectin) or act synergistically with TNF-α to up regulate I-CAM and E Selectin (Shutte et al, 1996 & Ward, 1996). IL-4 and IL-10 suppress TNF-α and can have a strong attenuating effect on TNF-α. Studies have shown that blocking IL-10 increased TNF-α production, neutrophil recruitment and the intensity of lung inflammation (Ward, 1996). Although the role of cytokines in the pathogenesis of ARDS has been widely recognized, their importance in the clinical diagnosis has not been clearly defined.

Recent studies have identified that the receptor for advanced glycation end products (RAGE) is activated by its ligands in many disorders including ALI/ARDS. RAGE and interaction with the high mobility group box-1 (HMGB-1)- one of its ligands- promotes local lung endothelial inflammation and evokes both local and systemic inflammation (Nakamura et al, 2011 & Wolfson et al, 2010). In vitro studies determined that RAGE is the primary receptor signaling HMGB-1 induced endothelial barrier disruption and endothelial gap formation in human pulmonary artery endothelial cells (Wolfson et al, 2010). Soluable RAGE (sRAGE) has also been noted in the plasma of patients with ARDS and it was investigated as a biomarker of severity and clinical outcomes in patients with ARDS. In addition sRAGE and HMGB-1 levels were elevated in non- survivors compared to survivors in ARDS (Nakamura et al, 2011). An analysis of biomarker levels in two randomized controlled trials of ventilator therapy for ALI was done and the biomarkers that were elevated were ICAM-1, von Willebrand factor, IL-8, soluble TNF receptor-1, and surfactant protein-D. It was concluded that combining three or more biomarkers may be useful for selecting a high risk ALI group of patients (Calfee et al, 2011). Biomarker identification of risk remains an area of intense research.

5. Non-inflammatory NCPE

Categories of NCPE that resolve more quickly than ARDS and NCPE due to infection, trauma or other medical illness are high altitude pulmonary edema (HAPE), Immersion pulmonary edema (SCUBA diving and swimming) and negative pressure pulmonary edema (NPPE). Most commonly the non-inflammatory forms of NCPE occur in baseline healthy people although there may be a predilection to development of pulmonary edema in some people. However, there is no known way to predict who will develop pulmonary edema and who will not in the same circumstances.

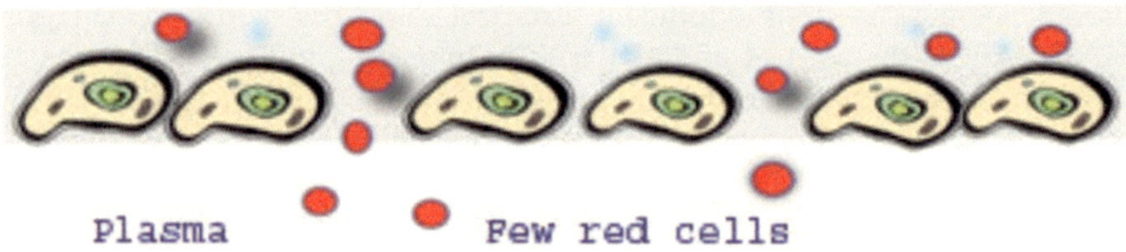

Fig. 3. Schematic representation of the endothelial barrier in Non-inflammatory Pulmonary Edema

Non- inflammatory pulmonary edema may have an element of hemorrhage leading to a pink frothy tint but will not initially have an inflammatory secretion of cells. The pulmonary edema resolves quickly and the endothelial barrier is thought to accommodate hydrostatic changes that resolve quickly compared to toxin mediated changes that heal slowly and may develop fibrinous changes.

6. HAPE

HAPE is a life threatening form of NCPE that has a rapid onset in healthy people who venture to elevations above 8200feet. This occurs when the lower barometric pressures result in hypoxia, usually less than 90% SPO_2 or 60 PaO_2. Studies done at high altitude on patients who developed HAPE and compared to those who did not, have shown that pulmonary artery pressures are elevated and lead to a protein rich and mildly hemorrhagic edema. Leukocytes, cytokines, nitric oxide metabolites and eicosanoids are normal when compared to control subjects who did not develop HAPE (Swenson et al, 2002). The mechanism of the increased pulmonary vasoconstriction and resulting increased pulmonary pressures is not resolved. The mechanism is thought to be increased pulmonary and arterial capillary pressures second to hypoxic pulmonary vasoconstriction. Another effect is a non-inflammatory increase in the permeability of the vascular endothelium. Some people are more susceptible to HAPE than others but the differentiating factors are not known. The most important treatment is to descend as soon as possible and provide oxygen therapy. Other treatments are Dexamethasone and nifedipine. Phosphodiesterase inhibitors are effective but the side effects worsen mountain sickness headaches (Maggiorini, 2010).

7. Immersion PE

Immersion PE that occurs in diving with self contained underwater breathing apparatus (SCUBA), and some triathlon athletes, combat swimmers (such as found in military missions) and breath hold divers is another type of non-inflammatory NCPE. Only about 1-2% of immersion divers develop PE and studies have not shown clearly what makes some people susceptible. One study did show that women, hypertension, fish oil and asthma may be factors that predispose to this condition (Miller III et al, 2010). The mechanism is poorly understood but reviews of cases have shown that the onset is rapid and that rapid improvement is also seen, similar to patients who develop HAPE (Slade et al, 2001). This observation lends credence to the probability that this is an acute but transient increase in pressure. The stress from the increased transalveolar pressure gradient that occurs with immersion is such that the non-cardiogenic capillary endothelium layer cell develops leaks (Slade et al, 2001). It has been shown that even asymptomatic dives result in an increased accumulation of extravascular lung water (Marinovic et al, 2010). They further demonstrated an increase in lung water, pulmonary artery pressure, NT-proBNP levels and decreased left ventricular contractility in healthy study volunteers who did not develop pulmonary edema. Immersion is known to increase preload and cold exposure increases both preload and afterload by vasoconstriction; it is possible that the changes could lead to damage in the pulmonary endothelium and lead to intrapulmonary redistribution of blood with regional overperfusion of some pulmonary capillaries and stress failure increasing capillary damage and permeability (Marinovic et al, 2010 & Pons et al, 1995). Hyperoxia and low tank pressures are other possible mechanisms that may damage the pulmonary endothelium and increase endothelial permeability the development of pulmonary edema in immersion PE.

8. Negative pressure pulmonary edema

Negative pressure pulmonary edema (NPPE) is pulmonary edema that occurs following an acute upper airway obstruction and may also be referred to as a post obstructive pulmonary edema. It often occurs in otherwise healthy patients. The most common cause is laryngospasm soon after extubation from an endo-tracheal intubation in about 0.1% in post anesthesia patients (Pathak et al, 2011). There are also case reports of NPPE after other causes such as foreign body, epiglottitis, tracheal secretions, upper airway tumors, obesity, obstructive sleep apnea, tumors (Fremont et al, 2007). Following an episode of obstruction of the airway there is a marked increase in negative intrathoracic pressure against the obstructed upper airway. The rapid increase in intrathoracic pressure causes a rise in venous return to the right heart, which increases pulmonary venous volume and pulmonary venous pressure which then increases the pulmonary capillary transmural pressure. Systemic pressures also rise due to catecholamine induced veno-constriction from anxiety, hypoxia and hypercarbia (Schwartz et al, 1999). Fremont et al have shown that the mechanism is due to hydrostatic changes with the fluid moving from high pressure in the pulmonary venous system to low pressure into the pulmonary interstitium and airspaces. Studies confirmed that the pulmonary edema fluid to plasma protein ratio were consistent with hydrostatic causes of acute fluid shifts and pulmonary edema. This causes an increase of blood flow (venous return) to the right heart increasing pulmonary venous pressure (Fremont et al, 2007). The treatment is resolving the obstruction, oxygen and either reintubation or if the patient is stable CPAP may be used. The issue is not volume overload and diuretics are not indicated (Kapoor, 2011).

9. Clinical manifestation of non cardiogenic pulmonary edema

Clinically non-cardiogenic pulmonary edema is a permeability edema. The Starling equation predicts that a change in permeability of the microvascular membrane will result in an increase in the amount of fluid and protein that leaves the vascular space and enters the interstitial space. When the interstitial fluid increases in the interstitium then the outward movement continues and fluid enters the alveolar spaces through the tight junctions of the epithelium. Many entities are associated with permeability edema manifested as ARDS, the most common entities are sepsis, pneumonia, multiple blood transfusions, gastric aspiration, trauma, drug overdose and pancreatitis. ~~and others.~~ Clinically NCPE prototype ALI/ARDS presents with progressive hypoxia and respiratory failure. Multi-organ failure is frequent and one of the reasons the mortality is so high. ARDS affects 200,000 people per year and has a mortality rate of 30-50%. This was initially described in the 1960s' by Petty and Ashbaugh (Ashbaugh et al, 1967). The diagnosis is made by four clinical criteria, acute onset of bilateral chest infiltrates, hypoxia, no evidence of left atrial hypertension (or clinical manifestations indicating left heart failure) and a ratio of arterial oxygen to fraction of inspired oxygen (PaO2/FIO2 ratio) of 201-300 for ALI and less than 200 for ARDS (Bernard et al, 1994 & The Acute Respiratory Distress Syndrome Network, 2000). Due to the profound respiratory failure most patients require mechanical ventilation and care in the intensive care unit (ICU). The best therapeutic approach for ARDS permeability edema is to find and treat the cause. There is no pharmacological treatment for ARDS, the only "treatment" that has emerged since it was first described in 1971 is the ARDS-net trial protocol of low tidal volume mechanical ventilation. This is a strategy that is called "lung-protective ventilation". The main benefit of lung-protective ventilation is to avoid further injury to the lungs from high tidal volumes often used for patients in the ICU as these large tidal volumes increase the injury and subsequently cause an increase in the permeability pulmonary edema in the injured lung. The standard tidal volumes used in ICU have been 10-15mg/kg for all mechanically ventilated patients, however, low tidal volumes of 6-8mg/kg are recommended for patients with ARDS. A mortality benefit was one of the primary outcomes demonstrated in the ARDS-net trial for patients with ARDS who are mechanically ventilated at these low tidal volumes (Matthay et al, 2002 & Marino 2007). Another aspect of NCPE and ARDS is heterogeneity of the lung parenchyma and the alveoli. The chest roentgenogram shows bilateral infiltrates that are difficult to distinguish from cardiogenic pulmonary edema and sometimes from pneumonia. The computed tomographic (CT) images are not necessarily diagnostic but in a patient with known ARDS shows that the lung edema and consolidation is not homogeneous but involves various lung regions, while other regions appear normal (Rouby et al, 2003). Alveolar over-distension from mechanical ventilation as well as repeated opening and collapse of the alveoli has been shown to cause lung injury initiating an increase in capillary stress and an increase in pro-inflammatory cytokine cascades (Matthay et al, 2002 & Slutsky &Tremblay, 1998). Hemodynamic evaluation of NCPE and ARDS requires careful ongoing evaluation, and may require monitoring cardiac filling pressures and cardiac output using a pulmonary artery catheter or currently, a non-invasive evaluation is more likely to be used. Diuretic therapy is then tailored to achieve the lowest cardiac filling pressures that do not compromise cardiac output and systemic oxygen transport. The nature of the lung interstitial infiltration is an inflammatory process, so that diuretic therapy to remove fluid does not remove the inflammation. Fluid treatment versus diuresis is not necessarily the goal of treatment in NCPE secondary to ARDS (Marino, 2007). Ultimately the treatment is supportive care using the appropriate ventilator strategies, promoting oxygenation, and treating the multi organ failure that is often contributes to the mortality. Histologically in this acute phase of lung injury there is widespread interstitial and alveolar edema with an abundance of neutrophils, erythrocytes, macrophages, cell debris, plasma proteins and strands of fibrin. At this phase there is injury to the capillary endothelium and denuding of the alveolar epithelium. If the patient survives this phase the pulmonary edema may completely resolve within a few months. Other patients with ALI/ARDS progress to a subacute phase over one to two weeks and may continue to have respiratory failure with hypoxia requiring mechanical ventilation. These patients develop fibrosis and capillary obliteration in the lungs, a condition called fibrosing alveolitis. These patients continue to progress with respiratory failure although they may recover from the initial event.

Progress from bench to bedside is being made; the mortality from NCPE and ALI/ARDS has improved from the initial 60% or more to 30-50%. The establishment of the NIH ARDS Network for clinical trials has improved the quantity and quality of large multicenter clinical trials for ALI/ARDS patients. New research is continuing and tools such as genetic analysis, genomics and proteomics may offer more value for patients in the future.

10. References

Abraham E. Neutrophils and acute lung injury. *Cr Care Med* 2003 Apr; 31(4 Suppl):S 195-9

Ashbaugh DG, Bigelow DB, Petty TL & Levine BE. Acute respiratory distress in adults. The Lancet, Sat 12 August 1967 *Crit Care Resusc* 2005 Mar;7(1):60-1

Bauer TT, Monton C, Torres A, Cabello H, Fellela X, Maldonado A, Nicolas JM & ZavalaE. Comparison of systemic cytokine levels in patients with acute respiratory distress syndrome, severe pneumonia and controls. *Thorax* 2000 Jan; 55(1):46-52

Bdeir, K, Higazi AA, Kulikovskaya I, Christofidou-Solomidou M, Vinogradov SA, Allen TC, Idell S Linzmeier R, Ganz T & Cines DB. Neutrophil α-Defensins Cause Lung Injury by Disrupting the Capillary Epithelial Barrier. *AJRCCM Am J Respir Crit Care Med* 2010 May;181(9): 935- 46

Bernard GR, Artigas A, Brigham KL, Carlet J, Falke D, Hudson L, Lamy M, LeGall JR, Morris A & Spragg R. Report of the American-European Consensus conference on acute respiratory distress syndrome: definitions, mechanisms, relevant outcomes, and clinical trial coordination. Consensus Committee. *J Crit Care* 1994 Mar;9(1):72-81

Blackwell TS, Blackwell TR, Holden EP, Christman BW & Christman JW. In vivo antioxidant treatment suppresses nuclear factor-kappa B activation and neutrophilic lung inflammation. *J Immuno.* 1996 Aug 15;157(4):1630-7

Braun, C, Hamacher J, Morel DR, Wendel A & Lucas R. Dichotomal Role of TNF in Experimental Pulmonary Edema Reabsorption. *J Immunol* 2005 Sep; 175(5):3402-8

Calfee CS, Ware LB, Glidden DV, Eisner MD, Parsons PE, Thompson BT & Matthay MA, National Heart, Blood, and Lung Institute Acute Respiratory Distress Syndrome Network. Use of risk reclassification with multiple biomarkers improves mortality prediction in acute lung injury. *Crit Care Med* 2011 Apr;39(4):711-7

Costello ML, Mathieu-Costello O & West JB. Stress failure of alveolar epithelial cells studied by scanning electron microscopy. *Am Rev Respir Dis* 1992 Jun;145(6):1446-55

Downey GP, Kong Q, Kruger J, Dedhar S & Cherapanov V. Regulation of Neutrophil Activation in Acute Lung Injury. *Chest* 1999 Jul;116(1suppl):46S-54S

Elia N, Tapponnier M, Matthay MA, Hamacher J, Pache JC, Brundler MA, Totsch M, DeBaetselier PD, Fransen L, Fukuda N, Morel DR & Lucas R. Functional identification of the alveolar edema reabsorption activity of murine tumor necrosis factor-alpha. *Am J Respir Crit Care Med* 2003 Nov;168(9):1043-50

Fein A, Grossman RF, Jones JG, Overland E, Pitts L, Murray JF & Staub NC. The value of edema fluid protein measurement in patients with pulmonary edema. *Am J Med* 1979 Jul;67(1):32-8

Folkesson HG & Matthay MA. Alveolar Epithelial Ion and Fluid Transport Recent Progess. *Am J Respir Cell Mol Biol* 2006 Jul;35(1):10-19Fremont RD, Kallet RH, Matthay MA & Ware LB. Postobstructive Pulmonary Edema: A case for Hydrostatic Mechanisms. *Chest* 2007 Jun;131;1742-46

Fukuda N, Jayr C, Lazrak A, Wang Y, Lucas R, Matalon S & Matthay MA. Mechanisms of TNF-α stimulation of amiloride sensitive sodium transport across alveolar epithelium. *Am J Physiol Lung Cell Mol Physiol* 2001 Jun; 280(6): L1258-65

Gantor CC, Jakob SM & Takala J. Pulmonary capillary pressure. *Minerva Anestesiol* 2006 Jan-feb;72(1-2):21-36

Geerts, Jorens, Willems, DeLey & Slegers. Natural inhibitors of neutrophil function in acute respiratory distress syndrome. *Crit Care Med* 2001 Oct;29(10):1920-24

Grommes J & Soehnlein O. Contribution of Neutrophils to Acute Lung Injury. *Mol Med* 2011 Mar;17(3-4)293-307

Hamacher J, Stammberger U, Roux J, Kumar S, Yang G, Xiong C, Schmid RA, Fakin RM, Chakraborty T, Hossain HM, Pittet JF, Wendel A, Black SM & Lucas R. The lectin like domain of tumor necrosis factor improves lung function after rat lung transplantation Potential role for a reduction in reactive oxygen species generation *Crit Care Med* 2010 Mar 38(3):871-8

Hasko G, Xu DZ, Lu Q, Nemeth, ZH, Jabush J, Berezina TL, Zaets SB, Csoka B & Deitch EA. Adenosine A2A receptor activation reduces lung injury in trauma/hemorrhagic shock. *Crit Care Med.* 2006 Apr;34(4): 1119-25

Holter JF, Weiland JE, Pacht ER, Gadek JE & Davis WB. Protein Permeability in the Adult Respiratory Distress Syndrome Loss of Size Selectivity of the Alveolar Epithelium. *J Clin Invest* 1986 Dec; 78(6): 1513-22

Hyers TM, Tricomi SM, Dettenmeier PA & Fowler AA. Tumor necrosis factor levels in serum and bronchoalveolar lavage fluid of patients with the adult respiratory distress syndrome. *Am Rev Respir Dis* 1991 Aug;144(2):268-71

Kaner RJ, Ladetto JV, Singh R, Fukuda N & Matthay MA, Crystal RG. Lung over-expression of the Vascular Endothelial Growth Factor Gene Induces Pulmonary Edema. *Am J Respir Cell Mol Biol* 2000 Jun; 22(6):657-664

Kapoor MC. Negative pressure pulmonary oedema. *Indian J Anaesth.* 2011 Jan; 55(1):10-1

Lucas R, Verin AD, Black SM & Catravas JD. Regulators of endothelial and epithelial barrier integrity and function in acute lung injury. *Biochem Pharmacol*2009 Jun 15;77(12): 1763-72

Maggiorini. Prevention and Treatment of High Altitude Pulmonary Edema. *Prog CardiovascDis 2010 May*-Jun;52(6):500-6Marino P. *The ICU Book third edition.* Lippincott Williams and Wilkins 2007 ISBN-13: 978-0-7817-4802-5

Marinovic, Ljubkovic, Obad, Breskovic, Salamunic, Denoble & Dujic. Assessment of Extravascular Lung Water and Cardiac Function in Trimix SCUBA Diving. *Med SciSports Exerc* 2010 Jun;42(6):1054-61

Nakamura T, Sato E, Fujiwara N, Kawagoe Y, Maeda S & Yamagishi S. Increased levels of soluble receptor for advanced glycation end products (sRAGE) and high mobility group box 1 (HMGB1) are associated with death in patients with acute respiratory distress syndrome. *Clin Biochem*2011 Jun;44(8-9): 601-4

Ono N, Mizuno R & Ohhashi T. Effective permeability of hydrophilic substances through walls of lymph vessels: roles of endothelial barrier. *Am J Physiol Heart Circ Physiol* 2005 Oct;289(4): H1676-82

Pathak V, Rendon IS & Ciubotaru RL. Recurrent Negative Pressure Pulmonary Edema. *Clin MedRes* 2011 Jun;9(2):88-91Petrache I, Birukova A, Ramirez SI, Garcia JG & Verin AD. The Role of the Microtubules in Tumor Necrosis Factor-α-Induced Endothelial Cell Permeability. *Am J Respir Cell Mol Biol* 2003 May;28(5):574-81

Pons, Blickenstorfer, Oechslin, Hold, Greminger, Franzeck & Russi. Pulmonary edema in healthy persons during scuba-Diving and swimming, *Eur Respir J*, 1995 May;8(5):762-7

Sartori C, Rimoldi SF & Scherrer U. Lung fluid movements in hypoxia. *Prog Cardiovasc Dis.* 2010 May;52(6):493-9

Schutte H, Lohmeyer, J, Rosseau S, Ziegler S, Siebert C, Kielisch H, Pralle H, Grimminger F, Morr H & Seeger W. Bronchoalveolar and systemic cytokine profiles in patients with ARDS, severe pneumonia and cardiogenic pulmonary edema. E*ur Respir J* 1996 Sep; 9(9):1858-67

Schwartz, Maroo, Malhotra & Kesselman. Negative Pressure Pulmonary Hemorrhage. *Chest* 1999; Apr;115(4):1194-97

Slade JB, Hattori T, Ray CS, Bove AA & Cianci P. Pulmonary Edema Associated with Scuba Diving: Case Reports and Review. *Chest* 2001Nov;120(5);1686-94

Slutsky AS, Tremblay LN. Multiple System Organ Failure Is Mechanical Ventilation a Contributing Factor? *Am J Respir Crit Care Med* 1998 Jun;157(6 Pt 1):1721-5

Staub NC, Hitoshi N & Pearce ML. Pulmonary edema in dogs, especially the sequence of fluid accumulation in lungs. *J Appl Physiol 1967* 22(2):227-240

Steinberg KP, Milberg JA, Martin TR,Maunder RJ, Cockrill BA & Hudson LD. Evolution of bronchoalveolar cell populations in the adult respiratory distress syndrome. *Am J Respir Crit Care Med* 1994 Jul;150(1):113-22

Swenson, Miggiorini, Mongovin, Gibbs, Greve, Mairbaurl & Bartsch. Pathogenesis of High Altitude Pulmonary Edema-Inflammation is not an etiologic Factor. *JAMA,* 2002 May; 287(17):2228-35

The Acute Respiratory Distress Syndrome Network. Ventilation with lower tidal volumes as compared with traditional tidal volumes for acute lung injury and the acute respiratory distress syndrome. *N Engl J Med* 2000 May;342(18):1301-8

Tzouvelekis A, Pneumatikos I & Bouros D. Serum biomarkers in Acute Respiratory Distress Syndrome: an ailing prognosticator. *Respir Res* 2005 Jun;6:62

Umapathy NS, Fan ZH, Zemskov EA, Alieva IB, Black SM & Verin AD. Molecular mechanisms involved in adenosine induced endothelial cell barrier enhancement. *Vascul Pharmacol2010 May;* 52(5-6):199-206

Ward PA. Role of Complement, Chemokines, and Regulatory Cytokines in Acute Lung Injury. *Ann NY Acad Sci.* 1996 Oct 31;796:104-12

Ware LB, Fremont RD, Bastarache JA, Calfee CS & Matthay MA. Determining the aetiology of pulmonary oedema by the oedema fluid-to-plasma protein ratio. *Eur Respir J* 2010 Feb;35(2): 331-7

Weiland JE, Davis WB, Holter JF, Mohammed JR, Dorinsky PM & Gadek JE. Lung neutrophils in the adult respiratory distress syndrome. *Am Rev Respir Dis* 1986 Feb;133(2):218-5

Wolfson RK, Chiang ET & Garcia JG. HMGB1 induces human lung endothelial cell cytoskeletal rearrangement and barrier disruption. *Microvas Res* 2011 Mar;81(2): 89-97

Ware LB & Matthay MA. Clinical practice. Acute pulmonary edema. *N Engl J Med*. 2005 Dec; 353(26):2788-96

Zimmerman GA & McIntyre TM. PAF, ceramide and pulmonary edema: alveolar flooding and a flood of questions. *Trends Mol Med*2004 Jun;10(6):245-8

25

High Altitude Pulmonary Edema

Zhou Qiquan and Luo Yongjun
Department of High Altitude Diseases, College of High Altitude Military Medicine, Third Military Medical University, Key Laboratory of High Altitude Medicine, Ministry of Education and Key Laboratory of High Altitude Medicine of PLA, Chongqing, China

1. Introduction

High altitude pulmonary edema (HAPE) is a form of high altitude idiopathy that occurs in a minority of people upon either the first or subsequent exposure to high altitudes. It is triggered by a shortage of oxygen and certain other predisposing factors, all of which lead to a sudden increase in pulmonary arterial pressure, increase in lung blood volume, disturbance of pulmonary circulation, and leakage of fluid in microcirculation into the pulmonary interstitium and alveoli. The clinical symptoms of this condition include dyspnea and hacking cough.

HAPE is a severe type of acute high altitude disease, typically occurring at altitudes above 4,000 meters. However, cases have been reported at altitudes as low as 2,261 meters in Xining, China. HAPE is a rapid-onset condition that can progress and change quickly, especially during the first stage of high altitude exposure, usually within a week, peaking within three days. According to a report based on 332 cases, 63% of HAPE patients presented symptoms within three days, and the fastest onset was after only a few hours. HAPE occurs mostly in unacclimatized sea-level residents when they first ascend to high altitudes or acclimatized individuals ascending from lower to higher altitudes. It can also occur in long-term high altitude residents or high altitude natives undertaking excessive physical activities or in those who return to high altitudes after living in low-altitude areas for a period of time. HAPE patients can recover after short-term treatment and continue to stay at high altitudes. However, improper treatment may lead to negative effects. The incidence rate is closely related to the altitude, rapidity of exposure, season, the individual's physical condition, and the intensity of activity.

2. Epidemiology

2.1 Incidence rate

1. Population Incidence

The incidence rate of HAPE varies significantly between China and the others country reports, for example it ranges between 0.15% and 9.9% in Chinese report. The incidence rate is higher in kids and teenagers than in adults. For instance, data collected from the Andes Mountain area of Peru reports that the incidence rate was 10% in children aged 2-12, 17% in teens aged 13-20, and 3% in adults over 21.

2. Hospitalization rate

Due to the differences in location and population served, different treatment facilities have reported rather different hospitalization rate. The Menon hospital, at an altitude of 3,450 meters, treated 101 HAPE patients over two years, accounting for 5-10% of all inpatients in the department of internal medicine; a hospital in Changdu (Tibetan), at an altitude of 3,200 meters, treated 33 HAPE patients over 11 years, accounting for 0.37% of all inpatients in the internal medicine department and 6.28% of all inpatients with high altitude diseases; the General Hospital of the Tibet Military Region, at an altitude of 3,658 meters, treated 2,853 HAPE patients from 1956 to 2005, accounting for 89.6% of all inpatients with high altitude diseases during the same time period.

3. Age Distribution

Reports from the Andes and Rocky Mountain areas show higher incidence in children, but occurrences in children below 2 years old are rare and the maximum age of all HAPE patients covered in these reports was found to be 53 years old. In the General Hospital of the Tibet Military Region, the youngest HAPE patient was 1 year old and the oldest one was 63 years old. We think that HAPE can occur at any age, but children and young adults are more susceptible.

4. Gender Differences

HAPE can occur in both males and females. Many reports show higher incidence in males, mainly because more males travel to high altitude areas. In mountaineering and high altitude medical research teams, male participants are more common, hence a higher reported incidence of HAPE in males. Horrobin et al. mentioned that in Kenyan mountain areas there were many female mountaineers, none of whom developed HAPE. However Hultgren et al. reported that among 97 lifelong mountain residents, HAPE occurred mainly in females.

5. Racial Differences

It has been shown that there is no significant difference in HAPE incidence between Peruvian Indians and Caucasians in the plateau areas of Peru. However, some have suggested that the Sherpa of Nepal have a lower HAPE incidence than the Indians of Peru. They point out that the Indians have only inhabited the Andes for about 10,000 years, whereas the Sherpa, originally from the Tibetan Plateau, have lived in high altitude areas for several tens of thousands of years. Therefore, the Sherpa may be more adapted to high altitudes environment than Peruvian Indians. Our investigation found that, on the Tibetan Plateau, HAPE incidence in native Tibetans was lower than in Han immigrants. In the 923 HAPE cases treated by the General Hospital of the Tibet Military Region over the past ten years, there was only one Tibetan patient. Recently we have retrospectively analyzed for severe acute mountain sickness of 3184 Inpatients cases in General Hospital of Tibet Military region Hospitalization from June 1956 to June 2005, and in which the incidence and clinical characteristics of native Tibetan plateau were analyzed.The results detected 24 cases of high altitude native Tibetan suffering severe cases of acute mountain sickness, high altitude pulmonary edema 21 cases and high altitude cerebral edema 3 cases in them, incidence of severe acute mountain sickness in native Tibetan population was 0.75% (24/3184).

6. First and Repeated Exposure to High Altitudes

Whether triggered by the patient's first or a subsequent exposure to high altitude, HAPE onset usually takes place between one and seven days, but it can start as early as three hours or as late as ten days after exposure. Occasionally, HAPE is triggered in high altitude residents by such factors as fatigue. For those who travel to high altitudes by plane, the typical time of HAPE onset is within three days. Data collected from Peru and the U.S. suggest that high altitude residents are likely to develop HAPE when returning to the plateau after spending typically one to three weeks on the plains. In Tibetan areas, HAPE tends to be triggered when residents spend typically three to six weeks on the plains before returning.

7. Mode of Transportation to High Altitude Area

Traveling to high altitude areas, whether on foot, by ground vehicle, or by airplane, can trigger HAPE. In recent years, as more people take airplane flights to the Tibetan Plateau, the number of HAPE patients who have arrived by plane has substantially increased. Among the 2,853 HAPE patients treated by the General Hospital of the Tibet Military Region between 1956 and 2005, 2,054 patients were traveled to Tibet by airplane.

8. Occupation and Labor Intensity

HAPE can occur in individuals of all occupations when they are exposed to high altitudes, but it is more common in those engaged in heavy physical labor. For instance, during the Qinghai-Tibet Highway, construction workers have a higher HAPE incidence than drivers, who in turn have a higher HAPE incidence than travelers taking rides. Those who are rapidly exposed to high altitudes and extreme fatigue are particularly susceptible to HAPE. Therefore, individuals engaged in physical activities at high altitudes, such as plateau mountaineering, alpine skiing, or traveling to high altitudes are all at risk for HAPE. In addition, HAPE is more likely to occur in young boys, as they tend to be more active and less willing to rest than young girls and adults.

9. Season of Onset and Changes in Climate

HAPE can occur in any season, but in general it is more common in the winter and spring. Earlier statistics from domestic show the onset of HAPE to be distributed mostly from November to March of the next year. More recent data suggest an increase in the prevalence of HAPE between January and October, mainly because there have been more people traveling to and from the plateau or engaging in high altitude activities during this period.

10. Upper Respiratory Tract Infection and Acute mild mountain sickness

Upper respiratory tract infection can also trigger HAPE. Among the 865 HAPE patients treated by a Tibetan hospital in Lhasa, 30% had already had a previous upper respiratory tract infection at the time of onset. It is suggested that upper respiratory tract infection may trigger HAPE because contracting an upper respiratory tract infection after reaching a high altitude substantially worsens the shortage of oxygen.

A minority of those who show Acute mild mountain sickness (AMMS) may develop HAPE without prompt treatment. Among the 230 HAPE cases reported by a hospital in southern Xinjiang, 112 (47%) started out with AMMS. From this it can be concluded that, when developing acute or even minor AMMS or upper respiratory tract infection, one should rest and receive immediate treatment to prevent the condition from progressing to HAPE.

11. Individual and Familial Susceptibility

It has been reported that there are patients who develop severe HAPE more than two times, up to four times. Analysis on the 923 HAPE cases treated by a hospital in Lhasa showed that 27% of the patients returning to high altitudes developed HAPE two or more times, two of them even seven times. In our clinical experience we have seen one worker developing HAPE eight times. It is worth pointing out that some HAPE patients, when returning to high altitudes from the plain, may still develop HAPE again even if they take active measures to prevent it, such as bed rest, oxygen inhalation, and medicine.

Some reports have shown that HAPE can co-occur in fathers and sons, brothers, and mothers and daughters. In Tibetan, Zhang reported HAPE occurring in three generations of one family, suggesting that familial and individual factors are involved in patients' susceptibility to HAPE. Animal studies have also shown species and individual differences in susceptibility to HAPE.

2.2 Fatality rate and cause of death

1. Fatality Rate

A collection of data showed that among 160 HAPE cases that occurred between 1958 and 1965 in China, the fatality rate was 9.4%. In recent years, due to substantial improvements in medical conditions and the promptness of treatment, the fatality rate has decreased significantly. For instance, among the 923 cases of HAPE treated by the General Hospital of the Tibet Military Region in the northern Tibetan plateau, the fatality rate was 0.33%.

2. Cause of Deaths

When treated promptly, most HAPE patients can recover in three to five days. However, death still occurs occasionally, and the causes can be generally summarized as belonging to one of the following categories: 1) Delay in diagnosis or treatment due to poor transportation and substandard medical conditions in remote areas. 2) Deterioration of the patient's general condition caused by undiagnosed and untreated complications such as heart failure, shock, massive pulmonary embolism, severe lung infection, and cerebral encephaledema/encephalorrhagia. 3) Severe HAPE may cause instant death, and co-occurring pulmonary embolisms or encephalorrhagia can also lead to death.

In summary, the incidence of HAPE is closely related to factors such as the mode of transportation to high altitude regions, the rapidity of exposure to high altitudes, the altitude itself, the medical support received, and individual susceptibility. Fatigue, upper respiratory tract infection, and excessive mental stress are all important triggers of HAPE. HAPE mostly occurs at altitudes above 3,000 meters because there are more immigrants at these altitudes. HAPE is not clearly correlated with age or gender. With the increasing of knowledge on HAPE and improvements to medical conditions, the fatality rate of HAPE has become extremely low.

3. Causes and predisposing factors

HAPE is a disease that occurs at high altitudes, its main cause being scarcity of oxygen. All factors that aggravate oxygen shortage in the body lower the body's tolerance to low oxygen levels, or add load to pulmonary circulation can trigger HAPE. The most common predisposing factors include cold, fatigue, and upper respiratory tract infection.

1. Cold

Cold is a basic feature of plateau weather. The temperature on the Tibetan Plateau is on average more than 20°C lower than the temperature at sea level on the same latitude. At night, wind blows downwards from the snow-covered mountaintops, further accelerating the drop in body surface temperature and making the night at high altitudes especially cold. Under external conditions, extreme coldness accompanied by wind and snow, the body will speed up its metabolism and consume more oxygen. At the same time, sympathetic excitability will become elevated, increasing the venous blood return from the peripheral veins, especially those on the surface of the skin, increasing the load of pulmonary circulation. In addition, pulmonary arterioles contract, inducing or aggravating pulmonary hypertension and eventually triggering HAPE.

2. Fatigue

Physical labor can increase oxygen demand ten times. Physical labor further aggravates oxygen shortage. In addition, physical labor at high altitudes increases the release of catecholamine, and hyperventilation can cause respiratory alkalosis, decrease the concentration of $PaCO_2$, and lead to venoconstriction in the systemic circulation and subsequent increases both in the cardiac output of the right side of the heart and in pulmonary blood volume. Physical labor may further increase the pulmonary arterial pressure and decrease the concentration of $PaCO_2$. Those who engage in excessive mental labor may also be susceptible to HAPE due to bodily fatigue.

3. Upper respiratory tract infection

Upper respiratory tract infection often causes fever, which increases oxygen consumption. If complicated by bronchitis, causing coughing and an increase in bronchial secretions, it will affect pulmonary ventilation and cause damage to the alveolar epithelia, impeding the generation of surface-active substances. According to statistics from Lhasa, 30% of HAPE cases were triggered by upper respiratory tract infections; data from southern Xinjiang showed 29%.

4. Excessive mental stress

Mental stress, anxiety, and fear can increase the release of catecholamine, which in turn increases pulmonary arterial pressure and triggers HAPE.

5. Rapidity of exposure to high altitudes

Among those who quickly enter the plateau areas by ground vehicle or by plane without adaptation trainings, the incidence of HAPE is substantially higher than in those who come by slower means. This is because rapid exposure to high altitudes leads to acute oxygen shortage, in which the body does not have enough time to adapt and shows extremely poor tolerance to low oxygen levels.

6. Sleep and hypnotic drugs

During sleep, the horizontal position of the body increases pulmonary blood volume (500 ml more than an upright position). The shallow breathing that takes place during sleep, especially the periodic or irregular breathing accompanied by temporary apnea can aggravate the oxygen shortage.

The incidence of HAPE mainly depends on the altitude, temperature, and adaptability of the body. High altitudes, low temperatures, and failure to acclimate are three basic factors that trigger HAPE. Individuals may not develop HAPE when only one factor is present. With two factors, the incidence rate is still not high. However, when all three factors are present, one is much more likely to develop HAPE. The incidence rate will increase further if there are other coexisting conditions. Those who are exposed to high altitudes without a thorough physical examination may have undetected organic cardiovascular diseases, organic diseases of the respiratory tract, liver, brain or kidney, malnutrition, or hypoproteinemia.

4. Pathogenesis

The incidence of HAPE is closely correlated with oxygen shortage at high altitudes. Currently, it is believed that the following processes are important: an excessive increase in the pulmonary arterial pressure, an increase in the permeability of the pulmonary capillaries, and impairment in alveolar epithelium water clearance. Among these three, an excessive increase in the pulmonary arterial pressure is the key link.

4.1 Excessive increase in the pulmonary arterial pressure

In 1904, Plumier et al. observed that low oxygen levels could lead to pulmonary hypertension. In 1964, Hultgnen performed right cardiac catheterization on four acute HAPE patients and found that in both the clinical and the recovery periods their pulmonary arterial pressures were significantly higher than that of control subjects at the same altitude, but their right arterial pressures, pulmonary venous pressures, and pulmonary capillary pressures were all essentially normal. There are several ways in which hypoxia that occurs at high altitudes can lead to pulmonary hypertension.

1. Pulmonary vasoconstriction caused by hypoxia

Hypoxic pulmonary vasoconstriction can redirect blood flow from low-oxygen alveolar regions to alveoli with higher oxygen content, which improves the ventilation/perfusion ratio and gaseous exchange, allows sufficient oxygenation of the blood, and increases arterial partial pressure of oxygen. However, pulmonary hypertension over a long period of time can also cause a series of pathophysiological changes and become an important pathologic basis of the initiation and development of HAPE.

Studies on the mechanisms of hypoxic pulmonary vasoconstriction have demonstrated that, at low oxygen levels, the calcium concentration and transmembrane inflow of calcium ions in the pulmonary arterial smooth muscle cells are both significantly increased. As hypoxia the distribution of ions across the membranes of the pulmonary arterial smooth muscle cells, calcium and sodium ions flow into the cells and potassium ions flow out, causing the resting membrane potential to decrease, approaching its excitation threshold. This depolarization of the pulmonary arterial smooth muscle cells leads to increased reactivity of the pulmonary vessels and increased tension in the pulmonary arterioles and pulmonary arteriolar contraction. Some investigators believe that hypoxia directly changes the transmembrane potential of the pulmonary artery smooth muscle cells, leading to calcium ion inflow and decrease of excitation threshold of these cells, which then causes the smooth muscles of the arterioles to contract. In addition, vasoactive substances such as prostaglandin, thromboxane A_2, angiotonin, and histamine may serve as regulators or synergists in hypoxic pulmonary vasoconstriction. However, persistent pulmonary hypertension caused by hypoxia may involve many vasoactive substances, the importance of each varying depending on the specific conditions.

Hypoxic pulmonary vasoconstriction doubtlessly leads to pulmonary hypertension. As to how the pulmonary hypertension causes HAPE, currently there are three hypotheses.

a. Regional maldistribution of blood flow. It has been proposed that when those who are sensitive to hypoxia at high altitudes are exposed to low-oxygen environments, their muscle arterioles contract rigorously and precapillary resistance increases, while their non-muscle arterioles expand under pulmonary hypertension. The sudden increase in the hydrostatic pressure in the afflicted areas, plus other factors, can cause HAPE. As the changes described above occur in some but not all pulmonary arterioles and capillaries, the pathological changes manifested in the HAPE are usually regional, in accordance with the patchy distributions of edema in HAPE observed via X-ray.

b. At high altitudes, as hypoxia leads to sudden increases in pulmonary arterial pressure, this high pressure in turn causes closed capillaries to instantly open. The abrupt increase in the capillary pressure then causes fluid to leak out.

c. It has been proposed that fluid does not leak out through the capillaries but rather directly through the walls of pulmonary arterioles under the pulmonary hypertension caused by hypoxia.

2. Increases in the resistance to pulmonary venous return

The left ventricle is a relatively large, muscular organ that needs to overcome the high pressure and high resistance of systemic circulation to pump blood. At high altitudes, when oxygen shortage is minor, the body can employ a series of adaptive mechanisms on levels ranging from the systemic to the cellular to alleviate the damage to myocardia caused by hypoxia. However, when oxygen shortage is severe (such as may occur in cases of rapid ascent, excessive physical activity, and severe cold), there is no time for the body to set up these adaptive mechanisms of antihypoxia on the cellular level. In this case, hypoxia will cause direct damage to myocardia, especially those on the left side of the heart. Although left heart failure is not the main cause of HAPE, in clinical situations, cardiac agents have proven to be effective to a certain extent. Animal studies have also shown that compensation in heart function can significantly affect the progress of hypoxic pulmonary hypertension.
When the myocardial damage induced by oxygen shortage exceeds a certain degree, the function of the left heart decompensates, causing an increase in the left ventricular end diastolic pressure (LVEDP) and in the left atrial pressure (LAP). This in turn boosts pulmonary hypertension and contributes further to the development of pulmonary edema. Pulmonary edema impedes gaseous exchange and oxygenation, and the resulting decrease in arterial partial pressure of oxygen further aggravates myocardial anoxia and damage. Increases in high altitude pulmonary blood volume cause an increase in the pulmonary venous resistance.

3. Increases in pulmonary circulation blood volume

Increases in pulmonary blood volume are another important factor that can elevate pressure in pulmonary circulation. It has been shown that 48-72 hours after healthy soldiers were airlifted from sea level to 3,658 meters, their pulmonary blood volumes increased by 82%. This is because oxygen shortage acts on the central nervous system and causes increased sympathetic excitability. Increased sympathetic excitability results in the large-scale release of catecholamines. At the same time, due to the increase in resistance in the peripheral vessels, the left ventricular load increases and cardiac output decreases while left atrial pressure increases. Pulmonary venous return is impeded, causing blood to fill the blood vessels of the lungs. The increased blood supply and reduced blood output in the pulmonary circulation increase pulmonary blood volume. The compensatory erythrocytosis and increase in both water and sodium retention caused by hypoxia increase blood volume in general, including pulmonary blood volume, which also leads to pulmonary edema.

4. Formation of micro-thrombi in the pulmonary vessels

The formation of micro-thrombi in the pulmonary circulation is a pathological feature of HAPE. Autopsies of HAPE patients have found extensive blockages by thrombi in the pulmonary capillaries and some in the branches of the pulmonary veins and arteries, demonstrating that the formation of thrombi in the pulmonary vessels is relatively important to the pathogenesis of HAPE. Due to extensive micro-thrombus formation in the pulmonary capillaries and in other organs such as the brain, the liver, the spleen, the kidney, and the intestine, it has been suggested that hypoxic pulmonary hypertension results from abnormal coagulation and general thrombus blockage of the pulmonary capillaries.

As to the mechanism by which micro-thrombi form in the pulmonary vessels, it is generally believed that as the levels of fibrinogen and anti-fibrinoclase released by the liver increase and levels of fibrinoclase activators released by the lung decrease, the resulting abnormal fibrinolysis is an important pathophysiological basis of the formation of micro-thrombi in the pulmonary vessels. Singh et al. proposed that hypoxia could lead to damage to the fibrinoclase system and that this damage might disturb the dynamic balance between the formation and dissolution of fibrin, causing fibrin to build up in the pulmonary vessels and hence cause the formation of micro-thrombi.

Studies have shown that during the initial stages of HAPE, there are substantial increases in the level of platelet factor 3, and in the release of ADP, resulting in decreased platelet mobility. They have also found that, in HAPE patients, the levels of plasma immunoglobulins, including IgG, IgA, and IgM, all increase significantly. IgG and IgM can adhere to the surface of platelets and change their electrophoretic mobility, increasing platelet adhesivity and release of ADP. ADP can promote the utilizing of platelet factor 3, which further speeds up the coagulation process. Imbalances in cellular immune function cause immune complexes to build up. As the immune complexes activate blood coagulation factors, they further aggravate blood clotting in the blood vessels. The aforementioned weakening of the cellular immune function co-occurs with a decrease in the dissolution activity of fibrin. When the dissolution activity of fibrin improves, cellular immune function also recovers. In addition, recent studies have found that the magnesium content of erythrocytes and leukocytes increases significantly in healthy individuals who adapt well to high altitudes, but in HAPE patients it decreases significantly. Magnesium can alleviate coagulation by expanding blood vessels, stabilizing fibrinogen and platelets, and accelerating the dissolution of fibrin.

4.2 Increases in the permeability of the pulmonary capillaries

It has been reported that when dogs were placed at a simulated altitude of 6,401 meters, the flow of lymph in the right lymphatic duct increased. After inhaling pure oxygen, lymph flow decreased, the lymphatic duct expanded, but there was no sign of blockage. The causes of lymph flow increase included increased pressure and increased permeability resulting from pores opening in the walls of the lymphatic ducts in a low-pressure, low-oxygen environment. When the dogs' arterial oxygen saturation dropped to 75% (corresponding to an altitude of 5,200 meters), the lymph flow began to increase. When the arterial oxygen saturation dropped to 52.5% (corresponding to an altitude of 6,100 meters), the lymph flow increased substantially. Once red blood cells enter the lymph, the capillaries are considered damaged. Schoene collected bronchoalveolar lavage fluid from HAPE patients in a lab at an altitude of 4,400 meters by branchofiberoscope. Component analysis showed elevated protein content, even higher than that in the edema fluid collected from adult respiratory distress syndrome (ARDS) patients. All these directly demonstrate that HAPE results from the leakage of fluid, protein, and even blood formed elements caused by the increased permeability of the pulmonary capillaries, suggesting that HAPE is a type of protein-rich, high-permeability pulmonary edema. In 1991, West JB et al. successfully simulated the pathophysiological process of HAPE in the laboratory by increasing the pulmonary arterial pressure of laboratory animals. He observed that when the rabbits' pulmonary capillary pressure reached 40 mmHg, the endothelia of the pulmonary capillaries and alveoli and sometimes even all the linings of the alveoli started to rupture.

The mechanisms by which the pulmonary capillary permeability increases may include the following factors.

1. Direct damage to the respiratory membrane structure

According to studies, under emergency conditions involving hypoxia, the endochylema of the pulmonary capillary and alveolar endothelial cells become condensed, causing the cells to shrink, which in turn expands the intercellular space of the alveolar capillary membranes and increases their permeability.

2. Decrease in secretion of alveolar surfactants

The alveolar surfactant is a type of phospholipin secreted by alveolar epithelial type II cells. When the lung tissues experience shortages of oxygen and blood, the normal metabolism of the alveolar epithelial type II cells is disturbed, and the secretion of this substance decreases. In high altitude, secretion of this substance may decrease, causing the permeability of the barrier between the capillaries and lung tissues to increase, leading to HAPE.

3. Increases in levels of acidic metabolites in local tissues

The anaerobic metabolism increases and the acidic metabolites accumulate, causing the physicochemical properties of the adhesion substance between the capillary endothelial cells to change and the basilar membrane to denature, which eventually leads to increased capillary permeability.

4. Respiratory tract infection

Any respiratory tract infection can directly damage the pulmonary capillaries and tissues through inflammatory metabolites and bacterial toxins, increasing their permeability. It is already known that hypoxia can induce inflammatory reactions involving immunocytes and epithelial cells, and therefore it can be deduced that high altitude hypoxia may induce the secretion of inflammatory cytokines, causing HAPE by producing pulmonary extravasation. To understand the relationship between inflammation and the pathogenesis of HAPE, researchers measured the levels of several inflammation mediators under hypoxia, including interleukin-6 (IL-6), interleukin -1 receptor antibody (IL-1ra), and C reactive protein (CRP). The moderate increase of these inflammatory markers reflects the presence of general local inflammation and suggests that inflammation may be involved in the pathogenesis of HAPE. Another study measured continuously the level of NO, a marker of respiratory inflammation, in the expiratory air of human subjects, and found that at 4,359 meters, the 13 subjects who were also HAPE patients among 28 subjects did not show trend of elevated NO levels during the clinical period, found the NO content in the expiratory air of subjects during their stay at high altitudes was 30% lower, indicating that respiratory tract infection does not precede HAPE.

5. Increases in plasma fibrinogen and the decreases in the dissolution activity of fibrin cause fibrin to accumulate in the pulmonary capillaries, forming thrombi that block them. This increases the permeability of the capillary walls.

4.3 Impairment of water clearance by the alveolar epithelium

HAPE results from unbalanced fluid secretion and reabsorption in the alveoli. In particular, the amiloride-sensitive epithelial sodium channel (ENaC) is involved in 40-60% of the re-absorption processes. It has also been found that β2 antagonist, which activates epithelial sodium channels (ENaC), also promotes water clearance in the lungs. In addition, *in vitro* studies have found that hypoxia inhibits Na+/K+-ATPase activity in alveolar epithelial type II cells as well as the co-transportation of Na, K, and Cl. This all suggests that hypoxia impedes the transmembrane re-absorption of water and sodium in epithelial cells.

4.4 Increases in sympathetic excitability

Studies have found that sympathectomy or blockage of cervical sympathetic nerves can eliminate HAPE. This suggests that the pathogenesis of HAPE is clearly related to sympathetic excitability. It has been found that the subjects' sympathetic excitability instantly increased at 3,500 meters, reaching a peak value within 24-72 hours, which is exactly the period of time during which HAPE is most likely to occur.

4.5 Individual susceptibility

Given the same conditions, the incidence of HAPE shows differences along racial, individual, and age lines. A study reported that among the 43 patients with recurrent HAPE, thirty-two developed HAPE 2 times, seven 3 times, three 4 times, and one 6 times. This shows that individual susceptibility is one of the factors for the incidence of HAPE. When comparing HAPE patients to normal subjects, researchers have found that the chest circumferences and chest anteroposterior diameters of acute HAPE patients are both longer than those of controls. In addition, there are more circular muscle fibers on the pulmonary arteriolar walls of the acute HAPE patients. Individual differences in internal factors such as the tissue structure of the pulmonary vessels and immune function status may lead to individual differences in sensitivity, tolerance to hypoxia, and other steps of the pathogenesis of HAPE.

In summary, the pathogenesis of HAPE is complex, involving many steps. Currently well-accepted factors include the following:

a. Hypoxia directly damages pulmonary capillary endothelial cells and expands or destroys the intercellular space, leading to general damage to the structure of the air-blood barrier, which causes blood plasma to leak directly into the alveolar space.
b. Hypoxia damages alveolar epithelial type II cells, diminishing their ability to secrete surfactants, leading to a decrease in alveolar surface tension, which causes the fluid and proteins in the pulmonary capillaries likely to leak out.
c. Hypoxia prompts the alveoli to release cytokines such as histamine, serotonin, interleukin-1, interleukin-6, leukotriene E4, tumor necrosis factor, and C-reactive protein, causing capillary permeability to increase.
d. Hypoxia prompts pulmonary arteriole constriction and an increase in vascular resistance, resulting in pulmonary hypertension. At the same time, sympathetic excitability increases and blood is redistributed, leading to an increase in pulmonary blood volume and body fluid retention, which causes capillary hydrostatic pressure to increase and fluid components to leak out, further aggravating HAPE.

5. Pathological changes

The pathological changes involved in HAPE mainly occur in the lungs. Visual inspections reveal increases in the volume, weight, and surface moisture of the two lungs and that the peripulmonary membrane has become stretched, rubbery, and dark red in color. When pressed, pink spumous fluid streams to the surface. Under optical microscope, expansion of the pulmonary capillaries is observed, with red blood cells accumulating inside and bleeding around the vessels. The middle layers of the muscular pulmonary arterioles thicken, the elastic layers appear serrated, and the arterioles muscularize. The pulmonary arterioles are expanded and interrupted and capillary thrombi are formed. The bronchioles and alveoli present hyaline membranous edema, and the alveolar ducts become filled with blended protein fluid or cluttered red blood cells. The capillaries in the alveolar septum expand, with blood accumulating inside and forming thrombi. Under electron microscope, unformed edema fluid with low electron concentration is observed inside the pulmonary alveolar space. Red blood cells accumulate, the capillaries in the alveolar septum expand, the intercellular space between endothelial cells enlarges, and the endothelial cells swell. The number of pinocytotic vesicles and some vacuolated were increased. The alveolar epithelial type I and type II cells swell, shedding surface microvilli. The perinuclear space of the alveolar epithelial type II cells expands, and the laminated bodies in their cytoplasts increase in number and show vacuolization.

6. Clinical manifestation

Like those of other types of acute pulmonary edema, the clinical manifestation of HAPE includes dyspnea, cyanopathy, cough, the production of large amounts of white or pink spumous phlegm when coughing, and moist rales in one or both lungs.

6.1 Symptoms

At the early stage, the most common symptoms of HAPE include severe headache, dyspnea, palpitations, shortness of breath, chest tightness, chest pain, panic, extreme fatigue, weakness, persistent dry cough, worsened nighttime insomnia, pale complexion, and moist, cold skin. As the condition progresses, the above symptoms worsen, and patients may experience severe dyspnea, an inability to lie flat, and coughing out spumous phlegm, which is initially white or faint yellow in color and later turns pink, in some worse cases gushing out of the mouth and nose. Most patients display dysphoria while a minority experience hypersomnia, in some cases accompanied by altitude coma.

6.2 Signs

One distinctive sign of HAPE is moist pulmonary rales. In severe cases, moist rales can be heard in all regions of both lungs along with wheezing and phlegm. The cardiac sound is often masked. In mild cases, moist rales can be heard at the base of one or both lungs. Most patients display cyanosis in the lips, nail beds, and parts of the face. Due to dyspnea, patients often take bed rest in a semi-reclining position. About two thirds of patients experience fever, usually at 37.5-39°C. If body temperature persists over 38.5°C, it usually indicates complicating upper respiratory tract infection. Signs also include increased heart rate, loud or splitting P2, and grade 2-3 systolic murmur in the apex region of the heart. Some patients exhibit sulcus terminalis cordis expansion, possibly with diastolic gallop, jugular vein distention, hepatosplenomegaly, and edema complicated in some cases by cardiac insufficiency. Compared to other acute pulmonary edemas, HAPE has the following distinctive clinical features:

a. At early stages, HAPE patients only show symptoms of mild AMS, such as headache, dizziness, palpitations, insomnia, anorexia, and nausea. As these can be early symptoms of HAPE, they must be addressed with caution. Pulmonary auscultation may show normal results, but X-ray examination will reveal typical infiltrated shadows.
b. In some patients, HAPE progresses very rapidly, with acute onset and severe symptoms. Patients experience extreme dyspnea, asphyxia, and rales in all lung regions, quickly reaching impending death status. They may exhibit bloody pleural fluid in one or both lungs before death.
c. Patients tend to have high blood pressure, fine pulse, tachycardia, loud or splitting P2, and either a mild systolic murmur or diastolic gallop in the apex region of the heart. Only a few also experience right heart failure.
d. Some patients mainly show neurological and psychiatric symptoms, which often include headache, vertigo, diplopia, vomiting, phrenitis, and irritation. A minority of patients exhibit symptoms of derangement, meningeal irritation, or even coma. Further examination typically reveals increased pressure in the cerebrospinal fluid and edema in the optic papilla. In these cases, encephaledema often co-occurs, as can be detected by encephalic CT or MRI examination.
e. At the onset of HAPE, there is usually no fever, but some patients show low fever and intolerance to coldness.

6.3 Diagnostic examination

a. Hemogram: The leukocyte count is typically normal or mildly increased; about 40% patients have a count over 10000/mm^3. The highest count recorded in our study was 64000/mm^3. The neutrophilic granulocyte count also increases mildly. If the leukocyte and neutrophilic granulocyte counts continue to rise, it usually indicates concurrent infection.
b. X-rays: HAPE patients often show unilateral or bilateral flake-like or cloudy shadows centered at the porta pulmonis, mostly in the right lung. A minority of patients show large patchy or butterfly/batwing shadows. The apex regions of the lung are usually clear. At early stages, there is only thickening of the lung markings, also called pulmonary interstitial edema.
c. Electrocardiography: Manifestations of HAPE on the electrocardiogram include nodal tachycardia, right axis deviation, right bundle branch blockage, sharply tented P waves or P pulmonale, T wave inversion, and ST segment depression.
d. Blood gas: HAPE patients show substantial decreases in levels of PaO_2 and SaO_2, which are not only lower than those of healthy controls but also significantly lower than those of mild AMS patients.
e. Pulmonary function: HAPE mainly features decreases in the expiratory flow rate or diffusion capacity.
f. Hemodynamics: The pulmonary arterial pressure and resistance to the pulmonary artery are significantly increased. Left atrial pressure remains normal. The pulmonary capillary wedge pressure and cardiac index remain normal or decrease slightly.

7. Clinical classification

Using clinical signs and symptoms and the results of diagnostic examination, HAPE can be classified into three types: mild, moderate, and severe.

1. Mild HAPE: Characterized by mild dyspnea, coughing, coughing out small amounts of spumous phlegm, focal moist rales at the base of one or both lungs, respiratory rate of 20-30 breaths/minute, pulse rate under 100 beats/minute, bilateral thickening of lung markings, or cloudy spots at the base of the lungs visible on sternal X-ray.
2. Moderate HAPE: Characterized by substantial dyspnea, chest pain, chest tightening, coughing out large amounts of white or pink spumous phlegm, moist rales at the base of both lungs spreading over other pulmonary regions, respiratory rate of 30-40 breaths/minute, pulse rate of 110-120 beats/minute, bilateral thickening of lung markings, and flake-like or cloudy shadows at the base of the lungs visible on sternal X-ray.
3. Severe HAPE: Characterized by polypnea, panic, inability to lie flat, coughing out large amounts of pink spumous phlegm, severe cough, considerable blowing systolic murmur upon examination of the apex region of the heart or pulmonary valve area, moist rales sounding like boiling water in all pulmonary regions, bilaterally symmetrical cloudy shadows centered at the porta pulmonis or bilaterally symmetrical butterfly/batwing shadows visible on sternal X-ray, heart enlargement, clear protruding of the pulmonary trunk, and in some cases signs of heart failure including jugular vein distention, hepatomegaly, and edema in both lower extremities.

8. Diagnosis and differential diagnosis

8.1 Diagnosis and diagnostic criteria

1. Clinical diagnostic criteria

In China, the clinical diagnosis of HAPE is mostly based on the clinical diagnostic criteria recommended in 1995 by the Chinese Medical Association's third national medicine academic seminar. These criteria have been approved by the International Society for Mountain Medicine. The criteria include the following:

a. Upon recent exposure to high altitudes (usually considered to be 3,000 meters or more above sea level), the subject experiences dyspnea at rest, chest stress and tightening, cough, coughing out white or pink spumous phlegm, malaise, or decreased activity.
b. There are unilateral or bilateral moist rales or wheezing sounds in the pulmonary field, central cyanosis, tachypnea, and tachycardia.
c. X-ray shows unilateral or bilateral flake-like or cloudy infiltrated shadows centered at the porta pulmonis, often scattered and irregularly distributed but sometimes fused into a large patch. The podoid is normal in most cases, but sometimes signs of pulmonary hypertension and right heart enlargement can also be observed.
d. Other cardiac and pulmonary diseases, such as myocardial infarction and heart failure are excluded by clinical and electrocardiographic examinations. Pneumonia is also excluded.
e. Symptoms quickly improve after bed rest, oxygen inhalation treatment, or descending to a lower altitude, and signs shown by X-ray disappear within a short period of time.

2. Criteria for early diagnosis

As we gain a deeper knowledge of HAPE and accordingly improve both protective and therapeutic measures, clinically typical HAPE cases have become rare. If we continue to refer to the previous diagnostic criteria, it will be difficult to identify HAPE patients. For this reason, we carried out a study funded by the National Sci-Tech Support Plan and proposed the following as the criteria for early diagnosis of HAPE:

a. Upon recent exposure to high altitudes (usually considered to be 3,000 meters or more above sea level), the at-rest subject experiences palpitations, chest tightening, dyspnea, and coughing with or without small amounts of white spumous phlegm.
b. There is local, unilateral or bilateral coarse breathing with or without focal moist rales. There is also central cyanosis, tachycardia (>100 beats/minute), and tachypnea (>24 breaths/minute).
c. Early routine X-ray examination shows a decrease in transmittance of the lungs, blurred or increased lung markings, and the presence of ground-glass opacity or small patchy shadows in the lung. CT scan shows increased number and thickening of lung markings, ground-glass opacity, nodular shadows, scattered or isolated alveolar edema on terminal bronchioles, and fine reticular shadows.
d. Routine blood examination shows increases in the leukocyte count and the proportion of neutrophilic granulocytes.
e. Arterial blood gas examination shows persistent hypoxemia accompanied by mild respiratory alkalosis.
f. Electrocardiographic examination shows nodal tachycardia, clockwise rotation, sharply tented P waves, and so on.
g. Ultrasonic cardiogram shows early, prominent, persistent pulmonary hypertension.
h. All symptoms quickly improve after treatment such as bed rest, oxygen inhalation, decreasing pulmonary arterial pressure, and diuresis.

It should be noted that criteria a-c must be met first. Conditions in d-h are then evaluated. The criteria are then combined collectively to produce an accurate early diagnosis. In clinical practice under aforementioned criteria, if we also refer to the severities of the condition and of the signs, the features and sizes of the shadows on the chest film, make proper diagnoses, and give prompt, effective, on-site treatment, it is completely possible that we will be able to keep early-stage HAPE under control.

8.2 Differential diagnosis

1. Adult respiratory distress syndrome

a. Differences in the cause of disease: The fundamental cause of HAPE is oxygen shortage at high altitudes and low pressure leading to disturbed pulmonary circulation and body fluid maldistribution, of which oxygen shortage is the cause. ARDS is the secondary lesion of the lung tissues directly or indirectly caused by trauma or severe infection, in which oxygen shortage is the consequence.
b. Differences in pathological changes: Both show high levels of permeability edema. However, HAPE features short duration, fibrosis of the interstitial tissues and alveolar walls, thickening of the interstitium, only mild hyperplasia in the epithelial cells of alveolar walls, and a full recovery without sequelae. ARDS may evolve into subacute and chronic conditions, such as alveolar wall fibrosis. Chronic patients may exhibit pathological changes in general bronchopneumonia, which can eventually lead to prominent fibrosis of the interstitium and the alveoli and the pathological changes of emphysema.
c. Differences in reaction to oxygen inhalation: After treatments such as oxygen inhalation and measures that decrease pulmonary arterial pressure, most HAPE patients can quickly improve and recover in 2-7 days. Only in rare cases will patients die, usually due to a long delay before treatment, extreme severity of the condition, or complication

by adult respiratory distress syndrome. ARDS usually features more severity and a longer duration, often with hemosputum or hemorrhagic sputum and unilateral or focal tubular sound with few moist rales. Oxygen inhalation, even high-pressure oxygen inhalation and assisted respiration, is often not effective. The fatality rate is relatively high, usually between 40% and 70%.

d. Differences in X-ray manifestations: HAPE often shows flake-like or cloudy shadows spreading outward from the porta pulmonis, mostly scattered at the middle and lower fields and rarely fused into large patch. The X-ray film of ARDS patients typically shows patchy shadow at the edges of the lungs, in server cases fused into a large patch. At the terminal stage, "white lung" is manifested, and the pulmonary shadows gradually disappear.

2. High altitude pneumonia

High altitude pneumonia and upper respiratory tract infection can trigger HAPE, and HAPE tends to be complicated by high altitude pneumonia. Therefore, we should carefully differentiate the two in both diagnosis and treatment.

a. Differences in cause: HAPE is caused by hypoxia under low-oxygen, low-pressure conditions at high altitudes. High altitude pneumonia is pulmonary inflammation caused by bacteria, viruses, allergies, or inhalation of hazardous substances such as kerosene or gasoline.
b. Differences in clinical manifestation: Both show increases in body temperature and hemogram. However, high altitude pneumonia usually has a rapid onset with chills and high fever. Body temperature reaches 39-40°C within hours and continues to rise, causing enecia. Both the leukocyte and the neutrophilic granulocyte counts increase significantly, reaching up to 20-30×10^{9}/L. Mostly neutrophilic granulocytes can reach more than 80%. There is also a left shift of nuclei, observable toxic granulations, and vacuoles in the cytoplasts. In comparison, HAPE patients usually do not have fever higher than 38.5^{o}C, and their leukocyte and neutrophilic granulocyte counts only increase slightly.
c. Differences in clinical signs: HAPE patients cough typical spumous hemosputum or pink spumous phlegm, which can gush out from mouth and nose when large amounts are present. High altitude pneumonia patients first cough mucus and then purulent or rusty sputum.
d. Differences in X-ray manifestation: HAPE often shows either intense shadows with different densities, shapes, and sizes, or spotty, flake-like, cloudy shadows. Lesion margins of HAPE were blurred and not constrained by the interlobar fissures. The above signs are widely scattered in both lungs. High altitude pneumonia shows increased numbers of lung markings and decreased transmittance of the lung fields at early stages. Later spotty, flake-like shadows of different sizes can be observed, sometimes fused into patchy shadow, but usually limited to one pulmonary lobe or one pulmonary segment.

9. Complications

9.1 High Altitude Cerebral Edema

High altitude cerebral edema (HACE) is a common complication of HAPE, as verified by clinical examinations, lab examinations, and autopsies. Because patients may have one or both of these two diseases, we should take great caution in diagnosis and treatment. HAPE patients often show signs and symptoms such as headache, vomiting, hypersomnia, and coma, which relate to increased intracranial pressure and cerebral edema. Fundus examination sometimes shows papilledema and fundus hemorrhage, and lumbar puncture often shows increased cerebrospinal fluid pressure. Such cases merit special attention during diagnosis and treatment.

Shortly after rapid exposure to a high altitude environment, blood within the body is redistributed via neural, fluid regulation. The vasomotion of the blood vessels in some organs undergo prominent changes resulting in large amounts blood moving to important organs, such as the lung, heart, and brain, ensuring their oxygen supply and normal function. However, if the blood flow volume, rate, and pressure in these organs become too high, disruption to microcirculation may occur. In particular, in the lung and brain, where low-pressure space is normally present, it can easily cause fluid to leak out into neighboring tissues, leading to edema. HAPE and HACE share some common pathogenesis, for the most part in the pathological changes in hemodynamics. HACE and HAPE may occur separately or jointly, sometimes in succession. Severe HAPE and large amounts of extravasation from the alveoli seriously impair oxygen uptake from the external environment, aggravating hypoxemia, which promotes the hemangiectasis of the cerebral blood-vessels via neuroendocrine regulation induced by severe hypoxia of the brain tissue. The resulting increase in cerebral blood flow and blood volume then further aggravates cerebral edema. However, HACE escalates the extravasation of pulmonary tissue and worsens HAPE via neural, fluid regulation. When HACE extends to the respiratory and cardiovascular centers of the medulla oblongata, respiration is inhibited and blood pressure drops, in severe cases leading to cerebral hernia, which can cause respiratory circulation failure or even sudden cardiac arrest, resulting in vicious circle. This is an important cause of death among patients with HAPE complicated by cerebral edema.

9.2 Cerebral infarction

Cerebral infarction is another common complication of HAPE, possibly induced by the following: 1) Acute erythrocytosis occurs due to excessive erythropoiesis triggered when the body is exposed to altitudes above a certain elevation. The compensatory erythrocytosis in the plasma leads to a significant increase in blood viscosity. Blood flow rate decreases and blood cells cluster together, resulting in increased contact between the platelets and the blood vessel walls, rendering the blood more likely to coagulate. 2) Wade et al. proposed that disturbances in cerebral circulation might play a major role in generating cerebral thrombosis. HAPE complicated with HACE is an important cause of disturbances in cerebral microcirculation, which slows down the blood flow and increases the blood viscosity of the patient, leading to cerebral thrombosis. 3) At high altitudes, the generation of blood coagulation factor in the plasma increases, creating a hypercoagulative condition. The blood of High altitude polycythemia (HAPC) patients is already in a hypercoagulative state, and second hyperfibrinolysis can easily occur. 4) HAPE patients have severe hypoxemia, which may result in damage to blood vessel endothelial cells. The above changes caused severe damage to the pulmonary capillary endothelial cells of HAPE patients, boosting platelet adhesion and activating the blood coagulation system, finally leading to cerebral thrombosis.

9.3 Multiple Organ Dysfunction Syndrome

Patients with HAPE complicated by cerebral edema are prone to multiple organ dysfunction syndrome (MODS). Patients show symptoms including headache, chest tightness, shortness of breath, nausea, aggravated vomiting, and abnormal psychological behavior. Auscultation can reveal aggravated pulmonary rales; fundus examination may show spotting or patchy bleeding in the retina and papilledema; there is gastrointestinal hemorrhage or fecal occult blood, hematuria, or proteinuria; chest X ray of most patients show enlarged hilar shadows, unilateral or bilateral cloudy shadows of uniform density in the lung field, in some cases fused into large, dense, patchy unilateral or bilateral shadows of uniform density; encephalic CT reveals decreased brain parenchymal density, narrowed bilateral cerebral ventricles, and the shallower, narrower sulci; laboratory examination will reveal increased leukocyte counts, often above $13.0\times10^9/L$, increased bleeding and clotting time, increased fibrinolytic activity, and increases in thromboxane B2, vWF, fibrinogen, tissue-type plasminogen activator and inhibitor in the plasma, increased levels of D-dimers, increased levels of alpha-granular membrane protein, significantly decreased levels of 6-keto-PGF1a and antithrombin III, and severe dysfunction of the coagulation and fibrolysis systems.

AMS complicated by MODS has been underemphasized and the diagnostic yield has been low. Our investigation shows that 2.5% of AMS cases are complicated by MODS, which is considerable. We need to improve early diagnosis and early detection because early treatment is crucial in reducing the fatality rate of AMS complicated by MODS.

10. Prevention and treatment

10.1 Prevention

1. Protection of susceptible populations from exposure to high altitudes

Physical examinations, especially inspections of cardiac and pulmonary functions, should be performed on individuals who are about to travel to high altitude areas. Those with heart and/or lung ailments should be advised against exposure to high altitudes.

2. Prevention of respiratory tract infection

Individuals with respiratory tract infections are more susceptible to HAPE at high altitudes. Those who catch upper respiratory tract infections before planned trips to high altitude areas should first seek treatment and only make the trip after full recovery. Prior to high altitude exposure, one should perform cold resistance exercises. After arrival, one should take active measures to keep warm and prevent respiratory tract infection.

3. Acclimatization to hypoxia

Prior to high altitude exposure, one should receive hypoxic training using masks or hypoxic respirators to increase the body's tolerance to hypoxia so as to promote high altitude acclimatization.

When possible, one should ascend to higher altitudes gradually and multisteply rather than rapidly ascend to higher altitudes to avoid body damage. Before traveling to high altitude regions, individuals should familiarize themselves with the climate characteristics and geological environment of the area and familiarize themselves with preventative treatments for high altitude diseases.

4. Reduction and control of activity level

During the first week of high-altitude exposure, one should take proper rest, reduce or avoid intense physical activity, avoid fatigue, and minimize oxygen consumption. Normal physical activity should be resumed only after the body is acclimatized to the hypoxic environment.

5. Administration of prophylactic medicine

a. Chinese traditional medicine
There are four courses of Chinese traditional medicines that may serve to prevent HAPE:
Compound codonopsis tablets: Take orally. Start 3 days before hypoxia exposure, 3-5 tablets/dose, 3 doses each day. Continue for 5-7 days after hypoxia exposure.
Ginseng and astragalus pollen tablets: Take orally. Start 3 days before high altitude exposure, 5 tablets/dose, 3 doses/day. Continue for 5-7 days after high altitude exposure.
Rhodiola rosea oral solution: Take orally. Start 3 days before high altitude exposure, 10 ml/dose, 3 doses/day. Continue for 5-7 days after high altitude exposure.
Compound rhodiola capsules: Take orally. Start 3 days before high altitude exposure, 2 capsules/dose, 3 doses/day, continue for 5-7 days after high altitude exposure.
b. Glucocorticoid preparations
Dexamethasone: Take orally. Start 1 day before high altitude exposure, 5 mg/dose, 3 doses/day. Continue for 2 days after high altitude exposure.
c. Carbonic anhydrase inhibitors
Nephramid (a.k.a. acetazolamide): Take orally. Start 1 day before high altitude exposure, 250 mg/dose, 3 doses/day. Take for 2-3 days.
Methazolamide (a.k.a. Ni Mu Ke Si): Take orally. Start 1 day before high altitude exposure, 25-50 mg/dose, 3 doses/day. Take for 2-3 days.
d. Calcium antagonists
Nifedipine: Take orally. Start 1 day before high altitude exposure, 10 mg/dose, 2 doses/day or sublingual administration 10 mg/dose, 3 doses/day. Take for 1-3 days.
e. Beta2- receptor stimulants
Salbutamol: Inhale. Start 1 day before high altitude exposure, 125 μg/dose, 2 doses/day. Continue for 2-3 days after high altitude exposure.
f. Phosphodiesterase inhibitors
Sildenafil: Take orally. Start 1 day before high altitude exposure, 50 mg/dose, 3 doses/day. Continue for 2-3 days after high altitude exposure.
Tadalafil: Take orally. Start 1 day before high altitude exposure, 10 mg/dose, 1 dose/day. Continue for 2-3 days after high altitude exposure.

10.2 Treatment

Accurate, effective early-stage treatment usually quickly improves symptoms. Therefore, early diagnosis and timely treatment are crucial to controlling the course of the disease and prognosis.

1. Oxygen inhalation or hyperbaric oxygen therapy

Oxygen inhalation can substantially decrease pulmonary arterial pressure in HAPE patients and quickly alleviate hypoxia and the series of clinical symptoms that it causes. HAPE

patients should in general use continuous administration of low-flow oxygen (4-6 L/minute). For patients with severe hypoxia, high-flow continuous oxygen may be administrated (8-10 L/minute) but for no longer than 24 hours in order to avoid oxygen toxicity. If the symptoms include excessive spumous phlegm, an appropriate amount of alcohol may be added to the oxygen humidifying containers for froth suppression.
Hyperbaric oxygen treatment can temporarily remove hypoxia for HAPE patients. Most patients show symptom improvement after 1-2 treatments and achieve recovery after 2-3 treatments. However, for a minority of patients, HAPE signs and symptoms worsen after departure from the hyperbaric oxygen chamber, which can be associated with disease severity variance and individual difference. Therefore, when treating HAPE patients with hyperbaric oxygen therapy, caution should be taken to acknowledge individual variability and monitor the severity of the condition.

2. Nitric oxide inhalation

Inhalation of low-concentration nitric oxide can quickly, selectively alleviate the pulmonary hypertension caused by hypoxia. The inhalation method is as follows: Mix 10 ppm nitric oxide with pure air and inhale through a nasogastric feeding tube at 3-5 L/minute, 30-60 minutes/treatment and 2-3 treatments/day. Patients with mild or moderate HAPE typically recover after 2-3 days. For severe HAPE patients, the duration and daily frequency of the inhalation treatments should be increased accordingly.
Inhaled nitric oxide can be oxidized into NO^{2-} and NO^{3-} in high-oxygen environments and can accumulate in the blood, which will damage the blood cells. For this reason, when treating HAPE patients with nitric oxide, simultaneous inhalation of high concentration oxygen should be avoided. Animal studies have shown that the effects of inhaling concentrations of nitric oxide ranging from 5-80 ppm on decreasing pulmonary arterial pressure are statistically the same.

3. Aminophylline

Aminophylline is the drug of choice for standard HAPE treatment. It can quickly diminish pulmonary arterial and vena cava pressure and decrease right atrial venous return volume. It can also be cardiotonic, diuretic and a smooth muscle relaxant and can reduce resistance in the systemic circulation, improving the heart function.
Regular dose: 0.25g diluted to 20ml 10-50% glucose, intravenously injected at an even speed. It can be repeated after 4-6 hours. For mild HAPE patients, administer 2 times/day. For severe patients, upgrade to 0.5g/administration, and increase the frequency of administration according to the severity.

4. Anticholinergic agents

Atropine and anisodamine can treat pulmonary vasospasms. They also decrease resistance in the pulmonary blood vessels, improve pulmonary microcirculation, keep pulmonary blood flow unimpeded, and prevent blood clotting and pulmonary thrombosis inside the blood vessels.
Regular dose: Atropine 2-5 mg/0.5hour. Anisodamine (654-2) 20-40 mg/0.5 hour, intravenous drip.

5. Dexamethasone

Dexamethasone can be used in both treating and preventing HAPE. Regular dose: 10 mg, IV injection, 2 times/day for no more than 3 days. For patients with comorbid conditions such as epilepsy, peptic ulcer, high blood pressure, or diabetes mellitus, dexamethasone should be taken with caution or contraindicated.

6. Diuretics

Nicorol: 10 mg IV injection, 1 dose/day; Nephramid: Take orally.250 mg/dose, 3 doses/day; Drugs that alleviate pulmonary hypertension: nifedipine: 10-20 mg/dose orally or sublingually, 2 doses/day. Sodium nitroprusside: IV drip, 10-20 mg/dose.

7. Cardiotonics

Cedilanid: IV injection, 0.4-0.8 mg. Strophanthin K: IV injection, 0.125-0.5 mg.

8. Sedatives

Morphine hydrochloride: 5-10 mg, subcutaneous injection. In severe cases, dilute 5 mg to 20 ml 10% glucose and administer IV injection. For some patients with anxiety symptoms, Valium may be used with caution, but its inhibitory effects on breathing should be monitored.

9. Antibiotics

HAPE is very likely to be complicated by pulmonary infection. When the two diseases co-occur, each aggravates the other and the situation becomes difficult to control. In treating HAPE, broad-spectrum antibiotics are usually used to prevent and treat infection. Patients with mild symptoms should take broad-spectrum antibiotics (e.g. amoxicillin, norfloxacin, trimethoprim and sulphame-thoxazole etc.) orally for anti-infection purposes, and control the intake of sodium chloride to avoid worsening the HAPE. The commonly used antibiotics include the following:

a. Amoxicillin: Take orally, 1g/dose, 3 doses/day.
b. Norfloxacin: Take orally, 0.2g/dose, 3 doses/day.
c. Trimethoprim and sulphame-thoxazole: Take orally, 1-2 tablets/dose, 2 doses/day, take orally.
d. Levofloxacin: Take orally, 0.1-0.2 g/dose, 2 doses/day.
e. Penicillin (still the first choice): 4,800,000-6,400,000 units diluted in 250-500 ml glucose or saline, IV drip, 1-2 times/day. Contraindicated in patients clinically significant allergy to penicillin.
f. Ampicillin sodium/sulbactam sodium: For mild infections, 1.5g/day in 2-3 IM injections. For moderate infections, 4-9g/day in 3-4 IM injections. For severe infections 9-12g/day in 2-3 IV drips.
g. Cefamezin: 2g/dose, 3 doses/day, IV drip.
h. Cefradine: 100-150 mg/kg/day, IV drip.
i. Lincomycin hydrochloride: 0.6g/dose, 1-2 doses/day, IV drip.
j. Ciprofloxacin Lactate: 0.2g/dose, 2 doses/day, IV drip.

10. Decent to lower altitude

When possible, patients should be quickly transferred to lower altitudes (below 3,000 meters) for further treatment. After leaving the hypoxic environment, the elevated pulmonary arterial pressure can quickly return to normal levels and the series of symptoms caused by hypoxia quickly disappear. However, descent treatment is only applicable in less remote areas within a relatively short amount of time. In remote mountain areas where transportation conditions are extremely poor and continuous oxygen supplies cannot be guaranteed in transit, it is for the best to administer on-site treatment.

When transferring patients to lower altitudes, the following should be noted: 1) Transportation utilities: fast, stable transportation utilities are preferable, e.g. helicopter, truck, heavy medical vehicle, small ambulance. 2) Accompanying crew: there should be one doctor and one nurse, or at least one medical professional who can perform effective treatment through the transfer. 3) The patient in should assume a semireclining position during descent to keep the airway clear. 4) Patients with high altitude coma should assume a semireclining position. Head movement and vehicle pitching should be minimized to prevent cerebral hernia. 5) The driver should proceed slowly when road conditions are rough so that the patient's position can remain relatively stable. 6) The accompanying crew should read and record vital signs and give effective treatment when needed. 7) If a patient passes away, the time and order of vital sign loss should be recorded and body position should respectfully be kept unchanged.

11. References

[1] Yu-Jing S,Ming-Wu F,Wen-Quan N,et al.Endothelial nitric oxide synthase gene polymorphisms associated with susceptibility to high altitude pulmonary edema in Chinese railway construction workers at Qinghai-Tibet over 4 500 meters above sea Level. Chin Med Sci J. 2010 Dec;25(4):215-22.

[2] Sonna LA. Pulmonary oedema at moderately high altitudes. Lancet 2002, 359(9303): 276-277.

[3] Grissom CK, Elstad MR. The pathophysiology of high altitude pulmonary edema. Wilderness Environ Med.1999,10(2):88-92.

[4] Bartsch P, Mairbaurl H, Maggiorini M, et al. Physiological aspects of high-altitude pulmonary edema. J Appl Physiol.2005,98(3):1101-10.

[5] Barry Brenner, David Cheng,Sunday Clark,et al.Positive Association between Altitude and Suicide in 2584 U.S. Counties. High Alt Med Biol.2011,12(1):1-5.

[6] Stewart J. Jackson, James Varley,et al. Incidence and predictors of acute mountain sickness among trekkers on Mount Kilimanjaro. High Alt Med Biol.2011,11(3):217-222.

[7] Schneider M, Bernasch D, Weymann J, et al.Acute mountain sickness: influence of susceptibility, preexposure, and ascent rate.Med Sci Sports Exerc. 2002,34(12):1886-91.

[8] Kao WF, Kuo CC, Hsu TF,et al. Acute mountain sickness in Jade Mountain climbers of Taiwan. Aviat Space Environ Med. 2002,73(4):359-62.

[9] Hackett PH, Rennie D, Levine HD. The incidence, importance and prophylaxis of acute mountain sickness.Lancet 1976,ii:1149-54.

[10] Honigman B, Theis MK, Koziol-McLain J,et al .Acute mountain sickness in a general tourist population at moderate altitudes.Ann Intern Med. 1993,118(8):587-92.

[11] Murdoch DR, Curry C.Acute mountain sickness in the Southern Alps of New Zealand.N Z Med J. 1998,111(1065):168-9.

[12] Ziaee V, Yunesian M, Ahmadinejad Z, et al .Acute mountain sickness in Iranian trekkers around Mount Damavand (5671 m) in Iran.Wilderness Environ Med. 2003,14(4):214-9

[13] Basnyat B, Subedi D, Sleggs J, et al .at 4300 m at Gosainkund in the Nepal Himalayas. Out of 5000 pilgrims, 228 were randomly chosen. Sixty-eight percent had AMS, Wilderness Environ Med.2000,11(2): 89-93.

[14] Ren Y, Fu Z, Shen W, et al.Incidence of high altitude illnesses among unacclimatized persons who acutely ascended to Tibet.High Alt Med Biol. 2010,11(1):39-42.

[15] Pratali L, Cavana M, Giardini G.High altitude pulmonary edema: the importance of early diagnosis. Recenti Prog Med. 2010 ,101(5):212-8.

[16] Stobdan T, Kumar R, Mohammad G, et al.Probable role of beta2-adrenergic receptor gene haplotype in high-altitude pulmonary oedema. Respirology. 2010,15(4):651-8.

[17] Gertsch JH, Seto TB, Mor J, et al.Ginkgo biloba for the prevention of severe acute mountain sickness (AMS) starting one day before rapid ascent.High Alt Med Biol. 2002,3(1):29-37.

[18] Maggiorini M, Bühler B, Walter M, et al.Prevalence of acute mountain sickness in the Swiss Alps.BMJ. 1990 Oct 13;301(6756):853-5.

[19] Maggiorini M. Prevention and treatment of high-altitude pulmonary edema.Prog Cardiovasc Dis. 2010,52(6):500-6.

[20] Scherrer U, Rexhaj E, Jayet PY, et al.New insights in the pathogenesis of high-altitude pulmonary edema.Prog Cardiovasc Dis. 2010,52(6):485-92.

[21] Fiore DC, Hall S, Shoja PAltitude illness: risk factors, prevention, presentation, and treatment. Am Fam Physician. 2010,82(9):1103-10.

[22] Stream JO, Grissom CK.Update on high-altitude pulmonary edema: pathogenesis, prevention, and treatment. Wilderness Environ Med. 2008,19(4):293-303.

[23] Gregorius DD, Dawood R, Ruh K, Nguyen HB.Severe high altitude pulmonary oedema: a patient managed successfully with non-invasive positive pressure ventilation in the Emergency Department. Emerg Med J. 2008,25(4):243-4.

[24] Fagenholz PJ, Gutman JA, Murray AF, et al.Treatment of high altitude pulmonary edema at 4240 m in Nepal. High Alt Med Biol. 2007,8(2):139-46.

[25] Suzhi Li,Bihai Zheng,Hongbing Wang,et al. The clinical characteristics of acute severe high-altitude diseases in indigenous Tibetans, Chin J Tuberc Respir Dis. 2006, 29(12):835-836

26

Mechanical Forces Impair Alveolar Ion Transport Processes – A Putative Mechanism Contributing to the Formation of Pulmonary Edema

Martin Fronius
Institute of Animal Physiology, Justus-Liebig-University Giessen
Germany

1. Introduction

The aim of this chapter is to highlight the importance of transepithelial ion transport processes for lung function in general and to focus on the impact of mechanical forces on pulmonary ion transport in particular. Linking mechanical forces with pulmonary ion transport derives from the fact that the lung is a dynamic organ as well as from several studies providing evidence that the amount of mechanical forces as used during artificial ventilation correlates with mortality rates in patients with respiratory failure such as ALI (acute lung injury) and ARDS (acute respiratory distress syndrome) (ARDS Network Investigators, 2000). In these patients the formation of pulmonary edema is a characteristic symptom (Frank and Matthay, 2003; Ricard et al., 2003) and the basic rationale behind this is, that mechanical perturbations cause epithelial leakage in response to mechanically induced damage of the epithelial layer. This damage is suggested to be a major cause for the formation of pulmonary edema as well as the inability to reabsorb the edema fluid. However, little is known whether or not mechanical forces may directly interfere with pulmonary ion transport processes and this represents a putative mechanism that facilitates the formation of pulmonary edema – in addition to damages of the epithelial layer.

2. Air breathing and pulmonary ion transport

The water land transition of tetrapods represents a fundamental process within vertebrate evolution that was accompanied by the development of lungs as gas exchanging structures. The major advantage of air breathing is the almost infinite access to oxygen, although this bears also some risks. The gas-exchanging structures must be moistened to facilitate oxygen solubility and the architecture of these structures must be adapted to the requirement of efficient gas exchange by diffusion. These problems were basically fixed by invagination of the gas-exchanging surface, protecting them from desiccation and from mechanical damage. Therefore, invagination could be considered as a basic improvement allowing the development of a highly conserved architecture of the air blood barrier that can be found within all air-breathing vertebrates. This architecture is referred to as the "three ply design" (Maina and West, 2005). The three layers of the air-blood barrier are represented by the

pulmonary epithelium, the basal lamina and the endothelium that forms the pulmonary capillaries. Although invagination and the development of the three ply design fixed a lot of problems, other challenges arose. To ensure a constant supply of oxygen as well as a continuous replacement of the breathing medium, ventilation mechanisms were needed. This was achieved by different strategies within the different vertebrate classes. Early tetrapods and amphibians ventilate their lungs by a buccal pump (Brainerd and Owerkowicz, 2006). In higher vertebrates ventilation occurs by a costal pump (Roux, 2002) where the movement of the ribs ensures aspiration of air. But independent of the strategy how the exchange of the breathing medium is accomplished, the gas-exchanging surface is permanently exposed to pollutions and pathogens that are omnipresent in the air supplied to the lungs.
It is also well known that the entire pulmonary epithelium is covered by a thin fluid layer (PLL: pulmonary liquid layer) (Daniels and Orgeig, 2003), that is of particular importance for the function of the lung. The PLL extends from the distal parts of the lung to the upper airways and consists of mucus, surfactant and periciliary fluid (Rubin, 2002) (Fig. 1). On the one hand the PLL is the first physical border that is exposed to the environment and the first line of host defense that absorbs pathogens. This is of particular importance in the airways, where the PLL is part of the innate immune system and crucial for protecting the host from the permanent exposure to pollutions and pathogens due to their removal by the mucociliary clearance (Welsh, 1987; Davis and Lazarowski, 2008).

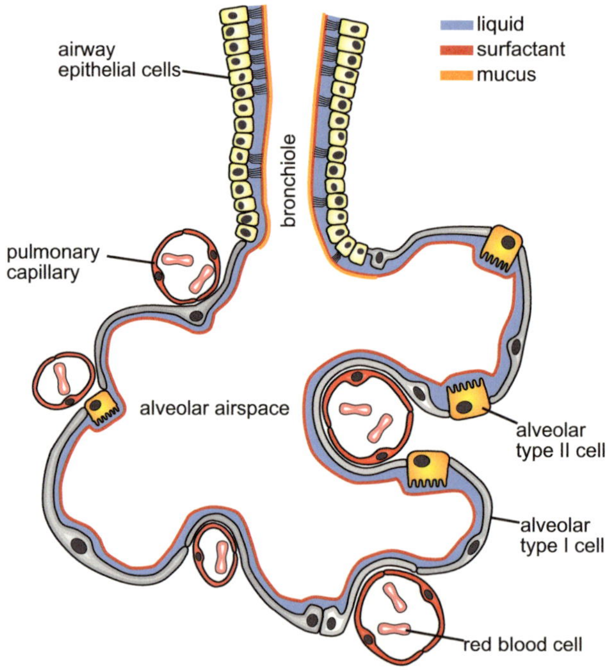

Fig. 1. Schematic drawing of the distal lung region. The distal lung is represented by respiratory bronchioles and terminal alveoli that are lined by a continuous layer of epithelial cells consisting of different cell types. The entire epithelium is further covered with a liquid film (PLL: pulmonary liquid layer) consisting of different layers. In the airways the PLL is composed from a liquid layer (periciliary fluid) and a layer of mucus and surfactant. In the alveolar regions the PLL consists of a liquid layer (alveolar fluid) and a surfactant layer.

On the other hand the height and volume of the PLL in the respiratory zone - primarily represented by the alveolar fluid - determines the distance of diffusion for the gases that is a limiting rate for the diffusion efficiency as defined by Fick's law of diffusion. Thus, increased fluid content in the alveolar region decreases oxygenation of the blood (Matalon and O'Brodovich, 1999; Matthay et al., 2000).

Therefore, the consistency as well as the volume of the PLL layer must be tightly regulated and controlled - in the airways as well as in the gas-exchanging region - to ensure effective host defense as well as effective gas exchange.

This principle becomes evident regarding pulmonary diseases that are associated with inappropriate fluid balance in the lung. For example hyperabsorption of water from the airspace increases the viscosity of the PLL and this interferes with the removal of inhaled pathogens due to impaired mucociliary clearance as observed in patients with cystic fibrosis (Fig. 2A) (Widdicombe et al., 1985; Riordan et al., 1989; Matsui et al., 1998). In contrast, too much fluid in the lung impairs gas diffusion and this can be observed in patients with pulmonary edema (Figure 2B) (Sznajder, 2001; Hoschele and Mairbaurl, 2003).

Thus, a defined content of water covering the pulmonary epithelia is a basic requirement for proper lung function and this depends on the development of appropriate ion transport processes accomplished by the pulmonary epithelia.

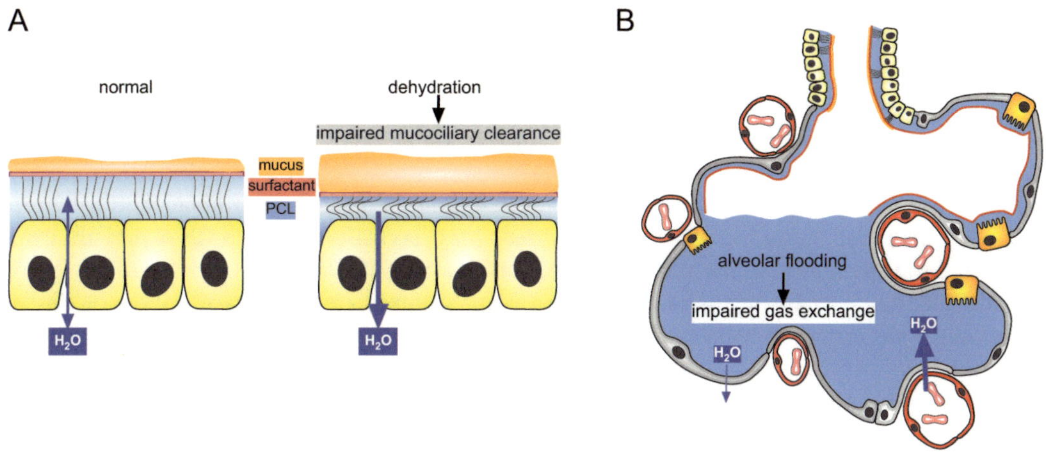

Fig. 2. Impaired epithelial fluid transport affects basic lung functions. A) Increased water reabsorption in the airways results in dehydration of the periciliary liquid layer (PCL) leading to an impaired mucociliary clearance and mucus accumulation within the airways. B) In the alveolar region an imbalance between fluid reabsorption and fluid infiltration leads to the formation of pulmonary edema that impairs the exchange of the breathing gases.

2.1 Transepithelial Na^+ and Cl^- transport are the main pathways to control the water content in the lung

Studying ion transport processes across pulmonary epithelia within the last decades improved our understanding how the fluid content in the lung is sustained. The basic principle of pulmonary water transport is ubiquitous - ions are transported across the epithelial layer and this generates transepithelial osmotic gradients that cause water diffusion across the epithelium (Sackin and Boulpaep, 1975). It is well accepted that pulmonary epithelia are Na^+ reabsorptive epithelia where active Na^+ reabsorption represents the bulk of transepithelial ion transport. Na^+ transport occurs via two steps: 1) Na^+ ions are taken up through epithelial Na^+ channels (ENaC) at the luminal side of the epithelial cells and are pumped out from the cells at the basolateral side by the Na^+/K^+ATPase. This process is suggested to be the principle mechanism for water reabsorption from the airspace into the body (Matthay et al., 2002). Another major component with significant impact on transepithelial water movement is represented by the transepithelial transport of Cl^-. In the airways it is well accepted that Cl^- is secreted via luminal Cl^- channels (Smith et al., 1982; Willumsen et al., 1989; Chambers et al., 2007). However the particular role of Cl^- channels Cl^- in alveolar epithelial cells remains unclear since there is evidence that Cl^- is secreted (McCray et al., 1993; Tizzano et al., 1994; Lazrak et al., 2002; Sommer et al., 2007), as well as absorbed (Fang et al., 2002; Fang et al., 2006). There are at least two different Cl^- channels identified in the apical membrane of pulmonary epithelial cells - the Ca^{2+} dependent Cl^- channel (TMEM16a) (Caputo et al., 2008; Schroeder et al., 2008; Yang et al., 2008) and the cAMP dependent CFTR Cl^- channel (Riordan et al., 1989; Welsh and Smith, 1993). In addition it might be noted that alveolar epithelial cells are characterized by a high water permeability (Folkesson et al., 1994; Dobbs et al., 1998) although the role of these proteins in pulmonary fluid handling is uncertain since no significant impact of aquaporins on alveolar clearance has been detected in transgenic (aquaporin deficient) animals (Verkman et al., 2000; Verkman, 2007).

However, the crucial importance of defined and regulated ion transport processes in the lung to control the water content is beyond dispute, since this was impressively confirmed by several studies using transgenic animal models with impaired ion channel functions. For example deletion of the α ENaC subunit in mice leads to early death due to the inability to reabsorb the alveolar fluid from the lungs after birth (Hummler et al., 1996). Interestingly, rescuing α ENaC expression in transgenic mice that were derived from α ENaC deficient mice demonstrated that these animals expressed decreased levels of ENaC mRNA and that this resulted in an increased susceptibility to the formation of pulmonary edema (Olivier et al., 2002). In addition overexpression of the β□ENaC subunit and hyperabsorption of Na^+ is associated with impaired mucociliary clearance resulting in a phenotype that is characteristic for cystic fibrosis (Mall et al., 2004). Recent studies established that mutations in the CFTR gene of pigs resulted in a cystic fibrosis like lung disease (Rogers et al., 2008; Stoltz et al., 2010).

3. Mechanical forces and breathing

Ventilation of the lungs due to the movement of the chest is associated with the appearance of physical forces. These forces are pressure (force per area), strain (deformation e.g. reasoned by the impact of pressure) and shear stress (movement of fluid at the cellular surface) (Fig. 3) (Wirtz and Dobbs, 2000). It might also be considered that due to the complex anatomy of the gas exchanging area it is difficult to estimate the distinct forces acting on individual cells (Liu et al., 1999) and that the local appearance of forces can be influenced by parameters like surfactants, focal adhesion molecules, the contractile machinery of the cells as well as the activity of molecular motor proteins within the cells (Fredberg and Kamm, 2006).

Although more or less all cell types within the lung are exposed to these physical stimuli the following section will focus on epithelial cells. Especially, the appearance and the reason for the stimuli as well as their impact on the pulmonary epithelial cells will be discussed.

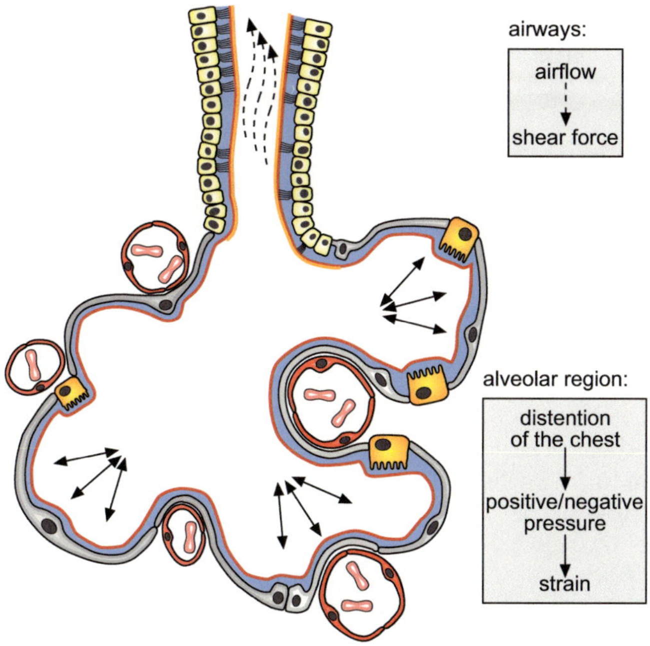

Fig. 3. Breathing is associated with the appearance of physical forces. Airway epithelial cells are primarily exposed to shear forces that are reasoned by the airstream flowing passing the surface of the airways. In the alveolar region the main physical force is strain due to the positive and negative pressure that are reasoned by the movement of the chest.

3.1 Pressure and strain in the lung

The appearance of pressure is the consequence of the movement of the chest. During inspiration and expiration epithelial cells are exposed to negative and positive pressures. This pressure is defined as transpulmonary pressure and resembles the pressure difference between the pressure in the pleural space and the atmospheric pressure (Fredberg and Kamm, 2006). During inspiration at rest the inflating pressure is approx. 5 cm H_2O and this can increase to approx. 30 cm H_2O at deep inspirations (Fredberg and Kamm, 2006). In the lung the appearance of pressure will always cause deformation of the cells due to the delicate anatomy and morphology of the alveolar structure. Therefore, increasing pressure is always associated with the appearance of strain. From this point of view, it seems obvious to consider that strain rather than pressure is the adequate stimulus acting on epithelial cells as a consequence of the breathing movements (Liu et al., 1999).

3.2 Shear stress in the lung

In addition to strain, the luminal surface of the epithelial cells is exposed to shear stress. Shear stress is defined by the tangential movement of particles (e.g. air or fluid) at the surface between different physical compartments. In the airways shear stress is primarily caused by the oscillating airflow passing the surface of the airway epithelial cells (Tarran et al., 2006). In the distal lung regions shear stress is a consequence of the movement due to distention, where the epithelial cell represents one compartment that is distended and the fluid of the PLL represents a static component of another compartment. Thus a relative

movement of the epithelial cell (with respect to the fluid) will cause shear stress at the luminal surface of the cells.
The next sections will focus on the impact of pressure and strain in particular on lung functions.

3.3 Strain is crucial for several functions of epithelial cells

It is well known that physical forces are important stimuli for distinct cellular functions of pulmonary epithelial cells (Fig. 4). An important indication for this is represented by the fact that development of the mammalian lung within the last third of gestation depends on breathing movements although the lungs are fluid filled (Kitterman, 1996). In animal models prevention of these breathing movements by spinal nerve sections resulted in retarded lung growth and development (Fewell et al., 1981). Further, *in vitro* studies demonstrated that distention of alveolar epithelial cells is an important trigger that affects alveolar cell differentiation. Mechanical distention of isolated and cultivated fetal alveolar cells promotes their differentiation to AT I cells whereas that lack of distention promotes the differentiation to ATII cells (Edwards, 2001).

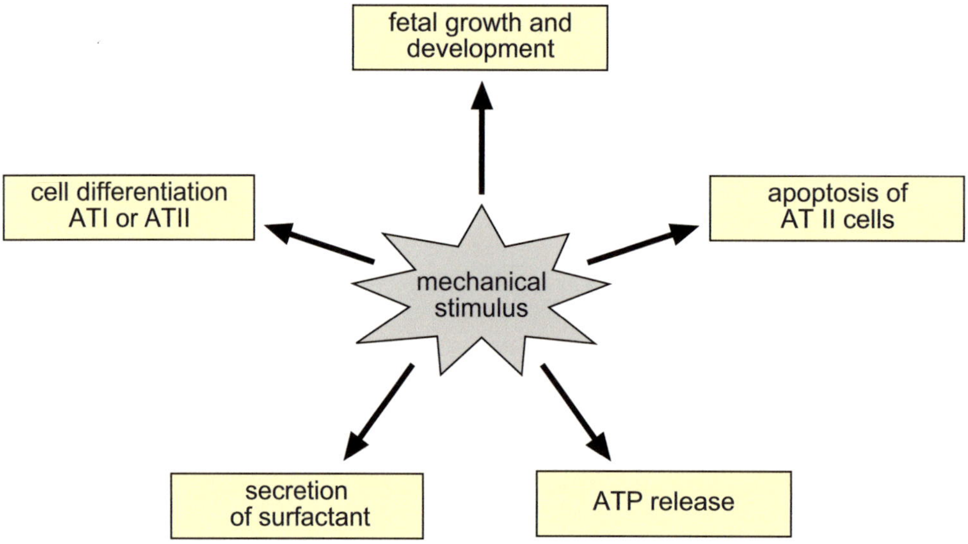

Fig. 4. Under normal breathing conditions mechanical stimuli are important for several functions of the lung.

Besides affecting cell differentiation and lung development there is also evidence for the contribution of physical stress as a factor that mediates production and secretion of surfactant proteins by ATII cells (Edwards et al., 1999) as well as by cultured H441 cells (Sanchez-Esteban et al., 1998). There is also evidence that mechanical forces induce apoptosis in ATII cells (Edwards et al., 1999; Hammerschmidt et al., 2007). In addition, different signaling mediators and ATP in particular are released in response to mechanical stress (Homolya et al., 2000; Okada et al., 2006; Button et al., 2007). The release of ATP offers the possibility to initiate a variety of different cellular reactions by acting on multiple purinergic receptors - including P2X, P2Y and P1 receptors (Leipziger, 2003; Bucheimer and Linden, 2004; Barth and Kasper, 2009). The relevance of purinergic signaling has been implicated by a study identifying alterations of transepithelial ion transport processes in airway epithelia in response to adenosine as a factor contributing to cystic fibrosis lung disease (Tarran et al., 2005; Tarran et al., 2006).

3.4 Deleterious effects of mechanical forces in the lung

Although, there is more than sufficient evidence that identifies mechanical stimuli as an important mediator for normal lung functions, a main reason for studying their effect in the lung arises from the hazardous effects that are caused by mechanical forces during artificial ventilation (Frank and Matthay, 2003; Ricard et al., 2003) (Fig. 5).

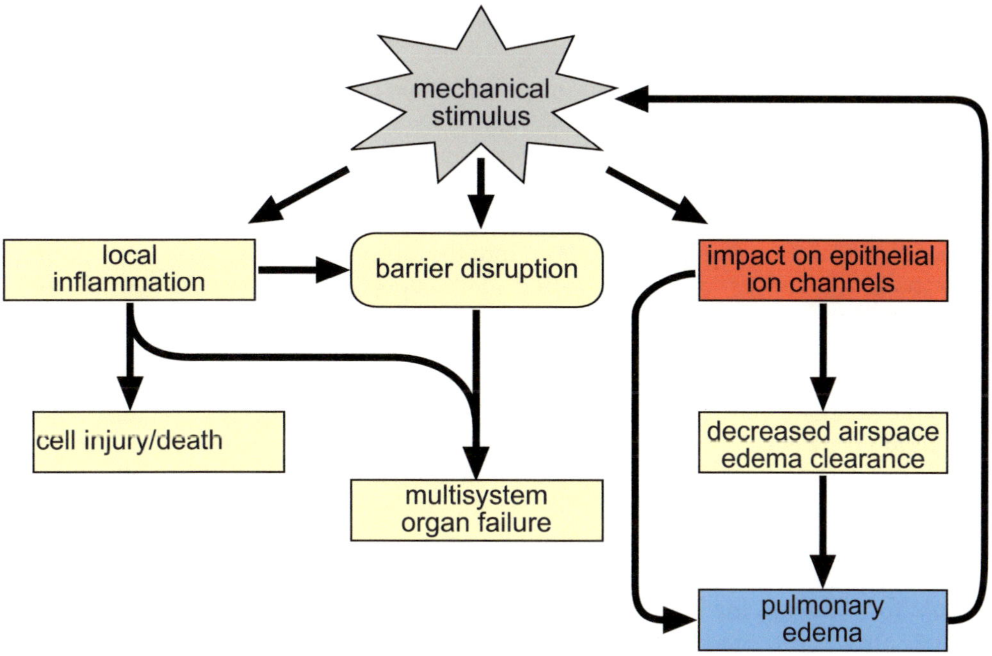

Fig. 5. Effect of deleterious physical forces related to ventilator induced lung injury. This scheme was modified from (Frank and Matthay, 2003) and extended by the potential interference of mechanical stimuli with the activity of epithelial ion channels. This represents a yet unidentified mechanism to improve the understanding how mechanical forces contribute to the formation and probably maintenance of pulmonary edema.

Artificial ventilation is a remedy of first choice for the treatment of patients with respiratory failure (e.g. acute lung injury (ALI); acute respiratory distress syndrome (ARDS)) (Ware and Matthay, 2000). However, the development of pulmonary edema due to fluid influxes into the airspace as well as the inability to resolve the edema fluid by decreased fluid reabsorption, is a major reason for the morbidity and mortality in these patients (Morty et al., 2007). The inability of the patients to resolve the edema fluid correlates with the mechanical ventilation duration times and mortality. High fluid clearance was associated with shorter durations of mechanical ventilation as well as with significantly decreased mortality rates (Sznajder, 2001; Ware and Matthay, 2001).
Considering the important role of pulmonary ion transport processes as discussed above, it is obvious that pulmonary edema are somehow related to alterations of pulmonary ion

transport processes (Matthay, 2002). Although changes of ion transport processes do not have to be causative for the development of pulmonary edema - there is sufficient evidence demonstrating that artificial ventilation worsens the situation in ALI/ARDS patients. This phenomenon has been termed ventilator induced lung injury (VILI) (Ricard et al., 2003) and is attributed to inappropriate ventilation strategies and thus the appearance of extensive physical forces (Fig. 5) (Plataki and Hubmayr, 2010).

This indication arises from the outcome of a multicenter trail study demonstrating a significantly reduced mortality in a group of patients that was ventilated with decreased tidal volumes (6 ml/kg) compared with high tidal volumes (12 ml/kg) (ARDS Network Investigators, 2000). Ventilation with decreased tidal volumes was also accompanied by the appearance of lower plateau pressures (ARDS Network Investigators, 2000) and this is associated with decreased mechanical forces.

However, regarding the symptoms observed in patients with ALI, ARDS and VILI there is an obvious connection between artificial ventilation and the development of pulmonary edema. There are two possible explanations reasonable for the development of pulmonary edema related to artificial ventilation:

1. Artificial ventilation causes ruptures and damages of the epithelial layer - enabling an uncontrolled influx of protein rich fluid into the airspace.
2. Mechanical forces as appearing during ventilation directly interfere with pulmonary epithelial ion transport processes

The first point has been extensively studied and there is no doubt that mechanical strain induced by artificial ventilation is a major reason for the development of pulmonary edema (Frank and Matthay, 2003). This is clearly indicated by the appearance of proteins in the edema fluid (Ware and Matthay, 2000). The second point is also obvious since a correlation between the ability to reabsorb alveolar fluid and the outcome of patients has been identified (Ware and Matthay, 2001). But for this instance, the mechanisms how artificial ventilation and thus mechanical forces interfere with ion transport processes are unknown.

3.5 Tools for studying the impact of mechanical forces on pulmonary ion transport

The first choice for studying functional epithelial ion transport is represented by electrophysiological Ussing chamber recordings. This technique was established by Hans Ussing during his studies on ion transport processes across the amphibian skin (Ussing and Zerahn, 1951). A major advantage as well as a prerequisite of this technique is the use of an intact epithelial layer consisting of differentiated polar cells. Although this technique is applicable for many freshly dissected epithelia including airway epithelia from mammals (Olver et al., 1975; Widdicombe and Welsh, 1980), the use of mammalian alveolar epithelium for elaborating this technique is not possible. This is due to the complex anatomy reasoned by miniaturization of the gas-exchanging region. Improved protocols and procedures for the isolation and cultivation of alveolar cells generally fixed this problem, but the use of isolated cells bears the risk of using cells with an artificial non-physiological phenotype. There is a bunch of studies published demonstrating that in isolated and cultivated cells the expression of ion transport proteins as well as their phenotype in terms of ion transport properties vary in dependence of the cultivation conditions used (Kunzelmann et al., 1996; Jain et al., 2001; Leroy et al., 2004; Dvorak et al., 2011). Further, these cells do not have their native surrounding (neighboring cells of different cell type, basal lamina etc.) that is important for the detection and transmission of forces. It remains also a challenge to expose these cultivated cells to defined physical forces (e.g. strain) to determine immediate changes of ion transport processes because usually the cells are cultivated on rigid polyester or polycarbonate membranes.

On the other hand pioneer studies addressing the function and relevance of pulmonary ion transport were performed on anaesthetized animals (Egan et al., 1976; Matthay et al., 1982). These studies identified the basic mechanisms of water and electrolyte transport by the alveolar epithelium. However, from such studies it is difficult to disentangle the particular ion conductances and to identify the specific ion transporting molecules that are involved in those processes.

3.5.1 Using native lung preparations for studying the impact of strain on pulmonary epithelial ion transport

Our lab has therefore established a native model for investigations of pulmonary ion transport. In accordance to Krogh's principle (Krebs, 1975) we decided to use lung preparations derived from the South African Clawed Frog *Xenopus laevis*. The alveolar epithelium of the *Xenopus* lung consists of one cell type referred to as pneumocytes (Meban, 1973). The anatomy and morphology of these cells is reminiscent to that of alveolar type I cells (Fischer et al., 1989), but they expose functional properties of alveolar type II cells as represented by the presence of lamellar bodies (Fischer et al., 1989). Most important, the *Xenopus* pneumocytes expose a Na^+ reabsorptive phenotype (Fischer et al., 1989; Kim, 1990; Fronius et al., 2003). In addition, expression and function of the CFTR Cl^- channel has been detected (Sommer et al., 2007). Recent studies identified the presence of the $Na^+/K^+/2Cl^-$ cotransporter, the function of a HCO_3^-/Cl^- exchanger (Berger et al., 2010) and evidence for basolateral Cl^- channels (Berger et al., 2011). Thus, the *Xenopus* pneumocytes exhibit the basic repertoire of ion channels and transporters that are supposed to be important in mediating the volume of the PLL.

The main advantage of this amphibian organ is its relatively simple sac-like structure. This feature is a prerequisite for dissecting a preparation that is suitable for Ussing chamber recordings. Comparable studies with other native lung preparations from higher vertebrates - and mammals in particular - are not possible, because of the growing complexity and miniaturization of the gas-exchanging region. In addition to establishing the use of *Xenopus* lung preparations for electrophysiological recordings, an Ussing chamber was developed that enables the exposure of the mounted pulmonary epithelium to mechanical forces. Mechanical forces are applied via an increased hydrostatic pressure and this is achieved by changing the outflow-height from the compartments Fig. 6.

4. Impact of strain on pulmonary ion transport in the *Xenopus* lung

Although the connection between high tidal volumes and pulmonary edema has been well established, little is known whether or not the underlying mechanisms can be attributed – at least partly – to a direct interaction of the mechanical forces with ion transport processes. Studies have been published providing evidence that high volume ventilation resulted in a decreased Na^+ transport due to a decreased Na^+/K^+-ATPase activity (Lecuona et al., 1999). Other studies demonstrated an increased Na^+/K^+-ATPase activity in response to cyclic stretch (Fisher and Margulies, 2002). Although these studies identified interference of strain with Na^+/K^+-ATPase activity, changes were observed hours after exposure to mechanical forces. So far little is known about a direct short-term effect of mechanical forces on ion transport processes in the lung.

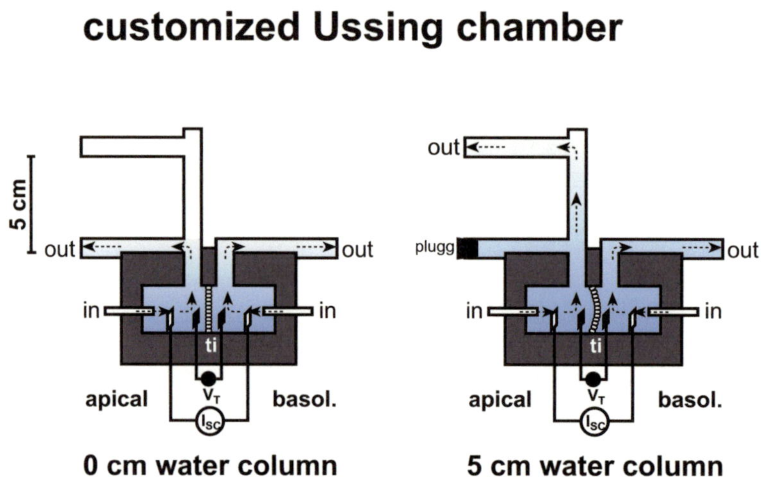

Fig. 6. Drawing of the Ussing chamber used to study the effect of mechanical forces on pulmonary epithelial ion transport (modified from (Bogdan et al., 2008)). Mechanical forces were applied by increasing the water column (5 cm water column) of the outflow. Both chamber compartments (apical, basolateral) were continuously perfused and the transepithelial short-circuit current (I_{SC}) and potential (V_T) was permanently monitored (ti: mounted tissue).

Using *Xenopus* lung preparations in combination with a customized Ussing chamber (Fig. 6) 5 cm hydrostatic pressure was applied from the apical side to mechanically challenge the tissue. Application of hydrostatic pressure was accompanied by immediate changes of the measured transepithelial short-circuit current (I_{SC}). The net effect induced by 5 cm H_2O was characterized by a decreased transepithelial current (Bogdan et al., 2008). Interestingly, the application of 5 cm H_2O from the basolateral side induced exactly the same response whereas the application of 5 cm H_2O synchronously from the apical and basolateral side did not cause any effect of the I_{SC} (Bogdan et al., 2008). These observations clearly demonstrate that the effective mechanical stimulus is strain and that it does not matter from which side the tissue is deflected.

In this setup a decreased transepithelial ion current is an indication for a decreased net reabsorption of ions from the apical to the basolateral side of the epithelium. Further, a reduced ion reabsorption reasoned by changes in ion transport processes will also reduce the osmoticaly driven water reabsorption from the airspace. This means that the changes of ion transport in the pulmonary epithelium observed with hydrostatic pressure decrease water reabsorption from the airspace and this represents a mechanism to facilitate the development of pulmonary edema - without affecting the integrity of the epithelial barrier that was assessed by determining the transepithelial electrical resistance.

4.1 Strain induces short-term activation of Na^+, K^+ and Cl^- channels

Further investigations using different ion channel inhibitors and substituting different ions from the perfusion solution revealed that the observed effect is reasoned by the activation of different ion channels and ion conductances resembled by:

1. activation of amiloride-sensitive Na^+ reabsorption
2. activation of an apical Cl^- secretion

3. activation of an apical K^+ secretion

Therefore, the inhibitory effect observed in the absence of drugs is an overlay of these three conductances (Fig. 7). Activation of Na^+ reabsorption as well as an increase of Cl^- secretion will produce an increase of the I_{SC}. In contrast to this, activation of apical K^+ channels will cause a decrease of the I_{SC}. Since the net pressure effect is an inhibition of the I_{SC}, the major response observed by the application of hydrostatic pressure is due to an activation of apical K^+ channels. Accordingly, the inhibitory effect of hydrostatic pressure should be prevented (or reversed → activation of the I_{SC}) following pre-incubation with K^+ channel inhibitors. And indeed this is exactly what we observed (Bogdan et al., 2008). Further, it has been found that the pressure-induced effect was largely prevented by glibenclamide (Bogdan et al., 2008), a compound that is a high affinity inhibitor of ATP-sensitive K^+ channels (K_{ATP}) (Nichols, 2006). Among other activating mechanisms, the activity of K_{ATP} channels is dependent on intracellular cyclic nucleotide levels and ATP in particular (Nichols, 2006). Interestingly, increased extracellular ATP concentrations were observed in response to the application of hydrostatic pressure and this represents a likely mechanism to explain our observations.

K_{ATP} channels are octameric complexes consisting of four pore forming Kir (inward rectifying K^+ channels) subunits and four associated SUR (sulfonylurea receptor) subunits (Nichols, 2006). In particular Kir channels are supposed to be involved in controlling the

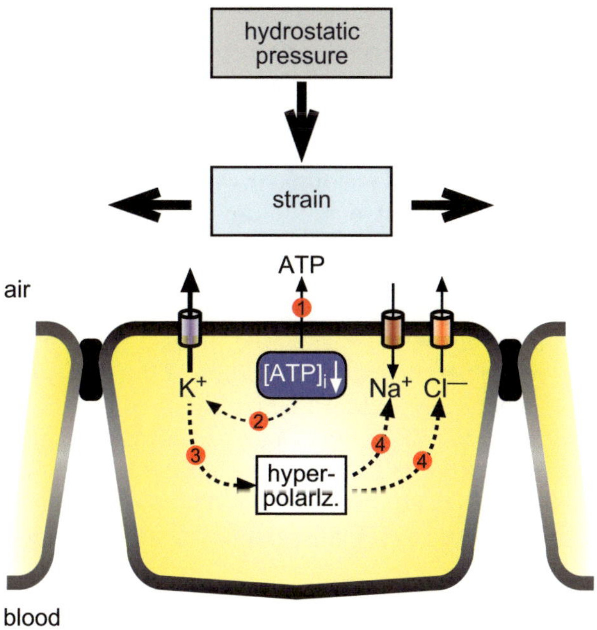

Fig. 7. Scheme illustrating the putative mechanism how hydrostatic pressure acts on epithelial ion transport processes in *Xenopus* lung epithelium (modified from Bogdan et al., 2008). The entire process could be initiated by the release of ATP via a yet unknown mechanism (1). The decrease of intracellular ATP levels ($[ATP]_i$) is likely to activate K_{ATP} channels (2). This will then cause the cell membrane potential to hyperpolarize (3) and subsequently facilitates the uptake of Na^+ via apical Na^+ channels (4) as well as the secretion of Cl^- via apical Cl^- channels.

membrane potential (Nichols, 2006) and this in turn enables the possibility to influence the driving forces for other conductances such as Na^+ and Cl^-. From this point of view it might be suggested that strain is primarily transduced in activation of K_{ATP} channels and that this in addition influences secondarily Na^+ and Cl^- transport as we observe by the application of hydrostatic pressure on *Xenopus* lung epithelia. Interestingly, increased ATP levels are also observed in rats ventilated with injurious ventilation parameters. In those experiments the increase of extracellular ATP concentrations was not reasoned by cell damage or cell lysis (Rich et al., 2003). These observations together with our findings indicate that the release of ATP (by a yet unidentified mechanism) might play a key role concerning the activation of ion channels in response to mechanical forces.
Last but not least it might be highlighted that the effect that was observed in response to the application of hydrostatic pressure (inhibition of the I_{SC}) represents a mechanism that impairs ion reabsorption from the alveolar airspace. This will result in a decrease osmotic gradient across the epithelial layer and will subsequently cause a reduction of fluid reabsorption from the airspace. Thus, this is a likely mechanism that impairs the resolution of pulmonary edema or maybe represents a mechanism that - among other incidents - initiates the formation of pulmonary edema in response to strain as induced by artificial ventilation.

5. Conclusions

The fact that mechanical forces directly affect pulmonary epithelial ion transport is important for future therapeutic options. On the one hand it further confirms the observations that modified ventilation strategies with low pressures and reduced volumes are beneficial for the outcome of patients with respiratory failure that are admitted to artificial ventilation. Therefore, the development of new ventilation strategies should be considered with the background that a minimum of mechanical stress should be used because this decreases interference with ion transport processes and this will preserve the ability of the epithelium for effective ion and water reabsorption.
On the other hand, it offers new therapeutic targets since we have evidence that K^+ channels and K_{ATP} channels in particular play a major role in the response observed by increased hydrostatic pressure. In our experiments, the inhibition of these channels has been identified to largely abolish the mechanically induced activation of K^+ channels and this would be beneficial to prevent the reduced ion transport absorption as that correlates with a decreased water reabsorption from the airspace. Another possibility in order to prevent the effects of strain on ion channels might be represented by the possibility to target the release of ATP, although the mechanisms of ATP release are still under debated.

6. Acknowledgements

The work was supported by the Deutsche Forschungsgemeinschaft (grant FR 2124 and the graduate program 455).

7. References

ARDS Network Investigators. (2000). Ventilation with lower tidal volumes as compared with traditional tidal volumes for acute lung injury and the acute respiratory distress syndrome. The Acute Respiratory Distress Syndrome Network. *N Engl J Med,* 342(18), 1301-1308, ISSN 0028-4793

Barth, K. & Kasper, M. (2009). Membrane compartments and purinergic signalling: occurrence and function of P2X receptors in lung. *FEBS J,* 276(2), 341-353, ISSN 1742-464X

Berger, J., Hardt, M., Clauss, W. G. & Fronius, M. (2010). Basolateral Cl- uptake mechanisms in Xenopus laevis lung epithelium. *Am J Physiol Regul Integr Comp Physiol,* 299(1), R92-100, ISSN 0363-6119

Berger, J., Richter, K., Clauss, W. G. & Fronius, M. (2011). Evidence for basolateral Cl- channels as modulators of apical Cl- secretion in pulmonary epithelia of Xenopus laevis. *Am J Physiol Regul Integr Comp Physiol,* 300(3), R616-23, ISSN 0363-6119

Bogdan, R., Veith, C., Clauss, W. & Fronius, M. (2008). Impact of mechanical stress on ion transport in native lung epithelium (Xenopus laevis): short-term activation of Na(+), Cl(-) and K(+) channels. *Pflugers Arch,* 456(6), 1109-1120, ISSN 0031-6768

Brainerd, E. L. & Owerkowicz, T. (2006). Functional morphology and evolution of aspiration breathing in tetrapods. *Respir Physiol Neurobiol,* 154(1-2), 73-88, ISSN 1569-9048

Bucheimer, R. E. & Linden, J. (2004). Purinergic regulation of epithelial transport. *J Physiol,* 555(Pt 2), 311-321, ISSN 0022-3751

Button, B., Picher, M. & Boucher, R. C. (2007). Differential effects of cyclic and constant stress on ATP release and mucociliary transport by human airway epithelia. *J Physiol,* 580(Pt. 2), 577-592, ISSN 0022-3751

Caputo, A., Caci, E., Ferrera, L., Pedemonte, N., Barsanti, C., Sondo, E., Pfeffer, U., Ravazzolo, R., Zegarra-Moran, O. & Galietta, L. J. (2008). TMEM16A, a membrane protein associated with calcium-dependent chloride channel activity. *Science,* 322(5901), 590-594, ISSN 0036-8075

Chambers, L. A., Rollins, B. M. & Tarran, R. (2007). Liquid movement across the surface epithelium of large airways. *Respir Physiol Neurobiol,* 159(3), 256-270, ISSN 1569-9048

Daniels, C. B. & Orgeig, S. (2003). Pulmonary surfactant: the key to the evolution of air breathing. *News Physiol Sci,* 18, 151-157, ISSN 0886-1714

Davis, C. W. & Lazarowski, E. (2008). Coupling of airway ciliary activity and mucin secretion to mechanical stresses by purinergic signaling. *Respir Physiol Neurobiol,* 163(1-3), 208-213, ISSN 1569-9048

Dobbs, L. G., Gonzalez, R., Matthay, M. A., Carter, E. P., Allen, L. & Verkman, A. S. (1998). Highly water-permeable type I alveolar epithelial cells confer high water permeability between the airspace and vasculature in rat lung. *Proc Natl Acad Sci U S A,* 95(6), 2991-2996, ISSN 0027-8424

Dvorak, A., Tilley, A. E., Shaykhiev, R., Wang, R. & Crystal, R. G. (2011). Do airway epithelium air-liquid cultures represent the in vivo airway epithelium transcriptome? *Am J Respir Cell Mol Biol,* 44(4), 465-473, ISSN 1044-1549

Edwards, Y. S. (2001). Stretch stimulation: its effects on alveolar type II cell function in the lung. *Comp Biochem Physiol A Mol Integr Physiol,* 129(1), 245-260, ISSN 1095-6433

Edwards, Y. S., Sutherland, L. M., Power, J. H., Nicholas, T. E. & Murray, A. W. (1999). Cyclic stretch induces both apoptosis and secretion in rat alveolar type II cells. *FEBS Lett,* 448(1), 127-130, ISSN 0014-5793

Egan, E. A., Nelson, R. M. & Olver, R. E. (1976). Lung inflation and alveolar permeability to non-electrolytes in the adult sheep in vivo. *J Physiol,* 260(2), 409-424, ISSN 0022-3751

Fang, X., Fukuda, N., Barbry, P., Sartori, C., Verkman, A. S. & Matthay, M. A. (2002). Novel role for CFTR in fluid absorption from the distal airspaces of the lung. *J Gen Physiol,* 119(2), 199-207, ISSN 0022-1295

Fang, X., Song, Y., Hirsch, J., Galietta, L. J., Pedemonte, N., Zemans, R. L., Dolganov, G., Verkman, A. S. & Matthay, M. A. (2006). Contribution of CFTR to apical-basolateral fluid transport in cultured human alveolar epithelial type II cells. *Am J Physiol Lung Cell Mol Physiol,* 290(2), L242-9, ISSN 1040-0605

Fewell, J. E., Lee, C. C. & Kitterman, J. A. (1981). Effects of phrenic nerve section on the respiratory system of fetal lambs. *J Appl Physiol,* 51(2), 293-297, ISSN 8750-7587

Fischer, H., Van Driessche, W. & Clauss, W. (1989). Evidence for apical sodium channels in frog lung epithelial cells. *Am J Physiol,* 256(4 Pt 1), C764-71, ISSN 1040-0605

Fisher, J. L. & Margulies, S. S. (2002). Na(+)-K(+)-ATPase activity in alveolar epithelial cells increases with cyclic stretch. *Am J Physiol Lung Cell Mol Physiol,* 283(4), L737-46, ISSN 1040-0605

Folkesson, H. G., Matthay, M. A., Hasegawa, H., Kheradmand, F. & Verkman, A. S. (1994). Transcellular water transport in lung alveolar epithelium through mercury-sensitive water channels. *Proc Natl Acad Sci U S A,* 91(11), 4970-4974, ISSN 0027-8424

Frank, J. A. & Matthay, M. A. (2003). Science review: mechanisms of ventilator-induced injury. *Crit Care,* 7(3), 233-241, ISSN 1364-8535

Fredberg, J. J. & Kamm, R. D. (2006). Stress transmission in the lung: pathways from organ to molecule. *Annu Rev Physiol,* 68, 507-541, ISSN 0066-4278

Fronius, M., Clauss, W. & Schnizler, M. (2003). Stimulation of transepithelial Na(+) current by extracellular Gd(3+) in Xenopus laevis alveolar epithelium. *J Membr Biol,* 195(1), 43-51, ISSN 0022-2631

Hammerschmidt, S., Kuhn, H., Gessner, C., Seyfarth, H. J. & Wirtz, H. (2007). Stretch-induced alveolar type II cell apoptosis: role of endogenous bradykinin and PI3K-Akt signaling. *Am J Respir Cell Mol Biol,* 37(6), 699-705, ISSN 1044-1549

Homolya, L., Steinberg, T. H. & Boucher, R. C. (2000). Cell to cell communication in response to mechanical stress via bilateral release of ATP and UTP in polarized epithelia. *J Cell Biol,* 150(6), 1349-1360, ISSN 0021-9525

Hoschele, S. & Mairbaurl, H. (2003). Alveolar flooding at high altitude: failure of reabsorption? *News Physiol Sci,* 18, 55-59, ISSN 0886-1714

Hummler, E., Barker, P., Gatzy, J., Beermann, F., Verdumo, C., Schmidt, A., Boucher, R. & Rossier, B. C. (1996). Early death due to defective neonatal lung liquid clearance in alpha-ENaC-deficient mice. *Nat Genet,* 12(3), 325-328, ISSN 1061-4036

Jain, L., Chen, X. J., Ramosevac, S., Brown, L. A. & Eaton, D. C. (2001). Expression of highly selective sodium channels in alveolar type II cells is determined by culture conditions. *Am J Physiol Lung Cell Mol Physiol,* 280(4), L646-58, ISSN 1040-0605

Kim, K. J. (1990). Active Na+ transport across Xenopus lung alveolar epithelium. *Respir Physiol,* 81(1), 29-39, ISSN 0034-5687

Kitterman, J. A. (1996). The effects of mechanical forces on fetal lung growth. *Clin Perinatol,* 23(4), 727-740, ISSN 0095-5108

Krebs, H. A. (1975). The August Krogh Principle: "For many problems there is an animal on which it can be most conveniently studied". *J Exp Zool,* 194(1), 221-226, ISSN 0022-104X

Kunzelmann, K., Kathofer, S., Hipper, A., Gruenert, D. C. & Gregner, R. (1996). Culture-dependent expression of Na+ conductances in airway epithelial cells. *Pflugers Arch,* 431(4), 578-586, ISSN 0031-6768

Lazrak, A., Thome, U., Myles, C., Ware, J., Chen, L., Venglarik, C. J. & Matalon, S. (2002). cAMP regulation of Cl(-) and HCO(-)(3) secretion across rat fetal distal lung epithelial cells. *Am J Physiol Lung Cell Mol Physiol,* 282(4), L650-8, ISSN 1040-0605

Lecuona, E., Saldias, F., Comellas, A., Ridge, K., Guerrero, C. & Sznajder, J. I. (1999). Ventilator-associated lung injury decreases lung ability to clear edema in rats. *Am J Respir Crit Care Med,* 159(2), 603-609, ISSN 1073-449X

Leipziger, J. (2003). Control of epithelial transport via luminal P2 receptors. *Am J Physiol Renal Physiol,* 284(3), F419-32, ISSN 1931-857X

Leroy, C., Dagenais, A., Berthiaume, Y. & Brochiero, E. (2004). Molecular identity and function in transepithelial transport of K(ATP) channels in alveolar epithelial cells. *Am J Physiol Lung Cell Mol Physiol,* 286(5), L1027-37, ISSN 1040-0605

Liu, M., Tanswell, A. K. & Post, M. (1999). Mechanical force-induced signal transduction in lung cells. *Am J Physiol,* 277(4 Pt 1), L667-83, ISSN 1040-0605

Maina, J. N. & West, J. B. (2005). Thin and strong! The bioengineering dilemma in the structural and functional design of the blood-gas barrier. *Physiol Rev,* 85(3), 811-844, ISSN 0031-9333

Mall, M., Grubb, B. R., Harkema, J. R., O'Neal, W. K. & Boucher, R. C. (2004). Increased airway epithelial Na+ absorption produces cystic fibrosis-like lung disease in mice. *Nat Med,* 10(5), 487-493, ISSN 1078-8956

Matalon, S. & O'Brodovich, H. (1999). Sodium channels in alveolar epithelial cells: molecular characterization, biophysical properties, and physiological significance. *Annu Rev Physiol,* 61, 627-661, ISSN 0066-4278

Matsui, H., Grubb, B. R., Tarran, R., Randell, S. H., Gatzy, J. T., Davis, C. W. & Boucher, R. C. (1998). Evidence for periciliary liquid layer depletion, not abnormal ion composition, in the pathogenesis of cystic fibrosis airways disease. *Cell,* 95(7), 1005-1015, ISSN 0092-8674

Matthay, M. A. (2002). Alveolar fluid clearance in patients with ARDS: does it make a difference? *Chest,* 122(6 Suppl), 340S-343S, ISSN 0012-3692

Matthay, M. A., Folkesson, H. G. & Clerici, C. (2002). Lung epithelial fluid transport and the resolution of pulmonary edema. *Physiol Rev,* 82(3), 569-600, ISSN 0031-9333

Matthay, M. A., Fukuda, N., Frank, J., Kallet, R., Daniel, B. & Sakuma, T. (2000). Alveolar epithelial barrier. Role in lung fluid balance in clinical lung injury. *Clin Chest Med,* 21(3), 477-490, ISSN 0272-5231

Matthay, M. A., Landolt, C. C. & Staub, N. C. (1982). Differential liquid and protein clearance from the alveoli of anesthetized sheep. *J Appl Physiol,* 53(1), 96-104, ISSN 8750-7587

McCray, P. B. J., Bettencourt, J. D., Bastacky, J., Denning, G. M. & Welsh, M. J. (1993). Expression of CFTR and a cAMP-stimulated chloride secretory current in cultured human fetal alveolar epithelial cells. *Am J Respir Cell Mol Biol,* 9(6), 578-585, ISSN 1044-1549

Meban, C. (1973). The pneumonocytes in the lung of Xenopus laevis. *J Anat,* 114(Pt 2), 235-244, ISSN 0021-8782

Morty, R. E., Eickelberg, O. & Seeger, W. (2007). Alveolar fluid clearance in acute lung injury: what have we learned from animal models and clinical studies? *Intensive Care Med,* 33(7), 1229-1240, ISSN 0342-4642

Nichols, C. G. (2006). KATP channels as molecular sensors of cellular metabolism. *Nature,* 440(7083), 470-476, ISSN 0028-0836

Okada, S. F., Nicholas, R. A., Kreda, S. M., Lazarowski, E. R. & Boucher, R. C. (2006). Physiological regulation of ATP release at the apical surface of human airway epithelia. *J Biol Chem,* 281(32), 22992-23002, ISSN 0021-9258

Olivier, R., Scherrer, U., Horisberger, J. D., Rossier, B C. & Hummler, E. (2002). Selected contribution: limiting Na(+) transport rate in airway epithelia from alpha-ENaC transgenic mice: a model for pulmonary edema. *J Appl Physiol,* 93, 1881-1887, ISSN 8750-7587

Olver, R. E., Davis, B., Marin, M. G. & Nadel, J. A. (1975). Active transport of Na+ and Cl- across the canine tracheal epithelium in vitro. *Am Rev Respir Dis,* 112(6), 811-815, ISSN 0003-0805

Plataki, M. & Hubmayr, R. D. (2010). The physical basis of ventilator-induced lung injury. *Expert Rev Respir Med,* 4(3), 373-385, ISSN 1747-6348

Ricard, J. D., Dreyfuss, D. & Saumon, G. (2003). Ventilator-induced lung injury. *Eur Respir J Suppl,* 42, 2s-9s, ISSN 0904-1850

Rich, P. B., Douillet, C. D., Mahler, S. A., Husain, S. A. & Boucher, R. C. (2003). Adenosine triphosphate is released during injurious mechanical ventilation and contributes to lung edema. *J Trauma,* 55(2), 290-297, ISSN 0022-5282

Riordan, J. R., Rommens, J. M., Kerem, B., Alon, N., Rozmahel, R., Grzelczak, Z., Zielenski, J., Lok, S., Plavsic, N., Chou, J. L. & et, a. (1989). Identification of the cystic fibrosis gene: cloning and characterization of complementary DNA. *Science,* 245(4922), 1066-1073, ISSN 0036-8075

Rogers, C. S., Stoltz, D. A., Meyerholz, D. K., Ostedgaard, L. S., Rokhlina, T., Taft, P. J., Rogan, M. P., Pezzulo, A. A., Karp, P. H., Itani, O. A., Kabel, A. C., Wohlford-Lenane, C. L., Davis, G. J., Hanfland, R. A., Smith, T. L., Samuel, M., Wax, D., Murphy, C. N., Rieke, A., Whitworth, K., Uc, A., Starner, T. D., Brogden, K. A., Shilyansky, J., McCray, P. B. J., Zabner, J., Prather, R. S. & Welsh, M. J. (2008). Disruption of the CFTR gene produces a model of cystic fibrosis in newborn pigs. *Science,* 321(5897), 1837-1841, ISSN 0036-8075

Roux, E. (2002). [Origin and evolution of the respiratory tract in vertebrates]. *Rev Mal Respir,* 19(5 Pt 1), 601-615, ISSn 0761-8425

Rubin, B. K. (2002). Physiology of airway mucus clearance. *Respir Care,* 47(7), 761-768, ISSN 0020-1324

Sackin, H. & Boulpaep, E. L. (1975). Models for coupling of salt and water transport; Proximal tubular reabsorption in Necturus kidney. *J Gen Physiol,* 66(6), 671-733, ISSN 0022-1295

Sanchez-Esteban, J., Tsai, S. W., Sang, J., Qin, J., Torday, J. S. & Rubin, L. P. (1998). Effects of mechanical forces on lung-specific gene expression. *Am J Med Sci,* 316(3), 200-204, ISSN 0002-9629

Schroeder, B. C., Cheng, T., Jan, Y. N. & Jan, L. Y. (2008). Expression cloning of TMEM16A as a calcium-activated chloride channel subunit. *Cell,* 134(6), 1019-1029, ISSN 0092-8674

Smith, P. L., Welsh, M. J., Stoff, J. S. & Frizzell, R. A. (1982). Chloride secretion by canine tracheal epithelium: I. Role of intracellular c AMP levels. *J Membr Biol,* 70(3), 217-226, ISSN 0022-2631

Sommer, D., Bogdan, R., Berger, J., Peters, D. M., Morty, R. E., Clauss, W. G. & Fronius, M. (2007). CFTR-dependent Cl- secretion in Xenopus laevis lung epithelium. *Respir Physiol Neurobiol,* 158(1), 97-106, ISSN 1569-9048

Stoltz, D. A., Meyerholz, D. K., Pezzulo, A. A., Ramachandran, S., Rogan, M. P., Davis, G. J., Hanfland, R. A., Wohlford-Lenane, C., Dohrn, C. L., Bartlett, J. A., Nelson, G. A. t., Chang, E. H., Taft, P. J., Ludwig, P. S., Estin, M., Hornick, E. E., Launspach, J. L., Samuel, M., Rokhlina, T., Karp, P. H., Ostedgaard, L. S., Uc, A., Starner, T. D., Horswill, A. R., Brogden, K. A., Prather, R. S., Richter, S. S., Shilyansky, J., McCray, P. B. J., Zabner, J. & Welsh, M. J. (2010). Cystic fibrosis pigs develop lung disease and exhibit defective bacterial eradication at birth. *Sci Transl Med,* 2(29), 29ra31, ISSN 1946-6234

Sznajder, J. I. (2001). Alveolar edema must be cleared for the acute respiratory distress syndrome patient to survive. *Am J Respir Crit Care Med,* 163(6), 1293-1294, ISSN 1073-449X

Tarran, R., Button, B. & Boucher, R. C. (2006). Regulation of normal and cystic fibrosis airway surface liquid volume by phasic shear stress. *Annu Rev Physiol,* 68, 543-561, ISSN 0066-4278

Tarran, R., Button, B., Picher, M., Paradiso, A. M., Ribeiro, C. M., Lazarowski, E. R., Zhang, L., Collins, P. L., Pickles, R. J., Fredberg, J. J. & Boucher, R. C. (2005). Normal and cystic fibrosis airway surface liquid homeostasis. The effects of phasic shear stress and viral infections. *J Biol Chem,* 280(42), 35751-35759, ISSN 0021-9258

Tizzano, E. F., O'Brodovich, H., Chitayat, D., Benichou, J. C. & Buchwald, M. (1994). Regional expression of CFTR in developing human respiratory tissues. *Am J Respir Cell Mol Biol,* 10(4), 355-362, ISSN 1044-1549

Ussing, H. H. & Zerahn, K. (1951). Active transport of sodium as the source of electric current in the short-circuited isolated frog skin. *Acta Physiol Scand,* 23(2-3), 110-127, ISSN 0001-6772

Verkman, A. S. (2007). Role of aquaporins in lung liquid physiology. *Respir Physiol Neurobiol,* 159(3), 324-330, ISSN 1569-9048

Verkman, A. S., Matthay, M. A. & Song, Y. (2000). Aquaporin water channels and lung physiology. *Am J Physiol Lung Cell Mol Physiol,* 278(5), L867-79, ISSN 1040-0605

Ware, L. B. & Matthay, M. A. (2000). The acute respiratory distress syndrome. *N Engl J Med,* 342(18), 1334-1349, ISSN 0028-4793

Ware, L. B. & Matthay, M. A. (2001). Alveolar fluid clearance is impaired in the majority of patients with acute lung injury and the acute respiratory distress syndrome. *Am J Respir Crit Care Med,* 163(6), 1376-1383, ISSN 1073-449X

Welsh, M. J. (1987). Electrolyte transport by airway epithelia. *Physiol Rev,* 67(4), 1143-1184, ISSN 0031-9333

Welsh, M. J. & Smith, A. E. (1993). Molecular mechanisms of CFTR chloride channel dysfunction in cystic fibrosis. *Cell,* 73(7), 1251-1254, ISSN 0092-8674

Widdicombe, J. H. & Welsh, M. J. (1980). Ion transport by dog tracheal epithelium. *Fed Proc,* 39(13), 3062-3066, ISSN 0014-9446

Widdicombe, J. H., Welsh, M. J. & Finkbeiner, W. E. (1985). Cystic fibrosis decreases the apical membrane chloride permeability of monolayers cultured from cells of tracheal epithelium. *Proc Natl Acad Sci U S A,* 82(18), 6167-6171, ISSN 0027-8424

Willumsen, N. J., Davis, C. W. & Boucher, R. C. (1989). Intracellular Cl- activity and cellular Cl- pathways in cultured human airway epithelium. *Am J Physiol,* 256(5 Pt 1), C1033-44, ISSN 0002-9513

Wirtz, H. R. & Dobbs, L. G. (2000). The effects of mechanical forces on lung functions. *Respir Physiol,* 119(1), 1-17, ISSN 0034-5687

Yang, Y. D., Cho, H., Koo, J. Y., Tak, M. H., Cho, Y., Shim, W. S., Park, S. P., Lee, J., Lee, B., Kim, B. M., Raouf, R., Shin, Y. K. & Oh, U. (2008). TMEM16A confers receptor-activated calcium-dependent chloride conductance. *Nature,* 455(7217), 1210-1215, ISSN 0028-0836

Part 6

Miscellaneous

27

Functional Evaluation in Respiratory Disorders

Cirelene Grobler, David M. Maree and Elvis M. Irusen
Pulmonology Division, University of Stellenbosch & Tygerberg Academic Hospital, Cape Town, South Africa

1. Introduction

In evaluating the respiratory system, many different tests are used and these can be divided into different categories based on the aspect of lung function they measure. Depending on availability and need, the tests can be complementary and yield results that allow deeper insight into respiratory function to understand disease processes and therapeutic interventions - both medical and surgical.

Categories of Pulmonary Function Tests
a. Airway Function
- Simple spirometry (VC, expiratory reserve volume {ERV}, inspiratory capacity {IC})
- Forced vital capacity (FVC, from which the Forced Expired Volume in the first second is derived- FEV1)
- Maximal inspiratory / expiratory pressures (MIP / MEP)
b. Lung volumes and ventilation
- Function residual capacity (FRC)
- Total lung capacity (TLC)
- Residual Volume (RV)
RV / TLC ratio
c. Diffusing Capacity Test
- Single breath (breath holding)
d. Blood gases and gas exchange tests
- Blood gas analysis and blood oximetry
- Pulse oximetry
e. Cardiopulmonary exercise tests
- Simple non-invasive tests
- Tests with exhaled gas analyses

Table 1. The categories of pulmonary function testing

1.1 Spirometry & other related tests

Spirometry is a physiological test that measures how an individual inhales or exhales volumes of air as a function of time. The primary signal measured may be volume or time. Spirometry is the pulmonary function test performed most often due to the large number of indications. "It is most often performed as a screening procedure because it may be the first test to indicate the presence of pulmonary disease"(Ruppel, 2009).

Indications for Spirometry

a. Diagnose the presence / absence of lung disease.
   1. History of pulmonary symptoms (dyspnoea, wheezing, cough, phlegm production, orthopnoea)
   2. Physical indicators (decreased breath sounds, chest wall abnormalities)
   3. Abnormal Laboratory findings (Chest x-ray or CT studies)

b. Quantify the extent of known disease on lung function
   1. Pulmonary disease (COPD, Asthma)
   2. Cardiac disease (Cardiac Failure)
   3. Neuromuscular disease (e.g. Guillain-Barrè syndrome)

c. Measure effects of occupational / environmental exposures

d. Determine beneficial / negative effects of therapy

e. Assess risk for surgical procedures
   1. Lung resection
   2. Thoracic procedures
   3. Pulmonary rehabilitation

f. Evaluate disability or impairment

g. Epidemiologic or clinical research involving lung health or disease.

Table 2. List of indications for spirometry (Ruppel, 2009)

> "Spirometry is recommended as the "gold standard" for the diagnosis of obstructive lung disease. However spirometry alone may not be sufficient enough to completely define the extent of disease, therapy response, preoperative risk, or level of impairment (Ruppel,2009)".

In view of the importance of spirometry in aiding an accurate diagnosis and monitoring changes that can be extremely subtle, a good quality spirometer is essential. As the machines become increasingly sophisticated and computerised, it is imperative that they meet the technical specifications so that are accurate and precise. These criteria are quite complex but are well laid out by the American Thoracic Society (ATS- Standardization of Spirometry, 1994 Update). Thus in purchasing or utilising such a device it is crucial that one obtains the manufacturer's guarantee that a reputable testing facility has checked that the spirometer meets and conforms with the ATS recommendations for accuracy and precision. Equally, a well trained pulmonary function technologist who understands the calibration and pitfalls of the testing can be invaluable.

> "The two most important measurements of spirometry are (1) **forced vital capacity (FVC)**, which is the volume delivered during an expiration made as forcefully and completely as possible starting from full inspiration, and the (2) **forced expiratory volume** in one second **(FEV_1)** of an FVC manoeuvre (ATS/ERS,2005)".

Another variable derived from spirometry is the slow **vital capacity (VC)**, which is the volume of gas measured from a slow, complete expiration after a maximal inspiration, without forced or rapid effort. The **Inspiratory capacity (IC)** and **expiratory reserve volume (ERV)** are subdivisions of the VC. The IC is the largest volume of gas that can be inspired from a resting expiratory level. ERV is the largest volume of gas that can be expired from the resting end-expiratory level. IC and ERV are used in the calculation of the **residual volume (RV)** and **total lung capacity (TLC)**. The RV is the volume of gas remaining in the lungs at the end of maximal expiration regardless of the lung volume at which exhalation was started. The TLC is the volume of gas contained in the lungs after maximal inspiration (ATS/ERS,2005).

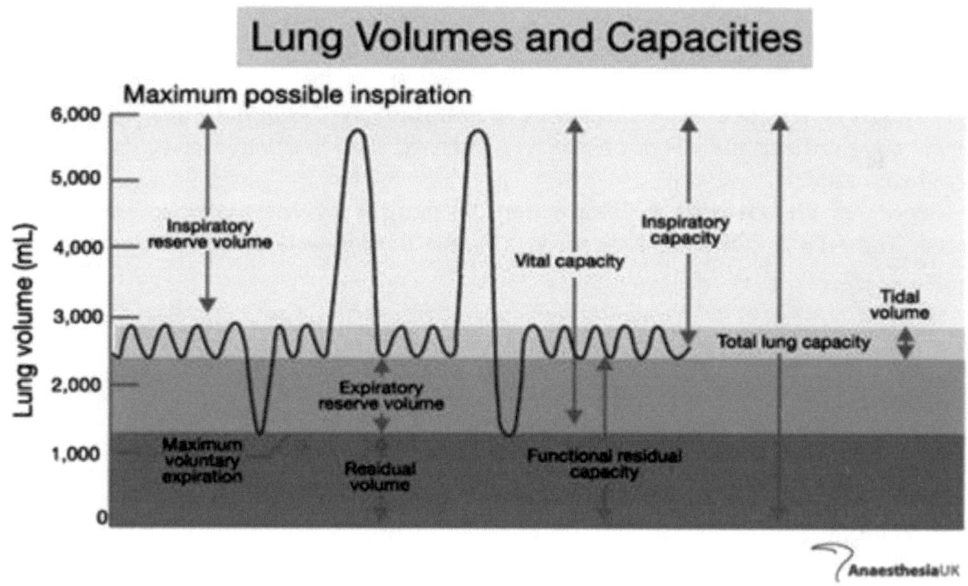

Fig. 1. A schematic presentation of the lung volumes and capacities.

Contraindications to Spirometry

- Myocardial infarction within the last month
- Recent stroke, eye surgery, thoracic / abdominal surgery
- Uncontrolled hypertension
- Known aortic, thoracic, cerebral aneurysm
- Recent pneumothorax
- Relative contraindications: chest, abdominal, facial pain, headache, stress incontinence, dementia, confusion

Table 3. A list of contraindications to spirometry (Ruppel,2009).

2. Flow-volume loop

This procedure is used to measure the FVC, FEV_1 and other forced expiratory flow volumes. This test is dependent on patient effort.

2.1 Significance and pathophysiology

2.1.1 Forced Vital Capacity

The FVC usually equals VC in healthy individuals and should be within 150ml of each other. The FVC and VC may differ if the patient's effort is variable or if significant airway obstruction is present (FEV_1 / FVC is less than 70%). The FVC may be lower than VC in patients with obstructive diseases as forced expiration can cause airway collapse. In these situations a slow VC (SVC) may be more accurate.

Healthy adults can expire their FVC within 4-6 seconds. Healthy children and adolescents may exhale their FVC in less than 4 seconds. Patients with severe obstruction may require 15 seconds or more to exhale completely.

2.1.2 Forced expiratory volume in the first second (FEV_1)

FEV_1 is reported as a volume, although it measures flow over a specific interval. FEV_1 may be reduced in either obstructive or restrictive patterns. The FEV_1 and FEV_1 / FVC ratio are the most standardized indices of obstructive diseases. An obstructive defect is defined best by a reduced ratio.

The severity of an obstructive disease may be gauged by the extent to which FEV_1 is reduced. The ATS / ERS 2005 Task force suggests the following classifications of severity (Ruppel, 2005):

Mild	FEV_1 > 70% predicted
Moderate	FEV_1 = 60% - 69% predicted
Moderately severe	FEV_1 = 50% -59% predicted
Severe	FEV_1 = 35% - 49% predicted
Very severe	FEV_1 < 35% of predicted

Once the VC is below normal, a concomitant restrictive defect may also be present, and this can be determined by further measurement of volumes, in particular TLC. Restrictive processes such as fibrosis, oedema, and obesity may all cause a decrease in FEV_1. Unlike the pattern seen in obstructive diseases, in which VC is preserved and FEV_1 reduced, in restriction VC and FEV_1 values are proportionally decreased.

The FEV_1 is the most widely used spirometric parameter, particularly for the assessment of airway obstruction. It is also used in conjunction with VC for simple screening, assessment of response to bronchodilators, and detection of exercise-induced bronchospasm.

2.1.3 FEV_1 / FVC ratio

The normal ratio expressed as a percentage for healthy adults is between 75% - 85%. This value can decrease with age, presumably because of gradual loss of lung elasticity. Diagnosis of an obstructive pattern based on spirometry should focus on three primary variables: FVC, FEV_1, and FEV_1 / FVC.

Examples of patterns seen in flow volume loops follow: The actual curve (with asterisks) is usually superimposed on the predicted as derived by the computer based on age, gender, height and ethnicity.

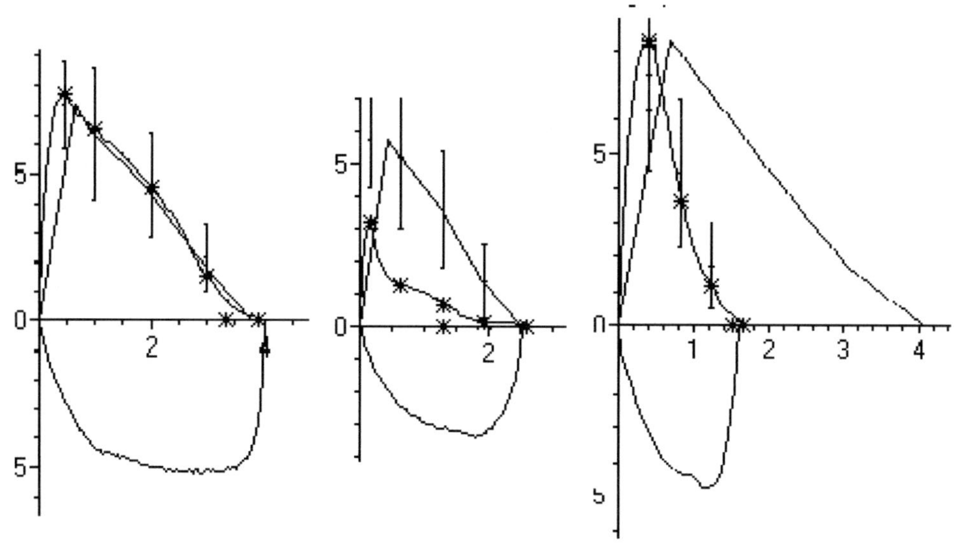

Normal curve　　Obstructive curve　　Restrictive curve

2.2 Reversibility testing

This is the determination of reversibility in airflow-limitation with drug administration and is commonly undertaken as part of lung function testing. The choice of drug, dose and mode of delivery is a clinical decision depending on what the clinician wishes to learn from the test. The aim is to determine whether the patient's lung function can be improved with therapy.

The subject first undergoes baseline lung function testing, preferably with no prior drug therapy. According to the ATS/ERS 2005 guidelines, short-acting inhaled drugs should not be used 4hr prior to testing and long-acting β-agonist bronchodilators or oral aminophylline should be stopped 12hr prior to testing. Smoking should be avoided for an hour or more prior to testing as well as throughout the duration of the test procedure.

2.2.1 Procedure (ATS/ERS, 2005)

1. The subject performs 3 acceptable tests, with acceptable repeatability of the two highest FEV_1, FVC and PEF as a baseline.
2. The drug administered (100ug Salbutamol) is inhaled in one breath to TLC from a valved spacer device. The breath is then held for 5-10 s before the subject exhales.
3. Three further doses of Salbutamol (total dose 400ug) are delivered at 30s intervals.
4. Step 1 is repeated 10 – 15 min after administration of a short acting β_2- agonists (and 30 min after short-acting anticholinergic agents).

2.2.2 Determination of reversibility

A positive response to bronchodilator therapy is when either the FVC or the FEV_1 of the post attempt improves by 12% and 200ml from the pre attempt.

1. BD response = $\frac{FEV_1(post) - FEV_1(pre)}{1} \times \frac{100}{1}$

2. BD response = $\frac{FVC\ (post)\ -\ FVC\ (pre)}{1} \times \frac{100}{1}$

2.2.3 Clinical significance

Reversibility of airway obstruction is considered significant for increases of greater than 12% and 200ml for either the FEV_1 or FVC. If the sGaw is assessed, an increase of 30%-40% is usually considered as significant. Some patients may show little or even no improvement in FEV_1, but have a significant improvement in their sGaw.

Increases greater than 50% in the FEV_1 may occur in patients with asthma. Patients with chronic obstructive pulmonary diseases may show little improvement in their flows. Failure to show a significant improvement after inhaled bronchodilator therapy does not exclude a response.

It has been erroneously extrapolated that reversibility testing can define a disease; this is not true (Richter & Irusen, 2008). Asthma can be irreversible on spirometry (especially when there is uncontrolled inflammation impairing bronchodilatation) and COPD can be spirometrically reversible in up to 50% of patients. (In this respect, the absolute volume of improvement is more important as it is easy to get a significant percentage change when one starts with a low baseline.)

3. Maximal inspiratory / expiratory pressure (MIP & MEP)

Forced manoeuvres during spirometry require the patient to give a maximal effort, yet it also requires that the patient should have normal muscle function. Muscle function is best assessed by measurement of maximal inspiratory and expiratory pressures. **Maximal inspiratory pressure (MIP)** is the lowest pressure developed during a forceful inspiration against an occluded airway. **Maximal expiratory pressure (MEP)** is the highest pressure that can be developed during a forceful expiratory effort against an occluded airway.

3.1 Significance and pathophysiology

MIP primarily measures inspiratory muscle strength. Healthy adults can generate inspiratory pressures greater than -50cmH_2O in women, and -75 cmH_2O in men (Ruppel, 2009). Decreased MIP is seen in patients with neuromuscular disease or diseases involving the diaphragm, intercostals or accessory muscles. MIP may also be decreased in patients with hyperinflation as in emphysema. MIP is sometimes used to assess patient response to strength training of respiratory muscles. It is also used in the assessment of respiratory muscle function in patients who need ventilatory support.

MEP measures the pressures generated during maximal expiration. Healthy adults can generate MEP values greater than 80 cmH_2O in women and greater than 100 cmH_2O in men (Ruppel, 2009). MEP may be decreased in patients with neuromuscular disorders, particularly those resulting in generalized muscle weakness.

Reduced MEP often accompanies increased RV as seen in emphysema. A low MEP is associated with inability to cough effectively.

Accurate measurement of MIP & MEP depends largely on patient effort. The best efforts should be reproducible within 20% or 10 cmH_2O, whichever is greater. Widely varying pressures for either MIP or MEP should be assessed carefully before interpretation.

4. Body plethysmography

The forces governing maximal airflow are the elastic recoil pressure of the lung and airway resistance upstream from the equal pressure point. **Airway resistance (Raw)** is the pressure difference per unit flow as gas flows into or out of the lungs. Raw is the difference between the mouth pressure and alveolar pressure, divided by flow at the mouth.
Airway conductance (Gaw) is the flow generated per unit of pressure drop across the airways. Gaw is not commonly reported as it changes with lung volume. Instead, specific airway conductance (sGaw), which is Gaw divided by the lung volume at which the measurement was made, is usually reported (Ruppel, 2009).
Spirometry may be performed with the patient in the plethysmograph. The pneumotachometer must be capable of accurately measuring the entire range of gas flows required.
Spirometry, lung volumes, and airway resistance can all be obtained in a single sitting using plethysmography.

4.1 The most common measurements made using a body plethysmograph are:

- Airway resistance (Raw).
- Lung Volumes:
  - VC= Volume measured from a maximal inspiration followed by a complete slow expiration.
  - FRC= It is the volume of air left in the lungs at the end of a quiet exhalation
  - IC = Maximal volume of air inspired from a resting expiratory level.
  - ERV= Maximal volume of air expired from a resting expiratory level
  - TGV= Is the absolute volume of gas in the thorax at any point in time and at any level of alveolar pressure
  - RV= Volume of air remaining in the lungs at the end of a maximal expiration.
  - TLC= Volume of gas that the lungs contain after maximal inspiration.
  - RV/TLC (must be in the range 20 - 35% in order to be normal)

4.2 Important derivatives

4.2.1 Thoracic Gas Volume (TGV)

The TGV is a quick and accurate means of measuring lung volumes. It can be used in combination with simple spirometry to derive all lung volume compartments. The plethysmograph's primary advantage is that it measures all gas in the thorax, whether in ventilatory communication with the atmosphere or not.

4.2.1.1 Clinical Significance

Normative data for TGV and pulmonary subdivisions allow definition of restrictive lung disease as distinct from obstructive, in the presence of a reduced VC. Definition of abnormally increased lung volumes in obstructive lung disease is a further appropriate clinical use of whole-body plethysmography. While lung volumes can be measured by gas dilution techniques, it is well known that dilution techniques measure only the volume of ventilated airspaces. Accordingly, when whole-body plethysmography is combined with dilution measures of lung volumes, the volume of trapped gas is estimated by the difference between FRCBox and dilutional FRCGas.

The ratio of FRCBox/FRCGas can be used as an index of gas trapping. This ratio is usually near 1.0 in patients with normal lungs, or even with restriction.

Values greater than 1 indicate gas volumes detectable by the plethysmograph but hidden to the gas techniques. Care must be taken that lung volumes determined by the 2 methods are reliable before the values can be expressed as a ratio. This ratio has been used to evaluate candidates for lung volume reduction surgery (LVRS). Lung volume reduction attempts to directly reduce gas trapping by removal of unperfused lung tissue. Patients with bullous emphysema may have a litre or more difference in TLC (Total Lung Capacity) when the methods are compared.

Some evidence suggests that in severe airway obstruction, FRC may actually be overestimated when the plethysmographic technique is used. This occurs primarily because PMouth may not equal alveolar pressure if the airways are severely obstructed. Rapid panting rates aggravate this inaccuracy.

4.2.2 RAW

Airway resistance (Raw) is the pressure difference per unit flow as gas flows into or out of the lungs. Raw is the difference between mouth pressure and alveolar pressure, divided by flow at the mouth. This pressure difference is caused primarily by the friction of gas molecules in contact with the airways.

4.2.2.1 Clinical Significance

The tracing labelled "(a)" displays a schematic sRaw loop in a normal patient during tidal breathing, which is shown after numerical software compensations to close the sRaw loop. Normal patients manifest a steep linear loop during tidal breathing without hysteresis. In contrast, during voluntary panting efforts, the upper and lower end portions of the loop may become slightly curvilinear.

The curvilinearity is in the form of a very slight "S" shape, analogous to that shown in tracing "(d)", but much less exaggerated. In normal patients during voluntary panting, the flattening of the sRaw loop at the upper right extremity (mid-inspiration) and at the lower left extremity (mid-expiration) of the loop are only barely visible, depending on the absolute value of flow rates achieved.

Tracing "(b)" is typical of patients with large (central) airway constriction that is relatively uniform (and not a localized stenosis) and without significant small airway obstruction. This might be seen in a patient with mild asthma.

It is well known that expiratory flow limitation and dynamic airway compression may occur during tidal breathing in COPD, and this contributes to the characteristic shape of the sRaw loop in tracing "(c)".

Tracing "(d)" shows the influence of a fixed or functional stenosis of the upper airways, for example laryngeal abnormality, or paralysis of one vocal cord. This type of "orifice" constriction manifests flow limitation during inspiration, such that, at sufficiently high flows, further increases in driving pressure do not result in any increase in airflow. This reflects localized upper airway obstruction, analogous to that which pertains in the maximal expiratory flow-volume curve. Thus, during forced expiration, when a critical driving pressure for expiratory airflow (intra-pleural pressure for forced expiration) is achieved, further increases in driving pressure do not cause any further increases in flow rate. A similar flow limitation may occur in the extra-thoracic airway during inspiration, as shown in the upper right portion of tracing "(d)".

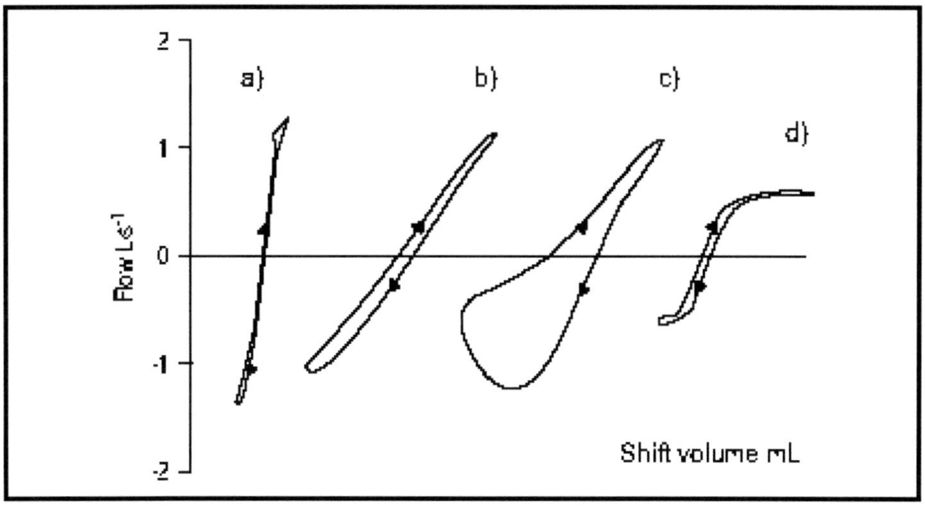

Fig. 2. A schematic presentation of the flow / volume shift measuring Raw

5. Functional Residual Capacity (FRC)

The FRC is the volume of air left in the lungs at the end of a quiet exhalation. There are 2 methods of measuring FRC which are (1) helium dilution and (2) the Nitrogen washout technique.

5.1 Helium dilution

The method for measuring lung volumes is based on the equilibration of gas in the lung with a known volume of gas containing helium. The test gas consists of air with added oxygen of 25–30%, but higher concentrations are acceptable.

5.1.1 Measurement technique (ATS / ERS, 2005)

Specific details of procedures will vary with different types of equipment and degrees of automation, but the basic procedure is as follows.

1. The equipment should be turned on and allowed an adequate warm-up time.
2. The equipment should be set up for testing, including calibration, according to manufacturer's instructions.
3. The patient should be asked if he/she has a perforated eardrum (if so, an earplug should be used).
4. The patient is seated comfortably, with no need to remove dentures. The procedure is explained, emphasising the need to avoid leaks around the mouthpiece during the test and to use a nose clip.
5. The patient breathes for 30–60 s on the mouthpiece to become accustomed to the apparatus and to ensure a stable end-tidal expiratory level.
6. The patient is turned "in" (i.e. connected to the test gas) at the end of a normal tidal expiration.
7. The patient is instructed to breathe regular tidal breaths.
8. The O_2 oxygen flow is adjusted to compensate for O_2 consumption (significant errors in the calculation of FRC can result if O_2 consumption is not adequately accounted for).

9. The helium concentration is noted every 15 s.
10. Helium equilibration is considered to be complete when the change in helium concentration is, 0.02% for 30 s. The test rarely exceeds 10 min, even in patients with severe gas-exchange abnormalities [9].
11. Once the helium equilibration is complete, the patient is turned "out" (i.e. disconnected from the test gas) of the system. If the measurements of ERV and IC are to be linked to the FRC measured, it should be ensured that the spirometer has an adequate volume for the full ERV and IVC manoeuvres (fig. 5).
12. At least one technically satisfactory measurement should be obtained. Due to the extra costs and time in making multiple measurements, and the relatively good inter-day variability in adults, two or more measurements of FRCHe need to be made only when necessitated by clinical or research need . If only one measurement of FRCHe is made, caution should be used in the interpretation. For younger children, however, it is recommended that at least two technically satisfactory measurements be performed. If more than one measurement of FRCHe is carried out, the value reported for FRCHe should be the mean of technically acceptable results that agree within 10%.

5.2 Nitrogen washout technique (ATS / ERS, 2005)

This technique is based on washing out the N_2 from the lungs, while the patient breathes 100% O_2. The initial alveolar N_2 concentration and the amount of N_2 washed out can then be used to calculate the lung volume at the start of washout. The technique originally utilized gas collections for a 7-min period, a period deemed adequate for washout of N_2 from the lungs of healthy subjects. The measurement technique should adhere to the following steps:

1. The equipment should be turned on and allowed an adequate warm-up time, with calibration as instructed by the manufacturer.
2. The patient should be asked if he/she has a perforated eardrum (if so, an earplug should be used).
3. The patient is seated comfortably, with no need to remove dentures. The procedure is explained, emphasizing the need to avoid leaks around the mouthpiece during the washout and using a nose clip.
4. The patient breathes on the mouthpiece for 30–60 s to become accustomed to the apparatus, and to assure a stable end-tidal expiratory level.
5. When breathing is stable and consistent with the end-tidal volume being at FRC, the patient is switched into the circuit so that 100% O_2 is inspired instead of room air.
6. The N_2 concentration is monitored during the washout. A change in inspired N_2 of .1% or sudden large increases in expiratory N_2 concentrations indicate a leak; hence, the test should be stopped and repeated after a 15-min period of breathing room air.
7. The washout is considered to be complete when the N_2 concentration is, 1.5% for at least three successive breaths.
8. At least one technically satisfactory measurement should be obtained. If additional washouts are performed, a waiting period of ≥ 15 min is recommended between trials. In patients with severe obstructive or bullous disease, the time between trials should be ≥ 1 h, if more than one measurement of $FRCN_2$ is made, the value reported for $FRCN_2$ should be the mean of technically acceptable results that agree within 10%. If only one measurement of $FRCN_2$ is made, caution should be used in the interpretation.

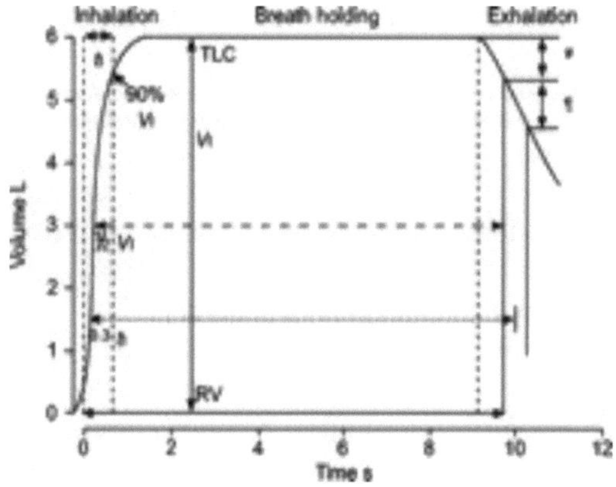

Fig. 3. A schematic presentation of the single breath DLCO manoeuvre

6. Diffusing capacity (DLCO)

6.1 Definition

DLCO measures the transfer of a diffusion-limited gas (CO) across the alveoli capillary membranes. DLCO is reported in millilitres of CO/minute/ml of Mercury at STPD.

6.2 Technique

CO combines with Haemoglobin (Hb) approximately 210 times more readily than O_2. In the presence of normal amounts of Hb and normal ventilator function, the primary limiting factor to diffusion of CO is the status of alveolocapillary membranes.

Diffusing capacity can be affected by factors that change the membrane component, as well as by alterations in Hb and in the capillary blood volume. DLCO is used to assess the gas exchange ability of the lungs, specifically oxygenation of mixed venous blood.

DLCO is used to evaluate pulmonary involvement in systemic diseases such as rheumatoid arthritis. DLCO measurements are often included in the evaluation of patients with obstructive lung disease such as emphysema.

DLCO may be indicated to monitor changes in lung function induced by drugs used to treat cardiac arrhythmias as well as changes caused by chemo and radiation therapy for lung cancer.

	Indications for DLCO
a.	Evaluate or follow the progress of parenchymal lung diseases
b.	Evaluate pulmonary involvement in systemic diseases
c.	Evaluate obstructive lung disease - Follow progression of disease - Differentiate types of obstruction - Predict arterial desaturation during exercise in COPD
d.	Evaluate cardiovascular diseases
e.	Quantify disability associated with interstitial lung disease
f.	Evaluate pulmonary haemorrhage, polycythemia, or left to right shunts (Increased DLCO)

Table 4. A list of DLCO indications (Ruppel, 2009)

The most commonly used method is the single-breath or breath-hold technique. The single-breath method is also the most widely standardized.

6.3 Significance and pathophysiology

The expected DLCO value in a healthy patient varies directly with the patient's lung volume. Women have slightly lower normal values, presumably because of smaller normal lung volumes. DLCO values can increase 2-3 times in healthy individuals during exercise in response to increased pulmonary capillary blood flow.

DLCO is often decreased in restrictive lung diseases, particularly those associated with pulmonary fibrosis. Fibrotic changes in the lung parenchyma are associated with asbestosis, berylliosis, and silicosis. Idiopathic pulmonary fibrosis, sarcoidosis, SLE, scleroderma are associated with a decreased DLCO. Inhalation of toxic gases causes alveolitis and a decrease in DLCO values.

A decrease in DLCO is more likely to be related to the loss of lung volume, alveolar surface area, or capillary bed than to thickening of the alveolocapillary membrane. DLCO also decrease when there is a loss of lung tissue or replacement of normal parenchyma by space occupying lesions such as tumours. DLCO may also be reduced in the presence of pulmonary oedema.

Low resting DLCO (less than 50-60 % of predicted) may indicate the need for assessment of oxygenation during exercise. DLCO is directly related to lung volume (V_A) in healthy individuals. DL / V_A relationship can be useful to differentiate whether decreased DLCO is the result of loss of lung volume or from some other causes.

In obstruction, low DLCO without reduction in V_A results in a low ratio. In a purely restrictive process, a decrease in DLCO reflects loss of V_A and the DL / V_A ratio is preserved.

Numerous other physiologic factors can influence the observed DLCO:

- Hb and Hct, COHb
- Alveolar P_{CO2}
- Pulmonary capillary blood volume
- Body position
- Altitude above sea level
- Asthma and obesity

6.4 Interpretive strategies (Ruppel, 2009)

- If DLCO is less than the lower limit of normal (LLN) after appropriate corrections, it's likely that a gas exchange abnormality exists. Evaluate DL / V_A
- If DL / V_A ratio is normal, reduced diffusing capacity is likely related to decreased lung volumes, parenchymal changes, pulmonary vascular disease or pulmonary hypertension. Consider clinical correlation.
- If DL / V_A ratio is decreased, reduced diffusing capacity is likely related to airway obstruction or increased dead space. Compare V_A and TLC; a large difference suggests uneven distribution of ventilation.
- If DLCO is increased after correction of Hb or altitude, consider possible causes of increased pulmonary blood volume, haemorrhage, obesity of left-to-right shunts. Also consider undiagnosed asthma.
- If DLCO is less than 50% of predicted, consider additional tests such as blood gases, exercise desaturation study.

7. Blood gases

Blood gas is the most basic test of lung function. Blood gas analysis is often done in conjunction with pulmonary function studies. Blood is drawn from a peripheral artery without being exposed to air (anaerobically). Blood gas analysis includes measurement of ph, pCO_2, and pO_2.
The same specimen may be used for blood oximetry to measure total Hb, oxyhaemoglobin (O_2Hb), carboxyhaemoglobin (COHb) and methaemoglobin (MetHb). Blood gas is the ideal measurement of pulmonary function because is assesses the two primary functions of the lung - oxygenation and carbon dioxide removal.

7.1 Indications

1. Evaluate adequacy of lung function
2. Determine the need for supplementary oxygen
3. Monitoring of ventilation
4. Document the severity of progression of known pulmonary disease
5. Provide data to correct or corroborate other pulmonary function measurements.

7.2 3 Most important variables in a blood gas result:

1. pH (7.35 - 7.45)
2. pCO_2 (4.67 - 6.00 kPa)
3. pO_2 (10.00 - 13.33 kPa)

7.3 Significance and pathophysiology

pH < 7.35 = Acidemia
pH > 7.45 = Alkalemia
Acid-base disorders arising from lung disease are often related to P_{CO2} and its transport as carbonic acid.

- Acid-base disorders -

	pH	*pCO_2*	*pO_2*
Metabolic acidosis	↓	*N*	↓
Metabolic alkalosis	↑	*N*	↑
Respiratory acidosis	↓	↑	*N*
Respiratory alkalosis	↑	↓	*N*
Compensatory Respiratory acidosis and metabolic alkalosis	*N*	↑	↑
Compensatory Metabolic acidosis and respiratory alkalosis	*N*	↓	↓
Combined Metabolic and Respiratory acidosis	↓	↑	↓
Combined Metabolic and Respiratory alkalosis	↑	↓	↑

Table 5. Three helpful parameters in interpreting a blood-gas result (in the simple uncompensated state- Ruppel, 2009)

pO_2 is the pressure of O_2 dissolved in blood. The amount of Hb and whether it is capable of binding O_2 has only a minimal effect on pO_2. Hypoxemia commonly results from inadequate or abnormal Hb. The severity of impaired oxygenation is indicated by the PaO_2 at rest. PaO_2 is a good index of the lungs 'ability to match pulmonary capillary blood flow with adequate ventilation.

Delivery of O_2 to the tissues however depends on Hb concentration and cardiac output as well as adequate gas transfer in the lungs. Because most O_2 transported is bound to Hb, there must be an adequate supply (12-15 g/dl) of functional Hb.

8. Pulse oximetry

SpO_2 estimates SaO_2 by analyzing absorption of light passing through a capillary bed, either by transmission or reflectance. Pulse oximetry is non-invasive.

8.1 Interfering factors

Motion artefact, shivering, bright ambient lightning, hypotension, low perfusion, hypothermia, vasoconstrictor drugs and dark skin pigmentation can confound.

8.2 Significance and pathophysiology

Most pulse oximeters are capable of accuracy of +/- 2% of actual saturation when SaO_2 is above 90%. Other uses of pulse oximetry are:

- Monitoring of O_2 therapy
- Ventilatory support
- Pulmonary / Cardiac rehabilitation
- Bronchoscopy
- Surgical procedures
- Sleep studies
- Cardiopulmonary exercise testing

Pulse oximetry may not be appropriate in all situations e.g. to evaluate hyperoxemia or acid-base status in a patient, a blood gas analysis is required. Measurement of O_2 delivery, which depends on Hb concentration, cannot be adequately assessed by pulse oximetry.

9. Six minute walk test (6MWT)

This is a simple exercise test used to assess the response to a medical or surgical intervention, but also been used to assess functional capacity as well as to estimate morbidity and mortality. This test doesn't require any sophisticated equipment.

INDICATIONS FOR THE SIX-MINUTE WALK TEST
Pre-treatment and post treatment comparisons
Lung transplantation / Resection
Lung volume reduction surgery
Pulmonary rehabilitation
COPD
Pulmonary hypertension
Heart failure
Cystic fibrosis
Heart failure
Peripheral vascular disease
Predictor of morbidity and mortality

Table 6. A list of indications for a six minute walk test (Ruppel, 2009)

Contraindications
Unstable angina during the previous month
Infarction during the previous month
A resting heart rate of more than 120,
Systolic blood pressure of more than 180 mm Hg,
Diastolic blood pressure of more than 100 mm Hg.

Table 7. A list of the contraindications of a six minute walk test (Ruppel, 2009)

Reasons for immediately stopping a 6MWT include the following:
1. chest pain,
2. intolerable dyspnoea,
3. leg cramps
4. staggering
5. diaphoresis
6. pale or ashen appearance.

Technicians must be trained to recognize these problems and the appropriate responses. If a test is stopped for any of these reasons, the patient should sit or lie supine as appropriate depending on the severity or the event and the technician's assessment of the severity of the event and the risk of syncope.The following should be obtained based on the judgment of the technician: blood pressure, pulse rate, oxygen saturation, and a physician evaluation. Oxygen should be administered as appropriate.

9.1 Equipment required

1. Countdown timer (or stopwatch)
2. Mechanical lap counter
3. Two small cones to mark the turnaround points
4. A chair that can be easily moved along the walking course
5. Worksheets on a clipboard
6. A source of oxygen
7. Sphygmomanometer
8. Telephone
9. Automated electronic defibrillator

9.2 Measurements (ATS / ERS 2002)

1. Repeat testing should be performed about the same time of day to minimize intraday variability.
2. A "warm-up" period before the test should not be performed.
3. The patient should sit at rest in a chair, located near the starting position, for at least 10 minutes before the test starts. During this time, check for contraindications, measure pulse and blood pressure, and make sure that clothing and shoes are appropriate. Complete the first portion of the worksheet
4. Pulse oximetry is optional. If it is performed, measure and record baseline heart rate and oxygen saturation and follow manufacturer's instructions to maximize the signal and to minimize motion artefact. Make sure the readings are stable before recording.

Note pulse regularity and whether the oximeter signal quality is acceptable. The rationale for measuring oxygen saturation is that although the distance is the primary outcome measure, improvement during serial evaluations may be manifest either by an increased distance or by reduced symptoms with the same distance walked. The SpO_2 should not be used for constant monitoring during the exercise. The technician must not walk with the patient to observe the SpO_2.

If worn during the walk, the pulse oximeter must be lightweight (less than 2 pounds), battery powered, and held in place (perhaps by a "fanny pack") so that the patient does not have to hold or stabilize it and so that stride is not affected.

5. Have the patient stand and rate their baseline dyspnoea and overall fatigue using the Borg scale
6. Set the lap counter to zero and the timer to 6 minutes. Assemble all necessary equipment (lap counter, timer, clipboard, Borg Scale, worksheet) and move to the starting point.
7. Instruct the patient as follows:
"The object of this test is to walk as far as possible for 6 minutes. You will walk back and forth in this hallway. Six minutes is a long time to walk, so you will be exerting yourself. You will probably get out of breath or become exhausted. You are permitted to slow down, to stop, and to rest as necessary. You may lean against the wall while resting, but resume walking as soon as you are able. You will be walking back and forth around the cones. You should pivot briskly around the cones and continue back the other way without hesitation. Now I'm going to show you. Please watch the way I turn without hesitation." Demonstrate by walking one lap yourself. Walk and pivot around a cone briskly. "Are you ready to do that? I am going to use this counter to keep track of the number of laps you complete. I will click it each time you turn around at this starting line. Remember that the object is to walk AS FAR AS POSSIBLE for 6 minutes, but don't run or jog. Start now or whenever you are ready."

THE BORG SCALE
0 Nothing at all
0.5 Very, very slight (just noticeable)
1 Very slight
2 Slight (light)
3 Moderate
4 Somewhat severe
5 Severe (heavy)
6
7 Very severe
8
9
10 Very, very severe (maximal)

Table 8. The Borg scale

At the beginning of the 6-minute exercise, show the scale to the patient and ask the patient this: "Please grade your level of shortness of breath using this scale." Then ask this: "Please grade your level of fatigue using this scale." At the end of the exercise, remind the patient of the breathing number that they chose before the exercise and ask the patient to grade their breathing level again. Then ask the patient to grade their level of fatigue, after reminding them of their grade before the exercise.

8. Position the patient at the starting line. You should also stand near the starting line during the test. Do not walk with the patient. As soon as the patient starts to walk, start the timer.
9. Do not talk to anyone during the walk. Use an even tone of voice when using the standard phrases of encouragement. Watch the patient. Do not get distracted and lose count of the laps. Each time the participant returns to the starting line, click the lap counter once (or mark the lap on the worksheet). Let the participant see you do it.
10. Post-test: Record the post walk Borg dyspnoea and fatigue levels and ask this: "What, if anything, kept you from walking farther?"
11. If using a pulse oximeter, measure SpO_2 and pulse rate from the oximeter and then remove the sensor.
12. Record the number of laps from the counter (or tick marks on the worksheet).
13. Record the additional distance covered (the number of meters in the final partial lap) using the markers on the wall as distance guides. Calculate the total distance walked, rounding to the nearest meter, and record it on the worksheet.

9.3 Interpretation

Most 6MWTs will be done before and after intervention, and the primary question to be answered after both tests have been completed is whether the patient has experienced a clinically significant improvement. With a good quality-assurance program, with patients tested by the same technician, and after one or two practice tests, short-term reproducibility of the 6MWD is excellent. It is not known whether it is best for clinical purposes to express change in 6MWD as

1. An absolute value,
2. A percentage change, or
3. A change in the percentage of predicted value.

Until further research is available, we recommend that change in 6MWD be expressed as an absolute value (e.g., the patient walked 50 m farther).

10. Stair climbing

In a setting where corridor length is limited, but a few flights of stairs are available, the stair climb is an ideal test as a primary screening test to decide if a patient can undergo thoracic surgery or needs additional testing e.g. Cardio Pulmonary Exercise Testing.

The stair climb as a test is easy to perform and easy to understand by patients as well as being safe. Minimal equipment and personnel is required. To do the test one instructs the patient to climb the flights of stairs at their fastest pace to a minimum ascent of +/- 20 metre. This climb is timed so as to calculate the speed of ascent, which correlates well with VO_2max measured during cycle ergometry. It was shown that climbing at a speed of ascent of

≥15m/min to an elevation of 20 metres accurately predicted a $VO_2max \geq 20ml/kg/min$. (Koegeleneberg, 2009)

11. Cardiopulmonary Exercise Testing (CPET)

Cardiopulmonary exercise testing is used to define work limitations. Cardiopulmonary variables are assessed in relation to the workload. The patterns of change in any particular variable are then compared with the expected normal response. The primary indications for performing this test are dyspnoea and exertion, pain (especially angina) and fatigue. Exercise induces airway narrowing in the majority of patients with asthma. Exercise-induced airway narrowing is called exercise- induced asthma (EIA) and exercise-induced bronchoconstriction (EIB).

Other indications include:

- Evaluation of exercise intolerance of level of fitness
- Exercise evaluation for cardiac or pulmonary rehabilitation
- Assess pre-operative risk, particularly lung resection or reduction.
- Assess disability, particularly related to occupational lung disease
- Evaluate therapeutic interventions such as heart or lung transplantation.

Exercise testing can detect the following:

- Presence and nature of ventilator limitation to work
- Presence and nature of cardiovascular limitations to work
- Extent of conditioning or de-conditioning
- Maximal tolerable workload and safe levels of daily exercise
- Extent of disability for rehabilitation purposes
- O_2 desaturation and appropriate levels of supplemental O2 therapy
- Outcome measurement after a treatment plan.

The preferred modes of exercise are the motor-driven treadmill with adjustable speed and grade or the electromagnetically braked cycle ergometer. Heart rate should be monitored from a three-lead electrocardiographic configuration as a minimum.

Alternatively, a pulse oximeter or other device able to reliably determine heart rate may be used. For those at higher risk for coronary artery disease, a 12- lead ECG configuration is advisable.

11.1 Treadmill protocol (ATS / ERS 1999)

The treadmill speed and gradient are chosen to produce 4–6 min of exercise at near-maximum targets with a total duration of exercise of 6–8 min. For children less than 12 yr of age, the time is usually 6 min; for older children and adults the time is usually 8 min. starting at a low speed and gradient, both are progressively advanced during the first 2–3 min of exercise until the heart rate is 80–90% of the predicted maximum. Ventilation rather than heart rate can be used to monitor exercise intensity. Ventilation should reach 40–60% of the predicted maximum voluntary ventilation (MVV, estimated as FEV1 x 35). The degree of physical fitness and body weight will strongly influence the grade and speed necessary to obtain the desired heart rate. A reasonable procedure is to quickly advance to a rapid, but comfortable, speed and then raise the treadmill slope until the desired heart rate or ventilation is obtained.

For older children and adults 8 min of exercise is usually required to elicit EIB when dry air temperature is inhaled. A treadmill speed greater than 3 mph (about 4.5 km/h) and a gradient greater than 15% or an oxygen consumption of 35 ml/min/kg or greater will usually achieve the target ventilation or heart rate in young healthy subjects. Nomograms have been proposed to predict speed and grade that will elicit the desired heart rate, but they have not been extensively validated. It may be preferable to use nomograms relating oxygen consumption per kilogram to speed and slope of the treadmill.
The test ends when the patient has exercised at the target ventilation or heart rate for at least 4 min. This usually requires a total of 6–8 min of exercise. The test may be terminated by the patient at any time.

11.1.1 Assessing the response

Forced expiratory volume in 1 s (FEV_1) is the primary outcome variable. Spirometry should be performed and evaluated as described earlier. One exception to ATS-recommended techniques for spirometry is allowed. If the only outcome variable to be used is the FEV_1, the duration of the expiration may be limited to 2–3 s. In all cases it is important to vigorously coach the patient to inhale fully even in the presence of chest tightness. Incomplete inhalations will result in false reductions in FEV_1.
If vocal cord dysfunction or other possible causes of central airway obstruction are suspected, full inspiratory and expiratory flow–volume loops should be obtained.
An appropriate post-exercise testing schedule is 5, 10, 15, 20, and 30 min after cessation of exercise. Some investigators include earlier measurements (1 and 3 min post-exercise) because severe EIB can sometimes be present at the cessation of exercise. Early recognition allows it to be dealt with promptly. If the FEV_1 has returned from its nadir to the baseline level or greater, spirometry testing may be terminated at 20 min post exercise. A β-agonist bronchodilator may be administered at any time to reverse the bronchoconstrictive response if the patient experiences appreciable dyspnoea, or if the FEV_1 has not recovered to within 10% of baseline when the patient is ready to leave the laboratory.
The presence of exercise-induced bronchoconstriction is defined by plotting FEV_1 as a percentage of the pre-exercise baseline FEV_1 at each post-exercise interval.
A decrease below 90% of the baseline FEV_1 (i.e., a 10% decrease) is a generally accepted abnormal response. Some authors suggest a value of 15% is more diagnostic of EIB, particularly if exercise has been performed in the field.

12. Bronchial provocation testing

Bronchial challenge testing is used to identify and characterize airway hyper-responsiveness. Challenge test may be performed in patients with symptoms of bronchospasm who have normal pulmonary function studies or uncertain results of bronchodilator studies. It can also be used to assess changes in hyper-reactivity of the airways or to quantify its severity.
Several commonly used provocative agents can be used to assess airway hyper reactivity. These include the following:

- Methacoloine challenge (increase parasympathetic tone in bronchial smooth muscle)
- Histamine challenge (trigger response producing bronchoconstriction)

- Exercise

FEV_1 is the variable most commonly used, although airway resistance and specific conductance can also be measured before and after testing.

12.1 Dosing protocols (ATS /ERS 1999)

1. Two-minute tidal breathing dosing protocol.
2. Five-breath dosimeter protocol.
   a. Set up and check the dosimeter.
   b. Prepare the following five concentrations of methacholine in sterile vials; place them in a holder; and store them in a refrigerator.
   c. Remove the vials from the refrigerator 30 min before testing, so that the contents warm to room temperature before use. Insert 2.0 ml of the first concentration into the nebulizer, using a sterile syringe. The patient is seated throughout the test.
   d. Perform baseline spirometry.
   e. Briefly open the dosimeter solenoid to make sure the nebulizer is nebulising.
   f. Ask the patient to hold the nebulizer upright with the mouthpiece in his/her mouth. Watch the patient during the breathing manoeuvres to ensure that the inhalation and breath hold are correct and that the nebulizer is not tipped.
   g. At end exhalation during tidal breathing (functional residual capacity), instruct the patient to inhale slowly and deeply from the nebulizer. Trigger the dosimeter soon after the inhalation begins; dosimeters may do this automatically. Encourage the patient to continue inhaling slowly (about 5 s to complete the inhalation) and to hold the breath (at total lung capacity, TLC) for another 5 s.
   h. Repeat step g for a total of five inspiratory capacity inhalations. Take no more than a total of 2 min to perform these five inhalations.
   i. Measure the FEV_1 at about 30 and 90 s after the fifth inhalation from the nebulizer. Obtain an acceptable-quality FEV_1 at each time point. This may require repeated attempts. Perform no more than three or four manoeuvres after each dose. It should take no more than 3 min to perform these manoeuvres. To keep the cumulative effect of methacholine relatively constant, the time interval between the commencements of two subsequent concentrations should be kept to 5 min.
   j. At each dose, report the highest FEV_1 from acceptable manoeuvres.
   k. If the FEV_1 falls less than 20%, empty the nebulizer, shake it dry, and trigger the dosimeter once to dry the nebulizer nozzle. Add 2.0 ml of the next higher concentration, and repeat steps g–j.
   l. If the FEV_1 falls more than 20% from baseline (or the highest concentration has been given), give no further methacholine, note signs and symptoms, administer inhaled albuterol, wait 10 min, and repeat the spirometry.

12.2 Interpretive strategies

1. Were there any factors present that could influence the result e.g. failure to withhold bronchodilators ?
2. Respiratory infection? If so interpret cautiously or not at all.
3. Were spirometric efforts repeatable and acceptable before and during the challenge? If not, interpret very cautiously or not at all.

4. For Metacholine or histamine challenge was there a 20% decrease after inhalant of dilatants. Is so, test result is positive.
5. Was there a 20% decrease of FEV1 after inhalation of agonist? If so, test result is likely positive and PC_{20} should be used to categorize the degree of hyper responsiveness.
6. Was there at least 35% decrease in SGaw (Preferably 50%)? If so, test result is likely positive
7. Were there signs of airway hyper reactivity (coughing, wheezing or shortness of breath)? If so, test suggests bronchial hyper responsiveness
8. Were the results borderline? If so, repeat the test.
9. Were symptoms present despite little or no change in FEV_1?
10. Consider additional measurements such as SGaw or related conditions such as vocal cord dysfunction.

13. Conclusion

There are a variety of tests, both simple and sophisticated, that allow greater insights into respiratory disease, functional impairment and suitability for operative intervention. Some of the tests are more complicated to perform and both improvement and deterioration in respiratory status can be subtle. For these reasons strict quality control, in terms of appropriately validated equipment, standardisation and trained and experienced personnel are mandatory. To ensure excellent quality results good patient co-operation is required as well. Disregard for these precautions can lead to diagnostic confusion, misclassification of improvement and deterioration or unnecessary further interventions. These can be costly and also result in needless morbidity and mortality. Thus a full understanding of the tests, their appropriateness and pitfalls can complement patient evaluation and result in greater diagnostic certainty and patient management.

14. References

American Thoracic Society: Standardisation of Spirometry; 1994 Update. *Am J Resir Crit Care Med* 1995; 152: 1107 - 1136.

Brunelli, A.,2008.Stair Climbing Test and Lung Surgery. *Respiration*, 2008;75:372-373

Crapo RO, Casaburi R, Coates AL, et.al. Guidelines for Metacholine and Exercise Challenge Testing - 1999. *Am J Respir Crit Care Med* 2000; 161: 309-329.

Crapo RO, Enright PL , Zeballos RJ. Guidelines for the Six-Minute Walk Test. *Am J Respir Crit Care* Med 2002; 166: 111-117.

Goldman MD , Smith HJ, Ulmer, WT. Whole Body Plethysmography. *Eur Respir Mon* 2005; 31: 15-43.

Koegelenberg CFN, Plekker D, Bolliger CT. Functional evaluation for treatment. *Eur Respir Mon* 2009; 44: 169–186.

Miller, M.R., Hankinson, J.Brusasco, V. Standardisation of Spirometry. Eur Respir J 2005; 26: 319-338.

Richter DC, Joubert JR, Nell H, Schuurmans MM, Irusen EM. Diagnostic value of post bronchodilator pulmonary function testing to distinguish between stable, moderate to severe COPD and asthma. Int J Chron Obstruct Pulmon Dis 2008; 3(4): 693–699.

Ruppel, G.L. 2009. Manual of Pulmonary Function Testing. Ruppel. G.L (ed.). 9th ed. St Louis Missouri: Mosby Elsevier. p.p.3,7-10,68-70,134,144-146,158,159,162-168,170-172,291

Wanger J, Clausen JL, Coates A. Standardisation of the Measurement of Lung Volumes. *Eur Respir J* 2005; 26: 511-522.

28

Novel Methods for Diagnosis of Pulmonary Microangiopathy in Diabetes Mellitus

Kalicka Renata and Kuziemski Krzysztof
Gdansk University of Technology, Department of Biomedical Engineering,
Medical University of Gdansk, Department of Allergology,
Poland

1. Introduction

Lung microangiopathy is a little known negative influence of diabetes mellitus on the functioning of the lungs. In current medical practice lung microangiopathy is diagnosed by comparing two measurements of lung diffusing capacity – one with the subject standing and one with the subject lying. The necessity to take two measurements is inconvenient.

In lung microangiopathy we observe a reduction of diffusing capacity, lung flow and volume. Diabetes is a chronic illness that can lead to diabetic angiopathy, a pathology of the blood vessels (arteries, veins and capillaries). There are two types of diabetic angiopathy: macroangiopathy (disease of the larger blood vessels) and microangiopathy (microvascular pathology). The examples of angiopathy include: neuropathy, nephropathy and retinopathy.

Current knowledge regarding diabetic lung microangiopathy is limited. Histopathological examination of lung biopsy samples is not a conclusive test of the consequences of diabetes (Dalquen, 1999). Animal experiments and post-mortem examinations have disclosed the influence of diabetes on the lung capillaries and alveolar-capillary membranes (Kida et al, 1993), (Kodolova et al, 1982) and (Popov& Simionescu, 1997). Histopathological tests have revealed the thickening of the alveolar and venous capillary walls (Matsubara& Hara, 1991) and (Weynand et al, 1999).

Lung diffusing capacity measurements illustrate the state of alveolar-capillary barrier (Goldman, 2003). These are measurements of diffusion across the alveolar-capillary membrane. For diagnosing microangiopathy, the lung diffusing capacity is measured in two body positions: standing (D_L^{standing}) and lying on the back (D_L^{lying}), (Strojek et al, 1993) and (Kuziemski et al, 2008). On account of the human anatomic structure, diffusing capacity depends on the body's position. For healthy subjects the diffusing capacity increases in the reclined position, $D_L^{\text{lying}} > D_L^{\text{standing}}$. The opposite is observed in the case of microangiopathic patients: the diffusing capacity decreases when the subject is lying $D_L^{\text{lying}} < D_L^{\text{standing}}$. This is the result of blood vessel damage and alveolar thickening caused by diabetes (Kuziemski et al, 2009). Only the fact that diffusing capacity increases or decreases in a given position is important as far as microangiopathy diagnosis is concerned.

Spirometry (measurement of the volume and flow of inhaled and exhaled air) is the most common pulmonary function test. It is helpful in diagnosing asthma, pulmonary fibrosis, cystic fibrosis, and COPD (Chronic Obstructive Pulmonary Disease).

Research (Goldman, 2003), (Kaminski, 2004) has shown that a single spirometry test does not provide sufficient information for a diagnosis of lung flow limitation and lung volume reduction caused by diabetes mellitus. Instead we need long-term observations of spirometry results to diagnose lung microangiopathy. Microangiopathy lung impairment is characterised by a decrease in spirometric parameters FVC (the maximum volume of air that can be exhaled or inspired during a forced manoeuvre) and FEV_1 (the forced expiratory volume during the first second of expiration) (Davis et al, 2004), (Litonjua et al, 2005), (Yeh et al, 2008).

A later study (Kuziemski et al, 2009) proved that a single spirometric test is insufficient to identify lung microangiopathy on account of functional reserve breathing. The reserves compensate, to some extent, the lung dysfunction, and thus the negative effect of diabetes is concealed until the effect reaches a higher level of impairment.

Since the direct measurements of pulmonary function are not conclusive and post-mortem autopsies do not serve the given patient, the diagnostics have to be based on such indirect results as spirometric measurements and modelling. It is probably also capable of revealing lung microangiopathy if the results are very carefully analysed.

Perfusion computed tomography (pCT) is a diagnostic method that enables the imaging of the organ and tissue. This is a powerful tool for diagnosing perfusion of internal organs such as the brain, liver, pancreas, spleen, kidneys and lungs (Alonzi & Hoskin, 2006), (Blomley et al, 1993), (Cao, 2011), (Eichinger et al, 2010), (Kuziemski et al, 2011). The method enables quantitative evaluation of circulation by determining changes in tissue during the flow of a contrast agent in the blood vessels. Changes, when compared to a normal tissue, can indicate tissue pathology. Lung pCT measurements can help in the diagnosis of cystic fibrosis (Eichinger et al, 2010) and diabetes (Kuziemski et al, 2011). It can also help to differentiate benign pulmonary nodules from lung cancer (Alonsi & Hoskin, 2006).

The technique of lung pCT involves the intravenous injection of a non-iodinated contrast agent and the sequential scanning of the diagnosed region of the chest. There are a number of pulmonary perfusion parameters, calculated pixel by pixel on the basis of raw CT data, which are next analysed in order to reveal differences between the normal and altered tissue. The most useful perfusion parameters are: blood volume (BV), blood flow (BF), mean transit time (MTT), time to peak (TTP) and permeability surface (PS) (Kuziemski et al, 2011).

The diagnosis of pulmonary function has to be based on indirect results, such as diffusing capacity, spirometry and pCT because direct assessment is difficult.

2. Materials

The tests were performed on a group of 72 diabetics. People with cardiovascular disease and smokers were not included in this group.

First the diabetics were tested for microangiopathy, by comparing diffusing capacity in standing and lying position, and on this basis they were split into two groups: $M^{angiop} = 44$ and $M^{non-angiop} = 28$, with and without microangiopathy respectively.

The spirometric tests were carried out on all the patients ($M = M^{angiop} + M^{non\text{-}angiop}$) to obtain the following spirometric parameters: FEV_1 (forced expiratory volume during the first second of expiration), FVC (the maximum volume of air that can be exhaled or inspired during a forced manoeuvre), PEF (peak expiratory flow), MEF_{50} (maximal instantaneous forced expiratory flow where 50% of the FVC remains to be expired), $MEF_{75/25}$ (maximal

mid-expiratory flow), IC (inspiratory capacity) and $FEV_1\%FVC$ (percentage relation of FEV_1 to FVC).
The pCT test was performed on a group of 18 subjects: 10 diabetics and 8 non-diabetic volunteers. The local perfusion parameters BF (blood flow), BV (blood volume), MTT (mean transit time) and PS (permeability surface) were obtained in selected regions of interest (ROI) in the artery and parenchyma.
The patients classified as suffering from microangiopathy had breathing impairment symptoms cause only by diabetes. They were all non-smokers and had not been diagnosed with any other acute or chronic respiratory disease.

3. Diffusing capacity

The quality of gas exchange in the lungs depends on the diffusing capacity $D_L[mol \cdot s^{-1} \cdot kPa]$. During the measurement of D_L (American Thoracic Society, 1995) a person takes a full inhalation of air mixed with small amounts of carbon monoxide and helium. The mixture is held in the lungs for a few seconds and then exhaled. The first part of the expired gas is discarded. The next portion, which includes gas from the alveoli, is collected. The D_L is determined by analyzing and comparing the concentrations of carbon monoxide and helium in the samples of the inhaled gas and the exhaled gas. The alveolar volume V_A is also determined in this test by using the single-breath helium dilution technique.

3.1 The oxygen pathway model

Fig. 1 shows oxygen diffusion. Oxygen transportation from the alveoli to erythrocytes, through the alveoli-capillary barrier, is presented as the flow f_{21} $[g\,s^{-1}]$. The blood saturation $S \in (0,1)$, (also given as $S \in (0,100\%)$) shows what part (percentage) of oxygen capacity (maximum amount of oxygen transported by the erythrocytes) is currently being transported in the blood. Poorly oxygenated blood enters the pulmonary artery and then, enriched in oxygen, flows out of the lung through the pulmonary vein. Lung arterial blood saturation S_A differs from lung venous blood saturation S_V, $S_A < S_V$.
Flows $f_{20}[g \cdot s^{-1}]$ and $f_{02}[g \cdot s^{-1}]$ represent the amount of oxygen in the blood flowing into the lung and flowing out of the lung. The oxygen diffusion model is:

$$\begin{cases} \dot{m}_1(t) = -f_{21}(t) + u(t), & m_1(0) \\ \dot{m}_2(t) = f_{21}(t) + f_{20}(t) - f_{02}(t), & m_2(0) \end{cases} \tag{1}$$

where the $m_1(t)[g]$ and $m_2(t)[g]$ are the O_2 masses in the alveoli and in the blood vessels respectively. The initial states $m_1(0)[g]$ and $m_2(0)[g]$ depend on oxygen partial pressure $P_1(0) = 13.32$ [kPa], $P_2(0) = 12.63$ $[kPa]$ and region volume $V_1 = V_A$, $V_2 = 10^{-4}[m^3]$, (Dalquen, 1999) ,West, 2008) and (Taylor et al, 1989). The alveolar volume $V_1 = V_A$ is measured during the diffusing capacity test. The relationship between the O_2 mass and the pressure is: $P_i(t) = RTm_i(t)/M_{O_2}V_i$, $i = 1,2$, where R $[N\,m\,K^{-1}\,mol^{-1}]$ is gas constant, T is absolute temperature and $M_{O_2}[g\ mol^{-1}]$ is the molecular mass. The mass diffusion, i.e. flow $f_{21}(t)$ via the membrane is caused by the concentration gradient $\Delta c = c_1 - c_2 > 0$, where $c_i(t) = m_i(t)/V_i$, $i = 1,2$:

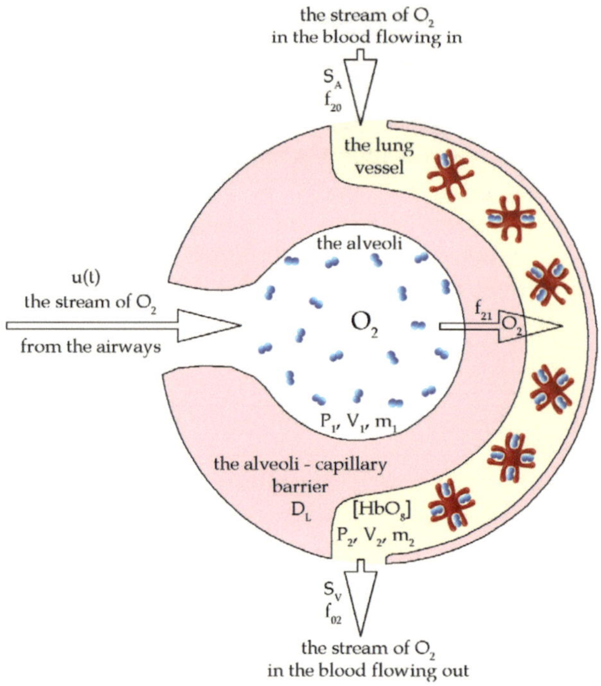

Fig. 1. The passage of oxygen from the airways to the lung vessels. The diffusing capacity D_L describes the condition of the alveoli-capillary barrier. The oxygen is bound in reversible bonds $[HbO_8]$ with the haemoglobin in the lung vessels

$$f_{21}(t) = D_L \cdot R \cdot T \cdot \left(\frac{m_1(t)}{V_1} - \frac{m_2(t)}{V_2} \right) \tag{2}$$

The signal $u(t)$ represents respiratory flow with the period T_p, the delay time t_0 [s] (the time the air passes through the airway to the alveoli) and the duty cycle d. The input amplitude $[g\ s^{-1}]$ depends on the organism's metabolic rate (MR), i.e. the organism's need for oxygen.

In medical practice, blood saturation S gives the basic information concerning the quantity of oxygen transported from the lungs to all the other organs. The kinetics of oxygen association with haemoglobin is described in Hill's equation (Khee-Shing, 2007):

$$S_V(t) = \frac{K \cdot (P_2(t))^n}{1 + K \cdot (P_2(t))^n} \tag{3}$$

where $P_2(t)$ is oxygen partial pressure in the blood, $n = 2.8$ is the Hill's constant and $K = 1.2256 \cdot 10^{-10}\ [1/(Pa)^n]$ is the association constant. The relationship between the endogenous inflow f_{20}, the outflow f_{02} and the organism's need for oxygen MR is as follows:

$$f_{20}(t) = f_{02}(t) - MR \tag{4}$$

while the outflow f_{02} depends on the blood velocity $\varphi[m^3s^{-1}]$, maximum erythrocyte oxygen capacity $\Phi[mol \cdot m^3]$ and venous blood saturation $S_V(t)$

$$f_{02}(t) = S_V(t) \cdot \varphi \cdot \Phi \cdot M_{O_2} \tag{5}$$

The elimination flow f_{02}, according to Hill's equation, is:

$$f_{02}(t) = \frac{c_{Hill}}{1+c_{Hill}} \cdot \varphi \cdot \Phi \cdot M_{O_2}, \quad c_{Hill} = K \cdot m_2^n(t) \cdot \left(\frac{R \cdot T}{M_{O_2} \cdot V_2} \right)^n \tag{6}$$

Taking into account (4), (5) and (6), the oxygen diffusion model is:

$$\begin{cases} \dot{m}_1(t) = -p_1 \cdot m_1(t) + p_2 \cdot m_2(t) + u_1(t), & m_1(0) \\ \dot{m}_2(t) = p_1 \cdot m_1(t) - p_2 \cdot m_2(t) - MR, & m_2(0) \end{cases} \tag{7}$$

where $u_1(t) = \frac{MR}{d} \cdot \sum_{i=0}^{\infty} \left[\mathbf{1}(i \cdot T_p - t_0) - \mathbf{1}((i \cdot T_p - t_0) - T_p \cdot d) \right]$.

The model parameters $p_1 = D_L \cdot R \cdot T / V_1$ and $p_2 = D_L \cdot R \cdot T / V_2$ can be estimated with the use of measurements D_L, V_1 and physiological constants R, T, V_2.
The example measurements (lying body position), $V_A^{non-angiop} = 5.42 \cdot 10^{-3}[m^3]$, $D_L^{non-angiop} = 1.54 \cdot 10^{-7}[mol \cdot s^{-1}Pa]$, $V_A^{angiop} = 5.71 \cdot 10^{-3}[m^3]$ and $D_L^{angiop} = 1.59 \cdot 10^{-7}[mol \cdot s^{-1}Pa]$ together with the constants: $V_2 = 0.10 \cdot 10^{-3}$ $[m^3]$ (blood volume in lung capillary vessels), $T = 293$ $[K]$ (absolute temperature) and $R = 8.314$ $[N \cdot m \cdot mol^{-1}K^{-1}]$ (gas constant), allow calculation of the example model parameter estimates:

$$\mathbf{p}^{angiop} = [p_1^{angiop}, p_2^{angiop}] = [5.6315 \cdot 10^{-2}, \ 3.3271]$$
$$\mathbf{p}^{non-angiop} = [p_1^{non-angiop}, p_2^{non-angiop}] = [6.2128 \cdot 10^{-2}, \ 3.9621]$$

The model parameter estimates have been calculated for all the $M = 72$ patients.

3.2 Statistical comparison of measurement and modelling results for microangiopathic and non- microangiopathic patients

Measurements were made for two groups of diabetic patients: ones with diagnosed microangiopathy and others with no microangiopathy. Lung microangiopathy was identified when $D_L^{\text{standing}} > D_L^{\text{lying}}$. This examination also gives the alveoli volume $V_A = V_1$. The null hypothesis H_0 assumes that the mean values in both groups of patients are the same. Calculated *ex post* significance level p is compared with *ex ante* significance level α (test-T). If a test of statistical significance gives *ex post* significance level p, which is lower than the α, the null hypothesis is rejected, alternatively we no grounds to reject this hypothesis. Table 1 and Table 2 show a statistical comparison of spirometry measurements and model parameters obtained from microangiopathic and non-microangiopathic patients. The results presented in Table 1 (H_0: $\bar{D}_L^{\text{lying}\,angiop} = \bar{D}_L^{\text{lying}\,non-angiop}$ is rejected and the conclusion is: $\bar{D}_L^{\text{lying}\,angiop} \neq \bar{D}_L^{\text{lying}\,non-angiop}$) suggest the possibility of diagnosing microangiopathy on the basis of D_L^{lying} only, instead of D_L^{lying} and $D_L^{standing}$. The lack of statistical significance for $D_L^{standing}$ means that it is not useful as an individual value for microangiopathy diagnosis.

	Microangiopathic		Non-microangiopathic		Statistical significance level p
	Mean value	Standard deviation	Mean value	Standard deviation	
$D_L^{standing}$	1.64 10^{-7}	0.14 10^{-7}	1.48 10^{-7}	0.11 10^{-7}	$p \geq 0.05$
$V_A^{standing}$	5.95 10^{-3}	0.21 10^{-3}	5.65 10^{-3}	0.21 10^{-3}	$p \geq 0.05$
D_L^{lying}	1.35 10^{-7}	0.06 10^{-7}	1.63 10^{-7}	0.14 10^{-7}	$p < 0.05$
V_A^{lying}	6.04 10^{-3}	0.27 10^{-3}	5.90 10^{-3}	0.40 10^{-3}	$p \geq 0.05$

Table 1. Statistical comparison of D_L and V_A. For D_L^{lying} *ex post* significance level is $p < \alpha$, $\alpha = 0.05$. The null hypothesis H_0: $\overline{D}_L^{lying\,angiop} = \overline{D}_L^{lying\,non-angiop}$ concerning equality of mean diffusing capacity values in both groups was rejected. D_L^{lying} allows us to distinguish between patients with and without microangiopathy, while the rest do not.

	Microangiopathic		Non-microangiopathic		Statistical significance level p
	Mean value	Standard deviation	Mean value	Standard deviation	
Measurements taken in standing body position					
p_1	$6.6176 \cdot 10^{-2}$	$0.4720 \cdot 10^{-2}$	$6.1900 \cdot 10^{-2}$	$0.2792 \cdot 10^{-2}$	$p \geq 0.05$
p_2	3.9330	0.3447	3.5301	0.2730	$p \geq 0.05$
Measurements taken in lying body position					
p_1	5.4339 10^{-2}	0.2233 10^{-2}	6.5672 10^{-2}	0.3139 10^{-2}	$p < 0.01$
p_2	3.2427	0.1551	4.0981	0.3518	$p < 0.01$

Table 2. Statistical comparison of p_1 and p_2. In the lying body position the ex post significance level is $p < \alpha$, $\alpha = 0.01$ and the H_0, concerning the equality of mean parameter values, is rejected. These parameters allow for a distinction to be made between patients with and without microangiopathy.

Next, the null hypothesis $H_0 = \overline{p}_i^{angiop} = \overline{p}_i^{non-angiop}$, $i = 1,2$ was tested (Table 2). The Kolmogorov-Smirnov test accepted the normality hypothesis concerning p_1 and p_2 at the significance level of $p < 0.01$. Therefore the mean values and standard deviations were calculated and the null hypothesis $H_0 = \overline{p}_i^{angiop} = \overline{p}_i^{non-angiop}$ was tested.

For p_1 and p_2, in lying body position, the *ex post* significance level $p < \alpha$, $\alpha = 0.01$ and so the H_0 was rejected. These parameters enable a distinction to be made between patients with and without microangiopathy.

In a standing body position ($p \geq 0.05$) the parameters p_1 and p_2 are not useful for microangiopathy diagnosis.

The results in Table 1 and Table 2 indicate the possibility of using a diagnostic test based on a single measurement D_L^{lying}, and also on the basis of modelling results p_1 .and p_2.

3.3 Binary classification on the basis of diffusing capacity measurement and modelling

Statistical analyses show that a single measurement D_L^{lying} and the model parameters p_1, p_2 contain information concerning lung microangiopathy. The question remains as to whether or not such values can be used for binary classification. Binary classification is the classifying of the members of mixed group $M = M^{angiop} + M^{non\text{-}angiop}$ into two subgroups, M^{angiop} and $M^{non-angiop}$, on the basis of whether or not they have microangiopathy. For this purpose an appropriate classification algorithm has to be chosen.

To select the best potential classification algorithm, statistical measures, sensitivity and specificity (Panzer, Blach & Griner, 1991) were considered. Sensitivity $Sens$ is the ability of a test to detect a disease when it is really present. Specificity $Spec$ is the ability to confirm the absence of a disease in patients when it is really absent.

$$Sens = \frac{True\ Positive}{True\ Positive + False\ Negative} \tag{8}$$

$$Spec = \frac{True\ Negative}{True\ Negative + False\ Positive} \tag{9}$$

The theoretically optimal prediction is: $Sens = 100\%$ (all the sick patients were identified as sick) and $Spec = 100\%$ (none of the healthy patients was identified as sick).

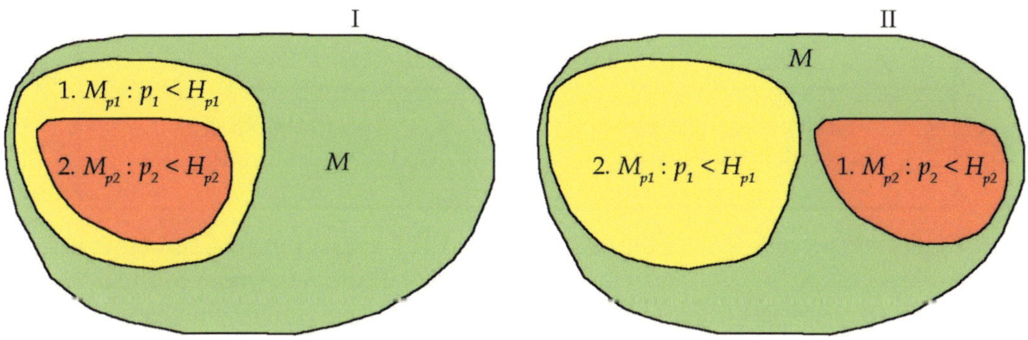

Fig. 2. Classification algorithms based on p_1 and p_2; I) M_{p_2} are classified as microangiopathic and $M - M_{p_2}$ are classified as non-microangiopathic, II) $M_{p_1} + M_{p_2}$ are classified as microangiopathic and $M - (M_{p_1} + M_{p_2})$ are classified as non-microangiopathic

For binary classification the discrimination levels (boundaries, diagnostic thresholds) H_{D_L}, H_{p_1} and H_{p_2} have to be calculated, respectively for D_L, p_1 and p_2. The discrimination levels classify the test result as positive or as negative. The parameter value where $Sens + Spec = \max$ was chosen as the parameter's diagnostic threshold.

Among different classification algorithms using p_1, p_2, H_{p_1} and H_{p_2} the best are the two shown in Fig. 2.

Classification algorithm	Wide range of anthropometric features, $M = 72$ (men and women, 21-69 y, 1.50-1.95m)		Narrowed range of anthropometric features $M_1 = 22$ (women, over 50 y, under 1.65 m)	
	$Sens[\%]$	$Spec[\%]$	$Sens[\%]$	$Spec[\%]$
I. p_1, p_2	50	84	62	87
II. p_2, p_1	76	50	79	80
D_L^{lying}	33	61	62	71

Table 3. Classification results obtained for entire group of $M = 72$ subjects and for the group of $M_1 = 22$ women, over 50 y, under 1.65 m. The best results are underlined.

Therefore the diagnostic procedure shown in Fig. 3 is recommend.

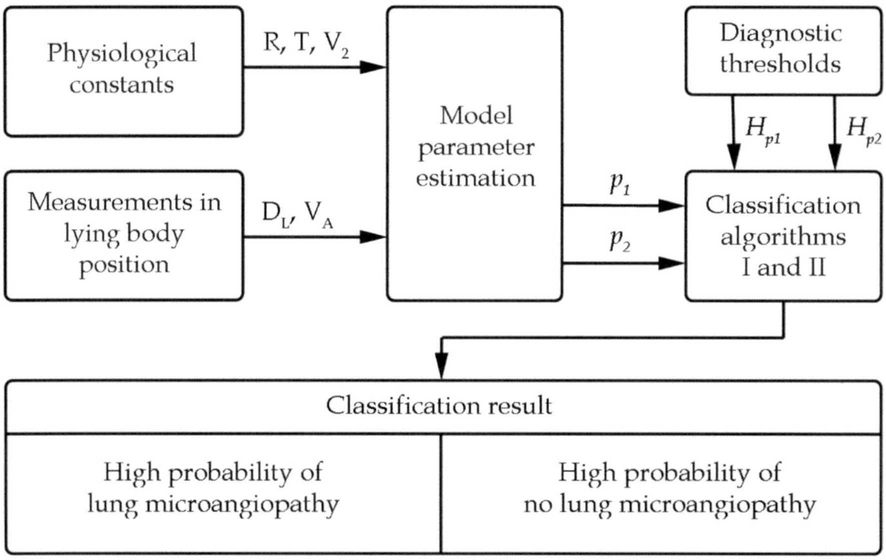

Fig. 3. Diagnostic procedure with the use of D_L^{lying}, V_A^{lying} measurements, constants R, T, V_2 and calculated p_1, p_2, H_{p_1} and H_{p_2}. For binary classification the more conclusive algorithms I) (with respect to $Spec$) and II) (with respect to $Sens$) are recommended.

The binary classification was performed for the $M = 72$ subjects. The results were compared with already known medical diagnoses of 44 microangiopathic patients and 18 patients with no microangiopathy. Then the sensitivity and the specificity were calculated according to equations (8) and (9), (Table 3). The larger the $Sens$ and $Spec$, the better. It seems reasonable to assume that results larger than 75% are satisfactory. Therefore an algorithm should be selected to fulfil this requirement, and not every entry in Table 3 does.

Diagnostic thresholds, calculated on the basis of $M = 72$ measurement data, are: $H_{p_1} = 5.80 \cdot 10^{-2}$, $H_{p_2} = 3.50$ and $H_{D_L} = 1.57 \cdot 10^{-7}$. The best statistical measures obtained are: $Sens = 76\%$ (algorithm II) and $Spec = 84\%$ (algorithm I). The results for D_L^{lying}, $Sens = 33\%$ and $Spec = 61\%$, are less than 75% and quite inadequate.

The thresholds established as common for the entire group did no take into account such important factors as age, height and gender. Therefore a subgroup $M_1 = 22$ was selected (women, over 50 years old and less than 1.65 m tall). Then the new diagnostic thresholds $H_{p_1} = 5.42 \cdot 10^{-2}$, $H_{p_2} = 3.06$, $H_{D_L} = 1.30 \cdot 10^{-7}$ and new *Sens* and *Spec* were calculated. As expected, both the new *Sens* and *Spec* were noticeably larger.
The diagnostic procedure in Fig. 3 uses D_L^{lying} and V_A^{lying} measurements, and R, T and V_2 physiological constants to calculate the p_1 and p_2 in a patient. Then algorithm I (with the most conclusive *Sens*) and algorithm II (with the most conclusive *Spec*) are applied together with H_{p_1} and H_{p_2} diagnostic thresholds to obtain a binary classification result.
This procedure produces one of two possible results: 1) high probability of lung microangiopathy or 2) high probability of no lung microangiopathy. This can serve as useful confirmation in a doctor's diagnosis.
The final decision is made by the doctor conducting the diagnosis, who can take into account this classification result along with other diagnostic data.

4. Spirometry

The most popular spirometry method is a dynamic one. The pneumotachometer (Miller, Harkinson&Brusasco, 2005) defines the volume $V(t)$ $[l]$ and airflow $Q(t)[ls^{-1}]$ during the inhalation and exhalation. The flow-volume curve $Q(V)$ is received on the basis of the spirometry measurements of $V(t)$ and $Q(t)$. Specific ventilation manoeuvres are required in the spirometric test. The measurement is preceded by a period of quiet breathing-in and out (Fry, Hyatt, 1960). Next the maximal breath-in and the maximal forced breath-out manoeuvres are performed as the important parts of the spirometric test.
The respiration parameters are defined on the basis of the volume–time curve $V(t)$ and the flow–volume curves $Q(V)$ (see Fig. 4 and Fig. 5), (Miller, Harkinson&Brusasco, 2005).
In medical practice two terms, volume and capacity, are used. The difference between them is based on the assumption that volume refers to lung volumes, while capacity refers to different combinations of lung volumes, usually in relation to inhalation and exhalation.
The relations between volumes and capacities are presented in equations (10).

$$\begin{aligned} TLC &= VC + RV \\ TLC &= IC + FRC \end{aligned} \tag{10}$$

The following respiratory parameters have been defined: TLC $[l]$ (Total Lung Capacity) is the volume of air in the lungs at the end of maximal inhalation; VC $[l]$ (Vital Capacity) is the maximum volume of air that can be exhaled or inhaled during either a forced (FVC) or a slow (VC) manoeuvre; RV $[l]$ (Residual Volume) is the volume of air remaining in the lungs after the maximal exhalation; IC $[l]$ (Inspiratory Capacity) is the maximal volume of air that can be inhaled from the resting expiratory level; FRC $[l]$ (Functional Residual Capacity) is the volume of air in the lungs at the resting end-expiration.
Also defined are the following respiratory parameters: FEV_1 $[l]$ the forced expiratory volume during the first second of expiration; FET $[s]$ the forced expiratory time; FIT $[s]$ the forced inspiratory time; PEF $[l\ s^{-1}]$ (Peak Expiratory Flow) and PIF $[l\ s^{-1}]$ (Peak Inspiratory Flow) are respectively the maximal expiratory and the maximal inspiratory flow

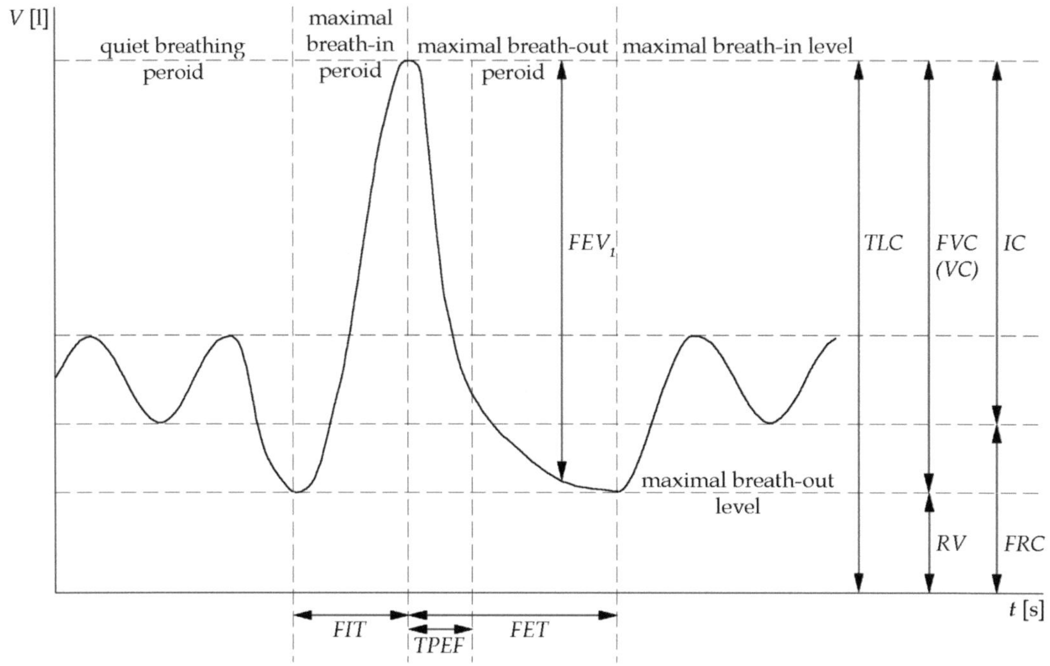

Fig. 4. The spirometry parameters defined on the basis of volume-time curve $V(t)$.

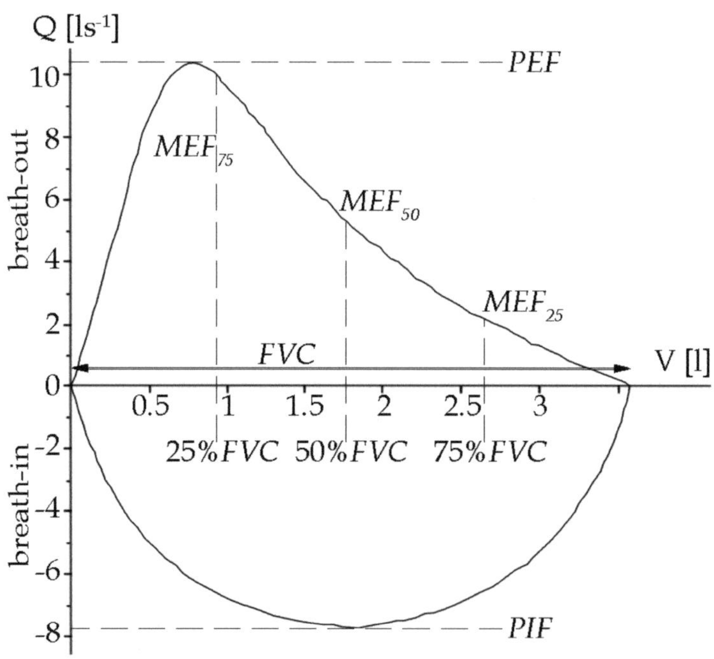

Fig. 5. The spirometric parameters defined on the basis of flow–volume curve $Q(V)$.

rates achieved; $TPEF$ $[s]$ the time of maximal expiratory flow; MEF_{75},MEF_{50},MEF_{25} $[l\,s^{-1}]$ maximal instantaneous forced expiratory flow where 75, 50, 25% of the FVC remains to be expired; $MEF_{75/25}$ $[l\,s^{-1}]$ is the maximal mid-expiratory flow and $FEV_1\%FVC$ is the percentage relation of FEV_1 to FVC.

The European Respiratory Society (Miller, Harkinson & Brusasco, 2005) has published the spirometric norms and the reference values for these spirometric parameters. The reference values of the respiration parameters, obtained for a representative healthy population, are used for the interpreting the spirometry data and making the diagnosis. The reference values depend on the patient's anthropometric data, such as age, height and gender. In some medical cases (asthma, pulmonary fibrosis, cystic fibrosis and COPD) the spirometric parameter boundary values have already been defined. However, as far as lung microangiopathy is concerned, this has not yet been done.

According to medical practice experience, lung microangiopathy is diagnosed on the basis of the following spirometric parameters: FEV_1, FVC, PEF, MEF_{50}, $MEF_{75/25}$, IC and $FEV_1\%FVC$. These spirometric parameters were collected from the $M = 72$ diabetic patients. However, a single spirometric test is not sufficient to diagnose the lung flow and volume reduction caused by microangiopathy; long term observation is necessary. Therefore one should consider an alternative method. By using the spirometric results in a statistical significance test, we can find the spirometric parameters that are most responsive to lung microangiopathy.

4.1 Spirometric parameters. Statistical comparison of results for microangiopathic and non- microangiopathic patients

Traditional spirometric parameters were tested for their ability to detect lung microangiopathy. The mean, standard deviation and the statistical significance level p for spirometric parameters are presented in Table 4.

	Microangiopathic		Non-microangiopathic		Statistical significance level p
	Mean spirometry parameter	Standard deviation	Mean spirometry parameter	Standard deviation	
FEV_1	2.970	0.699	2.919	0.832	$p \geq 0.05$
FVC	4.245	0.911	4.015	1.245	$p \geq 0.05$
PEF	9.175	1.545	11.621	1.914	$p \geq 0.05$
MEF_{50}	5.258	1.384	3.691	1.637	$p \geq 0.05$
$MEF_{25/75}$	2.896	1.051	2.853	1.206	$p \geq 0.05$
IC	3.182	0.706	3.275	1.097	$p \geq 0.05$
$FEV_1\%FVC$	70.731	7.482	73.621	8.880	$p \geq 0.05$

Table 4. Statistical comparison of spirometric parameters for microangiopathic and non-microangiopathic patients. In every case the *ex post* significance level $p > \alpha$, $\alpha = 0.05$, which means that H_0 concerning mean parameter value equality is not rejected. The parameters do not allow for a distinction to be made between patients with and without microangiopathy.

The parameters do not show statistical significance in detecting microangiopathy: *ex post* significance level p is larger than *ex ante* significance level $\alpha = 0.05$, which confirms the null hypothesis concerning equality of mean values for both groups. Therefore, none of spirometric parameters are useful in diagnosing microangiopathy.

4.2 Spirometry modelling

The maximal breathing-in flow was modelled by means of the sine function. The forced breathing-out flow was finally mimicked using the gamma variate function (Askey R.A.& Roy R,2007) - after testing a large group of prospective regression functions, such as exponentials, polynomials, etc (Kalicka et al, 2007).
The maximal inflow $Q_{in}(V)$ is modelled as follows:

$$Q_{in}(V) = A_{in} \cdot \sin(\varpi \cdot V),\ 0 \le V \le FVC \tag{11}$$

where A_{in} $[l\ s^{-1}]$ and ϖ $[l^{-1}]$ are model parameters and FVC is the forced vital capacity.
For modelling $Q_{out}(V)$ during the maximal outflow, the following gamma variate function is implemented:

$$Q_{out}(V) = K(V)^b e^{-V \cdot a},\ FVC \ge V \ge 0 \tag{12}$$

where $K[l\ s^{-1}]$, b and a $[l^{-1}]$ are model parameters.
The model consists of the equations (11) and (12). The model parameters are arranged into vector $\mathbf{p} = [p_i] = [A_{in}, \varpi, K, b, a]$, $i = 1 \div 5$. The parameter estimates were obtained using the least square procedure, according to the following:

$$\mathbf{p} = \arg\left[\min_{\mathbf{p}} \sum_{V=0}^{V_{\max}} \left(Q^{\text{model}}(V, \mathbf{p}) - Q^{\text{meas}}\left(V, \mathbf{y}^{\text{meas}}\right)\right)^2\right] \tag{13}$$

where $\mathbf{y}^{\text{meas}} = [y_j^{\text{meas}}] = [FEV_1, FVC, PEF, MEF_{50}, MEF_{25/50}, IC, FEV\%FVC]; j = 1 \div 7$ is vector of measurements and $V_{\max} = FVC$. The fitting procedure was executed separately to obtain A_{in}, ϖ and K, b, a based on the equations (11) and (12) respectively.
The parameter vector $\mathbf{p} = [A_{in}, \varpi, K, b, a] = [3.780, 1.030, 20.580, 0.772, 1.507]$ is an example of the model identification results. This was obtained from a 59-year-old woman suffering from lung microangiopathy. The spirometric parameters obtained from the patient were: $FEV_1 = 2.25$, $FVC = 2.84$, $PEF = 5.79 l/s$, $MEF_{50} = 3.47 l/s$, $MEF_{75/25} = 2.63 l/s$, $IC = 2.81$ and $FEV_1\%FVC = 78.95\%$.
Calculations of $\mathbf{p} = [A_{in}, \varpi, K, b, a]$ were performed for $M = 72$ diabetic patients. Fig. 6 shows an example of the model regression functions $Q_{in}(V)$ and $Q_{out}(V)$ drawn for the $\mathbf{p} = [A_{in}, \varpi, K, b, a] = [3.780, 1.030, 20.580, 0.772, 1.507]$. In Fig. 6 the $Q(V)$ spirometric test results have been added, for comparison.

4.3 Statistical comparison of modelling results for microangiopathic and non-microangiopathic patients

The mean parameter value and standard deviation were calculated separately for microangiopathic and non-microangiopathic patients (Table 5). The aim was to find out

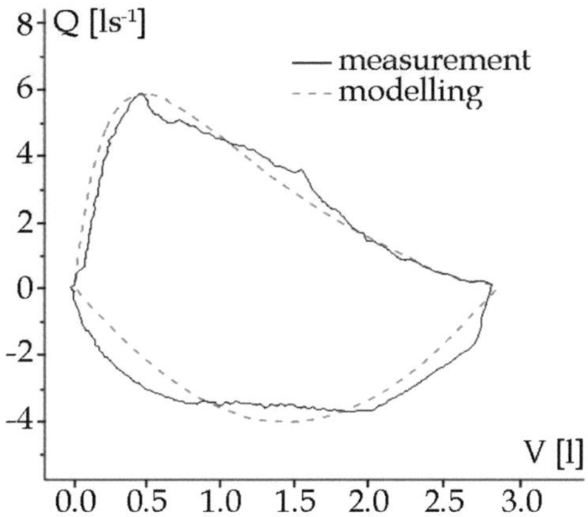

Fig. 6. An example result of the spirometric measurement and modelling of the flow–volume curve $Q(V)$.

	Microangiopathic		Non-microangiopathic		Statistical significance level p
	Mean model parameter	Standard deviation	Mean model parameter	Standard deviation	
A_{in}	5.92	1.72	5.88	2.20	$p \geq 0.05$
ϖ	0.78	0.17	0.82	0.22	$p \geq 0.05$
K	34.79	6.84	53.78	7.56	$p < 0.05$
b	1.193	0.83	1.58	1.06	$p \geq 0.05$
a	1.501	0.59	1.85	0.78	$p < 0.05$

Table 5. Statistical comparison of model parameters for microangiopathic and non-microangiopathic patients. For A_{in}, ϖ and b, the *ex post* significance level was $p > \alpha$, $\alpha = 0.05$, and thus the H_0, concerning mean parameter values equality, was not rejected – i.e. the parameters are not useful for diagnosis. However, parameters K and a are useful in distinguishing between patients with and without microangiopathy because the *ex post* significance level is $p < \alpha$, $\alpha = 0.05$.

whether or not the model parameters are helpful in distinguishing between microangiopathic and non-microangiopathic patients. For this purpose the null hypothesis $H_0 = \overline{p}_i^{angiop} = \overline{p}_i^{non-angiop}$, $i = 1,..,5$ was tested.

At first the normality hypothesis concerning the parameter estimates p_i was investigated, and the hypothesis was accepted (Kolmogorov-Smirnov test) at the significance level of $p < 0.05$. Then the mean values and standard deviations (Table 5) were calculated and statistical test-T was performed. For K and a the *ex post* significance level $p < \alpha$, $\alpha = 0.05$ and H_0 is rejected. The two model parameters K and a allow for a distinction to be made between patients with and without microangiopathy.

The remaining model parameters A_{in}, ϖ and a do not reveal the occurrence or absence of lung microangiopathy.

4.3 Binary classification on the basis of spirometric measurements and modelling

Binary classification algorithms, based on the model parameters K and a, were tested with discrimination levels H_K and H_a. The discrimination levels were first established for all $M=72$ subjects as $H_K=50.18$ and $H_a=1.72$. These discrimination levels correspond to the K and a values for which $Sens+Spec=\max$. The $M=72$ subjects were now divided into two groups on the basis of these discrimination thresholds.

Two algorithms, I and II (which gave the best results), were applied for binary classification. The algorithms are presented in Fig. 7. The binary classification decision was compared with previously known medical diagnoses, and then the $Sens$ and $Spec$ were calculated according to equations (8) and (9), (see Table 6).

None of the tested algorithms could produce simultaneously a large $Sens$ and a large $Spec$. Algorithm II gave the best $Sens=82\%$ and algorithm I gave the best $Spec=62\%$. Algorithm II accurately detected the majority of the microangiopathy cases ($Sens=82\%$), and only missed out on a few. Yet $Spec=50\%$ means algorithm II identified only 50% of the non-microangiopathic patients as non-microangiopathic and gave too many false alarms. This is an unacceptable result. Somewhat better $Spec=62\%$ was obtained with algorithm I but this was still not satisfactory. The most likely explanation for these poor results is the fact that the thresholds H_K and H_a are too general and do not take into consideration important anthropometric features.

Therefore the range of anthropometric features was made more specific ($M_1=22$ women, over 50 years old and under 1.65 m tall) and new diagnostic thresholds were calculated: $H_K=48.11$ and $H_a=1.68$. The new classification results are presented in Table 6.

This more accurate choice of the diagnostic thresholds gave much better results. The $Sens=100\%$ means that algorithm II identified all the sick patients as sick. This excellent result has been obtained for the sample $M_1=22$ selected from the general population and therefore should be treated with care. An another sample may give a somewhat different result but the great improvement is obvious.

The diagnostic procedure, utilising the algorithms I and II, is shown in Fig. 8.

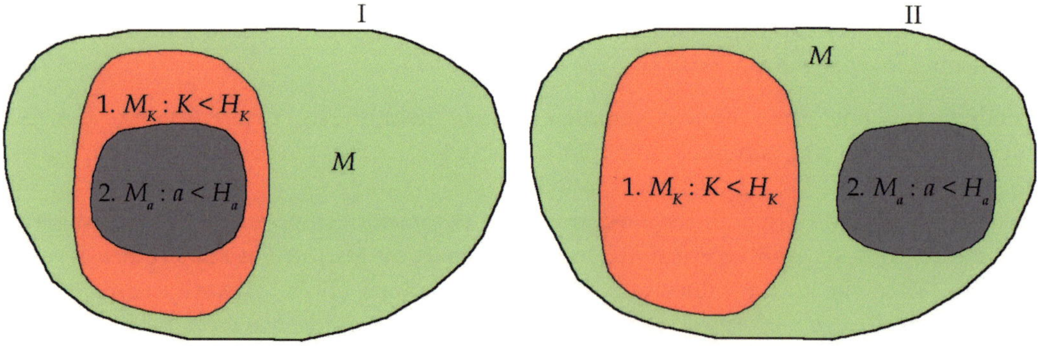

Fig. 7. Classification algorithms based on a and K; I) M_K are classified as microangiopathic and $M-M_K$ are classified as non-microangiopathic, II) M_a+M_K are classified as microangiopathic and $M-(M_a+M_K)$ are classified as non-microangiopathic

Classification algorithm	Full range of anthropometric features, $M = 72$ (men and women, 21-69 y, 1.50-1.95m)		Limited range of anthropometric features $M_1 = 22$ (women, over 50 y, under 1.65 m)	
	Sens[%]	*Spec*[%]	*Sens*[%]	*Spec*[%]
I. a, K	64	62	87	83
II. K, a	82	50	100	80

Table 6. Classification results obtained for entire group of $M = 72$ subjects and for the subgroup $M_1 = 22$ of women over 50 years old and under 1.65 m. The best results are underlined.

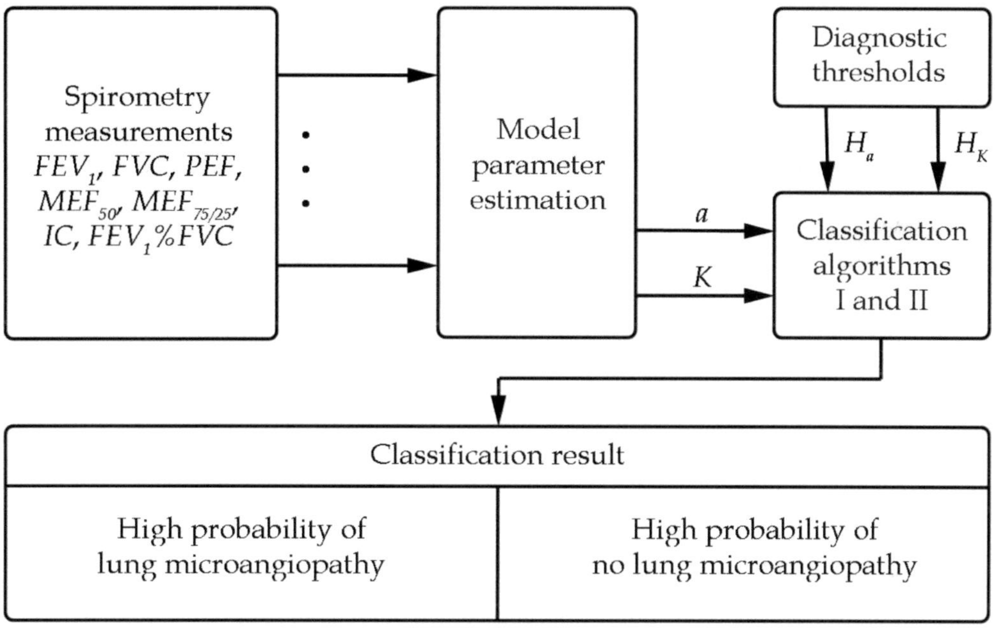

Fig. 8. Classification algorithms: I) M_K are classified as microangiopathic and $M - M_K$ as non-microangiopathic, II) $M_a + M_K$ are classified as microangiopathic and $M - (M_a + M_K)$ as non-microangiopathic

Applied with H_a and H_K, algorithm I gives the best (most conclusive) *Sens* classification result, while the algorithm II gives the best (most conclusive) *Spec* result.
This procedure gives one of two alternative results: 1) high probability of lung microangiopathy or 2) high probability of no lung microangiopathy. The final decision is made by the doctor.

5. Perfusion computed tomography (pCT)

Tests commonly used in clinical practice such as spirometry and lung diffusion capacity measurements are not considered precise enough to identify lung microangiopathy. There are very few publications in this field and most of them concern the decrease of diffusion

capacity in diabetics (Villa et al, 2004), (Goldman, 2003). Autopsies of patients who died of diabetes complications revealed a thickening in the basement membrane of alveolar capillaries and arterioles in the lungs as well as of the entire walls of pulmonary arterioles together with fibroblast proliferation (Weynand et al, 1999).
Impaired gas exchange in pulmonary alveoli results in the progressive reduction of reserves in small pulmonary vessels. For this reason lung perfusion in regions of lung microangiopathy may be diminished. Computed tomography of chest perfusion allows imaging of pulmonary vessels and parenchyma and may be useful in diagnosing pulmonary microangiopathy (Kuziemski et al, 2011).

5.1 Patients and study protocol

A group of 10 never-smoking diabetic adults and a control group of 8 non-diabetic volunteers were chosen. All participants had a similar body mass index and none of them suffered any disease that affected pulmonary function. The mean time from when diabetes mellitus was first diagnosed was 15.5 years. Nephropathy was diagnosed in 3 diabetics, retinopathy in 6 and polyneuropathy in 4. The question was whether or not they also suffered from lung microangiopathy. In the control group lung and cardio-vascular diseases were not diagnosed.
For all patients, spirometry and diffusing capacity tests were performed.
For the pCT tests a 64-row CT scanner GE - Light Speed VCT (GE Healthcare USA) was used. Pulmonary perfusion was evaluated after the intravenous administration of 40 ml of contrast at the rate of 4 ml/s. CT images were taken with 1 s resolution in the period of 40 s of a selected lung section (4 cm thick layer situated 2 cm below carina). Within this 4 cm thick segment, three cross-sections, anterior, medium and posterior, 5 mm thick each, were selected at uniform distances from each other. 6 ROIs were chosen in each of the cross-sections (18 ROIs in all, numbered ROI 3-ROI 20). The ROIs 3–20 were situated in the upper, medial and lower parts of the left and right lungs. The most vascularised areas of the lungs were left beyond the ROIs so as not to distort the evaluation of lung parenchyma.
The pCT measurements were performed using standard CT Perfusion 4 (GE Healthcare USA). The following perfusion parameters were calculated:

- $BV[ml/100g]$ - blood volume in 100g of lung tissue.
- $BF[ml/100g/\min]$ - blood flow through 100g of lung tissue in 1 minute.
- $MTT[\min]$ - mean transit time through the vascular system in selected region.
- $PS[ml/100g/\min]$ - permeability surface, the permeability of blood from intravascular to extravascular space, observed in 100g of lung tissue during 1 min.

5.2 pCT results

The example results of pCT scans, obtained from a 62 year old diabetic male, are shown in Fig. 9 a), b), c) and d). Perfusion parameters BF, BV, MTT and PS were calculated and mapped out on the lung cross-section. Analysis was made of the pulmonary artery - ROI 1, which represents the arterial input function, i.e. the flow blood into the pulmonary system.
In Fig. 9 the ROI 1 is marked with a circle. The calculated values of perfusion parameters (mean value for all pixels in the region and standard deviation of the mean) are displayed in the right lower corner of the scan.
Table 7 shows mean perfusion parameters *Avg* and standard deviation *Dev* in the ROI 1.

As the table shows, the obtained permeability surface *PS* for the impermeable pulmonary artery is equal to zero. The *Dev*, i.e. the disperse of parameter values within the ROI 1, is low, 4-7%.

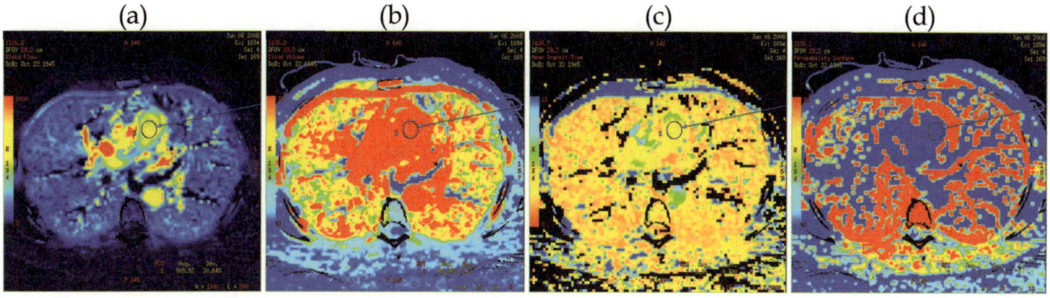

Fig. 9. The pCT scans (a) blood flow BF , (b) blood volume BV , (c) mean transit time MTT and (d) permeability surface PS for a 62 year old diabetic male.

Blood Flow *BF*		Blood Volume *BV*		Mean Transit Time *MTT*		Permeability Surface *PS*	
Avg	*Dev*	*Avg*	*Dev*	*Avg*	*Dev*	*Avg*	*Dev*
509.9	20.64	48.06	3.48	5.65	0.30	0	0

Table 7. Example results of perfusion parameters calculated as the mean values in the ROI 1 marked in Fig. 9. The calculated standard deviations *Dev* illustrates the distribution of test results within ROI 1.

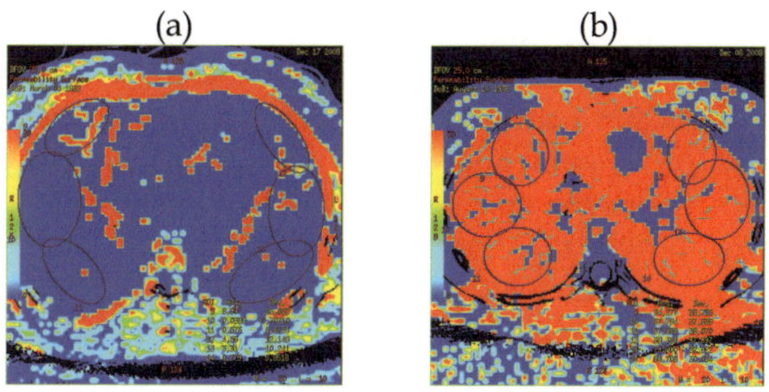

Fig. 10. The *PS* maps for (a) healthy subject and (b) diabetic subject. For example, in ROI 13 (right lower circle) $PS = 3.31$ for the healthy subject and $PS = 79.80$ for the diabetic subject. The measurements were obtained in the same location of the lung cross-section.

Fig. 10 shows PS maps obtained from a healthy patient and a diabetic patient. The qualitative comparison (amount of the red, permeable area) as well as the quantitative comparison (healthy patient $PS = 3.31$ and diabetic patient $PS = 79.80$) indicate damage to capillaries and pulmonary arterioles of the diabetic patient.

All perfusion parameters were calculated in 18 ROIs (3-20) in the parenchyma to discover whether parameter values depend on the location of tested lung cross-section. Statistical analysis revealed no correlation between perfusion parameter value and ROI location in the upper central or lower part of the lungs (Kuziemski et al, 2011). Therefore mean perfusion

parameters were calculated for all 18 ROIs. The results are shown in Table 8 (Kuziemski et al, 2011).
Here a noticeable increase was observed in the parenchyma perfusion parameter values of the diabetics with respect to control group, which may be due to diabetic mellitus.

$BF[ml/100g/\min] \pm Dev$		$BV[ml/100g] \pm Dev$		$PS[ml/100g/\min] \pm Dev$
Artery	Parenchyma	Artery	Parenchyma	Parenchyma
Diabetes 722.5±301.8	Diabetes 282.2±115.0	Diabetes 62.8±25.2	Diabetes 16.2±6.4	Diabetes 35.6±26.1
Control 681.7±133.2	Control 207.6±53.4	Control 61.0±5.9	Control 12.0±1.8	Control 8.6±4.8

Table 8. Mean parameters BF, BV and PS in the artery and parenchyma of the diabetics and of the control group. The calculated standard deviation Dev illustrates the distribution of test results in 18 ROIs (ROI 3 - 20, in upper, central and lower part of lungs) with respect to the mean of the eighteen results. No significant MTT differences were found.

Chest perfusion CT allows imaging of lung vessels and parenchyma, which is essential in diagnosing pulmonary angiopathy. The analyzed results are very new and currently not all that numerous. While this does not allow for a complex statistical analysis, the above preliminary results indicate the great potential of pCT tests in diagnosing lung microangiopathy.

5.3 Lung area extraction

Each pCT image (see Fig. 9) consists of the body cross-section, including the lungs, essential for medical diagnosis, the rest of the body and the background, which is unnecessary for lung diagnostics but was nevertheless included in the perfusion map calculations.
As computations of perfusion parameters involve complicated methods of signal processing, it is desirable that the distinction between diagnostically important regions (the lung cross-section) and other areas (background and the rest of body cross-section) is conducted before the process starts. This shortens the time needed to obtain parametric maps by omitting data processing from the area outside the lungs. It can also help avoiding false lung malfunction diagnoses, which can occur when the automatic methods of pathological changes wrongly interpret signals from areas outside the lungs as abnormal lung signals.
Literature describes many methods of lung area extraction from CT chest scans (Homma et al, 2009), (de Nunzio et al, 2011), (Vinhais & Campilho, 2006), (Zhou et al, 2004). Most methods are devoted to extracting the lung area from a single image. Some of these methods allow for neighbouring (upper and lower) slices to be analysed (Homma et al, 2009).
The lung extraction presented here was obtained using the two-step procedure. The objective of the preliminary processing was to define the rough mask, i.e. the border within which the lung contour is always contained during the pCT test while the lungs are breathing and the heart is beating. The lung and heart region contour pixels are subjected to the greatest changes. This behaviour can be utilised to detect the contours. It can be achieved by using a variability factor VF, which is defined as follows:

$$VF = \frac{x_{\max} - x_{\min}}{x_{median}} \tag{14}$$

where $x_{\max}$, $x_{\min}$ and x_{median} are respectively each pixel's maximum, minimum and median value. VF can be used to create a variability map, M_{VF}. Such a map is shown in Fig. 11.

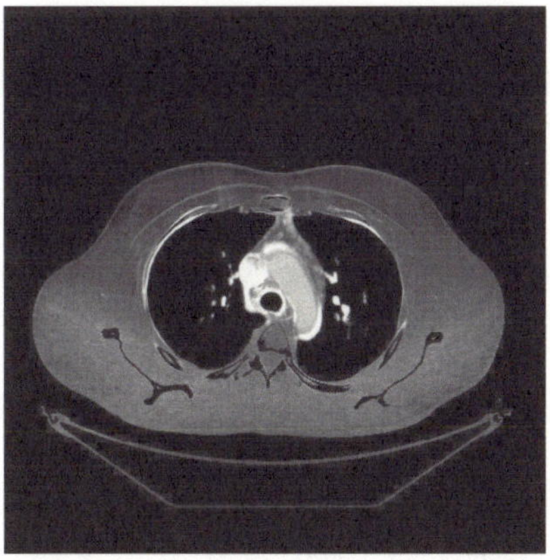

Fig. 11. Map M_{VF} of variability factor VF. The white areas are the most variable due to the breathing lungs and beating heart.

Then the final lung mask was obtained with the use of morphological operators (dilation, erosion, closing and opening) to extract lung cross-sections from the chest pCT.
Fig. 12 shows the BF, BV, MTT and PS maps of just the lungs, extracted using the mask. The lung mask was superimposed onto the calculated maps in Fig. 9.

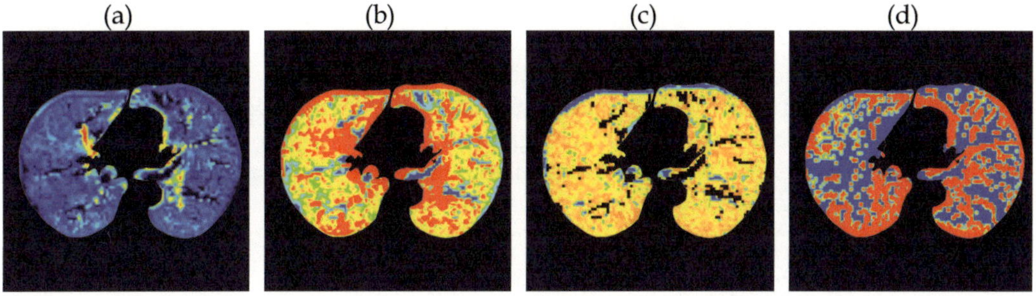

Fig. 12. Lung extraction. The pCT lung maps obtained for the scans in Fig. 9 (a) blood flow BF, (b) blood volume BV, (c) mean transit time MTT and (d) permeability surface PS.

Visual comparison of Fig. 9 and Fig. 12 shows just how much unnecessary computations are usually performed in areas outside the lungs. What is more, a clearly defined lung area allows for a much more accurate and reliable medical diagnosis.

6. Conclusion

Pulmonary diabetic microangiopathy has not yet been sufficiently studied and is difficult to diagnose. In clinical practice, lung microangiopathy is diagnosed by comparing two diffusing capacity measurements, taken with the patient standing up and lying down. Other methods to assist diagnosis of lung microangiopathy are needed.

The three methods presented here seem good enough to be competitive options to complement those currently used in medicine today.
Diffusing capacity measurement and modelling allows for the development of a procedure to enhance the diagnostic process. This procedure is based on a single diffusing capacity measurement taken from a patient lying down, together with a model of oxygen diffusion from the alveoli to the blood. The model parameters, calculated using routine medical test results and physiological constants, turned out to be useful for binary classification in lung microangiopathy diagnosis. Diagnostic thresholds were calculated. Next binary classification was performed, based on model parameters, and, for comparison, on the diffusing capacity test result. These results were compared with already known medical diagnoses. This allowed for the sensitivity and specificity to be calculated. The best binary classification results were $Sens = 79\%$ and $Spec = 87\%$, when based on model parameters, and, when based on diffusing capacity measurements, $Sens = 62\%$ and $Spec = 71\%$. These results show that for microangiopathy diagnosis the model parameters were more sensitive and more specific than the diffusing capacity measurements.
The next method to be examined for usefulness in lung microangiopathy diagnosis was spirometry. Statistical comparison of the spirometry parameters of microangiopathic and non-microangiopathic patients, revealed that such parameters do not allow for a distinction to be made between patients with and without microangiopathy. Therefore a spirometry model was developed and its parameters were tested for their ability to distinguish between microangiopathic and non-microangiopathic subjects. Two, out of five, model parameters were statistically significant and helpful in lung microangiopathy diagnosis. Diagnostic thresholds were calculated and binary classification was performed, based on the statistically significant model parameters. The best results were $Sens = 100\%$ and $Spec = 83\%$.
Both diagnostic procedures, the one based on the diffusing capacity and the one based on spirometric measurements and modelling, produce one of two possible results: 1) high probability of lung microangiopathy or 2) high probability of no lung microangiopathy.
Perfusion CT measurement seems to have considerable diagnostic potential with regard to lung microangiopathy. A study of lung tissue perfusion in diabetic patients in comparison with a group of healthy subjects showed an increase in the value of some parameters. These increased values may result from pulmonary microangiopathy. Further studies on the application of pCT in the detection of diabetes mellitus may not only improve diagnosis but also help us better understand pulmonary microangiopathy.

7. References

Alonzi R. & Hoskin P. Functional Imaging in Clinical Oncology: Magnetic Resonance Imaging- and Computerised Tomography-based Techniques, *Clin. Oncol.*, 18, 7, pp. 555-570, 2006

American Thoracic Society: Single-breath carbon monoxide diffusing capacity (transfer factor): recommendations for a standard technique - 1995 update. *Am. J. Respir. Crit. Care Med.*;152:2185-2198, 1995

Askey R.A., Roy R. Gamma function. In: *Digital Library of Mathematical Functions.* Edited by Olver FWJ, Lozier DM, Boisvert RF., N.I.S.T., 2007

Blomley M.J., Coulden R., Bufkin C., Lipton M.J.& Dawson P. Contrast bolus dynamic computed tomography for the measurement of solid organ perfusion. *Invest. Radiol.*, 28, pp. 72-77, 1993

Cao, Y. The Promise of Dynamic Contrast-Enhanced Imaging in Radiation Therapy, *Semin. Radiat. Oncol.*,21, 2, pp. 147-156, 2011

Dalquen, P. The lung in diabetes mellitus, *Respiration, International Journal of Thoracic Medicine*, Vol.66, No1, 1999

Davis A.W., Knuiman M., Kendall. P, Grange V. & Davis T. Glycemic exposure is associated with reduced pulmonary function in type 2 diabetes. *The Fremantle Diabetes Study. Diabetes Care*, 27:752–757, 2004

Eichinger M., Heussel C-P., Kauczor, H-U., Tiddens, H. & Puderbach, M. Computed Tomography and Magnetic Resonance Imaging in Cystic Fibrosis Lung Disease. *Jour. Magn. Reson. Imaging.*, 32, pp. 1370–1378, 2010

Fry D.L., Hyatt R.E. Pulmonary mechanics: a unified analysis of the relationship between pressure, volume and gas flow in the lungs of normal and diseased human subjects. Am. J. Med. 29:672-689,1960

Goldman D. Lung dysfunction in diabetes. *Diabetes Care.*;26:1913–1918, 2003

Kalicka R., Słomiński W.& Kuziemski K. Modelling of spirometry. Diagnostic usefulness of model parameters. *The IEEE Eurocon Conference*, 2137-2143, Warsaw 2007

Kaminski D., Spirometry and diabetes: Implications of reduced lung function. Diabetes Care; 27:837–838, 2004

Khee-Shing ML. Configuration of the haemoglobin oxygen dissociation curve demystified: a basic mathematical proof for medical and biological sciences undergraduates. *Advan Physiol Educ.*;31:198-201, 2007

Kida K., Utsuyama M., Takizawa T. & Thurlbeck W. Changes in lung morphologic features and elasticity caused by streptozotocin-induced diabetes mellitus in growing rats *Am. Rev. Respir. Dis.* 128:125–131, 1983

Kodolova I.M., Lysenko L.V.&Saltykov B.B. Changes in the lungs in diabetes mellitus. Arkh. Patol., 44:35-75, 1982

Kuziemski K., Górska L., Jassem E.& Madej-Dmochowska A. Lung microangiopathy in diabetes. *Pneumonol. Alergol. Pol.*;77:394-399, 2009

Kuziemski K., Górska L., Słomiński W., Kalicka R., Specjalski K.& Adamczyk-Bąk K., Sensitivity of DLCO for microangiopathy diagnosis. *Pneunomol. Alergol. Pol.* 76:43A, 2008

Kuziemski K., Pieńkowska J., Słomiński W., Specjalski K., Dziadziuszko K., Jassem E., Studniarek, M. Kalicka, R. & Słomiński J.M. Role of quantitative chest perfusion computed tomography in detecting diabetic pulmonary microangiopathy. *Diabetes Res. Clin. Pr.*, 91, pp. 80-86, 2011

Litonjua A., Lazarus R., Sparrow D., DeMolles D. & Weiss S: Lung function in type 2 diabetes: the Normative Aging Study. *Respir. Med.* 99:1583–1590, 2005

Matsubara T.& Hara F. The pulmonary function and histological studies of the lung in diabetes mellitus. *Journal of Nippon Medical School*;58:528–536, 1991

Miller M.R., Hankinson J. & Brusasco V. Standardisation of spirometry. *Eur. Respir. J.* 26:319-338, 2005

Panzer R.J., Black E.R. & Griner PF. Diagnostic strategies for common medical problems. Philadelphia: American College of Physicians, 1991

Popov D, Simionescu M. Alterations of lung structure in experimental diabetes, and diabetes associated with hyperlipidaemia in hamsters. *Eur. Respir. Journal.*;10:1850–1858, 1997

Strojek K., Ziora D., Sroczyński J.& Oklek K. Late lung symptoms of diabetes. *Pneunomol. Alergol. Pol.* 61:166, 1993.

Taylor AE, Rehder K, Hyatt RE & Parker JC. Clinical Respiratory Physiology. Emeryville: W.B.Saunders Company, 1989

Villa M.P., Montesano M., Barreto M., Pagani J., Stegagno M. & Multari G. Diffusing capacity for carbon monoxide in children with type 1 diabetes. *Diabetologia;* 47:1931–5, 2004

West JB., Respiratory physiology - the essentials. Philadelphia: Lippincott Williams & Wilkins, 2008

Weynand B., Jonckheere A. Frans &, Rahier J. Diabetes mellitus induces a thickening of the pulmonary basal lamina. *Respiration, International Journal of Thoracic Medicine.* 66:14–19, 1999

Yeh H., Punjabi N.M. & Wang N. Cross-sectional and prospective study of lung function in adults with type 2 diabetes: The Atherosclerosis Risk in Communities (ARIC) Study. *Diabetes Care;* 31:741–746, 2008

Homma, N., Shimoyama, S., Ishibashi, T., and Yoshizawa, M.: Lung Area Extraction from X-ray CT Images for Computer-aided Diagnosis of Pulmonary Nodules by using Active Contour Model, WSEAS Trans. Inf. Sci. Appl., 5, 6, pp. 746-755, 2009

de Nunzio, G., Tommasi, E., Agrusti, A., Cataldo, R., de Mitri, I., Favetta, M., Maglio, S., Massafra, A., Quarta, M., Torsello, M., Zecca, I., Bellotti, R., Tangaro, S., Calvini, P., Camarlinghi, N., Falaschi, F., Cerello, P., and Oliva, P.: Automatic Lung Segmentation in CT Images with Accurate Handling of the Hilar Region, *J. Digit. Imaging*, 24, 1, pp. 11-2, 2011

Vinhais, C., and Campilho, A.: Lung Parenchyma Segmentation from CT Images Based on Material Decomposition, *Lect. Notes Comput*. Sc., 4142, pp. 624-635, 2006

Zhou, X., Hayashi, T., Hara, T., Fujita, H., Yokoyama, R., Kiryu, T., and Hoshi, H.: Automatic recognition of lung lobes and fissures from multi-slice CT images, *Proceedings of SPIE*, 5370, pp. 1629-1633, 2004.

29

The Pneumoconioses

Nlandu Roger Ngatu[1], Ntumba Jean-Marie Kayembe[2], Benjamin Longo-Mbenza[2,3] and Narufumi Suganuma[1]
[1]*Kochi University Medical School, Kochi,*
[2]*University of Kinshasa, Kinshasa,*
[3]*Walter Sisulu University, Mtata,*
[1]*Japan*
[2]*Democratic Republic of Congo*
[3]*Republic of South Africa*

1. Introduction

1.1 Overview on pneumoconioses

Pneumoconiosis is an occupational lung disease caused by the exposure to dust. This section summarizes the generalities on pneumoconioses, including definitions, epidemiology and clinical manifestations of those occupational and environmental lung diseases. The most important step in the diagnosis of pneumoconiosis in to question the subject regarding specifics of the actual job and the minerals or materials involved in case of history of dust exposure. It is very important to seek a detailed account of workers' past employment, too; as some pneumoconioses develop after only a brief but intense dust exposure.

Lately, many cases have been linked to environmental exposure to dust. This suggests that pneumoconiosis is no more a pathology exclusively related to work. Clinicians and epidemiologists should keep in mind the fact that cigarette smoking has a devastating impact of the health of dust-exposed individuals. Rates of cigarette smoking as high as 80% have been recorded among miners and other dust-exposed populations (Baum et al, 1998; Hammond et al, 1979). Asbestos-related diseases, silicosis and coal worker's pneumoconiosis (CWP) are most predominant and widely investigated pneumoconioses.

Pneumoconioses have relatively specific radiologic features that are not well-known to most physicians. Radiological imaging plays an important role in the diagnosis of those occupational lung diseases, including asbestos-related diseases, Silicosis and coal worker's pneumoconiosis (Ngatu et al, 2010; Blum et al, 2008). This review is aimed at providing health care workers, especially clinicians, with basic and accurate knowledge on principal radiologic features often found on a pneumoconiotic chest radiograph that characterize each of the above mentioned lung diseases related to occupational or environmental exposure to dust.

1.2 Asbestosis and other asbestos-related diseases (ARDs)

1.2.1 Definitions and epidemiology

Asbestosis refers to the pneumoconiosis caused by inhalation of asbestos fibers. It is characterized by a slowly progressive, diffuse pulmonary fibrosis. Asbestos is a fibrous mineral whose specific properties have encouraged its use since ancient times, in particular for industrial applications since the 19th century (Tarres et al, 2009; American Thoracic Society [ATS], 2001). Few natural materials used in industry have been the subject of more epidemiological and pathological research than the fibrous mineral, asbestos. Asbestos fibers are divided into two categories based on fiber's shape:

- serpentine fibers (curly, long strands) of which chrisotile (white asbestos) is the most commercialized; it accounts for more than 90 percent of the asbestos produced in the United States;
- amphibole fibers (long and straight) which include amosite (brown asbestos), tremolite, crocidolite and other types of asbestos.

Of the different asbestos fibers used in industries, crocidolite (blue asbestos) is generally considered to be less toxic. The amphibole and amosite are reported to carry the greater risk of causing other asbestos-related diseases such as pleural plaque, mesothelioma and lung cancer. Exposed workers who have developed asbestosis are at risk of fatal complications (Wagner, 1997; Sichletidis et al, 2009; Mossman et al, 1990).

In patients with asbestosis, the chest radiograph usually shows small bilateral parenchymal opacities with a multinodular or reticular pattern that may be associated with pleural abnormalities. However, in some individuals with histopathologic evidence of pulmonary fibrosis, no interstitial abnormalities are found on the chest radiographs (Larson et al, 2010; Kipen et al, 1987). Other asbestos-related disorders are: pleural plaques, mesothelioma, diffuse pleural fibrosis, rounded atelectasia, benign asbestos-related pleural effusion and chronic bronchitis. In the course of asbestosis development, other radiographic features such as honeycombing changes and ground-glass opacities can be seen on the radiograph; they are well visualized on computed tomography (CT) and high resolution computed tomography (HRCT) scans.

It is estimated that approximately 27 millions workers in the United States received a significant exposure to asbestos during the middle of the last four decades of the twentieth century.

Pleural disease is one of the characteristics of asbestos exposure. Pleural plaques are present in about 50 percent of asbestos exposed individuals and most commonly involve the parietal pleura, while involvement of the visceral pleura is scarce. The histological examination of pleural plaque specimens shows the presence of predominant acellular bandles of collagen (Yang et al, 2010).

The prevalence of both pleural plaques and asbestosis is associated with "*time since the first exposure*" (TSFE) to asbestos, the "exposure intensity level", the "duration or cumulative exposure" to asbestos. Meanwhile, *time since the first exposure* seems to be the best predictor for pleural plaques related to asbestos exposure, whereas *cumulative exposure* to asbestos is reported to be a major determinant for asbestosis (American Thoracic Society [ATS], 2004; Schart, 1991). In a study conducted in Finish construction, shipyards and asbestos industry workers by Koskinen and coworkers (1998), a strong relationship was found between pleural plaques and *time since the first exposure* to asbestos. A recent study by Paris et al. (2009) showed for the first time, in a multivariate analysis, strong and independent correlations between *time since first exposure* and pleural plaques, and between *cumulative or level of exposure* with both pleural plaques and asbestosis, indicating that time and dose parameters should be included in the definition of high-risk populations in screening programs.

Malignant mesothelioma is an aggressive tumor that develops from the mesothelial cell of the pleura; it may also develop from the peritoneum, pericardium, or testicular tunica vaginalis.

The association between malignant mesothelioma and asbestos exposure has been well-known worldwide since the 1950s. Approximately, 90% of malignant mesothelioma cases are related to ealier exposure to asbestos and the risk of developing the disease is greater in case of exposure to the amphibole fibers in crocidolite and amosite, but serpentine fibers in chrysotile can also cause the disease with a relatively long latency period (30 years or more) (Fujimoto et al, 2010; Snashall et al, 2001). In Japan, one of the biggest consumers of asbestos in the last four decades of the twentieth century, the number of cases of malignant mesothelioma is shown to correlate with the amount of asbestos consumption and the country has been expected to confront an epidemic of asbestos-related malignancy (Suganuma et al, 2001; Takahashi, 1999).

The incidence of malignant pleural mesothelioma, an asbestos-related tumor, is increasing, with a median survival of seven to ten months; its clinical pattern usually involves substantial pain and dyspnea. The disease causes approximately 15,000 to 20,000 deaths per year worldwide (Pass et al, 2008).

Lung cancer can be consecutive to asbestos exposure. Clinician's search during risk assessment in patients with possible dust exposure may be hindered by the long latency period between the inhalation and the appearance clinical manifestions. In addition to its fibrogenic properties, asbestos is a first-level carcinogen and the most accepted oncological model is the dose-response without safety level (Rosell-Murphy et al, 2010; Goldberg et al, 1999). According to some previous studies, smoking increases the risk of lung cancer in asbestos exposed individuals by 50 - 90 times more than non-smokers (Valavanidis et al, 1996; Hartly et al, 2000).

A variety of occupational and nonoccupational settings can be source of exposure to asbestos:

- Manufacture of asbestos products
- Thermal and fire insulation
- Construction and demolition work
- Shipbuilding and repair
- Building maintenance and repair
- Plumbers and gasfitters
- Vehicle body builders
- Electricians
- Carpenters
- Mining...

Since a while, there is an increasing number of reports on cases of asbestos-related diseases in workers whose occupations have not been traditionally on the lists of occupational health specialists. Asbestosis and pleural plaques have been found in dentists and mechanics in Europe and the United States. And in some cases, these asbestos-related abnormalities are of unusual source of exposure.

Torbica and Krstev (2006) suggested that asbestos-related diseases in dentists might be linked to exposure to inorganic dust in the manufacturing of cobalt-chromium-molybdenum- based dental protheses. With the use of white asbestos-made lining material for casting rings in dentistry, dental technicians and dentists are potentially exposed to asbestos; and some cases of pleural plaques and malignant mesothelioma have been reported in a number of dentists after a relatively long period of work (35 to 45 years) (Choel et al, 2001; Reid et al, 1991; Sichletidis et at, 2009; Radi et al, 2002).

Similarly, pneumoconiosis may occur in mechanics. Most motor vehicles, from passenger cars to heavy duty trucks, have disc brakes on the front wheels and drum brakes on the rear

wheels which help control their movement. Asbestos containing brake lining is generally found in those vehicles, ranging from 35% to 65% of chrysotile contents. Their repair or replacement can be a source of exposure to asbestos (Gilles, 2005; Paustnebach et al, 2004; Kakooei et al, 2004).
According to previously published reports, the incidence of lung cancer and malignant mesothelioma in auto mechanics is higher than in the general population. In the Unites States, concentrations of airborne asbestos more than 300 times higher than the current permissible exposure limit (Occupational Safety and Health Agency, OSHA) of 0.1 fiber/cc were found (Levin et al, 1999; Lorimer et al, 1976; Rohl et al, 1976).

1.2.2 Clinical manifestations of asbestos-related diseases

For asbestosis, in general, the latency period between exposure and the appearance of symptoms is inversely proportional to the intensity of asbestos exposure. And the majority of patients remain asymptomatic for 20- 30 years after the first exposure, even though pleural plaque is present. The first symptom of asbestosis to appear is usually breathlessness with exertion. Dyspnea will follow as the disease progresses; however, cough, wheezing, sputum production are often present when the patient has a history of cigarette smoking.
With the progression of the disease, the patient will develop bibasilar crackles heard mostly at the end of inspiration, and clubbing. Pleural disease occurs earlier mostly within 15 years since the initial exposure to asbestos (Epler et al, 1982; Paris et al, 2009).

1.3 Silicosis

1.3.1 Definition and epidemiology

Silicosis is an interstitial pulmonary disease secondary to the inhalation of crystalline silica (silicon dioxide), usually in the form of quartz, and less commonly as cristobalite and tridymite. It is one of the world's oldest known occupational diseases characterized by irreversible, progressive lung disease. Crystalline silica has long been considered as the toxic form of silica; however, very little was known about the toxicity of amorphous silica until the very recent toxicological and mechanistic study in animals by Constantini and cowokers that revealed the fact that both crystalline and amorphous (which has been regarded as non-fibrogenic) silica are phagocytosed and are both toxic to alveolar macrophages and have similar pathway that lead to apoptosis.
Silica, the second most abundant element that forms the quarter part of the earth's crust, is an ubiquitous mineral in human environment. Thus, exposure to silicon dioxide and salts of silicic acid is a fact of life. However, intense exposure can lead to silicosis (Pascual et al, 2011; Wagner, 1995; Constantini et al, 2011; Baum et al, 1998). Silica is also bound to other minerals; it is then called silicate. Silicates are used in some industries; they include asbestos, talc (Mg3S4O10 (OH)2), and kaoline (Al2Si2O5(OH)4) [Gamble, 1986].
New cases of Silicosis are annually recognized worldwide. In the United States, up to 200,000 miners and 1.7 million non-mining workers have experienced significant occupational exposure to inhaled silica; and every year the country register between 3600 and 7300 new cases of Silicosis. The overall mortality attributable to Silicosis has decreased in the United states thanks to the improvement of workplace protection, compared to that of 30 years ago (3000 deaths a year) [Rosenman et al, 2003; CDC, 2008; NIOSH, 1999].
Silicosis can occur in many industries and work settings with evident dust exposure such as:

- Surface mining, underground mining.

- Quarrying
- Construction work, masonry.
- Sandblasting
- Foundry work
- Ceramics, etc.

The list is not complete; there are numerous other work sites with silica exposure, as free silica can be found anywhere. Mining and construction work that involve drilling, cutting, grinding or crushing the earth's crust or rocks are associated with high level of silica exposure. In several developing countries, in Africa and Asia particularly, mining and minerals processing industries represent the main source of income. It is common to find employers who fail to provide necessary personal protective materials to workers, putting them at high risk of occupational lung disease such as silicosis.

It is also obvious that, in some occupational settings, workers may be exposed to both silica and asbestos or other dust and develop what is called a mixed-dust pneumoconiosis (MDP). MDP is pathologically defined as an occupational lung disease that shows dust macules or mixed-dust fibrotic nodules, with or without silicotic nodules, in an individual with a history of exposure to mixed dust [Honma et al, 2004]. Radiologic features of MDP may include those related to exposure to silica and other fibrogenic duts such as silicates, metals, carbon.

1.3.2 Clinical manifestations of Silicosis

Clinical forms of Silicosis are described according to both their clinical and radiological manifestations. They are divided into:

- Simple Silicosis
- Acute Silicosis
- Chronic silicosis
- Accelerated silicosis

Simple Silicosis is characterized by the presence of small (less than 10 mm in diameter) opacities that are rounded in general, on the chest radiograph, and mostly without symptoms.

Acute Silicosis often occurs after weeks or a few years of an intense exposure to silica. The presence of silicotic nodules on the chest radiograph or computed tomography scan is the main radiologic manifestation.

Chronic silicosis usually appears 10 – 30 years after the initial exposure to silica and develops slowly. This clinical form often share the same radiographic feature with simple Silicosis; but in some cases silicotic nodules may coalesce and form a large opacity which represent a progressive massive fibrosis (PMF). Both accelerated and chronic silicosis have similar radiographic features. The only trait that differentiates them is the interval between the exposure to silica dust and the development of the disease symptoms.

Accelerated Silicosis occurs within ten years after initial exposure and is associated to high-level exposure to silica. Both chronic and accelerated Silicosis may be asymptomatic with the patient having only an abnormal chest radiograph consistent with Silicosis. However, symptomatic patients would present with a chronic cough and dyspnea on exertion. Later, symptoms will become severe with the worsening of the radiographic abnormalities. Crackles, rhonchi and or wheeze may be present in some patients.

The presence of large opacity or progressive massive fibrosis is always accompanied by the aggravation of patient's status and respiratory impairment. The presence of emphysema, air trapping on chest radiograph may be observed (Munakata et al, 1985). Progressive massive fibrosis (PMF) occurs when small rounded opacities enlarge progressively and coalesce to generate larger opacities (more than 10 mm in diameter). PMF, when it is present, its location is either the upper or the middle zone of the lung.

Malignancy represents one of the complications of Silicosis. The international Agency for Research on Cancer (IARC) determined in 1997 that there was evidence of carcinogenicity of crystalline silica (Scarselli et al, 2011). The relationship between silica exposure and lung cancer risk have been demonstrated in several studies. More than ten cohort studies have shown a standardized mortality ratio (SMR) between 1.37 and 3.70, and few reports showed stronger associations with highest risks and excess mortality from lung cancer among silicotics (Scarselli et al, 2011; Lacasse et al, 2005; Erren et a, 2009;Pelucchi et al, 2006).

This suggests that clinicians should keep in mind the relationship between a workplace with exposure to silica dust and the development of lung cancer. Ignoring this fact may mistakenly lead the clinician towards a wrong diagnosis of the patient's condition.

1.4 Coal worker's pneumoconiosis (CWP)

1.4.1 Definition and epidemiology

Coal worker's pneumoconiosis is defined as an occupational lung disease caused by the deposition of coal mine dust in the lung parenchyma and the reaction of tissues to its presence. Coal mining has been used as a source of fuel for hundreds of years, and it still remains a major industry in countries such as the United States, France, Germany, Australia, China, India and South Africa.

Recent researches suggest changes in terms of the epidemiology and clinical features of pneumoconiosis among underground coal miners that are characterized by an increase in the severity and rapid disease progression. Factors such as over-exposure to silica dust in coal mines, the increase in coal production and increasing hours of work are thought to be responsible of the current high prevalence and increased severity of the coal worker's pneumoconiosis (CDC, 2007; Laney, 2009; Antao, 2005).

Laney and Attfield's more recent work, conducted in the Unites States, demonstrated the role of size of mine as another factor that contribute to the high prevalence and fatality of disease observed the last decades. In their study, workers from small mines had a greater risk of coal worker's pneumoconiosis and progressive massive fibrosis than their large mines counterparts. Smaller mining operations often have limited capital to upgrade safety equipment, and dedicated safety and personnel are less likely to be available to workers. This influences the implementation of dust monitoring and control activities in the mines (Laney & Attfield, 2010].

1.4.2 Clinical forms of CWP

CWP comprises two clinical forms: the *simple* and *complicated* Coal worker's pneumoconiosis. Generally, simple CWP is not associated with symptoms. It is often characterized by a history of underground exposure of more than 10 years. As for silicosis, the early radiological features are small rounded opacities that first appear on upper lobes of the lung.

In contrast, complicated CWP is associated with symptoms and a marked impairment of lung function. Shortness of breath, cough and sputum production are common symptoms (Caplan, 1953). The pattern and severity of respiratory impairment in coal worker's pneumoconiosis are related to the levels of coal mine dust exposure, geologic factors, exposure to other respiratory hazards, and the immunologic response to dust (Shen et al, 2004).

2. Classification of High Resolution Computed Tomography (HRCT) scans and chest radiographs of pneumoconioses

2.1 Overview on the classification of pneumoconiotic HRCT scans

The use of Computed Tomography (CT) has revolutionized the radiologic diagnosis of chest diseases as compared with conventional radiography. However, the ability of CT scanners to evaluate pulmonary parenchymal abnormalities is limited because of their resolving power. With the introduction of High-Resolution Computed Tomography (HRCT) techniques, it became possible to perform images of the lung with excellent spatial resolution, providing anatomic detail similar to that available from gross pathologic specimens (Kusaka et al., 2005). Thus, HRCT increases the specificity in the diagnosis of lung diseases, including pneumoconioses. In addition, the early diagnosis of these chronic diseases allows an early care and avoidance of further exposure to the hazardous dusts. For that reason, the proposed International Classification of HRCT of pneumoconiosis is used in some developed countries (such as Japan, Germany and Finland) in the screening and surveillance programs; however, its acceptance by international health institutions might take a time.

The chest radiograph, which is easily accessible and cheaper, presently remains the unique internationally accepted diagnostic tool for pneumoconiosis. For this practical reason, in this chapter, we only present different parameters that are taken into account in the international classification of HRCT of pneumoconiosis.

This section summarizes briefly the information on the proposed international classification of HRCT of pneumoconiosis. Though it is not yet accepted by the International Labor Office (ILO), clinicians should have in mind the existence of this tool which, sooner or later could be of use worldwide.

The purpose of the international HRCT classification is to describe and code parenchymal and pleural manifestations of diffuse non-malignant occupational and environmental respiratory diseases. It is used for the screening (for early detection of pneumoconiosis) and surveillance and follow-up of the exposed individuals) (Kusaka et al., 2005).

In ***asbestosis***, the most common HRCT findings are centrilobular nodules on branching areas of high attenuation, and the thickened interlobular and intralobular lines, subpleural dot-like or curvilinear opacities and honeycombing predominantly distributed in the bases of the lungs. The interstitial fibrosis may also be manifested as traction bronchiectasis, honeycombing.

On the other hand, in case of *silicosis or CWP*, the common characteristic radiologic features on HRCT scan are small opacities predominantly distributed in the upper zones of the lung and, sometimes, images of progressive massive fibrosis (large opacity) (Aberle et al., 1988; Akira et al., 2002).

The reading sheet used in the coding system for CT or HRCT films of pneumoconiosis has the following main parameters to be reported: film quality, parenchymal abnormalities (small opacities, large opacity, emphysema, honeycombing, inhomogenous attenuation of lung parenchyma, pleural abnormalities) (Kusaka et al., 2005).

- *quality of the film*: four grades are considered, similarly to the ILO/ICRP (grade 1, 2, 3, 4; see ILO/ICRP).
- *parenchymal abnormalities*: the absence (No) or presence (Yes) of small opacities (rounded or irregular) has to be reported on the reading sheet; their overall distribution is recorded in a grading system for each side (right, left), according to each zone of the thorax (upper [U], middle [M] or lower [L]). In addition, the severity of the disease is also reported as follows:

0 = no definite opacities;

1=mild (present but only few small opacities);
2=moderate (numerous small opacities);
3=severe (very numerous small opacities and normal anatomical lung structure are poorly.
A number of additional parenchymal abnormalities have to be checked:

a. *inhomogenous attenuation* (absence [No] or presence [Yes] which may be due to the presence of *ground glass opacities* (GGO). When present on HRCT scan, the inhomogenous attenuation should be graded for each side and each zone for its extent as follows: 1=focal; 2=patchy; 3=diffuse.
b. *honeycombing* (HC): absence (No) or presence (Yes);
c. *emphysema*: absence (No) or presence (Yes) of emphysema has to be reported, and graded for right (R) and left (L) side, and for all zones as 1 (mild [up to 15% of area of one zone]), 2(moderate [15-30%]), 3(severe [more than 30%]).
d. *large opacity*: absence (No) or presence (Yes).

- *pleural abnormalities*: absence (No) or presence (Yes); two types of pleural abnormalities should be differentiated considering the CT appearance (parietal and visceral type). The parietal type refers to the flat thickening of the pleura, whereas the visceral type (diffuse pleural thickening) is associated with subpleural fibrosis or parenchymal bands (PB) and rounded atelectasis (RA). Their extent, width and location (medias- tinal, diaphragmatic,..) are also reported.
- *pleural calcifications*: their absence (No) or presence (Yes) should also be reported on the reading sheet.

Detailed information on the international classification of HRCT of pneumoconioses is available elsewhere (Kusaka et al., 2005).

2.2 The ILO International Classification of chest Radiographs of Pneumoconiosis (ILO/ICRP) and ILO/WHO global program for the elimination of Silicosis (ILO/WHO GPES)

The ILO 2000 International Classification of Radiographs of Pneumoconiosis (ILO/ ICRP) is used worldwide by experts to categorize conditions that are consistent with pneumoconiosis, with the use of a set of ILO standard films.

This international classification system was created with the purpose of coding anterio-posterior chest radiographs in a simple and reproducible manner; it provides a means for a systematic description and recording of radiographic abnormalities in the chest caused by the inhalation of dusts. It is useful in epidemiologic research, surveillance and medical checks of dust-exposed workers (Suganuma, 2001; International Labor Office [ILO], 2002). Chest radiographs of patients with silicosis, coal worker's pneumoconiosis asbestosis and other asbestos-related diseases can be interpreted and classified the same way anywhere in the world using the ILO/ICRP system. In this section, basics on the principal radiologic features of pneumoconioses and their characteristics are summarized. In order to fully understand the system, a special training is of utmost importance.

To classify a chest radiograph of a dust-exposed individual, there are four main points to be considered:

- Technical quality;
- presence (or absence) of parenchymal abnormalities consistent with pneumocoiosis;
- presence (or absence) of pleural abnormalities
- presence (or absence) of other abnormalities (represented by symbols on the reading sheet).

Technical quality There are four grades:
1. Good (**grade 1**);
2. Acceptable, with no technical defect (**grade 2**);
3. Acceptable, with some technical defect but still adequate for classification purposes (**grade 3**);
4. Unacceptable for classification purposes (**grade 4**).

A technical defect may be the presence of artifact, with poor contrast, under (light) or overexposed (dark) film or due to an improper position of the subject (overlapping of scapula, for example) or other defect. Artifacts can be interpreted as pathological abnormalities in case they mimic opacities, while the overlap of scapula (Fig. 1) can easily be interpreted as in-profile or face on plaque. An abnormal feature related to the lung parenchyma or pleura may be present on the chest radiograph, but hidden by the overlapping scapula. When a chest radiograph is qualified as unreadable, it is necessary that another one be indicated.

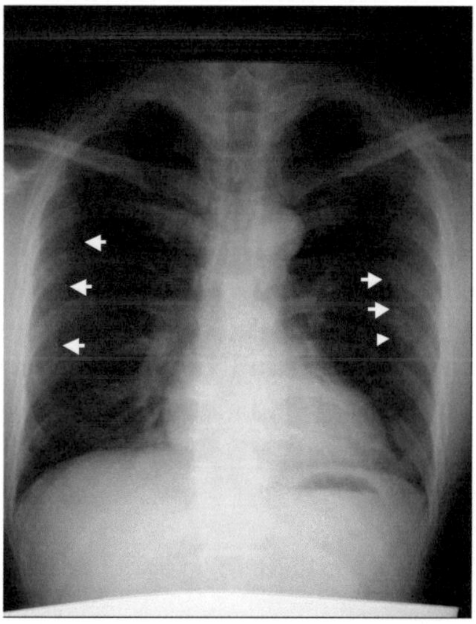

Fig. 1. Chest radiograph of poor quality showing overlapping scapula (white arrows) looking like pleural plaques on both right and left lung fields.
[Courtesy of Prof. Dr. Yukinori Kusaka, Asian Intensive Reading of Pneumoconiosis radiographs (AIR PNEUMO)]

2.2.1 Parenchymal abnormalities

They include two types of opacities: small and large opacities.

Small opacities are described by *profusion, affected lung zones,* the *shape* (rounded or irregular) and *size.*

- *Profusion* refers to the concentration of small opacities in the affected zones of the lung; the are four categories of profusion (0, 1. 2, 3) and 12 sub-categories of profusion (0/-; 0/0; 0/1; 1/1; 1/2; 2/1; 2/1; 2/2; 2/3; 3/2; 3/3; 3/+), where category 0 means the absence of small opacities or the presence of small opacities with a profusion lower than category 1, and category 3 has the highest profusion.

To classify the dust-exposed individual's chest radiograph, it has to be compared with the standard radiographs from ILO (known as ILO standard radiographs) which profusion seems to be closer to that in the worker's film. Standard radiographs provide examples of appearances classifiable as subcategory 0/0; 1/1; 2/2; 3/3.

- *Affected lung zone* is the area the lung where small opacities are seen; each lung field is divided into three zones (upper, middle, lower) by horizontal lines.
- *Shape and size* of small opacities are also recorded; for the shape, there are *rounded* and irregular (reticular) opacities. For *small rounded opacities*, there are three size ranges designated as **p** (diameter up to 1.5 mm), **q** (diameter exceeding 1.5 mm and up to 3 mm), **r** (diameter exceeding 3mm and up to 10 mm). Similarly, for *small irregular opacities*, the three sizes are denoted by the letters **s** (opacities with a width up to 1.5 mm), **t** (width exceeding 1.5mm and up to 3 mm), **u** (with a width exceeding 3mm and up to 10 mm). On each standard radiograph, the type of small opacities and their profusion are shown (for example: p/p, 2/2 which means 'small opacities of p type and profusion 2/2). However, some chest radiographs may show both small rounded and irregular opacities; this often happens in case the worker was exposed to silica and asbestos, for example (mixed-dust pneumoconiosis).

Large opacities are opacities whose longest diameter exceeds 10 mm. There are three categories of large opacities:

- category **A:** one large opacity with longest dimension up to 50 mm, or several large opacities with the sum of their longest dimension not exceeding about 50 mm;
- category **B**: longest diameter exceeding 50 mm, but not exceeding the equivalent area of the right upper zone; or several large opacities with the sum of their longest dimensions not exceeding the equivalent of the right upper zone (Fig. 2);
- category **C**: one large opacity which exceeds the equivalent area of the right upper zone, or several large opacities which, when combined, exceed the equivalent area of the right upper zone.

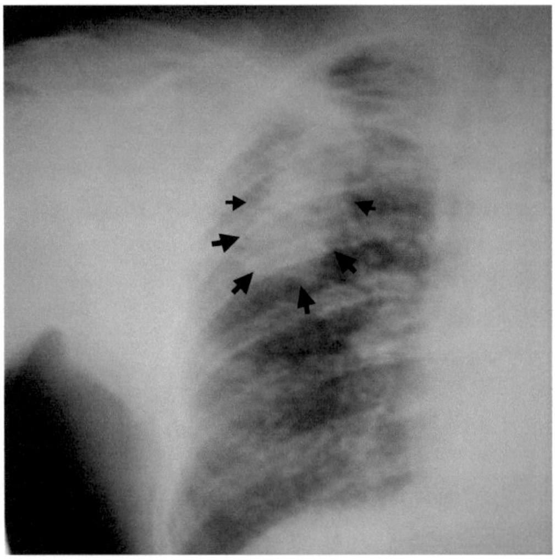

Fig. 2. Silicotic chest radiograph showing a large opacity of category B (black arrows) on the right upper zone. Numerous rounded opacities (q type) are present in all zones of the lung field. *(Courtesy of Dr Hisao Shida)*

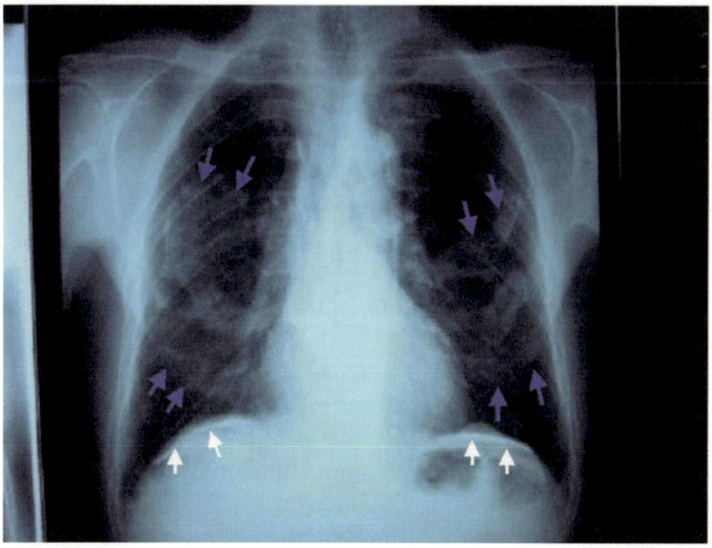

Fig. 3. Chest radiograph showing calcified diaphragmatic pleural plaques (white arrows) and face-on plaques (blue arrows) bilaterally. In this film, pleural plaques can also be seen in other site (mediastinal region bilaterally).
(Courtesy of Prof. Dr Yukinori Kusaka, AIR PNEUMO)

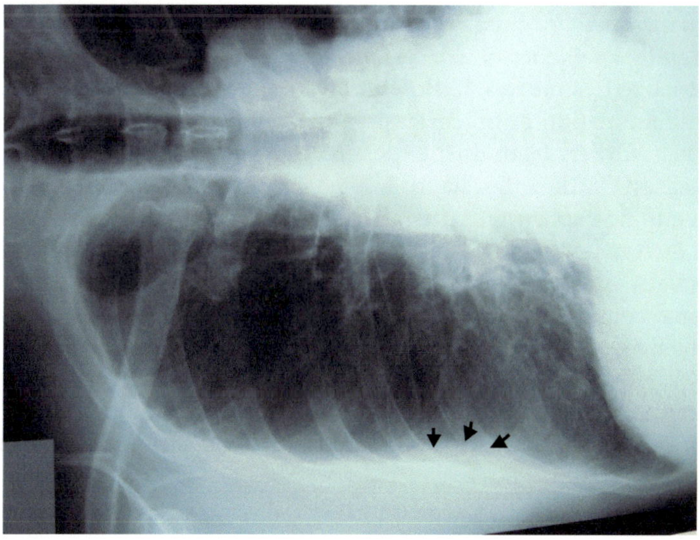

Fig. 4. Chest radiograph showing an in-profile pleural plaque (arrows) in asbestos-exposed worker.
(Courtesy of Dr Hisao Shida)

2.2.2 Pleural abnormalities

They comprise *pleural plaques* (localized pleural thickening), *costophrenic angle obliteration* and *diffuse pleural thickening* (DPT).

Pleural plaques may be located on the diaphragm, on the chest wall (in-profile or face-on plaques) and at other sites; they generally represent a thickening of the parietal pleura and are recoded as present or absent.
Other details regarding the site (right or left lung), presence or absence of calcification, width and extent of the plaque are recorded.

2.2.3 Costophrenic angle obliteration and diffuse pleural thickening

Costophrenic angle obliteration is recoded as present or absent. However, with the ILO classification, *diffuse pleural thickening* extending up to the lateral chest wall is recorded only in case of an obliterated costophrenic angle. All details are summarized in a single chest radiograph reading sheet (ILO, 2002).
The global program for the elimination of Silicosis (GPES) was adopted in 2003, Geneva, by a panel of experts in occupational health. It is aimed at establishing a wide international co-operation so as to eliminate Silicosis by the year 2030 (World Health Organization [WHO], 2003). GPES was established following recommendations of the twelfth session of the joint ILO/WHO Committee on occupational health in 1995, which indentified the global elimination of silicosis as a priority area for action in occupational health. The committee wanted countries to place it high on their agendas, with the belief that the experience gained through implementation of this program would provide a prevention model for other pneumoconioses and a proven system for the management of exposure to mineral dust.
The GEPS has two different approaches; the primary prevention of Silicosis that emphasizes the control of silica hazard at source using engineered methods of dust control, while the secondary prevention includes surveillance of the work environment to assess the efficacy of the implemented measures for dust exposure control, exposure evaluation by assessing health risk for workers and surveillance of workers' health for the early diagnosis of the disease.
In most industrialized countries, following recommendation of the ILO/WHO Global Program for the Elimination of Silicosis, pneumoconiosis prevention programs have been initiated to protect workers from dust exposure and the actual trend of show a decrease in number of new cases. On the other hand, in the majority of developing countries millions of workers continue to be exposure to dust. In order to reach the goal by 2030, each country should have its own national program. Unfortunately, the reality shows that there are still obstacles that might make it difficult to reach the GPES goal by 2030: one is the non adherence of some countries to the ILO/WHO program and, the insufficiency of qualified individuals in the interpretation of pneumoconiotic chest radiographs.
Under the ILO/WHO GPES, experts focused manly on secondary prevention, upgrading skills of occupational physicians in developing countries in using the ILO 2000 Classification of Radiographs of Pneumoconiosis (ILO 2000 ICRP) and strengthening national Silicosis elimination programs (Luton, 2007).

3. Short training on pneumoconiosis chest radiographs reading

3.1 Objective

The ILO classification system is an important tool for training occupational physicians in the diagnosis of pneumoconioses. Based on this ILO system, some countries have developed their own national program and produced necessary teaching materials. In the United States, the National Institute for Occupational Health (NIOSH) provides certification tests physicians, radiologists and other professionals in the field of occupational health through the B-readers system. And, since the year 2008, the Asian Intensive Reading of Pnemoconioses chest radiographs (AIR-PNEUMO) program started, organizing annual workshops and certification test for Asian countries and also Brazil. These programs contribute a lot for the achievement of the ILO/WHO Global Program for the Elimination of Silicosis, and also those dedicated to the elimination of asbestosis.

However, the number of physicians who have required skills to interpret pneumoconiotic radiographs remains insignificant in many regions of the world, as participation to ILO training course by physicians is quite costly and, moreover, the absence of local trainers constitutes a real obstacle. Countries that do not yet get involved in the ILO/WHO program are numerous. Despite the existence of institution such Air-pneumo, NIOSH and others, the elimination of silicosis may not be achieved by the year 2030 without involvement of governments and health authorities of all nations. Providing basic knowledge on pneumoconiosis to clinicians and those who are about to graduate from medical school would also be helpful for the diagnosis of pneumoconiosis, particularly in regions where occupational or environmental exposure to dust represent a real public health issue. Here is presented a short training on pneumocnioses and the evaluation of its potential to improve physicians' ability to detect main pneumoconiotic radiographic features on chest radiographs of dust-exposed individuals.

3.2 Differentiating normal and pneumoconiotic radiographs

Radiological imaging plays an important role in the diagnosis of pneumoconiosis. Although chest radiography has some limitations in terms of detecting earliest parenchymal and pleural abnormalities, it remains the most useful and universally accepted method for assessing pneumoconiosis; it is an easily accessible, cheap diagnostic tool (Takashima et al., 2007).

On a normal chest radiograph (Fig. 5), there are anatomical structures that resemble abnormal features and may lead the reader to wrong interpretation. The presence of lymph

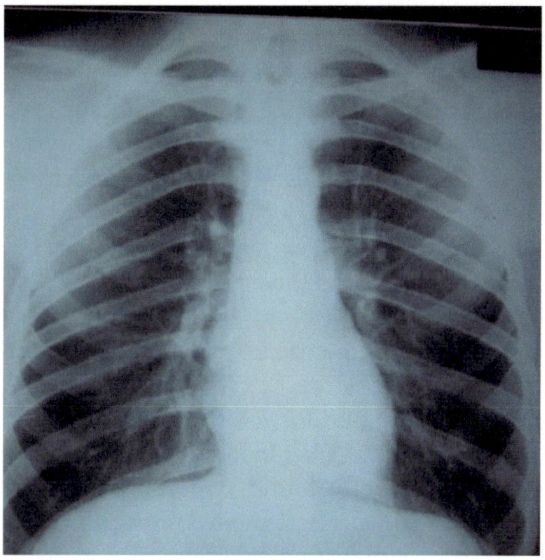

Fig. 5. Normal chest radiograph showing normal anatomical features. Note the presence of opacities that represent lymph nodes and blood vessels.
(Courtesy of Dr Hisao Shida)

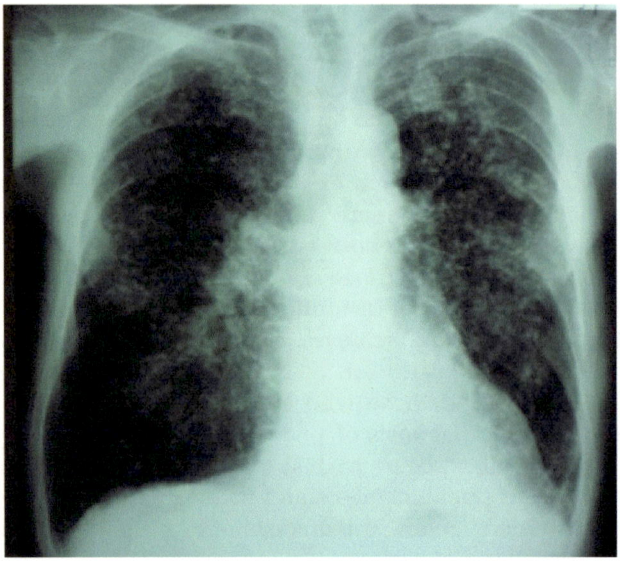

Fig. 6. Silicotic chest radiograph showing small rounded opacities of q type mostly, with involvement of all lung zones (upper, middle and lower zones). Coalescence of small rounded opacities is seen on the right upper zone.
(Courtesy of Dr Hisao Shida)

nodes, muscles (serratus anterior, oblique externus abdominis...), pleural fat's shadow and normal cross-section or tangential views of blood vessels can be interpreted as opacities or pleural plaques related to pneumoconiosis, for example. This poses a challenge during chest radiograph reading process and may lead to misclassification of conditions consistent with pneumoconioses (Ngatu et al, 2010; Jinkai et al, 2008).

For individuals who present with pneumoconiotic-like radiographic features, establishing the history of dust exposure is an important step towards the confirmation of the diagnosis. A silicotic or coal worker's pneumoconiosis' chest radiograph will often present small rounded opacities (opacities having a diameter up to 10 mm) as parenchymal abnormalities (Fig. 6). When they coalesce, small opacities form a large opacity (having a diameter > 10 mm). In addition, a silicotic radiograph may also show calcified lymph nodes (eggshell calcifications). In silicosis, small opacities are first localized on the upper zone of the lung, then will progress towards the middle and lower zones.

In contrast, a chest radiograph from an asbestosis patient will often present small irregular opacities (opacities having a longest dimension up to 10 mm) as parenchymal abnormalities (Fig. 7) and/or pleural plaque (s). Asbestosis small opacities appear on the lower zone of the lung, then later progress towards the middle and the upper lung zones. Other features may also be present such as diffuse pleural thickening, honeycombing changes.

The table below summarizes frequently found pneumoconiotic radiographic features for mineral dust-exposed subjects: their localization according to the type of pneumoconiosis, and their shape and size for small opacities (Table 1). It is important to know that individuals exposed to both silica and asbestos may develop a "Mixed Dust Pneumoconiosis (MDP); the radiograph may show a combination of features of silica, asbestos or other fibrogenic dusts related diseases.

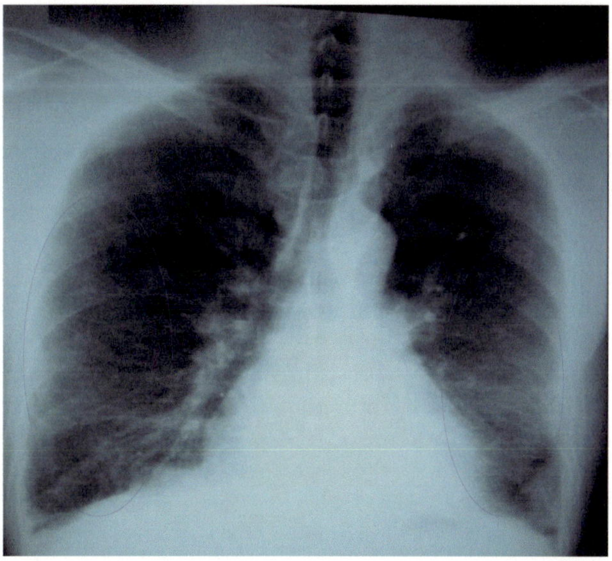

Fig. 7. Chest radiograph of asbestos-exposed worker showing the presence of small irregular opacities (of "t" type primarily and "s" type secondarily), predominantly on lower and middle lung zones. The right upper lobe is also involved. The profusion is 2/3. In addition, diffuse pleural thickening (DPT) is evident on the right and in-profile plaque on the left; also note the abnormal cardiac size. The film quality is of grade 2 (scapula overlap).
(Courtesy of Prof. Dr Yukinori Kusaka, AIR PNEUMO)

Occupational/environmental lung diseases			
Radiographic features		Silicosis	Asbestosis / Asbestos-related disease
First localisation		Upper zone	lower zone
Rounded opacities	Small opacities	often present	
Irregular opacities	Small opacities		often present
Large opacity		may be present **(category: A, B, C)**	
Pleural plaque			may be present **(face-on plaque and/ or In-profile plaque)**
Diffuse Pleural Thickening			may be present

Table 1. Summarized main radiographic findings related to silicosis and asbestos-related lung diseases

3.3 Implementation of the two-hour training session

3.3.1 Participants and methods

For the first reported training held in 2008, 102 Japanese physicians (72 males and 28 females; 2 to 44 years of experience) having different background (preventive medicine, internal medicine, psychiatrists, surgery, pediatrics) from different cities within the country. Participants were invited to the 2008 training session held in Kochi and Ehime prefecture through the staff of Japanese medical corporations, and the training session was conducted by a NIOSH-B reader from Kochi University Medical School, Japan.

We used three sets of chest radiographs were used, namely ILO/ICRP standard films, dust-exposed workers' chest radiographs and a set of twelve test films. ILO standard films were used to describe pneumoconiotic lung abnormalities (shape, size, profusion of small opacities; large opacities, pleural plaques) during the lecture. Dust-exposed workers' chest radiographs, having different radiographic features of pneumoconioses, were provided by the Japan Pneumoconioses Study Group (JPSG). In order to read them, each film was put side by side with the ILO standard whose profusion, for example, seems to be close to that of the patient.

Our intervention was aimed at improving inexperienced physicians' skill in reading pneumo-coniotic chest radiographs. Participants had to listen to a pre-session talk to remind them the abnormalities to be checked on each of patients' radiographs (before the main lecture); then, they take a pre-test as described in the protocol (Fig. 8). Each participant received a reading form that had a list of 12 radiograph numbers (from 1 to 12) and they had to check for the presence (Yes) or the absence (No) of parenchymal or pleural abnormalities consistent with pneumoconiosis (opacities and pleural plaques) for each chest radiograph. Classifying the radiographs using categories of profusion of small opacities, location, width or extent of pleural plaques was not indicated. The main lecture was given after the pre-test for two-hours; afterwards a post-test was organized using the same test films that were displayed on viewboxes in the lecture room.

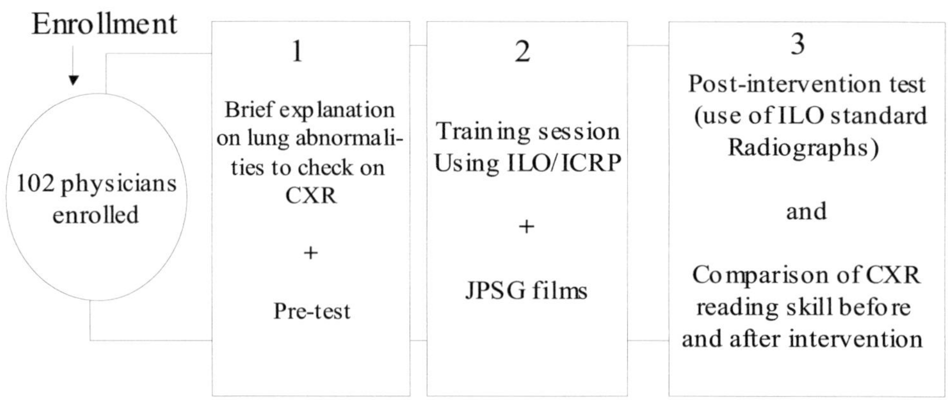

Fig. 8. Protocol of the intervention study (CXR: chest radiograph; JPSG: Japan pneumoconiosis study group)

3.3.2 Evaluation of physicians' reading skill and observed results

The reading forms were collected and managed by s staff who no relationship with any of the participant and all participants were anonymously coded for the analysis of the tests

(pre-test and post-test) results. The difference in the physicians' reading skill before and after the intervention was evaluated using McNemar's chi-square test.
The general trend was towards improvement in terms of physicians' ability to detect pneumoconiotic parenchymal and pleural abnormalities on the test-radiographs. Regarding the dectection of the presence of pneumoconiotic small opacities, a significant increase in the specificity score was observed, 65% in the pre-test and 73% in post-test ($p<0.0001$); whereas the sensitivity score remained high, 84% and 81% in pre- and post-test ($p>0.05$), respectively (Table 2). It is noticeable that the high sensitivity score in the pre-test was due to a high proportion of physicians who considered the normal radiographs to have pneumoconiotic opacities (false positive or over reading) in the pre-intervention test. The over reading of test radiographs was noticeable for the pre-intervention test for most of the readers.

Lung abnormality	Sensitivity		p	Specificity		p
	pre-test	post-test		pre-test	post-test	
Small opacitity	84%	81%	0.204	65%	73%	<0.0001
Pleural plaque	46%	60%	<0.0001	77%	79%	0.3339

p: p-value by McNemar's chi-square test.

Table 2. Overall distribution of the sensitivity and specificity scores of the participants for detecting pneumoconiotic small opacities and pleural plaques on chest radiographs

Group of readers	Lung abnormality	Sensitivity		p	Specificity		p
		pre-test	post-test		pre-test	post-test	
1. Internists	Small opacity	83%	78%	0.208	67%	76%	<0.01
	Pleural plaque	41%	61%	<0.0001	83%	80%	0.21
2. Other specialities	Small opacity	85%	83%	0.546	63%	71%	<0.01
	Pleural plaque	50%	59%	<0.05	72%	79%	<0.05

p: p-value by McNemar's chi-square test.

Table 3. Distribution of sensitivity and specificity scores of readers for detecting pneumoconiotic abnormalities according to medical specialty.

For pleural plaques, a marked increase in the sensitivity score was noted, 46% in pre-test and 60% in post-test ($p<0.0001$), while an improvement was also observed in the specificity score but not significantly (77% and 79% in pre and post-test, respectively) ($p>0.05$) as shown in Table 2.
When compared according their medical specialties, a relatively similar reading skill improvement was observed between internists and physicians from working in other departments. Higher scores of sensitivity for the detection of small opacities and specificity for plaques were found in internists, and a similar trend was also noted in the group of physicians from other specialties in which a significant improvement of specificity score for pleural plaques was found ($p<0.05$) in the post-test (Table 3) (Ngatu et al, 2010).
The lack of training for medical doctors in the diagnosis of occupational diseases is the main factor leading to the misdiagnosis of pneumoconiosis as either chronic bronchitis or

pulmonary tuberculosis (Murlidhar et al, 2005). One of the strong points of this training program is that, despite being carried out in relatively short time, it results in a noticeable improvement of physicians' ability to detect pneumoconiotic parenchymal and pleural abnormalities. Popularizing such program may contribute to the early diagnosis of pneumoconioses, improve their prognosis and give chances of survival for individuals with lung diseases related to dust exposure.

4. Conclusion

This review article provides basic knowledge on pneumoconioses and a practical approach that may help physcians to diagnose occupational lung disorders related to exposure to mineral dust. Meanwhile, a training with demonstrations on the pneumoconiotic chest radiograph reading process is of utmost importance. Holding regular short period training courses for physicians, and even medical students who are about to graduate, focusing on main radiolographic features of lung parenchymal and pleural abnormalities related to occupational or environmental exposure to dust, with the use of typical ILO standard films, will contribute to improving their skill in the diagnosis of pneumoconioses.

5. Acknowledgments

The authors thank Professor Yukinori Kusaka, Dr Hisao Shida and Dr Masanori Akira for providing materials used in this report.

6. References

[1] Baum, GL; Crapo, JD; Celli, BR & Karlinski, JB. (2008). Textbook of Pulmonary Diseases, 6th Edition. Lippincott-Raven Publishers, Philadelphia, 1998.

[2] Hammond, EC; Selikoff, IJ & Seidman, H. (1979). Asbestos exposure, cigarette smoking, and death rate. *Ann NY Acad Sci*, Vol.330, No?, (1979), pp.473-491.

[3] Ngatu, NR; Suzuki, S; Kusaka, Y; Shida, H; Akira, M & Suganuma, N. (2010). Effect of a Two-hour Training on Physicians' Skill in Interpreting Pneumoconiotic Radiographs. *J Occup Health*, Vol.52, (2010), pp.294-301.

[4] Blum, T; Kollmeier, J; Ott, S ; Serke, M ; Schonfeld, N & Bauer, T. (2008). Computed Tomography for diagnosis and grading dust-induced occupational lung disease. *Curr Opin pulm Med*, Vol.14, No (2008), pp.135-140.

[5] Tarres, J; Abos-Herrandez, R; Alberti, C et al. (2009). Asbestos-Related Diseases in a Population Near a Fibrous Cement Factory. *Arch Bronconeumol*, Vol.45, No9, (2009), pp.429-434.

[6] American Thoracic Society (ATS). (2004). Diagnosis and initial management of nonmalignant diseases related to asbestos. *Am J Respir Crit Care Med*, Vol.170, No?, (2004), pp.691.

[7] Snashall, D. & Patel, D.(2003). ABC of Occupayional and environmental Medicine. BMJ books, 2nd Ed., ISBN 0727916114, London.

[8] Wagner, GR. (1997). Asbestosis and silicosis. *Lancet*, Vol.349, (1997), pp.1311.

[9] Sichletidis, L.; Chloros, D.; Spyratos, D. et al. (2009). Mortality from occupational exposure to relatively Pure chrysotile: a 39-year study. *Respiration*, Vol.78, (2009), pp.63.
[10] Mossman, BT.; Bignon, J.; Corn, M. et al. (1990). Asbestos: scientific developments and implications for public health policy. *Science*, Vol.247, (1990), pp.294.
[11] Larson, TC. ; Meyer, CA.; Kapil, V. et al. (2010). Workers with Libby amphibole exposure: Retrospective identification and progression of radiographic changes. *Radiology*, Vol.255, (2010), pp.924.
[12] Kipen, HM.; Lilis, R. ; Suzuki, Y. et al. (1987). Pulmonary fibrosis in asbestos insulation workers with lung cancer: a radiological and histopathological evaluation. *Br J Ind Med*, Vol…, (1987), pp.44-96.
[13] Yang, HY.; Wang, JD.; Chen, PC.; Lee, JJ. et al. (2010). Pleural plaque Related to Asbestos Mining in Taiwan. *J Formos Med Assoc*, Vol.109, No12, (2010), pp.928-933.
[14] American Thoracic Society (ATS). (2004). Diagnosis and initial management of nonmalignant diseases related to asbestos. *Am J Respir Crit Care Med*, Vol.170, (2004), pp.691-715.
[15] Schwartz, DA. (1991). New developments in asbestos-induced pleural disease. *Chest*, Vol.99, (1991), pp.191-198.
[16] Koskinen, K; Zitting, A; Tossavainen, A et al. Radiographic abnormalities among Finish construction, shipyards and asbestos industry workers. Scand J Work Environ Health 1998; 24: 109-117.
[17] Paris, C; Martin, A; Thierry, S; Brochard, P et al. Pleural plaques and asbestosis: dose- and time-response relationships based on HRCT data. Eur Respir J 2009; 34: 72-79.
[18] Fujimoto, N.; Aoe, K.; Gemba, K; Kat,o K.; Yamazaki, K. & Kishimoto T. (2010). Clinical investigation of malignant mesothelioma in Japan. *J Cancer Res Clin Oncol, Vol.136,* (2010), p. 1755-1759.
[19] Suganuma, N.; Kusaka, Y.; Hiraga, Y. et al. (2001). Asbestos-Related Pleural Abnormalities Detected by Chest X-Ray: Fair Agreement with Detection by computed Tomography. J Occup Health, Vol.43, No, (2001), pp.365-370.
[20] Takahashi, K.; Huuskonen, M.; Tossavainen, A.; Higashi, T.; Okubo, T. & Rantanen, J. Ecological Relationship between Mesothelioma Incidence/Mortality and Asbestos consumption in Ten Western Countries and Japan. *J Occup Health*, Vol.41, No1, (1999), pp.8-11.
[21] Pass, HI; Wali, A; Tang, N; Ivanova, S; Harbut, M. et al.(2008). Soluble Mesothelin-related Peptide level Elevation in Mesothelioma Serum and Pleural Effusions. *Ann Thorac Surg*, Vol.85, No1, (January 2008), pp. 265-72.
[22] Rosell-Murphy, M.; Abos-Herranndiz, R,; Tarres, J. et al. (2010). Prospective study of asbestos-related diseases incidence cases in primary health care in an area of Barcelona province. *BMC Public Health*, Vol.10, *(April* 2010), pp.203.
[23] Goldberg M. (1999). Asbestos and Risk of cancer: exposure-effect relationships for occupationally exposed populations. *Rev Mal Respir*, Vol.16, No6, (December 1999), pp.278-85.
[24] Valavanidis, A; Balomenou, H; Macropoulou, I & Zarodimos, I.(1996). A study of the synergistic interaction of asbestos fibers with cigarette tar extracts for the

generation of hydroxyl 1 radicals in aqueous buffer solution. *Free Radic Biol Med,* Vol.20, No6, (May 1999), pp.853-858.

[25] Hartly PG & Schwartz DA. (2000). Occupational lung disease. In: Humes HD. *Kelly's Textbook of Internal Medicine* , Lippincott, Philadelphia, Philadelphia.

[26] Torbica, NO & Krstev, S. (2006). World at work: Dental laboratory technicians. *Occup Environ Med,* Vol.63, No2, (February 2006), pp.145-148.

[27] Choel, L; Grosgogeat, B; Bourgeois, D & Descotes, J. (2001). Occupational toxic risks in dental laboratory technicians. *J Environ Med,* Vol.1, No, (February 2001), pp.307-314.

[28] Reid, AS; Causton, BB; Jones, JSP & Ellis, IO. (1991). Malignant mesothelioma after exposure to asbestos in dental practice. *Lancet,* Vol.338, No8768, (September 1991), pp.696.

[29] Gilles, T. Automotive Chassis: Brakes, Steering & Suspension, Thomson Delmar Learning. A Division of Thomson Learning, Inc, USA.

[30] Paustenbach, DJ; Finley, BL; Lu, ET; Brorby, GP & Sheehan, PJ. (2004). Environmental and occupational health hazards associated with the presence of asbestos in brake linings and pads (1900 to present): a state-of-the-art review. J Toxicol Environ Health B Crit Rev, Vol.7, No1, (January-February 2004), pp.25- 80.

[31] Kakooei, H; Sameti, M & Kakooei, AA. (2007). Asbestos exposure during routine brake lining manufacture. *Ind health,* Vol. 45, No6, (December 2007), pp.787-792.

[32] Levin, JL; O Sulivan, MF; Corn, CJ; Williams, MG & Dodson, RF. (1999). Asbestos and small cell lung cancer in a clutch prefabricator. *J Occup Environ Med,* Vol.56, No9, (September 1999), pp.602-605.

[33] Lorimer, WV; Rohl, AN; Miller, A; Nicholson, WJ & Selikoff, IJ. (1976). Asbestos exposure of brake repair workers in the united States. *Mt Sinai J Med,* Vol. 43, No3, (May-June 1976), pp.207-218.

[34] Rohl, AN; Langer, AM; Wolff, MS & Weisman, I. (August 1976). Asbestos exposure during brake lining maintenance and repair. *Environ Resp,* Vol.12, No1, (August 1976), pp.110-128.

[35] Epler, GR; McLoud, TC & Gaensler, EA. (1982). Prevalence and Incidence of benign asbestos pleural effusion in a working population. *JAMA,* Vol.247, No5, (February 1982), pp.617-622.

[36] Paris, C; Thierry, S; Brochard, P et al. (2009). Pleural plaques and asbestosis: dose-and time-relatonship based on HRCT data. *Eur Respir J,* Vol.34, No1,(July 2009), pp.72-79.

[37] Gamble, JF. Silicate neumoconiosis. (1986). In: Occupational respiratory diseases, Merchant JA, (Ed), Publication No. DHHS (NIOSH) 86-102, Government Printing Office, Washington, DC, (1986). p.243.

[38] Rosenman, KD; Reilly, MJ & Henneberger, PK. (2003). Estimating the total number of newly-recognized silicosis cases in the United States. *Am J Ind Med,* Vol.44, No2, (August 2003), pp.141-147.

[39] Scarselli, A; Binazzi, F; Forastiere, F et al. (2011). Industry and job-specific mortality after occupational exposure to silica dust. *Occup Med (London)* (June 2011), doi: 10.1093/occmed/kqr060.

[40] Lacasse, Y; Martin, S; Simard, S et al. (2005). Meta-analysis of silicosis and lung cancer. Cand J Work Environ Health, Vol.31, No6, (December 2005), pp.450-458.

[41] Erren, TC; Glende, CB; Morfeld, P et al. (2009). Is exposure to silica associated with lung cancer in the absence of silicosis? A meta-analytical approach to an important public health question. Int Arch Occup Environ Health, Vol.82, No8, (August 2009), pp.997-1004.

[42] Pelucchi, C; Pira, E; Piolatto, G et al. Occupational silica exposure and lung cancer risk: a review of epidemiological studies 1996-2005. *Ann Oncol*, Vol.17, No7, (July 2006), pp.1039-1050.

[43] Centers for Disease Control and Prevention (CDC). (2008). Silicosis-related years of potential life lost before age 65 years—Unites States, 1968-2005. *MMWR Morb Mort Wkly Rep*, Vol.57, (2008), pp.771.

[44] National Institute for Occupational Health (NIOSH). (1999). Work-related lung disease surveillance report No. 200-105. DHHS (NIOSH), Cincinnati, OH, 1999.

[45] Honma, K.; Abraham, J.L.; Chiyotani, K. et al. (2004). Proposed criteria for mixed-dust pneumoconiosis: definition, descriptions, and guidelines for pathologic diagnosis and clinical correlation. Hum Pathol, Vol. 35, No12, (Dec. 2004), pp. 1515-23.

[46] Munakata, M; Homma, Y; Matsuzaki, et al. (1985). Rales in silicosis. A correlative study with physiological and radiological abnormalities. *Respiration*, Vol.48, No2, (February 1985), pp.140-144.

[47] Laney, AS & Attfield, MD. (2010). Coal worker's pneumoconiosis and progressive massive fibrosis are increasingly more prevalent among workers in small underground coal mines in the Unites States. *Occup Environ Med*, Vol.67, No6, (June 2010), pp.428-431.

[48] Caplan, A. (1958). Certain unusual radiological appearances in the chest of coal miners suffering from rheumatoid arthritis. *Thorax*, Vol.8, No1, (March 1953), pp.29-37.

[49] Shen, HN; Jerng, JS; Yu, CJ et al. (2004). Outcome of Coal Worker's Pneumoconiosis with Acute Respiratory Failure. *Chest*, Vol. 125, No3, (March 2004), pp.1052-1058.

[50] Kusaka, Y.; Hering, KG. & Parker, JE. (2005). *International Classification of HRCT for Occupational and Environmental Respiratory Diseases*. (1st Edition). Springer-Verlag, ISBN 4-431-23924-3, Tokyo.

[51] Aberle, D.R.; Gamsu, G.; Ray, C.S. et al. (1988). Asbestos-related pleural and parenchymal fibrosis: Detection with thin-section CT. Radiology, Vol. 166, (March 1988), pp. 729-734.

[52] International Labor Office (ILO). (2002). Guidelines for the use of the ILO international classification of radiographs of pneumoconioses, Revised Edition. ILO, Geneva.

[53] World Health Organization (WHO). (2003). The Global Occupational Health Network. Gohnet Newsletter, Available from http://www.who.int/occupational_healthPublications/newsletter/en/gohnet5e.pdf

[54] Luton, T. (2007). Silicosis: Educate, Eliminate, Eradicate. Available from: http://www.indianet.nl/pdf/silicosis.pdf

[55] Takashima, Y.; Suganuma, N.; Sakurazawa, H et al. (2007). A flat panel detector digital radiography and a storage phosphor computed radiography: screening for pneumoconioses. *J Occup Health*, Vol.49, pp.39-45.
[56] Jinkai, S.; Dong, W., Changshan, J et al. (2008). The value of high resolution computed tomography in the diagnosis of small opacities and complications of silicosis in mine machinery manufacturing workers compared to radiography. *J Occup Health*, Vol.50, pp.400-405.
[57] Murlidhar, V. & Kanhere, V. (2005). Asbestosis in an asbestos composite mil: a prevalence study. *Environ Health*, Vol.4, (2005), pp.24-30.

Lung Transplantation: Advances and Roadblocks in Treatment

Matthew T. Hardison[1] and J. Edwin Blalock[2]
[1]*Medical Genetics Laboratories, Department of Human and Molecular Genetics, Baylor College of Medicine*
[2]*Pulmonary, Allergy and Critical Care Medicine, Department of Medicine, University of Alabama at Birmingham*
United States of America

1. Introduction

The increasing population age, along with the prevalence of smoking and other environmental factors have contributed to a dramatic increase in the incidence of chronic pulmonary diseases with no known cures. Chronic obstructive pulmonary disease (COPD), lung cancer, and primary pulmonary hypertension are all conditions with well understood origins but few, if any therapeutic options. When taken in conjunction with the prevalence of genetic or poorly understood conditions such as cystic fibrosis (CF) and idiopathic pulmonary fibrosis (IPF) there is a large and growing cohort of patients that will eventually enter end-stage lung disease. The only currently available treatment option is lung transplantation which may potentially be extremely beneficial in terms of quality of life and life expectancy, although carries with it a vast array of considerations and complications. This chapter attempts to provide an account of the progress made in lung transplantation, complications associated with the procedure, current treatment for transplant associated conditions, and finally will discuss current research and possible future therapeutics.

2. History of lung transplantation

Lung transplantation remains the final therapeutic option for treatment of patients with diverse diagnoses of end stage lung disease. (Arcasoy and Kotloff 1999) This however, has not always been the case. It was only within the last three decades that the medical community achieved reproducible outcomes that translated into clinical improvement in the condition of the patient. Vladimir Demikhov is considered by some to be the founder of the field due to his work in animal models in the mid 20th century, but it wasn't until 1963 that the first attempt at human lung transplantation occurred. (Cooper 1969; Hardy et al. 1963) This early trial was in a prisoner with both terminal lung cancer, and severe emphysema. Unfortunately, the patient died a mere 18 days post-transplantation. (Cooper 1969) It was almost another two decades before the first successful heart-lung transplantation was performed resulting in the multi-year survival of the recipient. This 1981 triumph was followed up by a group out of Toronto that proved once and for all that the one-time pipe dream of regular lung transplantation in humans was, in fact, a reality. (Cooper et al. 1987)

It was in the early 1990s that a comparative "transplant boom" began and has since leveled off to the approximately 2,700/year lung transplants performed worldwide today. (Orens and Garrity 2009) The relatively limited number (compared to other whole organ transplant procedures) of lung transplantations is a factor of limited supply of acceptable organs and ability to procure donor tissue. (Dilling and Glanville 2011) Unfortunately, it is because of this dearth of patients that few multi-center trials have been performed to assist in the investigation of better pre-, peri-, and post-operative techniques. However, with the increase in surgeries seen in the 1990s, serious efforts at reducing the risk factors associated with lung transplantation were initiated.

3. Selection of candidates

The majority of this chapter will deal with the complications and efforts to reduce them post-transplantation, but we will briefly touch on steps that have been implemented to reduce risk exposure prior to surgery. These preventative steps begin with a strict limitation on those who are eligible for transplant. Typically, individuals 55 and older are considered unsuitable for operation; although the mean age of recipients has been steadily increasing (it is currently over 50). (Dilling and Glanville 2011) Multiple organ failure, history of non-compliance, active/recent cigarette smoking, and active cancer are all contraindications for enrolling a patient in the United Network for Organ Sharing (UNOS). (Maurer et al. 1998) One of the most important factors that clinicians must consider when evaluating a patient for transplantation is the infection state of the possible recipient. While most bacterial and/or viral colonizations are permissible, there are many transplant centers that refuse to operate on patients with unremitting infection with pan-resistant *P. aeruginosa* and *B. cepacia*. Even so, there is at least one group out of Canada that is willing to consider transplantation of this patient population. (Nash et al. 2010; Flume et al. 1994) Prior to 2005, the allocation of lungs in the United States was dependant solely on waiting time; those who had been on the list longer were given priority over newly enrolled patients. Unfortunately, this obviously created a selection bias against the acutely ill. In 2005 the Lung Allocation System underwent an overhaul, utilizing a Lung Allocation Score (LAS) to determine those patients that were both most in need of transplantation, and most likely to survive the surgery and excel in recovery. (Egan et al. 2006) The new LAS system includes a number of factors (age, 6 minute walk test, forced vital capacity (FVC), body mass index (BMI), etc) to determine the patient's predicted waitlist survival time. The LAS is equal to (Calculated 1 year survival benefit) - (Calculated 1 year waiting list survival). (Morton and Glanville 2009) Obviously, there are limitations to this type of allocation system; certain subjective metrics like functional status and diagnosis can affect the patient's LAS, but the new method of lung allocation appears to have had a beneficial effect on median survival time post-transplantation.

4. Selection of donor organs

4.1 Blood group matching and CMV status

All of the evaluations discussed above are recipient-focused mechanisms designed to facilitate better outcomes in lung transplantation, but perhaps some of the most important protocols in place are related to obtaining the most viable donor organ available. There are several factors that contribute to the difficulty of procuring optimal lungs. Due to the extremely limited time that lungs are able to endure ischemia (less than 6 hours), there is little opportunity to perform traditional human leukocyte antigen (HLA) matching. Physicians face an unfortunate catch-22; better HLA matching reduces incidence of chronic rejection, but increased ischemic time in turn leads to a higher propensity for rejection. (Brugiere et al. 2008) Blood groups, rather, are the primary method of histological matching, with consideration being given to size and cytomegalovirus (CMV) sero-status. However, this is somewhat disputed in a review of the heart-lung transplant patient population at Stanford. (Deuse et al. 2010) CMV sero-negative recipients are at a higher risk of developing CMV infection when miss-matched with sero-positive donors than those recipients that are already CMV sero-positive. CMV infection has shown to be immunomodulative; creating an increased risk of acute and chronic rejection, and infections. (Freeman 2009) Like other opportunistic infections, there is an increased risk of CMV disease with the use of immunosuppressive treatment, although CMV in turn increases the risk of rejection, defeating the intent of the immunosuppressive therapies. (Fishman et al. 2007) CMV infection is not only limited to lung transplant recipients and thus there have been significant efforts from all corners to establish a gold-standard of prevention and treatment for CMV disease in all transplant patients. In studies performed in kidney and liver recipients, investigators demonstrated a significant reduction in incidence of CMV disease and viremia, along with significant reduction in the number of opportunistic infections in patients treated with prophylactic valganciclovir. (Humar et al. 2010) Valganciclovir is currently considered the gold-standard in CMV prevention, but other DNA polymerase inhibitors, including ganciclovir and valacyclovir have been in use for several years with a smaller impact. (Zamora et al. 2004) Unfortunately, lung transplant recipients face a higher incidence of CMV infection than any other transplant patient population. This is for two primary reasons; first, CMV dormancy and recurrence have been shown to be higher in the lungs than anywhere else, and, unlike other whole organ transplant surgeries, there is a preponderance of lymphatic tissue transplanted with the lungs that contains further amounts of dormant virus. (Zamora, Davis, and Leonard 2005)

4.2 Other donor factors

Although blood group matching and CMV sero-status are two of the most important criteria when evaluating potential donor lungs, there are a multiple other factors surgeons must consider when assessing a possible donor organ. Traditionally it has been protocol to decline any lungs from donors positive for hepatitis B, even so, recent work has cracked open the door to this pool of donors, potentially increasing the donor pool and number of available organs. A 1-year longitudinal study showed no significant difference in survival of hepatitis B positive donor lung recipients compared to the hepatitis B sero-negative group. (Dhillon et al. 2009) The physicians must also take into account something as simple as time and distance when determining the possibility of performing the potentially life-altering operation. Lungs, like any other tissue, are susceptible to ischemia-reperfusion (IR) injury and the flood of damaging cytokines that go along with it. Primary graft dysfunction, which can occur in up to 20% of patients, has been directly attributed to IR injury. (Christie, Sager et al. 2005) In addition to this, the lungs are more readily affected by the abundance of fluids that are typically given in end of life situations. (Arcasoy and Kotloff 1999) Current thinking is that non-heart beating donors (NHBD) are ill suited for the harvesting of lungs due to the perceived damage that warm extended periods of ischemia would incur. This has been challenged, however by a group in Canada demonstrating no ill-adverse effects from the use of this here-to-for off-limits pool of potential donor candidates. They state that there is an ameliorative effect on the levels of inflammatory cytokines present in these lungs which off sets the perceived ischemic damage. (Cypel et al. 2009)

Donor age is another consideration that is factored in when considering possible transplantation. Not surprisingly, elevated donor age and increased ischemic times correlate with worse outcomes in transplant recipients. (Meyers and Patterson 2000) While not optimal, there is such a shortage of available donors, NHBDs over the age of 60 now represent over 10% of the NHBD donor population. (Ojo et al. 1999) There are several techniques available to try and optimize the donor lung, but most common are the use of vasopressin, and thyroid hormone. (Botha et al. 2008) Finally, brain dead (BD) donors represent a potential donor pool that presents its own unique set of possible complications. In animal models of BD, investigators observed a three fold increase in the blood volume in the pulmonary circulation within minutes after onset of BD. (Avlonitis et al. 2005) This, in concert with loss of sympathetic tone, contributes heavily to a rapid onset of pulmonary edema which in and of itself is enough to dissuade many surgeons from considering using the tissue. Furthermore, several groups have reported a significant increase in the concentrations of pro-inflammatory cytokines such as interleukin-1 (IL-1), IL-2, IL-6, and tumor necrosis factor-alpha (TNFα). (Skrabal et al. 2005; Pratschke et al. 2000; Shohami et al. 1994) Additionally, the neutrophil chemokine, IL-8, has also been demonstrated to be elevated in the lungs of BD lung donors. (Fisher et al. 1999) Increased neutrophil burden has been strongly associated with increased matrix-metalloprotease activity and possible exposure of the auto-antigen collagen V (Coll V). (Fisher et al. 2001; Hardison 2009) The exposure of Coll V directly correlates with the incidence of primary graft dysfunction. (Iwata et al. 2008)

All of the considerations discussed contribute to the limited number of lung transplants that are performed each year, but the lack of family consent is by far the largest obstacle to available donor organs. (Spital 2005) Since it is unlikely that an automatic-enrollment system similar to other countries is likely, it is vital that the best efforts are made to elucidate the mechanisms behind the numerous and varied complications inherent in lung transplantation by both basic scientists and clinicians alike. The litany of assessments and interventions discussed thus far are all employed to attempt to prevent the plethora of post-transplantation complications that can arise. The unfortunate reality is that while surgical techniques and medical therapeutics are far more advanced and elegant than when the initial forays in lung transplantation occurred, there is still ample room for improving the outcomes observed in lung transplant recipients. The remainder of this chapter will discuss post-transplantation complications, current therapies, recent research in the field, and the exciting possibilities for novel therapeutics that are on the horizon.

5. Post transplantation complications

Due to the myriad of risk factors associated with lung transplantation, it has one of the highest morbidity and mortality rates of any whole organ transplant procedure. (Trulock et al. 2007) Only recently has the mean survival time for transplant recipients risen to 5.7 years. (Ahmad, Shlobin, and Nathan 2011) There are four major causes of morbidity and mortality in all transplant recipients; primary allograft dysfunction, infection, acute rejection, and chronic rejection. These four primary causes are closely related; rather they exist on a spectrum with the incidence of chronic rejection (the most serious) rising with increasing occurrences of the PGD, infection and acute rejection.

5.1 Primary graft dysfunction

5.1.1 Characterization and etiology

Primary graft dysfunction (PGD) is defined as having a **PaO_2/Fi** O_2 of ≤ ~300 with radiographic infiltrates consistent with pulmonary edema. (Christie, Carby et al. 2005) PGD is further categorized into 3 gradations with Grades 1, 2 and 3 corresponding to **PaO_2/Fi** O_2 greater than 300, between 200 and 300, and less than 200, respectively. Clinically, PGD is simply a unique form of acute lung injury (ALI), presenting within 72 hours post-surgery with replete pulmonary infiltrates/edema and impaired compliance. These guidelines for evaluating PGD were initially put forth in 2005 by the International Society for Heart and Lung Transplantation (ISHLT) Working Group on PGD and later confirmed by a retrospective study of approximately 400 lung transplant recipients. This study demonstrated that PGD grade 3 did indeed correlate with the worst mortality. (Prekker et al. 2006) PGD can affect up to 25% of patients and correlates with much higher levels of mortality in the first 30 days. (Christie et al. 2005) The precise cause(s) of PGD are still unknown, but it is widely accepted that ischemia-reperfusion (IR) injury plays a major role in initiating the destructive process. It is in the ischemic period that reactive oxygen species (ROS) are produced in large quantities and directly damage the pulmonary epithelium and endothelium. (Tasoulis et al. 2009; de Perrot et al. 2003) This influx of ROS incites a pro-inflammatory cascade that activates both the innate and complement immune systems. (Carter, Gelman, and Kreisel 2008)

5.1.2 Risk factors for PGD

Advanced age of organ donors is strongly associated with increased incidence of PGD in lung transplant recipients. What is interesting is that no definitive studies have been performed that indicate that recipients' age play any role in the development of PGD. (Barr et al. 2005; Christie et al. 2003) Additionally, race (African-American), sex (female), and smoking history are all donor-dependent risk factors in the development of PGD. (Lee and Christie 2009) No conclusive studies of transplant recipients have explicitly delineated whether indication for transplantation correlates with development but it appears that idiopathic pulmonary fibrosis confers at least some increased risk of PGD. (Barr et al. 2005) Pulmonary arterial hypertension (PAH) has emerged as the only clinically measureable metric that correlates with the development of primary graft dysfunction. While the precise pathway of PAH to PGD is as yet unknown, multiple studies have demonstrated the relationship. (Whitson et al. 2006)

5.1.3 Treatment of PGD

Although over-used to the point of being a cliché, the maxim "an ounce of prevention is worth a pound of cure" is distinctly applicable to the treatment of primary graft dysfunction. Increasing emphasis is being placed on improved preservation of the donor organ. The main weapon in the clinician's arsenal of preservative techniques is induced hypothermia of the tissue. It has been demonstrated that by maintaining the organ at 4°C, the metabolic rate is drastically reduced compared to that of control temperature tissue. (de Perrot et al. 2005) Two methods of organ cooling are typically employed; core cooling and pulmonary arterial flush (PAF). (Okada and Kondo 2009) The core cooling method occurs prior to organ explantation and is initiated with cardio-pulmonary bypass to reduce the body temperature to ~14°C. Upon harvesting, the donor lungs are submerged in 4°C saline.

PAF is accomplished by instilling 60ml/kg into the pulmonary artery, there have been some recent studies investigating the effects of a dual flush with the addition of flushing the pulmonary veins as well. The hypothesis being that this would ensure the complete removal of micro-thrombi in the capillaries and result in a more equitable distribution of the preservative solution. (Struber et al. 2002) There are several different "recipes" of preservative solution but the first in wide use (Euro-Collins solution), with high a high K^+ and low Na^+ concentrations to mimic intracellular fluid, was originally developed for use in liver preservation. (Okada and Kondo 2009) Since then, more sophisticated preservation solutions have been developed and are in the process of being tested. The Okada group developed a solution termed extra-cellular phosphate buffered saline type 4 (Ep4) that included dextran 40. This solution was capable of preserving canine lungs for up to 96 hrs post-explantation. Dextran 40 appeared to exert an anti-coagulative effect, ostensibly by forming a protective coat on the endothelial surface. (Handa et al. 1989; Okada et al. 1997; Colombat et al. 2004)
Sadly, if efforts to prevent the development of primary graft dysfunction fail, the similarity to acute lung injury (ALI) and acute respiratory distress syndrome (ARDS) results in little that the clinician can do other than provide supportive care. Due to the increased concentration of pro-inflammatory cytokines in the pulmonary circulation it is of vital importance that fluid administration is closely monitored to decrease the risk of fulminant edema. (Shargall et al. 2005) In addition to the vigilance given to the administration of fluids in PGD patients, ventilator settings can play a major role in outcomes of those individuals. A multicenter, randomized, controlled trial demonstrated that lower tidal volumes, combined with elevated positive end expiratory pressure (PEEP) were significantly protective in individuals with ARDS. The authors of the study hypothesize that this was due to the decreased alveolar damage in the hyper-compliant lungs. (Petrucci and Iacovelli 2003)

5.1.4 Current research and future directions

Much of the current research in this area is focused on the development of better therapeutics and the identification of biomarkers in PGD to provide a deeper knowledge of the genetic and biochemical forces that are integral in the genesis of the condition. With the recent advances made in high through-put proteomics and DNA micro-array technology there are ample platforms to rapidly pursue numerous avenues of investigation in great detail.

5.1.4.1 Potential Biomarkers of PGD

A 2006 study by Kaneda et al, utilizing quantitative real time polymerase chain reaction (qPCR) revealed that the IL-6/IL-10 ratio in the donor lung was predictive of 30 day mortality in the transplant recipient. (Kaneda et al. 2006) Luminex analysis of blood samples from 25 Grade 3 PGD patients and 25 Grade 0 control patients by Hoffman, et al revealed a vastly different chemokine profile in the two population's plasma. Severe PGD patients had significantly elevated levels of monocyte chemotactic protein-1 (MCP1) and CXC motif ligand 10 (CXCL10) compared to controls. (Hoffman et al. 2009) The detection of novel biomarkers is not limited to new sophisticated techniques, more traditional approaches also have also yielded results. Indeed, a recent study by Diamond, et al, using a conventional "sandwich" enzyme linked immunosorbent assay (ELISA) provided evidence that increased Clara cell secretory protein 16 (CC16) was significantly associated with the development of PGD. (Diamond et al. 2011) There are numerous other studies that have produced a litany of possible biomarkers (soluble receptor for advanced glycosylation end-products (sRAGE), soluble P-selectin, Protein C, etc.) for primary graft dysfunction and that may one day provide the key to its early detection and prevention. (Kawut et al. 2009; Christie et al. 2007; Christie et al. 2009)

5.1.4.2 Novel/Future Therapeutics for PGD

The goal of those developing novel therapeutics for PGD is the prevention of the condition itself. A multi-center, randomized, placebo controlled trial by Keshavjee, et al showed a protective effect in the use of soluble complement receptor-1 (sCR1) resulting in decreased time to extubation and a trend toward abbreviated intensive care unit (ICU) stays. (Keshavjee et al. 2005) In an intriguing study by Eriksson, and colleagues, induced hypothermia appeared to be beneficial in case studies of PGD patients and was recapitulated in an animal model. (Eriksson and Steen 1998; Eriksson et al. 1999) Significant forays into the use of inhaled Nitric Oxide (iNO) as a therapeutic agent have also been made in recent years. There have been discordant results, however as to the efficacy, ranging from no change in outcomes to a decreased incidence of severe PGD and diminished concentrations of IL-6 and IL-8 in plasma compared to controls. (Meade et al. 2003; Ardehali et al. 2001) Due to the prevalence of PGD in lung transplant recipients, and the comparative lack of knowledge regarding the pathogenesis of this condition, it is reasonable to expect considerable resources to continue to be directed toward the investigation and prevention of this syndrome.

5.2 Infection

5.2.1 Characterization and etiology

Infection in post lung transplantation begins as any other infection, however with the host being in the unenviable position of possessing immune systems under active and permanent suppression, in addition to the mechanical and physiologic stress that is inherent to any major surgery. Infection is, in fact, the primary source of mortality in the first year post-transplant and continues to be a significant source of morbidity and mortality for the remainder of the recipient's life. (Corris and Christie 2008) Unlike all other solid organ transplants, the lungs are open to the external environment and all of the pathogens, both virulent and opportunistic, that entails. Furthermore, the denervation that is a necessary component of organ harvesting results in at least a temporary impairment in the cough reflex and thus diminished clearance. (Ahmad, Shlobin, and Nathan 2011) It is important to note that any infection, particularly recurrent infection, is a risk factor for the occurrence of rejection, both acute and chronic. Rapid identification of the pathogen and appropriate treatment is optimal to decrease morbidity and mortality in this patient population.

5.2.2 Bacterial infection

Bacterial infections are the most common type of infection in lung transplant recipients and occur in a bi-modal, temporal-dependant manner. Pulmonary bacterial infections are common both early, due to the previously mentioned impaired cough reflex and damaged lymphatic system, and late, as an element of chronic rejection. (Kramer et al. 1993) Due to the nature of the pre-transplant disease, those patients with cystic fibrosis (CF) are the most difficult to maintain in an infection free state. This is especially true in the individual with a single lung transplant due to the potential for colonization from the native lung. Interestingly, the CF patient population also has the best long-term results despite the proclivity towards infection. (Lease and Zaas 2010)

Pseudomonas aeruginosa is the most common bacterial organism isolated from the post-transplant lung. (Kramer et al. 1993) This opportunistic infection has a higher incidence in CF patients and has been estimated to be responsible for up to 33% of pneumonias in all transplant recipients. (Aguilar-Guisado et al. 2007; Campos et al. 2008) *P. aeruginosa* airway infection prior to transplant does not appear to demonstrate a predictive relationship for chronic rejection. However, this is not the case for colonization in the post-operative period. (Botha et al. 2008; Vos et al. 2008) *P. aeruginosa* infection is not limited to pneumonias; the pathogen has been reported to be responsible for nearly half of all post-transplant infections. (Valentine et al. 2008)

Mycobacterium is a designation indicating acid-fast bacteria that are capable of causing a wide range of diseases. Perhaps the most well known of these *M. tuberculosis*, has the robust cell wall that is a calling card of the classification, and helps to confer resistance to broad spectrum antibiotics. Although, not nearly as common as *P. aeruginosa* infection, *M. tuberculosis* colonization presents a unique set of treatment hurdles, especially in the presence of multi-drug resistant (MDR) strains. (Lee et al. 2003)

Opportunistic infections, hospital-acquired infections, and resistant strains of bacteria are all significantly more common in lung transplant recipients than the general population. *Staphylococci* strains have demonstrated a propensity for antibiotic resistance and this is only magnified in the already immunosuppressed transplant patient. Specifically, *S. aureus* is the second most common organism isolated from the airway, with multi-drug resistant *S. aureus* (MRSA) being extremely difficult to treat due to its almost pan-resistant nature. (Kotloff and Thabut 2011)

5.2.3 Treatment of bacterial infection

The treatment of infection in lung transplant recipients is a challenging task due to the patients' significant cocktail of immunosuppressive therapies. Many of these drugs, including cyclosporine and tacrolimus can be highly cross-reactive. There is unfortunately no "magic bullet" specific for transplant patients, the traditional regimen of broad spectrum antibiotics, with specific coverage for gram negative, acid-fast, etc. being added upon differential diagnosis.

5.2.4 Fungal infection

While colonization by widespread fungi such as *Aspergillus* and *Candida* is common, a much smaller percentage of patients will develop a clinically relevant fungal infection. (Singh 2003) *Aspergillus* and *Candida* are by far the most common, with *Cryptococcus* species and other molds playing a much smaller role. (Neofytos et al. 2010) The presence of foreign material (sutures) in the airway anastomosis, in addition to the inherent risk with ventilation, increases the risk of fungal infection in post-operative transplant patients.

5.2.5 Prevention/treatment of fungal infection

Similar to the treatment of bacterial infections, the therapeutic approach to fungal infection in lung transplant patients is primarily unchanged from the normal treatment options in other patients. Treatment regimens will typically consist of aerosolized Amphotericin B in the acute post-operative period, with voriconazole and itraconazole prophylactic treatment extending for up to a year post-transplantation. (Ahmad, Shlobin, and Nathan 2011)

5.2.6 Viral infection

As has previously been mentioned, the sero-status of cytomegalovirus (CMV) is an important factor in opting to transplant or harvest donor organs. CMV is by far the most common viral pathogen observed after lung transplant procedures, affecting at least a third of all patients. CMV usually presents with fever, exhaustion, and flu-like symptoms with associated leukopenia. (Snydman et al. 2011) Diagnosis of CMV syndrome is made with PCR evaluation of viral titers in peripheral blood. If CMV pneumonia is suspected, the definitive test must be performed on a biopsy specimen of the in tissue. (Kotton et al. 2010) CMV infection has been shown to predispose the patient to infection with other community acquired respiratory viruses (CARVs). (Sims and Blumberg 2011)

In a recent three year longitudinal study, Kumar et al showed the presence of virulent strains of H1N1 influenza, adenovirus, flu A, flu B, and rhinovirus in over half of transplant recipients. (Kumar et al. 2010) Diagnosis of these viral infections has become much more straightforward with the advent of qPCR to provide rapid evaluation of viral titer loads in bronchoalveolar lavage (BAL) fluid of patients. Antibody based assays are also available to determine the infection state of an individual, although these may vary from center to center.

5.2.7 Prevention/treatment of viral infection

Intravenous (IV) ganciclovir and the oral pro-drug valganciclovir are given prophylactically for anywhere from 6 to 12 months post-transplant. (Jaksch et al. 2009) CMV prophylaxis is standard protocol for all patients regardless of center and has been shown to be effective in reducing the CMV syndrome. (Palmer et al. 2010) Treatment for CARVs is dependant upon specific diagnosis of pathogen and strain and can include zanamivir, amantidine, oseltamivir, etc. (Ison and Michaels 2009) Unlike CMV therapy, prolonged treatment with these anti-virals is contraindicated for fear of contributing to the development of resistance.

5.3 Acute rejection

5.3.1 Characterization/etiology of acute rejection

Acute rejection (AR) presents clinically with non-specific symptoms including dyspnea, mild fever, malaise, cough, and leukocytosis. Although not present in all AR exacerbations, radiographic imaging may show mild pleural effusion, and interstitial opacities with a concurrent decline in oxygenation and spirometric measurements. (Millet et al. 1989; Otulana et al. 1990) AR is definitively diagnosed by BAL and TBB followed by histological analysis showing perivascular infiltrates. (Stewart et al. 2007) TBB may not always be possible due to patient status and thus AR is tentatively determined based upon clinical symptoms and radiologic evidence. Many transplant centers have post-transplant protocols that include routine monitoring by BAL which is also capable of confirming AR. (Chakinala et al. 2004) Most importantly, as indicated by the name, acute rejection is just that, a brief intermittent condition that is most often easily resolved with or without hospitalization.

Acute rejection is an extremely common complication of lung transplant patients, occurring in as many as 90% of lung recipients over their lifespan. (Arcasoy 2004) The incidence of AR is highest within the first year post-transplant, afflicting approximately one third of all patients. (Christie et al.) It is difficult to determine precise results in these retrospective studies due to the fact that AR can be clinically silent, only detectable upon transbronchiole biopsy (TBB). (Hopkins et al. 2002) The precise etiology of AR is still unknown but stratified risk appears to be heavily weighted toward donor-dependent factors in the immediate postoperative period, with recipient-dependent factors playing the predominant role after the first year. HLA-B mismatching, increasing donor age, non-O donor blood type, and increasing body-surface area (most likely corresponding to elevated BMI) all correspond with increased AR incidence. With a recipient history of diabetes, and recent transplant accounting for recipient driven risk in the intermediate and late phase AR. (Mangi et al. 2011)

The International Society for Heart-Lung Transplantation (ISHLT) has delineated the standard nomenclature to describe the various gradations of AR based solely on histological findings. Grade A0 is the absence of AR, no cellular infiltrates and healthy lung parenchyma. Grade A1 is characterized by patchy mononuclear cell infiltrates in alveolar parenchyma. Grade A2 is described as having more prevalent lymphocytic infiltrates centered in the perivascular area with the presence of some activated macrophages and eosinophils. Grade A3 features dense perivascular infiltrates, significant eosinophil presence, with the first observation of neutrophils in the intra-alveolar space. Grade A4 describes the finding of diffuse mononuclear infiltrates, pneumocyte damage, macrophage and neutrophil presence. (Stewart et al. 2007)

5.3.2 Treatment of acute rejection

Similar to many aspects of lung transplantation, treatment for AR varies dependant upon hospital setting with some centers opting to not treat AR considered to be <Grade A2. (Orens and Garrity 2009) In more severe cases however, conventional treatment consists of a hospital admission with a three day course of solumedrol followed by an oral prednisone taper. (Aboyoun et al. 2001; Yousem et al. 1994) Additional treatment with methotrexate, lymphoid irradiation, and antithymocyte globulin, among others, has been reported to be effective in alleviating the transient AR condition. (Hachem 2009)

5.3.3 Biomarkers of acute rejection

Although ISHLT has defined acute rejection based solely upon histological findings, there is significant effort to describe biomarkers specific to patients undergoing AR to better classify and determine treatment. A recent study by a group out of Copenhagen described elevated mRNA of the regulatory T cell (Treg) cytokine FoxP3, along with cytotoxic T cell-derived granzyme B in BAL fluid of patients in AR. (Madsen et al. 2010) A 2007 study by Lande et al describes the use of microarray analysis to observe relative gene expression levels of cytokines thought in be involved in acute rejection in the BAL fluid of AR patients. (Lande et al. 2007)

5.3.4 Novel/future therapeutics of acute rejection

Due to the incredible amounts of data generated by high through methods such as mass-spectrometry-assisted proteomics and gene microarray analysis there have never been more targets identified for the design of targeted therapeutics in acute rejection. The use of animal models of acute rejection have also significantly improved the ability to design and test novel therapeutics for acute rejection allograft rejection in lung transplantation.

Jung et al (2006) have developed a spontaneous model of acute rejection in rats by performing lung transplantation in a manner similar to that used in humans. By utilizing a small molecule, irreversible inhibitor of dipeptidylpeptidase IV (DPPIV/CD26) the investigators reduced the incidence of acute rejection, preserved lung function, and maintained normal histological structure in rat lung transplantees. (Jung et al. 2006) They previously published that DPPIV/CD26 was elevated in plasma of rats undergoing AR after cardiac transplant and hypothesize that the pulmonary protective effect is due to reducing the co-stimulatory effect of DPPIV/CD26 on T cells. (Korom et al. 1997) In a similar model, a group out of Fukouka, Japan employed a Janus kinase 3 (Jak3) inhibitor to prevent the development of AR. Jak3 is located at a biochemical bottleneck in the pathway of T cell clonal expansion. Higuchi, et al demonstrated a dose-dependant inhibition of the development of acute rejection by the AG490 in the experimental population. (Higuchi et al. 2005)

Animal models are not the only avenue available to scientists to pursue better methods of treating and preventing acute rejection. Investigators at the University Clinics of Leipzig reported a reduction in the incidence of acute rejection with preemptive administration of the traditional therapeutic methylprednisone. By simply giving bolus doses 2 hours prior to incision and immediately prior to completion of the transplant procedure they observed a significant improvement in outcomes. (Bittner et al. 2010)

Clearly this is not meant to be an exhaustive review of the potential novel therapeutics currently under development. We are merely presenting a representative sample indicating the myriad of pathways that are being studied to yield targeted countermeasures to acute rejection.

5.4 Chronic rejection (bronchiolitis obliterans syndrome)

5.4.1 Characterization/etiology of bronchiolitis obliterans syndrome

Chronic rejection, clinically termed bronchiolitis obliterans syndrome (BOS), is the primary source of morbidity and mortality seen in the lung transplant patient population. (Bando et al. 1995; Stewart et al. 2007) Due to the nature of BOS, primarily occurring irregularly in the small airways, diagnosis by transbronchial biopsy is ineffective. (Chamberlain et al. 1994) Diagnosis of BOS is difficult due to its similarities with other post-transplant complications. There are no tests to specifically determine BOS, rather, it is a diagnosis of exclusion. A persistent, unexplainable drop in forced expiratory volume in one second (FEV1) (~80% of baseline) with accompanying decline in FEV25-75 (less than or equal to 75% of baseline) is defined as BOS stage 0. (Belperio et al. 2009; Estenne et al. 2002) BOS is staged 0-3 based upon progressive declines in percent of expected FEV1.

BOS is unfortunately observed in over half of lung transplant patients who survive five years or more post-transplantation. (Bando et al. 1995) Chronic rejection initially presents clinically in a manner similar to that of other complications with dyspnea, cough, and progressive airway obstruction. (Estenne and Hertz 2002) X-ray analysis is often unremarkable, but computer assisted tomography (CT) may reveal air trapping and bronchiectasis. (Morrish et al. 1991)

BOS is characterized pathologically by a prominent neutrophilic component with a definite increase in pulmonary fibrosis and extra-cellular remodeling. (Billings et al. 2002; Boehler and Estenne 2003) The BAL fluid of the majority of BOS patients reveals chronic pulmonary neutrophilia. Indeed, when >20% of cells are neutrophils in BAL fluid patients fail to survive past 7 years post-transplant. (Neurohr et al. 2009) Unlike acute rejection, where the cellular infiltrates are centered around the vasculature, in BOS, the cells are located primarily in and around the airways with a striking increase in cell number and activation level of leukocytes. (Vanaudenaerde et al. 2008) The causes of BOS are only partially understood with much unknown about the exact causative events that lead to disease.

5.4.2 Risk Factors for bronchiolitis obliterans syndrome

What facts are known about the pathogenesis of BOS are the multiple risk factors that have been detailed via epidemiologic investigations. Both alloimmune and alloimmune-independent factors appear to play principle roles in the development of BOS. (Knoop and Estenne 2006) Primary graft dysfunction, along with gastroesophageal reflux (GER), and infection are all nonalloimmune factors that are associated with occurrence of BOS. (Estenne and Hertz 2002) CMV infection resulting in disease has been reported to enhance the relative risk of developing BOS, although there are conflicting reports regarding this. (Belperio et al. 2009) Alloimmune factors closely associated with BOS are recurrent, or persistent AR, and HLA mismatching. (Palmer et al. 2002)

5.4.3 Treatment of bronchiolitis obliterans syndrome

Currently there are no demonstrated effective treatments for BOS. Most present strategies rely on augmenting immunosuppression with the use of corticosteroids, cyclosporine, methotrexate, etc. (Date et al. 1998; Dusmet et al. 1996; Iacono et al. 1996) These, however have been met with little success. The majority of existing treatment methods rely on unproven, anecdotal evidence with few multi-center, randomized, controlled trials.

5.4.4 Current research and future directions in bronchiolitis obliterans syndrome

Our previously published hypothesis regarding the onset of BOS is that there is some initial insult (infection by CMV or other pathogens, inflammatory damage due to recurrent AR, etc.) that awakens the adaptive immune system to over-ride the potent cocktail of immunosuppressive drugs present. The adaptive immune (Type 1, and Type 2 T cells) further damages the transplanted organ by responding to the foreign epitopes innately present in the donor lung. This repeated damage induces a persistent release of pro-inflammatory cytokines that recruit neutrophils into the interstitium and airways where they remain and participate in a fibroproliferative and proteolytically destructive process. (Hardison et al. 2009)

5.4.4.1 Potential Biomarkers in Bronchiolitis Obliterans Syndrome

We, along with others, have reported on the activation of neutrophils by glutamate-leucine-arginine positive (ELR+) CXC chemokines such as IL-8. (Xu et al. 2011; Chakrabarti and Patel 2005) Upon activation, neutrophils degranulate which releases potent proteases such as matrix metalloproteinase-8, -9, and prolyl endopeptidase. (Xu 2011, O'Reilly 2010) It has been well established that collagen fragments are chemotactic to neutrophils, and in 1995, Pfister et al. were able to determine the sequence, proline-glycine-proline (Pro-Gly-Pro, PGP) confers chemotactic potential to collagen breakdown products. (Pfister et al. 1995) In a 2006 paper, our group demonstrated the mechanism by which PGP is able to attract neutrophils into tissue. PGP shares significant sequence and structural homology with almost all ELR+CXC chemokines, which act via CXC receptors 1 and 2 in human (CXCR1, CXCR2). We reported that PGP competes with the CXCR ligand, IL-8, for binding, causes chemotaxis in CXCR transfected cells and elicits a similar oxidative burst to IL-8 stimulation. (Weathington et al. 2006) Recently we have also published the step-wise manner in which it is produced. (Gaggar et al. 2008)

MMP-8 and -9 are capable of initially digesting collagen but are incapable of performing the final cleavage to PGP and a second step is necessary for the matrikine's production. Our lab demonstrated that the serine protease prolyl endopeptidase (PE) performs the final proteolysis. (Gaggar et al. 2008) PE cleaves after a proline in a peptide of ~100 amino acids or less.

We have reported the potential for PGP as a biomarker of disease in multiple chronic inflammatory lung diseases such as cystic fibrosis (CF), chronic obstructive pulmonary disease (COPD), and most relevant to this manuscript, BOS. (Gaggar et al. 2007; O'Reilly et al. 2009; Hardison et al. 2009) In matched BAL samples of patients obtained three months prior to, and concurrent with diagnosis of BOS, we described a temporal shift in the chemokine/matrikine profile. MMP-8, -9 and PE activities were increased in the samples collected at diagnosis of BOS compared to a transplant control population, and matched samples collected prior to confirmation of disease. By employing a previously published mass spectrometry technique, we detected measureable amounts of PGP in both pre- and post-diagnosis of BOS, however, there was a dramatic and significant increase in the levels observed in BAL fluid collected at the time of diagnosis. Through the use of neutralizing antibodies to IL-8 and PGP, first individually and then in concert, we demonstrated a shift from the relative importance of the classical PMN chemoattractant, IL-8, to the more novel molecule, PGP, upon diagnosis of BOS.

Clearly PGP is not the only molecule with the potential to serve as a novel biomarker for BOS diagnosis. There is a litany of research underway on a wide variety of proteins and cell types that may potentially one day play a role in the more precise classification of this condition. Endothelin-1, mesenchymal stromal cells, and serum KL-6 (a glycoprotein) have all been published as possible markers of disease progression. (Salama et al. 2011; Badri et al. 2011; Haberman et al. 2010)

5.4.4.2 Current Research in Bronchiolitis Obliterans Syndrome

Perhaps the most exciting development in the quest for reliable preventative therapy for BOS has been the recent establishment of reproducible rodent models of BOS which closely mimic human disease. The most recent model described by Jungraithmayr, et al., utilizing single lung transplantation, is a vast improvement over the traditional tracheal transplant which had the obvious limitation of leaving the native lung in the rodent. (Jungraithmayr et al. 2010) The Swiss group reports that a T cell response and cytokine presence, similar to that of humans with BOS, was observed. Another group, from the University of Pittsburgh, has developed a human-mouse chimeric model of BOS in which the allograft and immune effector cells are of human origin. (Xue et al. 2011) They state that the formation of chimeric allogenic T cells, and the resulting infiltration into small human airways is definitive in delineating the role T cells play in the development of BOS.

5.4.4.3 Future Therapeutics for Bronchiolitis Obliterans Syndrome

This is, in part, a continuation of the previous section due to the experimental nature of some of the procedures/drugs described herein. As was previously discussed, there is an association of GER and BOS incidence. A study out of Duke University describes improved pulmonary function in patients who underwent proactive treatment for GER. Surgical fundoplication was performed to reduce the possibility of bile aspiration and potential damage to the airway. (Davis et al. 2003) Additionally, a retrospective study of transplant recipients with BOS identified a possible advantage of treatment with Azithromycin (Az), though the mechanism of action remains unclear. (Jain et al. 2010) Patients with a higher initial neutrophil burden responded better to the treatment and had better outcomes. What is most interesting is the fact that azithromycin is a macrolide antibiotic, a class known to be

inhibitors of matrix metalloproteinases. It is possible that Az is preventing the generation of PGP and thus relieving some of the neutrophil burden associated with BOS.
A recent publication by our group in *Science* detailed a bi-functional enzyme, Leukotriene A4 Hydrolase (LTA4H), which serves to degrade PGP endogenously. This enzyme is present in both neutrophils and airway epithelium and is elevated in a mouse model of pulmonary infection and inflammation. (Snelgrove et al. 2010) Modulation of the activity of this important enzyme may provide a welcome opportunity to utilize patients' own biology to help resolve some of the destructive chronic neutrophilic inflammation seen in BOS. We have also described two specific inhibitors of PGP, arginine-threonine-arginine (RTR), and an all "D" isomer of PGP (DD-PGP) that are potent in preventing the mechanism of action of PGP *in vitro* and *in vivo*. (Jackson et al. 2011; van Houwelingen et al. 2008)

6. Conclusion

Even though long-term survival of lung transplant recipients has improved over time, the overall mortality rate in lung transplantation remains significantly higher than any other whole organ transplant population. The relatively recent advent of a more appropriate organ allocation system, along with improved ability to preserve donor organs has increased the pool of available organs to all-time highs. Even so, the number of actual lungs harvested each year compared to the estimated viable donor lungs is a small fraction of what is possible. With continued advancement in animal models, and description of biomarkers of the various complications associated with transplantation, there has been marked, if gradual, improvements in the therapeutic armament clinicians have at their disposal. It may yet be that lung transplantation one day be viewed as an early intervention in progressive irreversible pulmonary conditions such as idiopathic pulmonary fibrosis and confer a permanent, rejuvenative improvement in the lifespan and quality of life of such patients.

7. References

Aboyoun, C. L., M. Tamm, P. N. Chhajed, P. Hopkins, M. A. Malouf, S. Rainer, and A. R. Glanville. 2001. Diagnostic value of follow-up transbronchial lung biopsy after lung rejection. *Am J Respir Crit Care Med* 164 (3):460-3.

Aguilar-Guisado, M., J. Givalda, P. Ussetti, A. Ramos, P. Morales, M. Blanes, G. Bou, J. de la Torre-Cisneros, A. Roman, J. M. Borro, R. Lama, and J. M. Cisneros. 2007. Pneumonia after lung transplantation in the RESITRA Cohort: a multicenter prospective study. *Am J Transplant* 7 (8):1989-96.

Ahmad, S., O. A. Shlobin, and S. D. Nathan. 2011. Pulmonary complications of lung transplantation. *Chest* 139 (2):402-11.

Arcasoy, S. M. 2004. Medical complications and management of lung transplant recipients. *Respir Care Clin N Am* 10 (4):505-29.

Arcasoy, S. M., and R. M. Kotloff. 1999. Lung transplantation. *N Engl J Med* 340 (14):1081-91.

Ardehali, A., H. Laks, M. Levine, R. Shpiner, D. Ross, L. D. Watson, O. Shvartz, S. Sangwan, and P. F. Waters. 2001. A prospective trial of inhaled nitric oxide in clinical lung transplantation. *Transplantation* 72 (1):112-5.

Avlonitis, V. S., C. H. Wigfield, J. A. Kirby, and J. H. Dark. 2005. The hemodynamic mechanisms of lung injury and systemic inflammatory response following brain death in the transplant donor. *Am J Transplant* 5 (4 Pt 1):684-93.

Badri, L., S. Murray, L. X. Liu, N. M. Walker, A. Flint, A. Wadhwa, K. M. Chan, G. B. Toews, D. J. Pinsky, F. J. Martinez, and V. N. Lama. 2011. Mesenchymal stromal cells in bronchoalveolar lavage as predictors of bronchiolitis obliterans syndrome. *Am J Respir Crit Care Med* 183 (8):1062-70.

Bando, K., I. L. Paradis, S. Similo, H. Konishi, K. Komatsu, T. G. Zullo, S. A. Yousem, J. M. Close, A. Zeevi, R. J. Duquesnoy, and et al. 1995. Obliterative bronchiolitis after lung and heart-lung transplantation. An analysis of risk factors and management. *J Thorac Cardiovasc Surg* 110 (1):4-13; discussion 13-4.

Barr, M. L., S. M. Kawut, T. P. Whelan, R. Girgis, H. Bottcher, J. Sonett, W. Vigneswaran, D. M. Follette, and P. A. Corris. 2005. Report of the ISHLT Working Group on Primary Lung Graft Dysfunction part IV: recipient-related risk factors and markers. *J Heart Lung Transplant* 24 (10):1468-82.

Belperio, J. A., S. S. Weigt, M. C. Fishbein, and J. P. Lynch, 3rd. 2009. Chronic lung allograft rejection: mechanisms and therapy. *Proc Am Thorac Soc* 6 (1):108-21.

Billings, J. L., M. I. Hertz, K. Savik, and C. H. Wendt. 2002. Respiratory viruses and chronic rejection in lung transplant recipients. *J Heart Lung Transplant* 21 (5):559-66.

Bittner, H. B., M. J. Barten, C. Binner, S. Lehmann, J. Garbade, S. Hammerschmidt, H. Wirtz, and F. W. Mohr. 2010. Preoperative introduction and maintenance immunosuppression therapy of oral-only tacrolimus, mycophenolate mofetil and steroids reduce acute rejection episodes after lung transplantation. *Eur J Cardiothorac Surg* 38 (3):268-76.

Boehler, A., and M. Estenne. 2003. Post-transplant bronchiolitis obliterans. *Eur Respir J* 22 (6):1007-18.

Botha, P., L. Archer, R. L. Anderson, J. Lordan, J. H. Dark, P. A. Corris, K. Gould, and A. J. Fisher. 2008. Pseudomonas aeruginosa colonization of the allograft after lung transplantation and the risk of bronchiolitis obliterans syndrome. *Transplantation* 85 (5):771-4.

Botha, P., A. J. Rostron, A. J. Fisher, and J. H. Dark. 2008. Current strategies in donor selection and management. *Semin Thorac Cardiovasc Surg* 20 (2):143-51.

Brugiere, O., G. Thabut, C. Suberbielle, M. Reynaud-Gaubert, P. Thomas, C. Pison, C. Saint Raymond, J. F. Mornex, M. Bertocchi, C. Dromer, J. F. Velly, M. Stern, B. Philippe, G. Dauriat, G. Biondi, Y. Castier, and M. Fournier. 2008. Relative impact of human leukocyte antigen mismatching and graft ischemic time after lung transplantation. *J Heart Lung Transplant* 27 (6):628-34.

Campos, S., M. Caramori, R. Teixeira, J. Afonso, Jr., R. Carraro, T. Strabelli, M. Samano, P. Pego-Fernandes, and F. Jatene. 2008. Bacterial and fungal pneumonias after lung transplantation. *Transplant Proc* 40 (3):822-4.

Carter, Y. M., A. E. Gelman, and D. Kreisel. 2008. Pathogenesis, management, and consequences of primary graft dysfunction. *Semin Thorac Cardiovasc Surg* 20 (2):165-72.

Chakinala, M. M., J. Ritter, B. F. Gage, J. P. Lynch, A. Aloush, G. A. Patterson, and E. P. Trulock. 2004. Yield of surveillance bronchoscopy for acute rejection and lymphocytic bronchitis/bronchiolitis after lung transplantation. *J Heart Lung Transplant* 23 (12):1396-404.

Chakrabarti, S., and K. D. Patel. 2005. Regulation of matrix metalloproteinase-9 release from IL-8-stimulated human neutrophils. *J Leukoc Biol* 78 (1):279-88.

Chamberlain, D., J. Maurer, C. Chaparro, and L. Idolor. 1994. Evaluation of transbronchial lung biopsy specimens in the diagnosis of bronchiolitis obliterans after lung transplantation. *J Heart Lung Transplant* 13 (6):963-71.

Christie, J. D., M. Carby, R. Bag, P. Corris, M. Hertz, and D. Weill. 2005. Report of the ISHLT Working Group on Primary Lung Graft Dysfunction part II: definition. A consensus statement of the International Society for Heart and Lung Transplantation. *J Heart Lung Transplant* 24 (10):1454-9.

Christie, J. D., L. B. Edwards, P. Aurora, F. Dobbels, R. Kirk, A. O. Rahmel, J. Stehlik, D. O. Taylor, A. Y. Kucheryavaya, and M. I. Hertz. 2009. The Registry of the International Society for Heart and Lung Transplantation: Twenty-sixth Official Adult Lung and Heart-Lung Transplantation Report-2009. *J Heart Lung Transplant* 28 (10):1031-49.

Christie, J. D., L. B. Edwards, A. Y. Kucheryavaya, P. Aurora, F. Dobbels, R. Kirk, A. O. Rahmel, J. Stehlik, and M. I. Hertz. The Registry of the International Society for Heart and Lung Transplantation: twenty-seventh official adult lung and heart-lung transplant report--2010. *J Heart Lung Transplant* 29 (10):1104-18.

Christie, J. D., R. M. Kotloff, A. Pochettino, S. M. Arcasoy, B. R. Rosengard, J. R. Landis, and S. E. Kimmel. 2003. Clinical risk factors for primary graft failure following lung transplantation. *Chest* 124 (4):1232-41.

Christie, J. D., N. Robinson, L. B. Ware, M. Plotnick, J. De Andrade, V. Lama, A. Milstone, J. Orens, A. Weinacker, E. Demissie, S. Bellamy, and S. M. Kawut. 2007. Association of protein C and type 1 plasminogen activator inhibitor with primary graft dysfunction. *Am J Respir Crit Care Med* 175 (1):69-74.

Christie, J. D., J. S. Sager, S. E. Kimmel, V. N. Ahya, C. Gaughan, N. P. Blumenthal, and R. M. Kotloff. 2005. Impact of primary graft failure on outcomes following lung transplantation. *Chest* 127 (1):161-5.

Christie, J. D., C. V. Shah, S. M. Kawut, N. Mangalmurti, D. J. Lederer, J. R. Sonett, V. N. Ahya, S. M. Palmer, K. Wille, V. Lama, P. D. Shah, A. Shah, A. Weinacker, C. S. Deutschman, B. A. Kohl, E. Demissie, S. Bellamy, and L. B. Ware. 2009. Plasma levels of receptor for advanced glycation end products, blood transfusion, and risk of primary graft dysfunction. *Am J Respir Crit Care Med* 180 (10):1010-5.

Colombat, M., Y. Castier, G. Leseche, P. Rufat, H. Mal, G. Thabut, M. Fournier, O. Groussard, C. Degott, and A. Couvelard. 2004. Early expression of adhesion molecules after lung transplantation: evidence for a role of aggregated P-selectin-positive platelets in human primary graft failure. *J Heart Lung Transplant* 23 (9):1087-92.

Cooper, D. K. 1969. Transplantation of the heart and both lungs. I. Historical review. *Thorax* 24 (4):383-90.

Cooper, J. D., F. G. Pearson, G. A. Patterson, T. R. Todd, R. J. Ginsberg, M. Goldberg, and W. A. DeMajo. 1987. Technique of successful lung transplantation in humans. *J Thorac Cardiovasc Surg* 93 (2):173-81.

Corris, P. A., and J. D. Christie. 2008. Update in transplantation 2007. *Am J Respir Crit Care Med* 177 (10):1062-7.

Cypel, M., M. Sato, E. Yildirim, W. Karolak, F. Chen, J. Yeung, C. Boasquevisque, V. Leist, L. G. Singer, K. Yasufuku, M. Deperrot, T. K. Waddell, S. Keshavjee, and A. Pierre. 2009. Initial experience with lung donation after cardiocirculatory death in Canada. *J Heart Lung Transplant* 28 (8):753-8.

Date, H., J. P. Lynch, S. Sundaresan, G. A. Patterson, and E. P. Trulock. 1998. The impact of cytolytic therapy on bronchiolitis obliterans syndrome. *J Heart Lung Transplant* 17 (9):869-75.

Davis, R. D., Jr., C. L. Lau, S. Eubanks, R. H. Messier, D. Hadjiliadis, M. P. Steele, and S. M. Palmer. 2003. Improved lung allograft function after fundoplication in patients with gastroesophageal reflux disease undergoing lung transplantation. *J Thorac Cardiovasc Surg* 125 (3):533-42.

de Perrot, M., R. S. Bonser, J. Dark, R. F. Kelly, D. McGiffin, R. Menza, O. Pajaro, S. Schueler, and G. M. Verleden. 2005. Report of the ISHLT Working Group on Primary Lung Graft Dysfunction part III: donor-related risk factors and markers. *J Heart Lung Transplant* 24 (10):1460-7.

de Perrot, M., M. Liu, T. K. Waddell, and S. Keshavjee. 2003. Ischemia-reperfusion-induced lung injury. *Am J Respir Crit Care Med* 167 (4):490-511.

Demikhov, Vladimir. 1950. A new and simpler variant of heart-lung preparation of a warm-blooded mammal. *Bull Eksperimentalnoi Biologii i medicini* 24:383-390.

Deuse, T., R. Sista, D. Weill, D. Tyan, F. Haddad, G. Dhillon, R. C. Robbins, and B. A. Reitz. 2010. Review of heart-lung transplantation at Stanford. *Ann Thorac Surg* 90 (1):329-37.

Dhillon, G. S., J. Levitt, H. Mallidi, V. G. Valentine, M. R. Gupta, R. Sista, and D. Weill. 2009. Impact of hepatitis B core antibody positive donors in lung and heart-lung transplantation: an analysis of the United Network For Organ Sharing Database. *Transplantation* 88 (6):842-6.

Diamond, J. M., S. M. Kawut, D. J. Lederer, V. N. Ahya, B. Kohl, J. Sonett, S. M. Palmer, M. Crespo, K. Wille, V. N. Lama, P. D. Shah, J. Orens, S. Bhorade, A. Weinacker, E. Demissie, S. Bellamy, J. D. Christie, and L. B. Ware. 2011. Elevated plasma clara cell secretory protein concentration is associated with high-grade primary graft dysfunction. *Am J Transplant* 11 (3):561-7.

Dilling, D. F., and A. R. Glanville. 2011. Advances in lung transplantation: the year in review. *J Heart Lung Transplant* 30 (3):247-51.

Dusmet, M., J. Maurer, T. Winton, and S. Kesten. 1996. Methotrexate can halt the progression of bronchiolitis obliterans syndrome in lung transplant recipients. *J Heart Lung Transplant* 15 (9):948-54.

Egan, T. M., S. Murray, R. T. Bustami, T. H. Shearon, K. P. McCullough, L. B. Edwards, M. A. Coke, E. R. Garrity, S. C. Sweet, D. A. Heiney, and F. L. Grover. 2006. Development of the new lung allocation system in the United States. *Am J Transplant* 6 (5 Pt 2):1212-27.

Eriksson, L. T., R. Roscher, R. Ingemansson, and S. Steen. 1999. Cardiovascular effects of induced hypothermia after lung transplantation. *Ann Thorac Surg* 67 (3):804-9.

Eriksson, L. T., and S. Steen. 1998. Induced hypothermia in critical respiratory failure after lung transplantation. *Ann Thorac Surg* 65 (3):827-9.

Estenne, M., and M. I. Hertz. 2002. Bronchiolitis obliterans after human lung transplantation. *Am J Respir Crit Care Med* 166 (4):440-4.

Estenne, M., J. R. Maurer, A. Boehler, J. J. Egan, A. Frost, M. Hertz, G. B. Mallory, G. I. Snell, and S. Yousem. 2002. Bronchiolitis obliterans syndrome 2001: an update of the diagnostic criteria. *J Heart Lung Transplant* 21 (3):297-310.

Fisher, A. J., S. C. Donnelly, N. Hirani, M. D. Burdick, R. M. Strieter, J. H. Dark, and P. A. Corris. 1999. Enhanced pulmonary inflammation in organ donors following fatal non-traumatic brain injury. *Lancet* 353 (9162):1412-3.

Fisher, A. J., S. C. Donnelly, N. Hirani, C. Haslett, R. M. Strieter, J. H. Dark, and P. A. Corris. 2001. Elevated levels of interleukin-8 in donor lungs is associated with early graft failure after lung transplantation. *Am J Respir Crit Care Med* 163 (1):259-65.

Fishman, J. A., V. Emery, R. Freeman, M. Pascual, L. Rostaing, H. J. Schlitt, D. Sgarabotto, J. Torre-Cisneros, and M. E. Uknis. 2007. Cytomegalovirus in transplantation - challenging the status quo. *Clin Transplant* 21 (2):149-58.

Flume, P. A., T. M. Egan, L. J. Paradowski, F. C. Detterbeck, J. T. Thompson, and J. R. Yankaskas. 1994. Infectious complications of lung transplantation. Impact of cystic fibrosis. *Am J Respir Crit Care Med* 149 (6):1601-7.

Freeman, R. B., Jr. 2009. The 'indirect' effects of cytomegalovirus infection. *Am J Transplant* 9 (11):2453-8.

Gaggar, A., P. L. Jackson, B. D. Noerager, P. J. O'Reilly, D. B. McQuaid, S. M. Rowe, J. P. Clancy, and J. E. Blalock. 2008. A novel proteolytic cascade generates an extracellular matrix-derived chemoattractant in chronic neutrophilic inflammation. *J Immunol* 180 (8):5662-9.

Gaggar, A., Y. Li, N. Weathington, M. Winkler, M. Kong, P. Jackson, J. E. Blalock, and J. P. Clancy. 2007. Matrix metalloprotease-9 dysregulation in lower airway secretions of cystic fibrosis patients. *Am J Physiol Lung Cell Mol Physiol* 293 (1):L96-L104.

Haberman, B., M. L. Doan, E. O. Smith, M. G. Schecter, G. B. Mallory, and O. Elidemir. 2010. Serum KL-6 level and the development of bronchiolitis obliterans syndrome in lung transplant recipients. *Pediatr Transplant* 14 (7):903-8.

Hachem, R. R. 2009. Lung allograft rejection: diagnosis and management. *Curr Opin Organ Transplant* 14 (5):477-82.

Handa, M., S. Fujimura, T. Kondo, T. Ichinose, Y. Shiraishi, and T. Nakada. 1989. A study of preservation solution for 48- and 96-hour simple hypothermic storage of canine lung transplants. *Tohoku J Exp Med* 159 (3):205-14.

Hardison, M. T., F. S. Galin, C. E. Calderon, U. V. Djekic, S. B. Parker, K. M. Wille, P. L. Jackson, R. A. Oster, K. R. Young, J. E. Blalock, and A. Gaggar. 2009. The presence of a matrix-derived neutrophil chemoattractant in bronchiolitis obliterans syndrome after lung transplantation. *J Immunol* 182 (7):4423-31.

Hardison, MT, Jackson, PL, Blalock, JE, Gaggar, A. 2009. Protease Release from Neutrophils in Inflammation: Impact on Innate Immunity Seen in Chronic Pulmonary Disease. In *Handbook of Granulocytes: Classification, Toxic Materials Produced and Pathology*, edited by R. H. a. S. Kohlund: Nova Science Publishers.

Hardy, J. D., W. R. Webb, M. L. Dalton, Jr., and G. R. Walker, Jr. 1963. Lung Homotransplantation in Man. *JAMA* 186:1065-74.
Higuchi, T., T. Shiraishi, T. Shirakusa, S. Hirayama, H. Shibaguchi, M. Kuroki, M. Hiratuka, S. Yamamoto, and A. Iwasaki. 2005. Prevention of acute lung allograft rejection in rat by the janus kinase 3 inhibitor, tyrphostin AG490. *J Heart Lung Transplant* 24 (10):1557-64.
Hoffman, S. A., L. Wang, C. V. Shah, V. N. Ahya, A. Pochettino, K. Olthoff, A. Shaked, K. Wille, V. N. Lama, A. Milstone, L. B. Ware, J. Orens, A. Weinacker, E. Demissie, S. Bellamy, S. M. Kawut, W. W. Hancock, and J. D. Christie. 2009. Plasma cytokines and chemokines in primary graft dysfunction post-lung transplantation. *Am J Transplant* 9 (2):389-96.
Hopkins, P. M., C. L. Aboyoun, P. N. Chhajed, M. A. Malouf, M. L. Plit, S. P. Rainer, and A. R. Glanville. 2002. Prospective analysis of 1,235 transbronchial lung biopsies in lung transplant recipients. *J Heart Lung Transplant* 21 (10):1062-7.
Humar, A., Y. Lebranchu, F. Vincenti, E. A. Blumberg, J. D. Punch, A. P. Limaye, D. Abramowicz, A. G. Jardine, A. T. Voulgari, J. Ives, I. A. Hauser, and P. Peeters. 2010. The efficacy and safety of 200 days valganciclovir cytomegalovirus prophylaxis in high-risk kidney transplant recipients. *Am J Transplant* 10 (5):1228-37.
Iacono, A. T., R. J. Keenan, S. R. Duncan, G. C. Smaldone, J. H. Dauber, I. L. Paradis, N. P. Ohori, W. F. Grgurich, G. J. Burckart, A. Zeevi, E. Delgado, T. G. O'Riordan, M. M. Zendarsky, S. A. Yousem, and B. P. Griffith. 1996. Aerosolized cyclosporine in lung recipients with refractory chronic rejection. *Am J Respir Crit Care Med* 153 (4 Pt 1):1451-5.
Ison, M. G., and M. G. Michaels. 2009. RNA respiratory viral infections in solid organ transplant recipients. *Am J Transplant* 9 Suppl 4:S166-72.
Iwata, T., M. Chiyo, S. Yoshida, G. N. Smith, Jr., E. A. Mickler, R. Presson, Jr., A. J. Fisher, D. D. Brand, O. W. Cummings, and D. S. Wilkes. 2008. Lung transplant ischemia reperfusion injury: metalloprotease inhibition down-regulates exposure of type V collagen, growth-related oncogene-induced neutrophil chemotaxis, and tumor necrosis factor-alpha expression. *Transplantation* 85 (3):417-26.
Jackson, P. L., B. D. Noerager, M. J. Jablonsky, M. T. Hardison, B. D. Cox, J. C. Patterson, B. Dhanapal, J. E. Blalock, and D. D. Muccio. 2011. A CXCL8 receptor antagonist based on the structure of N-acetyl-proline-glycine-proline. *Eur J Pharmacol*. In Press.
Jain, R., R. R. Hachem, M. R. Morrell, E. P. Trulock, M. M. Chakinala, R. D. Yusen, H. J. Huang, T. Mohanakumar, G. A. Patterson, and M. J. Walter. 2010. Azithromycin is associated with increased survival in lung transplant recipients with bronchiolitis obliterans syndrome. *J Heart Lung Transplant* 29 (5):531-7.
Jaksch, P., B. Zweytick, H. Kerschner, A. M. Hoda, M. Keplinger, G. Lang, C. Aigner, and W. Klepetko. 2009. Cytomegalovirus prevention in high-risk lung transplant recipients: comparison of 3- vs 12-month valganciclovir therapy. *J Heart Lung Transplant* 28 (7):670-5.
Jung, F. J., L. Yang, I. De Meester, K. Augustyns, M. Cardell, S. Hillinger, P. Vogt, D. Lardinois, S. Scharpe, W. Weder, and S. Korom. 2006. CD26/dipeptidylpeptidase

IV-targeted therapy of acute lung rejection in rats. *J Heart Lung Transplant* 25 (9):1109-16.

Jungraithmayr, W., P. Vogt, I. Inci, S. Hillinger, S. Arni, S. Korom, and W. Weder. 2010. A model of chronic lung allograft rejection in the rat. *Eur Respir J* 35 (6):1354-63.

Kaneda, H., T. K. Waddell, M. de Perrot, X. H. Bai, C. Gutierrez, T. Arenovich, C. Chaparro, M. Liu, and S. Keshavjee. 2006. Pre-implantation multiple cytokine mRNA expression analysis of donor lung grafts predicts survival after lung transplantation in humans. *Am J Transplant* 6 (3):544-51.

Kawut, S. M., J. Okun, D. Shimbo, D. J. Lederer, J. De Andrade, V. Lama, A. Shah, A. Milstone, L. B. Ware, A. Weinacker, E. Demissie, and J. D. Christie. 2009. Soluble p-selectin and the risk of primary graft dysfunction after lung transplantation. *Chest* 136 (1):237-44.

Keshavjee, S., R. D. Davis, M. R. Zamora, M. de Perrot, and G. A. Patterson. 2005. A randomized, placebo-controlled trial of complement inhibition in ischemia-reperfusion injury after lung transplantation in human beings. *J Thorac Cardiovasc Surg* 129 (2):423-8.

Knoop, C., and M. Estenne. 2006. Acute and chronic rejection after lung transplantation. *Semin Respir Crit Care Med* 27 (5):521-33.

Korom, S., I. De Meester, T. H. Stadlbauer, A. Chandraker, M. Schaub, M. H. Sayegh, A. Belyaev, A. Haemers, S. Scharpe, and J. W. Kupiec-Weglinski. 1997. Inhibition of CD26/dipeptidyl peptidase IV activity in vivo prolongs cardiac allograft survival in rat recipients. *Transplantation* 63 (10):1495-500.

Kotloff, R. M., and G. Thabut. 2011. Lung transplantation. *Am J Respir Crit Care Med* 184 (2):159-71.

Kotton, C. N., D. Kumar, A. M. Caliendo, A. Asberg, S. Chou, D. R. Snydman, U. Allen, and A. Humar. 2010. International consensus guidelines on the management of cytomegalovirus in solid organ transplantation. *Transplantation* 89 (7):779-95.

Kramer, M. R., S. E. Marshall, V. A. Starnes, P. Gamberg, Z. Amitai, and J. Theodore. 1993. Infectious complications in heart-lung transplantation. Analysis of 200 episodes. *Arch Intern Med* 153 (17):2010-6.

Lande, J. D., J. Patil, N. Li, T. R. Berryman, R. A. King, and M. I. Hertz. 2007. Novel insights into lung transplant rejection by microarray analysis. *Proc Am Thorac Soc* 4 (1):44-51.

Lease, E. D., and D. W. Zaas. 2010. Complex bacterial infections pre- and posttransplant. *Semin Respir Crit Care Med* 31 (2):234-42.

Lee, J. C., and J. D. Christie. 2009. Primary graft dysfunction. *Clin Chest Med* 32 (2):279-93.

Lee, J., W. W. Yew, C. F. Wong, P. C. Wong, and C. S. Chiu. 2003. Multidrug-resistant tuberculosis in a lung transplant recipient. *J Heart Lung Transplant* 22 (10):1168-73.

Madsen, C. B., A. Norgaard, M. Iversen, and L. P. Ryder. 2010. Elevated mRNA levels of CTLA-4, FoxP3, and granzyme B in BAL, but not in blood, during acute rejection of lung allografts. *Transpl Immunol* 24 (1):26-32.

Mangi, A. A., D. P. Mason, E. R. Nowicki, L. H. Batizy, S. C. Murthy, D. J. Pidwell, R. K. Avery, K. R. McCurry, G. B. Pettersson, and E. H. Blackstone. 2011. Predictors of acute rejection after lung transplantation. *Ann Thorac Surg* 91 (6):1754-62.

Maurer, J. R., A. E. Frost, M. Estenne, T. Higenbottam, and A. R. Glanville. 1998. International guidelines for the selection of lung transplant candidates. The

International Society for Heart and Lung Transplantation, the American Thoracic Society, the American Society of Transplant Physicians, the European Respiratory Society. *Transplantation* 66 (7):951-6.

Meade, M. O., J. T. Granton, A. Matte-Martyn, K. McRae, B. Weaver, P. Cripps, and S. H. Keshavjee. 2003. A randomized trial of inhaled nitric oxide to prevent ischemia-reperfusion injury after lung transplantation. *Am J Respir Crit Care Med* 167 (11):1483-9.

Meyers, B. F., and G. A. Patterson. 2000. Current status of lung transplantation. *Adv Surg* 34:301-18.

Millet, B., T. W. Higenbottam, C. D. Flower, S. Stewart, and J. Wallwork. 1989. The radiographic appearances of infection and acute rejection of the lung after heart-lung transplantation. *Am Rev Respir Dis* 140 (1):62-7.

Morrish, W. F., S. J. Herman, G. L. Weisbrod, and D. W. Chamberlain. 1991. Bronchiolitis obliterans after lung transplantation: findings at chest radiography and high-resolution CT. The Toronto Lung Transplant Group. *Radiology* 179 (2):487-90.

Morton, J., and A. R. Glanville. 2009. Lung transplantation in patients with cystic fibrosis. *Semin Respir Crit Care Med* 30 (5):559-68.

Nash, E. F., A. Coonar, R. Kremer, E. Tullis, M. Hutcheon, L. G. Singer, S. Keshavjee, and C. Chaparro. 2010. Survival of Burkholderia cepacia sepsis following lung transplantation in recipients with cystic fibrosis. *Transpl Infect Dis* 12 (6):551-4.

Neofytos, D., J. A. Fishman, D. Horn, E. Anaissie, C. H. Chang, A. Olyaei, M. Pfaller, W. J. Steinbach, K. M. Webster, and K. A. Marr. 2010. Epidemiology and outcome of invasive fungal infections in solid organ transplant recipients. *Transpl Infect Dis* 12 (3):220-9.

Neurohr, C., P. Huppmann, B. Samweber, S. Leuschner, G. Zimmermann, H. Leuchte, R. Baumgartner, R. Hatz, L. Frey, P. Ueberfuhr, I. Bittmann, and J. Behr. 2009. Prognostic value of bronchoalveolar lavage neutrophilia in stable lung transplant recipients. *J Heart Lung Transplant* 28 (5):468-74.

O'Reilly, P., M. T. Hardison, P. L. Jackson, X. Xu, R. J. Snelgrove, A. Gaggar, F. S. Galin, and J. E. Blalock. 2010. Neutrophils contain prolyl endopeptidase and generate the chemotactic peptide, PGP, from collagen. *J Neuroimmunology* 217 (1-2):51-54.

O'Reilly, P., P. L. Jackson, B. Noerager, S. Parker, M. Dransfield, A. Gaggar, and J. E. Blalock. 2009. N-alpha-PGP and PGP, potential biomarkers and therapeutic targets for COPD. *Respir Res* 10:38.

Ojo, A. O., R. A. Wolfe, A. B. Leichtman, D. M. Dickinson, F. K. Port, and E. W. Young. 1999. A practical approach to evaluate the potential donor pool and trends in cadaveric kidney donation. *Transplantation* 67 (4):548-56.

Okada, Y., and T. Kondo. 2009. Preservation solution for lung transplantation. *Gen Thorac Cardiovasc Surg* 57 (12):635-9.

Okada, Y., A. M. Marchevsky, X. J. Zuo, J. A. Pass, R. M. Kass, J. M. Matloff, and S. C. Jordan. 1997. Accumulation of platelets in rat syngeneic lung transplants: a potential factor responsible for preservation-reperfusion injury. *Transplantation* 64 (6):801-6.

Orens, J. B., and E. R. Garrity, Jr. 2009. General overview of lung transplantation and review of organ allocation. *Proc Am Thorac Soc* 6 (1):13-9.

Otulana, B. A., T. Higenbottam, L. Ferrari, J. Scott, G. Igboaka, and J. Wallwork. 1990. The use of home spirometry in detecting acute lung rejection and infection following heart-lung transplantation. *Chest* 97 (2):353-7.

Palmer, S. M., R. D. Davis, D. Hadjiliadis, M. I. Hertz, D. N. Howell, F. E. Ward, K. Savik, and N. L. Reinsmoen. 2002. Development of an antibody specific to major histocompatibility antigens detectable by flow cytometry after lung transplant is associated with bronchiolitis obliterans syndrome. *Transplantation* 74 (6):799-804.

Palmer, S. M., A. P. Limaye, M. Banks, D. Gallup, J. Chapman, E. C. Lawrence, J. Dunitz, A. Milstone, J. Reynolds, G. L. Yung, K. M. Chan, R. Aris, E. Garrity, V. Valentine, J. McCall, S. C. Chow, R. D. Davis, and R. Avery. 2010. Extended valganciclovir prophylaxis to prevent cytomegalovirus after lung transplantation: a randomized, controlled trial. *Ann Intern Med* 152 (12):761-9.

Petrucci, N., and W. Iacovelli. 2003. Ventilation with lower tidal volumes versus traditional tidal volumes in adults for acute lung injury and acute respiratory distress syndrome. *Cochrane Database Syst Rev* (3):CD003844.

Pfister, R. R., J. L. Haddox, C. I. Sommers, and K. W. Lam. 1995. Identification and synthesis of chemotactic tripeptides from alkali-degraded whole cornea. A study of N-acetyl-proline-glycine-proline and N-methyl-proline-glycine-proline. *Invest Ophthalmol Vis Sci* 36 (7):1306-16.

Pratschke, J., M. J. Wilhelm, M. Kusaka, F. Beato, E. L. Milford, W. W. Hancock, and N. L. Tilney. 2000. Accelerated rejection of renal allografts from brain-dead donors. *Ann Surg* 232 (2):263-71.

Prekker, M. E., D. S. Nath, A. R. Walker, A. C. Johnson, M. I. Hertz, C. S. Herrington, D. M. Radosevich, and P. S. Dahlberg. 2006. Validation of the proposed International Society for Heart and Lung Transplantation grading system for primary graft dysfunction after lung transplantation. *J Heart Lung Transplant* 25 (4):371-8.

Salama, M., P. Jaksch, O. Andrukhova, S. Taghavi, W. Klepetko, and S. Aharinejad. 2011. Endothelin-1 is a useful biomarker for early detection of bronchiolitis obliterans in lung transplant recipients. *J Thorac Cardiovasc Surg* 140 (6):1422-7.

Shargall, Y., G. Guenther, V. N. Ahya, A. Ardehali, A. Singhal, and S. Keshavjee. 2005. Report of the ISHLT Working Group on Primary Lung Graft Dysfunction part VI: treatment. *J Heart Lung Transplant* 24 (10):1489-500.

Shohami, E., M. Novikov, R. Bass, A. Yamin, and R. Gallily. 1994. Closed head injury triggers early production of TNF alpha and IL-6 by brain tissue. *J Cereb Blood Flow Metab* 14 (4):615-9.

Sims, K. D., and E. A. Blumberg. 2011. Common infections in the lung transplant recipient. *Clin Chest Med* 32 (2):327-41.

Singh, N. 2003. Fungal infections in the recipients of solid organ transplantation. *Infect Dis Clin North Am* 17 (1):113-34, viii.

Skrabal, C. A., L. O. Thompson, E. V. Potapov, R. E. Southard, D. L. Joyce, K. A. Youker, G. P. Noon, and M. Loebe. 2005. Organ-specific regulation of pro-inflammatory molecules in heart, lung, and kidney following brain death. *J Surg Res* 123 (1):118-25.

Snydman, D. R., A. P. Limaye, L. Potena, and M. R. Zamora. 2011. Update and review: state-of-the-art management of cytomegalovirus infection and disease following thoracic organ transplantation. *Transplant Proc* 43 (3 Suppl):S1-S17.

Spital, A. 2005. Conscription of cadaveric organs for transplantation: a stimulating idea whose time has not yet come. *Camb Q Healthc Ethics* 14 (1):107-12.

Stewart, S., M. C. Fishbein, G. I. Snell, G. J. Berry, A. Boehler, M. M. Burke, A. Glanville, F. K. Gould, C. Magro, C. C. Marboe, K. D. McNeil, E. F. Reed, N. L. Reinsmoen, J. P. Scott, S. M. Studer, H. D. Tazelaar, J. L. Wallwork, G. Westall, M. R. Zamora, A. Zeevi, and S. A. Yousem. 2007. Revision of the 1996 working formulation for the standardization of nomenclature in the diagnosis of lung rejection. *J Heart Lung Transplant* 26 (12):1229-42.

Struber, M., J. M. Hohlfeld, T. Kofidis, G. Warnecke, J. Niedermeyer, S. P. Sommer, and A. Haverich. 2002. Surfactant function in lung transplantation after 24 hours of ischemia: advantage of retrograde flush perfusion for preservation. *J Thorac Cardiovasc Surg* 123 (1):98-103.

Tasoulis, M. K., O. Livaditi, M. Stamatakos, C. Stefanaki, P. Paneris, P. Prigouris, A. Flevari, N. Goutas, D. Vlachodimitropoulos, V. Villiotou, and E. E. Douzinas. 2009. High concentrations of reactive oxygen species in the BAL fluid are correlated with lung injury in rabbits after hemorrhagic shock and resuscitation. *Tohoku J Exp Med* 219 (3):193-9.

Trulock, E. P., J. D. Christie, L. B. Edwards, M. M. Boucek, P. Aurora, D. O. Taylor, F. Dobbels, A. O. Rahmel, B. M. Keck, and M. I. Hertz. 2007. Registry of the International Society for Heart and Lung Transplantation: twenty-fourth official adult lung and heart-lung transplantation report-2007. *J Heart Lung Transplant* 26 (8):782-95.

Valentine, V. G., R. W. Bonvillain, M. R. Gupta, G. A. Lombard, S. G. LaPlace, G. S. Dhillon, and G. Wang. 2008. Infections in lung allograft recipients: ganciclovir era. *J Heart Lung Transplant* 27 (5):528-35.

van Houwelingen, A. H., N. M. Weathington, V. Verweij, J. E. Blalock, F. P. Nijkamp, and G. Folkerts. 2008. Induction of lung emphysema is prevented by L-arginine-threonine-arginine. *FASEB J* 22 (9):3403-8.

Vanaudenaerde, B. M., W. A. Wuyts, N. Geudens, T. S. Nawrot, R. Vos, L. J. Dupont, D. E. Van Raemdonck, and G. M. Verleden. 2008. Broncho-alveolar lavage fluid recovery correlates with airway neutrophilia in lung transplant patients. *Respir Med* 102 (3):339-47.

Vos, R., B. M. Vanaudenaerde, N. Geudens, L. J. Dupont, D. E. Van Raemdonck, and G. M. Verleden. 2008. Pseudomonal airway colonisation: risk factor for bronchiolitis obliterans syndrome after lung transplantation? *Eur Respir J* 31 (5):1037-45.

Weathington, N. M., A. H. van Houwelingen, B. D. Noerager, P. L. Jackson, A. D. Kraneveld, F. S. Galin, G. Folkerts, F. P. Nijkamp, and J. E. Blalock. 2006. A novel peptide CXCR ligand derived from extracellular matrix degradation during airway inflammation. *Nat Med* 12 (3):317-23.

Whitson, B. A., D. S. Nath, A. C. Johnson, A. R. Walker, M. E. Prekker, D. M. Radosevich, C. S. Herrington, and P. S. Dahlberg. 2006. Risk factors for primary graft dysfunction after lung transplantation. *J Thorac Cardiovasc Surg* 131 (1):73-80.

Xu, X., P. L. Jackson, S. Tanner, M. T. Hardison, M. Abdul Roda, J. E. Blalock, and A. Gaggar. 2011. A self-propagating matrix metalloprotease-9 (MMP-9) dependent cycle of chronic neutrophilic inflammation. *PLoS One* 6 (1):e15781.

Xue, J., X. Zhu, M. P. George, M. M. Myerburg, M. W. Stoner, J. W. Pilewski, and S. R. Duncan. 2011. A human-mouse chimeric model of obliterative bronchiolitis after lung transplantation. *Am J Pathol* 179 (2):745-53.

Yousem, S. A., T. Martin, I. L. Paradis, R. Keenan, and B. P. Griffith. 1994. Can immunohistological analysis of transbronchial biopsy specimens predict responder status in early acute rejection of lung allografts? *Hum Pathol* 25 (5):525-9.

Zamora, M. R., R. D. Davis, and C. Leonard. 2005. Management of cytomegalovirus infection in lung transplant recipients: evidence-based recommendations. *Transplantation* 80 (2):157-63.

Zamora, M. R., M. R. Nicolls, T. N. Hodges, J. Marquesen, T. Astor, T. Grazia, and D. Weill. 2004. Following universal prophylaxis with intravenous ganciclovir and cytomegalovirus immune globulin, valganciclovir is safe and effective for prevention of CMV infection following lung transplantation. *Am J Transplant* 4 (10):1635-42.

31

Bronchial Atresia

Lirios Sacristán Bou and Francisco Peña Blas
Hospital General de Tomelloso & Centro de Salud de Monforte del Cid
España

1. Introduction

Bronchial atresia is an interesting congenital abnormality because of its variable appearance and its semblance to certain acquired diseases. It is characterized by a branching mass formed by mucus that dilates the proximal bronchi to the atretic segment. The distal lung to atresia can develop normally but it shows a paucity of blood vessels and is hyperinflated due to unidirectional collateral air drift through intraalveolar pores of Kohn, bronchoalveolar channels of Lambert and interbronchiolar pores of Martin from the adjacent normal lung. These collateral communications act as a check-valve mechanism allowing the air to enter but not to leave the distal lung.

More than 150 cases of bronchial atresia have been reported since 1953, when it was first described by Ramsay & Byron. The exact mechanism that ends in bronchial atresia is still unknown, but there are two hypotheses about the pathogenesis which have in common that they should occur before birth because the bronchial pattern to the site of stenosis is entirely normal. Many of the most relevant case reports and published series of cases are reviewed in this chapter to update our knowledge of bronchial atresia. They have been obtained as the result of a bibliographical research at Pubmed; ninety five articles were found using the Medical Subject Headings (MeSH) thesaurus descriptors congenital and bronchial atresia.

2. Pathogenesis

Bronchial buds appear in the fifth week of gestation and then complete branching takes place in the sixteenth week. Although bronchial atresia is associated with a decreased amount of alveoli, the number of airways is not reduced.

Congenital bronchial atresia pathogenesis is not completely understood, but there are two pathogenic hypotheses. The first one proposes that proliferating cells at the distal tip of the developing bud are disconnected from the normal branch at any time from the fifth to the sixteenth weeks by a still unknown agent (Bucher et al., 1961; Kuhn et al., 1992).

The other one postulates that focal ischemic insults at the fifth week or later result in necrosis and obliteration of the already completed bronchus (Reid, 1977 or Waddell et al., 1965). The experiment of Louw & Barnard (1955), in which they tied off a mesenteric arterial branch in puppies two weeks before birth, showed that atresia may result from a vascular occlusion and develop late in intra-uterine life. Their findings favour vascular occlusion rather than a failure of growth as the cause.

The pulmonary arterial development is closely associated with the developing lung bud. The primitive pulmonary artery is already present as a major branch and grows toward the lung bud. Subsequently, it gives off a branch to accompany each airway branch in the preacinar region. Pulmonary vascular abnormalities have been documented in bronchial atresia (Ko et al., 1998; Lacquet et al., 1971).

3. Respiratory symptoms and epidemiology

Bronchial atresia has a male predominance, with an estimated prevalence of 1.2 cases per 100,000 males and 0.6 cases per 100,000 females - a male: female ratio of 2:1.

About two thirds of the reported patients were asymptomatic before diagnosis and occurred as an incidental radiological discovery. It is usually diagnosed in the second or third decade of life, and the diagnosis is infrequent during childhood. One third of patients may present with cough, shortness of breath and recurrent infections and less frequently with refractory wheezing, haemoptysis, chest pain, or pneumothorax (Agarwal et al., 2005; Kameyama et al., 2006; Morikawa et al., 2005 (Table 1).

Asymptomatic	58.00%
Recurrent Infection	21.00%
Dysnea	14.00%
Coughing	6.00%

Table 1. Frequency of symptoms from more to less frequent (Jederlinic et al., 1987).

The bronchi involved in this congenital anomaly are the apico-posterior segment of left upper lobe, right upper lobe, right middle lobe and right lower lobe, in decreasing order of frequency (Acosta Gordillo et al., 2005; Psathakis et al., 2004).

4. Imaging techniques for the diagnosis

Currently clinicians have lot of many imaging techniques at their disposal for the investigation of patients with this congenital anomaly.

4.1 Plain Chest Radiography

The radiographic findings mirror the pathologic changes.

On chest radiography the typical finding of a mucocele is that of a nodule or a shadow-like mass close to the hilum, with well-defined margins, presenting as a tubular, round, ovoid or branching structure (Sacristán Bou et al., 2010) (Fig 1). A mucocele with an air-fluid level is considered by some authors as a variance of congenital bronchial atresia (Matsushima et al., 2003).

The branching bronchocele mimics a glove-finger shadow, but is not pathognomonic of bronchial atresia.

It has been proposed that the impacted mucous can also liquefy producing the radiological sign of an air-fluid level-mimicking a cavitatory lesion. When the hyperinsuflated area gets

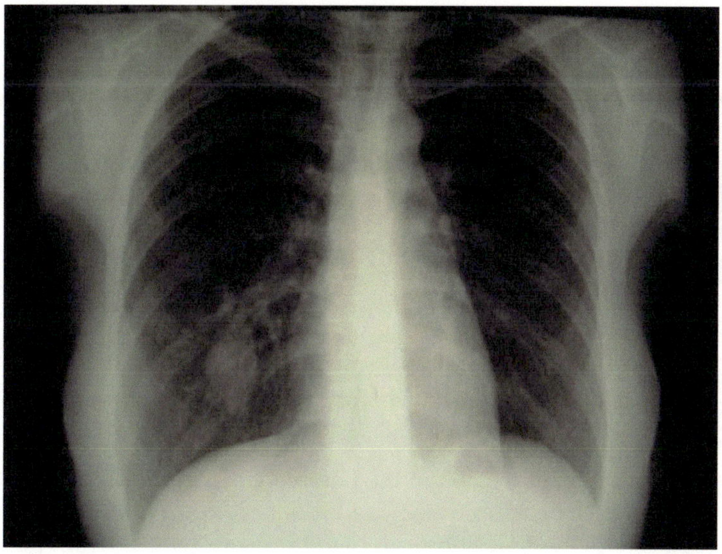

Fig. 1. Polylobulated round mass near to the hilum in the right lower lobe (Sacristán Bou et al., 2010).

infected and presents as a pneumonia, the walls of bronchoceles develop tiny breaks that enables the air to enter in its lumen (Psathakis et al., 2009; Rahalkar et al., 2005).

Occasionally, the dilated bronchi may appear as purely air-filled, lucent bands of odd shapes (Nussbaumer-Ochsner & Kohler, 2011; Van Klaveren et al., 1992).

The distal lung is always distended, forming the apex of a roughly triangular zone of hyperlucency of the lung parenchyma (due to oligoemia and hyperinflation). On radiography obtained at expiration, obstructive emphysema is obvious, however, the synchronous appearance of both the mucocele and lung hyperlucency is only seen in 69% of cases (Jederlinic et al., 1987).

Sometimes bronchial atresia is associated with other congenital anomalies like pectum excavatum (Van Klaveren et al., 1992).

4.2 Computed Tomography (CT) and High-Resolution Computed Tomography

Computed tomography is the procedure of choice for the diagnosis and study of congenital bronchial atresia.

The bronchocele presents as a round/ovoid/branching structure near the hilum, with or without a fluid level, without contrast enhancement and it exhibits a density between 10 to 25 Hounsfield Units due to mucoid material. Computed tomography allows characterization of the lack of communication between the mucocele and hilum (Fig. 2).

High resolution techniques can display the characteristic features of the mucocele, being more sensitive than the plain chest radiography to show oligaemia, reduced caliber of the pulmonary vessels, hyperinflation of the lung parenchyma (Fig. 2), small mucoceles invisible to conventional radiography, associated mass effect and even calcification (Kinsella et al., 1992 and Primetis et al., 2011).

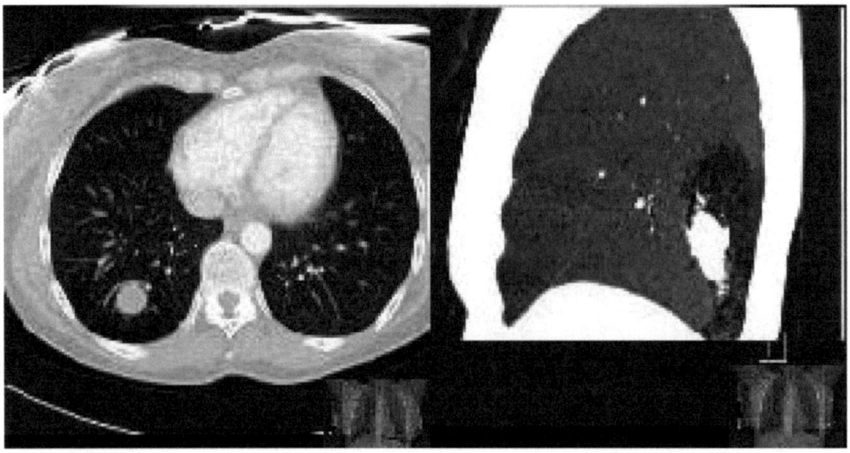

Fig 2. Polilobulated round mass located in the posterobasilar right subsegmental bronchi with a distal segmental area of radiolucency and lack of communication between the mucocele and hilum on high-resolution computed tomography (Sacristán Bou et al., 2010).

4.3 Magnetic Resonance Imaging (MRI)

MRI shows a very high signal intensity within the bronchocele on T1W and T2W modes due to mucoid contents; however, it cannot depict regional air-trapping (Matsushima et al., 2003) and it does not have the same sensivity as computed tomography to evaluate the lung parenchyma (Naidich et al., 1988). So this technique has a limited role in the diagnosis of congenital brochial atresia, although a small number of case reports have dealt specifically with differential diagnosis and have established its value.

Magnetic resonance imaging seem to be useful for the evaluation of either anomalous vessels or fluid collections that are usually associated with pulmonary abnormalities (Cohen et al., 1987).

5. Bronchoscopy

Before the advent of computed tomography, the diagnosis of bronchial atresia was made by bronchography, which allowed confirmation of the atretic segmental bronchus showing non-filling of the involved bronchus.

Flexible-bronchoscopy identifies blind-ending bronchi. In clinical practice however, any absence of a segmental or sub-segmental bronchus that is found by chance during bronchoscopy in the absence of the characteristic radiographic features may be considered as a normal anatomic variance of the bronchial tree rather than a bronchial atresia.

In the majority of the cases therefore, congenital bronchial atresia remains a radiological diagnosis.

Some authors suggest that similar findings could be found in other disorders as well, such as lung cancer or bronchial adenoma (Jeung et al., 2002; Woodring, 1990). The role of bronchoscopy is to exclude these disorders and demonstrate the patency of the central bronchi, especially in doubtful cases (Daoud et al., 2001; Ward &, Morcos, 1999).

6. Lung function tests

Pulmonary function tests do not aid in diagnosis. They are normal in comparison with the magnitude of the radiological abnormality. The most interesting point is the normal physiological dead space that implies air trapping in the emphysematous area as a result of collateral ventilation that causes the inflation.

7. Differential diagnosis

The singular finding of a dilated bronchus due to mucoid impaction (bronchocele) can be seen in a variety of conditions apart from bronchia atresia. It is important to differentiate between congenital and acquired causes of obstruction (Table 2).

7.1 Congenital obstructive illnesses

7.1.1 Lung Aplasia

Pulmonary agenesis refers to undeveloped pulmonary vessels, bronchi, and parenchyma. It may be unilateral or bilateral. In unilateral aplasia, the remaining lung contains twice as much alveoli as normal, but has normal bronchi. Although aplasia does not have the same structures, it has a rudimentary bronchus.

Pulmonary aplasia (agenesis) is thought to result from the negative effects that occur in the 4th week of fetal life. Although its etiology is not fully understood, Vitamin A or folic acid deficiency or the use of salicylates may be responsible. The incidence in males and females and the occurrence of the anomaly in the right or left lung are about the same. Hypoplasia and aplasia are often observed together with other malformations (diaphragm defects, kidney anomalies, extrapulmonary sequestration, muscular or skeletal system defects). Nearly one-third of the patients have congenital heart diseases. Although the most common is the atrial septal defect, ventricular septal defect, patent ductus arteriosus, or aorta coarctation can also be observed. Clinical findings change with the presence of comorbid anomalies and their severity. Recurrent infections can increase respiratory dysfunction. Although patients with unilateral lung aplasia (agenesis) are believed to die usually in the neonatal period, there are patients who live up to adulthood, some of whom are completely asymptomatic. In the diagnosis of this condition, methods such as contrast-enhanced CT, bronchography, bronchoscopy, pulmonary angiography, and magnetic resonance imaging are also employed.

7.1.2 Congenital Lobar Emphysema

A congenital lobar emphysema (CLE) refers to an over inflation of one or more lung lobes presumably due to various factors including a possible obstructive check valve mechanism at the bronchial level. It is more common in males and often detected in neonates or identified during in utero ultrasound. Anomalies are rather infrequent. Patients will typically have respiratory distress within the first 6 months of life.

CLE almost always involves one lobe, with rates of occurrence as follows: 41% left upper lobe, 34% right middle lobe, 21% right upper lobe. Congenital lobar emphysema has two forms of presentation: hypoalveolar: fewer than the expected number of alveoli, and polyalveolar: greater than the expected number of alveoli.

There are many presumed mechanisms for progressive overdistension of a lobe including obstruction, cartilage deficiency, dysplasia, immaturity and idiopathic. It can be associated with cardiac anomalies such as: a ventricular septal defect, patent ductus arteriosus and tetralogy of Fallot. Congenital lobar emphysema appears in the immediate postpartum period.

Radiography of the chest in anteroposterior and lateral projections identifies the involved lobe, the degree of involvement, and the effect on surrounding structures. If a decubitus position radiograph is obtained, the involved lung does not collapse. Computed tomography scanning can provide details about the involved lobe and its vascularity, as well as information about the remaining lung. MRI can be used as an adjunctive modality to evaluate vascular supply and distribution to the involved lobe but is not routinely employed. In congenital lobar emphysema, the abnormal lobe usually has a normal vascular supply.

7.1.3 Congenital Cystic Adenomatoid Malformation (CAM)

The first cystic adenomatoid malformation (CAM) was described as a distinct entity by Ch'in and Tang in 1949. CAM is a developmental hamartomatous abnormality of the lung, with adenomatoid proliferation of cysts resembling bronchioles. CAM represents approximately 25% of all congenital lung lesions (Colin et al., 2006).

CAM is subdivided into three major types:

- Type I lesions, the most common, are composed of 1 or more cysts measuring 2-10 cm in diameter. Larger cysts are often accompanied by smaller cysts, and their walls contain muscle, elastic, or fibrous tissue. Cysts are frequently lined by pseudostratified columnar epithelial cells, which occasionally produce mucin. Mucinogenic differentiation is unique to this subtype of CAM.
- Type II lesions are characterized by small, relatively uniform cysts resembling bronchioles. These cysts are lined by cuboid-to-columnar epithelium and have a thin fibromuscular wall. The cysts generally measure 0.5-2 cm in diameter.
- Type III lesions have the appearance of solid masses without obvious cyst formation although adenomatoid cysts can be detected microscopically.

CAM receives its blood supply from pulmonary circulation and is not sequestered from the tracheobronchial tree. However, type II and III lesions can occasionally coexist with extralobar sequestration, and in such cases, they may receive a systemic arterial supply. CAM may also occur in combination with a polyalveolar lobe. This is a form of congenital emphysema with an increased number of alveoli with normal bronchi and pulmonary vasculature. CAM usually occurs early in fetal life, whereas the polyalveolar lobe occurs later.

Prenatal ultrasonography is accurate in diagnosing CAM. Prenatally diagnosed lesions may be asymptomatic at birth (71%), and they have normal radiographic findings (57%). A concurrent sequestration may not be identified. Usually, radiographic findings are apparent in a symptomatic individual, but they may not be as apparent in an asymptomatic child.

Most often, the diagnosis can be made by using plain radiographs. CT scans may be used for confirmation and when planning surgery. Overlapping CT features exist among cases of CAM, pulmonary sequestration, bronchogenic cyst, and other foregut malformations.

7.1.4 Bronchogenic cysts

Bronchogenic cysts are part of a spectrum of congenital abnormalities of the lung including pulmonary sequestration, congenital cystic adenomatoid malformation and congenital lobar hyperinflation (emphysema). There exists a predilection in all of them for the left upper lobe that could be due to the embryologic instability of this area (Sadler, 1990).

Although relatively rare, cysts represent the most common lesion of the mediastinum. In infants and small children, these cysts can be life threatening when they compress vital structures. In particular, subcarinal cysts can pose life-threatening airway compromise. In infants, the initial presentation may be respiratory distress. More than one half of patients are asymptomatic.

These are usually found using antenatal ultrasonography or routine chest radiography and during evaluations for gastro-intestinal or cardiac symptomatology. Bronchogenic cysts are the result of anomalous development of the ventral foregut; they are usually single but may be multiple and can be filled with fluid or mucus. They have been found all along the tracheoesophageal course, in perihilar or intraparenchymal sites, with a predilection for the area around the carina. Those in the mediastinum frequently attach to, but do not communicate with, the tracheobronchial tree. Bronchogenic cysts have also been described in more remote locations, including the interatrial septum, neck, abdomen, and retroperitoneal space. Chest pain and dysphagia are the most common symptoms in adults with bronchogenic cysts; in infants, symptoms are most often produced as a result of airway or esophageal compression.

Bronchogenic cysts are usually an incidental finding, and differentiating them from other pathologic conditions is important. On conventional radiographs, the appearances of mediastinal or lung masses are nonspecific and should be evaluated further using computed tomography (CT) scanning or magnetic resonance imaging (MRI). Intrapulmonary cysts are difficult to diagnose and must usually be aspirated to confirm the diagnosis.

7.1.5 Anomalous pulmonary venous return

Abnormal development of the pulmonary veins may result in either partial or complete anomalous drainage back into the systemic venous circulation. Three major clinical patterns of total anomalous pulmonary venous return (TAPVR) are seen: severe pulmonary venous obstruction; early heart failure; mildly symptomatic or asymptomatic.

7.1.6 Pulmonary sequestration

Pulmonary sequestration is a cystic or solid mass composed of nonfunctioning primitive tissue that does not communicate with the tracheobronchial tree and has an anomalous systemic blood supply rather than the pulmonary circulation. In 15-20% of cases multiple feeding vessels may be present. The two forms of pulmonary sequestration are intrapulmonary, which is surrounded by normal lung tissue, and extrapulmonary, which has its own pleural investment. Demonstration of a dominant feeding vessel, usually from the aorta or its major vessels, and venous drainage to the pulmonary veins suggests the diagnosis. Other congenital malformations may be present.

Chest radiographs can provide a reasonable diagnostic clue to pulmonary sequestration. A mass in the posterobasal segment of the lung in young patients with recurrent, localized pulmonary infections is suggestive of pulmonary sequestration. Computed tomography scanning, angiography, magnetic resonance imaging or bronchography may be helpful in excluding other diagnoses. CT scans have 90% accuracy in the diagnosis of pulmonary sequestration. Arteriography is helpful in differentiating the lesion from other abnormalities of the lung, such as pulmonary arteriovenous fistulae. Magnetic resonance angiography can provide information similar to that on CT scans.

7.1.7 Cystic Fibrosis (CF)

The name cystic fibrosis refers to the characteristic scarring (fibrosis) and cyst formation within the pancreas, first recognized in the 1930s. Difficulty breathing is the most serious symptom and results from frequent lung infections that are treated with, though not cured by, antibiotics and other medications. A multitude of other symptoms, including sinus infections, poor growth, diarrhea, and infertility result from the effects of CF in other parts of the body.

CF is caused by a mutation in the gene for the protein: the cystic fibrosis transmembrane conductance regulator (CFTR). This gene is required to regulate the components of sweat, digestive juices, and mucus. Although most people without CF have two working copies of the CFTR gene, only one is needed to prevent cystic fibrosis. CF develops when neither gene works normally and therefore has autosomal recessive inheritance.

Individuals with cystic fibrosis can be diagnosed before birth by genetic testing, or by a sweat test in early childhood. Ultimately, lung transplantation is often necessary as CF worsens. CF mainly affects the lungs, pancreas, liver, intestines, sinuses, and sex organs.

7.2 Acquired obstructive illnesses

7.2.1 Allergic bronchopulmonary aspergillosis (ABPA)

Allergic bronchopulmonary aspergillosis (ABPA) can be classified as an eosinophilic hypersensitivity disease. It appears concomitantly in patients with long standing asthma, and occasionally in patients with cystic fibrosis. Rarely, it can appear in patients with no other identifiable pulmonary illness. In general, patients are diagnosed before the age of 40 years.

Clinically, patients have atopic symptoms and they present with recurrent chest infection. A clinical staging system has been developed: Stage I Acute, Stage II Remission, Stage III Recurrent Exacerbation, Stage IV Steroid-Dependent Asthma and Stage V Pulmonary Fibrosis.

Laboratory findings include elevated Aspergillus specific IgE, elevated precipitating IgG against Aspergillus, peripheral eosinophilia and positive skin test.

In patients with ABPA radiological findings will be reversible after appropriate treatment or may show progression from multi-focal and non-segmental consolidations to pulmonary fibrosis and central varicose type of bronchiectasis (stage V).

7.2.2 Other causes

Bronchial obstruction may be due to many acquired conditions including inflammatory diseases (broncholithiasis and foreign body aspiration), benign neoplastic processes (bronchial hamartoma, lipoma, and papillomatosis) and malignancies (bronchogenic carcinoma, carcinoid tumor, and metastases) (Gipson et al., 2009; Wilson et al., 2009). They can even take place after a segmentectomy as a surgical complication (Okuda et al., 2006).

All these situations can produce an appearance of a round, oval or branching (glove-finger shadow) type of bronchocele. Most of these conditions can be differentiated by appropriate history (as all will be symptomatic), the progressive nature of the disease, imaging techniques, bronchoscopy and biopsy.

Congenital obstructive illnesses	**Bronchopulmonary anomalies:** Lung Aplasia Bronchial atresia Lobar emphysema Cystic adenomatoid malformation Bronchogenic cysts **Vascular anomalies:** Anomalous pulmonary venous return **Combined lung and vascular anomalies:** Brochopulmonary sequestration **Genetic diseases:** Cystic fibrosis
Acquired obstructive illnesses	**Infectious diseases:** Allergic bronchopulmonary aspergillosis (ABPA) Tuberculous bronchoestenosis **Inflammatory diseases:** Broncholithiasis, foreign body aspiration **Benign neoplastic processes:** Bronchial hamartoma, lipoma, papillomatosis. **Malignancies:** Bronchogenic carcinoma, carcinoid tumor, metastases **Surgery complication:** Lung segmentectomy

Table 2. The differential diagnosis of bronchial atresia.

8. Treatment of bronchial atresia

Treatment of bronchial atresia is controversial. The majority of patients are asymptomatic and therefore no treatment is necessary. It is currently felt that surgical excision should be reserved for patients with secondary complications to the atretic bronchus, such as infection or significant compromise of adjacent lung parenchyma. However, some physicians advocate performing surgery on all patients because a definitive diagnosis could only be made by exeresis of the lung (Cohen et al., 1987). Lobar resection and segmentectomy have been used to preserve as much normal lung parenchyma as possible to maintain pulmonary function (Miyahara et al., 1999; Pamer et al., 2008).

9. Prenatal bronchial atresia

Antenatal ultrasonography can raise the suspicion of bronchial atresia in the prenatal period by the presence of a hyperechogenic mass at the hilum of the lung which corresponds to a mucocele (Kamata et al., 2003; McAlister et al., 1987). Those hyperechogenic lesions are more likely to regress compared with cystic or mixed lesions (Hadchouel et als. 2011a, 2011b).

The routine use of prenatal steroids for microcystic congenital cystic adenomatoid malformation seemed to enhance regression (Curran et al., 2010). There are no documented cases on regression of bronchial or lobar bronchial atresia. Despite the lack of evidence, it would be advisable to follow an expectant management (Bonnefoy et al., 2011).

10. Diagnostic algorithm

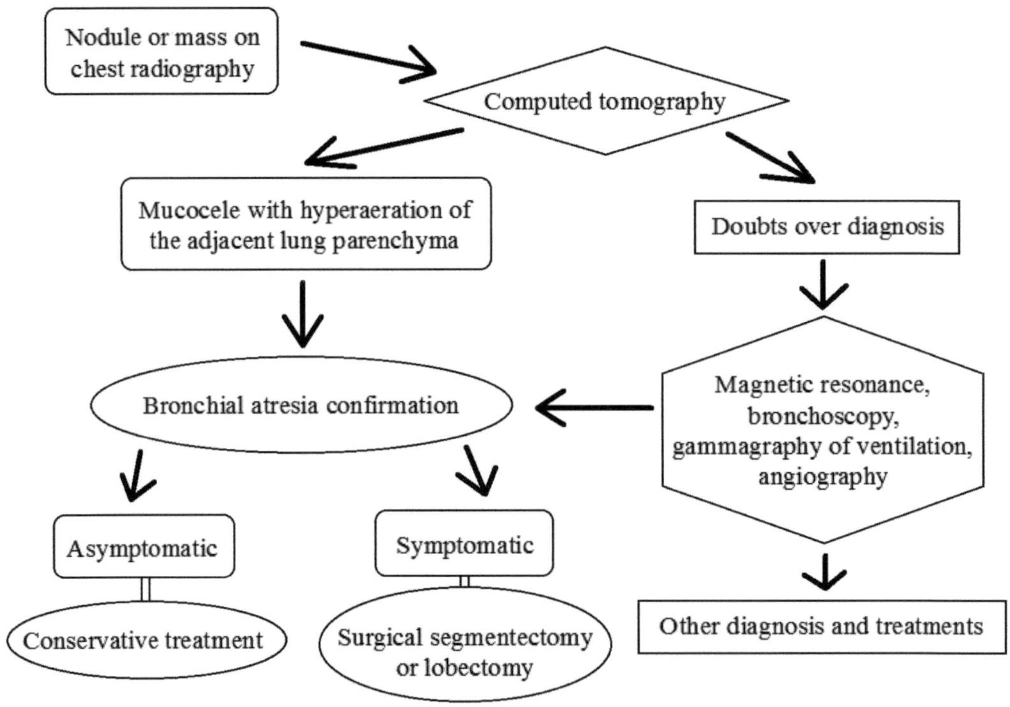

Fig. 3. Diagnostic algorithm in suspected bronchial atresia.

11. State of art during the last three years

Due to a wave of new interest in bronchial atresia among clinicians, there have been many more articles and case descriptions published in the last three years than previously. The aim of this section is to summarize the main aspects of these reports.

- In asymptomatic patients the bronchial atresia is usually found by chance on a radiographic image as described by Psathakis et al. (2009) and Sacristán Bou et al. (2010), or sometimes because a patient refers to a shoulder ache, as Hooker & Hendriksz (2011) show.
- Nussbaumer-Ochsner & Kohler (2011) report a 31-year-old HIV-positive man who presented with a history of chronic dry cough. They describe the finger-in-glove sign, a radiographic feature that refers to mucoid impaction in central airways.
- Some surgeons like Cappeliez et al. (2009) or Zribi et al. (2011) think that bronchial atresia may lead to infectious complications and, in the long term, to damage to the adjacent lung parenchyma. Therefore, a surgical resection may be necessary. The first group of surgeons reported their experience with three patients (two lobectomies and one segmentectomy) and the second group with six.
- Niimi & Gotoh (2010) present the rare case of pneumothorax due to the perforation of bullae associated with congenital bronchial atresia in a 25-year-old woman that complained of right chest pain and shortness of breath. A lateral segmentectomy was successfully performed by thoracoscopy-assisted limited thoracotomy. Diagnosis of congenital bronchial atresia and subpleural bullae were confirmed by pathological examination.
- Discioscio et al (2010), Shimizu et al (2010) and Siddiqui et al. (2011) describe several anomalies associated with bronchial atresia like anomalous pulmonary venous return, congenital cystic adenomatoid malformation or right-sided descending aorta.
- Jung et al. (2011) published a case report of a woman with diagnosis of bronchial atresia in whom the conversion of epidural analgesia to epidural anesthesia for cesarean delivery failed during labor, needing the application of general anesthesia for a successful delivery.

12. Conclusions

Bronchial atresia is a congenital abnormality with characteristic radiological features: a nodule or a mass like a shadow close to the hilum, with well-defined margins, presenting as a tubular, round, ovoid or branching structure and distal oligaemia and hyperinflation.

When it is required to do differential diagnosis over bronchial obstruction, bronchial atresia should be kept in mind.

Knowledge of this condition in patients with suspected bronchial obstruction would avoid unnecessary surgery. Currently, surgical excision is reserved only for patients with secondary complications to the atretic bronchus. Most surgeons try to preserve as much normal lung parenchyma as possible to maintain pulmonary function, whilst others prefer to resect the atretic segment.

13. References

Acosta Gordillo, L.; Márquez Fernández, J. & Medina Gil, M.C. Asymptomatic congenital bronchial atresia in a 10-year-old boy. *Anales de Pediatría*, Vol. 62, No.4, (April 2005), pp. 386-388, ISSN 1695-4033

Agarwal, P.P.; Matzinger, F.R. & Seely, J.M. An unusual case of systemic arterial supply to the lung with bronchial atresia. *American Journal of Roentgenology*, Vol.185, No.1, (July 2005), pp. 150-153, ISSN 0361-803X

Amin, M.U.; Rahim, A. & Nafees, M. Mucocoele formation due to congenital bronchial atresia-a rare cause of solitary pulmonary nodule. *Journal of the Pakistan Medical Association*, Vol.57, No.2, (February 2007), pp. 98-101, ISSN 0030-9982

Bonnefoy, C.; Blanc, P. & Coste, K. Prenatal diagnosis of lobar bronchial atresia. *Ultrasound in Obstetrics & Gynecology*, Vol.37, No.1, (January 2011), pp. 110-112, ISSN 0960-7692

Bucher, U. & Reid, L. Development of the intrasegmental bronchial tree: the pattern of branching and development of cartilage at various stages of intra-uterine life. *Thorax*, Vol.16, (September 1961), pp. 207-218, ISSN 0040-6376

Cappeliez, S.; Lenoir, S. & Validire, P. Totally endoscopic lobectomy and segmentectomy for congenital bronchial atresia. *European Journal of Cardio-Thoracic Surgery*, Vol.36, No.1, (July 2009), pp. 222-224, ISSN 1010-7940

Ch'in, K.T. & Tang, M.Y. Congenital adenomatoid malformation of one lobe of lung with general anasarca. *Archives of Pathology*, Vol.48, No.3, (September 1949), pp. 221-229, ISSN 0361-7017

Cohen, M.D.; Scales, R.L. & Eigen, H. Evaluation of pulmonary parenchymal disease by magnetic resonance imaging. *The British Journal of Radiology*, Vol.60, No.711, (March 1987), pp. 223-230, ISSN 0007-1285

Colin, A.A.; Reid, L.M. & Kozakewich, H.P. Bronchial atresia is common to extralobar sequestration, intralobar sequestration, congenital cystic adenomatoid malformation, and lobar emphysema. *Pediatric and Developmental Pathology*, Vol.9, No.5, (September-October 2006), pp. 361-373, ISSN 1093-5266

Curran, P.F.; Jelin, E.B. & Rand, L. Prenatal steroids for microcystic congenital cystic adenomatoid malformations. *Journal of Pediatric Surgery*, Vol.45. No.1, (January 2010), pp. 145-150, ISSN 0022-3468

Daoud, B.; Moncada, R. & Ali, J. Lung mass in a smoker. *Chest*, Vol.119. No.3, (March 2001), pp. 947-949, ISSN 0012-3692

Cohen, A.M.; Solomon, E.H. & Alfidi, R.J. Computed tomography in bronchial atresia. *American Journal of Roentgenology*, Vol.135, No.5, (November 1980), pp. 1097-1099, ISSN 0361-803X

Discioscio, V.; Feraco, P. & Bazzocchi, A. Congenital cystic adenomatoid malformation of the lung associated with bronchial atresia involving a different lobe in an adult patient: a case report. *Journal of Medical Case Reports*, Vol.28, No.4, (May 2010), pp. 164, ISSN 1752-1947

Gipson, M.G.; Cummings, K.W. & Hurth, K.M. Bronchial atresia. *Radiographics*, Vol.29, No.5, (September-October 2009), pp. 1531-1535, ISSN 0271-5333

Hadchouel, A.; Benachi, A. & Delacourt, C. Outcome of prenatally diagnosed bronchial atresia. *Ultrasound in Obstetrics & Gynecology*, Vol.38, No.1, (July 2011), pp. 119-120. ISSN 0960-7692

Hadchouel, A.; Benachi, A. & Revillon, Y. Factors associated with partial and complete regression of fetal lung lesions. *Ultrasound in Obstetrics & Gynecology*, Vol.38, No.1, (July 2011), pp. 88-93, ISSN 0960-7692

Hooker, I.D. & Hendriksz, T.R. A woman with an abnormality in the lung. *Nederlands Tijdschrift voor Geneeskunde*, Vol.155, No.8, (June 2011), pp. A1170, ISSN 0028-2162

Jederlinic, P.J.; Sicilian, L.S. & Baigelman, W. Congenital bronchial atresia. A report of 4 cases and a review of the literature. *Medicine*, Vol.66. No.1, (January 1987), pp. 73-83, ISSN 0025-7974

Jeung, M.Y.; Gasser, B. & Gangi, A. Bronchial carcinoid tumors of the thorax: spectrum of radiologic findings. *Radiographics*, Vol.22, No.2, (March-April 2002), pp. 351-365, ISSN 0271-5333

Jung, H.J.; Kim, J.B. & Im, K.S. Failure of epidural analgesia converted to epidural anesthesia for cesarean delivery in a patient with bronchial atresia in labor. *The Journal of Obstetrics and Gynaecology Research*, Vol.37, No.6, (June 2011), pp. 613-616, ISSN 1341-8076

Kamata, S.; Sawai, T. & Usui, N. Case of congenital bronchial atresia detected by fetal ultrasound. *Pediatric Pulmonology*, Vol.35, No.3, (March 2003), pp. 227-229, ISSN 8755-6863

Kameyama, K.; Okumura, N. & Kokado, Y. Congenital bronchial atresia associated with spontaneous pneumothorax. *The Annals of Thoracic Surgery*, Vol.82, No.4, (October 2006), pp. 1497-1499, ISSN 0003-4975

Kinsella, D.; Sissons, G. & Williams, M.P. The radiological imaging of bronchial atresia, *The British Journal of Radiology*, Vol.65, No.776, (August 1992), pp. 681-685, ISSN 0007-1285

Ko, S.F.; Lee, T.Y. & Kao, C.L. Bronchial atresia associated with epibronchial right pulmonary artery and aberrant right middle lobe artery. *The British Journal of Radiology*, Vol.71, No.842, (February 1998), pp. 217-220, ISSN 0007-1285

Kuhn, C. & Kuhn, J.P. Coexistence of bronchial atresia and bronchogenic cyst: diagnostic criteria and embryologic considerations. *Pediatric Radiology*, Vol.22, No.8, (June 1992), pp. 568-570, ISSN 0301-0449

Lacquet LK, Fornhoff M, Dierickx R & Buyssens N (1971). Bronchial atresia with corresponding segmental pulmonary emphysema. *Thorax*, Vol.26, No.1, (January 1971), pp. 68-73, ISSN 0040-6376

Louw, J.H. & Barnard, C.N. Congenital intestinal atresia; observations on its origin. *Lancet*, Vol.269, No.6899, (November 1955), pp. 1065-1067, ISSN 0140-6736

Matsushima, H.; Takayanagi, N. & Satoh, M. Congenital bronchial atresia: radiologic findings in nine patients. *Journal of Computer Assisted Tomography*, Vol.27, No.1, (January-February 2003), pp. 103, ISSN 0363-8715

McAlister, W.H.; Wright, J.R. Jr. & Crane, J.P. Main-stem bronchial atresia: intrauterine sonographic diagnosis. *American Journal of Roentgenology*, Vol.148, No.2, (February 1987), pp. 364-366 , Vol.135, No.5, (November 1980), pp. 1097-1099, ISSN 0361-803X

Miyahara, N.; Eda, R. & Makihara, S. Bronchial atresia with transient spontaneous disappearance of a mucocele. *Internal Medicine*, Vol.38, No.12, (December 1999), pp. 974-978, ISSN 0918-2918

Morikawa, N.; Kuroda, T. & Honna, T. Congenital bronchial atresia in infants and children. *Journal of Pediatric Surgery*, Vol.40, No.12, (December 2005), pp. 1822-1826, ISSN 0022-3468

Murat, A.; Ozdemir, H. & Yildirim, H. Bronchial atresia of the right lower lobe. *Acta Radiologica*, Vol.46. No.5, (August 2005), pp. 480-483, ISSN 0001-6926

Naidich, D.P.; Rumancik, W.M. & Ettenger, N.A. Congenital anomalies of the lungs in adults: MR diagnosis. *American Journal of Roentgenology*, Vol.151, No.1, (July 1988), pp. 13-19 , ISSN 0361-803X

Niimi, T. & Gotoh, M. Pneumothorax secondary to congenital bronchial atresia. *Kyobu Geka*, Vol.63, No.4, (April 2010), pp. 324-327, ISSN 0021-5252

Nussbaumer-Ochsner, Y. & Kohler, M. Finger-in-glove sign in bronchial atresia. *Thorax*, Vol.66. No.2, (February 2011), pp. 182, ISSN 0040-6376

Okuda, M.; Huang, C.L. & Masuya, D. Lobar bronchial atresia demonstrating a cystic lesion without overinflation. *European Journal of Cardio-Thoracic Surgery*, Vol.30, No.2, (August 2006), pp. 391-393. ISSN 1010-7940

Pamer, M.J. & Lenhardt, R. Bronchial Atresia With Mucoceles and Concurrent Sinus Mucoceles: First Reported Case and a Review of the Literature. *Clinical Pulmonary Medicine*, Vol.15, No.2, (March 2008), pp. 122-125, ISSN 1068-0640

Pedicelli, G.; Ciarpaglini, L.L. & De Santis, M. Congenital bronchial atresia (CBA). A critical review of CBA as a disease entity and presentation of a case series. *La Radiologia Medica*, Vol.110. No.5-6, (November-December 2005), pp. 544-553, ISSN 0033-8362

Primetis, E.; Koureas, A. & Dalakidis, A. Congenital bronchial atresia with a calcified mucocele. *Respiration*, Vol.81, No.6, (June 2011), pp. 511-522, ISSN 0025-7931

Psathakis, K.; Lachanis, S. & Kotoulas, C. The prevalence of congenital bronchial atresia in males. *Monaldi Archives for Chest Disease*, Vol.61, No.1, (January-March 2004), pp. 28-34, ISSN 1122-0643

Psathakis, K.; Eleftheriou, D. & Boulas, P. Congenital bronchial atresia presenting as a cavitary lesion on chest radiography: a case report. *Cases Journal*, Vol.2, No.1, (January 2009), pp. 17, ISSN 1757-1626

Rahalkar, A.M.; Rahalkar, M.D. & Rahalkar, M.A. Pictorial Essay: All About Bronchial Atresia. *The Indian Journal of Radiology and Imaging*, Vol.15, No.3, (June 2005), pp. 389-393, ISSN 0971-3026

Ramsay, B.H. & Byron, F.X. Mucocele, congenital bronchiectasis, and bronchogenic cyst. *The Journal of thoracic surgery*, Vol .26, No.1, (July 1953), pp. 21-30, ISSN 0096-5588

Reid, L. 1976 Edward B.D. Neuhauser lecture: The Lung: Growth and Remodeling in Health and Disease. *American Journal of Roentgenology*, Vol.129, No.5, (November 1977), pp. 777-788, ISSN 0361-803X

Sacristán Bou, L.; Martín Serrano, C. & Romero Candeira, S. Bronchial atresia together with a gonadal teratoma: what is the relationship? *Archivos de Bronconeumología*, Vol.46, No.5, (May 2010), pp. 278-279, ISSN 0300-2896

Sadler, T.W. & Langman, J. (1990). *Langman`s medical embryology* (6th edition), Williams & Wilkins, ISBN 978-068-3074-93-2/0683074938, Baltimore, United States.

Shimizu, K.; Masuda, K. & Hebisawaa, A. A surgical case of congenital bronchial atresia with right-sided descending aorta. *Nihon Kokyuki Gakkai Zasshi*, Vol.48, No.3, (March 2010), pp. 210-213, ISSN 1343-3490

Siddiqui, T.S.; Ul Haq, I. & Rehman, B. Bronchial atresia with partial anomalous pulmonary venous return. *Journal of the College of Physicians and Surgeons--Pakistan*, Vol.21, No.6, (June 2011), pp. 362-363, ISSN 1022-386X

Van Klaveren, R.J.; Morshuis, W.J. & Lacquet, L.K. Congenital bronchial atresia with regional emphysema associated with pectus excavatum. *Thorax*, Vol.47, No.12, (December 1992), pp. 1082-1083, ISSN ISSN 0040-6376

Waddell, J.A.; Simon, G. & Reid, L. Bronchial Atresia of the left upper lobe. *Thorax*, Vol.20, (May 1965), pp. 214-218, ISSN ISSN 0040-6376

Ward, S. & Morcos, S.K. Congenital bronchial atresia--presentation of three cases and a pictorial review. *Clinical Radiology*, Vol.54, No.3, (March 1999), pp. 144-148, ISSN 0009-9260

Wilson, E.P.; Patel, J. & Logalbo, F. An Adult Case of Bronchial Atresia Mimicking Pulmonary Embolism. *Clinical Pulmonary Medicine*, Vol.16, No.1, (January 2009), pp. 57-59, ISSN 1068-0640

Woodring, J.H. Unusual radiographic manifestations of lung cancer. *Radiologic Clinics of North America*, Vol.28, No.3, (May 1990), pp. 599-618, ISSN 0033-8389

Zribi, H.; Brian, E. & Lenoir, S. Congenital bronchial atresia in adults. *Revue des Maladies Respiratoires*, Vol.28, No.5, (May 2011), pp. 672-676, ISSN 0761-8425

32

A Case of Adult Congenital Cystic Adenomatoid Malformation of the Lung with Atypical Adenomatous Hyperplasia

Ho Sung Lee[1], Jae Sung Choi[1], Ki Hyun Seo[1], Ju Ock Na[1], Yong Hoon Kim[1], Mi Hye Oh[2] and Sung Shick Jou[3]
[1]Department of Internal Medicine Diagnostic
[2]Department of Pathology and [3]Department of Radiology
Soonchunhyang University College of Medicine, Cheonan
Korea

1. Introduction

Congenital cystic adenomatoid malformation of the lung is a rare disease that shows multiple cystic lesions in pulmonary tissues in the development process. It was first described by Chin et al.[1] in 1949 and its incidence is known to be 1:25,000 to 1:35,000[2]. With the development of prenatal diagnosis, this disease can be diagnosed in 60% and detected within 2 years because of such symptoms as respiratory distress by compression of surrounding lung tissues immediately after birth and repeated respiratory infections in infancy. Among adults, it is detected accidentally on X-ray or by such symptoms as pneumonia, pneumothorax, and hemoptysis. In Korea, the first case in a 28 year-old woman was reported by Geun-Heung Ki et al.[3] in 1989. Since then, about 25 adult cases were reported until 2006.

Atypical adenomatous hyperplasia is pathologically defined as the proliferation of atypical cuboidal or columnar cepithelial cells which are typically 5 mm or smaller in size along the alveolus or respiratory bronchiole[4,5]. In 1999, the WHO classified this disease as a precancerous lesion together with squamous dysplasia and diffuse idiopathic pulmonary neuroendocrine cell hyperplasia[5]. It is known to be found in about 12% of lung cancers and highly correlated with glandular cancer[6].

2. Case

Patient: O-Back Kim, Female, 37

Current case history: The patient had been treated in a private clinic due to purulent sputum and cough and hemoptysis which had started two weeks before transfer to our hospital.

Past case history: The patient had been treated for hyperthyroidism from 1999 to 2003.

Examination findings: Vital signs were stable. Chest examination detected reduced bilateral breathing sounds only.

Laboratory findings: The peripheral blood examination found 13.2 g/dL of hemoglobin, 39.5 % of hematocrit, 5210 /mm^3 of white blood cells (neutrophils 43%, lymphocytes 44.5%, monocytes 9.2%), and 255,000 /mm^3 of platelets. The results of serum biochemical examination, hepatitis marker test, urinalysis, mycoplasma antigen test, and pulmonary function test were normal. The thyroid function test found minor hypothyroidism with 8.72 nIU/ml of thyroid stimulating hormone (TSH), 0.894 ng/dl and 1.19ng/ml of free T4 and T3 respectively. The results of the sputum culture and bronchial washing cytodiagnosis were also negative. The results of arterial blood gas analysis which was conducted in atmosphere were 7.407 of pH, 41.2 mmHg of carbon dioxide tension, 82.6 mmHg of oxygen tension, 25.4 mEq/L of bicarbonates, and 96.2% of oxygen saturation. The tumor marker test result was also normal with 1.49 ng/mL of CEA and 1.57 ng/mL of cyfra 21-1.

Chest radiology: The chest X-ray showed a 2.5cm cavitating lesion in the left upper zone. (Figure 1).

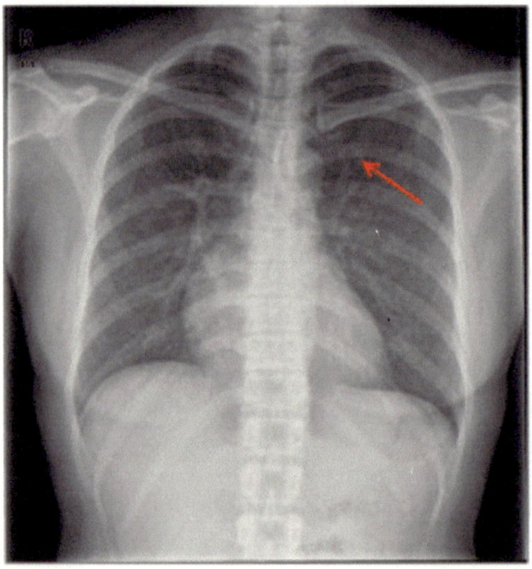

Fig. 1. Chest PA shows cavitatory lesion in the left upper zone

On the second day after hospitalization, the chest CT showed a diffuse ground glass appearance and cystic lesions that spread in a branching pattern were found in the left lung (Figure 2).

Clinical progress: The patient received symptomatic therapy as there were no features of infection. The bronchial endoscopy did not reveal any lesions. The bronchoalveolar lavage fluid test found 82% of macrophages, 8% of neutrophils, 0.5% of eosinophils, and 9.5% of lymphocytes. Endobronchial lung biopsy was performed at the left lower lobe and only chronic inflammatory changes were noted. On the 9th day after hospitalization, a wedge resection of the top section of the left upper lobe was performed. On the 20th day after hospitalization, the patient was discharged with no complications.

Biopsy: The microscopic findings of the resected lung showed cystic lesions of various sizes. The cells covering them were diverse, including ciliated pseudostratified columnar cells, monolayer columnar cell, and cuboid cells, which corresponded to type 2 of the congenital cystic adenomatoid malformation(Figure 3).

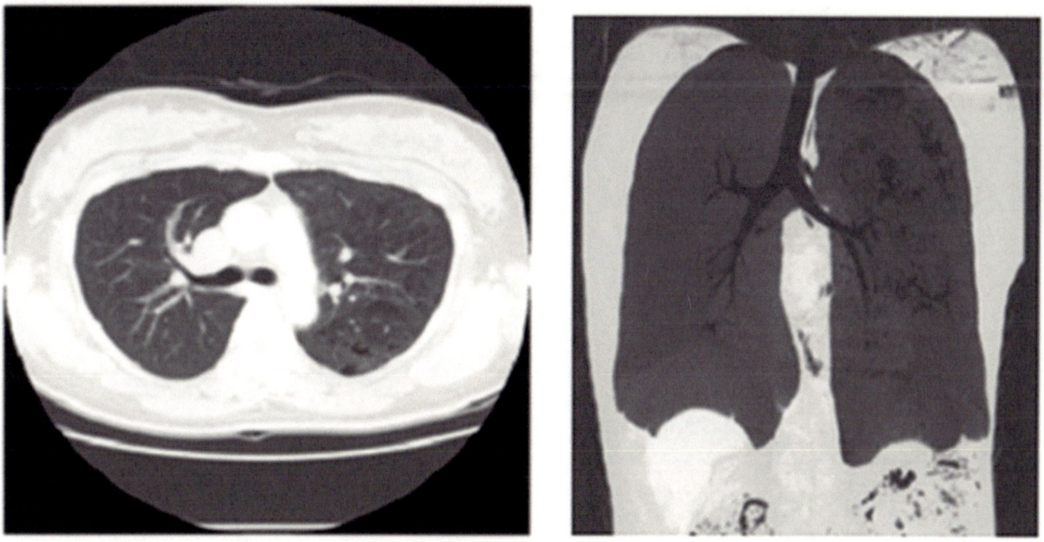

Fig. 2. Chest CT shows diffuse ground glass opacity and multiple branching cystic lesion in left lung

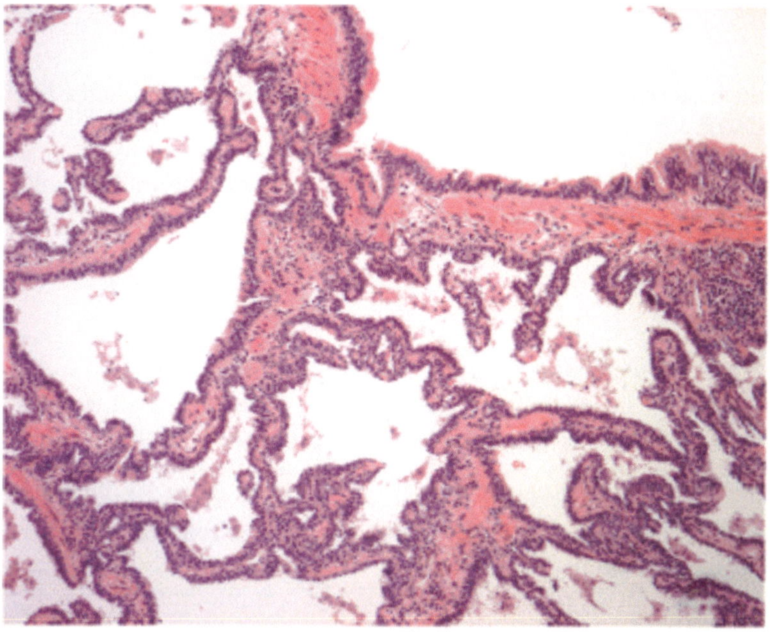

Fig. 3. The lining cells are pseudostratified ciliated columnar cells to columnar and cuboidal cells like bronchiolar epithelial cells (H&E, x100).

As there were minor atypical nuclei locally and linear structures filled with mucus in the cytoplasm, it looked similar to the mucoid bronchioloalveolar carcinoma, but because their sizes were all smaller than 5mm, they were judged to be atypical adenomatous proliferation (Figure 4).

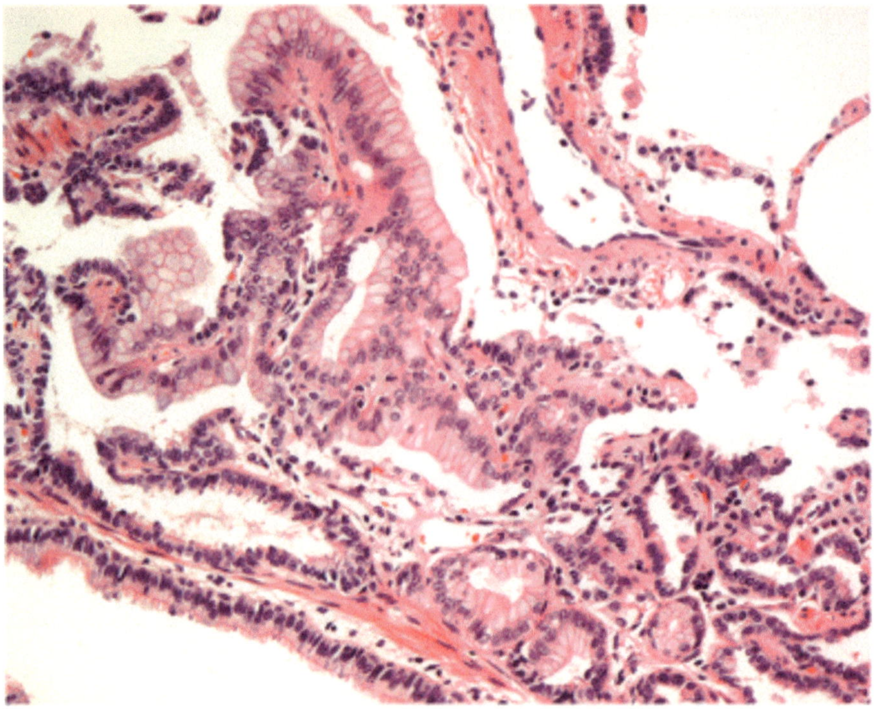

Fig. 4. Focal mucinous epithelial lesion with mild atypism is revealed in the intervening parenchyma (H&E, x200).

Treatment and progress: After discharge, the patient was transferred to another hospital at her request; As it was checked, she was being followed up with chest CT every 3 months with no specific treatment.

3. Discussion

The congenital cystic adenomatoid malformation of the lung is very rare and its incidence is known to be 1:25,000 - 1:35,000[2]. The cause is not known, but two hypotheses have been suggested: cessation in the development of the lung tissues and no development of aveoli during the development process of the respiratory system[7,8]. The time when the malformation occurs is estimated to be between 5 and 6 weeks before the lobe divides and prechondrial tissues are formed in the bronchus. It has been reported that it causes stillborn and premature infants. Immediately after birth, respiratory distress is frequent in most cases, and as the baby grows, repeated infections and pneumothorax are more frequent than respiratory distress. Accompanying malformations include kidney growth failure, diaphragmatic hernia, jejunul atresia, and colon growth failure[1]. A histological characteristic is the arrangement of polyp-shaped cysts of various sizes in the bronchial epithelium or simple columnar epithelium with no cartilaginous tissues or inflammatory reaction. Stoker et al. classified them based on size and pathological findings into type I (only a few large thick walled cyst), type II (numerous, evenly spaced cyst, less than 1cm), and type III (less numerous, firm and bulky masses) in 1977. In 1994, they re-classified them into 5 types based on bronchial invasion: type 0 (bronchial), type I (bronchial/bronchiolar), type II (bronchiolar), type III (bronchiolar/alveolar), and type IV (peripheral). In 1994, they reported that type I was the most frequent at 50 - 70% and type III showed the worst prognosis. Radiographic diagnoses include chest X-ray test, CT, and prenatal ultrasonography. Among them, chest CT can observe lesions that contain cysts with multiple large and small thin walls. It must be differentiated from pneumonia accompanied by pneumatosis, pulmonary sequestration, congenital lobar emphysema, and bronchiectasis. Definite diagnosis is only possible by pathological tests. Some claim that it is associated with malignant tumors of the lung. There was a report of pulmonary rhabdomyosarcoma in 22-month old boy, and several papers reported the accompaniment of mucoid bronchioloalveolar carcinoma in adults and children[3,9]. Hence, Ioachimescu et al.[9] recommended surgical removal even if there were no symptoms, because it may become malignant.

Pathological findings in this patient were accompanied by atypical adenomatous hyperplasia. Atypical adenomatous hyperplasia is pathologically defined as the proliferation of atypical cuboidal epithelial cells or columnar epithelial cells along the alveolus or respiratory bronchiole[4]. Their sizes are mostly 5 mm or smaller, although a size of 19mm has been reported. As it is difficult to differentiate from bronchioloalveolar carcinoma, one researcher suggested 5 mm as the reference size for differentiation. It occurs in up to 5% of normal people and is usually asymptomatic. It is known to develop in 2.9% of total population and increases to 10 - 23.2% in lung cancer [11,12,13,14,15]. The recent diagnostic rate is increasing due to low dose chest CT as a lung cancer screening test. Although there are no specific CT findings, the most frequent finding are nodules with a good boundary accompanied by a ground glass apperance[10]. In 1999, the WHO classified this disease as a precancerous lesion together with squamous dysplasia and diffuse idiopathic pulmonary neuroendocrine cell hyperplasia[5]. Chapman et al.[6] analyzed the pathological findings of 554 patients with primary lung cancer and found that atypical adenomatous hyperplasia was accompanied in 67 cases (12.1%), and that the percentage of glandular cancer was the highest (glandular cancer 23.2%, giant cell undifferentiated cancer 12.5%, epithelial carcinoma 2.2%). There are many different opinions among pathologists and no established views on the differentiation level of atypical adenomatous hyperplasia, classification based on this, and its relationship with adenocarcinoma. However, there are some reports related to morphological changes of the nuclei, expression of Ki-67 and p53, and K-ras mutation, which are expected to be helpful for better investigation of the characteristics of atypical adenomatous hyperplasia as a precancerous lesion[5,10]. As there are no principles in therapy yet, careful follow-up is needed.

Although there is controversy about the treatment of this patient, the authors believe that pneumonectomy of the left lung will be necessary because the patient has both congenital cystic adenomatoid malformation which can be accompanied by bronchioloalveolar carcinoma and atypical adenomatous hyperplasia which is a precancerous lesion.

After a literature review, it is believed that this is the first case report of congenital cystic adenomatoid malformation accompanied by atypical adenomatous hyperplasia.

4. References

Brambilla, E. et al.(2001). The new World Health Organization classification of lung tumours. *Eur Respir J*, Vol.18, No.6, (Dec2001), pp.1059-1068. ISSN 1182-9087

Chapman, AD. & Kerr, KM.(2000). The association between atypical adenomatous hyperplasia and primary lung cancer. *Br J Cancer,* Vol. 83, No.5,(Sep2000), pp. 632-636, ISSN 1094-4604

Chin, KY. & Tang, MY.(1949). Congenital adenomatoid malformation of one lobe of a lung with general anasarca. *Archives of Pathology,* Vol.48, No.3,(Sep1949), pp.221-229, ISSN 0361-7017

Ioachimescu, OC., Mehta, AC.(2005). From cystic pulmonary airway malformation, to bronchioloalveolar carcinoma and adenocarcinoma of the lung. *Eur Respir J,* Vol.26, No.6, (Dec2005), pp. 1181-1187. ISSN 1631-9347

Kawakami, S. et al.(2001). Atypical adenomatous hyperplasia of the lung: correlation between high resolution CT findings and histopathologic features. *Eur Radiol,* Vol.11, No.5, (2001), pp.811-814. ISSN 1137-2613

Kerr, KM.(2001). Pulmonary preinvasive neoplasia. *J clin Pathol,* Vol.54, No.4, (April2001), pp. 257–271, ISSN 1130-4841

Kim, JI. et al.(2004). Congenital cystic adenomatoid malformation of the lung presenting as Hemoptysis in 49-year-old woman: a case report. *Korean J Crit Care Med,* Vol.19, No.2,(Dec 2004), pp.139-142
<http://search.koreanstudies.net/search/result_kiss.asp>

Nakahara, R. et al.(2001). Atypical adenomatous hyperplasia of the lung: a clinicopathological study of 118 cases including cases with multiple atypical adenomatous hyperplasia. *Thorax,* Vol.56,No.4, (April2001), pp.302-205. 1125-4822

Shackelford, GD., & Siegel, MJ.(1989). CT apperance of cystic adenomatoid malformations. *J Comput Assist Tomogr,* Vol.13, No.4, (Jul1989), pp. 612-616. ISSN 274-5778

Stocker, JT.(1994) Congenital and developmental diseases. In: *Pulmonary Pathology 2nd ed,* Dali DH, Hammar SP, (Ed),155-90, 978-078-1782-08-1, New york, Springer-verlag Weng S et al.(1990). Multiple atypical hyperplasia of type II pneumocytes and bronchioloalveolar carcinoma. *Histopathology,* Vol.16,No.1,(Jan1990), pp.101-103. ISSN 230-7410

Stocker, JT. et al.(1977). Congenital cystic adenomatoid malformation of the lung : Classification and morphologic spectrum. *Hum Pathol,* Vol.8, No.2,(Mar1977) pp.155-171. ISSN 85-6714

Takigawa, N. et al. (1999). Clinical investigation of atypical adenomatous hyperplasia of the lung, *Lung cancer,* Vol.25,No.2, (Aug1999), pp.115-121. ISSN 1047-0845

Weng, S. et al.(1990). Multiple atypical hyperplasia of type II pneumocytes and Bronchioloalveolar carcinoma. *Histopathology,* Vol.16, No.1,(Jan1990), pp.101-103. ISSN 230-7410

Yokose, T. et al.(2000). High prevalence of atypical adenomatous hyperplasia of the lung in autopsy specimens from elderly patients with malignant neoplasms. Lung cancer, Vol.29, No.2, (Aug2000), pp. 125-130. ISSN 1096-3842

Yokose, T. et al.(2001). Atypical adenomatous hyperplasia of the lung in autopsy cases. *Lung cancer,* Vol.33, No.2-3, (Aug2001), pp.155-161. ISSN 1155-1410